KOCHAR'S

CLINICAL MEDICINE FOR STUDENTS

FIFTH EDITION

KOCHAR'S

CLINICAL MEDICINE FOR STUDENTS

FIFTH EDITION

EDITOR-IN-CHIEF

DARIO M. TORRE, MD, MPH, FACP

Associate Professor of Medicine
Medical College of Wisconsin/Zablocki VA Medical Center
Medicine Clerkship Director
Milwaukee, Wisconsin

EDITORS

GEOFFREY C. LAMB, MD, FACP

Associate Professor of Medicine
Division of General Internal Medicine
Associate Director, Joint Quality Office
Froedtert Hospital and Medical College of Wisconsin
Milwaukee, Wisconsin

JEROME J. VAN RUISWYK, MD, MS, FACP

Associate Professor of Medicine
Medical College of Wisconsin
Associate Chief of Staff for Clinical Affairs
Zablocki VA Medical Center
Milwaukee, Wisconsin

RALPH M. SCHAPIRA, MD, FACP, FCCP

Professor and Vice-Chairman of Medicine
Medical College of Wisconsin
Chief of Medicine
Zablocki VA Medical Center
Milwaukee, Wisconsin

CONSULTING EDITOR

MAHENDR S. KOCHAR, MD, MS, MACP, FRCP (LONDON)

Professor of Medicine
Senior Associate Dean, Graduate Medical Education
Medical College of Wisconsin
Milwaukee, Wisconsin

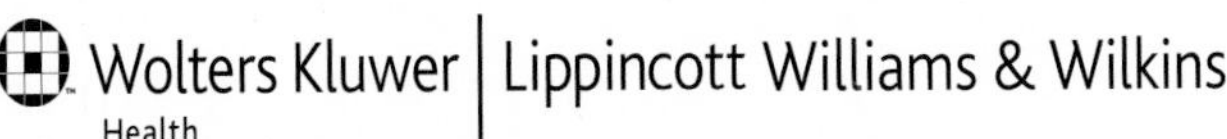

Philadelphia • Baltimore • New York • London
Buenos Aires • Hong Kong • Sydney • Tokyo

Acquisitions Editor: Nancy Anastasi Duffy
Associate Managing Editor: Liz Stalnaker
Marketing Manager: Jennifer Kuklinski
Design Coordinator: Teresa Mallon
Associate Production Manager: Kevin Johnson
Compositor: Maryland Composition

351 West Camden Street
Baltimore, MD 21201

530 Walnut Street
Philadelphia, PA 19106

Printed in China

Library of Congress Cataloging-in-Publication Data

Kochar's clinical medicine for students / editor in chief, Dario M. Torre ; editors, Geoffrey C. Lamb, Jerome Van Ruiswyk, Ralph M. Schapira ; consulting editor, Mahendr S. Kochar.—5th ed.
p. ; cm.
Rev. ed. of: Kochar's concise textbook of medicine / editor-in-chief, Kesavan Kutty. 4th ed. c2003.
ISBN-13: 978-0-7817-6699-9
1. Clinical medicine. 2. Internal medicine. I. Torre, Dario M. II. Kochar's concise textbook of medicine. III. Title: Clinical medicine for students.
[DNLM: 1. Clinical Medicine. 2. Internal Medicine. 3. Primary Health Care. WB 115 K756 2008]
RC46.T328 2008
616—dc22

2007031544

The publishers have made every effort to trace the copyright holders for borrowed material. If they have inadvertently overlooked any, they will be pleased to make the necessary arrangements at the first opportunity.

To purchase additional copies of this book, call our customer service department at **(800) 638-3030** or fax orders to **(301) 223-2320.** International customers should call **(301) 223-2300.**

Visit Lippincott Williams & Wilkins on the Internet: http://www.LWW.com. Lippincott Williams & Wilkins customer service representatives are available from 8:30 am to 6:00 pm, EST.

11 12 13 14
3 4 5 6 7 8 9 10

To Alessia, innocent rainbow, beautiful, eternal flower in the garden of my life.
Dario Torre

To students, who always challenge and inspire their teachers.
Geoffrey Lamb, Jerome Van Ruiswyk, Ralph Schapira, Mahendr Kochar

FOREWORD

Twenty-five years of Kochar!

Following the 4th edition of *Kochar's Concise Textbook of Medicine*, faculty and students around the country can now welcome its new incarnation, *Kochar's Clinical Medicine for Students*, reconceived in its overall structure and rewritten in every detail. The new *Kochar* helps students meet the core tenet of professionalism in internal medicine—fulfilling a duty of expertise for each and every patient—but also moves with its students into the 21st century. The principles and the insistence on rigor in the clinical essentials are the same, but these days, we all learn in new ways, and we access information differently. The new *Kochar* is true to the basics, while adapting itself to the needs of a new generation.

From the beginning, Dr. Kochar conceived a book that could be read by students during their 3rd year clerkship. Throughout its earlier editions, *Kochar* has prided itself on providing exactly the information that students and residents needed to take care of their patients, in a way that they could quickly access and effectively apply. In a word, it was "concise." The new edition does this today, and to the same high standards as the previous four editions, as would be expected of a text in use in medical schools throughout the country.

Under the general editorship of Dr. Dario Torre, it is almost entirely rewritten, brought up-to-date in every respect. He and the section editors and faculty of the Medical College of Wisconsin have done right by their readers. The table of contents reflects the curriculum guide of the Clerkship Directors in Internal Medicine and the website of the United States Medical Licensing Examination.

There has been a growing national consensus in medical education that every graduating student should have mastered basic clinical skills, and the 5th edition of *Kochar* opens with an entirely new section, "Key Manifestations and Presentations of Disease." This section describes all the key symptoms and findings that clinicians look for in patients, and links these to a basic understanding of physiology. All by itself, this section could be used in introduction to clinical medicine and basic "doctoring" courses throughout the country. The section editor, also Dr. Torre, and chapter authors have created something that covers all the common problems, while still remaining concise. In other words, it contains all the basics, with just the right amount of material for which all students can be held accountable.

The "Diseases and Disorders" section is organized by traditional organ systems. Every chapter has been rewritten in detail, and the majority of authors are new to the 5th edition. While maintaining the goals of clarity and conciseness, the level of expertise is appropriate for residents in internal medicine and family medicine, and this edition keeps faith with the view of Dr Kochar that general medicine and primary care are essential to the practice of every specialty and subspecialty. A new "Ambulatory Medicine" section of 18 chapters, edited by Dr. Jerome Van Ruiswyk, has been developed for those clerkships that have also an ambulatory component.

Finally, this edition of *Kochar* is linked to an interactive website, which supplements each section's description with multimedia materials, images, and demonstrations of findings in support of the text. For instance, cardiology is supported with multiple EKGs, dermatology with striking images. Students will also appreciate the interactive online multiple-choice questions.

Innovation and tradition are the hallmarks of the new *Kochar*. The new General Editor for this edition is Dr. Dario Torre, Associate Professor of Medicine and Internal Medicine Clerkship Director at the Medical College of Wisconsin. Dr. Geoffrey Lamb has written several sections and joins the group as Associate Editor. Two editors remain from the 4th edition: Dr. Jerome Van Ruiswyk, in writing the new section on "Ambulatory Medicine", one which we can ask all students to read at the start of their ambulatory rotations with adult patients, and Dr. Ralph Schapira's guidance is retained throughout, especially in the Pulmonary section. Although he is no longer an editor, the presence of Dr. Kesavan Kutty, editor of the 2nd, 3rd and 4th editions, is gratefully retained in the section chapter on tuberculosis.

The editors and authors of the new *Kochar* have thought carefully about what essential knowledge and skills students still need in the contemporary world of medicine—high speed, information-dense and less time than ever between students and patients. But as Dr. Kochar wrote in 1982, "there is only one way to learn clinical medicine, and that is at the bedside," where everything is anchored in the students' own experience with their patients. The new *Kochar's Clinical Medicine* will keep them on course.

Louis N. Pangaro, MD, FACP
Vice Chair for Educational Programs
Department of Medicine
Uniformed Services University of the Health Sciences
F. Edward Hébert School of Medicine
Past President, Clerkship Directors of Internal Medicine

PREFACE

"Few will be found to doubt the importance of books as means to. . .the end of all study—the capacity to make a good judgment," Sir William Osler.

The acquisition of knowledge is essential to creating diagnostic hypotheses and achieving a solution to the patient's clinical problem. With that in mind, we have developed the 5th edition of *Kochar's Clinical Medicine for Students* to link theoretical information more closely to the practice of medicine. Although direct patient experience is an irreplaceable way to develop the practice of medicine and patient care, theoretical knowledge is still an essential component of the learning process. Formal knowledge, which can be acquired from a book, serves as the basis for the application of knowledge in the context of the clinical practice, allowing the student to continuously learn from their experiences.

This edition of *Kochar's* has undergone major changes and a significant transformation to meet the current needs of students in the health professions, in particular the needs of medical students in their third and forth years of medical school.

The conceptual framework behind the development of this book was based on the ADDIE instructional model: Assessment of the learners' needs, Development, Demonstration, Implementation, and Evaluation of each section of the book. This process occurred constantly throughout the manuscript process, to ensure the creation of a text that was centered on the actual needs of the student.

The 5th edition has been substantially revised, reorganized, and updated. Because the duration of courses or clerkships in medical schools is restricted, we decided to include only a selected number of key topics, which were chosen from two sources: Clerkship Directors in Internal Medicine (CDIM) core medicine clerkship curriculum guide, created by a national consensus of clerkship directors and academic general internists from the Society of General Internal Medicine (http://www.im.org/CDIM), and from USMLE™ Step II Clinical Knowledge (CK) content outline (www.usmle.org).

We also recognized that it was important not only for students to learn the typical presentation and diagnosis of common diseases, but also to recognize patients presenting with a specific complaint or finding, for which the generation of diagnostic hypotheses and their evaluation is essential. Finally, it was important to introduce a brief ambulatory medicine section to correspond to the ambulatory component included in many medicine clerkships.

Another innovation of this edition is the collaborative effort between general internists and subspecialists; every chapter was written and reviewed by both groups. We believe that this cooperation will ensure accuracy, readability, and a more appropriate depth of content for medical students. In particular, the depth and relevance of content and the language used throughout the book were specifically revised. Additionally, 3rd and 4th year medical students acting as reviewers were involved in the development of the book from the beginning. Their feedback was most helpful, and their comments and suggestions were incorporated into the editing process.

The organization and presentation of the material is divided into three sections: the diagnostic and clinical approach to common presenting complaints with particular attention to elements of the differential diagnosis; disease and disorders frequently encountered in medicine, formally described in a logical and structured manner; and principles of ambulatory medicine. This organization of content yields a broad, yet still selective, number of topics and approaches in inpatient and outpatient settings. We have organized the material so that it will make sense to 3rd year medical students who need to gain an understanding and knowledge of medicine, and to 4th year medical students who want to further their knowledge for clinical problem solving as well as prepare for the USMLE™ Step II Clinical Knowledge exam. We also intend this book to be a resource for nurse practitioners and physician assistants who would like to review in a rapid and concise manner a number of medicine topics.

A strong electronic component has been added to this edition of *Kochar's*. This content is well organized and easy to access on the Lippincott Williams & Wilkins website called The Point. The Point is an electronic interactive platform that provides students and instructors not only access to the additional online material, but also the ability to interact with each other during the length of the course if they wish to do so. The electronic content includes more than 30 additional chapters and approximately 300 multiple-choice questions with detailed explanations. To help students prepare for end-of-clerkship exams, such as the NBME Medicine subject test (also known as the "Shelf exam"), these questions have been divided into three practice shelf exams. The three exams rigorously follow the NBME medicine subject test blueprint available at the official NBME website. Each of the three tests contains the same percentage of organ system-based questions currently present on the NBME Medicine subject test. Tables and images of electrocardiograms and x-rays are also available on The Point, as well as a bibliography and suggested readings.

The editorial team has also undergone changes with Dr. Torre, new Editor-in-Chief, and Dr. Lamb joining Drs. Van Ruiswyk and Schapira who were editors of the 4th edition. Dr. Kochar, Founder and Editor-in-Chief of the first two editions of the book, serves as a consulting editor. We truly hope that students, who are the brightest hope for the healing and comfort of those who suffer, learn from this book. Our greatest wish is that this book will ultimately improve the practice of medicine by linking this theoretical information to clinical practice. If learning is a lifelong process and not a destination, let us begin this journey with you!

Dario Torre
Geoffrey Lamb
Jerome Van Ruiswyk
Ralph Schapira

ACKNOWLEDGMENTS

We express our appreciation to the contributors and their office staff who have worked diligently and patiently in getting their literary contributions into our hands on time. The Editorial Staff at Lippincott Williams & Wilkins, including Dona Balado, Nancy Duffy, Liz Stalnaker, Jennifer Kuklinski, and Catherine Noonan.

We would also like to take this opportunity to thank Dr. G. Richard Olds, The John and Linda Mellowes Professor and Chairman, Department of Medicine, Medical College of Wisconsin, and Dr. Lee A. Biblo, Professor and Vice-Chairman, Department of Medicine, Medical College of Wisconsin, for their emphatic and unyielding support of this book and their enthusiasm that served to inspire each of its contributors and members of the editorial team.

Thank you to Dr. Ann B. Nattinger, Professor and Chief, General Internal Medicine, Department of Medicine, Medical College of Wisconsin, for your enthusiastic support of this project, which served to inspire and energize the authors.

We would also like to offer our sincere thanks to Dr. Piero Antuono who gave generously of his time as a reviewer. His expertise and careful eye ensured a continued high standard of quality and his efforts are greatly appreciated by our team.

The editors would like to extend their deepest gratitude to Kenneth Howe, MA, for his outstanding organizational skills. Ken combines an easy and approachable manner with a tireless work ethic, both of which served to keep us focused, organized, and motivated so we could meet our highest expectations for this book. His efforts are very much appreciated by the Editorial team.

We gratefully acknowledge the contributions of Dr. Mahendr Kochar whose gentle encouragement and quiet leadership helped us to bring forth our best effort.

We thank the following medical student reviewers from the Medical College of Wisconsin class of 2007 and 2008 for their contribution to this book. Their feedback, ideas, and critiques have been essential for the development of the fifth edition of *Kochar's Clinical Medicine for Students.*

Class of 2007

Anderson Bauer
Elizabeth Becherer
Elizabeth Berdan
Nicole Collins
Shana Elman
Erica Fallon
Damian Kosempa
Andrew Palisch
David Pugh
Charlene Vander Zanden

Class of 2008

Robert Beyer
Kyle Blake
Jared Burton
Mary Castillo
Shaun Corbett
Jennifer Fancher
Ethan Handler
Jeehea Haw
Pardis Javadi
Jessica Lambert
Samantha Lewis
Eileen Lorenz
Christine Palmer
Khanh Pham
Payal Potnis
Andrea Rock
Stephanie Siehr
Michael Stoesz
Rachel Thompson
Christopher Vaughan

ACKNOWLEDGMENTS

We express our appreciation to the contributors and their office staff who have worked diligently and patiently in getting their literary contributions into our hands on time. The Editorial Staff at Lippincott Williams & Wilkins, including Donna Balado, Nancy Duffy, Liz Stalnaker, Jennifer [illegible] and Catherine Noonan.

We would also like to take this opportunity to thank Dr. G. Richard Olds, The John and Linda Mellowes Professor and Chairman, Department of Medicine, Medical College of Wisconsin, and Dr. Lee A. Biblo, Professor and Vice Chairman, Department of Medicine, Medical College of Wisconsin, for their emphatic and unwavering support of this book and their enthusiasm that served to inspire each of its contributors and members of the editorial team.

Thank you to Dr. Ann B. Nattinger, Professor and Chief, General Internal Medicine, Department of Medicine, Medical College of Wisconsin, for your enthusiastic support of this project, which served to inspire and energize the authors.

We would also like to offer our sincere thanks to Dr. Pietro Antonio who gave generously of his time as a reviewer. His expertise and careful eye ensured a continued high standard of quality and his efforts are greatly appreciated by our team.

The editors would like to extend their deepest gratitude to Kenneth Rowe, MM, for his outstanding organizational skills. Ken combines an easy and approachable manner with a tireless work ethic, both of which served to keep us focused, organized, and motivated so we could meet our highest expectations for this book. His efforts are very much appreciated by the Editorial team.

We gratefully acknowledge the contributions of Dr. Mahendr Kochar whose gentle encouragement and quiet leadership helped us to bring forth our best effort.

We thank the following medical student reviewers from the Medical College of Wisconsin class of 2007 and 2008 for their contribution to this book. Their feedback, ideas, and critiques have been essential for the development of the fifth edition of *Kochar's Clinical Medicine for Students.*

Class of 2007	Class of 2008	
Anderson Bauer	Robert Beyer	Samantha Lewis
Elizabeth Bechtler	Kyle Blake	Eileen Lorenz
Elizabeth Beedan	Jared Burton	Christine Palmer
Nicole Collins	Mary Carrillo	Khanh Pham
Sirina Ehrom	Shaun Corbett	Payal Patel
Erica Fallon	Jennifer Fenchler	Andrea Rock
Damian Kosempa	Ethan Handler	Stephanie Sucher
Andrew Pallisch	Jessica Haw	Michael Specz
David Pugh	Pardis Javadi	Rachel Thompson
Charlene Vander Zanden	Jessica Lambert	Christopher Vaughan

CONTRIBUTORS

John W. Adamson, MD, FACP (Hematology)
Chief of Hematology
Professor of Medicine
Division of Hematology
Medical College of Wisconsin
Milwaukee, Wisconsin

William Anderson, MD (Ambulatory Medicine)
Staff Psychiatrist
Mental Health Division
Zablocki VA Medical Center
Milwaukee, Wisconsin

Raj Bhargava, MD, FACP, FAAP (Key Manifestation)
Clinical Assistant Professor of Medicine
Medical College of Wisconsin
Professional Internal Medicine Services, SC
St. Joseph Regional Medical Center
Milwaukee, Wisconsin

Lee Biblo, MD (Cardiology)
Vice-Chairman for Clinical Activities
Professor of Medicine
Department of Medicine
Medical College of Wisconsin
Milwaukee, Wisconsin

Diane Book, MD (Neurology)
Assistant Professor of Neurology
Department of General Neurology
Medical College of Wisconsin
Milwaukee, Wisconsin

Ty Carroll, MD (Endocrinology)
Clinical Instructor
Chief Resident
Department of Medicine
Medical College of Wisconsin
Milwaukee, Wisconsin

John Charlson, MD (Hematology & Oncology)
Assistant Professor of Medicine
Department of Medicine
Medical College of Wisconsin
Milwaukee, Wisconsin

Christopher Chitambar, MD, FACP (Oncology)
Professor of Medicine
Division of Neoplastic Diseases
Department of Medicine
Medical College of Wisconsin
Milwaukee, Wisconsin

Asriani (Ria) Chiu, MD, FACP (Allergy & Clinical Immunology)
Assistant Professor of Pediatrics and Medicine
Division of Allergy and Immunology
Medical College of Wisconsin
Chief, Section of Allergy
Zablocki VA Medical Center
Milwaukee, Wisconsin

Mary Cohan, MD (Geriatrics)
Assistant Professor of Medicine
Division of Geriatrics & Gerontology
Department of Medicine
Medical College of Wisconsin
Milwaukee, Wisconsin

Sumanth Daram, MD (Allergy & Clinical Immunology)
Assistant Clinical Professor
Medical College of Wisconsin
St. Joseph's Hospital
Milwaukee, Wisconsin

Susan Davids, MD (Infectious Diseases)
Assistant Professor of Medicine
Department of Medicine
Medical College of Wisconsin
Milwaukee, Wisconsin

Kathryn Denson, MD (Geriatrics)
Assistant Professor of Medicine
Division of Geriatrics and Gerontology
Department of Medicine
Medical College of Wisconsin
Milwaukee, Wisconsin

Steve Denson, MD (Rheumatology)
Assistant Professor of Medicine
Division of Geriatrics and Gerontology
Department of Medicine
Medical College of Wisconsin
Milwaukee, Wisconsin

Edmund H. Duthie, Jr., MD (Geriatrics)
Professor of Medicine
Chief, Geriatrics and Gerontology
Department of Medicine
Medical College of Wisconsin
Froedtert Hospital
Zablocki VA Medical Center
Milwaukee, Wisconsin

Michael Earing, MD (Cardiovascular Diseases)
Assistant Professor of Pediatrics and Medicine
Medical College of Wisconsin
Milwaukee, Wisconsin

Janet Fairley, MD (Dermatology)
Professor of Dermatology
Chief of Dermatology
Medical College of Wisconsin
Zablocki VA Medical Center
Milwaukee, Wisconsin

Deidre Faust, MD (Rheumatology)
Clinical Assistant Professor of Medicine
Medical College of Wisconsin
Milwaukee, Wisconsin

Karen Fickel, MD (Ambulatory Medicine)
Assistant Professor of Medicine
Director, Sargeant Internal Medicine Clinic
Medical College of Wisconsin
Milwaukee, Wisconsin

José Franco, MD (Gastroenterology & Hepatology)
Associate Professor of Medicine
Division of Gastroenterology and Hepatology
Medical College of Wisconsin
Milwaukee, Wisconsin

Michael O. Frank, MD, FACP (Infectious Diseases)
Associate Professor of Medicine
Division of Infectious Diseases
Director, Residency Program
Department of Medicine
Medical College of Wisconsin
Milwaukee, Wisconsin

Virginia Gennis, MD (Behavioral Medicine)
Assistant Professor of Medicine
Department of Medicine
Medical College of Wisconsin
Milwaukee, Wisconsin

Richard Gibson, MD (Behavioral Medicine)
Assistant Professor of Psychiatry
Department of Psychiatry
Medical College of Wisconsin
Zablocki VA Medical Center
Milwaukee, Wisconsin

Amandeep Gill, MD (Key Manifestation)
Hospitalist
Department of Medicine
Medical College of Wisconsin
Milwaukee, Wisconsin

Jerome Gottschall, MD (Hematology)
Professor of Pathology
Department of Pathology
Medical College of Wisconsin
Milwaukee, Wisconsin

Paul Halverson, MD, FACP (Rheumatology)
Professor of Medicine
Division of Rheumatology
Department of Medicine
Medical College of Wisconsin
Milwaukee, Wisconsin

Avery Hayes, MD (Key Manifestation)
Assistant Professor of Medicine
Department of Medicine
Medical College of Wisconsin
Milwaukee, Wisconsin

Shibin Jacob, MD (Key Manifestation & Nephrology)
Hospitalist
Department of Medicine
Medical College of Wisconsin
Milwaukee, Wisconsin

Safwan Jaradeh, MD, FACP (Neurology)
Professor and Chairman of Neurology
Department of Neurology
Medical College of Wisconsin
Milwaukee, Wisconsin

Jasna Jevtic, MD (Infectious Diseases)
Assistant Professor of Medicine
Department of Medicine
Medical College of Wisconsin
Milwaukee, Wisconsin

Albert Jochen, MD (Endocrinology)
Associate Professor of Medicine
Division of Endocrinology, Metabolism &
Clinical Nutrition Department of Medicine
Medical College of Wisconsin
Zablocki VA Medical Center
Milwaukee, Wisconsin

James Kleczka, MD, FACC (Cardiology)
Assistant Professor of Medicine
Medical Director, Cardiology Inpatient Services & CICU
Division of Cardiology
Department of Medicine
Medical College of Wisconsin
Milwaukee, Wisconsin

Robert Krippendorf, MD (Dermatology)
Assistant Professor of Medicine
Department of Medicine
Medical College of Wisconsin
Milwaukee, Wisconsin

Kesavan Kutty, MD, FACP, FCCP (Pulmonary Disease & Critical Care)
Professor of Medicine
Department of Medicine
Chairman of Medicine
St. Joseph Regional Medical Center
Milwaukee, Wisconsin

Geoffrey C. Lamb, MD (Cardiology)
Associate Professor of Medicine
Department of Medicine
Medical College of Wisconsin
Milwaukee, Wisconsin

Gunnar Larson, MD (Psychiatry)
Assistant Professor of Psychiatry
Department of Psychiatry
Medical College of Wisconsin
Zablocki VA Medical Center
Milwaukee, Wisconsin

Jon Lehrmann, MD (Psychiatry)
Assistant Professor of Psychiatry
Department of Psychiatry
Medical College of Wisconsin
Zablocki VA Medical Center
Milwaukee, Wisconsin

Ann Maguire, MD, MPH (Key Manifestation)
Assistant Professor of Medicine
Department of Medicine
Medical College of Wisconsin
Milwaukee, Wisconsin

Bob Maglio, MD (Ambulatory Medicine)
Assistant Professor of Medicine
Department of Medicine
Medical College of Wisconsin
Milwaukee, Wisconsin

Ellen McCarthy, MD (Nephrology)
Associate Professor of Medicine
Division of Nephrology & Hypertension
Department of Medicine
University of Kansas Medical Center
Kansas City, Kansas

Theodore MacKinney, MD, MPH, FACP (Ambulatory Medicine)
Assistant Professor of Medicine
Department of Medicine
Medical College of Wisconsin
Milwaukee, Wisconsin

Julie Mitchell, MD, MS (Key Manifestation & Ambulatory Medicine)
Assistant Professor of Medicine
Department of Medicine
Medical College of Wisconsin
Milwaukee, Wisconsin

Marcos Montagnini, MD (Key Manifestations & Geriatrics)
Assistant Professor of Medicine
Division of Geriatrics & Gerontology
Department of Medicine
Medical College of Wisconsin
Milwaukee, Wisconsin

Tayyab Mohyuddin, MD (Cardiology)
Assistant Professor of Medicine
Hospitalist
Department of Medicine
Medical College of Wisconsin
Milwaukee, Wisconsin

Martin Muntz, MD (Neurology)
Assistant Professor of Medicine
Department of Medicine
Medical College of Wisconsin
Milwaukee, Wisconsin

Joan Neuner, MD (Ambulatory Medicine)
Assistant Professor of Medicine
Department of Medicine
Medical College of Wisconsin
Milwaukee, Wisconsin

Kendall Novoa-Takara, MD (Ambulatory Medicine)
Assistant Professor of Medicine
Department of Medicine
Medical College of Wisconsin
Milwaukee, Wisconsin

Gwen O'Keefe, MD (Key Manifestation)
Assistant Professor of Medicine
Department of Medicine
Medical College of Wisconsin
Milwaukee, Wisconsin

Irene O'Shaughnessy, MD, FACP (Endocrinology)
Professor of Medicine
Associate Chief of Endocrinology
Division of Endocrinology, Metabolism & Clinical Nutrition Department of Medicine
Medical College of Wisconsin
Milwaukee, Wisconsin

Jenny Petkova, MD (Hematology & Oncology)
Assistant Professor of Medicine
Department of Medicine
Medical College of Wisconsin
Milwaukee, Wisconsin

Kurt Pfeifer, MD (Gastroenterology & Hepatology)
Assistant Professor of Medicine
Department of Medicine
Medical College of Wisconsin
Milwaukee, Wisconsin

Vishal Ratkalkar, MD, FACP (Cardiology)
Clinical Assistant Professor of Medicine
St. Joseph's Hospital
Milwaukee, Wisconsin

Robert Riniker, MD (Nephrology)
Assistant Professor of Medicine
Department of Medicine
Medical College of Wisconsin
Milwaukee, Wisconsin

Elizabeth Russell, MD (Key Manifestation)
Assistant Professor of Medicine
Department of Medicine
Medical College of Wisconsin
Milwaukee, Wisconsin

Kia Saeian, MD (Gastroenterology & Hepatology)
Assistant Professor of Medicine
Director, GI Endoscopy Laboratory
Division of Gastroenterology and Hepatology
Department of Medicine
Medical College of Wisconsin
Milwaukee, Wisconsin

Linus Santo Tomas, MD (Pulmonary Disease & Critical Care)
Assistant Professor of Medicine
Division of Pulmonary/Critical Care
Department of Medicine
Medical College of Wisconsin
Milwaukee, Wisconsin

Virginia Savin, MD (Nephrology)
Professor of Medicine
Division of Nephrology
Department of Medicine
Medical College of Wisconsin
Milwaukee, Wisconsin

Ralph M. Schapira, MD, FACP, FCCP (Pulmonary Disease & Critical Care)
Professor and Vice-Chairman of Medicine
Medical College of Wisconsin
Chief of Medicine
Zablocki VA Medical Center
Milwaukee, Wisconsin

Siddhartha Singh, MD (Pulmonary Disease & Critical Care)
Assistant Professor of Medicine
Department of Medicine
Medical College of Wisconsin
Milwaukee, Wisconsin

Christopher Sobczak, MD (Ambulatory Medicine)
Assistant Professor of Medicine & Pediatrics
Departments of Medicine & Pediatrics
Medical College of Wisconsin
Milwaukee, Wisconsin

Heather L. Toth, MD (Key Manifestation)
Assistant Professor of Medicine & Pediatrics
Departments of Medicine & Pediatrics
Medical College of Wisconsin
Milwaukee, Wisconsin

Dario M. Torre, MD, MPH, FACP (Key Manifestations)
Associate Professor of Medicine
Medicine Clerkship Director
Department of Medicine, VA Medical Center
Medical College of Wisconsin
Milwaukee, Wisconsin

Jerome J. Van Ruiswyk, MD, MS, FACP (Ambulatory Medicine & Geriatrics)
Associate Professor of Medicine
Department of Medicine
Medical College of Wisconsin
Associate Chief of Staff for Clinical Affairs
Zablocki VA Medical Center
Milwaukee, Wisconsin

Jeff Wesson, PhD, MD (Nephrology)
Assistant Professor of Medicine
Division of Nephrology
Department of Medicine
Medical College of Wisconsin
Zablocki VA Medical Center
Milwaukee, Wisconsin

Jeffrey Whittle, MD, MPH (Ambulatory Medicine)
Associate Professor of Medicine
Department of Medicine
Medical College of Wisconsin
Milwaukee, Wisconsin

Krista Wiger, MD (Gastroenterology & Hepatology)
Assistant Professor of Medicine
Department of Medicine
Medical College of Wisconsin
Milwaukee, Wisconsin

Priya Young, MD (Dermatology)
Assistant Professor of Dermatology
Department of Dermatology
Medical College of Wisconsin
Milwaukee, Wisconsin

Jennifer R. Zebrack, MD, FACP (General Internal Medicine)
Associate Professor of Medicine
Division of General Internal Medicine
University of Nevada School of Medicine
Reno, Nevada

Monica Ziebert, MD, DDS (Key Manifestation)
Assistant Professor of Medicine
Department of Medicine
Medical College of Wisconsin
Milwaukee, Wisconsin

CONTENTS

Foreword *vii*

Preface *ix*

Acknowledgments *xi*

Contributor *xiii*

I Key Manifestations and Presentations of Diseases—Dario Torre

1. Abdominal Pain 2
JOSÉ FRANCO

2. Acid-Base Disorders 7
MONICA ZIEBERT

3. Acute Gastrointestinal Bleeding 13
MONICA ZIEBERT

4. Altered Mental Status 19
JULIE MITCHELL and DARIO TORRE

5. Anemia 25
GWEN O'KEEFE and DARIO TORRE

6. Chest Pain 31
DARIO TORRE

7. Cough 37
SHIBIN JACOB and AMANDEEP GILL

8. Diarrhea 41
DARIO TORRE and JOSÉ FRANCO

9. Dizziness and Vertigo 48
AVERY HAYES

10. Dyspnea 54
ANN MAGUIRE

11. Dysuria 61
JULIE MITCHELL

12. Edema 68
ANN MAGUIRE

13. Fever and Rash 72
HEATHER TOTH

14. Fever and Fever of Unknown Origin 76
JASNA JEVTIC

15. Headache 80
RAJ BHARGAVA

16. Heart Sounds and Murmurs 86
GEOFFREY C. LAMB and DARIO TORRE

17. Hematuria 94
AVERY HAYES

18. Hemoptysis 98
AMANDEEP GILL and SHIBIN JACOB

19. Jaundice 101
MONICA ZIEBERT

20. Joint Pain 109
ELIZABETH RUSSELL

21. Nausea and Vomiting 116
MONICA ZIEBERT

22. Seizures 121
GEOFFREY C. LAMB and DARIO TORRE

23. Shock 125
ANN MAGUIRE

24. Syncope 130
ANN MAGUIRE

25. Thrombocytopenia 137
GWEN O'KEEFE and DARIO TORRE

26. Weight Loss 141
MARCOS MONTAGNINI

II Diseases and Disorders

Cardiology—Geoffrey C. Lamb

27. Coronary Artery Disease 148
JAMES KLECZKA

28. Heart Failure 169
GEOFFREY C. LAMB

29. Cardiomyopathies/Myocarditis 178
TAYYAB MOHYUDDIN

30. Valvular Heart Disease 186
GEOFFREY C. LAMB

31. Pericardial Disease 197
VISHAL RATKALKAR

32. Arrhythmias 204
LEE BIBLO

33. Atrial Fibrillation 216
LEE BIBLO

34. Aortic Dissection 220
JAMES KLECZKA

Pulmonary—Ralph Schapira

35. Bronchial Asthma 226
LINUS SANTO TOMAS

36. Chronic Obstructive Pulmonary Disease 232
LINUS SANTO TOMAS

37. Interstitial Lung Disease 239
LINUS SANTO TOMAS

38. Pleural Effusions 243
SIDDHARTHA SINGH

39. Pneumothorax 247
SIDDHARTHA SINGH

40. Obstructive Sleep Apnea 250
SIDDHARTHA SINGH

41. Venous Thromboembolic Disease 252
SIDDHARTHA SINGH

42. Asbestosis 259
RALPH SCHAPIRA

43. Tuberculosis 261
KESAVAN KUTTY

44. Sarcoidosis 266
LINUS SANTO TOMAS

45. The Solitary Pulmonary Nodule 269
LINUS SANTO TOMAS

Rheumatology—Deidre Faust, Paul Halverson, and Steve Denson

46. Osteoarthritis 274
STEVEN DENSON and PAUL HALVERSON

47. Rheumatoid Arthritis 279
DEIDRE FAUST and PAUL HALVERSON

48. Systemic Lupus Erythematosus 288
DEIDRE FAUST and PAUL HALVERSON

49. Polymyositis and Scleroderma 294
STEVEN DENSON and PAUL HALVERSON

50. Sjögren's Syndrome 298
STEVEN DENSON and PAUL HALVERSON

51. Seronegative Spondyloarthropathies 300
STEVEN DENSON and PAUL HALVERSON

52. Wegener's, Polyarteritis Nodosa, Polymyalgia Rheumatica, and Temporal Arteritis 305
STEVEN DENSON and PAUL HALVERSON

53. Gout and Other Crystal-induced Synovitis 310
DEIDRE FAUST and PAUL HALVERSON

54. Infectious Arthritis 314
STEVEN DENSON and PAUL HALVERSON

Infectious Diseases—Michael Frank

55. Pneumonia 320
JASNA JEVTIC

56. Urinary Tract Infection 328
JASNA JEVTIC

57. Cellulitis 333
SUSAN DAVIDS

58. Meningitis and Encephalitis 337
MICHAEL FRANK

59. Sepsis Syndrome 343
JASNA JEVTIC

60. Endocarditis 349
JASNA JEVTIC

61. Osteomyelitis 358
SUSAN DAVIDS

62. Syphilis 362
SUSAN DAVIDS

63. HIV Infection 366
MICHAEL FRANK

Endocrinology—Irene O'Shaughnessy and Albert Jochen

64. Diabetes Mellitus and Hypoglycemia 378
JENNIFER ZEBRACK

65. Disorders of Parathyroid, Calcium, Vitamin D, and Metabolic Bone Diseases 391
JENNIFER ZEBRACK

66. Thyroid Diseases 401
TY CARROLL

67. Anterior Pituitary Diseases 413
TY CARROLL

68. Posterior Pituitary Diseases (Diabetes Insipidus/Syndrome of Antidiuretic Hormone) 421
TY CARROLL

69. Diseases of the Adrenal Glands 427
JENNIFER ZEBRACK and ALBERT JOCHEN

Gastroenterology—Kia Saeian

70. Peptic Ulcer Disease 442
KRISTA WIGER

71. Gastroesophageal Reflux Disease 450
KURT PFEIFER

72. Biliary Disorders 454
KIA SAEIAN

73. Hepatitis 463
KIA SAEIAN

74. Cirrhosis 475
JOSÉ FRANCO

75. Pancreatitis 482
KRISTA WIGER

76. Inflammatory Bowel Disease 490
KURT PFEIFER

77. Diverticular Disease of the Colon 497
KURT PFEIFER

78. Bowel Obstruction 500
KURT PFEIFER

Nephrology—Virginia Savin

79. Acute Renal Failure 504
ROBERT RINIKER

80. Chronic Renal Failure 512
SHIBIN JACOB and VIRGINIA SAVIN

81. Glomerulonephritis 520
VIRGINIA SAVIN

82. Nephrotic Syndrome 528
ROBERT RINIKER

83. Acute Interstitial Nephritis 531
VIRGINIA SAVIN

84. Polycystic Kidney Disease 533
ELLEN MCCARTHY

85. Nephrolithiasis 535
JEFFREY WESSON

86. Fluid and Electrolyte Disorders 539
VIRGINIA SAVIN

87. Hypertensive Emergencies 550
SHIBIN JACOB and VIRGINIA SAVIN

Hematology—John Adamson

88. Acute Leukemias 556
JOHN CHARLSON

89. Myeloproliferative Disorders 561
JOHN CHARLSON

90. Iron Deficiency Anemia 569
JOHN CHARLSON and JENNY PETKOVA

91. B_{12} Deficiency and Other Megaloblastic Anemias 573
JOHN CHARLSON

92. Anemia of Chronic Disease 575
JOHN CHARLSON

93. Sickle Cell Disease 577
JENNY PETKOVA

94. Thalassemias 580
JENNY PETKOVA

95. Hereditary Spherocytosis 585
JENNY PETKOVA

96. Autoimmune Hemolytic Anemia 588
JENNY PETKOVA

97. ITP/TTP/HUS 593
JENNY PETKOVA

98. Disseminated Intravascular Coagulation 599
JENNY PETKOVA

99. Hemophilia/von Willebrand Disease 602
JENNY PETKOVA

Oncology—Christopher Chitambar

100. Multiple Myeloma 612
JOHN CHARLSON

101. Lymphomas 617
JOHN CHARLSON

102. Breast Cancer 624
JOHN CHARLSON

103. Colon Cancer 631
JENNY PETKOVA

104. Lung Cancer 635
JOHN CHARLSON

105. Cervical, Endometrial, and Ovarian Cancers 639
JENNY PETKOVA

106. Prostate Cancer 647
JENNY PETKOVA

Neurology—Martin Muntz, Safwan Jaradeh, and Diane Book

107. Ischemic Stroke 652
DIANE BOOK and MARTIN MUNTZ

108. Intracerebral and Subarachnoid Hemorrhage 660
DIANE BOOK and MARTIN MUNTZ

109. Seizures 665
MARTIN MUNTZ and DIANE BOOK

110. Headaches 668
MARTIN MUNTZ and DIANE BOOK

111. Normal Pressure Hydrocephalus 671
MARTIN MUNTZ and DIANE BOOK

112. Parkinson's Disease 673
MARTIN MUNTZ and SAFWAN JARADEH

113. Peripheral Neuropathy 677
MARTIN MUNTZ and SAFWAN JARADEH

114. Multiple Sclerosis 680
MARTIN MUNTZ and SAFWAN JARADEH

115. Amytrophic Lateral Sclerosis 684
MARTIN MUNTZ and SAFWAN JARADEH

116. Guillain-Barré Syndrome 686
MARTIN MUNTZ and SAFWAN JARADEH

117. Myasthenia Gravis 689
MARTIN MUNTZ and SAFWAN JARADEH

Psychiatry—Jon Lehrmann

118. Depression 696
KIMBERLY STONER and JON LEHRMANN

119. Anxiety Disorders 702
KIMBERLY STONER and GUNNAR LARSON

120. Schizophrenia 707
KIMBERLY STONER and GUNNAR LARSON

121. Eating Disorders 711
KIMBERLY STONER and JON LEHRMANN

Dermatology—Priya Young, Robert Krippendorf, and Janet Fairley

122. Psoriasis 718
ROBERT KRIPPENDORF, PRIYA YOUNG, and JANET FAIRLEY

123. Seborrheic Dermatitis 720
ROBERT KRIPPENDORF, PRIYA YOUNG, and JANET FAIRLEY

124. Impetigo 721
ROBERT KRIPPENDORF, PRIYA YOUNG, and JANET FAIRLEY

125. Dermatophytosis 723
ROBERT KRIPPENDORF, PRIYA YOUNG, and JANET FAIRLEY

126. Acne 728
ROBERT KRIPPENDORF, PRIYA YOUNG, and JANET FAIRLEY

127. Basal Cell Carcinoma, Actinic Keratoses, Squamous Cell Carcinoma, and Malignant Melanoma 732
ROBERT KRIPPENDORF, PRIYA YOUNG, and JANET FAIRLEY

128. Urticaria 738
ROBERT KRIPPENDORF, PRIYA YOUNG, and JANET FAIRLEY

III Ambulatory Medicine—Jerome Van Ruiswyk

129. Disease Prevention and Screening 742
JEROME VAN RUISWYK

130. Smoking Cessation 749
ROBERT MAGLIO

131. Substance Abuse 753
KIMBERLY STONER and WILLIAM ANDERSON

132. Obesity 757
JENNIFER ZEBRACK

133. Hypertension 761
JEFF WHITTLE

134. Dyslipidemias 776
KAREN FICKEL

135. Osteoporosis 783
JOAN NEUNER

136. Back Pain 787
KENDALL NOVOA-TAKARA

137. Knee, Shoulder, and Other Regional Musculoskeletal Syndromes 792
JEROME VAN RUISWYK

138. Upper Respiratory Tract Infection 801
ROBERT MAGLIO

139. Sexually Transmitted Diseases 805
CHRISTOPHER SOBCZAK

Women's Health Issues

140. Menstrual Concerns and Menopause 814
JULIE MITCHELL and JENNIFER ZEBRACK

141. Polycystic Ovary Syndrome and Hirsutism 820
JENNIFER ZEBRACK and JULIE MITCHELL

142. Contraception 823
JENNIFER ZEBRACK and JULIE MITCHELL

Geriatrics

143. Falls 830
MARCOS MONTAGNINI

144. Delirium and Dementia 834
JEROME VAN RUISWYK and EDMUND DUTHIE

145. Urinary Incontinence 840
MARY COHAN and KATHRYN DENSON

146. Benign Prostatic Hypertrophy 843
JEROME VAN RUISWYK

Online Chapters

Diseases and Disorders (Part II)

Cardiology—Geoffrey C. Lamb

E1. Congenital Heart Disease in Adults
MICHAEL G. EARING

E2. Electrocardiography
GEOFFREY C. LAMB

Pulmonary—Ralph Schapira

E3. Pulmonary Function Testing
RALPH SCHAPIRA

E4. Cystic Fibrosis and Bronchiectasis
RALPH SCHAPIRA

E5. Pulmonary Hypertension
RALPH SCHAPIRA

E6. Adult Respiratory Distress Syndrome
RALPH SCHAPIRA

E7. Mycoses
RALPH SCHAPIRA

Endocrinology—Ty Carroll

E8. Thyroid Cancer
TY CARROLL

Gastroenterology—Kia Saeian

E9. Benign and Malignant Liver Tumors
KIA SAEIAN

E10. Nonalcoholic Steatshepatitis and Nonalcoholic Fatty Liver Disease
DARIO TORRE

E11. Pancreatic Cancer
KIA SAEIAN

Hematology—John Adamson

E12. Leukopenia
JENNY PETKOVA

E13. Reactive Leukocytosis
JENNY PETKOVA

E14. Eosinophilia
JENNY PETKOVA

E15. Blood Transfusion
JENNY PETKOVA, JOHN CHARLSON, and JEROME GOTTSCHALL

E16. Heparin Induced Thrombocytopenia
JENNY PETKOVA

Nephrology—Virginia Savin

E17. Acid-Base Disorders
VIRGINIA SAVIN

E18. Renal Tubular Acidosis
VIRGINIA SAVIN

Psychiatry—Jon Lehrmann

E19. Somatoform Disorders
JEROME VAN RUISWYK and JON LEHRMANN

E20. Substance Abuse
JEROME VAN RUISWYK and JON LEHRMANN

Dermatology—Priya Young and Robert Krippendorf

E21. General Approach to Dermatologic Disorders
ROBERT KRIPPENDORF

E22. Dermatitis and Eczema
ROBERT KRIPPENDORF, PRIYA YOUNG, and JANET FAIRLEY

E23. Vitiligo
ROBERT KRIPPENDORF, PRIYA YOUNG, and JANET FAIRLEY

E24. Herpes
ROBERT KRIPPENDORF, PRIYA YOUNG, and JANET FAIRLEY

E25. Common Warts
ROBERT KRIPPENDORF, PRIYA YOUNG, and JANET FAIRLEY

E26. Eryspipelas
ROBERT KRIPPENDORF, PRIYA YOUNG, and JANET FAIRLEY

E27. Scabies
ROBERT KRIPPENDORF, PRIYA YOUNG, and JANET FAIRLEY

Allergy and Clinical Immunology—Sumanth Daram and Asriani Chiu

E28. Anaphylaxis
SUMANTH DARAM and ASRIANI CHIU

E29. Drug Allergy
SUMANTH DARAM and ASRIANI CHIU

Ambulatory Medicine—Jerome Van Ruiswyk

E30. Chronic Pain
THEODORE MACKINNEY

E31. Red Eye
JEROME VAN RUISWYK

E32. Benign Breast Problems
JULIE MITCHELL and JENNIFER ZEBRACK

E33. Preconception Care and Issues in Pregnancy
JULIE MITCHELL and JENNIFER ZEBRACK

E34. Functional Decline in Elderly Patients
KATHRYN DENSON and MARY COHAN

I

Key Manifestations and Presentations of Diseases

Dario Torre

CHAPTER 1

Abdominal Pain

José Franco

Abdominal pain is one of the most common indications for patients seeking health care. It is a cause of significant morbidity and mortality. Annual costs are in the billions of dollars as a result of direct health costs, as well as indirect costs through lost wages and productivity.

Although abdominal pain can be classified as acute or chronic, this chapter will focus only on acute pain.

DIFFERENTIAL DIAGNOSIS

The most common causes that should be included in the differential diagnosis of acute abdominal pain are listed in Table 1.1.

Abdominal pain typically can be divided into visceral, somatoparietal, and referred pain syndromes (Fig. 1.1). Visceral pain is typically dull and poorly localized to one of three regions: the epigastric, periumbilical, or lower midabdomen regions. The patient tends to complain of nausea and frequently has emesis. Attempts to relieve the pain by changes in position are rarely successful. Somatoparietal pain develops when there is peritoneal wall irritation, frequently from progressive inflammation of involved viscera. Due to greater innervation relative to viscera, somatoparietal pain is better localized and tends to be "sharper." Unlike visceral pain, the patient prefers to remain motionless. Referred pain is felt at sites distant from the involved organs and is the result of convergence of visceral afferent and somatic neurons from different locations.

Gastroenteritis is most commonly the result of a virus. The patient characteristically complains of nonfocal, crampy abdominal pain that is mild to moderate in intensity and temporally progresses over days before peaking and resolving. Associated symptoms include low-grade fevers, nausea, emesis not related to meals, and diarrhea. Examination reveals generalized tenderness without evidence of guarding or rebound. With more severe cases, there is evidence of dehydration that may manifest as sunken eyes, dry mucous membranes, skin tenting, and orthostatic hypotension.

Appendicitis typically begins with vague periumbilical pain associated with nausea and occasionally vomiting, which progresses over the course of 6 to 10 hours to a more intense and localized pain in the right lower quadrant. Symptoms are not consistently associated with meals. Low-grade fevers are common. The presence of involuntary guarding and rebound pain are peritoneal signs and, along with high fevers, suggest perforation.

Biliary colic is the result of intermittent obstruction of the cystic duct by calculi. The pain is dull and is localized to the right upper quadrant and epigastric region. The duration typically is 6 to 8 hours and may be preceded by a fatty meal. Associated symptoms include nausea, emesis, and occasionally low-grade fevers. Between pain episodes, the patient may be asymptomatic for days to years.

Cholecystitis is caused by persistent obstruction of the cystic duct by calculi, which causes symptoms similar to those of biliary colic but differs in that symptoms persist beyond the 6- to 8-hour

TABLE 1.1 Differential diagnosis of acute abdominal pain

Gastroenteritis
Appendicitis
Biliary colic
Cholecystitis
Pancreatitis
Diverticulitis
Small bowel obstruction
Perforated peptic ulcer
Mesenteric ischemia
Ruptured abdominal aortic aneurysm

period. The pain can be localized to the epigastric area and right upper quadrant or radiate toward the right scapular region (Chapter 72).

Pancreatitis typically presents with epigastric pain that progresses in severity over the course of hours to days. Although initially described as vague, the pain becomes more localized, unrelenting, and is associated with radiation to the back. Associated symptoms include nausea, vomiting, and fever. Although symptoms are generally progressive, they most commonly worsen with meals. Examination varies depending on severity but may include hypoactive bowel sounds, guarding, and rebound. Intra-abdominal bleeding into the pancreatic bed, in very severe cases, may manifest with periumbilical (Cullen's sign) or flank (Gray-Turner's sign) ecchymoses (Chapter 75).

Diverticulitis is an infection of colonic diverticula. It is most commonly seen in elderly patients and usually involves the sigmoid colon. The pain is initially poorly localized to the lower mid-abdomen and is described as dull. With progression of symptoms, over hours to days, localization to the left lower quadrant occurs. Associated nausea, vomiting, and fever are common. Examination reveals tenderness, guarding, and possibly a palpable mass (Chapter 77).

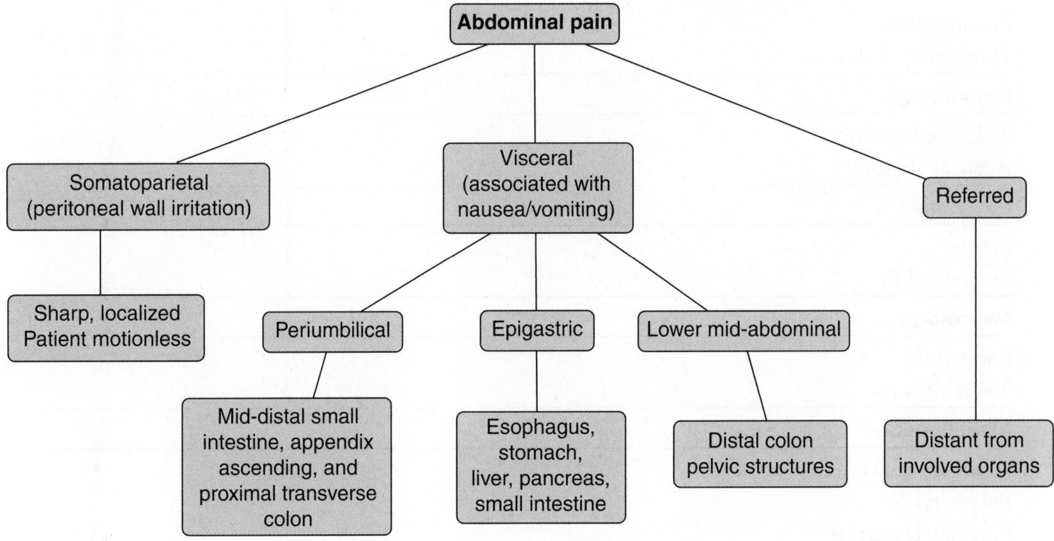

Figure 1.1 • Types of abdominal pain.

Small bowel obstruction in adults is most commonly the result of intra-abdominal adhesions from previous surgeries. Depending on the site of obstruction, the patient may complain of epigastric (upper small bowel obstruction) or periumbilical (distal small bowel obstruction) pain that is frequently described as crampy. Emesis of bilious or feculent material is common. Examination reveals distension, diffuse tenderness, and hyperactive bowel sounds. Peritoneal symptoms typically are absent. Low-grade fever may be present.

Perforated peptic ulcer most commonly occurs in the proximal portion of the duodenum. The pain is severe and initially localized to the epigastric region; however, gastric and intestinal contents quickly spread down the right pericolic gutter, leading to diffuse peritonitis. Examination frequently reveals hypotension, tachycardia, involuntary guarding, abdominal rigidity, and rebound (Chapter 70).

Mesenteric ischemia typically is seen in patients with compromised intestinal circulation such as those with cardiac arrhythmias, peripheral vascular disease, and hypercoagulable states. These conditions predispose patients to acute arterial and venous insufficiency. The pain is poorly localized to the epigastric and periumbilical regions and is frequently described as having developed suddenly. A detailed history, however, will reveal preceding milder pain that worsens with meals and is suggestive of pre-existing ischemia. Examination will reveal an uncomfortable patient with relatively benign findings seemingly out of proportion to the severe subjective complaints. Evidence of gastroin-

TABLE 1.2 Differential diagnosis of nonabdominal causes of adominal pain

Cardiac
Myocardial ischemia
Myocarditis
Endocarditis
Thoracic
Esophagitis
Esophageal spasm
Esophageal rupture
Pneumonia
Pneumothorax
Pulmonary embolism
Hematologic
Sickle cell anemia
Acute leukemia
Infections
Herpes
Osteomyelitis
Neurologic
Radiculitis
Tabes dorsalis
Miscellaneous
Muscular contusion
Porphyria
Psychiatric disease

testinal bleeding is common. If bowel infarction has occurred, vital signs are unstable with hypotension and tachycardia being present.

Abdominal aortic rupture is a rapidly occurring event. Patients present with acute midabdominal pain that is described as "tearing." The patient is typically hemodynamically unstable with hypotension and tachycardia. Femoral pulses are diminished to absent and skin mottling is present. Nonabdominal causes of abdominal pain should also be considered in the differential diagnosis (Table 1.2).

EVALUATION

Evaluation of the patient with acute abdominal pain involves a thorough but rapid history and examination.

Subjective characterization of pain is highly variable and frequently unreliable. There are significant variations in patients' perception of pain based on age, sex, ethnicity, and previous pain experience. Pain scales, including those assigning numerical values, have not been validated and should be avoided as a diagnostic tool.

Changes in the quality and severity of abdominal pain over time are frequently helpful in determining the etiology. Pain that progresses over hours to days and resolves spontaneously over similar time periods is suggestive of gastroenteritis. If family members and close encounters of the patient have similar symptoms, this also suggests gastroenteritis. Pain whose presence and intensity waxes and wanes over days to weeks is suggestive of biliary colic. Pain that is progressive over time without waxing and waning, unless medical intervention is provided, could indicate diverticulitis, pancreatitis, and cholecystitis. Pain that develops acutely, frequently without prodromal symptoms, and rapidly progresses in minutes to an hour is seen in perforated peptic ulcer disease and ruptured abdominal aortic aneurysm.

Factors that lead to the development or exacerbation of pain are also helpful in determining the cause of abdominal pain. Symptoms that develop upon swallowing suggest an esophageal source. Pain that decreases with flatus or bowel movements suggests a colonic source and, less frequently, small bowel disease. Pain associated with any movement suggests peritonitis, whereas musculoskeletal pain may be caused by fatigue but no particular bodily movement.

SPECIFIC DISORDERS

Gastroenteritis is self-resolving in the majority of patients and can be managed conservatively without the need for extensive evaluation. When there is evidence of volume depletion, biochemical testing should include complete blood count with differential, electrolytes, and renal functions, which may show leukocytosis with left shift, hypokalemia, and prerenal azotemia, respectively. In addition, urinalysis to evaluate for urinary tract causes of pain, including infection, should be obtained. Abdominal imaging is rarely helpful.

Appendicitis should be evaluated with a complete blood count including differential, which will show leukocytosis with a left shift; a chemistry panel, which frequently reveals acidosis, multiple electrolyte disorders, and renal dysfunction; and urinalysis to evaluate for a urinary tract process. Computed tomography should be performed because it will reveal an inflamed appendix and occasional pericecal fluid collections.

Biliary colic should be evaluated with an abdominal ultrasound, which will reveal gallstones. Laboratory evaluation is typically unremarkable but may rarely reveal cholestatic liver tests with an elevated alkaline phosphatase and bilirubin.

Acute cholecystitis will result in inspiratory arrest on palpation of the right subcostal region (Murphy's sign). Radiographic evaluation most commonly includes ultrasound, which will reveal the presence of stones and, occasionally, gallbladder wall edema and pericholecystic fluid. Cholescintigraphy will demonstrate failure of the gallbladder to take up contrast. Biochemical testing reveals leukocytosis with a left shift and frequently mild transaminase, alkaline phosphatase, and bilirubin elevation.

Pancreatitis is evaluated with amylase and lipase testing and a liver panel. Cholestasis suggests gallstone pancreatitis. There is typically leukocytosis with a left shift and, in more severe cases, a metabolic acidosis. Imaging traditionally includes computed tomography, which serves multiple purposes including the exclusion of other abdominal pathology, staging the pancreatitis, and determining if complications such as necrosis and abscess are present.

Diverticulitis will occasionally result in a palpable left lower quadrant mass. Laboratory testing will reveal leukocytosis with possible left shift and pyuria if the involved segment is adjacent to the ureter or bladder. Computed tomography is the most useful imaging study when evaluating the patient with diverticulitis because it provides localization as well as identification of possible abscess or fistula.

Small bowel obstruction on auscultation will reveal increased high-pitched bowel sounds separated by episodes of relative quiet. Radiographic evaluation should include plain abdominal imaging, which confirms the diagnosis (air-fluid levels) as well as localizes the site of obstruction. In atypical cases, oral contrast studies with barium as well as computed tomography are helpful in confirming the diagnosis. Laboratory testing reveals mild leukocytosis and, in patients with significant vomiting, electrolyte disorders and prerenal azotemia may be present.

Perforated peptic ulcer disease is most commonly due to nonsteroidal anti-inflammatory agents in the elderly. Examination reveals diffuse peritonitis with a rigid board-like abdomen. Plain abdominal radiographs or computed tomography will reveal free air. Upper gastrointestinal series with water-soluble contrast will reveal the site of perforation if initial imaging is inconclusive. Upper endoscopy should be avoided in patients with suspected perforation. Laboratory testing will typically reveal leukocytosis with a left shift as well as a metabolic acidosis.

Mesenteric ischemia most commonly occurs in specific subgroups as previously described. A high index of suspicion is necessary because the abdomen is frequently soft and nondistended in some patients. The development of peritoneal symptoms suggests bowel infarction. Laboratory testing includes leukocytosis with a left shift, metabolic acidosis, and elevated lactic acid levels. Selective mesenteric angiography is the diagnostic study of choice and also offers therapeutic options.

Ruptured abdominal aortic aneurysm is a catastrophic event typically occurring in patients with atherosclerotic disease. The patient will present in hemodynamic shock. Laboratory testing demonstrating acidosis suggests lack of tissue perfusion. Numerous studies including ultrasound and computed tomography are helpful, but mortality remains high.

CHAPTER 2

Acid-Base Disorders

Monica Ziebert

Acid-base disorders are common and their consequences can be serious and even life threatening. They require precise diagnosis and treatment of the underlying conditions. There are four types of acid-base disorders: metabolic acidosis, metabolic alkalosis, respiratory acidosis, and respiratory alkalosis. Clinically, the disorders can present as simple (one disorder present) or mixed (more than one disorder present at the same time).

DIFFERENTIAL DIAGNOSIS

The common causes of acid-base disorders are listed in Table 2.1.

Metabolic Acidosis

In metabolic acidosis, there is a primary decrease in the serum bicarbonate (HCO_3). The clinical presentation depends on the cause but all patients with a severe metabolic acidosis can present with Kussmal breathing, very deep and rapid breathing, hypotension from a depressed myocardium, and vasodilation that results from acidemia. The causes of metabolic acidosis are classified according to the presence of a high anion gap or a normal anion gap. The anion gap refers to the difference between the serum concentrations of sodium (Na) and the major measured anions, chloride (Cl) and HCO_3. A normal anion gap is approximately 12 mEq/L ($\pm$ 2). In patients with a normal gap acidosis, as the bicarbonate decreases, the chloride will increase and the anion gap will be maintained. For example, a typical normal gap acidosis patient would present with Na 140 mEq/L, HCO_3 16 mEq/L, Cl 113 mEq/L, and an anion gap of 11 mEq/L. In patients with an elevated anion gap acidosis, the bicarbonate decreases and the anion gap increases reflecting an increase in unmeasured anions. For example, a typical anion gap acidosis would present with a Na 140, HCO_3 16, Cl 105, and an anion gap of 20 mEq/L. Several disorders and medications and toxins can cause an anion gap acidosis.

Advanced renal failure is the most common cause of metabolic anion gap acidosis in the outpatient setting. When kidney function deteriorates (creatinine >3.0 mg/dL), sulfates, phosphates, and metabolic waste products accumulate. Patients often complain of constitutional symptoms such as fatigue, nausea, and anorexia. Serum HCO_3 rarely decreases below 12 and the anion gap characteristically remains <20 mEq/L.

Lactic acidosis is the most common cause of metabolic anion gap acidosis in the hospitalized setting. Lactic acidosis develops secondary to tissue hypoperfusion most commonly from septic shock. Patients with septic shock will classically present with fever, tachypnea, tachycardia, and hypotension. Medications, including metformin in the setting of renal failure and antiretroviral therapy, can also lead to lactic acidosis. Serum lactate levels can confirm lactic acidosis.

Ketoacidosis elevates the anion gap secondary to the overproduction of the ketoacids, acetoacetic acid, and β-hydroxybutyric acid. Ketoacidosis typically occurs in three settings: diabetic ketoacidosis, starvation ketoacidosis, and alcoholic ketoacidosis. Diabetic ketoacidosis (DKA) occurs primarily in patients with compete insulin deficiency such as type 1 diabetes mellitus but it also occurs in type 2

TABLE 2.1 Common causes of acid-base disorders

Normal anion gap
Diarrhea Renal tubular acidosis (RTA) Ureteral diversions Early renal insufficiency
High anion gap
Ketoacidosis
Diabetic ketoacidosis Starvation Alcoholic
Lactic acidosis **Uremia** **Medications and toxins**
Salicylate toxicity Ethylene glycol (↑ osmolar gap) Methanol (↑ osmolar gap)
Gastrointestinal (GI) losses
Vomiting Nasogastric suction Laxative abuse
Renal losses
Loop or thiazide diuretics Mineralocorticoid excess Posthypercapnic alkalosis High-dose intravenous penicillin
Hypokalemia **Administration of alkali (antacids)** **Respiratory Acidosis**
Respiratory control center depression
Medications and toxins Trauma Sleep apnea Hemorrhage Stroke
Neuromuscular disease
Amyotrophic lateral sclerosis Guillain-Barré Polio
Chest wall
Flail chest Muscular dystrophy

(*continued*)

TABLE 2.1 Common causes of acid-base disorders (*continued*)

Lung disease
Chronic obstructive pulmonary disease
Asthma
Pulmonary edema from congestive heart failure
Pneumonia
Pleural diseases
Effusions
Pneumothorax
Respiratory Alkalosis
Hypoxemia
High altitude
Anemia
Pulmonary disorder
Pulmonary embolism
Pulmonary edema
Interstitial lung disease
Pneumonia
Mechanical ventilation
Central nervous system disease
Cerebrovascular accident
Tumor
Infection
Drugs
Salicylates
Catecholamines
Progesterone
Fever or sepsis
Pregnancy
Hepatic failure

diabetes mellitus. DKA can be triggered by infection, hyperglycemia from noncompliance with medications, and severe emotional stress. DKA can also be the initial presentation for a new-onset type 1 diabetes mellitus patient. Patients with DKA can present with a variety of symptoms including severe thirst, polyuria, fever, nausea, vomiting, and abdominal pain. Serum HCO_3 is markedly depressed in DKA. Serum and urine ketones will be elevated. Alcoholic ketoacidosis occurs in the setting of chronic alcoholism when alcohol intake is suddenly reduced. Patients can present with DKA-like symptoms including vomiting, dehydration, and abdominal pain. Acidosis may be as severe as DKA. Glucose, however, will be normal or low. Starvation ketoacidosis occurs in the setting of prolonged fasting and the acidosis is mild.

Ingestion of salicylates and the volatile alcohols, ethylene glycol (antifreeze), and methanol (wood alcohol) is associated with a high anion gap metabolic acidosis. Patients with salicylate toxicity will also have a concurrent respiratory alkalosis caused by direct stimulation of the the medullary respiratory center. If suspected, salicylate levels should be ordered. Methanol and ethylene glycol produce a concurrent osmolar gap. The osmolar gap is the difference between the measured and calculated serum osmolarity; it is found by using this formula:

$$\text{Calculated serum osmolarity} = 2\text{Na} + (\text{glucose}/18) + (\text{blood urea nitrogen}/2.8)$$

The normal osmolar gap is <10 mOsm/kg. A higher osmolar gap indicates the possible presence of volatile alcohols; if suspected, individual levels can be obtained.

The differential for the most common causes of a normal or nonanion gap metabolic acidosis includes diarrhea, renal tubular acidosis (RTA), and early renal insufficiency. Diarrhea results in gastrointestinal tract loss of HCO_3 and the diagnosis is usually obvious from the history. Patients will also have hypokalemia secondary to loss of potassium from the gastrointestinal tract. RTA can cause acidosis through impaired hydrogen ion excretion or through renal loss of HCO_3<online E.17>. There are three types of RTA: type 1, type 2, and type 4. (Note: there is no type 3 RTA!).

Type 1 (distal) RTA can be associated with a number of disorders including Sjogren's syndrome. Type 2 (proximal) RTA can be observed in patients with multiple myeloma and Fanconi's syndrome. Type 4 (hyporenin hypoaldosterone) RTA is most often seen in diabetic patients and in association with medications such as nonsteroidal anti-inflammatory drugs, angiotensin-converting enzyme inhibitors, cyclosporine, and heparin. Type 4 RTA is also associated with hyperkalemia, whereas types 1 and 2 are associated with hypokalemia. Less common causes of a normal gap metabolic acidosis include loss of HCO_3 through surgical ureteral diversions to the intestine, pancreatic fistulas, or biliary drainage to the intestines.

Metabolic Alkalosis

In metabolic alkalosis, there is a primary increase in HCO_3. In general, the clinical presentation of severe metabolic alkalosis can include severe cramping, paresthesias, and even seizures. Most typically, metabolic alkalosis is asymptomatic or the presenting symptoms are related to the underlying conditions. The most common causes include gastrointestinal hydrogen ion loss through vomiting or nasogastric tube drainage and renal hydrogen loss secondary to diuretic use. Loop diuretics in particular can also lead to another cause, contraction alkalosis. This occurs during aggressive diuresis for edema when there is a loss of a large quantity of bicarbonate-free fluid. Posthypercapnic alkalosis occurs when patients with prolonged CO_2 retention are quickly returned to a normal pCO_2. This can occur during mechanical ventilation.

Respiratory Acidosis

In respiratory acidosis, there is a primary increase in the pCO_2 level. In general, the clinical presentation of a respiratory acidosis depends on the severity and duration (acute vs. chronic) and the underlying condition. Severe acute respiratory acidosis can present with dyspnea and anxiety or irritability that can progress to delirium and a somnolence known as carbon dioxide narcosis. Chronic respiratory acidosis is associated with headache, tremor, sleep disturbances, and daytime somnolence. The common causes of respiratory acidosis include lung disease, obstructive sleep apnea, neuromuscular disease, and medications that depress the respiratory control center. Chronic respiratory acidosis typically occurs in patients with severe, longstanding chronic obstructive pulmonary disease or obstructive sleep apnea.

Respiratory Alkalosis

In respiratory alkalosis, there is a primary decrease in the pCO_2 level. The clinical presentation of respiratory alkalosis can include dizziness, syncope, altered mental status, perioral and extremity paresthesias, and even arrythmias and seizures in severe cases.

Respiratory alkalosis is very common in hospitalized patients as it occurs in fever, sepsis, and mechanical ventilation. Central nervous system disease ranging from infection to malignancy can also produce sustained hyperventilation and respiratory alkalosis. Salicylate toxicity is the most common cause of medication associated respiratory alkalosis. Salicylates directly stimulate the medullary respiratory center resulting in hyperventilation. (Remember: salicylates also cause a high anion gap metabolic acidosis!)

EVALUATION

The diagnosis and the management of the cause of an acid-base disorder require a detailed history and physical examination and a stepwise approach to the arterial blood gases (ABG) (Fig. 2.1).

First, check the pH and draw conclusions. A normal pH range is 7.38 to 7.42. If the pH is <7.38, then the primary disorder is an acidosis, either respiratory or metabolic or both. There might also be an alkalosis present. If the pH is >7.42, then the primary disorder is an alkalosis, either

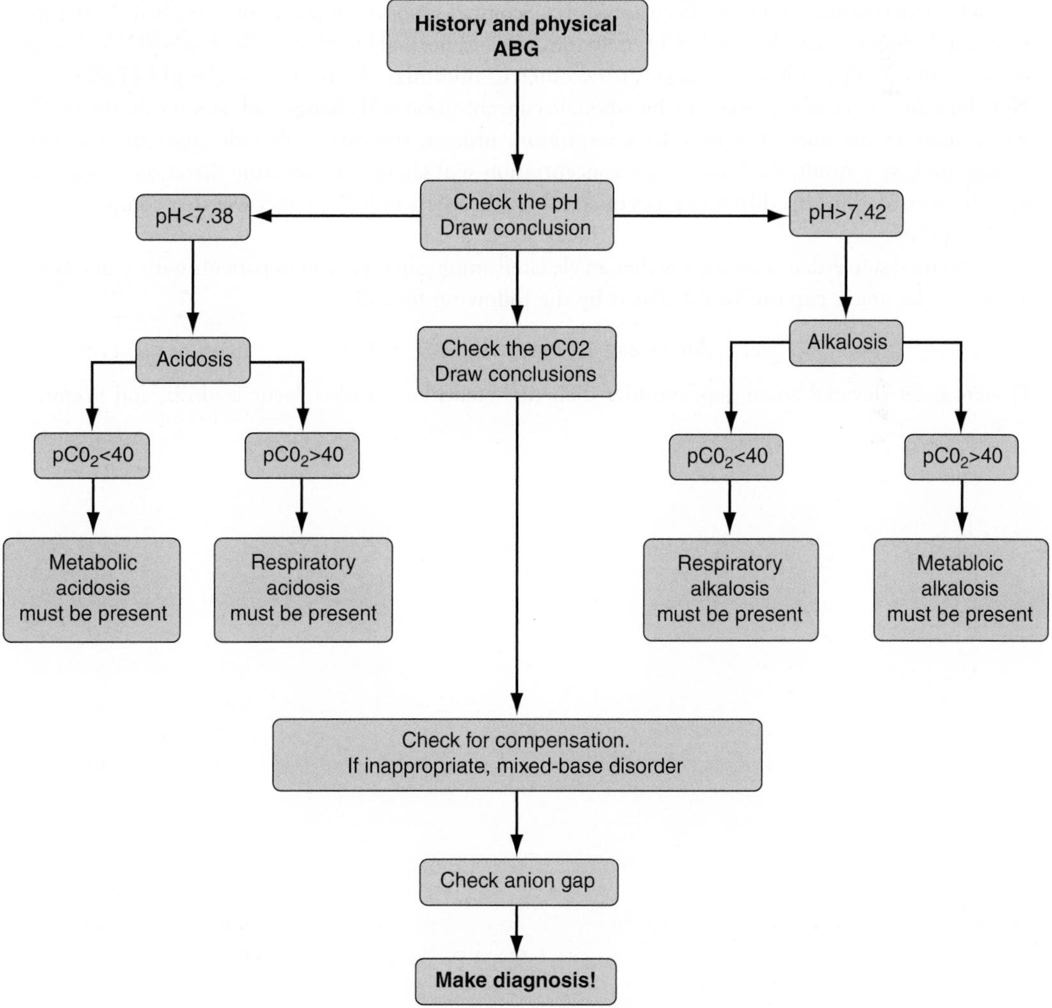

Figure 2.1 • Approach to the evaluation of acid-base disorders.

TABLE 2.2 Understanding compensation of acid-base abnormalities

Diagnosis	pH	Original Change	Compensation Change
Metabolic acidosis	<7.38	HCO_3 <24	pCO_2 <40
Metabolic alkalosis	>7.42	HCO_3 >24	pCO_2 >40
Respiratory acidosis	<7.38	pCO_2 >40	HCO_3 >24
Respiratory alkalosis	>7.42	pCO_2 <40	HCO_3 <24

respiratory or metabolic or both. There might also be an acidosis present. If the pH is normal, then either there is no acid-base disorder or there is a mixed acid-base disorder.

Second, evaluate the pH in light of the pCO_2. If pH is <7.38 and pCO_2 is <40 mm Hg, then metabolic acidosis must be present. If pH is <7.38 and pCO_2 is >40 mm Hg, then respiratory acidosis must be present. If pH is >7.42 and pCO_2 is <40 mm Hg, then respiratory alkalosis must be present. If pH is >7.42 and pCO_2 is >40 mm Hg, then metabolic alkalosis must be present.

Third, determine if there has been appropriate compensation. Compensation is the body's attempt to maintain homeostasis. Normal pCO_2 is 40 mm Hg and normal bicarbonate is 24 mEq/L. A change in one system will result in a change in the other to minimize the impact on the pH (Table 2.2). Note how in a metabolic process the bicarbonate concentration will change and, as a result, the pCO_2 will change in the same direction. In a respiratory process, the carbon dioxide concentration will change and, as a result, the bicarbonate concentration will change in the same direction. Formulas have been created for the different types of acid-base disorders to help predict whether compensation is appropriate.

The final step is determining whether an elevated anion gap is present in patients with a metabolic acidosis. The anion gap can be calculated by the following formula:

$$\text{Anion gap} = \text{Na} - (\text{HCO}_3 + \text{Cl})$$

If there is an elevated anion gap, consider diabetic ketoacidosis, toxins, lactic acidosis, and uremia.

CHAPTER 3

Acute Gastrointestinal Bleeding

Monica Ziebert

Acute gastrointestinal (GI) bleeding is a common medical condition associated with high morbidity and mortality. Patients who have acute and overt bleeding from the GI tract will present in one of three ways (Table 3.1). *Hematemesis* is vomiting red blood or blood that has been altered by gastric acid. Hematemesis is commonly described as "coffee-ground emesis." It usually represents bleeding from the upper GI tract. *Melena* is black, tarry, foul-smelling stool. Melena represents bleeding from a source anywhere in the upper GI tract, small intestine, or right colon. Approximately 60 mL of blood are required to produce a single black stool. *Hematochezia* is the passage of bright red or maroon blood or blood clots from the rectum. It usually represents bleeding from the lower GI tract. It is important to note, however, that stool color is not an absolute indicator of the GI bleed location. A very brisk and massive bleed in the proximal upper GI tract can present as hematochezia.

All acute, overt GI bleeding is considered major when accompanied by hemodynamic instability.

DIFFERENTIAL DIAGNOSIS

The most common causes of acute GI bleeding are listed in Table 3.2. They are divided into upper GI causes and lower GI causes. Upper GI bleeding is arbitrarily defined as bleeding from a source proximal to the ligament of Treitz. Lower GI bleeding is defined as bleeding from a source distal to the ligament of Treitz. Lower GI bleeding includes both the colon and small intestine, but nearly 95% of cases arise from the colon.

The history and physical examination will provide information on the cause of the GI bleed as well as the severity and duration of bleeding. Important historical clues include the presence of abdominal pain, orthostatic symptoms, history of liver disease, previous history of GI bleeding, alcohol use, and nonsteroidal anti-inflammatory drug (NSAID) use. On examination, look for signs of hemodynamic instability and shock by assessing for orthostatic hypotension and skin pallor. The patient may also present stigmata of liver disease (e.g., jaundice, ascites, spider angiomata, and gynecomastia) and stool color on rectal exam should be sought.

Upper GI Bleeds

Bleeding peptic ulcers (either duodenal or gastric) are the most common cause of upper GI bleeds, accounting for approximately 50% of the cases. They have an acute mortality rate of 6% to 10%. Patients present with hematemesis or melena. Hematochezia may be a presenting feature if bleeding is rapid and massive. Patients with duodenal ulcers often complain of a sharp, burning, or gnawing epigastric pain that occurs hours after eating and wakes the patient from sleep. Pain is often relieved by food. Patients with gastric ulcers also present with epigastric pain but the pain is often made worse by food. Weight loss may occur in patients with gastric ulcers secondary to food aversion. The risk factors for bleeding peptic ulcers include NSAID use, *Helicobacter pylori* infection, and stress from critical illness. On examination, epigastric tenderness is the most frequent finding. The

TABLE 3.1 Clinical presentation of acute gastrointestinal bleeding

Clinical presentation	Location
Hematemesis	Proximal to the ligament of Treitz
Melena	Upper gastrointestinal tract to the right colon
Hematochezia	Entire gastrointestinal tract, usually lower

rectal examination will show melena or bright red blood depending on the severity of the bleed (Chapter 70).

Esophageal variceal bleeding accounts for approximately 10% to 30% of all upper GI bleeds. Esophageal varices located in the distal 5 cm of the esophagus are the most common site of bleeding. Esophageal varices are a complication of portal hypertension and portosystemic shunting of blood that develops as a consequence of cirrhosis from any cause, most commonly alcoholic liver disease or chronic active hepatitis. Varices are present in 50% of patients with cirrhosis but it is important to remember that more than half of GI bleeds in patients with portal hypertension are from nonvariceal causes. Patients present with painless sudden onset large-volume hematemesis of bright red blood or clots. It is not uncommon for patients to present with concurrent hematochezia. Patients usually have a history of GI bleeding. On examination, there are usually physical signs of hemodynamic instability ranging from orthostatic hypotension to shock. Patients may have the stigmata of chronic liver disease. Although variceal bleeding will spontaneously stop in 50% of the cases, continued bleeding is associated with a high mortality of nearly 80% (Chapter 74).

Erosive esophagitis from chronic gastroesophageal reflux can cause significant GI bleeding. Patients present with hematemesis and have a history of heartburn. Examination findings are nonspecific.

Gastric erosions (hemorrhagic or erosive gastropathy) are superficial mucosal erosions. They are

TABLE 3.2 Common causes of acute gastrointestinal bleeding

Upper gastrointestinal bleeding	Lower gastrointestinal bleeding
Peptic (gastroduodenal) ulcers	Diverticulosis
Esophageal varices	Angiodysplasia
Gastric erosions (Hemorrhagic or erosive gastropathy)	Colitis • Inflammatory • Ischemic • Infectious
Erosive esophagitis	Malignancy or polyp
Mallory-Weiss tear	Hemorrhoids and anorectal fissures
Less common: • Dieulafoy's lesion • Aortoenteric fistula • Malignancy • Vascular lesions	Less common: • Postpolypectomy • Aortocolic fistula • NSAID-induced colitis • Vasculitis

NSAID, nonsteroidal anti-inflammatory drug.

an uncommon cause of acute severe GI bleeding and more commonly result in chronic blood loss. They are strongly associated with NSAID, aspirin, and alcohol use. Gastric erosions can also develop as a result of stress in hospitalized patients who have undergone major surgery or experienced severe trauma, major burns covering greater than one third of body area, or life-threatening medical illness. Patients will present with hematemesis, usually coffee-ground emesis, or melena. Patients may present with or without associated epigastric discomfort. Examination findings are nonspecific.

A Mallory-Weiss tear is a longitudinal laceration at the gastroesophageal junction or gastric cardia. Patients classically present with hematemesis (which may be severe) preceded by vomiting, retching, or coughing and often associated with heavy alcohol use. A Mallory-Weiss tear can also be a complication of upper GI endoscopy. Examination findings are nonspecific. Generally, the bleeding stops spontaneously.

Less common but dangerous causes of acute GI bleeding include Dieulafoy's lesion and sequelae from an aortoenteric fistula. A Dieulafoy's lesion occurs when an aberrant submucosal arteriole bleeds upon erosion of the overlying mucosa. Dieulafoy's lesions are found throughout the GI tract but most commonly in the proximal stomach. Patients present classically with recurrent, painless, and massive hematemesis. A history of alcohol abuse or NSAID use is usually absent. Examination findings include signs of hemodynamic instability from the massive bleeding but are otherwise nonspecific.

Rupture of an aortoenteric fistula is a rare but disastrous occurrence. Fistulae can be classified as primary when they are due to atherosclerosis or secondary when they are a consequence from aortic aneurysm reconstructive surgery. In the latter case, aortoenteric fistulae can form between small bowel lumen and a synthetic graft from an aortic aneurysm repair. Patients may present with a small "herald" bleed prior to the massive and usually fatal bleed.

Lower GI Bleed

Diverticulosis accounts for nearly 50% of the causes of lower GI bleeds. A diverticulum is a sac-like protrusion from the colonic wall. Over time, the diverticulum continues to herniate and eventually the surrounding vasa recta (at the neck or dome) become susceptible to rupture. Diverticula are most commonly found in the left colon. Patients typically present with large-volume, painless hematochezia. Some patients may also complain of bloating and cramping. Diverticular bleeding typically occurs in the absence of diverticulitis. Risk factors for diverticular bleeding include lack of dietary fiber, aspirin or NSAID use, advanced age (the mean age for diverticular bleeds is the sixth decade), and constipation. On examination, physical findings are nonspecific because patients rarely have pain or signs of peritoneal inflammation. Diverticular bleeding stops spontaneously in a majority of cases but rebleeding occurs in up to 25% of patients (Chapter 77).

Angiodysplasia is an acquired vascular anomaly characterized by dilated, tortuous submucosal blood vessels lined by endothelial cells, but no smooth muscle cells. Angiodysplasia presents as painless hematochezia or melena and most often originates from the ascending colon or cecum. In contrast to diverticulosis in which bleeding is arterial, bleeding from angiodysplasia is venous. Therefore, it tends to be less massive. Angiodysplasia is responsible for approximately 20% of cases of lower GI bleeding in the general population but has a higher prevalence in patients over age 65. Angiodysplasia is associated with aortic stenosis (Heyde's syndrome) and chronic renal failure. Physical examination findings are nonspecific. Like diverticular bleeding, rebleeding is common and occurs in up to 80% of untreated patients.

Colitis is simply a colonic mucosal inflammation in response to acute injury. Colitis can be infectious, ischemic, or inflammatory in origin. The clinical presentation is similar in all types of colitis. Patients classically present with hematochezia (with or without diarrhea), abdominal pain, and fever. The clinical setting should be the first clue to diagnosis. For infectious colitis, the history may include symptoms developing after ingesting a contaminated food or following previous antibiotic use. The most common organisms associated with food poisoning include invasive bacteria such as *Campylobacter*, *Salmonella*, and *Shigella* and bacteria that produce cytotoxins such as *Escherichia coli* (serotype O157:H7). *Clostridium difficile* is associated with previous antibiotic use and also produces a cytotoxin. On examination, patients with infectious colitis can have severe abdominal pain with peritoneal signs suggesting a surgical abdomen. Routine stool cultures and toxin assays will identify the most common causes of infectious colitis. Ischemic colitis usually occurs in elderly patients with associated hypotension, heart failure, or arrhythmia. On examination, patients may be hypotensive and will have severe lower abdominal tenderness. Often, physical signs of peritonitis are seen. Inflammatory colitis is due to either Crohn's disease or ulcerative colitis (Chapter 76). On examination, there may be abdominal distention and tenderness. Fever, tachycardia, and hypotension are associated with severe disease. Inflammatory colitis is associated with extracolonic manifestations such as arthritis, skin changes, or evidence of liver disease.

Hemorrhoid bleeding presents as hematochezia with rectal pain made worse with bowel movements, straining, or sitting. Less commonly, patients will present with painless bleeding. Patients will note bright red blood on the toilet paper or coating the stools. The presentation is similar whether the bleeding arises from external (located below the dentate line) or internal hemorrhoids (located above the dentate line). On rectal examination, bleeding hemorrhoids can be directly observed and palpated in almost all patients with external hemorrhoids. Internal hemorrhoidal bleeding may require anoscopy for visualization. Examination is often difficult secondary to the pain. Severe GI bleeding is unusual from hemorrhoids.

Malignancy or polyps are a relatively uncommon cause of acute GI bleeding. The bleeding has a tendency to be low grade and recurrent. Patients can present with either hematochezia, which suggests a left-sided large bowel neoplasm, or melena, which suggests a right-sided large bowel malignancy. Patients often have a history of anemia. Other presenting symptoms and physical examination findings depend on the location of the tumor. Right-sided neoplasms tend to have few localizing symptoms or examination findings. Left-sided neoplasms can have associated obstructive symptoms, change in stool caliber, tenesmus, and change in bowel habits. A rectosigmoid lesion may be detected on rectal exam.

EVALUATION

The initial evaluation of an acute GI bleed requires assessment of hemodynamic stability and an identification of risk factors for mortality from an acute GI bleed (Table 3.3). Blood loss of less than 500 mL rarely causes systemic signs but greater volumes result in symptomatic orthostatic hypotension. When blood loss is greater than 25% of blood volume, shock may ensue. All patients with GI bleeding should immediately receive two large-bore (18 gauge) catheters or a central venous line for intravenous access. Patients should be stabilized with fluid replacement or blood transfusions. Coagulopathy or

TABLE 3.3 Risk factors for gastrointestinal bleed mortality
Advanced age
Hemoglobin decrease of at least 2 g/dL
Transfusion requirement greater than 2 units packed red blood cells
Shock or orthostatic hypotension
Comorbid illnesses (e.g., cirrhosis, coronary artery disease)
In-hospital bleed
Bright red hematemesis in patients with liver cirrhosis

American College of Physicians. Philadelphia, PA; 2006 (www.acpmedicine.com).

electrolyte disturbances should be corrected. Patients with overt major bleeding should have intensive care monitoring. Once a patient is stabilized, further diagnostic evaluation can be done.

The hemoglobin level will assess the severity of the bleed and serve as a baseline to monitor for rebleeding. An important caveat in the setting of an acute, rapid GI bleed is that the initial hemoglobin may not accurately reflect the magnitude of blood loss as it takes approximately 8 hours for equilibration with extravascular fluid. Other essential laboratory tests include a basic chemistry for electrolytes, blood urea nitrogen (BUN), and creatinine. An increased BUN/creatinine ratio greater than 25:1 suggests an upper GI source. The BUN increases due to breakdown of blood products to urea by intestinal bacteria and when there is a concomitant reduction in the glomerular filtration rate.

Patients can undergo endoscopy (either esophagogastroduodenoscopy [EGD] or colonoscopy) for both diagnostic and therapeutic purposes. Endoscopy is highly sensitive and specific for locating bleeding lesions in the GI tract (Fig. 3.1). If a patient remains hemodynamically unstable, then endoscopy must be done urgently and EGD is the first choice regardless of whether a patient presents with hematemesis, melena, or hematochezia. If the EGD is negative and the patient presents with hematochezia, then colonoscopy is indicated. If the colonoscopy is negative, then enteroscopy can be performed to look at the upper portions of the small intestine (proximal jejunum). If the EGD is

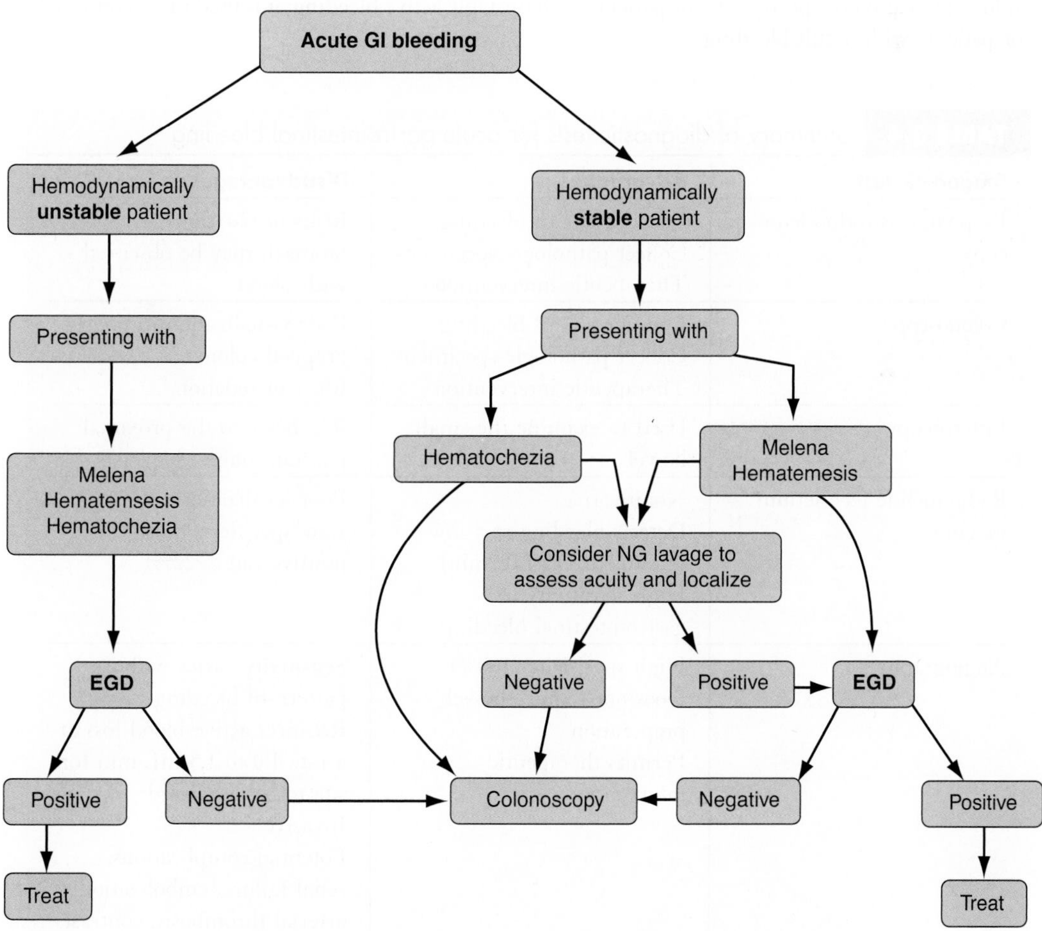

Figure 3.1 • Approach to the evaluation of acute gastrointestinal bleeding. (Adapted from American College of Physicians. Philadelphia, PA; 2006 [www.acpmedicine.com]).

negative and the patient presents with hematemesis, then enteroscopy can be performed. If enteroscopy is negative, then angiography or surgery is needed to localize the bleeding source.

If a patient is hemodynamically stable, then the choice for the initial endoscopic procedure will be based on the type of presenting GI bleed. Stable patients can undergo nasogastric or gastric lavage if there is uncertainty about the location of the bleeding source. There are two important points to remember about the use of lavage. First, a negative lavage does not rule out an upper GI bleed as it could suggest the bleeding has temporarily stopped or arises beyond a closed pylorus. Second, in patients with hematochezia, a nasogastric lavage can be used to confirm an upper very brisk bleed as opposed to a lower GI source. If the patient is stable and presents with hematochezia and the nasogastric lavage is negative for blood, then colonoscopy is performed. If the colonoscopy is negative, then enteroscopy is performed. If a patient is stable and presents with hematemesis or melena, then EGD is performed. If the EGD is negative, then enteroscopy is performed. If enteroscopy is negative, then other diagnostic tests, including angiography and radionuclide imaging (tagged red blood scans), may reveal the source of the bleed (Table 3.4).

Angiography requires active blood loss of approximately 1.0 to 1.5 mL/minute for a bleeding site to be visualized, whereas a tagged red blood scan requires bleeding rates as low as 0.1 to 0.5 mL/min. GI studies with barium are contraindicated in patients with acute upper or lower GI bleeds because they will interfere with endoscopy, angiography, or surgery, if required. Video-capsule endoscopy is also not appropriate for patients with unstable active bleeding; it is used more commonly for patients with occult bleeding.

TABLE 3.4 Summary of diagnostic tests for acute gastrointestinal bleeding

Diagnostic test	Advantages	Disadvantages
Esophagogastroduodenoscopy	Localize site of bleeding Collect pathologic specimens Therapeutic intervention	Risks of sedation Stomach may be obscured with blood
Colonoscopy	Localize site of bleeding Collect pathologic specimens Therapeutic intervention	Poor visualization in poorly prepped colon Risks of sedation
Enteroscopy	Used to examine the small bowel	Reaches into the proximal jejunum only
Radionuclide technetium imaging	Noninvasive Detects bleeding at a low rate (0.1 to 0.5 mL/min) High sensitivity for gastrointestinal bleeding	Poor localization Low specificity (false-positive rate ~22%)
Angiography	High specificity (100%) Does not require bowel preparation Permits therapeutic intervention	Sensitivity varies with pattern of bleeding Requires active blood loss at a rate 1.0 to 1.5 mL/min for site to be visualized Invasive Potential complications: renal failure, embolization, arterial thrombosis, contrast reaction

CHAPTER 4

Altered Mental Status

Julie Mitchell and Dario Torre

Altered mental status is a broad term purposefully encompassing any disorder that causes a change in mental functioning, with decreased mental clarity, reduced reasoning, and diminished thinking process. The term *consciousness* implies both a normal level of alertness and normal mental functioning in other domains (particularly thought process). Altered mental status occurs in about 10% of hospitalizations, and 30% to 50% of hospitalizations of patients over the age of 65 years. It may range from acute confusion, delirium, or dementia.

Acute confusion refers to a global loss of mental functioning (usually including orientation, attention, memory, thought process, and consciousness). Commonly, patients present as disoriented, not able to hold attention, slow in action and words, and with a decreased level of alertness. Language may be rambling and disorganized.

Delirium refers to a rapidly developed state of "clouded consciousness," often waxing and waning. Delirium is a kind of acute confusion state that connotes agitated behavior, sometimes with hallucinations, other misperceptions, or tremor.

Dementia is a chronic process of reduced cognition in all areas, but primarily with memory problems (such as word-finding, comprehension, and recognition difficulties and disorganization) while attention and alertness are preserved until late stages. Compared to delirium, the confusion associated with dementia is fairly constant from day to day. Compared to acute confusion, dementia is chronic and progressive. Dementia may co-exist with a superimposed confusion or delirium (Chapter 144).

DIFFERENTIAL DIAGNOSIS

The differential diagnosis of altered mental status include: neurological, metabolic, psychiatric, systemic, and drug/medications (Table 4.1).

Neurological Abnormalities

These may include meningitis, cerebrovascular accident (CVA), intracranial bleeding, subdural hematoma, normal pressure hydrocephalus (NPH), and seizures (Chapters 107 to 117).

1. The presence of fever, nuchal rigidity, and altered mental status suggest meningitis.
2. Vomiting, headache, and hemiplegia can be manifestations of intracerebral hemorrhage.
3. A sudden onset of severe headache, transient loss of consciousness, vomiting, and a past history of hypertension may be consistent with subarachnoid hemorrhage.
4. CVA patients will present with hemiparesis, sensory loss, aphasia, and visual changes, but less commonly with an altered mental status. Subdural hematoma is suggested by a history of trauma, accompanied by headache and confusion.
5. NPH is characterized by a triad consisting of ataxia, confusion, and urinary incontinence.
6. A previous history of seizures, decreased level of responsiveness, fecal or urinary incontinence, evidence of tongue biting, and a postictal period that may last minutes to hours may be present.

TABLE 4.1 Differential diagnosis of acute altered mental status

Condition	Mechanism causing altered mental status
Neurological processes	
Mass (tumor, metastases, abscess, or hematoma) or mass effect (edema) with increased intracranial pressure	Compression, herniation, hydrocephalus, hemorrhage
Subdural hematoma	Injury, hemorrhage, herniation
Aneurysm, hemorrhage	Hemorrhage, herniation
Encephalitis, meningitis	Inflammation
Vasculitis	Inflammation
Seizures (status epilepticus or postictal state)	Low blood flow, neuron dysfunction
Metabolic processes	
Drug overdose or withdrawal (alcohol, sedatives, opiates, psychotropics, anticholinergics, corticosteroids, digoxin)	Toxin to neurotransmission
Liver failure	Ammonia as toxin
Renal failure	Uremia as toxin
Hypo- or hypernatremia, hypercalcemia, dehydration, acidosis, alkalosis	Maintenance of electrolyte charge, osmolarity
Diabetes (ketoacidosis, nonketotic hyperosmolar hyperglycemia, or hypoglycemia)	Maintenance of electrolyte charge, osmolarity, low glucose
Addisonian crisis, hypo- and hyperthyroidism	Required cofactors for neuron function
Profound nutritional deficiency (thiamine or vitamin B12)	Required cofactors for neuron function
Psychiatric processes	
Affective disorders	
Mania and bipolar illness	
Schizophrenia	
Fugue (psychogenic amnesia)	
Systemic processes	
Severe infection (sepsis, pneumonia, urinary tract infection in elderly)	Low blood flow from vasodilatation, bacterial toxins
Respiratory failure	Hypoxia, hypercarbia
Heart failure (myocardial infarction, arrhythmia)	Low blood flow, hypoxia
Hypertensive encephalopathy	Low blood flow, hypoxia
Drugs/medications	
Sedative	
Narcotics	
Anticholinergics	

Metabolic Abnormalities

Metabolic abnormalities may include:

1. Electrolyte abnormalities such as hypo-hypernatremia or hypercalcemia as well as marked acidemia or alkalemia
2. Encephalopathy secondary to severe liver disease (presence of asterixis or flapping tremor), renal failure (uremia), and sever hypoxia or hypercapnia
3. Endocrine abnormalities such as thyroid storm manifested by hyperthermia, marked agitation, tachycardia, or myxedema coma characterized by hypothermia, stupor, and respiratory depression
4. Adrenal crisis (Chapter 69) precipitated by infection or trauma and accompanied by hypotension, nausea, vomiting, and abdominal pain
5. Hyperglycemia caused by hyperosmolar nonketotic coma (Chapter 64) or hypoglycemia (nausea, sweating, hunger, and lightheadedness)
6. Severe nutritional deficiency
   a. Vitamin B12 deficiency may present with changes in mental status such as dementia, personality changes, memory loss, and megaloblastic anemia.
   b. Thiamine deficiency can be the cause of Wernicke-Korsakoff syndrome (Korsakoff's psychosis manifests with confabulation and impaired short-term memory).

Psychiatric Abnormalities

Psychiatric processes can masquerade as confusion or delirium.

1. Affective disorders (anxiety, grief, and depression) often clinically present with mood and affect changes as well as preserved orientation and attention (particularly if the patient is pressed to perform).
2. Mania often clinically presents with constantly increased alertness and distractibility as well as hyperactivity, elevated mood, pressured speech, and delusions.
3. Schizophrenia often clinically presents as psychosis (hallucinations and delusions) as well as intact consciousness, orientation, and attention.

Systemic Abnormalities

1. Infection: particularly in the elderly, urinary tract infection or pneumonia may cause altered mental status.
2. Severe anemia (hematocrit <30%)
3. Hypoxia due to cardiopulmonary disease (chronic obstructive pulmonary disease or myocardial infarction)
4. Cerebral vasculitides (Systemic Lupus Erythmatosus (SLE), Polyarteritis nodosa, amiloidosis, Behchet's disease [Chapters 42 and 58], hypertensive encephalopathy) caused by cerebral edema due to a severe elevation of blood pressure (usually diastolic blood pressure >120 mm Hg). Other symptoms may include headache, nausea, vomiting, papilledema, and seizures.

Drugs or Medications

1. Sedative hypnotics, narcotics, and anticholinergic drugs by overdoses or withdrawal may all cause change in mental status.
2. Alcohol withdrawal generally occurs 6 to 48 hours after cessation and may present with fever, tachycardia, hypertension, agitation, and seizures. Thiamine deficiency in alcoholics and in malnourished patients may cause Wernicke's encephalopathy (confusion, nystagmus, ophthalmoplegia, and ataxia).

TABLE 4.2 Physical examination findings, vital signs, and their diagnostic significance in patients with altered mental status

Finding	Suggests
Focal neurologic signs	
Hemiparesis	Stroke (but consider hypoglycemia in elderly)
Neck stiffness	Meningitis, subarachnoid hemorrhage
Gait disturbance	Hydrocephalus
Any asymmetry in cranial nerve, cerebellar, strength, or sensation testing	Focal central nervous system lesion
Nonfocal neurologic signs	
Tremor	Metabolic encephalopathy
Asterixis (flapping tremor elicited when arms, wrists, and hands extended)	Metabolic encephalopathy (typically liver disease), especially when bilateral
Myoclonus	Metabolic encephalopathy (typically renal disease)
Spontaneous movements in patient with reduced alertness	
Prolonged twitching of finger, foot, face	Seizure
Outturned leg at rest	Hemiparesis
Nature of respirations in patient with reduced alertness	
Shallow, slow breathing	Metabolic cause
Rapid, deep breathing (Kussmaul)	Metabolic or brainstem cause
Cyclic shallow to deep breathing with apnea (Cheyne-Stokes)	Metabolic or diffuse bilateral hemisphere lesions
Vital signs	
Fever	Infection (systemic, meningitis), heat stroke, anticholinergic overdose
Hypothermia (<31°C induces coma)	Outside temperature, alcoholic, or drug toxicity, hypoglycemia, heart failure, hypothyroidism
Markedly high blood pressure	Hypertensive encephalopathy, hemorrhage, hydrocephalus, acute trauma
Low blood pressure	Alcohol or drug toxicity, internal bleeding, myocardial infarction, sepsis, Addisonian crisis
Fundus	
Papilledema	Increased intracranial pressure
Exudate, hemorrhage, vessel-crossing changes	Hypertensive encephalopathy
Other	
Petechiae	Bleeding diathesis leading to intracranial hemorrhage
Periorbital ecchymosis	Skull fracture (trauma)

(*continued*)

TABLE 4.2 Physical examination findings, vital signs, and their diagnostic significance in patients with altered mental status (*continued*)

Finding	Suggests
Posturing	
Flexion of elbows and wrists with arm supination (decorticate)	Severe bilateral damage above midbrain
Extension of elbows and wrists with arm pronation (decerebrate)	Damage in midbrain metabolic cause (e.g., hypoxia) or acute bilateral hemisphere lesion
Pupillary reflexes (use bright light in dim room)	
Symmetric, reactive, 2.5 to 5 mm	Intact midbrain and cranial nerve III
Bilateral, reactive, 1 to 2.5 mm	Metabolic cause, hydrocephalus, or thalamic lesion
Bilateral, reactive, <1 mm (pinpoint pupils)	Narcotic toxicity, acute pons lesion
Single, nonreactive, >5 mm	Herniation or ipsilateral midbrain lesion
Reflexive eye movements	
Full and conjugate oculocephalic movements (eyes move loosely in opposite direction of head as it is turned to the side; i.e., eyes continue to look forward)	Intact brainstem, but bilateral hemisphere damage or metabolic cause of coma
Abnormal oculoenchaphalic reflex (eyes move with head to side, "doll's eyes")	Brainstem damage or reflex suppression by drugs (confirm with oculovestibular testing)
Oculovestibular reflex (eyes move toward ear when stimulated with cold water irrigation)	Reflex present indicates intact brainstem, absent indicates brainstem damage

EVALUATION

A careful history and physical examination should be performed. Ask about the circumstances (trauma) and timing of onset of confusion, associated symptoms (weakness, headaches, convulsions, dizziness, diplopia [double vision], nausea, and vomiting), social history (alcohol and other drug use), medications (including over-the-counter), and past medical history (liver, kidney, lung, and heart diseases; seizure; and stroke). A complete general medical examination is important. A detailed neurologic examination is paramount in any case of altered mental status and any focal neurological sign should be sought (Table 4.2).

Usually, a comprehensive metabolic panel (including renal function, electrolytes, liver function tests, and calcium), complete blood count, urinalysis, urine culture, a urine toxic screen, chest x-ray, blood culture, electrocardiogram, and arterial blood gas is a reasonably complete evaluation in an elderly patient developing altered mental status. Stroke is a rare cause of acute mental status change (<10%), as are seizures in persons without history and meningitis. Thus, head imaging is indicated with focal neurological findings.

A lumbar puncture should be performed when meningitis is suspected, if fever exists without explanation, or when subarachnoid hemorrhage is strongly suspected and the patient has a normal head computed tomography (CT) scan. An electroencephalogram can be helpful in the evaluation

TABLE 4.3 Laboratory and imaging evaluation of altered mental status

Disease	Test	Comment
Intercerebral hemorrhage, subarachnoid hemorrhage, subdural hematoma, normal pressure hydrocephalus	CT/MRI imaging	CT helpful to detect intracerebral and subarachnoid bleeding
Hypo-hypernatremia, hypercalcemia, hyper-/ hypoglycemia, uremia, severe liver disease	Comprehensive metabolic panel (electrolytes, calcium, glucose, blood urea nitrogen, creatinine), liver function tests	Hypercalcemia may be caused by malignancy or hyperparathyroidism
Anemia, infection	Complete blood count, blood cultures	Infections may include urinary tract infection, pneumonia, endocarditis
Meningitis	Lumbar puncture	Cerebrospinal fluid analysis needed
Seizures	Electroencephalogram	Low specificity, most helpful in unconscious patients with status epilepticus
Drug overdose, intoxication, withdrawal	Toxicology screen	Alcohol blood level, urine screen for benzodiazepine, narcotics, cocaine
Acid-base disorders	Arterial blood gas	Evaluation of acidemia or alkalemia, hypoxemia, and hypercapnia
Myocardial infarction, tachyarrhythmia, bradyarrhythmias	Electrocardiogram	ST-T changes, supraventricular tachycardia, heart block
Thyroid disease, adrenal insufficiency	Thyroid-stimulating hormone, FT3, FT4, morning cortisol levels (cosyntropin test)	Thyroid storm, myxedema coma, adrenal crisis
Vitamin B12 deficiency	Methylmalonic acid and homocysteine levels	More common in elderly patients

of seizures; however, it is nonspecific and might be abnormal in encephalopathy, migraine headaches, or with use of medications.

Noncontrast head CT is the study of choice to evaluate patient for intracerebral hemorrhage and subarachnoid hemorrhage. Noncontrast head CT has greater sensitivity in the diagnosis of subarachnoid bleed in the first 12 hours after the event. However, for the diagnosis of CVA, sensitivity of noncontrast head CT is greater after 24 hours. A head CT can also detect the presence of NPH; however, magnetic resonance imaging (MRI) is a more accurate imaging test. Newly developed brain MRI can be particularly accurate in the diagnosis of CVA in the early hours (Table 4.3).

CHAPTER 5

Anemia

Gwen O'Keefe and Dario Torre

Anemia is a frequent laboratory finding in medical patients, often incidentally found during evaluation for other conditions. It is defined as hemoglobulin <13.5 g/dL or hematocrit <41.0% in men and <12.0 g/dL or <36.0%, respectively, in women. Approximately 5% of the population will have values out of the range of "normal" without true abnormalities. Women and black men have values that are typically 1 to 2 g/dL lower than in white men.

Only occasionally do patients present with symptoms related to low blood counts. Signs and symptoms of acute blood loss will develop with rapid losses of 10% to 15% of total blood volume, but in chronic blood loss, patients may not present with symptoms until the hemoglobin is 50% of normal because of mechanisms that allow compensation over time. Such mechanisms involve increased cardiac output and shift of the oxygen-hemoglobin dissociation curve to the right, leading to increased oxygen (O_2) delivery and shunting of O_2 from organs rich in blood supply (kidneys, gastrointestinal tract, skin).

DIFFERENTIAL DIAGNOSIS

The differential diagnosis of anemia is quite broad and extensive, but is initially narrowed when the red cell indices are evaluated. One preferred way to categorize anemias is by the mean corpuscular volume (MCV), the key measure of the size of the cells (Table 5.1). All causes of anemia can be found in one of three categories: microcytic, normocytic, and macrocytic.

An additional classification of anemia, based on a defect in formation, survival, and maturation of red cells, includes three major classes: decreased production (hypoproliferative bone marrow), increased peripheral destruction (hemolysis or blood loss), and a defect in red cell maturation (ineffective erythropoiesis).

A complete history and physical examination can often provide clues to the cause of anemia. The patient's background and ethnic origin can provide clues to the presence of inherited hemoglobinopathies (sickle cell anemia, thalassemia major), toxic exposures (due to medications such as metotrexate or other chemotherapeutic agents), and nutritional deficits (such as poor intake of iron, B_{12}, or folate). History of travel in areas where malaria is endemic may be a clue to the diagnosis of hemolytic anemia caused by infection. The occurrence of episodes of anemia, precipitated by drugs such as sulfanomides or antimalarials, suggests glucose-6-phosphate dehydrogenase deficiency. The presence of hereditary anemia associated with pain crises (acute chest syndrome, bone and joint pain due to vaso-occlusive episodes), splenomegaly early in the disease, and inability to concentrate urine (hyposthenuria) suggests sickle cell anemia.

Blood loss is the most common cause of anemia, and one of the most common causes of iron deficiency anemia. Blood loss may be caused by gastrointestinal bleeding (manifested by hematemesis and or melena), trauma, genitourinary (presenting with menometrorrhagia or hematuria), postsurgical blood loss, and (less commonly) bleeding due ruptured spleen or retroperitoneal bleed.

Symptoms such as onset of new fatigue or dyspnea, or noticeable bleeding, can help determine

TABLE 5.1 Anemia: classification by microcorpuscular volume

Microcytic (MCV <80 fL)	Normocytic (MCV 80 to 100 fL)	Macrocytic (MCV >100 fL)
Iron deficiency	Anemia of chronic disease	B12, folate deficiency
Thalassemias	Anemia of renal disease	Myelodysplastic syndrome
Anemia of chronic disease	Hemolytic anemias	hypothyroidism liver disease
Sideroblastic anemias Medications Toxins Lead poisoning	Iron deficiency (early stage)	Toxins, medications Hydroxiurea Azidovidine Alcohol Methotrexate

the timing of onset of anemia. Obtaining old values for comparison can help to determine if a slightly low value is the norm for that patient or date the onset of the anemia.

On physical examination start with examination of vital signs; hypotension and tachycardia may be signs of acute blood loss or very severe levels of anemia. Orthostatic hypotension will be present when the anemia overcomes the body's compensatory mechanisms in chronic states or severe blood loss in acute bleeding. Most patients with chronic anemia will have normal vital signs. Pale mucous membranes, particularly in the palmar creases, suggest hemoglobin <10 mg/dL. The presence of purpura may indicate anemia associated with thrombotic thrombocytopenic purpura or hemolytic uremic syndrome (Chapter 97). Splenomegaly is found in immune hemolytic anemia, hereditary spherocytosis, thalassemia major, leukemia, lymphoma, and myelofibrosis. Icterus may indicate hemolysis. A systolic "flow" murmur due to a hyperdynamic left ventricle may be best heard at the second left intercostal space. Koilonychia (spooning of nails), glossitis, and pica (craving for ice) can indicate iron deficiency. History of dementia, ataxia, and neurologic abnormalities such as paresthesias, decreased vibration, and proprioception may reflect vitamin B12 deficiency. Guaiac-positive stool suggests a gastrointestinal source of bleeding.

Microcytic Anemias

In microcytosis, the ferritin level should be checked. A ferritin level <10 ng/ml is very specific for iron deficiency states, the most common cause of microcytic anemia. A low ferritin level is diagnostic and can be reinforced by the aforementioned peripheral smear findings.

The two other most common causes are thalassemias (Chapter 94), either alpha or beta. These are diagnosed by hemoglobin electrophoresis and anemia of chronic disease (although this is usually a normocytic anemia). Rarely, sideroblastic anemia is found.

Normocytic Anemias

Anemia of chronic disease (Chapter 92) can be associated with low iron and transferrin saturations, but is distinguished by normal or high ferritin levels from iron deficiency. It is thought to be due to a cytokine-mediated process that interferes with erythropoietin production and leads to altered iron homeostasis (Chapter 90). Anemia of chronic disease is frequently found in patients with diabetes, chronic infections, inflammatory diseases, or malignancies. The peripheral smear is usually normal.

Anemia of renal disease is manifested by a normal peripheral smear and a normal or low erythropoietin level in the presence of anemia. Even mild to moderate renal insufficiency may be associated with anemia.

TABLE 5.2 Classification of hemolytic anemias

Intracorpuscular defect	
Disorders of the red cell membrane	Hereditary spherocytosis
Disorders resulting from enzyme abnormalities	Glucose-6-phosphate dehydrogenase deficiency Pyruvate kinase deficiency
Hemoglobinopathies	Sickle cell disease Thalassemias Hemoglobin C disease
Acquired	Paroxysmal nocturnal hemoglobinuria
Extracorpuscular defect (all are acquired)	
Immune	Autoimmune hemolytic anemia • Warm-antibody type • Cold-antibody type • Mixed • Drug mediated
Nonimmune	Resulting from chemical and physical damage Resulting from infections with microorganisms • Malaria • Bartonella • Babesia • Clostridium perfringens Drug induced

Hemolytic anemias (Table 5.2) are a group of diseases characterized by decreased erythrocyte survival time followed by anemia unless compensated by increased bone marrow production. Several general clues suggest hemolytic anemia: unexplained drop in the hemoglobin, sustained reticulocytosis, and elevated serum lactate dehydrogenase (LDH). Decreased haptoglobin levels are common and free serum hemoglobin can be present with intravascular red cell destruction (Table 5.3). Hemolytic anemias may show peripheral smear evidence of hemolysis: schistocytes and helmet cells in microangiopathic hemolytic anemia, spherocytes in hereditary spherocytosis (Chapter 95) or in autoimmune hemolytic anemia.

Primary Bone Marrow Disorders

There are several types of primary disorders that affect the bone marrow. Often the complete blood count will demonstrate abnormalities in all cell lines (white blood cells and platelets). Infiltrative processes may show immature myeloid cells and nucleated red cells in the peripheral smear; these disorders include myelofibrosis or metastatic cancer involving the bone marrow. Other classifications of primary disorders include primary bone marrow failure—exhibited as pure red cell aplasia or aplastic anemia—and may include abnormalities of platelets and white blood cells as well. Myelodysplastic syndrome (Chapter 89) may exhibit an increased red cell distribution width (RDW) and various other cellular abnormalities. A bone marrow biopsy is necessary to make the final diagnosis of a primary bone marrow disorder.

Macrocytic Anemias

The first step in macrocytic anemia is to eliminate drugs and other toxic exposures as causes. The list if drugs that may cause macrocytosis is long, but the most common offenders include azidovidine,

TABLE 5.3 Laboratory findings in hemolytic anemia

Feature	Finding	Comment
Degree of anemia	Variable	Hemoglobulin ranges from 11 to 12 g/dL in chronic compensated hemolytic anemia to <2 g/dL in severe cases
Type of anemia	Normocytic normochromic	Can be macrocytic due to reticulocytosis
Morphology	Variable	Spherocytosis in hereditary spherocytosis and autoimmune hemolytic anemia Sickle cells in sickle cell disease Target cells in thalassemias Schistocytes in microangiopathy
Reticulocytosis	Frequent	Sensitive but not specific for hemolysis
Normoblasts	Variable	Frequent in brisk hemolysis
Serum lactate dehydrogenase	Increased	Nonspecific for hemolytic anemia
Serum hemoglobin	Variable	Increased in intravascular hemolysis
Serum haptoglobin	Low	Specific for hemolysis if no severe decompensated liver disease (haptoglobin is synthesized in the liver)
Urinary hemoglobin	Variable	Present and confirms intravascular hemolysis
Splenomegaly	Frequent	Present if red blood cells are destroyed primarily by phagocytosis in the splenic reticuloendothelial system

hydroxyurea, methotrexate, trimethoprim (in Bactrim), and alcohol. The second most common cause is a nutritional deficiency, namely vitamin B12 and/or folate deficiency (Chapter 91). The serum folate level is easily raised by recent dietary intake of folate, so the homocysteine level can be used to document folate deficiency. The homocysteine level is raised in low folate states as the metabolic conversion to methionine requires folate. Similarly, vitamin B12 levels are usually low in deficient states. If falsely low levels are suspected, methylmalonic acid levels can be obtained; a normal level makes B12 deficiency unlikely.

EVALUATION

Initial laboratory evaluation should include (Fig. 5.1):

1. A complete blood count containing hemoglobin, hematocrit, red cell indices (MCV, MCHC, and MCH) white blood cell count and differential, and platelet count
2. A reticulocyte count
3. A careful examination of the peripheral smear
4. Iron studies

The reticulocyte count is the percentage of total red cells that are reticulocytes (usually 0.5% to 1%). A more useful and accurate estimate of the reticulocytes response produced by the bone marrow is

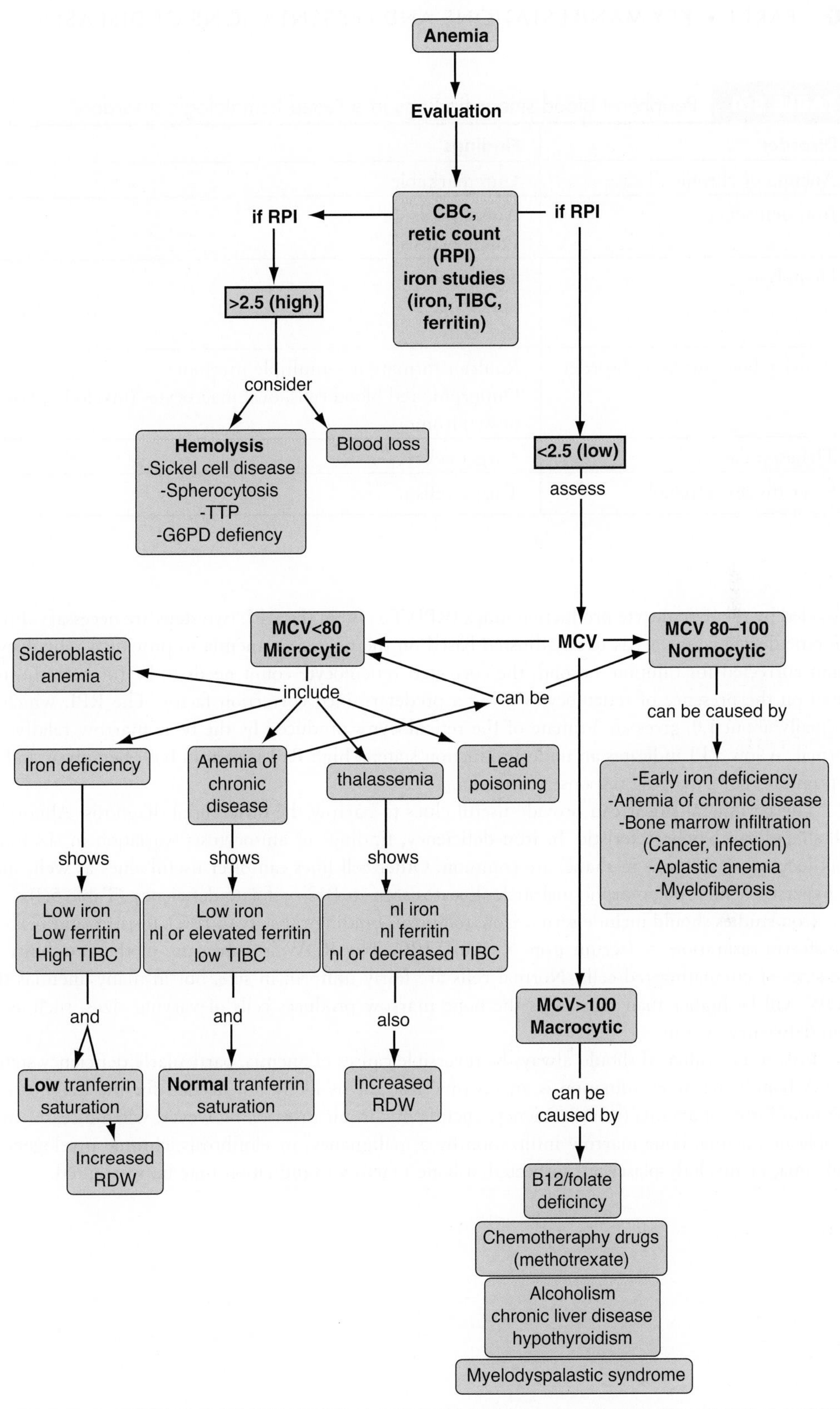

Figure 5.1 • Approach to diagnosis of anemia.

TABLE 5.4 Peripheral blood smear findings in selected hematologic disorders

Disorder	Findings
Anemia of chronic disease	Unremarkable
Iron deficiency	Anisocytosis Poikilocytosis
Hemolysis	Schistocytes Spherocytes Bite cells
Primary bone marrow disorder	Rouleau formation—multiple myeloma Dimorphic red blood cells, oval macrocytes (myelodysplastic syndrome)
Thalassemia	Target cells
Liver disease, ethanol	Target cells

provided by the reticulocyte production index (RPI).To obtain the RPI, two steps are necessary. First, the reticulocyte count needs to be adjusted based on the degree of anemia to provide a reticulocyte count corrected for dilution. Second, the corrected reticulocyte count needs to be further adjusted based on the presence of reticulocytes using a predetermined correction factor. The RPI, which is normally about 1.0, gives an estimate of the reticulocytes produced by the bone marrow relative to normal. A low RPI indicates an underproduction state; a high RPI is seen in both hemolysis and in appropriate bone marrow response to anemia.

The peripheral smear can provide useful clues to narrow the differential diagnosis. Abnormal cell shapes can be characteristic. In iron deficiency, findings of anisocytosis (variation in size) and poikilocytosis (variations in shape) are common. Other cell lines can offer useful clues as well, such as hypersegmented polymorphonuclear leukocytes seen in B12 or folate deficiency (Table 5.4).

Iron studies should include serum iron, total iron-binding capacity (TIBC), ferritin, and percent transferrin saturation = (serum iron × 100)/TIBC. The RDW is a measure of the variability of the sizes of circulating red cells. Normal cells are fairly uniform in size, but in many anemias the RDW will be higher than normal as the bone marrow produces cells of varying sizes, such as in iron deficiency anemia.

First to be evaluated should always be reversible causes of anemia, particularly deficiency states.

A bone marrow examination is an invasive test and is likely not needed for the diagnosis of common forms of anemia (iron deficiency, anemia of chronic disease). However, when diseases such as aplastic anemia, bone marrow infiltration by a malignancy, myelofibrosis, chronic myelogenous leukemia, or myelodysplasia are suspected, a bone marrow examination may be warranted.

CHAPTER 6

Chest Pain

Dario Torre

Chest pain is one of the most common complaints in primary care and emergency medicine. In the outpatient setting, musculoskeletal problems are the most common cause of chest pain. In patients presenting to the emergency room with chest pain, approximately half have coronary artery disease, either myocardial infarction or unstable angina.

DIFFERENTIAL DIAGNOSIS

The differential diagnosis of chest pain ranges from life-threatening conditions to more benign etiologies (Tables 6.1, 6.2, and 6.3).

Cardiac

Ischemic heart disease can present with pressure, tightness, or heaviness (see Chapter 27). Pain can radiate to the jaw, shoulders, or back. At times, the pain may also be described as burning or aching. It typically is located in the retrosternal area and generally may last 10 to 30 minutes. Ischemic chest pain is often related to exertion or emotional stress, typically relived by rest, and may be accompanied by dyspnea, diaphoresis, and nausea. Epigastric distress may represent an uncommon presentation of ischemic heart disease. Chest pain lasting a few seconds usually is not of cardiac origin. Patients with diabetes, women, or the elderly may present with atypical symptoms, such as dyspnea in the absence of chest pain. The physical examination may show tachycardia and elevated blood pressure. An S4 may be heard during angina attacks and an S3 may be present if congestive heart failure ensues (Chapter 28).

Acute pericarditis may also cause chest pain that typically is located in the retrosternal area. The pain is worsened by cough, deep inspiration (pleuritic pain), and supine position; it is relieved by the patient sitting up and leaning forward. A history of a recent viral infection may precede the occurrence of pericarditis. Physical examination may reveal the presence of a pleural rub and tachycardia. A pericardial rub may be present in 85% of the cases (see Chapter 31).

Aortic dissection typically presents with severe, sharp, or "tearing" abrupt-onset chest pain, often radiating to the back or to the abdomen. Hypertension is an important risk factor. On physical examination, aortic dissection may present with elevated blood pressure (49%), presence of a differential in blood pressure (31%; defined as >20 mm Hg difference between the right and left arm), or an early diastolic murmur due to acute aortic insufficiency (28%) when the dissection involves the ascending aorta and extends into the aortic valve (Chapter 34).

Aortic stenosis can present with chest pain that typically occurs on exertion. Dyspnea, palpitations, and exertional syncope (due to a diminished cardiac output) may also be presenting symptoms of aortic stenosis. On physical examination, a harsh crescendo-decrescendo systolic murmur with radiation to the carotids is best heard at the second right intercostal space (Chapter 30).

Cocaine-induced chest pain has become more common in the last several years, particularly among young people. The risk of a cocaine-related myocardial infarction is highest in the first 60

TABLE 6.1 Differential diagnosis of chest pain by system

System	Differential diagnosis
Cardiac	Ischemic heart disease Acute pericarditis Aortic dissection Aortic stenosis Cocaine-induced
Gastrointestinal	Gastroesophageal reflux disease Esophageal spasm Dysmotility Cholecystitis Peptic ulcer disease Pancreatitis
Psychosomatic	Panic attack Anxiety Depression
Pulmonary	Pulmonary embolus Pneumonia Pneumothorax
Musculoskeletal	Costochondritis Fibromyalgia Arthritis
Miscellaneous	Herpes zoster

TABLE 6.2 Important questions to characterize chest pain

P	Provocative Palliative	What activities precipitate pain? What alleviates pain?
Q	Quality	Describe pain and any associated symptoms, such as difficulty breathing, nausea, vomiting, diaphoresis.
R	Region Radiation	Where is the pain located? Does pain radiate and, if so, where?
S	Severity	Describe intensity of pain.
T	Timing Time	How long does the pain last each episode? How long since episodes first began?

TABLE 6.3 Clinical and diagnostic features of chest pain

Condition	Pain features	Physical examination	Electrocardiogram	Chest x-ray
Stable angina	Substernal pressure, tightness, ache, heaviness after exertion, lasting 10 minutes or more, relieved by rest	Normal or S4, murmur may be present	ST depression, T-wave abnormalities	May be normal
Unstable angina	Substernal pressure or tightness at rest lasting 10 to 20 minutes occasionally relieved by nitroglycerin	Normal or S4, murmur may be present	ST depression, T-wave abnormalities	May be normal
Myocardial infarction	Substernal pressure or tightness with radiation to left or both arms or neck, lasting >30 minutes	Normal or S4, murmur may be present, S3 if congestive heart failure present	ST elevations in contiguous leads with reciprocal changes	May be normal unless congestive heart failure is present
Pericarditis	Sharp, pleuritic, in the left precordial area, may last hours or days, relieved by sitting upright	± Pericardial rub	Diffuse ST elevations	
Aortic dissection	Abrupt onset of severe tearing pain radiating to the back	Blood pressure differential upper extremities, murmur of aortic insufficiency	LVH may be present	Widened mediastinum
Anxiety/panic attacks	Sharp, stabbing, variable length	Normal cardiovascular exam	Normal	Normal
Pneumonia	Sharp, sudden onset accompanied by fever, dyspnea	Crackles, egophony	Normal	Evidence of consolidation
Pulmonary embolism	Abrupt onset, accompanied by dyspnea	Right ventricle heave, tachycardia, right-sided S3	Tachycardia, RVH, RAD	May be normal, atelectasis
Costochondritis	Sharp pain, lasting seconds or hours, worsened by palpation or movement	Chest tenderness may be present	Normal	Often normal
Pneumothorax	Abrupt onset, accompanied by dyspnea	Absent breath sounds on the affected side, hyper resonant to percussion	Tachycardia	Collapsed lung
GERD	Burning or epigastric pain, relieved by antacids or proton pump inhibitors	Normal	Normal	Normal

GERD, gastroesophageal reflux disease; LVH, left ventricular hypertrophy; RAD, right axis deviation; RVH, right ventricular hypertrophy; ST, sinus tachycardia.

minutes after cocaine use. Patients with cocaine-related myocardial infarction or ischemic heart disease can present similar to those with ischemic heart disease. They typically complain of substernal chest pain, nausea, vomiting, diaphoresis, and/or headache. Physical examination may reveal severe hypertension, dyspnea, and or pupillary constriction.

Gastrointestinal

Gastroesophageal reflux disease (GERD) is a common gastrointestinal cause of chest pain, which can mimic anginal pain. GERD causes a burning substernal chest pain, which may last minutes, hours, or weeks; it may resolve either spontaneously or with medications (antacids, H2 blockers, proton pump inhibitors). It is often worsened by lying down, fatty meals, alcohol, or nonsteroidal anti-inflammatory drugs (e.g., ibuprofen). GERD may wake the patient from sleep. Other symptoms may include chronic cough, sore throat, and hoarseness (Chapter 71).

Esophageal spasm may cause a squeezing chest pain that may be indistinguishable from anginal pain. The physical examination may show wheezing, halitosis, dental erosions, and pharyngeal erythema.

Chest pain may also result from abdominal diseases such as cholecystitis, pancreatitis, or peptic ulcer diseases, although concomitant abdominal pain is often present. Chest pain associated with the aforementioned conditions often occurs after meals and is not associated with exertion. Acute cholecysticitis can present with right shoulder pain; however, abdominal discomfort is a more common presentation. On physical examination, patients may exhibit abdominal tenderness on palpation of epigastric or right upper quadrant abdominal regions.

Pulmonary

Pulmonary embolism may present with sudden-onset pleuritic chest pain, dyspnea, and less commonly with cough and hemoptysis. A number of risk factors should be considered to determine the likelihood of this diagnosis such as recent surgery, recent immobilization (>4 weeks), history of deep vein thrombosis, and malignancy. On physical examination, tachycardia and tachypnea may be present as well as wheezing, a right ventricular heave due to right ventricular hypertrophy, and dilatation as a result of pulmonary hypertension (Chapter 41).

Pneumonia presenting with pleuritic chest pain often is associated with fever, cough productive of purulent sputum, chills, and dyspnea. The physical examination may show wheezing or crackles, egophony (E to A change), and increased tactile fremitus (Chapter 55).

Pneumothorax should be considered in any patient who complains of sudden onset of pleuritic chest pain and unexplained acute dyspnea. The physical examination includes tachypnea, decreased or loss of breath sounds on the affected side, and hyperresonance to percussion (Chapter 39).

Musculoskeletal

Costochondritis or costochondral pain is the most common cause of musculoskeletal chest pain in the outpatient setting. Chest pain of musculoskeletal origin may last few seconds or hours to weeks, and has an insidious onset. It can be sharp, localized, or diffuse. The pain may be worsened by movement of the trunk, deep breathing, or arm movement. On physical examination, musculoskeletal chest pain may be reproducible by chest palpation. The reproducibility of the pain by chest palpation does not definitively exclude life-threatening causes of chest pain such as ischemia; however, it reduces the likelihood of a myocardial infarction. Chest pain in a dermatome distribution may suggest herpes zoster, even though skin lesions may not yet have appeared. Other causes may include arthritis or fibromyalgia, the latter being more common in women then men. The presence of trigger points (pressure points that elicit pain upon palpation) in the upper chest increases the likelihood of fibromyalgia. Often, cardiovascular examination is normal.

Psychosomatic

Panic attack, severe anxiety, and depression (Chapters 118 and 119) may represent almost 10% of causes of acute chest pain presenting to the emergency departments. The chest pain in such patients may be described as sharp or stabbing, and may last a few minutes or hours. Patients may complain of sweating, trembling or shaking, sensations of shortness of breath or smothering, a feeling of choking, nausea, abdominal distress, or lightheadedness. On physical examination, tachycardia and tachypnea may be present, whereas the rest of the cardiovascular and pulmonary examination is often unremarkable (Tables 6.2 and 6.3).

EVALUATION

The evaluation of chest pain has a dual purpose of (a) identifying the correct diagnosis and (b) eventually assessing the severity of disease and/or the need for immediate intervention.

Cardiac

Ischemic chest pain should be evaluated with an electrocardiogram (ECG) and serum cardiac markers if there is suspicion of an acute coronary syndrome (ACS, which includes in its definition myocardial infarction and unstable angina). A normal ECG markedly reduces the likelihood of a myocardial infarction; however, 20% of patients presenting with chest pain and a normal ECG may still have unstable angina. An abnormal ECG that shows at least 1 mm sinus tachycardia (ST) elevation or tachycardia (ST) depression is very suggestive of acute coronary syndrome. Troponin serum markers have shown high accuracy in predicting the diagnoses of myocardial injury. These markers can be found in the blood 3 to 12 hours after a myocardial infarction and up to 7 to 11 days after myocardial necrosis. If ACS is suspected, the evaluation may also include a chest x-ray (CXR) and possibly an echocardiogram. A CXR may yield relevant information by helping in the diagnosis of other cardiovascular etiology of chest pain (e.g., aortic dissection) as well as the diagnosis of pulmonary (e.g., pneumothorax or pneumonia) or musculoskeletal causes of chest pain. An echocardiogram may reveal the presence of significant valvular causes of chest pain. A cardiac stress test can be performed for patients at low risk of ischemic heart disease (patients with normal ECG, at least one risk factor for coronary artery disease, atypical chest pain, and normal cardiac enzymes).

In acute pericarditis, an ECG should also be obtained. It typically shows diffuse ST elevations without reciprocal changes. A CXR and a transthoracic echocardiogram (TTE) may be helpful if there is suspicion of a significant pericardial effusion or pericardial tamponade.

Aortic dissection should be evaluated first with a CXR, which may show a widened mediastinum (85% of cases). A normal ECG in a patient with abrupt onset of tearing chest pain should raise the suspicion for aortic dissection. The ECG may be useful to exclude other life-threatening causes of acute chest pain such as ischemic heart disease and/or pericarditis (ECG evidence of left ventricular hypertrophy may be found in aortic dissection as a result of long standing hypertension). A chest computed tomography scan, transesophageal echocardiogram, angiography of the aortic root, and magnetic resonance imaging can be used to confirm the diagnosis.

Aortic stenosis evaluation entails the identification of a diamond-shaped systolic ejection murmur best heard in the second right intercostal space with the patient supine. A transthoracic echocardiogram can be used to detect the severity of the valvular disease, if present. Cocaine-related chest pain should be evaluated with an ECG and serum cardiac markers. Troponin concentrations should be measured. A previous history of cocaine use should be sought. Serum creatine kinase may be measured and found to be elevated as a result rhabdomyolysis (muscle breakdown). A urine drug screen should be ordered to identify cocaine as a possible cause of chest pain.

Pulmonary

Pneumothorax or pneumonia should initially be evaluated with a CXR to detect the presence of a collapsed lung or an infiltrate, respectively. A complete blood count should be ordered in the evaluation of pneumonia to detect the presence of an elevated white cell count. A helical or CT scan of the chest or a ventilation perfusion (V/Q) scan with or without duplex of lower extremities is indicated to diagnose pulmonary embolism when the suspicion is moderate to high. A blood D-dimer level should be ordered when the clinical suspicion of pulmonary embolism is low due to its high negative predictive value; it is high in patients with deep venous thrombosis.

Gastrointestinal

GERD and esophageal dysfunction (esophageal spasm) are often diagnosed after the exclusion of cardiac causes. Esophageal disease can be evaluated with a symptomatic response to acid suppression therapy (proton pump inhibitors or H2 antagonists,) followed by esophageal pH monitoring if symptoms persist. Endoscopy should be considered in patients who are unresponsive to medical treatment and those at risk for Barrett's esophagus with long-standing history of GERD (premalignant lesion).

Musculoskeletal

Costochondritis or costochondral pain and arthritis can be evaluated with a CXR. If symptoms persist, a CT of the chest or bone scan may be helpful. If a systemic rheumatologic disorder is suspected, tests such as complete blood count, rheumatoid factor, antinuclear antibody, and urinalysis may be part of the evaluation.

Psychosomatic

Panic attacks, anxiety, or depression as a cause of chest pain can be suspected by the presence of symptoms such as shaking, dizziness, hyperventilation (which may be a cause of ST depression on ECG), previous history of anxiety or depression, and the absence of confirmatory markers for the aforementioned etiologies of chest pain. No specific diagnostic or laboratory test is helpful in this diagnosis; this is often a diagnosis of exclusion after other causes of chest pain have been evaluated and excluded.

CHAPTER 7

Cough

Shibin Jacob and Amandeep Gill

Cough is an explosive expiration that provides a normal protective mechanism for clearing the tracheobronchial tree of secretions and foreign material. Cough is also one of the most common complaints for which patients seek medical care. It can have a profound impact on quality of life for a variety of reasons including discomfort from the cough itself, interference with normal lifestyle, and concern for the cause of the cough, especially fear of cancer. Based on duration of symptoms, cough is broadly divided into acute (<3 weeks), subacute (3 to 8 weeks), and chronic (>2 months) (Fig. 7.1).

DIFFERENTIAL DIAGNOSIS

Estimating the duration of cough is the first step in narrowing the differential diagnosis. Because all cough is acute at the time of onset, the differential diagnoses is determined by the time at presentation. It is possible to diagnose the cause of chronic cough about 90% of the time, which leads to specific therapies in about 85% to 98% of cases.

Acute Cough

Acute cough is often caused by upper respiratory infections such as the common cold, acute bacterial sinusitis, pertussis, exacerbations of chronic obstructive pulmonary disease, allergic rhinitis, and rhinitis due to environmental allergies. Viral infections of the respiratory tract account for cough in about 83% patients in the first 48 hours and about 26% on day 14. Prolonged exposure to any airway irritants can also lead to airway inflammation, which can then trigger cough; the initial mechanism may go unnoticed.

Acute cough can also be the presenting manifestation of pneumonia, left ventricular failure, asthma, or conditions that predispose patients to the aspiration of foreign matter. It is especially important to have a high index of suspicion for these disorders in elderly patients, because classic signs and symptoms may be nonexistent or minimal.

Subacute Cough

For a cough that began with an upper respiratory tract infection and has lasted for 3 to 8 weeks, the most common conditions to consider are postinfectious cough, bacterial sinusitis, and asthma. Postinfectious cough is defined as cough that begins with an acute respiratory tract infection that is not complicated by pneumonia. This usually resolves without treatment. It may result from postnasal drip or clearing of the throat due to rhinitis, tracheobronchitis, or both, with or without transient bronchial hyperresponsiveness.

Chronic Cough

Chronic cough can be caused by a variety of different diseases, although a few diagnoses account for 95% of patients. These include postnasal-drip syndromes, asthma (Chapter 35), gastroesophageal

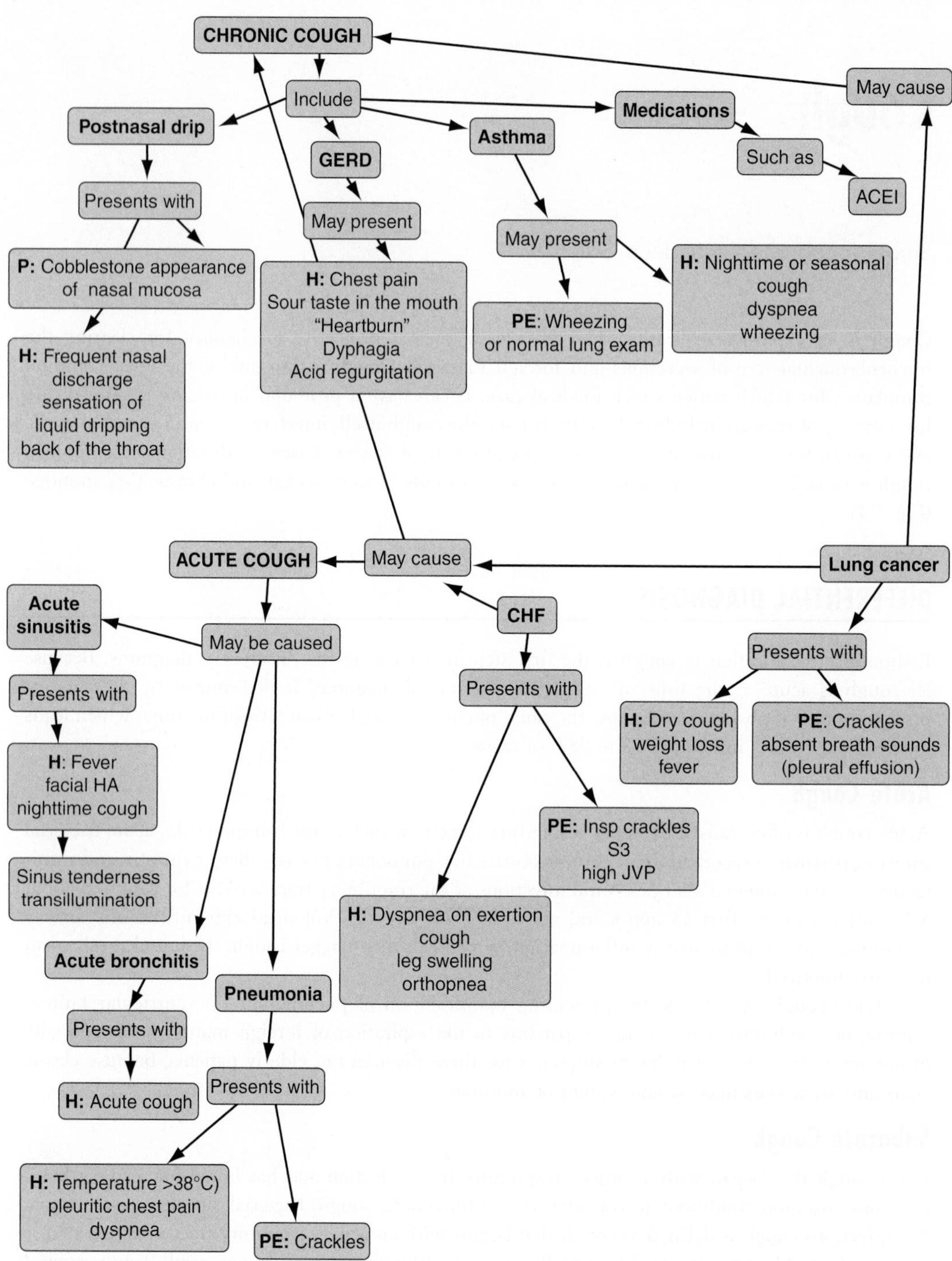

Figure 7.1 • Chronic cough. ACEI, angiotensin-converting enzyme inhibitors; CHF, congestive heart failure; GERD, gastroesophageal reflux disease; HA, headache; JVP, jugular venous pressure.

TABLE 7.1 Causes of acute and chronic cough

Acute cough	Chronic cough
	Most common
Acute bronchitis	Postnasal drip
Acute sinusitis	Gastroesophageal reflux disease
Chronic obstructive pulmonary disease	**Less common**
Asthma exacerbation	Medications (ACE inhibitor)
Allergic rhinitis	Lung cancer
Whooping cough (Pertussis)	Bronchiectasis
	Interstitial lung disease
	Congestive heart failure
	Chronic obstructive pulmonary disease
	Whooping cough

reflux disease, and chronic bronchitis. The differential diagnosis of postnasal-drip syndrome includes sinusitis and various types of rhinitis, including nonallergic, allergic, postinfectious, vasomotor, drug induced, and environmental-irritant induced. These can occur alone or in combination. Chronic bronchitis (Chapter 36) can be caused by cigarette smoking, other irritants, bronchiectasis, or eosinophilic bronchitis. Angiotensin-converting enzyme (ACE) inhibitors can be associated with cough approximately 10% of the time. In the remaining 5% of patients, the differential diagnosis includes bronchogenic carcinoma, lung metastatic cancer, sarcoidosis, and left ventricular failure (Table 7.1).

EVALUATION

The character of the cough (e.g., paroxysmal, loose and self-propagating, productive, or dry), the quality of the sound (e.g., barking, honking, or brassy), and the timing of the cough (e.g., at night or with meals) have not been shown to be diagnostically useful.

In acute cough with symptoms suggestive of viral rhinosinusitis (common cold), diagnostic testing is not indicated because of low yield. It is diagnosed when patients present with an acute respiratory illness characterized by symptoms and signs related primarily to the nasal passages as rhinorrhea, sneezing, nasal obstruction, and postnasal drip, and when a chest examination is normal. Such cases, although common, can be clinically indistinguishable from bacterial sinusitis.

Subacute cough is evaluated in much the same way as chronic cough, if it is not associated with obvious respiratory infection.

When faced with chronic cough, physicians can narrow the list of possible diagnoses by reviewing the patient's history and physical examination and focusing on the most common causes of chronic cough (i.e., postnasal drip syndrome, asthma, gastroesophageal reflux disease [GERD], ACE inhibitor use); obtaining a chest radiograph; and determining whether the symptoms conform to the clinical profile that is usually associated with a diagnosis of postnasal drip syndrome, asthma, GERD, chronic bronchitis, or combination of these. A normal radiograph in an immunocompetent patient, or a radiograph that shows no abnormality other than one consistent with an old and unrelated process, makes postnasal-drip syndrome, asthma, GERD, chronic bronchitis, and eosinophilic bronchitis likely and bronchogenic carcinoma, sarcoidosis, tuberculosis, and bronchiectasis unlikely.

Asthma is best diagnosed by spirometry accompanied by drug therapy or provocation. If signs of obstruction are present at baseline, a bronchodilator is administered. If the baseline is normal, a methacholine "challenge" is performed. A negative result of methacholine challenge rules out asthma as a cause of chronic cough, whereas a positive response or a response to bronchodilator therapy is virtually diagnostic. The methacholine challenge test is also positive in the presence of ACE inhibitor–induced cough and can be used for confirmation when this diagnosis is in question.

CHAPTER 8

Diarrhea

Dario Torre and José Franco

Diarrhea is an exceedingly common complaint that one may encounter in daily practice both in the clinic and hospital settings. Diarrhea is defined as a stool amount >300 g/day on a high-fiber diet (>200 g/day on a typical Western diet); however, it frequently is used as a general term to describe loose, watery, or frequent stools (more than three per day). Diarrheal diseases represent one of the leading causes of death worldwide, particularly among children in developing countries.

DIFFERENTIAL DIAGNOSIS

In the differential diagnosis of diarrhea, two main conceptual frameworks help in generating a diagnostic hypothesis: duration of symptoms (acute vs. chronic) and pathophysiologic mechanism (osmotic, secretory, inflammatory, malabsorptive, decreased absorptive surface, and abnormal motility) (Fig. 8.1).

According to the duration of symptoms, diarrhea is most commonly defined as:

- Acute: ≤14 days
- Persistent: >14 days
- Chronic: >30 days

Acute Diarrhea

Ninety percent of acute diarrhea cases are infectious in etiology (Table 8.1). The remainder of cases are caused by medications, toxin ingestions, and ischemia.

INFECTIOUS DIARRHEA

Infectious diarrhea usually is acquired by transmission through the fecal-oral route, most commonly by ingesting food or water contaminated by human or animal feces. The major causes include viral, bacterial, and (less commonly) protozoal pathogens.

Viral infections are the most common and usually self limited, lasting 1 to 3 days. Noroviruses are the most common cause of nonbacterial diarrhea in the United States. Outbreaks typically occur in the winter months and are responsible for the epidemic form of family and community-wide outbreaks of acute explosive vomiting and diarrhea. The illness usually lasts 24 to 48 hours, occurring among school-aged children and both child and adult family contacts of the index patients. Worldwide, rotaviruses are the most common cause of diarrhea in infants and children, although adults may be affected with mild symptoms.

Bacterial pathogens more commonly cause severe diarrhea and are more likely to be associated with bloody diarrhea. Nontyphoidal salmonellae are the leading cause of foodborne disease in the United States, associated with ingestion of poultry, eggs, and milk products. Serotypes *Salmonella enteritides* and *Salmonella typhimurium* are the most commonly identified. Risk factors for infection include young age, altered intestinal flora due to antibiotic use or surgery, and inflammatory bowel disease.

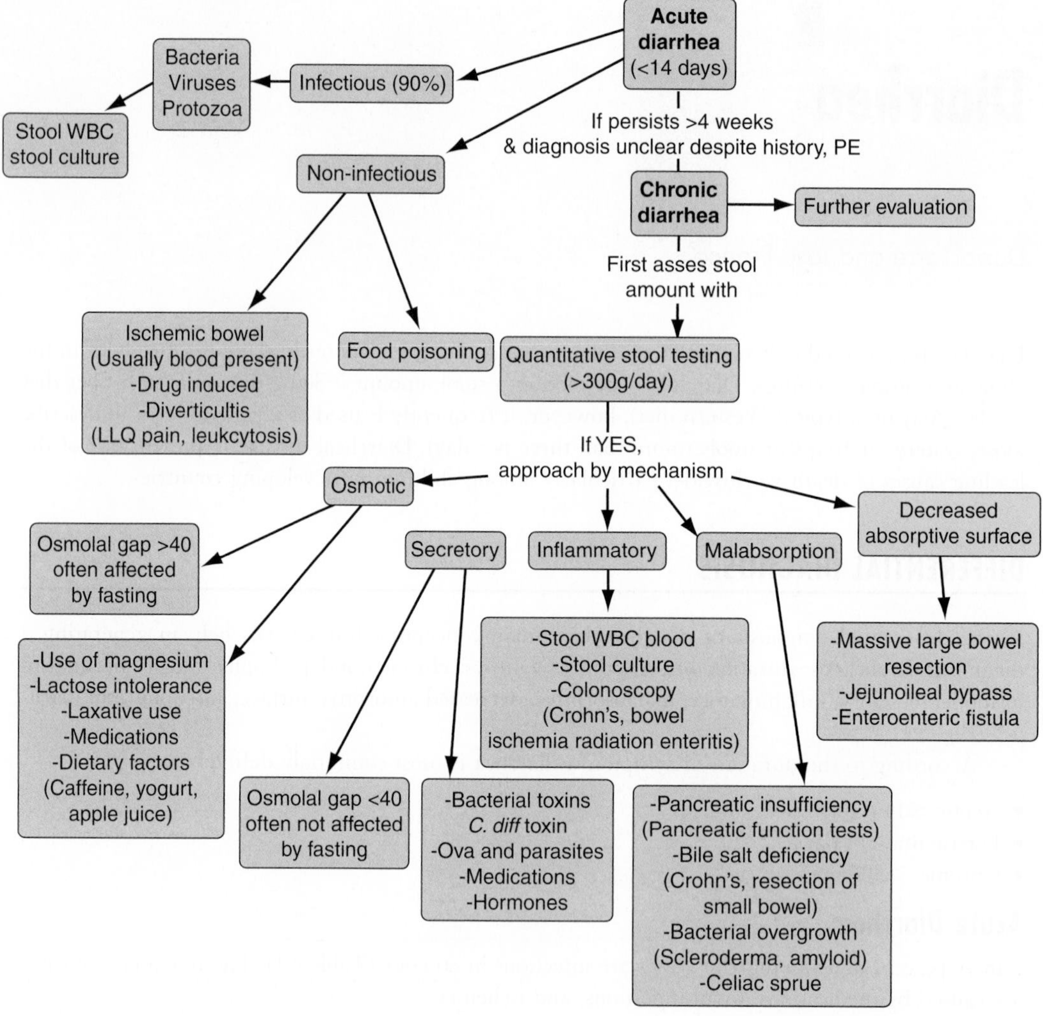

Figure 8.1 • Differential diagnosis and evaluation of diarrhea.

Campylobacter is the second most common cause of foodborne disease in the United States. Commonly associated with undercooked poultry, diarrhea caused by this organism can be watery or hemorrhagic. *Campylobacter* has also been linked causally with the development of reactive arthritis and Guillain-Barré syndrome.

Shigella classically causes dysenteric or bloody diarrhea. Transmission can occur both from person to person and as a foodborne disease. Enterohemorrhagic *Escherichia coli* (EHEC), most commonly O157:H7, is a common cause of infectious colitis. The usual route of transmission is ingestion of undercooked ground beef. The EHEC organisms and *Shigella* may be complicated by the development of the hemolytic-uremic syndrome and thrombotic thrombocytopenic purpura.

Clostridium difficile diarrhea is an important cause of diarrhea particularly among hospitalized patients. It causes a toxin-mediated enteric disease. The major risk factors are advanced age, hospitalization, and exposure to antibiotics. The antibiotics most frequently implicated are clindamycin, extended-spectrum penicillins, and cephalosporins, although any antibiotics can predispose to the infection. In the appropriate clinical setting, findings that are suggestive of *Clostridium difficile* infec-

TABLE 8.1 Differential diagnosis of acute diarrhea

Virus
Norovirus
Rotavirus
Adenovirus
Astrovirus
Human immunodeficiency virus
Bacteria
Escherichia coli
Salmonella
Shigella
Campylobacter
Clostridium difficile
Protozoa
Giardia lamblia
Cryptosporidium
Entamoeba histolytica

tion are leukocytosis, low serum albumin, fecal leukocytes, and in severe cases, direct visualization of pseudomembranes on endoscopic evaluation of the colon.

Protozoa can cause infection both in the immunocompetent and immunocompromised, although they tend to be self-limited in the former. *Giardia lamblia* is one of the most common gastrointestinal parasites in the United States. *G. lamblia* causes both epidemic and sporadic disease and is an important cause of waterborne and foodborne diarrhea and day-care center outbreaks. Infection with *Cryptosporidium* presents as a severe dehydrating but self-limited diarrheal illness in immunocompetent hosts. In immunocompromised hosts, it may have a more prolonged and severe course. It has been shown to be the causative agent responsible for several waterborne community outbreaks in the United States. Person-to-person transmission is also common, particularly among household members, sexual partners, children in daycare centers and their caretakers, and healthcare workers. Intestinal amebiasis is caused by *Entamoeba histolytica*. In the United States, amebiasis is mainly seen in migrants from and travelers to endemic countries. Institutionalized patients and sexually active homosexuals are also at increased risk of infection. Symptoms range from mild diarrhea to severe dysentery producing abdominal pain, diarrhea, and bloody stools.

NONINFECTIOUS CAUSES OF ACUTE DIARRHEA

Medication side effects are the most common noninfectious cause of acute diarrhea. The more frequently incriminated medications include antibiotics (penicillin), cardiac antiarrhythmics (quinidine), diuretics, antihypertensives (calcium channel blockers), nonsteroidal anti-inflammatory drugs, colchicine antidepressants (fluoxetine, sertraline), chemotherapeutic agents, bronchodilators, antacids (containing magnesium), and laxatives. Factitious or surreptitious diarrhea may be caused by voluntary laxative or diuretic abuse to achieve weight loss (anorexia nervosa) or other secondary gains.

Vascular insufficiency leading to ischemic colitis may also present as acute lower abdominal pain associated with watery or, more frequently, bloody diarrhea. Acute diarrhea may also accompany colonic diverticulitis, graft-versus-host disease, and systemic compromise including after ingestion of toxins such as organophosphate insecticides, amanita and other mushrooms, arsenic, and preformed environmental toxins in seafood, such as ciguatera and scombroid.

Chronic Diarrhea

Diarrhea lasting >4 weeks is defined as chronic diarrhea. In contrast to acute diarrhea, most of the causes of chronic diarrhea are noninfectious; the cause usually can be determined by a thorough history and basic stool studies. Large-volume diarrhea suggests a small bowel or proximal colonic etiology, whereas frequent small-volume stools may be more common with diseases affecting the distal colon or rectal area.

The presence of chronic bloody diarrhea associated with oral ulcers and erythema nodosum (painful, erythematous nodules on the anterior surfaces of both legs) raises suspicion for inflammatory bowel disease (IBD) (Chapter 76). Diverticular disease and ischemic colitis may also present with bloody diarrhea. Steatorrhea (voluminous, greasy, foul-smelling stools), weight loss, dermatitis herpetiformis (pruritic, papulovesicular rash located on the trunk and over the external surface of the extremities), and a positive family history for gluten sensitivity suggests celiac disease (celiac sprue).

Osmotic diarrhea occurs when ingested, osmotically active solutes draw fluid towards the intestinal lumen to exceed the resorptive capacity of the colon. Osmotic diarrhea stops with 48 hours fasting or with stoppage of the offending agent. One of the most common causes of osmotic chronic diarrhea in adults is lactase deficiency.

Secretory diarrheas result from alterations in fluid and electrolyte transport across the enterocolic mucosa with an excess of water. It usually presents as painless watery diarrhea that persists with fasting. Diarrhea may be caused by bacterial toxins (*C. difficile* colitis), enteropathogenic viruses, medications, and hormones such as serotonin, histamine, gastrin, and prostaglandins. Zollinger Ellison syndrome (gastrinoma), characterized by multiple peptic ulcers and diarrhea, is the result of excess secretion of gastrin. The watery diarrhea of hypokalemia achlorhydria syndrome, also called pancreatic cholera, results from vasoactive intestinal peptide (VIP) secretion from a pancreatic lesion (VIPoma). Carcinoid tumors can cause chronic diarrhea though the secretion of histamine and serotonin, whereas medullary carcinoma of the thyroid may cause diarrhea through the production of histamine and prostaglandins.

Inflammatory diarrheas, caused by mucosal ulceration and inflammation, are generally associated with pain, fever, bleeding, or other symptoms (systemic manifestation). The presence of fecal leukocytes on stool analysis is characteristic of inflammatory bowel disease (IBD), a common cause of inflammatory diarrhea.

Malabsorption-related diarrhea causes greasy, foul-smelling diarrhea associated with weight loss and nutritional deficiencies due to malabsorption of essential nutrients and vitamins. The mechanism may be a combination of osmotic and secretory components. Quantitatively, steatorrhea is defined as stool fat exceeding 7 g/day on a nonrestricted diet.

Diarrhea resulting from decreased absorptive surface or decreased contact time may be seen with extensive bowel resection or use of laxatives, respectively. Laxatives shorten intestinal transit time and result in excess water remaining in the stool, causing a watery diarrhea. Finally, it is important to remember that more than one pathophysiologic mechanism may be implicated in diarrheal diseases. (Table 8.2)

EVALUATION

First and foremost, diarrhea must be differentiated from other entities that may mimic the symptoms. Pseudodiarrhea is the frequent passage of small volumes of stool, and can be evaluated with a 48- to 72-hour quantitative stool collection while the patient is on a regular diet and not using antidiarrheal agents. If stool weight is <200 g/day, then the diagnosis of diarrhea should not be entertained.

TABLE 8.2 Classification of diarrhea by pathophysiologic mechanism

Classification of diarrhea by pathophysiologic mechanism
Osmotic diarrhea
Mg, SO_4, PO_4 ingestion Carbohydrate malabsorption
Malabsorption-related diarrhea
Intraluminal maldigestion (pancreatic exocrine insufficiency from chronic pancreatitis, bacterial overgrowth, liver disease) Mucosal disease (celiac sprue, Whipple's disease, infections, scleroderma, ischemia, diabetes, hyperthyroidism, hypoparathyroidism) Bile salt deficiency (cirrhosis, Crohn's disease, ileal resection, bacterial overgrowth)
Inflammatory diarrhea
Inflammatory bowel disease • Ulcerative colitis • Crohn's disease • Diverticulitis Infectious diseases • Tuberculosis • Yersiniosis • Cytomegalovirus • Herpes simplex virus Ischemic colitis Radiation colitis Neoplasm • Colon cancer • Lymphoma
Secretory diarrhea
Bacterial, viral, protozoal infections Exogenous stimulant laxatives Endogenous laxatives (malabsorption of bile salts from ileitis) Hormone-producing tumors (carcinoid, VIPoma, medullary cancer of thyroid, mastocytosis, gastrinoma) Villous adenoma (secretion of potassium)
Diarrhea due to abnormal intestinal motility
Bowel obstruction or fecal impaction Diabetes, Addison's disease, hyperthyroidism Laxatives Irritable bowel syndrome Parkinson's disease
Diarrhea due to decreased absorptive surface
Small or large bowel resection Enteroenteric fistulas

TABLE 8.3 Clinical characteristics associated with severity of diarrheal illnesses
Profuse watery diarrhea with signs of hypovolemia
Passage of many small volume stools containing blood and mucus
Bloody diarrhea
Temperature ≥38.5°C (101.3°F)
Passage of at least six unformed stools per 24 hours or a duration of illness >48 hours
Severe abdominal pain
Recent hospitalization or use of antibiotics
Diarrhea in the elderly (≥70 years of age) or the immunocompromised patients

A medical evaluation is always indicated in patients with relatively severe illness, as suggested by one or more of characteristics in Table 8.3.

The initial clinical evaluation of the patient with diarrhea should focus on gathering data about the onset, duration, characteristic of stools (color, consistency, presence of blood), and presence of associated symptoms such as abdominal pain, nausea, vomiting, and fever. Other pertinent questions should be asked regarding residency, occupational exposure, recent and remote travel, pets, hobbies, recent food consumption, hospitalization, and antibiotic use. Signs of volume depletion (dry mucosa, flat jugular vein, orthostatic hypotension) should be sought. A complete abdominal exam should be carried out to detect clues related to the cause of diarrhea. Inspection may reveal a scar indicating a previous bowel resection; tenderness in the left lower quadrant may be consistent with diverticulitis. A nodular liver, caput medusae, and ascites may suggest cirrhosis. One of the easiest ways to differentiate osmotic and secretory diarrheas is to fast the patient for 48 hours and assess the effect on stool output. When diarrhea ceases with fasting, an ingested agent is likely to be the cause; if diarrhea persists unabatedly with fasting, a dietary nutrient is not likely to be the cause.

The timing of exposure should also be assessed as it frequently gives clues to the cause. Symptoms that begin abruptly (within 6 hours) suggest ingestion of a preformed toxin of *Staphylococcus aureus* or *Bacillus cereus*. Symptoms that begin between 8 to 14 hours suggest infection with *Clostridium perfringens*. Symptoms that develop more insidiously (>14 hours) can result from viral or bacterial infection (e.g., contamination of food with enterotoxigenic or enterohemorrhagic *E. coli*).

Stool examination is also an important part of the evaluation. Cultures for bacterial agents (*Salmonella, Shigella, Campylobacter*), *C. difficile* colitis toxin, and examination for ova and parasites should be performed. Presence of leukocytes in the stool suggests an inflammatory cause such as IBD or infection.

A 72-hour fecal fat analysis may be performed if malabsorption or pancreatic insufficiency is suspected (values >7 g/day indicate malabsorption). The measurement of an osmolal gap may help to differentiate osmotic diarrheas (>125 mOsm/kg) from other types of diarrhea (<50 mOsm/kg in secretory diarrhea). The osmotic gap is calculated from electrolyte concentrations in stool water by the following formula:

$$290 - 2(Na^{+} + K^{+})$$

A complete blood count may reveal leukocytosis (suggesting inflammation or infection) and anemia (bloody diarrhea). If surreptitious laxative abuse is suspected, urine and stool analysis should be performed. Stool testing can detect almost all types of laxatives (bisacodyl, senna, magnesium-containing laxative, castor oil, and mineral oil). Urine testing, currently the most sensitive screening test, can detect the aforementioned laxatives except castor and mineral oil. Phenolphthalein-containing laxatives, no longer available over the counter, can be detected by adding NaOH or KOH to observe a color change to reddish-purple.

If the diagnosis is still not apparent, then referral to a gastroenterologist is warranted. Additional tests such as colonoscopy, upper gastrointestinal endoscopy, or other more specialized tests (lactose breath test for lactose insufficiency, bentiromide and secretin test for pancreatic insufficiency) may be needed to determine the diagnosis.

CHAPTER 9

Dizziness and Vertigo

Avery Hayes

Dizziness is one of the most common complaints in clinical practice and affects approximately 20% to 30% of the general population. This symptom is responsible for numerous visits to emergency departments and outpatient clinics. Ongoing dizziness can lead to a loss of function, falls, and injuries. Balance-related falls account for more than one half of all accidental deaths in the elderly. Dizziness is a nonspecific symptom and may be used by the patient to describe a number of different experiences. Because the differential diagnosis is broad, the evaluation of the dizzy patient can be both overwhelming and time consuming.

DIFFERENTIAL DIAGNOSIS

Dizziness may be classified into four broad categories based on clinical characteristics, which will provide for more accurate diagnosis (Table 9.1):

1. **Vertigo** (Table 9.2) is the illusory sensation of spinning or motion. The patient may feel as if their body or the environment is in motion. Vertigo may be peripheral in etiology, due to disorders of the vestibular end organs (semicircular canals and utricle), eighth cranial nerve, or the vestibular nuclei. Central causes of vertigo include ischemia or damage to brainstem structures, or the cerebellum.
2. **Presyncope** is the sense of impending loss of consciousness due to impaired cerebral blood flow, or anoxia, which often implies an underlying cardiovascular, metabolic, or hematologic disorder.
3. **Disequilibrium** is a sense that one is about to fall, often associated with motor or sensory dysfunction resulting in the inability to maintain balance and gait.
4. **Lightheadedness** describes other nonspecific symptoms related to multiple sensory disturbances, psychiatric illness, and medication side effects that alter the sensorium.

Vertigo

A crucial aspect of the evaluation of vertigo is to differentiate peripheral from central causes (Table 9.3. The latter have more serious consequences and require emergent evaluation and treatment. The clinical presentation, nature of the nystagmus, and presence of associated neurologic signs and symptoms may help distinguish vertigo of peripheral and central etiologies. Peripheral causes of vertigo often present as abrupt, intense attacks, which last several seconds to minutes, and are accompanied by nausea and vomiting. Vertigo due to central causes may occur with a more gradual onset but have a prolonged duration of symptoms. The intensity of symptoms may be less severe with central causes but often the patient may be unable to stand or walk. Nystagmus associated with peripheral vertigo can be decreased with visual fixation and is typically unidirectional (horizontal with a rotary component). Nystagmus that is purely vertical is due to a central cause. During cases of prolonged vertigo, nystagmus from peripheral causes is diminished by compensation and generally does not last longer than 48 hours.

TABLE 9.1 Differential diagnosis of dizziness

Dizziness subtype	Type of sensation	Temporal characteristics	Differential diagnosis
Vertigo	Spinning or motion	Episodic or continuous	Benign paroxysmal positional vertigo Ménière's disease Labyrinthitis Vertebrobasilar ischemia Cerebellar infarction or hemorrhage
Presyncope	Faint feeling, as though one were about to pass out	Episodic, may last seconds, may be relieved by recumbent position	Dehydration Ischemic heart disease Obstructive cardiac lesions Cardiac arrhythmia Neurocardiogenic syncope Anemia Hypoglycemia or hyperglycemia Infection
Disequilibrium	A sense of unsteadiness of the lower extremities	Constant but may fluctuate in intensity	Multiple sensory deficits including peripheral neuropathy and vision loss
Lightheadedness	Nonspecific		Psychiatric conditions including anxiety, depression, panic attacks, and agoraphobia Hyperventilation Medications

TABLE 9.2 Differential diagnosis of vertigo

Peripheral vertigo	Central vertigo
Benign paroxysmal positional vertigo Cerebellar hemorrhage or infarct Acute vestibular neuritis Labyrinthitis Acoustic neuroma Ménière's disease	Brainstem ischemia Vertebrobasilar insufficiency

TABLE 9.3 Characteristics of peripheral and central vertigo

Characteristics	Peripheral	Central
Severity	Severe	Mild
Onset	Sudden	Gradual
Duration	Seconds to minutes	Weeks
Positional	Yes	No
Fatigable	Yes	No
Associated symptoms	Auditory	Neurological and visual
Nystagmus	Horizontal	Vertical

From Chawala N, Olshaker JS. Diagnosis and management of dizziness and vertigo. *Med Clin North Am* 2006;90:291–304, with permission.

Because brainstem structures subserve many neurologic functions, infarcts causing vertigo will also have neighborhood effects due to injury to other cranial nerve nuclei, long motor, or sensory tracts. Common presentations are summarized in Table 9.4. Lateral medullary infarcts cause vertigo by infarction of the vestibular nuclei. Associated symptoms and signs include Horner's syndrome, ipsilateral facial numbness, diplopia, dysphagia, or contralateral limb numbness. Patients with cerebellar infarcts have signs such as dysmetria, past-pointing, or dysdiadochokinesis. Vertigo associated with transient ischemic attack due to vertebrobasilar artery (VBA) insufficiency is associated with additional symptoms such as diplopia, transient blindness, drop attacks, or dysarthria. Stroke in the VBA distribution may have a wide range of findings depending on the branch affected and collateral blood supply. Symptoms include hearing loss, ophthalmoplegia, blindness, sensory loss, and ataxia. Other processes affecting the cerebellum such as hemorrhage may present with headache, severe gait ataxia, or depressed levels of consciousness. The cerebellum may also be involved in demyelinating disorders such as multiple sclerosis.

Peripheral causes of vertigo are more common than central etiologies. Benign paroxysmal positional vertigo (BPPV) is the most common cause of peripheral vertigo. This condition occurs when debris form the utricle forms a plug and circulates within the endolymph of the semicircular canals. This clot is thought to act as a plunger and induce a push-and-pull force on the cupula, creating asymmetric impulses between both ears that result in vertigo and nystagmus. Most patients describe episodes of vertigo that are triggered by changes in head position, such as looking up or rolling over

TABLE 9.4 Stroke syndromes associated with vertigo

Site (artery)	Clinical presentation
Labyrinth (internal auditory artery)	Tinnitus, hearing loss
Lateral medullary infarct (vertebral artery, posterior inferior cerebellar artery)	Horner's syndrome, cranial nerves V and VII, crossed sensory loss
Lateral pontomedullary infarction (anterior inferior cerebellar artery)	Horner's syndrome, cranial nerves V and VII, crossed sensory loss, hearing loss
Cerebellum (posterior and anterior inferior cerebellar arteries, superior cerebellar artery)	Limb dysmetria, ataxia

From Delaney K. Bedside diagnosis of vertigo: value of the history and neurologic examination. *Acad Emerg Med* 2003;10:1388–1395, with permission.

in bed. Attacks are usually sudden in onset and generally last less than 60 seconds. BPPV is characterized by fatigability. The patient will develop tolerance to repeated head movements, causing a reduction in continued symptoms.

Labyrinthitis and vestibular neuritis are characterized by inflammation; either the canals of the inner ear, vestibular nerve, or nuclei can be affected. Both syndromes can follow a viral upper respiratory infection. Patients usually present with severe vertigo, nausea, and vomiting. Symptoms usually last from days to weeks. The vertigo gradually subsides as the inflammation resolves and central compensatory mechanisms evolve. Otitis media may cause a suppurative labyrinthitis due to bacterial spread form the middle ear through a ruptured membrane or perilymph fistula. These patients appear acutely ill and present with hearing loss and fever in addition to nausea, vomiting, and vertigo. Ramsay-Hunt syndrome is caused by *Varicella zoster* and is a variant of vestibular neuritis with involvement of the cranial nerves VII and VIII, causing facial paresis, tinnitus, hearing loss, and vertigo.

Ménière's disease is due to an increase in the volume of endolymph, causing distention of the endolymphatic system. The classic triad is vertigo, tinnitus, and fluctuating sensorineuronal hearing loss. Attacks of vertigo are abrupt and may last from minutes to hours. Attacks also vary in intensity and may be associated with aural fullness or pain. Symptoms can be unilateral or bilateral.

Acoustic neuroma is a benign tumor composed of Schwann cells of the vestibular nerve. Patients often present with tinnitus and hearing loss. These tumors are slow growing and central compensation leads to less severe vertigo. Enlargement of the tumor within the cerebellopontine angle causes compression of the adjacent cranial nerves and brainstem, and may result in facial anesthesia and weakness.

Presyncope

As noted above, presyncope is the sensation that one is about to lose consciousness. Often, this is a milder manifestation of an event that ultimately could result in true syncope. The differential diagnosis and evaluation are the same as for syncope (Chapter 24).

Disequilibrium

Dysequilibrium syndrome should be suspected when a patient feels unsteady, as though they are about to fall. This sensation is particularly prominent following a sudden change in position or with loss of visual cues, as when getting on or off an elevator. This phenomenon is triggered by loss of sensory inputs that cue the brain to position or the loss of musculoskeletal function interfering with the minor readjustments in position to maintain balance.

Disequilibrium can be seen in association with a number of disorders including peripheral neuropathy, visual impairment, severe arthritis, and Parkinson's disease. It is particularly common in patients with long-standing diabetes who may have several of these issues present simultaneously.

Lightheadedness

A substantial number of patients with dizziness describe relatively vague symptoms that are difficult to verbalize. Oftentimes these are characterized as a sensation of being lightheaded or floating. A majority of these patients have an underlying psychological issue including anxiety, depression, or increased stress. Physical examination is usually unremarkable. In some of these patients, subclinical hyperventilation may play a role.

EVALUATION

Some patients may not be able to give an accurate history; therefore, the physical examination not only serves to differentiate peripheral from central causes of vertigo, but also helps to evaluate for causes of dizziness other than vertigo. Vital signs should be measured, including orthostatic blood pressure.

Physical examination should include a complete eye, ear, nose, and throat examination (looking for nystagmus, asymmetry, or defects in the pupillary reactivity and extraocular movements) and a funduscopic examination to check for papilledema. Inspection of the tympanic membranes should be performed to evaluate for scarring, fluid, or infection. If hearing loss is detected, the Weber and Rinne tuning fork examinations can differentiate between conductive and sensorineural hearing loss. Auscultation for carotid bruits and cardiac examination should be performed to evaluate for potential sources of emboli or obstructive cardiac lesions. A thorough neurological examination is important, including examination of motor strength and sensation, cranial nerves, cerebellar function, Rhomberg's test, and gait.

The Dix-Hallpike maneuver is used to diagnose BPPV (Fig. 9.1). The patient is seated upright on the examining table with the head held in the hands of the examiner for support. The patient's head is turned 45 degrees toward the side being tested. The patient is rapidly lowered to a supine position with the head hanging below the level of the examining table. The patient should be reminded

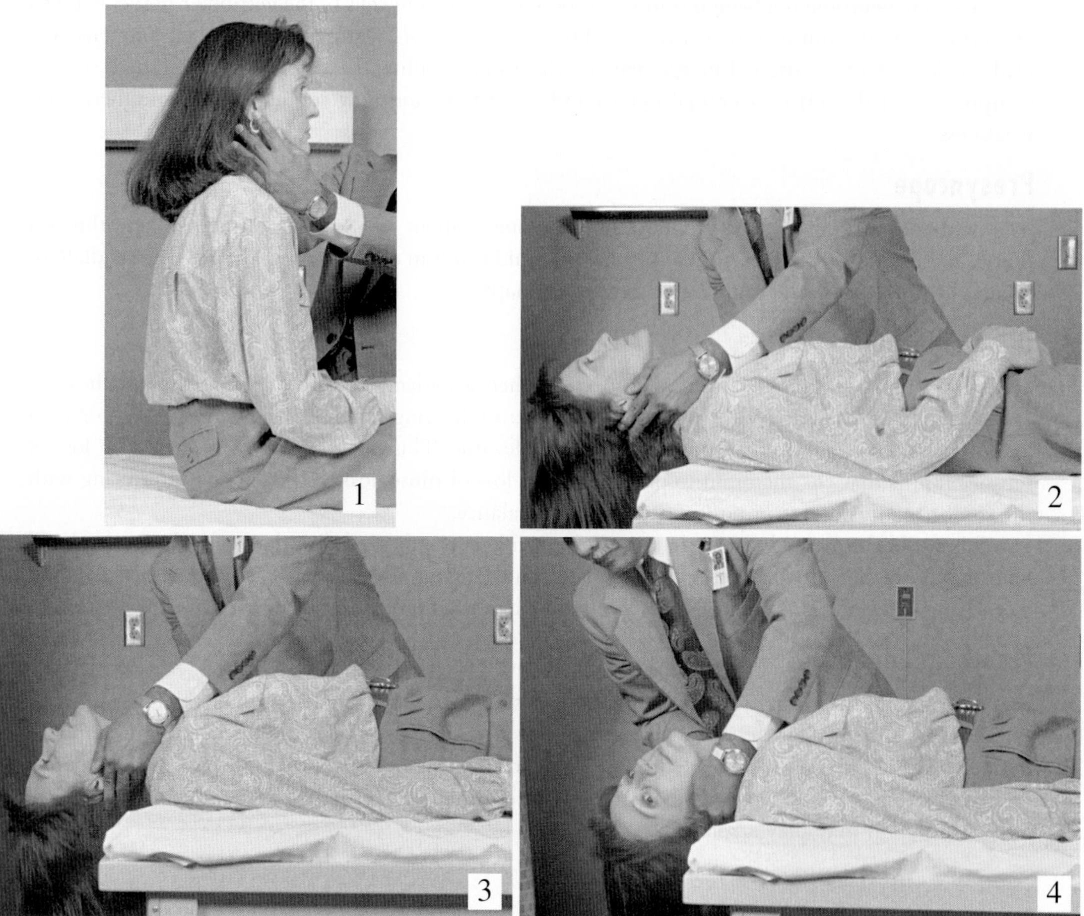

Figure 9.1 • Dix-Hallpike maneuver. The patient is positioned with the head hanging 30 to 45 degrees over the table edge first in the midline, which is repeated with the head rotation to right and left. Frames one through four show the procedure in sequence.

to keep the eyes open because it is critical to see if vertigo occurs. After a short period of latency, a positive test is indicated by a burst of torsional-vertical nystagmus (the upper poles of the eyes beat torsionally toward the ground) associated with vertigo. The vertigo typically lasts between 20 to 40 seconds and is pathognomonic of the posterior canal variant of BPPV.

If disequilibrium is suspected, it can be helpful to perform a finger touch test. The physician attempts to reproduce the symptom by having the patient turn or change position quickly. In the presence of the symptom, the patient is asked to touch the examiner's finger with their own. If the symptoms improve dramatically, it is very suggestive of disequilibrium.

If the complaint is lightheadedness, the patient should be asked to deliberately hyperventilate. If the symptoms are reproduced, this can help confirm the diagnosis and be used as a tool to reassure the patient.

Laboratory tests may not be helpful if the dizziness is caused by vertigo, but may indicate another cause. Complete blood counts, basic metabolic panel, and thyroid function tests may indicate the presence of anemia, electrolyte abnormalities, hypoglycemia, dehydration, or thyrotoxicosis causing symptoms. Electrocardiography may show signs of atrial fibrillation or ischemia.

Electronystagmography is an examination that records eye movements in response to vestibular, visual, cervical, caloric, rotational, and positional stimulation, and may be used to assess vestibular function. Audiologic evaluation can be performed if indicated to evaluate for patterns of hearing loss.

Patients with suspected central cause of vertigo require cranial imaging with either computed tomography (CT) or magnetic resonance imaging (MRI). CT will identify cerebellar hemorrhage or infarction and suggest the presence of tumor, but lacks the sensitivity to detect small infarcts in the brainstem. MRI has superior sensitivity and will identify small lesions including infarcts, tumors, and plaques. Magnetic resonance angiography will visualize the intracranial vasculature, including the vertebrobasilar system. Patients suspected of having an infarct should also be evaluated for a source of thromboembolism, including electrocardiogram to rule out atrial fibrillation and echocardiogram with a bubble study to evaluate for intracardiac shunt.

CHAPTER 10

Dyspnea

Ann Maguire

Dyspnea is one of the most common symptoms encountered in outpatient practice and hospital settings and is the primary diagnosis for millions of patient visits each year. The American Thoracic Society defines dyspnea as "a subjective experience of breathing discomfort." The development of dyspnea is a complex phenomenon that results from derangements in oxygenation, carbon dioxide, or acid-base balance. Hypoxia, hypercapnia, and a low pH trigger chemoreceptors in the medulla, carotid, and aortic bodies. These in turn trigger an effort to increase ventilation, which then stimulates mechanoreceptors throughout the airways, lungs, and chest wall. These receptors signal the central nervous system in a manner that conveys the individual's sensation of shortness of breath.

DIFFERENTIAL DIAGNOSIS

Dyspnea can be either acute or chronic and it may be caused by pulmonary disorders, cardiac disorders, or a diverse group of other causes (Table 10.1). The most common causes of dyspnea are asthma, chronic obstructive pulmonary disease (COPD), interstitial lung disease, and cardiomyopathy, but deconditioning is a major contributing factor in all patients with chronic dyspnea. Many individuals who suffer from chronic dyspnea have multiple causes.

Pulmonary Disorders

Obstructive lung disease due to asthma or COPD is a common cause of acute and chronic dyspnea. Individuals will often report a sensation of tightness in the throat or chest and a feeling that they cannot get enough air. Symptoms may be triggered by exercise, cold air, or viral upper respiratory tract infection. Smokers with COPD often report chronic cough with sputum production. Common physical findings include wheezing or, in severe cases, a generalized decrease in breath sounds and prolongation of forced expiration due to the severity of the bronchoconstriction. In cases of established obstructive lung disease, patients may report a decrease in their peak flow as measured by a handheld peak flow meter and relief of symptoms with increased use of a beta-agonist bronchodilator.

Tracheal obstruction is another important cause of dyspnea. Acute obstruction due to laryngeal edema secondary to allergy, bacterial epiglottitis, or viral croup can be life threatening and requires immediate attention. In addition to visible signs of respiratory distress such as tachypnea and diaphoresis, patients will exhibit stridor. Chronic causes of upper airway obstruction include vocal cord dysfunction, multinodular goiter, and neoplastic processes that may lead to fixed airway obstruction. In some cases, patients report more difficulty breathing when they are supine.

Emphysema, in the absence of airway obstruction, causes chronic dyspnea and hypoxia by reducing alveolar oxygen exchange. Affected individuals usually report an extensive smoking history or are found to have an inherited deficiency in the α-1 antitrypsin enzyme that is involved in maintaining alveolar elasticity. Common findings on examination include pursed lip breathing, resting tachypnea, diminished breath sounds, barrel-shaped chest, hyperresonance to percussion, and decreased precor-

TABLE 10.1 Differential diagnosis of dyspnea

Pulmonary causes	Cardiac causes	Other causes
Asthma	Coronary syndromes	Respiratory muscle weakness
Chronic obstructive pulmonary disease	Valvular disorders	Myasthenia gravis
Tracheal obstruction	Cardiomyopathy	Guillain-Barré syndrome
Emphysema	Pericardial disorders	Anemia
Interstitial lung disease		Metabolic acidosis
Pulmonary hypertension	Arrhythmias	Diabetic ketoacidosis
Pulmonary embolism	Congestive heart failure	Salicylates
Pneumonia		Pregnancy
Pleural effusion		Psychiatric disorders
Pneumothorax		Anxiety Panic disorder Musculoskeletal Kyphoscoliosis

dial heart sounds. Note that most smokers with emphysema do share some features of COPD (Chapter 36).

Interstitial lung disease (Chapter 37) is a cause of chronic dyspnea. Numerous pulmonary and systemic disorders have been known to cause interstitial lung disease, including granulomatous disorders such as sarcoidosis, connective tissue disorders including rheumatoid arthritis and scleroderma, lung injury due to dust inhalation including asbestosis and silicosis, and idiopathic pulmonary fibrosis. Most patients report gradual progressive dyspnea, dry cough, and chest pain that may be pleuritic. It is critical to obtain a history of exposure to possible offending agents. Physical findings include tachypnea, "dry" rales on auscultation, and finger clubbing. Patients with connective tissue disease may also have arthritis, malar rash, or erythema nodosum.

Primary pulmonary hypertension, a disorder predominantly affecting women in their 30s and 40s, is rare. Pulmonary hypertension is most often a manifestation of another disease process. Examples include COPD, interstitial lung disease, massive obesity, congenital heart disease, sleep apnea, and pulmonary embolism. Physical findings often found among patients with pulmonary hypertension include right ventricular heave, prominent jugular venous "a-wave" pulsations, loud P_2 (pulmonic valve closure), right-sided third or fourth heart sound, ankle edema, and pulsatile liver or tender hepatomegaly.

Pulmonary embolism is a common diagnosis that is often associated with acute dyspnea. However, chronic venous thromboembolic disease, characterized by embolization of multiple small thrombi, can also lead to chronic shortness of breath and exercise intolerance. Pulmonary embolism causes dyspnea by increasing pulmonary vascular resistance. Hypoxia is due to atelectasis, increased V/Q mismatch, and decreased cardiac output. In many cases, patients with pulmonary embolism will have a predisposing risk factor for deep vein thrombosis if there is not an identifiable peripheral clot. In severe or acute cases, presentation may include chest pain, hypotension, cor pulmonale, and even sudden death. Physical findings suggestive of pulmonary hypertension previously described may be present. Subacute presentations are more likely to be associated with an increase in baseline chronic dyspnea without other classic features, making this diagnosis difficult to distinguish from a worsening of baseline heart failure or lung disease. A history of hemoptysis or severe pleuritic chest pain suggests pulmonary infarct may be present. Physical findings may include low-grade fever, pleural friction rub, or findings of ipsilateral consolidation or effusion; however, in many cases the physical examination is unrevealing (Chapter 41).

Pneumonia is a frequent cause of acute dyspnea. A detailed discussion of the organisms causing community-acquired and nosocomial pneumonia can be found in Chapter 55. Additional symptoms include fever, chills, pleuritic chest pain, and cough, which may or may not be productive. Physical examination may be helpful in identifying the extent of the infection. Inspiratory rales, wheezes, and bronchial breath sounds are often present. Dullness to percussion, increased tactile fremitus, egophony with "E" to "A" changes, and whispering pectoriloquy are found in patients with lobar consolidation (Chapter 55).

Pleural effusion is an abnormal accumulation of fluid in the pleural space. It can be caused by an imbalance of hydrostatic and oncotic pressures (transudate), an inflammatory process, or another disorder of the pleura (exudate). In addition to dyspnea, patients may report the presence of a nonproductive cough and chest pain that can be either pleuritic or nonpleuritic. Physical findings of pleural effusion are decreased tactile fremitus, dullness to percussion, and decreased breath sounds on auscultation (Chapter 38).

Pneumothorax usually presents as dyspnea that is acute in onset. Traumatic or iatrogenic causes are often seen in individuals who have suffered penetrating or blunt injury to the chest, or among those who have recently undergone invasive medical procedures.

Spontaneous pneumothorax is more difficult to diagnose. Populations at increased risk for primary spontaneous pneumothorax include tall, thin men and cigarette smokers. Secondary spontaneous pneumothorax has been associated with many pulmonary disorders. Common examples include emphysema, cystic fibrosis, lung abscess, tuberculosis, and sarcoidosis. In addition to dyspnea, sudden onset of chest pain is the symptom most often reported by patients with pneumothorax. Physical findings include diminished to absent breath sounds over the affected lungs, decreased tactile fremitus, and hyperresonance to percussion. Tension pneumothorax is a respiratory emergency and is often manifested by tachypnea, tachycardia, distended neck veins, and hypotension (Chapter 39).

Cardiac Disorders

Coronary syndromes including stable angina, unstable angina, and myocardial infarction often present with dyspnea as one of the primary symptoms. The dyspnea is usually exertional and may be associated with chest pain, diaphoresis, and nausea. In many cases, the dyspnea and other symptoms are relieved by rest. Physical examination is often nonspecific; however, an S4 may be present during acute ischemic attacks. If the myocardial ischemia is severe and involves a large area of the myocardium, which affects cardiac output, then left ventricular dysfunction and congestive heart failure may ensue. Common findings include rales on auscultation of the lungs, tachycardia, or the presence of a third or fourth heart sound (Chapter 28).

Cardiomyopathy is one of the most common causes of acute and chronic dyspnea. The cardiomyopathies are primary myocardial diseases affecting the structure and function of heart muscle. All three subgroups (dilated, restrictive, and hypertrophic) can cause dyspnea. Dyspnea initially may be exertional; however, in severe cases patients experience symptoms at rest as well as orthopnea and paroxysmal nocturnal dyspnea. Most patients demonstrate some signs and symptoms of heart failure including tachycardia, low blood pressure, atrial S4 and ventricular S3 gallops, and systolic murmurs associated with mitral and tricuspid regurgitation caused by ventricular dilation (Chapter 29).

Valvular disorders are frequent causes of acute and chronic dyspnea. Aortic stenosis, mitral regurgitation, aortic regurgitation, and mitral stenosis are those most often encountered. When these disorders develop acutely, they are always poorly tolerated due to acute ventricular dysfunction and the respiratory distress can be quite severe. When valvular disorders are chronic, the most common symptom is exertional dyspnea. In most cases, the valvular disorder leads to ventricular dysfunction and ultimately congestive heart failure. The triad associated with aortic stenosis of moderate to severe degree includes syncope on exertion, chest pain, and congestive heart failure. Cardiac auscultation is characterized by a harsh systolic ejection murmur best heard at the second left intercostal space (Chapter 30).

Pericardial disorders can result from diverse causes. The acute and chronic inflammation leads to fluid accumulation and, in some cases, fibrous adhesions that can obliterate the pericardial space. The resulting pericardial tamponade or restrictive pericarditis can cause dyspnea by impairing ventricular filling and reducing cardiac output. In addition to dyspnea, patients may report chest pain that is dull or sharp. Less than one third of patients have an identifiable pericardial friction rub on auscultation. When fluid accumulation is rapid, tamponade may follow. Associated findings on physical examination include tachypnea, tachycardia, hypotension, narrow pulse pressure, neck vein distension, pulsus paradoxus (a fall in systolic blood pressure on inspiration), and muffled heart sounds (Chapter 31).

Other Causes of Dyspnea

Respiratory muscle weakness due to neuromuscular disorders or abnormal respiratory mechanics may also cause chronic dyspnea. Myasthenia gravis is a common autoimmune disorder that involves the formation of antibodies against acetylcholine receptors. As the disease progresses, it leads to respiratory muscle weakness and ultimately respiratory failure (Chapter 117). Guillain-Barré syndrome (acute inflammatory demyelinating polyneuropathy) causes rapid distal and proximal muscle weakness that may affect respiration (Chapter 116). Individuals with severe kyphoscoliosis experience chronic dyspnea due to limited chest wall and diaphragmatic mobility.

Anemia results in limited serum oxygen carrying capacity and is an important cause of chronic dyspnea. Additional symptoms include dizziness, fatigue, and cold sensitivity. On physical examination, patients may have tachycardia, heart murmurs, pallor, and other findings specific to the cause of the anemia.

Metabolic acidosis triggers an increase in ventilatory effort that is perceived as dyspnea by the central nervous system. Pregnancy can also lead to a sensation of dyspnea, termed physiologic dyspnea, through hormonal changes (hyperventilation due to increased progesterone) and the effect of the gravid uterus on respiratory mechanics. Psychosomatic disorders such as generalized anxiety disorder and panic disorder are commonly associated with complaints of dyspnea; however, this is often a diagnosis of exclusion.

EVALUATION OF DYSPNEA

The timely evaluation of dyspnea involves an initial determination of the severity and need for immediate intervention or close monitoring. This requires initial assessment of vital signs and oxygenation status. Once the need for emergent stabilization is addressed, then the focus becomes pursuit of the diagnosis.

The first step is to distinguish between pulmonary, cardiac, neuromuscular, metabolic, and psychological causes (Fig. 10.1). Oftentimes, this distinction can be determined rapidly from the history of present illness, past history, and initial physical examination, but on occasion further testing is required.

Such tests should include a chest x-ray, electrocardiogram, and a pulse oximeter. The chest x-ray is useful for identifying conditions involving the lung tissue and adjacent structures such as pneumonia, pneumothorax, pleural effusion, and congestive heart failure. An electrocardiogram can be useful to identify arrhythmias or acute ischemia. Most medical settings have ready access to a pulse oximeter. The pulse oximeter measures oxygen saturation of the hemoglobin. Low oxygen saturation generally indicates a relatively acute decline in oxygenation and identifies a patient in

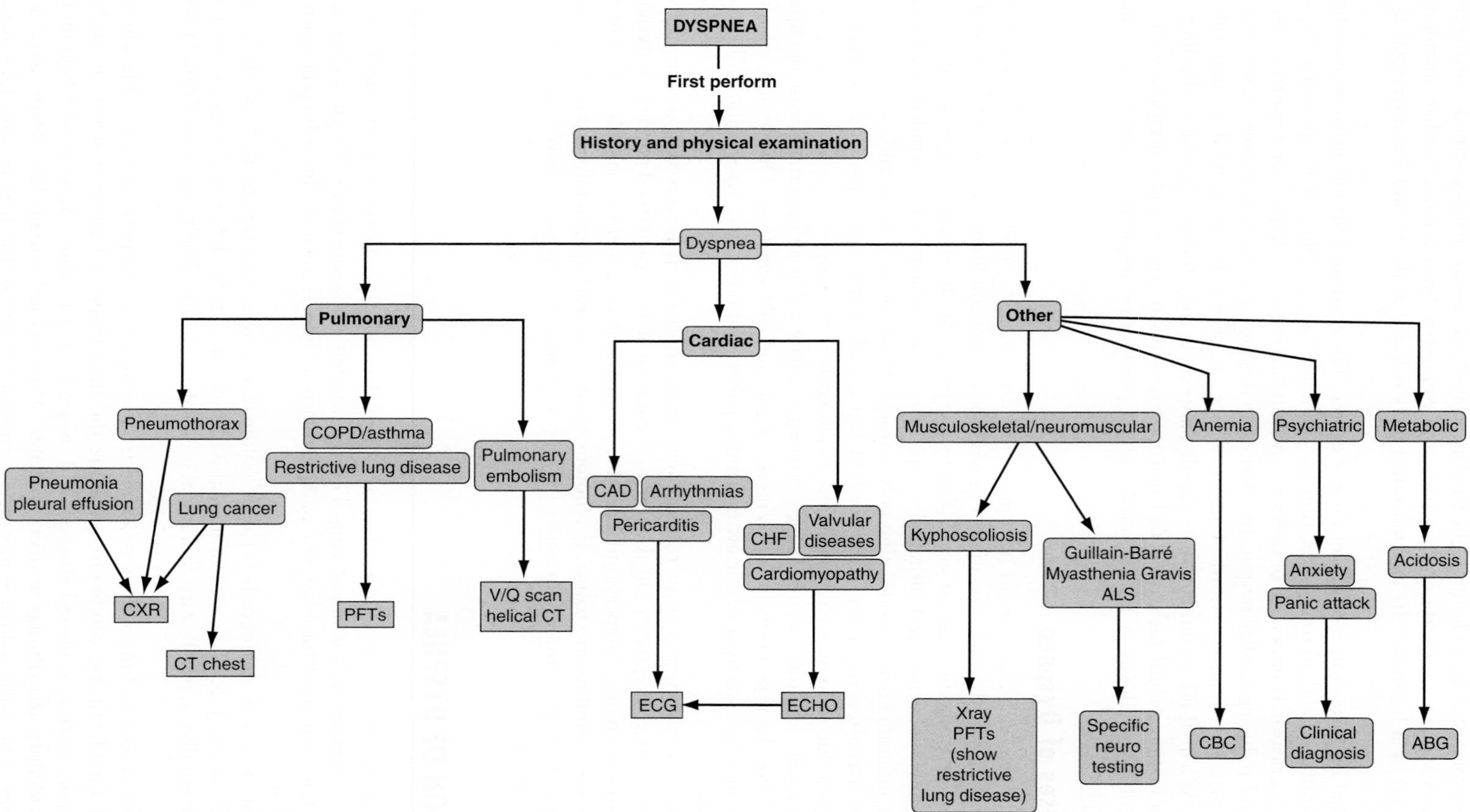

Figure 10.1 • Differential diagnosis and evaluation of dyspnea. ABG, arterial blood gas; ALS, amyotrophic lateral sclerosis; CAD, coronary artery disease; CBC, complete blood count; ECHO, echocardiogram; PFTs pulmonary function tests.

need of close observation and supplemental oxygen therapy. This is usually associated with a primary pulmonary process, congestive heart failure, increased ventilation perfusion mismatch, or mechanical hypoventilation. The pulse oximeter does not assess ventilation status and may not identify patients who are hyperventilating to maintain their oxygenation status or who are developing respiratory failure with a high carbon dioxide level. Also, the pulse oximeter reading may be inaccurate in the setting of anemia, poor perfusion, pigmented skin, and nail polish.

An arterial blood gas is the best test for assessing ventilation, oxygenation, and acid-base status. Review of the PCO_2, PO_2, HCO_3, and O_2 saturation may be the only clues available to identify hyperventilation, respiratory failure, pulmonary embolism, or an acid-base disorder.

If the nature of the underlying problem remains uncertain, some preliminary laboratory tests can be helpful. A complete blood count can identify anemia and an elevated white blood cell count may be a marker for underlying infection. Electrolytes may reveal a low bicarbonate level, which can be a marker for a metabolic acidosis or hyperventilation; a high bicarbonate level may be indicative of compensation for CO_2 retention. An elevated anion gap may be indicative of a metabolic acidosis.

At this stage, most causes of dyspnea can be sorted into the broad categories of pulmonary, cardiac, or other disorders. Recognize that in many patients more than one factor may be playing a role and a high threshold of suspicion must be maintained.

Pulmonary Disorders

Asthma and COPD should be evaluated with measurement of pulmonary function tests. A decrease in peak flow or FEV1/FVC ratio $<70\%$ is consistent with the presence of obstructive lung disease. The presence of hypercapnia and acidosis will impact management. In some cases, a chest x-ray is helpful in identifying the presence of additional pulmonary pathology (e.g., pneumonia). Infection is a common cause of COPD exacerbations. Sputum gram stain and culture may be helpful in making decisions about antibiotic therapy; however, the result of the Gram stain specimen is rarely used as the only decisive factor for antibiotic use. A chest x-ray should be obtained in the presence of fever, pleuritic pain, or abnormal auscultatory findings on lung examination, which may suggest the presence of pneumonia.

When tracheal obstruction is suspected, chest x-ray and, in most cases, computed tomography (CT) scan of the neck and chest is needed to identify the source of the obstruction. Direct laryngoscopy is the only way to definitively evaluate for vocal cord dysfunction or other forms of dynamic airway obstruction. When emphysema is the suspected cause of dyspnea, the initial evaluation should also include an assessment of oxygenation. Pulmonary function testing including spirometry and lung volumes will help assess the severity of disease. When dyspnea is acute, a chest x-ray to exclude infection or pneumothorax is warranted. CT scan of the chest will help assess the extent of the parenchymal lung disease, but often does not aid in management of acute exacerbations.

When pulmonary hypertension is suspected, a careful evaluation to exclude underlying disorders is critical. Pulmonary function testing to identify COPD, echocardiogram to confirm the presence of congenital heart disease, overnight polysomnography to diagnose sleep-disordered breathing, or studies to confirm the presence of pulmonary embolism are needed. Patients in whom primary pulmonary hypertension is suspected must undergo right heart catheterization to confirm the diagnosis. In some cases a tissue diagnosis may be in order. A helical CT scan of the chest or a ventilation perfusion (V/Q) scan with or without duplex of lower extremities is indicated to diagnose pulmonary embolism when the suspicion is moderate to high. A blood D-dimer level should be ordered when the clinical suspicion of pulmonary embolism is low because of its high negative predictive value.

Pneumonia, pleural effusion, and pneumothorax are often diagnosed based simply on the combination of physical examination and chest x-ray. In some cases, if concern remains high and these are equivocal, it may be necessary to follow this with a computed tomography scan of the chest to identify an infectious process that does not manifest as a lobar infiltrate or a small effusion or pneumothorax.

Cardiac Disorders

Ischemia due to coronary syndromes must be quickly ruled out whenever it is the suspected cause of dyspnea. The evaluation should begin with an electrocardiogram. When the symptoms are acute, measurement of cardiac enzymes is very important. Patients with chronic exertional dyspnea of potential cardiac etiology should undergo exercise or pharmacologic stress testing. When the symptoms are acute, decisions about stress testing versus immediate cardiac catheterization should be made in consultation with a cardiologist (Chapter 27).

Evaluation of suspected cardiomyopathy, valvular disorders, and pericardial disorders must include a transthoracic echocardiogram, especially if an electrocardiogram or chest x-ray show evidence of cardiomegaly and congestive heart failure.

Other Causes of Dyspnea

Dyspnea due to respiratory muscle weakness from a neuromuscular disorder or peripheral neuropathy may be suspected from the initial chest x-ray and arterial blood gas. Patients who are experiencing respiratory failure from either cause will often exhibit decreased lung volumes and evidence of compensated respiratory acidosis. Pulmonary function testing with special attention to lung volumes and measurement of negative inspiratory force is helpful in assessment when patients with neuromuscular disease are likely to require ventilatory support. An electromyelogram is needed to differentiate neuromuscular disorders such as myasthenia gravis from peripheral neuropathies including Guillain-Barré syndrome. Kyphoscoliosis is usually evaluated with plain radiograph of the thorax and spine. If this is thought to be the cause of chronic dyspnea, pulmonary function tests to evaluate lung mechanics are very useful.

Anemia is common and frequently found among patients with dyspnea (Chapter 5). It is recommended that before attributing the patient's dyspnea to anemia alone, a careful search be undertaken to exclude pulmonary and cardiac causes of dyspnea.

Metabolic acidosis due to diabetic ketoacidosis or lactic acidosis is a frequent cause of dyspnea in the acute inpatient or emergency department setting and should be suspected in the presence of decreased serum bicarbonate on initial laboratory evaluation. An arterial blood gas and further evaluation to identify the underlying cause of the acidosis is critical to the treatment of the patient.

Pregnancy and psychiatric disorders are usually obvious when present; however, caution should be used before attributing acute dyspnea to these diagnoses. A full investigation to exclude other potential causes should be undertaken.

CHAPTER 11

Dysuria

Julie Mitchell

Dysuria is the sensation of pain, discomfort, or burning during or just after urination. It is common: for example, the 2-year prevalence of dysuria among women is as high as 25% and the prevalence of perineal pain among men is about 5% to 10%. About 10% of women have a urinary tract infection (UTI), the most common cause of dysuria, in a given year.

DIFFERENTIAL DIAGNOSIS

Because many of the clinical features of dysuria vary according to sex, the differential diagnosis of dysuria should be approached according to gender (Table 11.1).

Dysuria in Women

Dysuria occurs either with inflammation or infection of the urinary tract, or because of urine contact with an inflamed vulva or vagina (Table 11.2). In women, at least half of cases of dysuria are due to a UTI, which is a bacterial infection of the urethra (urethritis), bladder (cystitis), or kidneys (pyelonephritis). Pyelonephritis is an "upper tract" infection and, although less common, is more serious (Chapter 56).

Sexually transmitted infections (STIs) can cause dysuria, either by urethral infection, vaginitis, or vulvar lesion. Chlamydia and gonorrhea infections can have wide clinical presentations from no symptoms, to cervicitis (infection of the cervix), to pelvic inflammatory disease. *Trichomonas* infection usually presents as vaginitis or occasionally cystitis. Herpes virus infection causes urethritis and painful (usually vulvar) ulcers.

Vaginitis (inflammation of the vagina) is also an important cause of dysuria (Table 11.3). Common causes are yeast vaginitis (generally due to *Candida*) and bacterial vaginosis (a decrease in lactobacilli flora and an increase in other bacteria such as *Gardnerella*). Atrophic vaginitis can cause dysuria in older women.

Interstitial cystitis is a syndrome of chronic bladder pain and urinary frequency, sometimes accompanied by dysuria. It is more common in women and the prevalence approximates 50 in 100,000. Vulvovaginal irritation may occur without infection: either from chemical exposure (soaps, aerosol deodorants, or douching), trauma (iatrogenic instrumentation or domestic violence), foreign body (e.g., retained tampon), or urolithiasis (note urethral stones are much less common than kidney or bladder stones).

The history of a dysuria patient should include accompanying urinary symptoms (urgency, frequency, and upper tract symptoms), vaginal symptoms (women may not volunteer these if not asked) and pelvic pain, sexual history (such as history of STI, number of partners, use of contraception, and type of contraception), trauma history, and use of vaginal products (commonly obtained over the counter). Past medical history should focus on previous UTIs, function and anatomy of the urinary tract, and conditions causing immunosuppression.

TABLE 11.1 Etiology of dysuria in women and men

Category	Examples	Risk factors	Key elements of the history (in addition to dysuria)	Key elements of the exam
UTI: lower tract	Urethritis Cystitis	Sexually active, older, and catheterized women; men with enlarged prostates and catheters	Frequency, urgency Suprapubic pain Hematuria	Normal
UTI: upper tract	Pyelonephritis	Immunosuppression, urinary tract abnormality, nephrolithiasis, instrumentation, diabetes, pregnancy	Lower tract symptoms Fever Flank pain Nausea, vomiting	CVA tenderness
STI	Urethritis Cervicitis Vaginitis PID	Sexually active men and women without use of condom, those with history of STI	Vaginal/penile discharge No hematuria Pelvic pain: think PID	Erythema Discharge Tenderness Herpetic ulcer
Vaginitis	Bacterial vaginosis Yeast vaginitis Trichomonas Atrophic vaginitis	Female sex (Table 11.2)	Discharge Pruritus	Erythema Discharge Tenderness
Dermatitis	Irritant Allergic	Use of vaginal products (e.g., deodorants, douches) or pads (e.g., with perfumes or in the setting of incontinence)	Vaginal irritation Vulvar irritation Pruritus	Erythema Edema Evidence of product
Trauma	Iatrogenic (procedural) Domestic violence	History of procedures, catheter, violence	Vaginal irritation Vulvar irritation	Evidence of trauma
Urolithiasis		History of stones	Colicky pain	Normal
Interstitial cystitis		Female sex	Chronic symptoms Pelvic pain	Normal

Prostatitis	Acute Chronic Noninfectious	Male sex BPH or other obstructive uropathy	Frequency, urgency Pelvic or rectal pain Fever	Tender boggy prostate
Benign prostatic hypertrophy		Male sex	Frequency, urgency Nocturia Obstructive symptoms	Enlarged prostate Distended bladder
Bladder cancer		Male sex, tobacco use	Hematuria	Normal
Epididymitis	STI UTI	Male sex, STI risks After trauma, sexual activity, or heavy lifting	Severe pain in scrotum, may radiate to flank	Tenderness
Other	Behçet's syndrome Lichen planus Pemphigus		Specific to diagnosis	Specific to diagnosis

BPH, benign prostatic hypertrophy; CVA, costovertebral angle; PID, pelvic inflammatory disease; STI, sexually transmitted infection; UTI, urinary tract infection.

TABLE 11.2 Frequency distribution of etiologies of dysuria in women

Cause of dysuria	Diagnosis frequency among women with dysuria
UTI: cystitis	50% to 60% 90% if no vaginal symptoms
UTI: pyelonephritis	<5%
STI: *Chlamydia* urethritis	5% to 20%
STI: Gonorrhea urethritis	<5% ~10% in inner city
Vaginitis: *Candida*, bacterial vaginosis, or *Trichomonas*	50% to 70% if vaginal symptoms <10% if no vaginal symptoms

STI, sexually transmitted infection; UTI, urinary tract infection.

Because classic UTI symptoms in combination with an absence of signs and symptoms of STI, vaginitis, or complicated UTI predict a UTI 90% of the time, a physical examination is not always required when the history taking is complete. However, a physical should include a pelvic examination and examination for costovertebral angle tenderness.

Dysuria in Men

In men, dysuria occurs with inflammation or infection of the urinary tract, including the urethra, bladder, prostate, kidney, and epididymis. Table 11.1 lists specific causes of dysuria within broad categories. The most common cause of dysuria in men is due to infection: older men are more likely to have a UTI, namely prostatitis, and younger men are more likely to have an STI. UTIs in men generally result in urethritis, prostatitis (inflammation or infection of the prostate), or pyelonephritis. STIs in men generally result in urethritis and, less frequently, epididymitis.

Prostatitis can be acute (symptoms lasting days) or chronic (symptoms lasting months). Chronic prostatitis can evolve from acute prostatitis or can be an asymptomatic (or low symptom) chronic insidious or relapsing condition. Nonbacterial prostatitis is a chronic syndrome of the irritative symptoms (dysuria, urgency, frequency, and nocturia) and pelvic pain without demonstration of a bacterial cause.

Benign prostatic hypertrophy (BPH) can lead to dysuria from inflamed urethral mucosa where it is distended (proximal to the prostate-induced obstruction) or compressed (at the prostate due to increased fibromuscular tone). BPH is common in older men: up to 50% of men older than 60 years have some urinary symptoms.

Less common causes of dysuria in men are urolithiasis and bladder cancer.

As in women, the history should include accompanying urinary symptoms (frequency, urgency, and upper-tract symptoms), pelvic pain, and sexual history (such as history of STI, number of partners, gender of partner[s], and use of condoms). Men should also be asked about obstructive symptoms: difficulty starting (hesitancy) or maintaining (intermittency) urine stream, prolonged dribbling at the end of the stream, and the sensation of incomplete bladder emptying. PMH should focus on previous UTIs, function and anatomy of the urinary tract, presence of BPH, and conditions causing immunosuppression.

Men with dysuria should have a physical examination, including rectal (assessing prostate), genital (assessing for urethral irritation, discharge, skin lesions, and scrotal tenderness), abdominal (for bladder distension, a sign of obstruction), and an examination for costovertebral angle tenderness.

TABLE 11.3 Evaluation of vaginal discharge

Diagnosis	Historical elements suggestive of diagnosis (in addition to discharge)	Signs suggestive of diagnosis	Wet mount and KOH preparation	Diagnosis frequency in women with discharge
Yeast Vaginitis	Pruritus Discomfort Dysuria Previous yeast infection, antibiotic use, immunosuppression	Discharge: thick, clumpy, adherent Erythema Edema pH 4 to 4.5	Budding yeast and hyphae with KOH (sensitivity 40% to 80%)	10% to 40%
Bacterial vaginosis	Malodor No pruritus	Discharge: off-white, thin, homogenous pH >4.5	Whiff test[a] Clue cells (>20%)[b]	20% to 50%
Trichomonas	Pruritus Dysuria Dyspareunia Malodor STI risks	Discharge: yellow-green, frothy Erythema pH 5 to 6	Trichomonads (sensitivity 50% to 70%) Can also order DNA probes	5% to 30%
Atrophic vaginitis	Postmenopausal Dryness Dyspareunia Petechiae Spotting (rare)	Vulvovaginal thinning (decreased rugae) Erythema pH 5 to 7	Increased polymorphonuclear leukocytes	Rare

[a]Positive whiff test is the presence of amine odor with the addition of KOH.
[b]Clue cells are squamous epithelial cells with adherent bacteria blurring cell borders.
KOH, potassium hydroxide solution.

EVALUATION

Women

An algorithm for evaluation of dysuria is shown in Figure 11.1. History and physical examination are the most important elements as previously described.

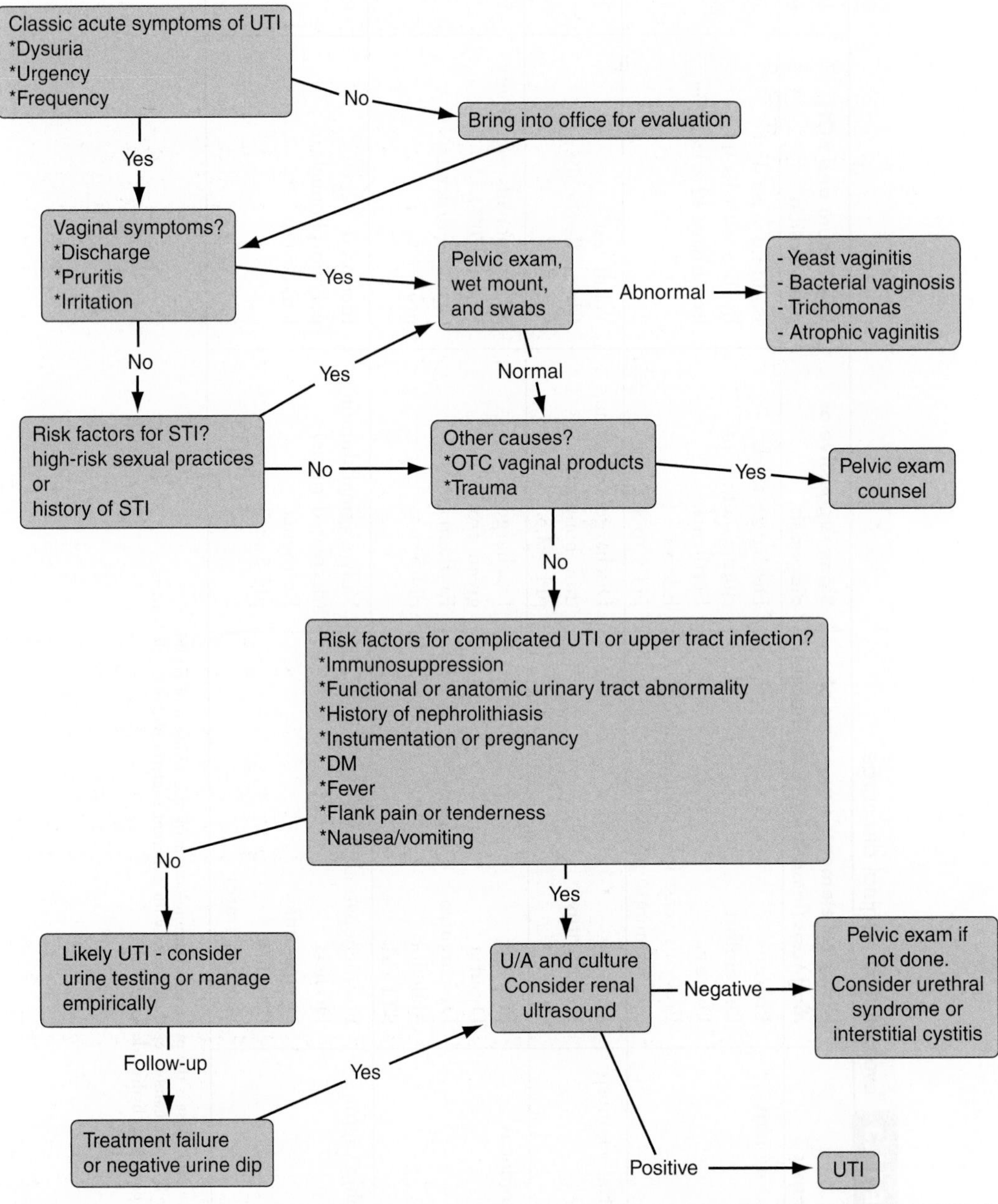

Figure 11.1 • Dysuria in women. DM, diabetes mellitus; OTC, over the counter; STI, sexually transmitted infection; U/A, urinalysis; UTI, urinary tract infection.

Men

Men with dysuria should have urine testing. Urine dipstick testing can be done quickly and conveniently in the office. This test is also less expensive than urinalysis with microscopy. Defining a positive dipstick test as positive nitrite or positive leukocyte esterase, the sensitivity of this test for a UTI is 75% and specificity is 80%. In comparison, a microscopic urine examination has a sensitivity to pyuria (more than 2 to 5 white cells per high power field) of 95% and a specificity of 70%); for visible bacteria, its sensitivity is 40% to 70% (specificity 85% to 95%). Young men, men with STI risk factors, and men with penile discharge should be tested for STIs (Chapter 139).

For men with urine tests not suggestive of infection and negative STI testing, any localizing physical examination finding should be evaluated: tenderness on genital examination indicates testicular ultrasound, distended bladder indicates a test for outlet obstruction (such as ultrasound). For men with hematuria, a urology referral for cystoscopy is indicated. Men with obstructive symptoms and a large prostate may be treated empirically for BPH and observed. Urine cultures can demonstrate notable bacterial counts even when urinalysis is normal (false-negative rate of about 5%); therefore, urine culture should be ordered when the history or examination suggests infection.

CHAPTER 12

Edema

Ann Maguire

Edema is generally defined as an increase in interstitial fluid volume that results in some degree of palpable swelling. Edema can be either pitting or nonpitting; in most cases, it is first detected in the lower extremities. Generalized edema usually becomes clinically apparent when extracellular fluid volume expands by about 5 L, corresponding to a 10-lb weight gain due to sodium and water retention. Localized edema is more likely to be nonpitting and is typically caused by a focal obstructive or inflammatory process. The balance of hydrostatic and oncotic pressure in the vascular system and interstitial space creates an environment that allows normal movement of water and diffusible solutes from the vascular space at the arteriolar end of the capillaries and a return at the venous end by way of the lymphatics. Edema occurs when there is an increase in vascular hydrostatic pressure, a decrease in vascular oncotic pressure, or some local process obstructing venous or lymphatic return.

DIFFERENTIAL DIAGNOSIS

Generalized Edema

The causes of generalized edema can be broadly organized according to six major categories: cardiac, hepatic, renal, medications, nutritional deficiency, and myxedema. The causes of localized edema involving the dependent limbs or periorbital tissues will be discussed separately (Table 12.1).

CARDIAC CAUSES

Cardiac edema usually reflects right heart failure; it is gravity-dependent and therefore is first noted in the feet and ankles of ambulatory patients. Right heart failure and edema usually develop late in heart disease. The cause of cardiac edema is most often congestive heart failure (CHF) due to either systolic or diastolic dysfunction (Chapter 28). The edema associated with CHF is due to a decrease in cardiac output leading to a decrease in the effective plasma volume and activation of the renin-angiotensin systems. These hormonal changes result in renal vasoconstriction and increased sodium and water retention with subsequent increased capillary hydrostatic pressure. Constrictive pericarditis and pulmonary hypertension can also cause edema by decreasing cardiac output and activating the same mechanisms. Cardiac edema is generally symmetric, pitting, and most obvious in the distal lower extremities. In more chronic cases, the edema can become extensive, progressing to anasarca involving the proximal lower extremities and abdominal wall. Cardiac edema is often also associated with other symptoms of heart failure and fluid overload including dyspnea, basilar rales, jugular venous distension, hepatomegaly, and x-ray findings consistent with pulmonary vascular congestion and pleural effusions.

HEPATIC CAUSES

Cirrhosis (Chapter 74) is the primary cause of edema in patients with liver disease. Portal systemic pressure is increased due to the obstruction of hepatic venous outflow caused by hepatic damage.

TABLE 12.1 Differential diagnosis of generalized edema
Cardiac
Heart failure due to systolic or diastolic dysfunction Primary pulmonary hypertension Constrictive pericarditis
Hepatic
Cirrhosis with portal hypertension
Renal
End-stage renal failure Nephrotic syndrome
Medications
Calcium channel blockers
Nutritional deficiency
Hypoalbuminemia (malnutrition)
Myxedema
Hypothyroidism

This decrease in venous return leads to a reduction in effective arterial blood volume stimulating sodium and water retention. The decreased plasma oncotic pressure due to cirrhosis-related hypoalbuminemia further exacerbates this process and combines to stimulate the renin-angiotensin-aldosterone system resulting in additional sodium and water retention. Ascites, fluid accumulation in the peritoneal cavity, is the hallmark of cirrhosis-related edematous patients; however, in advanced cirrhosis generalized edema may develop, particularly when serum albumin is <3.5 mg/dL. Edema is usually dependent edema in the lower extremities, but patients who are bedridden may have significant presacral edema. Tense abdominal ascites may increase intra-abdominal pressure, decreasing venous return from the lower extremities and further worsening lower extremity edema. Patients with peripheral edema related to cirrhosis and portal hypertension often demonstrate other manifestations of chronic liver disease. The presence of ascites may be detected by "shifting dullness" to percussion of the abdomen or a "fluid wave" due to free-flowing ascites. Other findings include gynecomastia, testicular atrophy, jaundice, hepatomegaly, splenomegaly, caput medusa, spider angiomata, palmar erythema, and encephalopathy.

RENAL CAUSES

Edema is a common physical finding in patients with chronic renal insufficiency. At first, the reduction in glomerular filtration rate results in increased renal retention of sodium and water through stimulation of the renin-aldosterone system. In end-stage renal disease, oliguria and anuria prevents renal elimination of water. Patients with acute glomerulonephritis and nephrotic syndrome (Chapter 82) may also be edematous; however, they are likely to have larger amounts of proteinuria and worse secondary hypoalbuminemia as a cause of the edema. Patients with edema due to chronic renal insufficiency often have laboratory evidence of renal disease including elevated serum creatinine and urea nitrogen, hyperkalemia, hyperphosphatemia, hypocalcemia, and metabolic acidosis.

MEDICATIONS

Several classes of medications have been associated with edema as an undesirable side effect. Vasodilating antihypertensives, including calcium channel blockers and direct vasodilators such as hydralazine and minoxidil, are among those most likely to cause peripheral edema. The dihydropyridine calcium channel blockers including nifedipine and amlodipine appear to be more likely than other calcium channel blockers to cause edema. Hormones such as estrogens, testosterone, and corticosteroids have been shown to cause peripheral edema, most likely due to vasodilatation or increased sodium and water retention. Nonsteroidal anti-inflammatory drugs inhibit prostaglandins and can cause deterioration in renal function through renal vasoconstriction and increased sodium retention, which leads to increased edema, particularly in patients with cirrhosis or chronic renal insufficiency.

NUTRITIONAL DEFICIENCY

Hypoalbuminemia due to severe protein malnutrition can be a significant contributing factor to edema in many patients. Protein-losing enteropathy and other malabsorptive states such as chronic pancreatitis, which lead to serum albumin <3.5 mg/dL, are potential causes. Susceptible patients include those with underlying disorders of swallowing or mental status in whom maintenance of adequate nutrition is a problem. Individuals with large soft-tissue wounds, chronic infections, and metastatic cancer are also at risk for poor nutrition and hypoalbuminemia.

MYXEDEMA

Hypothyroidism (Chapter 66) causing myxedema is a common cause of nonpitting edema. Myxedema is typically noted in the pretibial region and may sometimes be associated with periorbital puffiness. Patients demonstrating myxedema may also have other manifestations of hypothyroidism including cognitive impairment, coarsening of hair, bradycardia, fatigue, dyspnea, constipation, and depression. Laboratory abnormalities include elevated thyroid-stimulating hormone, low free T4, anemia, and hypercholesterolemia.

Idiopathic Edema

Idiopathic edema is a clinical syndrome occurring most commonly among women. In many patients, it is associated with abdominal distension and diurnal variations in weight that may vary by several pounds from morning to evening. The most likely cause is increased capillary permeability; however, there may be some contribution from chronic stimulation of the renin-angiotensin-aldosterone system. This syndrome differs from the cyclic edema experienced by many women related to estrogen-induced sodium and water retention. In some cases, the use of diuretics can exacerbate the edema by causing mild hypovolemia and further renin stimulation.

Localized Edema

The differential diagnosis of localized edema includes obstructive processes causing limb edema and inflammatory processes causing increased capillary permeability and localized edema of a different nature. In most cases, this edema is nonpitting.

Obstructive processes causing limb edema can be either venous or lymphatic and include venous insufficiency due to deep venous thrombosis or more superficial thrombophlebitis, lymphadenopathy or pelvic masses inhibiting lower extremity venous return, congenital or primary lymphatic obstruction, and neoplasm with surgery- and radiation-associated inflammatory changes that impede lower extremity venous return. Infectious diseases such as lymphangitis and filariasis are also known to cause limb edema.

Other causes of localized edema that do not appear to involve an entire limb include burns, cellulitis, and angioedema. Inflammation due to infection or other tissue injury causes increased capillary permeability and interstitial edema. In such patients, the edema is usually nonpitting and the history and visible erythema suggest these diagnoses.

EVALUATION

The clinical evaluation of a patient with edema should begin with a careful history of the symptom. Particular attention should be paid to the onset, duration, and distribution of the edema. After excluding burns, cellulitis, and angioedema, most patients require further evaluation to differentiate generalized edema due to a systemic process from obstructive edema involving the lower extremities only and to identify a specific cause.

Frequently patients with generalized edema due to cardiac, hepatic, or renal disease have worse symptoms in the lower extremities; therefore, a standardized approach to all patients is appropriate. Additional history with particular attention to known diagnoses of CHF, cirrhosis, and renal insufficiency as well as a complete medication list should be obtained. All patients should undergo laboratory testing including a measurement of serum creatinine, liver function testing, and albumin. Urinalysis with screening for albuminuria is also recommended.

In many cases, the physical examination and review of initial laboratory testing will help to identify the cause of generalized edema. Physical findings of CHF and pulmonary edema on chest x-ray support cardiac causes. The serum albumin can be very helpful in differentiating cardiac causes of edema in which serum albumin is usually normal from hepatic or renal causes in which hypoalbuminemia is often present. Stigmata of chronic liver disease, coagulopathy, and the presence of abdominal ascites will make cirrhosis a likely diagnosis. Significant elevation of serum creatinine often points to chronic renal insufficiency. Hyperlipidemia and large proteinuria suggest nephrotic syndrome. Among patients with normal serum albumin, myxedema due to hypothyroidism should be excluded with thyroid-stimulating hormone testing. Discontinuation of calcium channel blockers, other vasodilators, and (when permissible) hormones and corticosteroids may help to establish these agents as the cause of edema. Finally, if patients have been using loop or thiazide diuretics for a long period of time to manage mild idiopathic edema, a trial period without therapy and with a low-sodium diet is appropriate.

When the major systemic causes of edema have been excluded, it is appropriate to evaluate for the presence of obstructive causes of lower extremity edema. Often the edema is nonpitting. Onset can be acute or chronic depending on the cause. Deep venous thrombosis is more likely when the edema is asymmetric and associated with lower extremity pain and erythema. Some patients may have identifiable risk factors for thrombosis. Venous Doppler ultrasonography is the preferred test for establishing this diagnosis. If pelvic lymphadenopathy or other mass is suspected, contrast-enhanced computed tomography scan of the pelvis is appropriate.

If there is suspicion that there is progression of lower extremity edema in patients who have an established diagnosis of venous or lymphatic obstruction, it may be necessary to repeat ultrasound or computed tomography scanning.

CHAPTER 13

Fever and Rash

Heather Toth

Fever is a common cause of physician visits. Fever and rash are important clinical findings for a clinician to consider when seeing patients in the primary care setting.

DIFFERENTIAL DIAGNOSIS

The differential diagnosis is extensive and includes infection, hypersensitivity disorders, malignancies, collagen vascular diseases, and others.

When encountering a patient with a fever and rash, a detailed history and physical examination are essential to lead the clinician to the appropriate diagnosis or the need for additional tests or studies. A thorough history, including questions such as "Who first noticed the rash?", "What did the rash initially look like?", and "Why do you think you have the fever and rash?" may give essential clues to the diagnosis. Other important history components to inquire about include any sick contacts, animal exposure, travel, and sexual history. Also, underlying medical illnesses should be elicited in the history, such as diabetes mellitus, alcoholism, drug abuse, or any chronic medical illness. A description of the rash itself can be helpful for the differential diagnosis. This should include a general description of the rash, such as maculopapular, vesicular, or petechial. For example, the varicella zoster virus ("chickenpox") classically presents with vesicles (see Color Plate 1). A hemorrhagic or petechial rash cautions the physician to the possibility of meningococcal disease, which is a medical emergency (see Color Plate 2).

The location and type of rash are also important diagnostic clues for the differential diagnosis of fever and rash (Table 13.1). Systemic lupus erythematous may present with a "malar rash" present over the nasal bridge and cheeks. Urticarial rashes may be caused by an allergy to a medication, chemical, or other exposure.

Infection

Viruses such as Ebstein-Barr virus (EBV), enterovirus, measles, and rubella typically cause a maculopapular rash. Ebstein-Barr virus is the virus responsible for mononucleosis. The clinical presentation includes malaise, fever, sore throat with lymphadenopathy, and possible splenomegaly. Measles is transmitted via respiratory droplets and causes a prodrome of fever, coryza (acute rhinitis), cough, and conjunctivitis. Koplik spots, which are tiny white spots inside of the cheeks, are pathognomonic for measles. Other viruses, such as varicella zoster (chickenpox) and herpes simplex virus may cause a vesicular rash (see Color Plate 3). Herpes zoster, the clinical reactivation of a prior varicella zoster infection, resembles herpes simplex in a dermatomal distribution (see Color Plate 4). Patients typically note a prodrome (early symptoms) of burning or pain prior to the appearance of the vesicular rash.

Bacterial infections such as meningococcemia (*Neisseria meningitidis*) may be characterized by a prodrome of fever, headache, malaise, and sore throat. On examination, the patient may have a petechial rash of the skin and mucous membranes. The rash first appears on the lower extremities, but quickly progresses. Gonococcemia is caused by the gram-negative bacteria *Neisseria gonorrhea*

TABLE 13.1 Differential diagnosis of fever and rash by description or location of the rash

Rash	Differential Diagnosis
Type	
Maculopapular	Viruses (Epstein-Barr virus, cytomegalovirus, enterovirus, human immunodeficiency virus, measles, rubella, parvovirus B19, human herpes virus 6) Bacteria (salmonella, secondary syphilis, mycoplasma)
Vesicular	Varicella zoster (see Color Plate 1) Herpes simplex and herpes zoster (see Color Plates 3 & 4)
Petechial/purpuric	Meningococcemia (*Neisseria meningitides*; see Color Plate 2) Gonococcemia (*Neisseria gonorrhea*) Rocky Mountain spotted fever (*Rickettsia rickettsii*) Endocarditis (*Streptococcus viridans*) Vasculitis (systemic lupus erythematosus, Henoch-Schönlein purpura)
Diffuse erythroderma	Toxic shock (secondary to Group A *Streptococcus* or *Staphylococcus aureus*) Scarlet fever (Group A *Streptococcus*)
Well-demarcated erythema	Cellulitis Erysipelas Necrotizing fasciitis
Target lesion (erythema chronicum migrans)	Lyme disease (see Color Plate 5)
Hemorrhagic ulcers with gangrenous centers (ecthyma gangrenosum)	*Pseudomonas aeruginosa*
Urticarial	Viruses (Epstein-Barr, hepatitis B) Mycoplasma Parasites Drug reaction (see Color Plate 6) Insect bites
Location	
Rash present on palms and soles	Coxsackie (see Color Plate 7) Syphilis (see Color Plate 8) Rocky Mountain spotted fever
Involvement of mucous membranes	Coxsackie A virus (vesicular pharyngitis) Measles (Koplik spots: white/bluish lesion noted on buccal mucosa near lower molars) Group A *Streptococcus* (palatal petechiae)

and presents with fever, arthralgias (typically large joint involvement), and a rash. It is a sexually transmitted infection with the highest incidence in young adults aged 15 to 28 years.

Another common etiology to keep in mind when evaluating a patient with a well-demarcated rash and fever is cellulitis. This is an acute infection typically caused by bacterial skin flora such as *Streptococcus* or *Staphylococcus*, sometimes noted after minor trauma to the skin. The involved area is erythematous, swollen, and warm. Erysipelas is a specific cutaneous inflammatory disease caused by beta-hemolytic streptococci and characterized by hot, red, well-demarcated, raised firm borders. Necrotizing fasciitis is the rapidly progressing necrosis of soft tissue and is a medical emergency requiring immediate surgical debridement and antibiotics.

Rickettsial illnesses such as Rocky Mountain spotted fever and Lyme disease may present with fever and a characteristic rash. Lyme disease is caused by the spirochete *Borrelia burgodorferi* and is transmitted via ixodid ticks. The rash typically begins as an erythematous lesion that expands with central clearing (erythema migrans, Color Plate 5). Arthralgias, myalgias, and headache may be noted. Most regions in the United States are now affected, but it is still most common in the mid-Atlantic, northeastern, and north central regions of the United States. Rocky Mountain spotted fever has a prodrome of fever, chills, headache, arthralgias, and myalgias, and a red macular rash appears first on the ankles and wrists and spreads toward the thorax. The rash may progress to petechial in appearance.

Parasitic infections may also cause a fever and rash, although uncommonly encountered in the United States. Some examples include leishmaniasis and trypanosomiasis. If a patient presents with a history of foreign travel, it is important to assess for type of travel, accommodations, and exposure.

Hypersensitivity Disorders

Hypersensitivity disorders are divided into four types, but all may have fever and skin manifestations. When obtaining the history, it is important to ask about current and prior exposure to the allergen(s). It sometimes may be difficult to elicit a specific etiology when the patient may have been exposed to multiple allergens. If the etiology is unclear, a logbook may be helpful to have the patient journal the exposures over time. Also, the physical examination at the time of allergen exposure is most useful to help classify the rash. The rash may be urticarial with or without angioedema or may be a diffuse classic "drug rash" (see Color Plate 6). Serum sickness (Type III hypersensitivity) is characterized by fever, dermatitis, and arthralgias. Drugs that have been implicated in the development of serum sickness–like reactions include procainamide, sulfonamides, and hydralazine. If the history and physical examination are consistent with anaphylaxis, pay close attention to the vital signs as hypotension/shock may occur from systemic vasodilation.

Malignancies and Collagen Vascular Diseases

Malignancies and collagen vascular diseases may also present with fever and rash. Patients with a malignancy may have nonspecific constitutional symptoms that indicate a systemic effect of the disease, which include fever, fatigue, weight loss, or night sweats. Lymphomas, leukemias, gastric carcinoma (associated with acanthosis nigricans [pigmented lesion]) may present with fever and rash.

Collagen vascular diseases or vasculitis may also present with constitutional symptoms that include fever and rash. Systemic lupus erythematosus (Chapter 48) can present with fever and discoid (raised patches with keratotic scaling), malar rash (facial erythema-sparing the nasolabial folds), or photosensitivity. Scleroderma may exhibit fever accompanied by skin induration, telangiectasias, and Raynaud's phenomena. Henoch-Schönlein purpura may show fever and purpuric lesions on the lower extremities, arthralgias, and abdominal pain.

Other Disorders

Other disorders present with constitutional symptoms such as fever and rash. Sarcoidosis (erythema nodosum, subcutaneous nodules, and lupus pernio; Chapter 44), inflammatory bowel disease (erythema nodosum, pyoderma gangrenosum; Chapter 76), Stills' disease or juvenile rheumatoid arthritis (evanescent rash), porphyria cutanea tarda (bullae on sun-exposed skin), and Whipple's disease (fever, steatorrhea, and hyperpigmentation) should also be included in the differential diagnosis of fever and rash.

EVALUATION

Evaluation including laboratory or radiological studies of a patient with fever and rash will depend greatly on the history and physical examination. Specific laboratory studies may not be necessary for illnesses such as varicella zoster virus or coxsackie when the history and physical examination obtained are classic for the disease. The presence of a petechial rash/purpura or fever of unknown origin suggest vasculitis. Further workup such as blood cultures, urine cultures, cerebral spinal fluid analysis, viral studies, and immunologic studies will depend upon the presenting history, physical examination, and differential diagnoses entertained.

CHAPTER 14

Fever and Fever of Unknown Origin

Jasna Jevtic

NORMAL BODY TEMPERATURES

Body temperature, normally set around 37°C (98.6°F), varies greatly. The hypothalamus is the thermoregulatory center maintaining the temperature of internal organs, great vessels, and aortic blood between 37°C and 38°C. Esophageal and tympanic membrane temperatures are closest to that of aortic blood, but rectal temperature is about 0.5°C higher, presumably due to higher metabolism. Oral and axillary temperatures are about 0.25°C and 1.0°C lower than core temperature, respectively. Skin temperature is even lower. Body temperature is lowest in the early morning and highest in the late afternoon, with the variation not usually exceeding ±0.6°C (1°F). Individuals maintain body temperature at slightly above or below the so-called normal of 37°C (98.6°F). However, temperature exceeding 37.8°C (100.2°F) is considered abnormal.

FEVER AND HYPERTHERMIA

Fever is a body temperature above that seen in normal diurnal variation and is sustained by normal thermoregulatory mechanisms. The primary initiating event is the release of endogenous pyrogens (i.e., interleukins 1 and 6, interferon, tumor necrosis factor), which cause fever and a number of other systemic changes collectively called acute phase responses. These involve alterations in leukocytes, liver protein synthesis, serum iron, hormone metabolism, and other phenomena. These changes and the behavioral and autonomic responses are outlined in Table 14.1.

Fever has some beneficial effects, such as enhanced stress response modulated by glucocorticoids; increased neutrophil counts, opsonins, and complement components; as well as enhanced T-lymphocyte activation and expansion of lymphocyte clones.

Although fever is a regulated response, hyperthermia is dysregulated and caused by a dysfunction of excessive heat production, decreased heat loss, and malfunction of the thermoregulatory center. Several causes of hyperthermia are listed in Table 14.2.

Heat stroke is usually precipitated by exercise in very hot climates. The onset is minutes to hours after exposure; the patient presents with severe hyperthermia (105°F), altered mental status, and tachycardia. Neuroleptic malignant syndrome (NMS) occurs hours to days after ingestion of neuroleptic drugs (haloperidol [Haldol] is one of the most common drugs implicated); its presentation includes hyperthermia, rigidity, altered mental status, and rhabdomyolysis.

FEVER OF UNKNOWN ORIGIN

While fever is a common sign of infection, sometimes the actual cause of the infection is difficult to identify. When this happens, the cause is often a transient viral illness. Occasionally, febrile states

TABLE 14.1 Systemic aspects of fever

Behavioral responses	Acute phase responses	Autonomic
Seek warmth	↑ White blood cell count	↓ Skin blood flow
Anorexia	Liver protein changes	↑ Pulse and blood pressure
Malaise	↓ Serum iron Altered hormone metabolism (glucocorticoids, aldosterone, vasopressin, growth hormone)	↓ Sweating

last longer and become difficult clinical problems. Fever of unknown origin (FUO) is defined as a prolonged febrile illness, lasting at least 3 weeks, with temperatures of at least 38.3°C (101°F), and no diagnosis after 1 week of evaluation in the inpatient setting or a similar intensive outpatient workup.

DIFFERENTIAL DIAGNOSIS

The differential diagnosis of FUO includes predominantly neoplastic disease (31%), infections (30%), collagen-vascular diseases (16%), and miscellaneous (3% to 10%), which all together can account for 80% to 90% of FUO. In 10% of cases, however, no diagnosis is made. Causes of FUO are listed in Table 14.3.

Neoplastic disease is a common cause of FUO. A number of primary or metastatic tumors cause fever, but some are more prone to do so than others. Occult lymphoma, particularly in the retroperitoneal area, may present with weight loss, anorexia, and fever, but usually without hepatosplenomegaly. Another common cause of FUO is renal cell carcinoma, which may be difficult to localize and diagnose because hematuria may be absent. Metastatic cancer to the liver is more common

TABLE 14.2 Causes of hyperthermia

Excessive heat production	Diminished heat loss	Hypothalamic dysfunction
Exertional hyperthermia	Heat stroke	Neuroleptic malignant syndrome
Status epilepticus	Neuroleptic malignant syndrome	Cerebrovascular accident
Thyrotoxicosis	Dehydration	Trauma
Pheochromocytoma	Autonomic dysfunction	Encephalitis
Malignant hyperthermia of anesthesia		
Neuroleptic malignant syndrome		

TABLE 14.3 Causes of fever of unknown origin

Common	Uncommon
Infections	**Collagen vascular diseases**
Pelvic abscess	Giant cell arteritis abscesses
Intra-abdominal	Periarteritis nodosa
Extrapulmonary tuberculosis	Adult Still's disease
Neoplastic diseases	Systemic lupus erythematosus
Renal cell carcinoma	Rheumatoid arthritis
Lymphoma	**Miscellaneous**
Metastatic cancer to liver	Familial Mediterranean fever
Miscellaneous	Hyperthyroidism
Drug fever	Pheochromocytoma
Alcoholic hepatitis	Subacute thyroiditis
Cirrhosis	Cyclic neutropenia
	Recurrent pulmonary embolism
	Factitious fever

than primary liver tumors, but both may cause FUO. Usually, these pose no diagnostic problems unless liver function abnormalities are absent. Other neoplasms causing FUO include leukemias, pancreatic carcinoma, atrial myxoma, and central nervous system tumors.

Although infections continue to cause a substantial proportion of FUO, the types of infections that cause FUO have changed over the years. For instance, bacterial endocarditis is currently a less common etiology of FUO, in part due to blood cultures becoming a common part of the evaluation of fever.

Common infectious causes today include intra-abdominal (i.e., hepatic, periappendiceal, pericolic, perinephric, splenic) and pelvic abscesses. Dental or brain abscesses are less common. Tuberculosis (Chapter 43) is another common cause of FUO, particularly when extrapulmonary sites (i.e., meningeal, miliary and renal) are involved. Less common infectious causes include enteric fever, human immunodeficiency virus (HIV) infection, osteomyelitis, toxoplasmosis, endocarditis due to fastidious or nonculturable organisms, relapsing fever, leptospirosis, malaria, fungal infections, and others.

Because of improved diagnostic techniques, certain collagen vascular disorders have become less common causes of FUO. For example, serologic testing has improved the detection of systemic lupus erythematosus and rheumatoid arthritis, reducing the likelihood of their presenting as an FUO. Both diseases, however, may still be rare causes of FUO. Many rheumatic and vasculitic diseases causing FUO lack specific diagnostic tests and thus require a diagnostic tissue biopsy. Examples include giant cell arteritis, periarteritis nodosa, and other vasculitides, such as Takayasu arteritis.

Drug fever tops the list of miscellaneous causes of FUO. Drugs usually cause fever by acting as a foreign antigen, sensitizing T cells, and leading to endogenous pyrogen release. Common offenders are antibiotics, particularly beta-lactams and sulfonamides, analgesics, diuretics, hypnotics, anticonvulsants, and antiarrhythmics. Intermittent eosinophilia and elevated liver enzyme levels may be seen. Some drugs (i.e., penicillin, isoniazid, salicylates, phenytoin, thiouracil, iodides, and methyldopa) are notable for causing fever without other clinical signs. Alcoholic and granulomatous hepatitis are liver diseases that cause FUO and can be confirmed by liver biopsy.

EVALUATION

FUO, as the name implies, is a diagnostic challenge even to an astute clinician. Close attention must be paid to the history. Recent abdominal or pelvic surgery (abscess), exposure to tuberculosis, history of a heart murmur (risk factor for endocarditis), or history of high-risk behavior (unsuspected HIV infection) are examples of historical clues that require further exploration. In addition to an examination of specific complaints, contacts, or exposures, the patient's medications should be checked. Drug fever may follow even years of use, so that the diagnosis is usually made by exclusion (i.e., withdrawing the drug and observing).

A detailed physical examination should follow, especially pursuing clues from the history. Of particular importance are the cardiac, abdominal, lymph node, and musculoskeletal examinations. Useful findings are heart murmur (suggests endocarditis or atrial myxoma), hepatomegaly, lymphadenopathy (suggests infection or lymphoma), and spinal tenderness (suggests vertebral osteomyelitis or epidural abscess).

Routine laboratory studies, such as a complete blood count, can give some clues. For instance, leukopenia might suggest lymphoma; eosinophilia may be consistent with lymphoma or drug fever; and a lymphocytosis might suggest infectious mononucleosis (especially if the peripheral smear shows atypical lymphocytes). Noninvasive imaging tests for FUO evaluation include ultrasound, computed tomography (CT), magnetic resonance imaging (MRI), and radionuclide scans. Abdominal or pelvic abscesses and retroperitoneal lymphoma are readily detected by CT or MRI.

In certain settings, invasive tests are required to make a specific diagnosis. Physical findings such as tenderness over the temporal arteries in the right clinical setting might suggest giant cell arteritis, but temporal artery biopsy is required for definitive diagnosis. In another setting, the finding of a liver mass on CT scan might indicate the need for a biopsy to direct definitive therapy.

CHAPTER 15

Headache

Raj Bhargava

Headaches remain one of the most common and frustrating symptoms. It occurs at any age and is more common in women. Any first and persistent headache after the fifth decade generally requires full workup. A recent survey revealed that 28 million people suffer from migraines alone, half of them undiagnosed. Headaches account for 3% of office visits to primary care offices. The most common headaches are migraines, tension headaches, and cluster headaches. Less than 5% of headaches are secondary to significant underlying diseases.

DIFFERENTIAL DIAGNOSIS

Headaches can be classified into two main categories: primary and secondary (Table 15.1). Secondary headaches are headaches that may be caused by specific underlying conditions. Thus, it is important to investigate for secondary origins of headaches when formulating a differential diagnosis. A thorough history combined with a careful general and neurologic physical examination are the most useful tools when diagnosing a headache. Historical and physical examination findings suggesting a serious underlying cause of headache should be sought.

A complete physical examination should focus on blood pressure, bruits in head/neck, palpation of the head and neck for tenderness over temporal arteries, and nuchal rigidity. The fundus should be examined for papilledema, which is a sign of increased intracranial pressure. The examination should also include a complete neurological assessment including gait and balance.

Common Primary Headache Syndromes

Common primary headache syndromes are detailed in Tables 15.2 and 15.3.

MIGRAINE HEADACHES

Migraine headaches are more common in women with onset at a young age and strong family history. Migraines without aura are classified as common migraines; those with a preceding aura are called neurologic migraine. They typically present with unilateral or bilateral throbbing headache with a recurrent pattern. Onset is usually gradual with moderate to severe intensity, lasting for several hours. Frequently, migraines are preceded by auras consisting of scotomata, flashing lights, and anxiety, and are associated with nausea/vomiting, photophobia, and phonophobia.

TENSION HEADACHES

Tension headaches have variable predisposing factors. They are usually bilateral and tend to wax and wane but have characteristic pressure/tightening in forehead, temporal, or nuchal areas. They can last for days or even weeks, but patients are usually able to remain active. Typically, these are not accompanied by auras or other neurological symptoms. They may be associated with depression or anxiety disorders.

TABLE 15.1 Classification of headache

Primary headaches: benign/recurrent without underlying pathology
Migraine Tension headache Cluster headache Others: medication overuse headache (acetaminophen, aspirin, butalbital-caffeine, opioids); temporomandibular joint dysfunction syndrome
Secondary headaches: have serious underlying pathology
Subarachnoid hemorrhage Intracranial bleed Subdural hematoma Cerebral venous thrombosis Stroke Brain tumors Brain abscess Meningitis/encephalitis Temporal arteritis/giant cell arteritis Pseudotumor cerebri (papilledema, normal neural imaging, elevated cerebrospinal fluid pressure) Hypertensive crisis (hypertensive encephalopathy) Carotid or vertebral artery dissection Narrow angle glaucoma

TABLE 15.2 Risk factors and triggers for primary headaches

Cluster headache
Genetic predisposition Alcohol
Migraine headache
Caffeine intake/withdrawal Alcohol Oral contraceptives Cold stimulus Tension Foods (cheese, red wine) Bright lights
Tension headache
Psychological: depression, anxiety, phobia, somatization, conversion disorders, Fatigue Tension

TABLE 15.3 Key features of three common primary headache syndromes

Feature	Migraine headache	Tension headache	Cluster headache
Predisposing factors	Female:male, 3:1 Peak age, 25 to 55 years Strong family history	More common in female adults	Male:female, 6:1 Peak age, 20s and 30s Genetic predisposition
Characterization	60% unilateral; 40% bilateral Stable, recurrent pattern, self-limiting gradual onset, with crescendo buildup, pulsating (75%), throbbing, moderate to severe intensity aggravated by physical activity Duration, 4 to 72 hours	Bilateral Waxes and wanes, pressure/tightening, can be infrequent, frequent, or chronic; patient remains active for the most part Variable duration, less than 15 days per month	Always unilateral around eye/temple Begins quickly, peaks in minutes, deep/continuous, explosive in quality, 1 to 8 episodes daily, episodic/circadian pattern Duration 15 to 180 minutes; clusters may last weeks to months
Associated symptoms	Nausea/vomiting Photophobia/phonophobia	Fatigue, symptoms of depression or anxiety	Ipsilateral autonomic features, stuffy nose, Horner's syndrome, rhinorrhea, sweating, lacrimation, conjunctival congestion, eyelid edema

CLUSTER HEADACHES

These headaches are more common in males, with a peak incidence in the 20s and 30s. There is a genetic predisposition. They have a rapid onset usually at night, have no warning signs, and occur several times a day, lasting 15 minutes to 3 hours per episode. The pain is unilateral, continuous, and excruciating. Clusters may last weeks or even months followed by a remission period ranging from 6 months to a year. They are usually associated with ipsilateral autonomic features like nasal congestion, Horner's syndrome, sweating, lacrimation, and conjunctival congestion.

Secondary Headache Syndromes

SUBARACHNOID HEMORRHAGE

The main clinical characteristic of this headache is the sudden onset of a stabbing pain. It is often associated with a decreased level of consciousness rather than focal neurological signs. This type of headache is often accompanied by signs of meningeal irritation (neck stiffness and photophobia). It usually results from blood in the subarachnoid space due to leaking of an aneurysm or arteriovenous malformations. Prompt intervention is required as this is a medical emergency (Chapter 108).

HEADACHE DUE TO SPACE-OCCUPYING LESIONS

This type of headache is due to tumor, abscess, or intracranial hemorrhage that results in increased intracranial pressure. Suggestive symptoms include headache upon waking in the morning, vomiting, seizures, progressive focal motor or sensory symptoms and signs, visual or hearing loss, diplopia, or gait abnormalities. Pituitary adenomas may be associated with hyper- or hyposecretion of hormones.

HEADACHE DUE TO INFECTION

Headaches can be caused by intracranial infections, meningitis, encephalitis, or human immunodeficiency virus infection. These headaches are usually associated with fever along with nuchal rigidity, altered mental status, photophobia, seizures, behavioral changes, and focal motor abnormalities (Chapter 58).

HEADACHES DUE TO STROKE

These headaches are usually present in the setting of focal neurological deficits due to the underlying vascular process resulting in cerebral edema, intracranial hypertension, and vasospasm. They are often associated with fluctuating neurological deficits.

HEADACHES DUE TO TEMPORAL/GIANT CELL ARTERITIS

These headaches commonly affect women over the age of 50 years, are frequently temporal in location, and are often associated with visual changes/blindness, tenderness over the temporal area/temporal artery and are often associated with very high sedimentation rate. There is an association between temporal arteritis and polymyalgia rheumatica.

EVALUATION

Evaluation of headache involves a comprehensive history to determine risk factors, triggers, location, and frequency, which will determine the headache type. Imaging of the brain is usually unnecessary in the vast majority, but critical when underlying secondary causes are suspected due to focal features of the headache or findings on examination.

The general approach in evaluating a headache patient involves (i) exclusion of signs and symptoms suggestive of underlying systemic organic disease; (ii) assessing severity and type of primary

TABLE 15.4 Clinical features and causes of headaches

Clinical feature	Diseases
History	
Sudden onset	Subarachnoid hemorrhage Venous sinus thrombosis Hypertensive emergencies
"Worst headache ever"	Subarachnoid hemorrhage
Presence of concomitant infection	Meningitis Acute sinusitis Brain abscess Systemic infection
Altered mental status	Meningitis/encephalitis Subarachnoid hemorrhage
Headache with exertion, sexual activity, cough, or valsava	Intracranial mass lesion
Immunocompromised host	Toxoplasmosis Brain abscess Meningitis
New headache in age >50 years	Intracranial mass lesion Temporal arteritis
Impaired vision	Narrow angle glaucoma Pseudotumor cerebri Temporal arteritis
Trauma	Hydrocephalus Subdural hematoma
Physical examination	
Focal neurologic findings (asymmetric pupils, pronator drift, extensoplantar response [Babinski])	Intracranial hemorrhage Space-occupying lesion Tumor, abscess, fungal mass Intraparenchymal hemorrhage Carotid or vertebral artery dissection
Meningeal signs	Meningitis/encephalitis
Papilledema	Intracranial mass lesion Hypertensive encephalopathy Pseudotumor cerebri Subdural hematoma Subarachnoid hemorrhage

headache by using history as primary diagnostic tool; (iii) assessing the necessity for imaging/lumbar puncture; (iv) and assessing for the need to consult a neurologist.

Symptoms of serious underlying pathology (secondary headaches) include sudden onset of severe new headache after the age of 40 years, a history of altered level of consciousness, progressive worsening of neurological status, occipital-nuchal radiation, prior/coexistent infectious illness, onset with exertion, and immune deficiency.

Physical findings suggestive of underlying pathology include fever, toxic appearance, nuchal rigidity, presence of papilledema, localizing/focal neurological deficits, decreased level of consciousness (drowsy/confused/memory loss), chronic myalgia, arthralgia, malaise, progressive loss of vision, weakness/loss of balance/coordination, and tender/pulsatile cranial arteries (see Table 15.4).

Imaging studies of the brain are indicated in the presence of unexplained underlying disease and unexplained abnormal neurological examination. They are also indicated for new onset of headache after age of 40 years, presence of orbital bruit, or headache triggered by cough, exertion, or sexual activity. Imaging for primary headaches is usually not necessary unless they present with atypical features or there has been a significant change in the pattern, frequency or severity of previous headaches. Usually a computed tomography scan is adequate; however, magnetic resonance imaging or angiography studies are preferred if vascular or posterior fossa lesions are suspected. Blood tests are often not helpful. Erythrocyte sedimentation rate (ESR) can be useful when temporal arteritis is suspected; ESR >60 mm/hour is an indication for further workup for cerebral vasculitis.

Lumbar puncture is indicated and is diagnostic when central nervous system infection is suspected. It is also indicated in a small number of patients with suspected subarachnoid hemorrhage when a computed tomography scan of the head is negative and clinical suspicion remains high. It always important to exclude the presence of increased intracranial pressure (no papilledema, normal is head computed tomography scan) to prevent cerebral herniation prior to performing a lumbar puncture.

CHAPTER 16

Heart Sounds and Murmurs

Geoffrey C. Lamb and Dario Torre

Auscultation of heart sounds is an important part of the internist's diagnostic armamentarium. Careful listening with the diaphragm and bell in an organized fashion can reveal useful clues to the nature of myocardial or valvular dysfunction. Heart sounds are generated by the opening and closing of the heart valves, turbulence in blood flow, and vibrations in the support structures of the heart.

DIFFERENTIAL DIAGNOSIS

First Heart Sound (S_1)

The first heart sound, S_1, signals the beginning of ventricular systole and is generated by mitral and tricuspid valve closure. It is loudest over the apex and is heard best by using the diaphragm of the stethoscope because its pitch, although relatively high, is lower than S_2.

The intensity of S_1 is determined primarily by valve mobility, force of ventricular contraction, and most importantly, the velocity of valve closure (Table 16.1).

S_1 is louder in mitral stenosis, a short PR interval, and tachycardia. S_1 is softer when there is a long PR interval or with acute aortic regurgitation. S_1 may vary in intensity from beat to beat in atrial fibrillation, reflecting variable contractility.

Second Heart Sound (S_2)

Evaluation of S_2 is a key component of the cardiac physical examination. S_2 is best heard at the left upper sternal border (over the base of the heart). The closure of the aortic (A_2) and pulmonic (P_2) valves at end-systole generates S_2. Abnormalities of S_2 relate primarily to alterations in intensity or timing.

A_2 is the louder component and is audible at all locations on the chest wall. In normal subjects, P_2 is heard only at the upper left sternal border and is always less audible than A_2 at this location. An audible P_2 at the apex is an abnormal finding and strongly suggests pulmonary hypertension.

The timing, or splitting, of S_2 varies with the phases of respiration (Fig. 16.1). Normally, the split widens during inspiration and narrows during expiration. Wide splitting of S_2 during expiration with further widening during inspiration (i.e., a widely split S_2 having normal respiratory variation) occurs when P_2 is delayed (e.g., right bundle branch block) or with early A_2 (e.g., mitral regurgitation).

Fixed splitting of S_2 occurs when the right ventricle (RV) cannot augment its stroke volume (e.g., in right heart failure) or when respiration-induced changes in filling, and hence stroke volumes, are similar in both ventricles (e.g., in atrial septal defect).

Paradoxical splitting of S_2 occurs typically in conditions that delay the onset of left ventricle (LV) depolarization and thus LV ejection (e.g., in left bundle branch block) or those that delay aortic valve closure (e.g., in severe aortic stenosis).

In paradoxical splitting of S_2, A_2 follows P_2 during expiration and gets closer to P_2 during inspiration. Normally the interval from A_2 to P_2 would lengthen during inspiration. In paradoxical splitting, the interval shortens during inspiration; hence the name.

TABLE 16.1 Factors affecting intensity of first and second heart sounds

	S_1	S_2	
		A_2	P_2
Increased	Short PR interval (160 ms) Mitral stenosis Hyperdynamic states Tachycardia	Systemic HTN Hyperdynamic states Aortic dilation	Pulmonary HTN Atrial septal defect
Decreased	Long PR interval (>200 ms) Poor LV systolic function LBBB	Calcific aortic stenosis Aortic regurgitation	Pulmonic stenosis

A_2, aortic component of second heart sound; HTN, hypertension; LBBB, left bundle branch block; P_2, pulmonic component of second heart sound; LV, left ventricle.

Diastolic Sounds

A ventricular gallop (S_3) sound occurs in early diastole; it corresponds to the end of the rapid filling phase in the LV. It is a low-frequency sound, best heard with the bell of the stethoscope lightly applied to the apex (LV S_3) or left lower sternal border (RV S_3) best heard in the left lateral decubitus position.

The S_3 is caused by interplay between ventricular filling and ventricular compliance. An S_3 will be intensified by maneuvers that enhance ventricular filling and lessened by maneuvers that diminish venous return. A nonphysiologic S_3 is associated with abnormally high LV filling pressures, low cardiac output, and a dilated, poorly contractile LV (e.g., congestive heart failure) (Table 16.2).

A pericardial knock, a higher-pitched diastolic sound, occurs earlier (closer to A_2) than the usual S_3 and is heard in patients with constrictive pericarditis.

Atrial gallop (S_4) is a dull, low-frequency sound that precedes S_1 and is best heard over apex with the bell of the stethoscope in the left lateral position. The S_4 is attributed to forceful atrial contraction to fill a noncompliant or stiff ventricle. An S_4, although abnormal, is quite common in older adults. The S_4 disappears in atrial fibrillation (Table 16.2).

Mitral opening snap (OS) is a sharp, high-frequency sound heard best over the left lower sternal border in patients with mitral valve stenosis. It is attributed to the sudden arrest of a rapidly opening mitral valve that is stenotic but pliable.

Systolic Sounds

Ejection click (EC) is a sharp, high-frequency sound audible immediately after S_1 over the entire precordium and varies little with respiration. They occur in aortic and pulmonary valvular stenoses.

Nonejection clicks are associated with mitral valve prolapse. They are high-frequency sharp clicks occurring over the apex or left lower sternal border. These may occur as isolated findings or be followed by late systolic murmurs. Maneuvers such as squatting and gripping one's hand move a midsystolic click later toward S_2, whereas standing and performing the Valsalva maneuver moves the click earlier toward S_1.

Heart Murmurs

A prolonged series of audible vibrations constitute a heart murmur. Heart murmurs are traditionally classified as systolic, diastolic, or continuous (Fig. 16.2; Tables 16.3 and 16.4). During auscultation of a murmur, its timing in the cardiac cycle in relation to S_1 and S_2, intensity, quality (e.g., blowing, harsh, rumbling), duration, and radiation (e.g., to the neck, axilla, or back) should be defined.

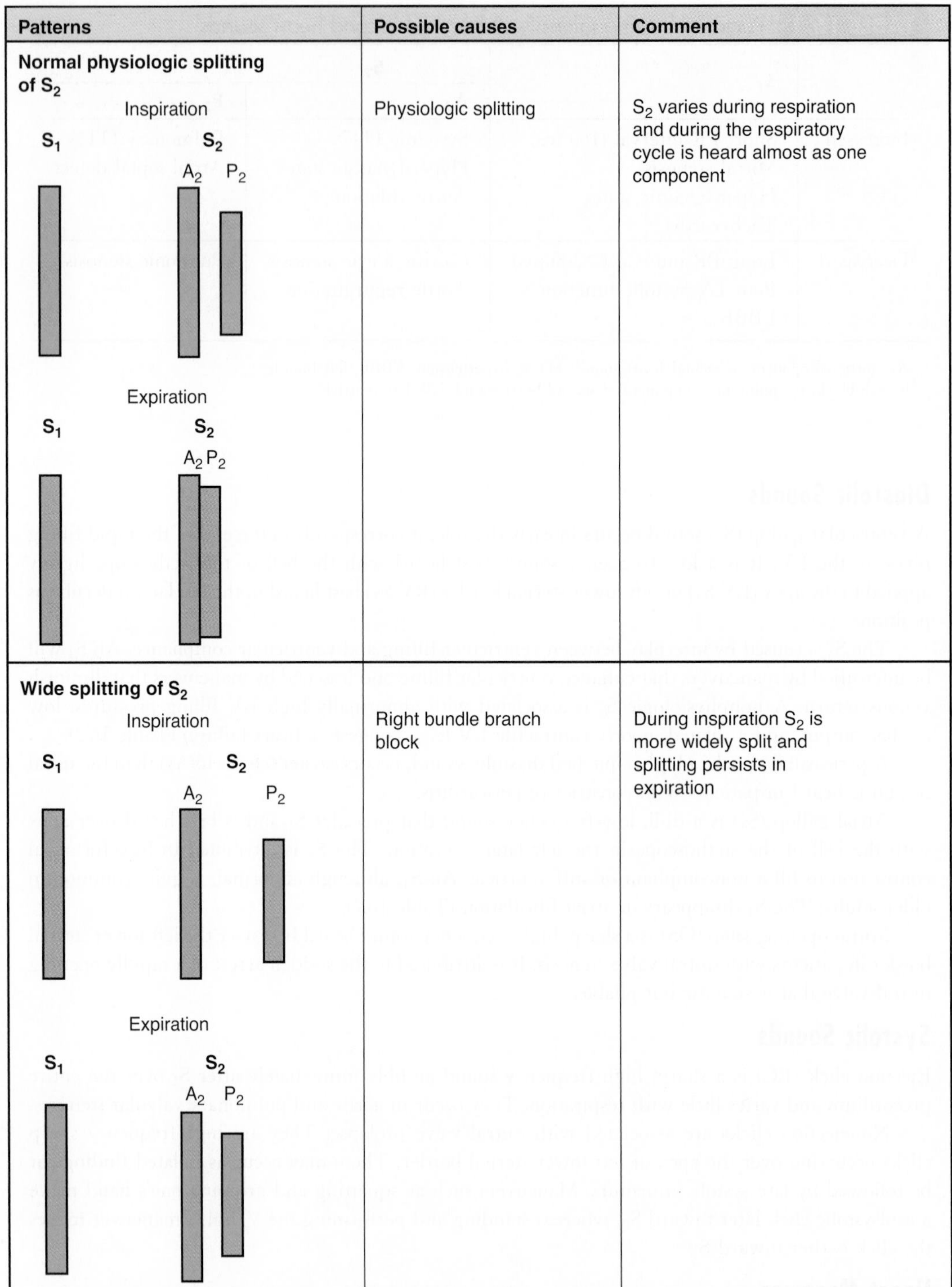

Patterns	Possible causes	Comment
Normal physiologic splitting of S_2 Inspiration: S_1 S_2 (A_2 P_2) Expiration: S_1 S_2 (A_2 P_2)	Physiologic splitting	S_2 varies during respiration and during the respiratory cycle is heard almost as one component
Wide splitting of S_2 Inspiration: S_1 S_2 (A_2 P_2) Expiration: S_1 S_2 (A_2 P_2)	Right bundle branch block	During inspiration S_2 is more widely split and splitting persists in expiration

Figure 16.1 • Splitting patterns of the second heart sound. *(continued)*

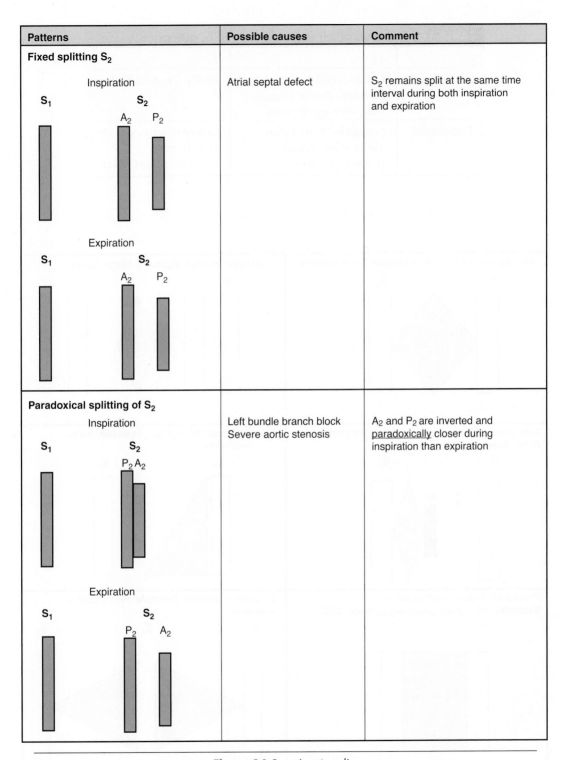

Patterns	Possible causes	Comment
Fixed splitting S_2 Inspiration: S_1, S_2 (A_2, P_2) Expiration: S_1, S_2 (A_2, P_2) 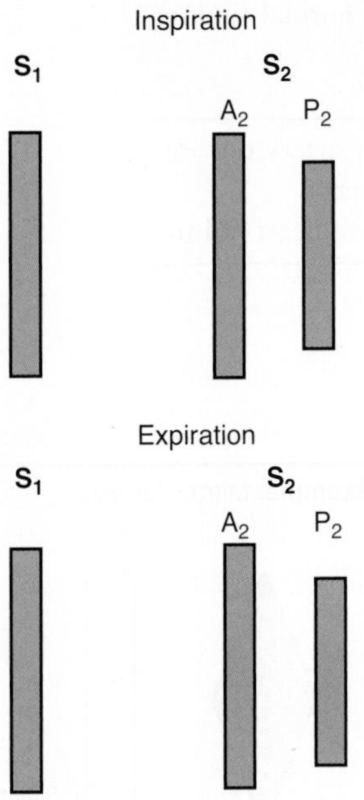	Atrial septal defect	S_2 remains split at the same time interval during both inspiration and expiration
Paradoxical splitting of S_2 Inspiration: S_1, S_2 (P_2 A_2) Expiration: S_1, S_2 (P_2, A_2) 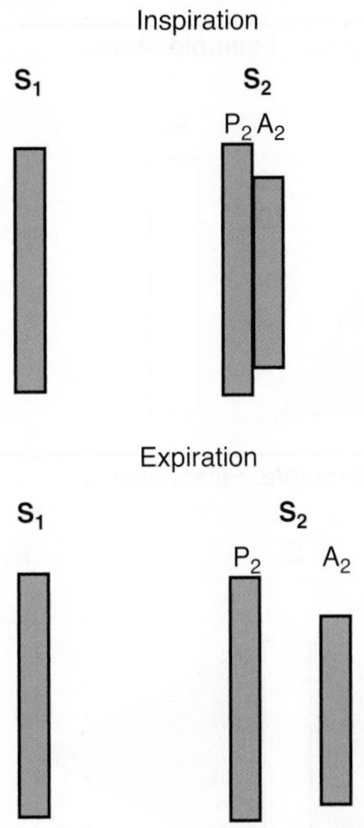	Left bundle branch block Severe aortic stenosis	A_2 and P_2 are inverted and paradoxically closer during inspiration than expiration

Figure 16.1 • *(continued)*

TABLE 16.2 Causes of left ventricular S_3 and S_4 gallops

	S_3	S_4
Physiological	Children and young adults Common during pregnancy Rare after age 40 years	Rarely a normal finding
Pathological	Congestive heart failure Mitral regurgitation Aortic regurgitation	Coronary artery disease Hypertension Congestive heart failure

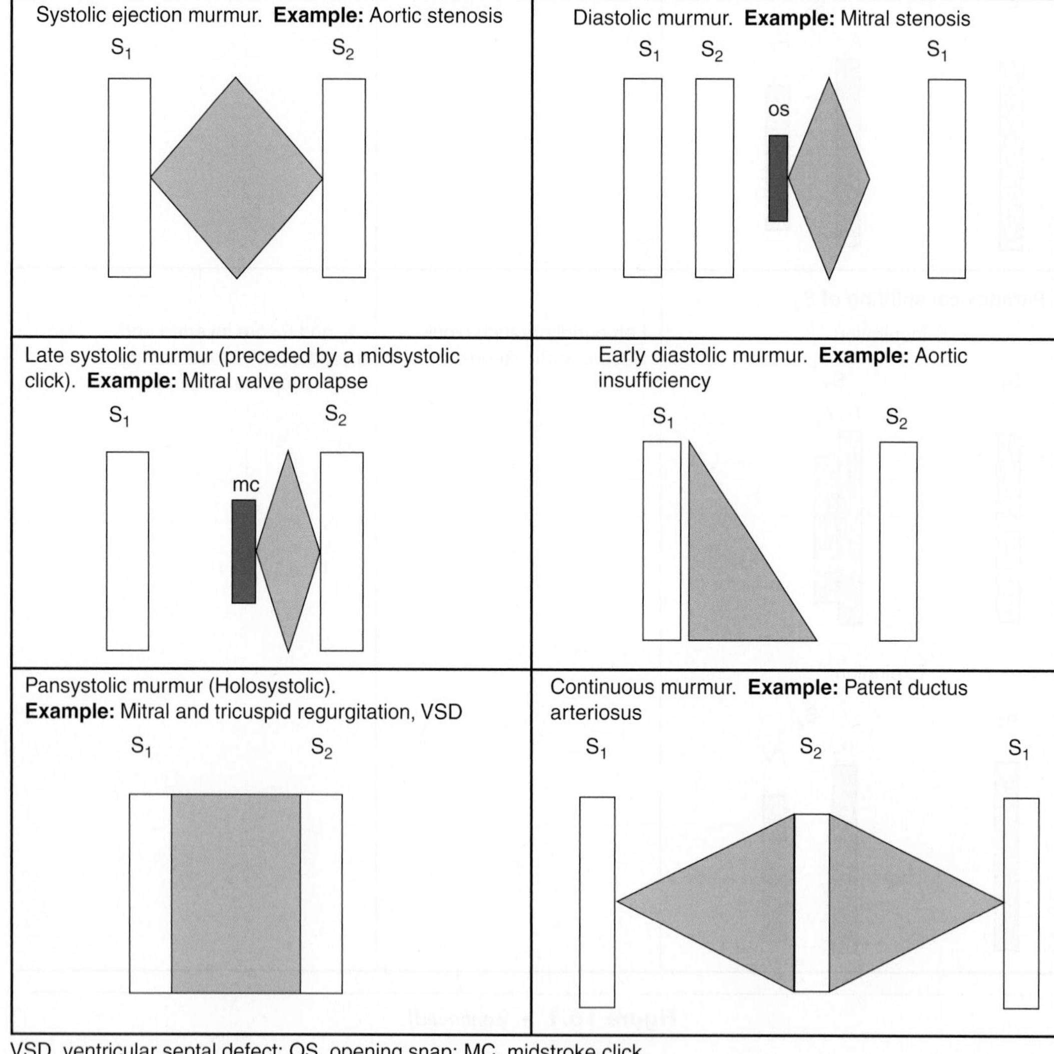

VSD, ventricular septal defect; OS, opening snap; MC, midstroke click.

Figure 16.2 • Heart murmurs and related disease.

TABLE 16.3 Overview of murmurs and their characteristics

Timing	Example	Heard best	Radiation	Bedside maneuvers	Added sounds
Systolic					
Pansystolic	Mitral regurgitation	Apex	Axilla or back	↑ Handgrip squatting	S_3 or S_4
	VSD	LLSB		Handgrip ↑ Squatting	Thrill
	Tricuspid regurgitation	LLSB	Neck	↑ With inspiration	
Midsystolic	Aortic stenosis	Second IS		↓ With standing	S_4
	HCM	Apex, LLSB		↑ Valsalva, standing	S_4
Late systolic	Mitral valve prolapse	Apex, LLSB		Occurs earlier with Valsalva and standing	Midsystolic click
Diastolic					
Early diastolic	Aortic insufficiency	LSB, third IS		Best heard with patient sitting, leaning forward, in forced expiration	S_3
Middiastolic rumble (low pitched)	Mitral stenosis	Apex, with the bell		Best heard with patient in LLD position	Opening snap (best heard with the diaphragm)
Continuous					
Systolic-diastolic	PDA	Left first and second IS LSB			Thrill

HCM, Hypertrophic cardiomyopathy; IS, intercostal space; LLD, left lateral decubitus; LLSB, left lower sternal border; LSB, left stemal border; PDA, patent doctus arteriosus; VSD, Ventricular septal defect.

TABLE 16.4 Classification, description, and causes of heart murmurs

Innocent murmurs	Systolic ejection murmur (not associated with any other abnormal cardiovascular findings). Caused by vibrations and turbulant blood flow across vessels or valves.
Systolic murmurs	**Systolic ejection murmurs (midsystolic; crescendo-decrescendo)** Aortic stenosis Pulmonic stenosis Malformed but nonstenotic aortic valve (aortic sclerosis) **Pansystolic murmurs** Mitral and tricuspid regurgitation Mitral valve prolapse (late systolic) Ventricular septal defect
Diastolic murmurs	**Early** (onset with A_2 or P_2; decrescendo; high-pitched) Aortic regurgitation **Middiastolic** (begin after S_2; low-pitched rumble) Mitral stenosis **Continuous** (systolic/early diastolic; peak late systole) Patent ductus arteriosus

Murmur intensity is described by a grading system (I through VI) (Table 16.5). Most innocent murmurs are grades I or II. With a grade III murmur, one should initiate a search for pathology. Although some systolic murmurs may be innocent, all diastolic and continuous murmurs are abnormal and pathological.

SYSTOLIC MURMURS

Systolic murmurs are categorized according to their duration and relationship to S_1 and S_2. The most important point to ascertain is whether the systolic murmur extends to S_2 (Fig. 16.2).

Ejection murmurs usually are crescendo-decrescendo in shape and end prior to S_2. Regurgitant or pansystolic murmurs are usually of more uniform intensity and extend to or even through S_2.

A midsystolic ejection murmur begins at the time of semilunar valve opening, following S_1. These murmurs are classically diamond-shaped (crescendo-decrescendo) and end before S2. The

TABLE 16.5 Grading system for murmur intensity

Grade	Description
I/VI	Very faint; barely audible
II/VI	Soft but readily audible
III/VI	Moderately loud; no palpable thrill
IV/VI	Very loud; palpable thrill present
V/VI	Louder; palpable thrill present; still requires a stethoscope on the chest to be heard
VI/VI	Audible with stethoscope close to, but not touching, chest; thrill present

most common type of midsystolic ejection murmur is the flow murmur, which arises owing to the normal turbulence of aortic blood flow during systolic ejection.

The classic pathologic midsystolic ejection murmur (Fig. 16.2) is aortic stenosis. Regurgitant or pansystolic murmurs begin with S_1 and extend to S_2. The resulting murmur is classically high frequency, blowing in quality (not harsh), and relatively uniform in intensity. All pansystolic murmurs are pathologic. The classic pathologic pansystolic murmur example is mitral regurgitation.

Late systolic murmurs occur in the latter part of systole, well after S_1 and end in or after A_2. The classic pathologic late systolic murmur example is that of mitral valve prolapse (a midsystolic click may precede the murmur). All late systolic murmurs are pathologic.

DIASTOLIC MURMURS

Early diastolic regurgitant murmurs are heard with aortic and pulmonic regurgitation (Table 16.5). These murmurs are classically decrescendo because the regurgitant flow between the aorta and left ventricle (or pulmonary artery and right ventricle) decreases throughout diastole. The murmur of aortic regurgitation can be easily missed on auscultation. It is best heard with the patient sitting up and leaning forward, with breath held in expiration.

Middiastolic murmurs are caused by increased diastolic flow across mitral and tricuspid valves. Classically, the murmur of mitral stenosis (Chapter 30) follows the opening snap of the mitral valve and then diminishes in intensity, only to increase again at the end of diastole (presystolic accentuation if patient is in sinus rhythm). These murmurs are of low frequency and are heard best with the bell of the stethoscope with the patient in the left lateral decubitus position.

CONTINUOUS MURMURS

Continuous murmurs occur when a large and persistent pressure difference throughout the cardiac cycle exists. This may occur between two communicating chambers or vessels with no intervening valve or across a severely stenosed segment of an artery. The classic example of a continuous murmur is that of patent ductus arteriosus. It begins in systole and continues without interruption throughout diastole, with a peak at S2.

Pericardial Friction Rub

A pericardial friction rub is a scratching sound heard over the precordium in acute pericarditis. Faint rubs are best heard with the patient sitting up and leaning forward; they may occur intermittently. Friction rubs may be triphasic with systolic, diastolic, and presystolic components. The systolic component is loudest and virtually always present. All three components are present in only about 50% of cases (Chapter 31).

EVALUATION

Physical Maneuvers

Certain physical maneuvers can profoundly affect murmur intensity by acutely changing loading conditions (Table 16.4). These maneuvers can augment the intensity of soft murmurs or gallops and aid in the differential diagnosis of various murmurs.

Diagnostic Tests

If the diagnosis is uncertain following physical examination or if a lesion is suspected that requires more definitive evaluation (Chapters 29, 30, and 31), further testing is indicated. An electrocardiogram may be useful to assess chamber size and provide useful diagnostic clues. A transthoracic echocardiogram is typically the test of choice. It can characterize ventricular motion and size, valvular characteristics and many pericardial disorders. Cardiac catheterization is indicated if the need for surgery is contemplated or if other tests are not definitive in an ill patient.

CHAPTER 17

Hematuria

Avery Hayes

Hematuria is generally defined as three or more red blood cells (RBCs) per high-power field on microscopic evaluation. The overall prevalence of asymptomatic microscopic hematuria varies from 0.19% to 21%, depending on the age of the population examined. Blood in the urine can originate anywhere along the urinary tract and, whether gross or microscopic, may be a sign of serious disease. Gross hematuria typically causes the patient to seek prompt medical attention, whereas microscopic hematuria is often discovered incidentally on urinalysis.

DIFFERENTIAL DIAGNOSIS

Causes of hematuria can be classified as glomerular (Chapter 81), which usually causes microscopic hematuria, or nonglomerular, which usually causes gross or macroscopic hematuria.

Glomerular hematuria may result from primary renal disease or be related to a systemic illness (Table 17.1). Glomerular bleeding may present with asymptomatic microscopic or macroscopic (i.e., gross) hematuria. Findings in support of glomerular bleeding include the presence of red-cell casts, dysmorphic red blood cells (characterized by an irregular outer cell membrane), or acanthocytes (ring-formed erythrocytes with the membrane protrusions attached). Associated hypertension, proteinuria, or elevated serum creatinine may also indicate a glomerular source.

Nonglomerular hematuria (Table 17.2) can be differentiated in renal and extrarenal sources. Renal cell carcinoma presents with painless hematuria in 40% to 50% of cases.

Renal cell cancer accounts for 2% of all cancers. It occurs more frequently in men, with peak incidence in the seventh and eighth decades of life. Higher rates occur in North Americans and Scandinavians. Cigarette smoking doubles the risk. Obesity is also a risk factor, particularly in women. The most common presentations of renal cell cancer are painless hematuria (50% to 60% of patients), abdominal pain (40%), and a palpable mass in the flank or abdomen (30% to 40%). This classic triad only occurs in about 10% of patients. However, gross painless hematuria should alert one to consider renal cell carcinoma. Other nonspecific signs include fever, night sweats, weight loss, and malaise.

Von Hippel-Lindau disease is a familial multiple cancer syndrome where there is a predisposition to a variety of neoplasms including renal cell cancer, renal cysts, retinal hemangiomas, hemangioblastomas of the cerebellum and spinal cord, pheochromocytoma, and pancreatic carcinomas and cysts.

Bladder cancer is the fourth most commonly diagnosed malignancy in the United States. Risk factors include advanced age, cigarette smoking (three- to fivefold increased risk), heavy phenacetin use, previous treatment with cyclophosphamide, and occupational exposure to arylamines, which are chemicals used in leather, dye, and rubber manufacturing. Hematuria is the presenting symptom in up to 85% of patients with bladder cancer and can manifest as microscopic or macroscopic hematuria, which may be intermittent in nature. Patients may experience urinary frequency or urgency. Hepatomegaly or supraclavicular adenopathy may be present with metastatic disease. Lymphedema of the lower extremities may occur as a result of locally advanced tumors or spread to pelvic lymph nodes.

TABLE 17.1 Glomerular causes of hematuria

Primary glomerulonephritis	Secondary glomerulonephritis
Immunoglobulin A nephropathy Hereditary nephritis (Alport's syndrome)	Systemic lupus erythematosus Systemic infections (poststreptococcal, bacterial endocarditis, or other bacteria, viral or protozoal infections)
Membranoproliferative	Systemic vasculitis Wegener's granulomatosis Cryoglobulinemia Churg-Strauss syndrome Henoch-Schönlein purpura Polyarteritis nodosa Hypersensitivity vasculitis
Rapidly progressing glomerulonephritis Goodpasture antiglomerular basement membrane disease Focal glomerulosclerosis	Hemolytic-uremic syndrome Thrombotic thrombocytopenic purpura

TABLE 17.2 Nonglomerular causes of hematuria

Renal	Extrarenal
Acute tubular necrosis	Nephrolithiasis
Polycystic kidney disease	Lower urinary tract infections (cystitis, prostatitis, epididymitis, and urethritis)
Solitary renal cyst	Benign prostatic hypertrophy
Infection (pyelonephritis, tuberculosis)	Bladder cancer
Interstitial nephritis	Prostate cancer
Renal cell cancer	Urethral stricture
Vascular disease	Inflammation: drug or radiation induced
Arteriovenous malformations	Metabolic conditions: hypercalciuria, hyperuricuria
Malignant hypertension	
Renal artery or vein thrombosis	
Sickle cell disease	Vigorous exercise Sexual intercourse Menstrual contamination Mild trauma Indwelling catheters

Patients with nephrolithiasis (Chapter 85) may present with acute colicky, severe low back or flank pain radiating to the inguinal region, associated with microscopic or macroscopic hematuria.

Infections anywhere along the urinary tract may cause hematuria. Pyelonephritis may present with fever, chills, or flank pain. Physical examination may reveal costovertebral angle tenderness.

Cystitis and prostatitis may present with dysuria, increased urinary frequency, or other irritative voiding symptoms with lower abdominal or suprapubic tenderness. The prostate may feel enlarged, tender, or boggy. Epididymitis causes testicular pain and swelling.

Traumatic catheter insertion or prolonged exercise may cause nonpersistent hematuria.

EVALUATION

The evaluation of hematuria should begin with a detailed medical history including occupation, recreational, and radiation exposures, and all medications. Oral anticoagulants, such as warfarin, do not generally cause hematuria de novo; these patients need to be evaluated for another underlying cause.

A dipstick (a strip embedded with reagents) and microscopic examination (urinalysis) of the urine sediment should be performed. A urinalysis, which includes microscopic examination of urine and sediment, is used to detect red blood cells, white blood cells, casts, and crystals and is the gold standard to detect the presence of hematuria. If blood is found on the dipstick but no red blood cells are found in the microscopic analysis of urine sediment, the presence of hemoglobin or myoglobin should be suspected. This may indicate the presence of rhabdomyolysis.

Patients with clinical manifestations of glomerular disease such as hypertension and edema, and urinary abnormalities such as red blood cell casts, proteinuria, and decreased glomerular filtration rate should undergo additional evaluation for potential causes of glomerular disease. Renal biopsy may be needed, especially if renal function is abnormal, to establish a diagnosis and begin treatment if necessary. A complete blood count and sedimentation rate are very helpful.

Many patients with vasculitis syndromes may have leukocytosis, anemia of chronic disease, and an elevated sedimentation rate. Serologic evaluation includes measurement of antiglomerular basement membrane antibodies, which may indicate Goodpasture's syndrome. Titers for antinuclear antibodies and anti-DNA antibodies are elevated in systemic lupus erythematosus (SLE). Cryoglobulins are cold precipitable antibodies, which may be present in malignancy, rheumatic disease, and hepatitis C infection. Antineutrophil cytoplasmic antibodies (ANCA) are specific for antigens in the cytoplasmic granules of neutrophils and monocyte lysosomes. There are two main types: cytoplasmic (c-ANCA), which is present in 90% of patients with Wegener's granulomatosis, and perinuclear (p-ANCA), which is associated with polyarteritis nodosa and Churg-Strauss syndrome. Complement levels are low in SLE, cryoglobulinemia, subacute bacterial endocarditis, acute poststreptococcal disease, and membranoproliferative glomerulonephritis. Complement levels are normal in systemic vasculitis, immunoglobulin A nephropathy, and idiopathic rapidly progressive glomerulonephritis.

Blood cultures may be positive with bacterial endocarditis. Antistreptolysin O titers may be elevated in poststreptococcal illness. If urinalysis shows evidence of infection, the patient should be treated accordingly and repeat urinalysis performed 4 to 6 weeks later to document resolution. If traumatic urinary catheter insertion or prolonged exercise is suspected to be the cause, a clean-catch voided urine specimen should be repeated. If repeat urinalysis is negative, then no further workup is needed.

If nonglomerular causes of hematuria are suspected, radiologic evaluation of the urinary tract is warranted to identify the site of urinary tract bleeding.

Helical or spiral computed tomography (CT) is now considered the test of choice to evaluate hematuria. CT has the highest efficacy for the wide range of possible underlying abnormalities and the use of CT may shorten the duration of the diagnostic evaluation. CT protocol begins with a noncontrast study, especially when nephrolithiasis is suspected. For detecting renal stones, CT has sensitivity of 94% to 98%, compared with 52% to 59% for intravenous urogram, and 19% for ultrasound. Subsequent administration of contrast provides good visualization of small masses within the kidney and collecting system. CT also provides additional information regarding renal and perirenal inflammation, and visualizes other organs and blood vessels.

Magnetic resonance imaging provides excellent imaging of the upper urinary tract but is limited by cost and availability and is not appropriate for initial testing.

Ultrasound is also a good study for evaluating renal lesions and can distinguish between solid and cystic masses. It can also identify hydronephrosis. It may, however, miss small lesions less than 3 cm. Ultrasound is the least expensive modality and does not expose the patient to intravenous contrast. Excretory urography (previously known as an intravenous pyelogram) has long been used and can visualize the entire upper urinary tract. It is excellent for detecting filling defects in the ureters, but has limited sensitivity in detecting renal masses less than 3 cm and cannot distinguish solid from cystic masses.

Cystoscopy may be indicated in patients older then 50 years of age, with other risk factors for bladder cancer such as heavy smoking, dye exposure, or frequent phenacetin use. Cystoscopy may also be warranted in patients with persistent unexplained hematuria, inconclusive radiologic tests (CT or ultrasound), and negative urine cytology. Direct visualization of the bladder with cystoscopy is the most reliable way to identify transitional cell carcinoma of the bladder, and biopsy of a suspected lesion is required. Urine cytology can be performed on voided specimens or bladder washings obtained during cystoscopy. The sensitivity is highest for high-grade lesions and carcinoma in situ.

CHAPTER 18

Hemoptysis

Amandeep Gill and Shibin Jacob

Hemoptysis (expectoration of blood) is one of the most alarming symptoms of respiratory disease. Its extent varies from scant blood streaking of sputum to frank expectoration of large amounts of fresh blood. Massive hemoptysis is variably defined as bleeding from 100 mL/day to 1,000 mL/day. Because patient descriptions of the amount of bleeding are often not accurate and it is historically difficult to quantify the bleeding, a more useful and practical definition of massive hemoptysis is any amount of bleeding that causes a drop in oxygenation or hemodynamic instability. Asphyxiation from airway occlusion and alveolar flooding is an important mechanism that contributes to the mortality of this condition. Fortunately, the incidence of massive hemoptysis is only about 5%.

DIFFERENTIAL DIAGNOSIS

The differential diagnosis of hemoptysis includes airway diseases, lung parenchymal causes, vascular causes, and miscellaneous causes (Table 18.1).

It is very important to differentiate true hemoptysis from bleeding originating from a nasopharyngeal or gastrointestinal source. Bleeding from the lungs usually is bright red, is often frothy, may be mixed with sputum, and often occurs in the setting of pre-existing lung disease. Bleeding from the gastrointestinal tract may be accompanied by nausea/vomiting, is mixed with food, consists of altered blood, and may occur in the setting of known cirrhosis or peptic ulcer disease. Despite these clinical clues, it is often not possible to clearly demarcate the two categories, especially because expectorated blood may be swallowed or vomited blood may be aspirated into the airways.

Airway Diseases

Bronchitis, both acute and chronic, is probably the most common cause of hemoptysis in the United States today. The extent of bleeding is usually mild but may be significant because the bronchial arteries are part of the systemic circulation rather than pulmonary circulation, which is low pressure. Symptoms consist of upper respiratory infection and cough productive of mucoid or mucopurulent sputum tinged with blood. Fever may or may not be present and physical findings are usually scant, but scattered rhonchi may be heard. The chest radiograph is usually normal.

Bronchiectasis is one of the most common causes of massive hemoptysis worldwide, but in the United States its incidence has diminished over the last few decades; this is due to early treatment of lower respiratory infection with better antibiotics and a decline in tuberculosis cases. The patient usually gives a long history of chronic cough and copious purulent phlegm production along with past episodes of hemoptysis. Physical examination reveals clubbing and prominent chest findings consisting of scattered crepitations and rhonchi. There may also be evidence of right-sided heart failure (cor pulmonale) in the form of elevated jugular venous pulses, ejection pulmonary murmurs, and leg edema. In children and younger patients, cystic fibrosis has to be kept in the differential diagnosis. In asthma (Chapter 35) patients, allergic bronchopulmonary aspergillosis (ABPA) is an important cause of bronchiectasis.

TABLE 18.1 Differential diagnosis of hemoptysis by source

Airways	Lung parenchyma
Bronchitis[a]	Pneumonia[a]
Bronchiectasis[a]	Lung abscess[a]
Cystic fibrosis	Mycetoma (fungus ball)[a]
Bronchogenic carcinoma[a]	Tuberculosis[a]
Endobronchial metastases	Lung contusion
Foreign body aspiration	Lupus pneumonitis
	Goodpasture's syndrome
	Wegener's granulomatosis
Cardiovascular	**Miscellaneous**
Pulmonary embolus/infarction[a]	Anticoagulant therapy
Congestive heart failure[a]	Thrombocytopenia
Mitral stenosis	Pulmonary endometriosis
Aortic aneurysm	
Pulmonary arteriovenous malformation	

[a]Common cause.

Bronchogenic carcinoma (Chapter 104) remains an important cause of hemoptysis but the extent of bleeding is typically not massive. Patients are usually smokers and older than 45 years of age. A history of new cough or change in character of chronic cough may be elicited, along with weight loss or anorexia. Physical findings in early cases are scant; chest radiographs may be normal or show subtle findings easily missed by the clinician. Endobronchial metastases typically present in patients with established tumors, especially in patients with recent or remote history of breast cancer, renal cancer, melanoma, or sarcoma. Physical findings and chest radiographs are usually normal and the diagnosis is usually made by invasive methods.

Foreign body aspiration is an uncommon cause of hemoptysis. It usually occurs in children or mentally disabled adults. The history of the actual aspiration episode is usually not forthcoming. Based on the size of the aspirated material and its lodgement in the tracheobronchial tree, patients may present with recurrent breathlessness or lung infections. Examination may reveal signs of atelectasis and reduced air entry. If radiopaque, the aspirated foreign body is easily detected on the chest radiograph.

Lung Parenchymal Diseases

Pneumonia/lung abscess (Chapter 55) is an important cause of moderate hemoptysis especially in necrotizing lung infections. The history will consist of fever, pleuritic chest pain, and blood mixed with significant amounts of mucopurulent phlegm. In lung abscess, the sputum may be foul smelling, indicating anaerobic bacterial infection. Physical findings will consist of bronchial breath sounds, increased vocal resonance, and pleural rubs.

Tuberculosis (Chapter 43) is still an important worldwide cause of hemoptysis. In acute tuberculosis, the bleeding is usually scant, but in reactivation tuberculosis (especially cavitary disease) the amounts may be massive. Pre-existing cavities may develop mycetoma (fungus ball), which can cause fatal hemoptysis. Even when adequately treated with antimycobacterial drugs, areas of localized bronchiectasis may persist, causing recurrent episodic hemoptysis over years.

Immunological diseases are also well-known causes of hemoptysis. Concurrent renal disease and hemoptysis may indicate a renopulmonary disease such as Goodpasture's syndrome, Wegener's granulomatosis (Chapter 52), or systemic lupus erythematosus (Chapter 48).

Cardiovascular Diseases

Pulmonary embolism (Chapter 41) with infarction is another cause of frank hemoptysis without mucoid or purulent phlegm and is often associated with pleuritic chest pain and breathlessness. There may be predisposing factors to the above condition, such as recent surgery (especially orthopedic surgery), recent immobilization (>4 weeks), prior history of deep venous thrombosis, and malignancy. On physical examination, tachycardia and tachypnea are usually present, with an occasional pleural rub.

Left ventricular failure (Chapter 28) is an important cause of pink frothy hemoptysis. Cardiac examination usually reveals an S3 sound, basilar crepitations, and in the case of mitral stenosis, a middiastolic murmur at the apex. Chest radiology is usually quite suggestive of congestive heart failure and may consist of cardiomegaly and pulmonary vascular changes, including Kerley B lines at the lung bases.

Miscellaneous Diseases

Systemic coagulopathy and hemorrhagic diathesis are important causes of mild to moderate hemoptysis. Patients presenting are usually known to have an identifiable cause such as severe thrombocytopenia.

EVALUATION

Because hemoptysis is potentially a serious condition, all patients must be urgently and thoroughly examined and evaluated.

First the patient's oxygenation and hemodynamic status must be established by assessing pulse oximetry, arterial blood gas if needed, and blood pressure. If hemoptysis is ongoing and massive, the patient must be immediately transferred to the intensive care unit because he or she may need emergent tracheal or selective bronchial intubation. If hemoptysis is mild with mere streaking of sputum and the patient is otherwise stable, he or she may be observed on the general medical unit. Initial laboratory results must include a complete blood count, coagulation studies, urinalysis, and renal function parameters.

A chest radiograph must be obtained to determine the presence of pulmonary infiltrate, masses, or pulmonary vascular changes. If sputum is being produced with blood, it must be sent for culture, cytology, and acid fast staining/culture.

High-resolution computed tomography scans of the chest are very helpful in revealing changes missed on chest radiograph, such as localized bronchiectasis. If the patient is a smoker and older than 45 years of age, flexible bronchoscopy is indicated to rule out early lung cancer. Bronchoscopy can be both diagnostic and therapeutic to stop ongoing bleeding by local measures. Despite all these investigations, in a substantial percentage of patients (up to 20% in some studies), the cause of hemoptysis remains unidentifiable.

CHAPTER 19

Jaundice

Monica Ziebert

Jaundice (or icterus) is the yellow discoloration of tissue due to deposition of bilirubin secondary to an elevated serum bilirubin level. Jaundice is caused by liver disease, biliary tract obstruction, hemolysis, and abnormal bilirubin metabolism. An elevated serum bilirubin level of approximately 3.0 mg/dL (normal <1.5 mg/dL) will usually result in scleral icterus, a tissue that has a high affinity for bilirubin. Jaundice can also be detected at this level under the tongue and along the tympanic membranes. As the bilirubin level rises, the skin will become jaundiced; in certain causes of jaundice, the urine can become dark, described as tea or cola colored.

Bilirubin is primarily a product of hemoglobin breakdown from old red blood cells. It is measured as indirect (unconjugated), direct (conjugated), and total. Unconjugated bilirubin is always bound to albumin, will not be filtered by the kidney, and as a result will not be found in the urine. The serum bilirubin level reflects the balance between bilirubin production and hepatic or biliary removal. Jaundice occurs when this balance gets perturbed from either overproduction of bilirubin, impaired uptake, conjugation or excretion of bilirubin, or impaired secretion of bile into the bile ducts from damage to the liver (hepatocellular) or the biliary system (intrahepatic or extrahepatic cholestasis).

DIFFERENTIAL DIAGNOSIS

The causes of jaundice can be classified according to the type of hyperbilirubinemia (unconjugated or conjugated) and the pathophysiologic mechanism (see Table 19.1).

Unconjugated Hyperbilirubinemia

The most common causes of jaundice within this category are hemolytic disorders, ineffective erythropoiesis, medications, and inherited disorders. Patients will present with mild jaundice, elevated indirect (unconjugated) bilirubin, and normal stool and urine color.

Increased Bilirubin Production

The inherited disorders that cause jaundice from hemolysis include hereditary spherocytosis, sickle cell anemia, and glucose-6-phosphate dehydrogenase deficiency. In these conditions, the serum bilirubin rarely exceeds 5 mg/dL. Higher levels can occur in sickle cell patients experiencing an acute crisis or in patients with concomitant cholelithiasis. Patients with chronic hemolysis are more likely to develop black pigmented gall stones. Acquired hemolytic disorders include hemolytic-uremic syndrome, paroxysmal nocturnal hemoglobinuria, and immune hemolysis. Abdominal or back pain may occur in patients with acute, massive hemolytic crises. Ineffective erythropoiesis occurs with vitamin B12, folate, and iron deficiencies.

Impaired Hepatic Bilirubin Uptake

The medications most commonly associated with jaundice caused by unconjugated hyperbilirubinemia are rifampin, ribavirin, and probenecid.

TABLE 19.1 Causes of jaundice by pathophysiologic mechanism

Unconjugated hyperbilirubinemia	Conjugated hyperbilirubinemia
Increased bilirubin production • Inherited hemolytic disorders (sickle cell anemia, spherocytosis, G-6-PD deficiency) • Acquired hemolytic disorders • Ineffective erythropoiesis (severe iron, B12, or folate deficiencies) • Hematoma resorption Impaired hepatic bilirubin uptake • Medications (rifampin, probenecid, ribavirin) • Congestive heart failure • Portosystemic shunts Impaired bilirubin conjugation • Crigler-Najjar types I/II • Gilbert's syndrome	Impaired secretion Extrahepatic cholestasis • Choledocholithiasis • Malignancy (cholangiocarcinoma, gallbladder and pancreatic cancer) • Primary sclerosing cholangitis • AIDS cholangiopathy • Acute and chronic pancreatitis • Benign strictures • Parasitic infections (Ascaris lumbricoides) Intrahepatic cholestasis • Viral hepatitis • Alcoholic hepatitis • Nonalcoholic fatty liver disease • Primary biliary cirrhosis • Medications (herbal, estradiol, anabolic steroids, erythromycin) • Sepsis and hypoperfusion • Infiltrative diseases (amyloidosis, lymphoma, sarcoidosis, tuberculosis) • Total parental nutrition • Postoperative • Pregnancy Hepatocellular injury • Viral hepatitis • Medications (acetaminophen, isoniazid) • Alcohol • Toxins (vinyl chloride, kava kava, wild mushrooms) • Wilson's disease • Autoimmune hepatitis • End-stage liver disease Inherited conditions • Dubin-Johnson syndrome • Rotor's syndrome

Impaired Bilirubin Conjugation

The most common inherited condition associated with jaundice from impaired conjugation is Gilbert's syndrome, with a reported incidence between 3% and 7% of the population. Impaired bilirubin conjugation is due to reduced bilirubin uridinediphosphoglucuronate (UDP) glucuronosyltransferase activity. The serum levels of bilirubin often fluctuate in Gilbert's syndrome and jaundice may be identified only in periods of fasting.

Conjugated Hyperbilirubinemia

The most common causes of jaundice are a result of conjugated hyperbilirubinemia from impaired secretion due to cholestasis (retention of bile in the liver), hepatocellular injury, or inherited conditions. In this category, jaundice seldom occurs as an isolated event and most often indicates a serious, systemic illness. Patients, however, may not relate jaundice to other symptoms so the history, physical examination, and diagnostic tests will be crucial in order to narrow the differential diagnosis.

Extrahepatic cholestasis is known as biliary obstruction and is due to conditions that block biliary flow. Patients will present with jaundice, elevated conjugated and unconjugated, bilirubin light (clay colored) stools and dark (cola or tea colored) urine from the presence of conjugated bilirubin in the urine. The elevated serum bilirubin will be accompanied by an elevated alkaline phosphatase as a marker for cholestasis. The differential diagnosis of jaundice due to extrahepatic cholestasis includes choledocholithiasis, malignancy (intrinsic and extrinsic tumors), primary sclerosing cholangitis (PSC), acquired immunodeficiency syndrome (AIDS) cholangiopathy, pancreatitis, medications, strictures after invasive procedures, and parasitic infections.

Patients with choledocholithiasis (common bile duct gallstones) can present with jaundice and pruritus. If the obstruction of the common bile duct is gradual then patients will have few other symptoms. However, these patients often present with symptoms from complications of the obstruction including ascending cholangitis or pancreatitis. Patients with ascending cholangitis have the characteristic presentation of jaundice, biliary colic, and fevers with chills (Charcot's triad). Pancreatitis should be suspected in patients who develop a steady, boring pain in the epigastrium or left upper quadrant pain with radiation to the back and prolonged nausea and vomiting.

Malignancy causes jaundice from compression of the bile ducts. The most common cause of extrinsic compression is carcinoma of the head of the pancreas. Patients present with jaundice, weight loss, and the insidious onset of a gnawing abdominal pain radiating from epigastrium to the back. Cholangiocarcinoma is an adenocarcinoma of the extrahepatic bile ducts. Patients will present with painless jaundice, pruritus, and weight loss. Physical examination findings include hepatomegaly and a palpable, distended gallbladder (Courvoisier's sign). Cancer of the gallbladder presents with jaundice, weight loss and a palpable right upper quadrant mass, but unlike cholangiosarcoma, there is accompanied unrelenting right upper quadrant pain.

PSC is a disorder characterized by a progressive obliterative process involving the extrahepatic bile ducts. PSC can be associated with inflammatory bowel disease. Patients present with jaundice, pruritus, right upper quadrant abdominal pain and even, acute ascending cholangitis. AIDS cholangiopathy is a disorder that results in bile duct lesions and a clinical presentation similar to PSC. Infectious organisms include Cryptosporidium, cytomegalovirus, and human immunodeficiency virus (HIV) itself are felt to be the culprits in the pathogenesis.

Patients with acute pancreatitis from nongallstone causes can present with a transient jaundice that usually resolves in 4 to 5 days after the acute event. Patients with chronic pancreatitis can present with jaundice due to chronic inflammation of the common bile duct. These patients also have a characteristic deep-seated, persistent epigastric pain, and steatorrhea. Benign strictures of the extrahepatic ducts can arise from previous interventions like endoscopic retrograde cholangiopancreatography (ERCP) or surgery. Patients can present with jaundice from biliary obstruction or cholangitis as long as 2 years after the intervention. Parasitic infections including nematodes and trematodes cause jaundice. Ascaris lumbricoides is a large roundworm that migrates from the small intestine to the biliary tree and obstructs the extrahepatic biliary ducts. Clonorchis sinensis is a fluke that resides in the biliary ducts and gallbladder. Infection is associated with symptoms similar to acute pancreatitis or cholelithiasis and complications such as ascending cholangitis and cholangiocarcinoma.

Intrahepatic Cholestasis

Patients with jaundice due to intrahepatic cholestasis present in a similar manner as extrahepatic cholestasis except that the bile ducts are patent. With intrahepatic cholestasis, the elevated serum bilirubin and alkaline phosphatase may also be accompanied by varying degrees of elevated transaminases, aspartate aminotransferase (AST), and alanine transferase (ALT).

The differential diagnosis of jaundice due to intrahepatic cholestasis includes viral hepatitis, alcoholic hepatitis, nonalcoholic fatty liver disease (NAFLD), primary biliary cirrhosis (PBC), medications, toxins, sepsis, total parental nutrition (TPN), liver infiltrative processes, postoperative state, and pregnancy.

Viral hepatitis (Chapter 73) can present with jaundice and pruritus due to cholestasis. Patients may also have low-grade fever, anorexia, and myalgias, but it is usually difficult to distinguish viral hepatitis from other causes of cholestasis on presentation. Risk factor assessment can provide important clues. Patients should be asked about exposure to contaminated food, travel history, high-risk sexual activity, intravenous drug use, transfusions before 1990, and tattoos.

Patients with alcoholic hepatitis present with jaundice, fever, malaise, and tender hepatomegaly in the setting of alcohol dependency. The transaminases AST and ALT will also be elevated in a characteristic pattern of an AST-to-ALT ratio of greater than 2. Because cirrhosis can already exist, complications of portal hypertension, such as ascites, varices, and encephalopathy may also be present.

Patients with NAFLD present with signs and symptoms related to one of the underlying causes such as diabetes, obesity, short bowel syndrome, medications, and toxins. Patients with NAFLD may present with no symptoms and mild elevations of alkaline phosphatase or the aminotransferases or jaundice with fulminate hepatic failure from medications and toxins.

Primary biliary cirrhosis (Chapter 74) is characterized by chronic inflammation of the intrahepatic biliary ducts. Patients are often diagnosed when an elevated alkaline phosphatase is noted on routine laboratory testing and are initially asymptomatic. Jaundice and pruritus develop months or years later. Common physical examination findings are xanthomas and moderate to severe hepatomegaly. Diagnostic laboratory tests include positive antimitochondrial antibodies.

Medications most likely to cause jaundice secondary to intrahepatic cholestasis include anabolic steroids, ethinyl estradiol, and herbal medicines. Sepsis leads to jaundice secondary to hypotension and release of bacterial endotoxins.

Total parental nutrition can cause jaundice from cholestasis after about 2 weeks of therapy. Risk factors for this complication include previous history of liver disease and the concomitant use of hepatotoxic drugs.

Infiltrative diseases that cause jaundice include amyloidosis, sarcoidosis, and lymphoma. Although they have a variety of extrahepatic manifestations, they can all be associated with jaundice and gradual deterioration of liver function. The diagnosis of these disorders as a cause of jaundice often depends on the presence of associated clinical findings or ultimately a liver biopsy.

Postoperative jaundice is quite common and is due to increased unconjugated bilirubin availability from transfusions and hematoma resorption in the setting of risk factors such as renal insufficiency, hypotension, and hypoxia. Pregnancy is associated with serious causes of jaundice including intrahepatic cholestasis of pregnancy, acute fatty liver, and the HELLP (hemolysis, elevated liver tests, low platelets) syndrome. Intrahepatic cholestasis of pregnancy occurs in the first trimester and can be associated with premature births and still births. Acute fatty liver of pregnancy and the HELLP syndrome are potentially fatal conditions.

Hepatocellular Injury

The differential diagnosis for jaundice due to hepatocellular injury includes viral hepatitis, alcohol, medications (i.e., isoniazid, valproic acid, phenytoin) or environmental toxins, Wilson's disease, and autoimmune hepatitis.

Viral hepatitis and alcohol can cause jaundice from either intrahepatic cholestasis or hepatocellular injury. Clinically, it is difficult to distinguish many of these conditions from cholestatic causes. In acute hepatocellular injury, however, AST and ALT are elevated, along with the elevations in serum conjugated bilirubin and alkaline phosphatase. In chronic hepatocellular injury, the liver enzymes may normalize as the injury progresses to cirrhosis and end-stage liver disease. At this time, the patient will present with the stigmata of liver disease including spider angiomata, ascites, palmar erythema, gynecomastia, and caput medusa.

Medications that cause acute hepatocellular injury may include phenytoin, isoniazid, valproic acid, and sulfonamides. Toxins causing liver injury may include poison mushroom and carbon tetrachloride.

Wilson's disease is a rare autosomal recessive disease that results from a defect in copper transport. Patients present with either psychiatric symptoms, neurologic symptoms such as dystonia or Parkinsonism, or one of four types of hepatic injury including an acute hepatitis, parenchymal liver disease, cirrhosis, or fulminant hepatitis with jaundice. On physical examination, Kayser-Fleischer rings (subtle golden deposits around the periphery of the cornea) may be present. Obtaining a serum ceruloplasmin level and urinary copper level can aid in the diagnosis.

Autoimmune hepatitis is a chronic disorder that results in cirrhosis and liver failure. Patients are typically young to middle-aged women who present with acute or insidious onset jaundice, fatigue, malaise, anorexia, and arthralgias. Many of these symptoms are indistinguishable from the presentation of viral hepatitis. Diagnosis is aided by the presence of antinuclear antibodies, specifically antismooth muscle antibodies.

Fulminant hepatic failure is acute onset of hepatocellular dysfunction characterized by jaundice, coagulopathy, and encephalopathy in the absence of previously established liver disease. Common causes include acetaminophen toxicity (most common cause) and acute hepatitis A or B.

Inherited Conditions

The inherited causes of jaundice due to conjugated hyperbilirubinemia, like Dubin-Johnson and Rotor's syndrome, are very rare and benign. Patients with both of these conditions present with asymptomatic jaundice.

EVALUATION

The evaluation of the patient with jaundice requires an assessment of the severity of the presentation and the simultaneous determination of the likely diagnosis.

A thorough history and physical examination along with immediate measure of the total and conjugated (direct) bilirubin and liver enzymes will provide clinical clues that can lead to the diagnosis or direct further appropriate testing (Fig. 19.1).

The urgency of the evaluation of the patient with jaundice will depend on the severity of the presenting symptoms. Jaundice that is associated with alarm symptoms such as fever, right upper quadrant abdominal pain, altered mental state, epistaxis, gingival bleeding, back pain, or pregnancy should raise the concern for very serious, potentially life-threatening illness. These conditions include massive hemolysis, ascending cholangitis, and fulminant hepatic failure.

History should include information on hepatitis risk factors (transfusions before 1990, sexual promiscuity, and intravenous drug use), medications (including prescribed, herbal, and over the counter), travel history, HIV status, exposure to toxins, alcohol use, and personal or family history of hemolytic disorders. Presenting symptoms and risk factors that suggest an obstructive etiology include severe pain, weight loss, history of gallstones, and prior biliary tract surgery. Symptoms that suggest hepatocellular injury include viral prodrome of malaise, anorexia, and fatigue, and exposures such as alcohol and new medications. An appreciation of the role of the postoperative state, sepsis, the use of TPN, and pregnancy are also important in the work up of jaundice. Helpful physical examination findings include the signs of chronic liver disease, a Courvoisier sign, Kayser-Fleischer rings (Wilson's disease), and xanthomas in (PBC).

Screening laboratory tests include the total bilirubin, conjugated (direct) bilirubin, unconjugated

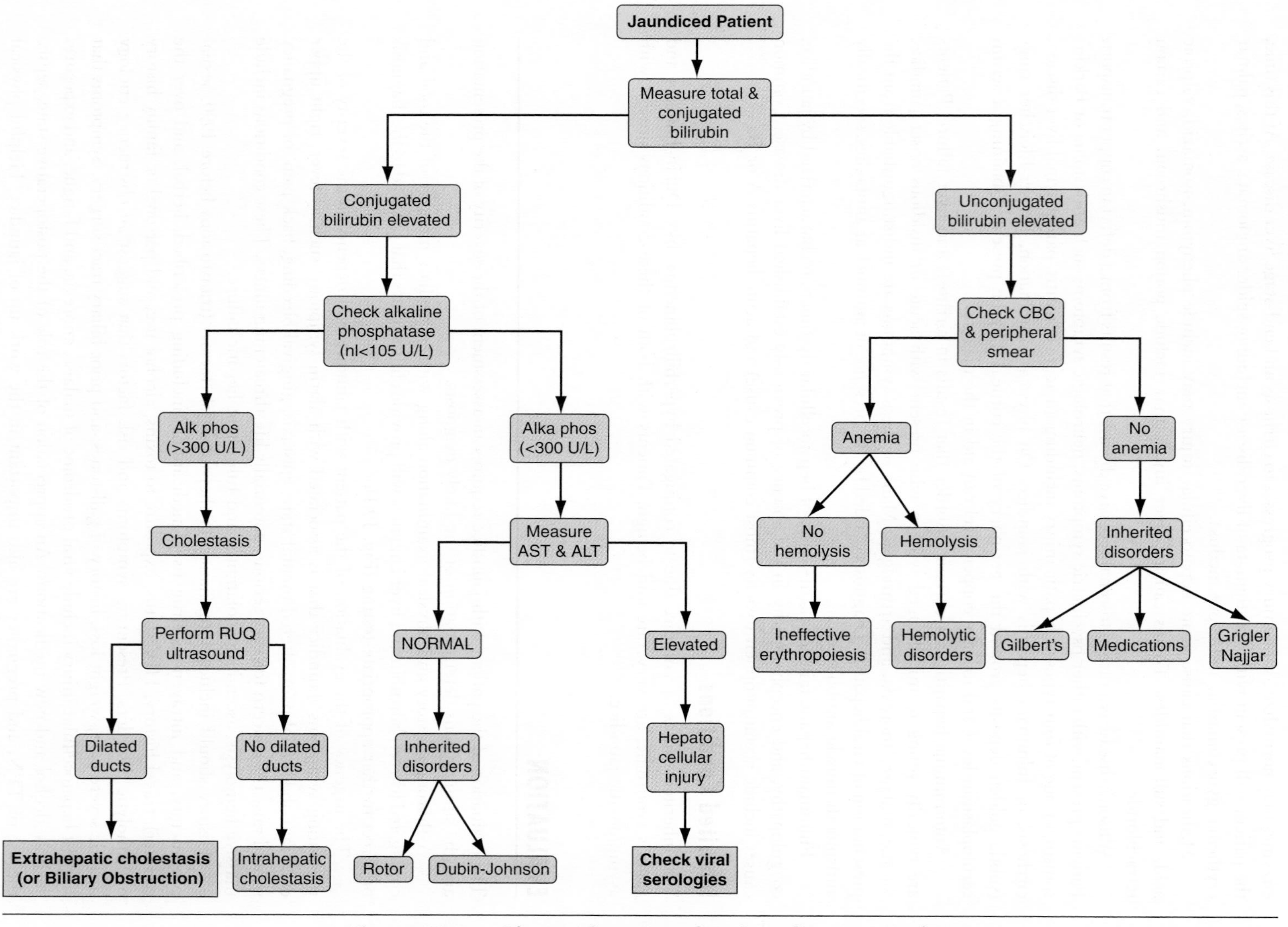

Figure 19.1 • Diagnostic approach to jaundice. *(continued)*

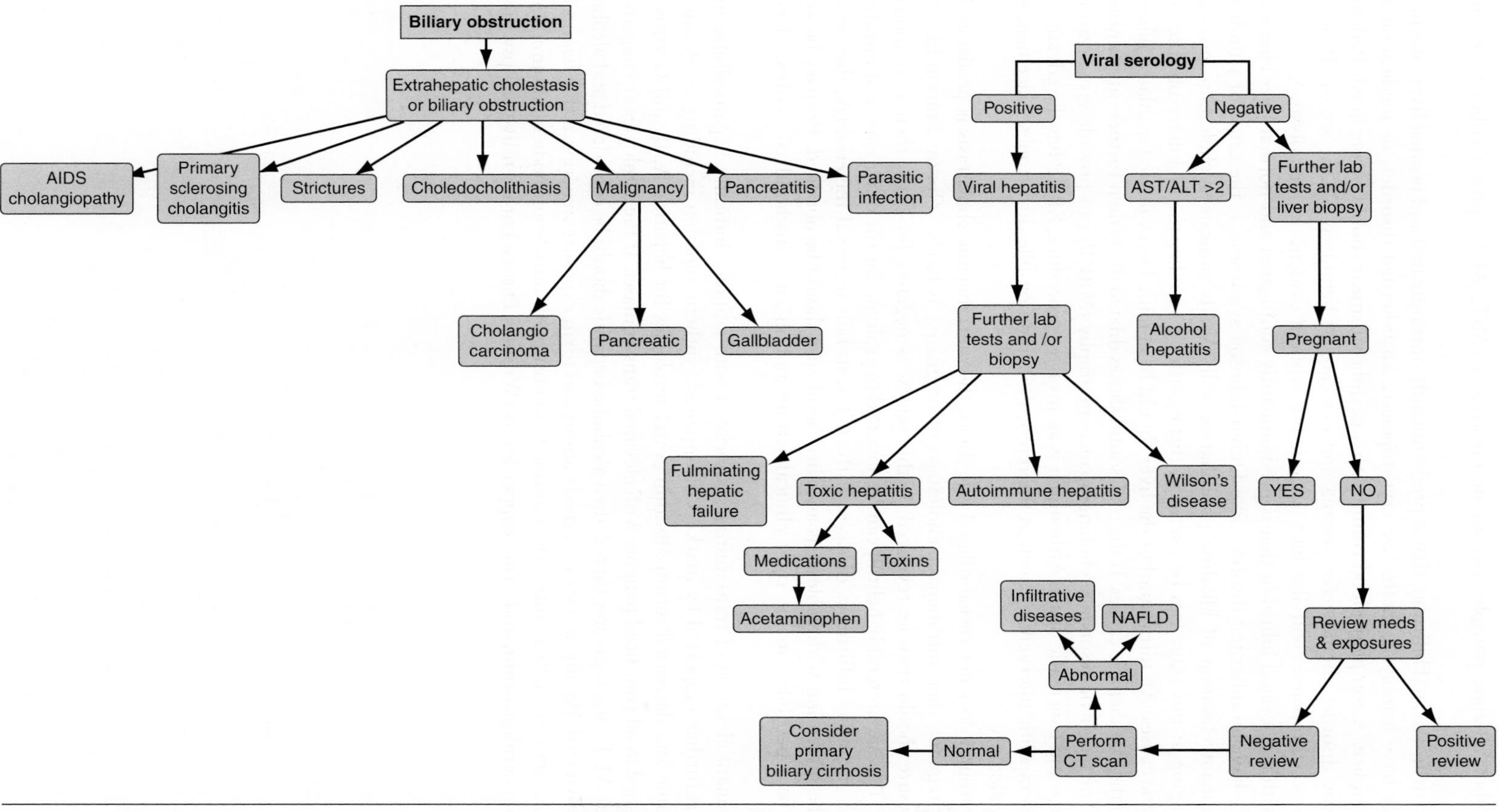

Figure 19.1 • *(continued)*

(indirect) bilirubin, alkaline phosphatase, aminotransferases (AST, ALT), prothrombin time, and albumin.

Patients with an elevated bilirubin that is predominantly unconjugated and normal liver enzymes will most likely have hemolysis, ineffective erythropoiesis, an inherited disorder, or medication as the cause of jaundice. A complete blood count with a peripheral smear should be obtained. Patients with a hemolytic disorder should have anemia and evidence of hemolysis on the smear. Patients with ineffective erythropoiesis will also have anemia but without evidence of hemolysis.

Patients with an elevated bilirubin that is predominantly conjugated and normal liver enzymes will most likely have an inherited disorder like Dubin-Johnson syndrome as the cause of jaundice.

A predominant elevation of alkaline phosphatase will usually indicate a cholestatic process. Diagnostic imaging at this stage can be useful in distinguishing extrahepatic or biliary obstruction from intrahepatic causes. An ultrasound of the liver should be obtained to evaluate for dilated biliary ducts as seen in the extrahepatic causes. If the ultrasound shows dilated ducts then further intervention with an ERCP or magnetic resonance cholangiopancreatography (MRCP) can provide visualization of the biliary tree and pancreatic ducts. Although it is an invasive procedure, ERCP has the advantage of providing therapeutic intervention such as the removal of common bile duct stones, placement of stents, and papillotomy.

If the ultrasound does not reveal dilated bile ducts, then intrahepatic cholestasis is probable. If the patient is pregnant, then intrahepatic cholestasis of pregnancy is likely. The medication history and toxin exposure should then be reviewed. If this review is negative for clues, then a computed tomography (CT) scan, preferably helical, can be obtained to evaluate for the other causes of intrahepatic cholestasis including infiltrative diseases. If the CT scan fails to reveal the etiology, then viral hepatitis may be presenting with cholestasis and viral serologies should be obtained. Primary biliary cirrhosis may be a possibility in the right clinical setting and an antimitochondrial antibody level will be helpful.

A predominant elevation of transaminases associated with jaundice indicates hepatocellular injury, and this is further supported by markers of impaired synthetic function including an elevated prothrombin time and decreased serum albumin. Viral serologies for hepatitis A, B, and C viruses should be obtained in all jaundiced patients with elevated transaminases. If the serologies are negative and the AST-to-ALT ratio is greater then 2, then alcoholic hepatitis should be considered and alcohol use should be reviewed. Finally, a review of medications and toxin exposure may reveal the diagnosis or further laboratory tests such as antinuclear antibodies antismooth muscle antibodies (autoimmune hepatitis), serum ceruloplasmin, and urine copper levels (Wilson's Disease) or even liver biopsy may be needed.

CHAPTER 20

Joint Pain

Elizabeth Russell

Joint pain or inflammation is associated with a large differential diagnosis. Attention to the number and distribution of painful joints and to features of disease evolution help distinguish categories of disease. Laboratory tests and imaging studies are often used as diagnostic adjuncts but do not replace a careful history and physical examination. The review of systems and physical examination are the most useful diagnostic maneuvers in diagnosing systemic disorders associated with joint pain because this information will uncover patterns of disease that will facilitate diagnosis.

DIFFERENTIAL DIAGNOSIS

The first determination is to identify whether the joint itself is the source of pain or an adjacent structure such as adjacent tendons, bursae, or bones. A careful physical examination may help distinguish between true articular and periarticular processes. For example, passive range-of-motion testing should not be painful in periarticular disorders, whereas recruitment of the affected muscle or tendon will reproduce the pain. Bone disorders are suspected when pain is reproduced with weight bearing.

Joint pain in a normal joint is termed arthralgia. Patients with arthralgia complain of pain in the joint but have no objective evidence of inflammation (warmth, redness, tenderness, and swelling) and no evidence of joint derangement.

Joint pain in an abnormal joint is termed arthritis (Fig. 20.1).

Inflammatory and Noninflammatory Arthritis

Noninflammatory arthritis is typical of osteoarthritis, anatomic derangements, metabolic disturbances, and endocrine diseases such as hypothyroidism (Table 20.1). Synovial fluid from patients with arthralgia or noninflammatory arthritis is noninflammatory (i.e., less than 2,000 white blood cells [WBC] per squared centimeter). The distinction between inflammatory and noninflammatory joint pain is critical in developing a differential diagnosis. Noninflammatory joint diseases are seldom urgent and workup can usually proceed on an outpatient basis.

Inflamed joints are warm, swollen, and tender and synovial fluid from such joints reveals WBC counts greater than 2,000. This represents true synovitis where the synovial lining of the joint becomes inflamed and thickened. Patients with joint inflammation complain of pain with any movement of the joint and note morning stiffness correlated with the extent of inflammation. The examination of patients with inflammatory joint problems reveals tenderness over the joint line, thickening of the lining (synovium), warmth and effusion, and patient reluctance to move the joint either passively or actively. Inflammatory joint processes are associated with autoimmune, infectious, and crystalline disorders. On the other hand, many disorders associated with inflammatory joint pain may be life- or organ-threatening and require urgent assessment in the hospital. Such diseases include endocarditis, septic arthritis, and vasculitis. Usually other clues of the systemic nature of the process will be present. Fever is a key clue and febrile patients with inflamed joints should be admitted for culturing and possible treatment with antibiotics while evaluation proceeds.

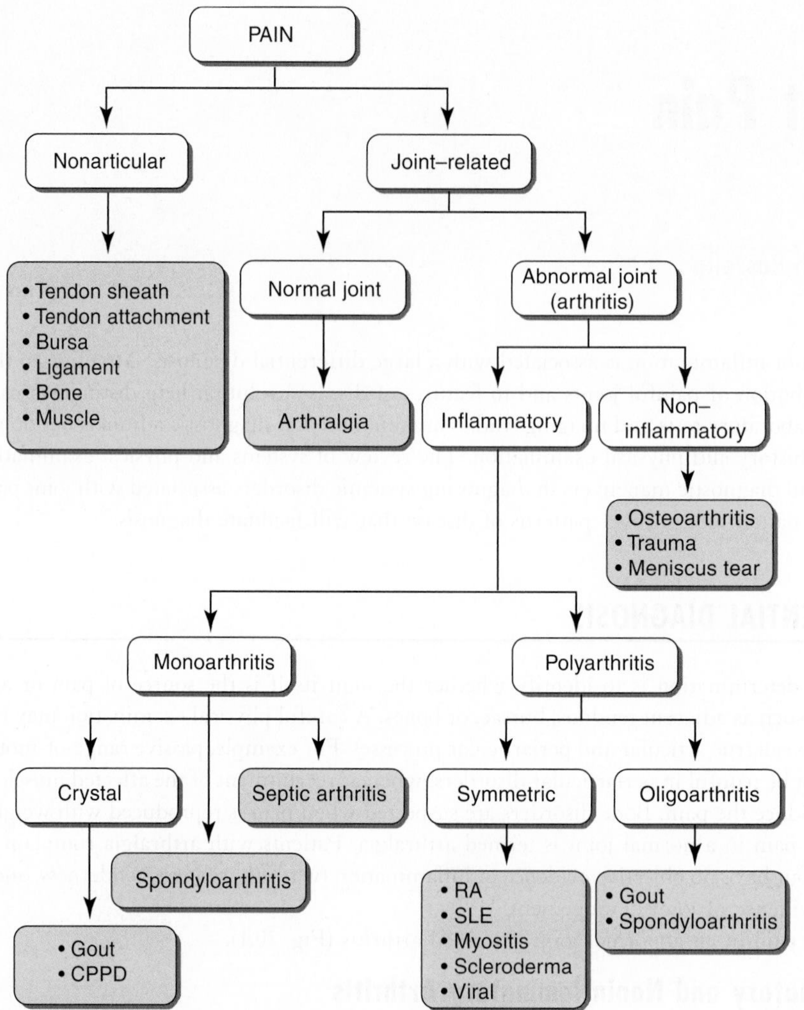

Figure 20.1 • Diagnostic algorithm of joint-related pain. CPPD, calcium pyrophosphate disease; RA, rheumatoid arthritis; SLE, systemic lupus erythematosus.

Pattern of Joint Involvement

The pattern of involvement of joints and duration of symptoms are quite useful in further distinguishing the cause of the problem.

Monoarthritis denotes involvement of just one joint. Acute inflammatory monoarthritis should be considered to be related to infection (septic joint), trauma (hemarthrosis), or crystal diseases (gout, pseudogout) until proven otherwise. Chronic inflammatory monoarthritis is more typical of a lingering adventitious infection such as Lyme disease, fungal infection, or mycobacterial infection. Acute and chronic noninflammatory monoarthritis is typical for osteoarthritis, internal derangement of a joint or adjacent bone, and local tumors.

Polyarthritis (Fig. 20.2) denotes involvement of more than one joint and is further subdivided into oligoarthritis (four or fewer joints involved) and polyarthritis (more than four joints). Inflammatory oligoarthritis is typical of a subgroup of autoimmune diseases called spondyloarthritis such as psoriatic

TABLE 20.1 Differential diagnosis of monoarticular and oligoarticular arthritis

Noninflammatory
Trauma
Osteoarthritis
Meniscus/ligament tear
Inflammatory
Gout
Pseudogout
Septic joint
Spondyloarthritis
Reactive arthritis
Reiter's syndrome
Psoriatic arthritis
Rheumatoid arthritis, lupus (unusual)

arthritis. Often the lower extremity joints are involved in spondyloarthritis and inflammation may be episodic and migratory in its pattern. A migratory inflammation of just a few joints is also typical of reactive arthritis. Any sequence of a few joints can be involved in reactive arthritis, which includes rheumatic fever and Whipple's disease. Rarely, an autoimmune polyarthritis will present initially as a monoarthritis or oligoarthritis.

Patients presenting with a polyarthritis constitute a large group with diverse diagnostic possibilities. The history and physical examination will be the most useful maneuvers to clarify the diagnosis. In addition, the pattern of joint involvement can be very useful. For instance, rheumatoid arthritis (RA) usually involves the wrists and metacarpophalangeal joints and does not involve the distal interphalangeal (DIP) joints whereas osteoarthritis, psoriatic arthritis, and gout often involve the DIP joints. The presence or absence of inflammation further assists in narrowing the differential diagnosis. Osteoarthritis can be polyarticular but there is seldom intense inflammation, whereas joints affected with RA are quite inflamed.

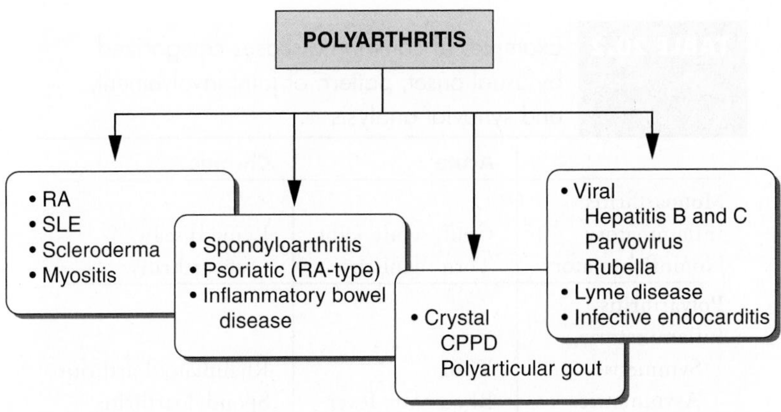

Figure 20.2 • Possible causes of polyarthritis. RA, rheumatoid arthritis; SLE, systemic lupus erythematosus.

Onset and Timing of Joint Pain

The onset of the joint pain can be quite useful in diagnosis. Few processes will begin and develop to full intensity within hours. A hemarthrosis from trauma to the joint can result in bleeding that visibly distends and inflames the joint within minutes of the injury. Gout or calcium pyrophosphate disease (CPPD) are crystal deposition diseases that often develop intense inflammation overnight. Rheumatic fever can have an associated reactive oligoarthritis that migrates daily. However, subacute processes develop over days to weeks and include most bacterial infections that develop crescendo inflammation over several days. Most viral infections fall into this category too, as well as many of the autoimmune diseases like RA, which develops additively over weeks with progressively more joints involved. Noninflammatory polyarthritides that fall into the subacute category of onset include posttraumatic osteoarthritis and arthritis related to adjacent bone disorders such as tumors. Lastly, chronic arthritis denotes the development of symptoms over months to years. Examples of chronic monoarthritis include adventitious infections such as tuberculosis, fungi, or Lyme disease. Reaction to an internal derangement of a joint (such as a torn meniscus of the knee) can result in a noninflammatory chronic monoarthritis. Chronic noninflammatory polyarthritis includes such entities as osteoarthritis, arthropathies associated with endocrine disorders (acromegaly, thyroid disease), and metabolic disorders such as hemochromatosis and chronic tophaceous gout.

Categorizing monoarthritis, oligoarthritis, or polyarthritis as acute, subacute, or chronic and either inflammatory or not will help focus the differential diagnosis (Table 20.2). In addition, noting the course of the illness is revealing. Disorders that are typically episodic (typified by "attacks") include gout, CPPD, and spondyloarthritis (such as Reiter's disease). Diseases often associated with a migratory joint inflammation include bacterial endocarditis, rheumatic fever, reactive arthritis of any infectious etiology, and the spondyloarthritides. RA is often additive (gradually increasing numbers of joints involved), whereas polyarthritis associated with viral infection typically develops synchronously in all affected joints. Lastly, symmetry of joint involvement is another clue to the origin of the process. The inflammatory polyarthritis of RA is usually symmetric, whereas that of spondyloarthritis is not.

When considering whether arthralgia or true synovitis is part of systemic disease, the differential diagnosis should address possibilities in the six pathophysiologic categories: neoplastic, infectious, metabolic, toxic, autoimmune, and traumatic. Keeping the differential open at the onset of evaluation makes it less likely that a closed inventory will be created, inadvertently excluding the accurate diagnosis. Traumatic processes are usually obvious but occult stress fractures can present as "joint" pain. Neoplastic processes are rare and more likely in adults with a single, chronically painful joint and local tumors are more likely than metastatic disease.

TABLE 20.2 Examples of common diseases categorized by usual onset, pattern of joint involvement, and synovial analysis

	Acute	Chronic
Monoarthritis		
Inflammatory	Gout, septic joint	Lyme disease
Noninflammatory	Torn meniscus	Osteoarthritis
Polyarthritis		
Inflammatory		
Symmetric	Viral	Rheumatoid arthritis
Asymmetric	Rheumatic fever	Spondyloarthritis
Noninflammatory	Drug-induced	Thyroid disease

Infectious arthritis is most often a monoarthritis and staphylococcus accounts for 75% of cases. The next most common pathogens are streptococcus (15%) and gonococcus (particularly in young, sexually active patients). Occasionally, multiple joints may be septic, which is more common when pathogen seeding is hematogenous (e.g., bacterial endocarditis) or in severely immunocompromised patients (e.g., patients receiving organ transplants). Most viral infections present as acute polyarthritis (e.g., parvoB19, hepatitis, and echovirus) but other pathogens like treponemes, spirochetes, fungi, and mycobacteria often present as a chronic monoarthritis. Toxic etiologies for joint pain usually result in arthralgia rather than arthritis and numerous medications can cause arthralgias (e.g., bisphosphonates). Most metabolic disturbances, such as vitamin C deficiency, also result in arthralgia but occasionally manifest as noninflammatory polyarthritis. Most autoimmune diseases develop patterns of organ inflammation that allow specific diagnosis and most are associated with some type of inflammatory arthritis.

EVALUATION

The patient's history is particularly useful in establishing a diagnosis of a systemic disease in association with the patient's joint pain. As noted above, the nature of the onset, evolution, and distribution of joints involved will be valuable in guiding the differential diagnosis. In addition, the presence of joint stiffness lasting more than 20 minutes in the involved joint(s) is historical evidence that suggests an inflammatory state. Complaints of joint stiffness after prolonged immobility ("gelling phenomenon"), however, suggest noninflammatory degenerative arthritis. The historical presence of fever, fatigue, and joint swelling and warmth all suggest an inflammatory process. The presence or absence of other symptoms from the review of systems will point to patterns of organ involvement that will assist diagnosis. Family history is often positive for other autoimmune diseases in patients with connective tissue diseases, although exact genetic transmission is still poorly understood. Social history is useful to detect travel that might expose the patient to certain infections (e.g., Lyme disease) as well as to note occupations that may result in injury (e.g., painting and rotator cuff injury) (Table 20.3).

The physical examination of the joints should include inspection and palpation of all joints. Bony malalignment is often testimony to bone distortion (e.g., bone erosions from RA) or capsular disruption (e.g., joint dislocation). Tenderness and warmth are expected with inflammation. Synovial effusions are detected by palpation for fluctuance within the joint. Chronicity of an inflammatory

TABLE 20.3 Review of systems for clues to specific rheumatic diseases

Systemic	Fever, weight loss
Mucocutaneous	Rash, ulcers, nodules, sun sensitivity, alopecia, oral or genital sores
Head and neck area	Red painful eyes, dry eyes or mouth, jaw claudication
Cardiopulmonary	Pleurisy, cough, dyspnea, Raynaud's phenomenon, edema, claudication
Gastrointestinal	Dysphagia, abdominal pain, diarrhea, bloody stools
Genitourinary	Dysuria, bloody or cloudy urine, urethral discharge
Musculoskeletal	Weakness, myalgias, arthralgias; joint swelling, pain, warmth, redness, or decreased motion
Neurologic	Numbness, paraesthesias, urinary or fecal incontinence, radicular pain, weakness, exercise-induced pain or weakness, seizures, cranial or peripheral nerve abnormalities, visual disturbance, headache, vertigo

process can be gauged by feeling a thickening of the capsule/synovium of a joint. Although adjacent structures such as tendons and bursae can be palpated directly, tendon inflammation is better assessed by selective recruitment of the tendon in question and noting pain. Passive range of motion is often preserved in tendonitis, whereas inflammatory processes within the joint will result in splinting of both passive and active range of motion. A full physical examination will examine for other organ system involvement that will speak to a systemic disorder outside of the joints. This is critical in assessing the patient with polyarthritis. For instance, the inflammatory symmetric polyarthritis of RA can be identical to that of systemic lupus erythematosus (SLE) but the presence of rash, Raynaud's syndrome, hair loss, and sun sensitivity would alert the physician to possible SLE and would not be seen in RA.

Arthrocentesis is the process of aspirating synovial fluid from a joint for analysis (synovial analysis). The appearance of the fluid can provide clues to the diagnosis: noninflammatory fluid is clear and cloudy fluid suggests a high leukocyte count (WBC) that typifies inflammatory states. A WBC greater than 2,000 is arbitrarily used as the cutoff for inflammatory synovial fluid, but exact white cell counts cannot make a specific diagnosis. In general, however, very high white cell counts are more likely to occur in infections. The synovial fluid should have a Gram stain performed as well as cultures in cases of suspected septic arthritis. Compensated light microscopy is done to evaluate for crystals and this test is diagnostic in cases of suspected gout or pseudogout (CPPD). Presence of blood in the synovial fluid can exist in cases of crystalline diseases and can also be a clue to internal derangement or to fractures through the joint line wherein fat globules are also seen. Arthrocentesis is the diagnostic test for septic arthritis and crystal diseases like gout and all patients with an acute monoarthritis need to have arthrocentesis performed to analyze joint fluid for crystals, cell count, and culture. It is less mandatory diagnostically in cases of polyarthritis but recommended in new patients with RA to dispel confusion with polyarticular gout or whenever the diagnosis remains unclear. Rarely, synovial biopsy is used in evaluation of a chronic monoarthritis after synovial analysis, laboratory work, and imaging have failed to make a diagnosis. Synovial biopsy is useful in diagnosing chronic infections like tuberculosis.

Serologic studies are often ordered in cases of polyarthritis. Rheumatoid factor (RF) and anticitrullinated cyclic protein antibodies (CCP) are adjuncts to the diagnosis of RA. The rheumatoid factor is an antibody to the Fc portion of immunoglobulin G and occurs in about 80% of cases. The newer CCP antibody is felt to be slightly more sensitive and specific for RA and will be positive earlier. Neither test is sufficient for diagnosis because neither is 100% specific; both can occur in other types of arthritis and in chronic inflammatory states.

The antinuclear antibody (ANA) is used as a screening test for the autoimmune diseases. A positive ANA is found in 5% to 15% of normal people, which can also be induced by drugs (e.g., procainamide). The ANA is positive in 95% of patients with SLE, which makes it a useful screening test but also not sufficient for diagnosis because it is found in many other connective tissue diseases (Table 20.4). The ANA becomes significant when other features suggesting SLE or another connective tissue disease are present clinically. Other serologic tests are then done that are more specific for a particular disease such as anti–double-stranded DNA for SLE or anticentromere antibody for limited scleroderma. Serum complement determinations help in assessing whether the patient's disease is causing activation of the complement system. This is common in infections, SLE, vasculitis, and disorders associated with circulating immune complexes like cryoglobulinemia in hepatitis C virus (Table 20.4).

Other laboratory tests that are useful in diagnosing diseases associated with joint pain include the serum uric acid in patients suspected to have gout. However, the serum uric acid cannot be used to diagnose gout because fluctuations in serum uric acid may not correlate with clinical gout. Asymptomatic but chronically high uric acid values (hyperuricemia) are common in the population. However, gout is a clinical syndrome of intense joint inflammation during supersaturation of the synovial fluid, and demonstration of monosodium urate crystals in the synovial fluid is diagnostic.

TABLE 20.4 Antinuclear antibodies: frequency of positive finding in rheumatic diseases (%)

Antibody	SLE	Scl	CREST	PM/DM	RA	DLE	MCTD	SS
ANA	>95	95	95	20–50	15–35	>95	>95	75
Antinative DNA	50							
Smith	40							
Ribonucleoprotein	40	15	10	15			>95	15
Centromere			50					
Histones	30				<20	>95		
Scl-70		40	15					
SS-A/Ro	25[a]			10	10			50
SS-B/La	15							25
PM-1				30–50				

[a]Positive in subacute cutaneous lupus, in which ANA may be negative. SS-A/Ro positive patients usually have secondary Sjogren syndrome.
ANA, antinuclear antibody; CREST, *c*alcinosis, *R*aynaud's syndrome, *e*sophageal dysmotility, *s*clerodactyly, *t*elangiectasia; DLE, drug-induced lupus; DM, dermatomyositis; MCTD, mixed connective tissue disease; PM, polymyositis; RA, rheumatoid arthritis; Scl, diffuse scleroderma; SLE, systemic lupus erythematosus; SS, Sjogren's syndrome.

The erythrocyte sedimentation rate has little specificity but provides a quantification of ongoing inflammation. It is expected to be elevated in many inflammatory and infectious states but is used to help establish the diagnosis and to monitor treatment in polymyalgia rheumatica and in temporal arteritis. It is of little use diagnostically but is often followed in other autoimmune diseases as an additional marker of disease activity.

Plain radiography seldom assists in diagnosis of acute arthritis with the exception of those joints associated with fractures and other adjacent bone abnormalities. Tendon or cartilage calcification is seen in connection with calcific tendonitis or pseudogout respectively and in such cases a causal relationship is inferred in the appropriate clinical setting of acute peri- or monoarthritis. Radiography is more useful in chronic arthritis where bone remodeling occurs. When bone erosions of inflammatory disorders like RA occur, then a degenerative or noninflammatory process like osteoarthritis can be excluded. In addition, bony erosions can be monitored over time during treatment.

Magnetic resonance imaging is useful in visualizing both intra-articular soft tissues (e.g., torn meniscus of knee) and extra-articular tissues (e.g., tendon inflammation). Other modalities such as ultrasound, computed tomography scans, angiography, and nuclear medicine are used in specific clinical situations.

CHAPTER 21

Nausea and Vomiting

Monica Ziebert

Nausea is the subjective disagreeable sensation of the need to vomit that may or may not result in vomiting. Vomiting (emesis) is the forcible expulsion of the upper gastrointestinal contents through the mouth. This is different from regurgitation, which is the passive passage of the gastric contents into the mouth. Vomiting is controlled by the vomiting center in the medulla and is triggered by afferent neural pathways from the gastrointestinal (GI) tract in response to distention, mucosal injury, peritoneal irritation or infection. Other non-GI sources of input include the cerebral cortex, when noxious thoughts, emotional experiences, sights, or smells provoke vomiting. The vestibular apparatus signals the vomiting center during motion sickness and inner ear disorders. Finally, the chemoreceptor trigger zone within the medulla provides input to the vomiting center in response to bloodborne stimuli (such as drugs, toxins, and metabolic disorders) provoke vomiting.

DIFFERENTIAL DIAGNOSIS

There are a myriad of causes of nausea and vomiting, which can be included in the differential diagnosis. They range from mild, quickly resolving illnesses to serious, life-threatening conditions. The causes can be classified according to conditions within the GI tract and conditions outside the GI tract (Table 21.1).

The history and physical examination provide clinic clues that will narrow the large differential diagnosis associated with the causes of nausea and vomiting (Table 21.2). The history should reveal information on symptom characteristics such as severity, duration of symptoms, frequency, provocative features such as relationship to meals and medications, and the quality and quantity of vomits. Acute onset of nausea and vomiting in the setting of severe abdominal pain usually points to a gastrointestinal cause such as obstruction or peritoneal irritation from one of the inflammatory conditions (appendicitis, cholecystitis, and pancreatitis). Acute symptoms without abdominal pain can be due to gastroenteritis, medications, central nervous system (CNS) conditions like hemorrhage and infection, and myocardial infarction.

Chronic nausea and vomiting can occur in GI conditions associated with impaired motor function (dysmotility), CNS diseases, and systemic illnesses ranging from malignancy to endocrinopathies. Intermittent and recurrent symptoms suggest cyclic vomiting syndrome, a rare disorder of unknown etiology but strongly related to migraine headaches. Nausea and vomiting that occurs mostly in the morning favors pregnancy, alcohol use, uremia, and increased intracranial pressure. Provocative features such as knowing the relationship of symptoms to eating can be helpful. The onset of nausea and vomiting immediately after eating strongly suggests an eating disorder, whereas postprandial symptom onset can point to obstruction or gastroparesis. In gastroparesis, patients will also often complain of early satiety. The vomitus might even contain ingested food from the previous day. Small bowel obstruction is associated with large volumes of bilious emesis with colicky periumbilical pain. Other important distinguishing quality features of the vomitus are whether it is feculent or projectile. A feculent vomitus occurs in a distal small bowel obstruction while projectile vomiting

TABLE 21.1 Causes of nausea and vomiting

Conditions within the GI tract	Conditions outside the GI tract	
Obstructive • Pyloric obstruction • Small bowel obstruction • Colonic obstruction Enteric infections • Viral gastroenteritis • Bacterial gastroenteritis • Hepatitis Inflammatory diseases • Cholecystitis • Pancreatitis • Appendicitis Impaired motility • Gastroparesis • Intestinal pseudo-obstruction • Functional dyspepsia • Gastroesophageal reflux • Irritable bowel syndrome Malignancy • Pancreatic cancer • Metastatic disease • Radiation therapy Mucosal injury • Peptic ulcer disease • Gastritis • Esophagitis	Pregnancy • Hyperemesis gravidarum Cardiopulmonary disease • Myocardial infarction • Cardiomyopathy Labyrinthine diesease • Motion sickness • Viral Labyrinthitis • Malignancy Intracerebral disorders (increased intracranial pressure) • Brain tumor • Hemorrhage • Abscess • Pseudotumor cerebri Seizure disorders Demyelinating diseases Migraine CNS infections • Meningitis • Encephalitis Cyclic vomiting syndrome Psychiatric illness • Anorexia and bulimia • Depression • Anxiety • Psychogenic	Medications • Cancer chemotherapy • Antibiotics • Digoxin • Oral hypoglycemics • Oral contraceptives • Nonsteroid anti-inflammatory drugs • Beta blockers • Opioids • Theophylline • Iron supplements Toxins • Ethanol Endocrine/metabolic disease • Uremia • Liver failure • Ketoacidosis • Thyroid and parathyroid disease • Adrenal insufficiency Nephrolithiasis (renal colic) Postoperative vomiting

Adapted from Kaspar DL. *Harrison's Principles of Internal Medicine,* 16th ed. New York: McGraw-Hill, 2004. With permission.

occurs in pyloric (or gastric outlet) obstruction or in intracerebral process causing increased intracranial pressure. Pyloric obstruction may also produce a sensation of epigastric fullness, blunt pain, nausea, and weight loss and can lead to the vomiting of food consumed even days before.

The identification of associated symptoms can be the key to further narrowing the differential. Neurologic symptoms such as vision changes, headache, photophobia, and vertigo will point to a CNS or labyrinthine cause. The presence of other GI symptoms like constipation and diarrhea can be important. For example, diarrhea along with nausea and vomiting suggests gastroenteritis. The presence of constipation can lead to a consideration of colon obstruction or pseudo-obstruction. The latter condition is impaired motility of either the small bowel and colon resulting retention of food residue, abdominal distention, pain, and altered bowel movements. Pseudo-obstruction can be idiopathic or caused by inherited conditions or systemic diseases including a malignant or paraneoplastic process.

TABLE 21.2 Clinical clues associated with the causes of nausea and vomiting

Clinical clues → Possible cause of nausea and vomiting

Duration

Acute onset →	GI tract:	Non-GI tract:
	Obstruction	Toxins and medications
	Gastroenteritis	Meningitis
	Inflammatory condition	CNS hemorrhage
		Myocardial infarction

Quality

Bilious → Small bowel obstruction
Feculent → Small bowel obstruction or rarely colonic
Projectile → Pyloric obstruction or intracerebral condition
Hematemesis → Peptic ulcer disease, esophageal varices, esophagitis (GERD), Mallory-Weiss tear
Partially digested food → Gastroparesis or pyloric obstruction

Quantity

Large volumes → Small bowel obstruction

Frequency

Only in the morning → Pregnancy, intracerebral condition, uremia, and alcohol use
Recurrent and intermittent → Cyclic vomiting syndrome

Provocative features

Immediately after eating → Eating disorder (bulimia)
>1 hour after eating → Gastroparesis or pyloric obstruction
While a passenger in car → Motion sickness
Recumbent posture → Intracranial involving the posterior fossa
After taking medications → Medications
Recent picnic with potato salad → Bacterial gastroenteritis ("food poisoning")

Associated symptoms

Crampy, colicky pain → Obstructive conditions
Abdominal pain relieved with vomiting → Pyloric obstruction
Bloating → Colonic obstruction or pseudo-obstruction
Epigastric pain radiating to back → Pancreatitis
Right upper quadrant abdominal pain → Cholecystitis
Right lower quadrant abdominal pain→ Appendicitis
Abdominal pain radiating to groin → Nephrolithiasis (renal colic)
Jaundice, dark urine, light stools → Hepatitis or choledocholithiasis
Constipation → Colonic obstruction or pseudo-obstruction
Diarrhea, myalgia, headache → Viral gastroenteritis
Chest pain and diaphoresis →Myocardial infarction
Headache → Migraine, meningitis, gastroenteritis, or intracerebral process
Neck stiffness, photophobia, altered mental status → Meningitis
Vertigo and ataxia → Labyrinthitis
Vertigo and tinnitus → Ménière's disease
Altered mental status → CNS infection or toxin ingestion
Missed menstrual period → Early pregnancy

(continued)

TABLE 21.2 Clinical clues associated with the causes of nausea and vomiting (*continued*)

Clinical clues → Possible cause of nausea and vomiting
Associated comorbid conditions
Diabetes → Ketoacidosis or gastroparesis
History of abdominal surgery → Small bowel obstruction
Heart disease → Myocardial infarction
Kidney disease → Uremia
Peptic ulcer disease → Pyloric obstruction
Pregnancy → Hyperemesis gravidarum, acute fatty liver, HELLP syndrome
Migraine headaches → Cyclic vomiting syndrome
Physical exam findings
Fever → Infection or inflammatory conditions
Quiet bowel sounds → Pseudo-obstruction
High-pitched bowel sounds → Mechanical obstruction
Succussion splash → Pyloric obstruction
Tympanic abdomen → Obstructive conditions
Rebound and guarding → Inflammatory disorders
Papilledema → Intracerebral disorders
Nystagmus → Labrynthine disorder
Kernig and Brudzinski signs → Meningitis
Tachycardia, gallops, edema → Cardiomyopathy
Dental enamel erosion → Bulimia

Adapted from Tierney LM, Henderson M. *The Patient History: Evidence-based approach.* New York: McGraw-Hill, 2004.

Nausea and vomiting are also associated with many medications and co-existing medical conditions ranging from pregnancy to diabetes mellitus. Pregnancy is associated with hyperemesis gravidum, severe nausea, and vomiting occurring in the first trimester. Two other conditions associated with nausea and vomiting and pregnancy, acute fatty liver and HELLP (hemolysis, elevated liver tests, low platelets) syndrome, occur in the second and third trimester. Diabetics are prone to an impaired motility disorder known as gastroparesis or chronic delayed gastric emptying.

Pyloric (or gastric outlet) obstruction in adults is most commonly associated with peptic ulcer disease.

The physical examination should be guided by the information from the history. If a GI tract cause is suspected, then a focused abdominal and rectal exam will be essential. For example, bowel sounds may be quiet or absent in patients with a pseudo-obstruction, whereas high-pitched bowel sounds could suggest an early mechanical bowel obstruction. A distended and tympanic abdomen suggests a bowel obstruction. Tenderness to palpation with rebound or guarding raises the strong possibility of an inflammatory disorder with associated peritoneal signs. A succussion splash can be heard during auscultation of the abdomen in patients with a gastric outlet obstruction or gastroparesis when the patient is passively shaken. Rectal examination can reveal melena or hematochezia to suggest GI hemorrhage from a specific cause like peptic ulcer disease (PUD) or gastritis or from a complication of vomiting like a Mallory-Weiss tear. If a non-GI tract cause is suspected, then the physical examination findings should complement the history. For example, in patients with a suspected intracerebral condition caused by increased intracranial pressure, the neurologic examination may reveal papilledema, focal neurologic deficits, or visual field cuts. For example, pseudotumor cerebri is a condition affecting obese young women and characterized with intracranial hypertension not caused by a mass. Patients present with headache, nausea, and pulsatile tinnitus. On examination, they will universally have papilledema and many will have a sixth nerve deficits.

EVALUATION

The evaluation of nausea and vomiting begins with an assessment of the acuity and severity of symptoms and any immediate complications. Certain causes and complications of nausea and vomiting are emergencies and as such must be recognized immediately in order that urgent diagnostic tests and therapy are provided. These conditions include obstruction, intra-abdominal perforation, peritonitis, myocardial infarction, CNS infection, intracranial hemorrhage, toxic ingestion, aspiration, and gastrointestinal hemorrhage.

Severe or protracted nausea and vomiting can present with orthostatic hypotension and lethargy secondary to dehydration and electrolyte disturbances such as hypokalemia, azotemia, or metabolic alkalosis. These also must be addressed as soon as possible.

In the nonurgent presentation of nausea and vomiting, the findings from the thorough history and examination will point to a gastrointestinal or nongastrointestinal cause and guide the selection of appropriate tests such as routine hematologic tests, biochemical screening, drug levels, toxicology, imaging (plain abdominal radiograph, ultrasounds, computed tomography scans, magnetic resonance imaging), gastric emptying studies, and endoscopy.

CHAPTER 22

Seizures

Geoffrey C. Lamb and Dario Torre

A seizure or "convulsion" is a paroxysmal event due to an abnormal, excessive, electrical discharges from a locus of neurons in the brain. Up to 10% of the population will have at least one seizure during their lifetime, with the highest incidence occurring in early childhood and late adulthood.

The occurrence of a seizure does not necessarily imply epilepsy. *Epilepsy* is a general term describing a group of disorders in which a person has recurrent seizures due to a chronic, underlying process, independent of toxins, metabolic disorders, or acute injury. There are many forms and causes of epilepsy, but true epilepsy affects less than 2% of the population.

DIFFERENTIAL DIAGNOSIS

Seizures may be either partial (synonymous with focal) or generalized (Table 22.1). Partial seizures are those in which the seizure activity is restricted to isolated areas of the cerebral cortex. Generalized seizures involve diffuse regions of the brain simultaneously (Chapter 109).

Disorders that must be differentiated from a seizure include syncope, migraine, transient ischemic attack, psychogenic seizures (nonepileptic seizure), and panic attacks (Table 22.2). Once it has been determined that the event is truly a seizure, then it is important to differentiate between the multiple neurologic and systemic disorders that can lead to a seizure (Fig. 22.1).

EVALUATION

An in-depth history is the most important and essential feature in the evaluation of any seizure. Questions should be focused on the symptoms before, during, and after the episode in order to discriminate a seizure from other paroxysmal events. Seizures frequently occur out-of-hospital and the patient may be unaware of the ictal (during the seizure) and immediate postictal phases; thus, witnesses to the event should be interviewed carefully.

A common diagnostic challenge is distinguishing tonic–clonic seizure from syncope (Table 22.2). Tonic–clonic seizure and syncope can both be characterized by loss of consciousness and a fall. Muscle twitching can also be seen in some episodes of syncope. Syncope is suggested by an onset while the patient is erect and by a brief duration (10 seconds), flaccid muscle tone during the event, pale color, cold and clammy skin, or electrocardiographic abnormalities. Tonic–clonic seizure is suggested by an onset while the patient is asleep or awake and in any posture, duration of 1 minute or longer, increased muscle tone during the event, incontinence, biting of the tongue, flushed color, hot and sweaty skin, effortful respiration, or a family history of seizures.

TABLE 22.1 Classification of seizures

I. Generalized seizures (bilaterally symmetrical and without local onset)
  A. Tonic, clonic, or tonic–clonic (grand mal)
  B. Absence (petit mal)
    1. With loss of consciousness only
    2. Complex—with brief tonic, clonic, or automatic movements
  C. Lennox-Gastaut syndrome
  D. Juvenile myoclonic epilepsy
  E. Infantile spasms
  F. Atonic (astatic, akinetic) seizures (sometimes with myoclonic jerks)
II. Partial, or focal, seizures (seizures beginning locally)
  A. Simple (without loss of consciousness or alteration in psychic function)
    1. Motor–frontal lobe origin (tonic, clonic, tonic–clonic; jacksonian; benign childhood epilepsy; epilepsia partialis continua)
    2. Somatosensory or special sensory (visual, auditory, olfactory, gustatory, vertiginous)
    3. Autonomic
    4. Pure psychic
  B. Complex (with impaired consciousness)
    1. Beginning as simple partial seizures and progressing to impairment of consciousness
    2. With impairment of consciousness at onset
III. Special epileptic syndromes
  A. Myoclonus and myoclonic seizures
  B. Reflex epilepsy
  C. Acquired aphasia with convulsive disorder
  D. Febrile and other seizures of infancy and childhood
  E. Hysterical seizures

Risk factors for seizures include a history of febrile seizures, earlier undiagnosed episodic spells, and family history of seizures. Epileptogenic factors such as prior head trauma, stroke, tumor, or vascular malformation should be identified. Precipitating factors such as sleep deprivation, systemic diseases, electrolyte or metabolic derangements, acute infection, drugs that lower the seizure threshold, or alcohol or illicit drug use should also be identified.

A physical examination is performed to look for signs of disorders associated with seizures, including signs of head trauma and infections of the ears or sinuses (which may spread to the brain). The presence of abnormal neurological signs (hemiparesis, ataxia, sensory loss) may suggest brain tumor, encephalitis, or vascular malformation. The presence of hepatomegaly may suggest alcohol abuse with resulting alcoholic encephalopathy, abnormal lung findings, and weight loss (wheezing, crackles) may raise suspicion for lung cancer with metastatic brain disease. Café au lait spots may indicate congenital neurologic disease such as tuberous sclerosis.

The electroencephalogram provides three types of information: confirmation of the presence of abnormal electrical activity, information about the type of seizure disorder, and the location of the seizure focus. It is customary to perform electroencephalographic studies 48 hours or more after a suspected seizure, because obtaining an electroencephalogram shortly after a seizure may yield misleading findings due to the postictal period. The electroencephalogram should include

TABLE 22.2 Disorders and clinical features that may help distinguish seizures from other disorders

Disorder	Clinical presentation	Comment
Seizure	Prolonged LOC (minutes) Prolonged recovery Onset abrupt or preceded byaura Usually not related to posture Urinary incontinence: sometimes	Aura: bad smell, déjà-vu Postictal state: headache, drowsiness may last minutes to hours
Syncope	Brief LOC (seconds) Rapid recovery Onset may be sudden or preceded by premonitory symptoms Urinary incontinence: rare May be related to posture	Premonitory symptoms: lightheadedness, nausea, sweating, dizziness
TIA	Rare LOC Onset abrupt Neurological deficits 5 to 20 minutes	Neurological deficits: (hemiparesis, aphasia, monocular blindness)
Migraine	Rare LOC History of migraine Occasional neurological deficits Onset variable with aura Severe headaches	Aura: flashing lights, visual field deficits, hemisensory loss
Psychogenic seizures	Epilepsy may be concomitant History of psychiatric illness Lack of response to antiepileptic drugs Social and environmental triggers	It may be difficult to distinguish from complex partial seizures due shared behavioral features (anxiety, fear, depression)
Panic attacks	Brief LOC History of psychiatric illness Hyperventilation Palpitations, trembling, dizziness	LOC may be secondary to severe hyperventilation

LOC, loss of consciousness.

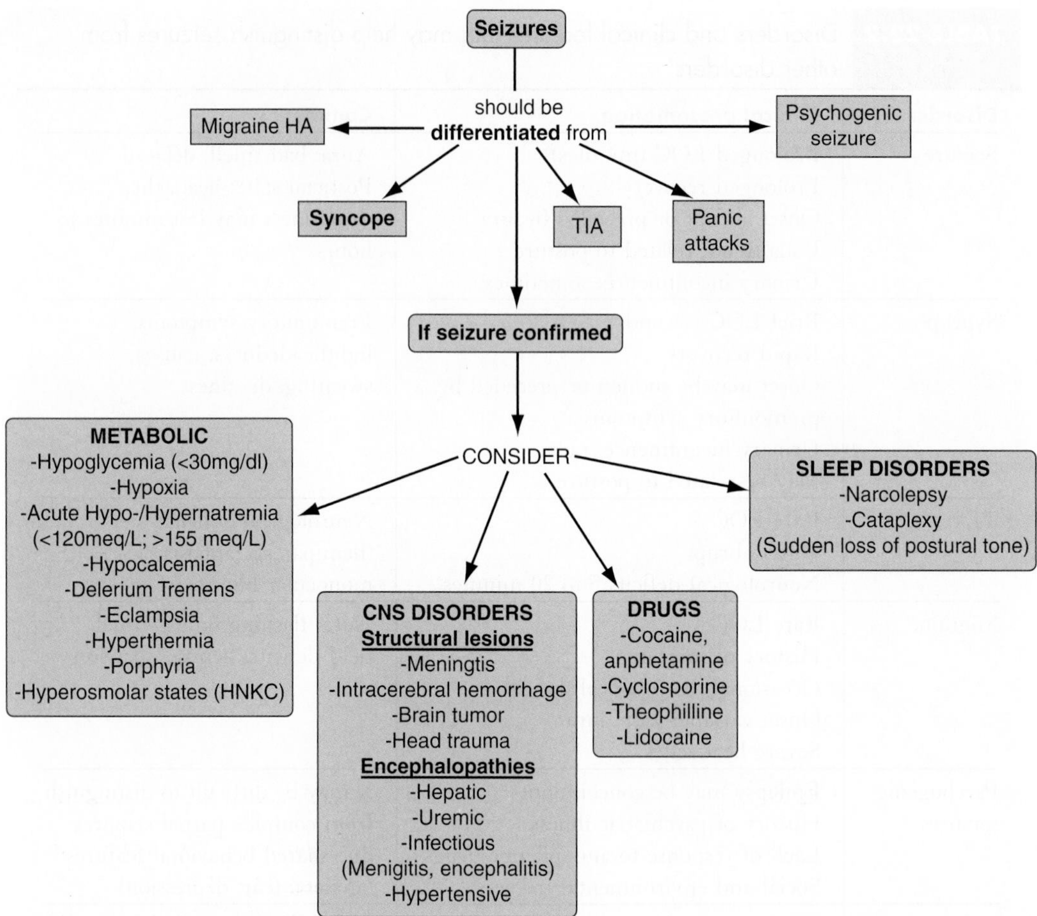

Figure 22.1 • Differential diagnosis of seizures. CNS, central nervous system; HA, headache; HNKC, hyperosmolar nonketotic coma; ICH, intracerebral hemorrhage; TIA, transient ischemic attack.

recordings during sleep, photic stimulation, and hyperventilation, because certain types of paroxysmal activity are most likely to occur under these conditions.

Laboratory studies performed to look for metabolic causes of a newly diagnosed seizure disorder include electrolyte and liver function tests in all patients. A screening test for toxic substances is performed if alcohol or drug abuse or withdrawal is suspected, and a lumbar puncture is performed if infection or cancer is suspected. Neuroimaging should be performed immediately in patients who are suspected to have a structural lesion. These include patients who have new focal deficits, a persistently altered mental status (with or without intoxication), fever, recent trauma, persistent headache, or a history of cancer or anticoagulant therapy and those who are immunosuppressed (cancer, human immunodeficiency virus).

CHAPTER 23

Shock

Ann Maguire

Shock is more than a symptom; it is a clinical syndrome resulting from inadequate tissue perfusion and oxygenation. Hypotension (mean arterial pressure <60 mm Hg in previously normotensive persons) is the finding most commonly associated with shock. Mortality rates for patients presenting with shock range from 40% to 80%.

The pathophysiology of circulatory shock is complex. Tissue hypoperfusion causes cellular injury and creates an imbalance between tissue oxygen supply and demand. In addition to causing tissue hypoxia and cell death, hypoperfusion results in the production of inflammatory mediators and other hormonal changes that affect the ability of vascular smooth muscle to constrict. The final common pathway for all forms of long-lasting severe shock appears to be vasodilation that is nonresponsive to vasopressor drugs. The resulting prolonged tissue hypoperfusion ultimately causes irreversible cell death and organ failure.

DIFFERENTIAL DIAGNOSIS

There are numerous ways to classify the processes leading to shock. Understanding the underlying cause of shock is critical to initiating the proper therapy. Shock can be categorized broadly into three types: hypovolemic shock (preload failure), vasodilatory shock (afterload failure), and cardiogenic shock (pump failure). Symptoms common to all causes of shock include hypotension, tachycardia, oliguria, and altered mental status. Many patients also experience hypoxia, hepatic dysfunction, and bowel ischemia due to prolonged hypotension (Table 23.1).

Hypovolemic Shock

Hypovolemic shock is one of the most common forms of shock. Hypovolemia causes a loss of ventricular filling (also known as decreased preload), which leads to a drop in cardiac output and subsequent vasoconstriction and increased systemic vascular resistance (SVR). The pulmonary capillary wedge pressure (PCWP) as measured by a pulmonary artery catheter is always low in such patients.

Hypovolemic shock can be either hemorrhagic or nonhemorrhagic. In hemorrhagic hypovolemic shock, patients who have lost 20% of their overall blood volume will begin to show symptoms including cool extremities, increased capillary refill time, diaphoresis, collapsed veins, and anxiety. Moderate blood loss (20% to 40% of blood volume) can be associated with the same symptoms plus tachycardia, tachypnea, oliguria, and postural hypotension. Patients who have suffered severe blood loss (>40% blood volume) demonstrate hemodynamic instability including hypotension, marked tachycardia (heart rate >120 bpm), and alterations in mental status including agitation, confusion, and obtundation. Nonhemorrhagic hypovolemic shock is associated with loss of plasma volume due to extravascular fluid sequestration such as that seen in massive ascites, very large gastrointestinal losses from diarrhea or vomiting, excessive urinary losses due to polyuria from diabetes insipidus or osmotic diuresis due to severe hyperglycemia, and excessive insensible volume losses often associated

TABLE 23.1 Differential diagnosis of shock

Hypovolemic
Hemorrhage
Diarrhea
Vomiting
Polyuria
Hyperthermia
Vasodilatory
Sepsis
Neurogenic
Hypoadrenal
Anaphylactic
Trauma
Pancreatitis
Burns
Toxins/medications
Cardiogenic
Myopathic
Arrhythmic
Mechanical
Extracardiac (obstructive) tension pneumothorax

with hyperthermia or heat stroke. As in all forms of shock, the onset of mental status changes is a very ominous sign and can indicate imminent death.

Vasodilatory Shock

Vasodilatory shock is caused by a loss of vascular tone (afterload failure) in the arteries and to a lesser extent veins and is associated with both low SVR and normal to low PCWP. Cardiac output is often elevated initially, but in prolonged shock it will later decrease. Causes of vasodilatory shock include: sepsis, neurogenic injury, adrenal crisis, anaphylaxis, pancreatitis, trauma, and severe burns.

Septic shock is best understood as tissue hypoperfusion in the setting of an infection-induced syndrome that includes the presence of two or more of the following features of systemic inflammation: fever or hypothermia, leukocytosis or leukopenia, tachycardia, and tachypnea. Sepsis occurs most frequently among immunocompromised patients. Infections are most often caused by gram-negative bacteria including *Escherichia coli*, *Klebsiella*, *Proteus*, and *Pseudomonas*. Gram-positive cocci (*Staphylococcus* and *Streptococcus*) and gram-negative anaerobes (*Bacteroides*) are less common causes of shock. Endotoxins released by gram-negative bacteria in particular cause adult respiratory distress syndrome, thrombocytopenia, and neutropenia in addition to decreasing myocardial contractility. Oliguric renal failure and lactic acidosis are also common.

Neurogenic shock is caused by the disruption of sympathetic vasomotor input and can be associated with central nervous system (CNS) injuries such as severe closed head trauma or high cervical spinal cord injury. Unlike most other forms of shock, neurogenic shock does not cause peripheral vasoconstriction. Therefore, extremities remain warm and appear well perfused.

Adrenal crisis or hypoadrenal shock occurs in settings in which unrecognized adrenal insufficiency complicates the patient's response to the stress induced by acute illness or major surgery. The normal response to illness, surgery, or trauma is a hypersecretion of cortisol that helps to maintain vascular tone. Patients with idiopathic adrenal atrophy, Addison's disease, or other systemic illnesses such as tuberculosis, metastatic carcinoma, and amyloidosis are prone to this form of shock.

Anaphylaxis, trauma, pancreatitis, severe burns, medication overdose, and toxins are known causes of shock in which the patient's medical history and circumstances surrounding the presentation may be the most important factors in making a diagnosis.

Cardiogenic Shock

Cardiogenic shock (pump failure) is defined by a primary decrease in cardiac output in the presence of adequate intravascular volume. The low output produces vasoconstriction, increase in SVR and high PCWP. The causes of cardiogenic shock can be divided into four categories: myopathic, arrhythmic, mechanical, and extracardiac (obstructive). Cardiomyopathy due to ischemia (Chapter 29), including myocardial infarction, is the most common cause of cardiogenic shock. Other myopathic causes include significant cardiac contusion, severe ischemic heart disease, or end-stage dilated cardiomyopathy. Patients may present with shock secondary to right heart failure in the setting of right ventricular infarct or severe pulmonary hypertension. The most common sign of left heart failure is pulmonary congestion. Both atrial and ventricular arrhythmias either bradycardic or tachycardic can produce shock by decreasing cardiac output. Valvular heart disease including acute mitral regurgitation, acute aortic insufficiency, and critical aortic stenosis can cause shock. Ventricular septal defects or ruptured aneurysms are also potential causes. Extrinsic factors that reduce myocardial compliance include pericardial tamponade (muffled heart sounds, pulsus paradoxus), tension pneumothorax (neck vein distension, asymmetric breath sounds, and tracheal deviation), and massive pulmonary embolism (chest pain, hypercoagulable states, hypoxia).

EVALUATION

The clinical progression of circulatory shock is summarized in Table 23.2. Some patients can present with a picture of clinical shock with a "normal" blood pressure, especially if prior hypertension has

TABLE 23.2 Clinical stages of circulatory shock

	Stage I (preshock)	Stage II (organ hypoperfusion)	Stage III (end-organ failure)
Mental state	Clear but distress present	Confusion, restlessness	Apathy, agitation, or coma
Skin	Pale and cool	Cool and clammy	Cool, cyanotic, and mottled
Peripheral vasoconstriction	Mild	Marked	Intense
Blood pressure	Normal or slightly low	Hypotension	Undetectable by cuff
Urine output	Oliguria	Oliguria	Anuria
Heart rate	Tachycardia	Tachycardia	Tachycardia
Other	Tachypnea, respiratory alkalosis	Respiratory failure, lactic acidosis, possible angina	Severe metabolic acidosis, multiple organ failure

From Teba L, Banks DE, Balaan MR. Understanding circulatory shock. Is it hypovolemic, cardiogenic, or vasogenic? *Postgrad Med* 1992;91:124, with permission.

been present. Conversely, a systolic blood pressure below 90 mm hg is not necessarily shock because end-organ hypoperfusion also should be present, manifested by general fatigue and weakness and features of hypoperfusion of the kidneys, central nervous system, and skin.

Most specialists use a pulmonary artery catheter placed percutaneously via the subclavian or jugular vein to assess the hemodynamic profiles of patients in shock and to classify them according to three broad categories: hypovolemic, cardiogenic, and vasodilatory. The procedure involves the measurement of the following key parameters: central venous pressure, PCWP, cardiac index, left ventricle stroke work index, SVR, and total O_2 consumption index or venous O_2 concentration (Fig. 23.1).

The evaluation of shock must include a thorough physical examination since the mental status changes often associated with shock make it difficult to obtain a detailed medical history. A review of medical records is essential to identify valuable information that might point toward a specific cause of shock. Examples of such historical clues include food and medication allergies and recent ingestions, recent changes in medications, potential acute or chronic drug intoxication, pre-existing

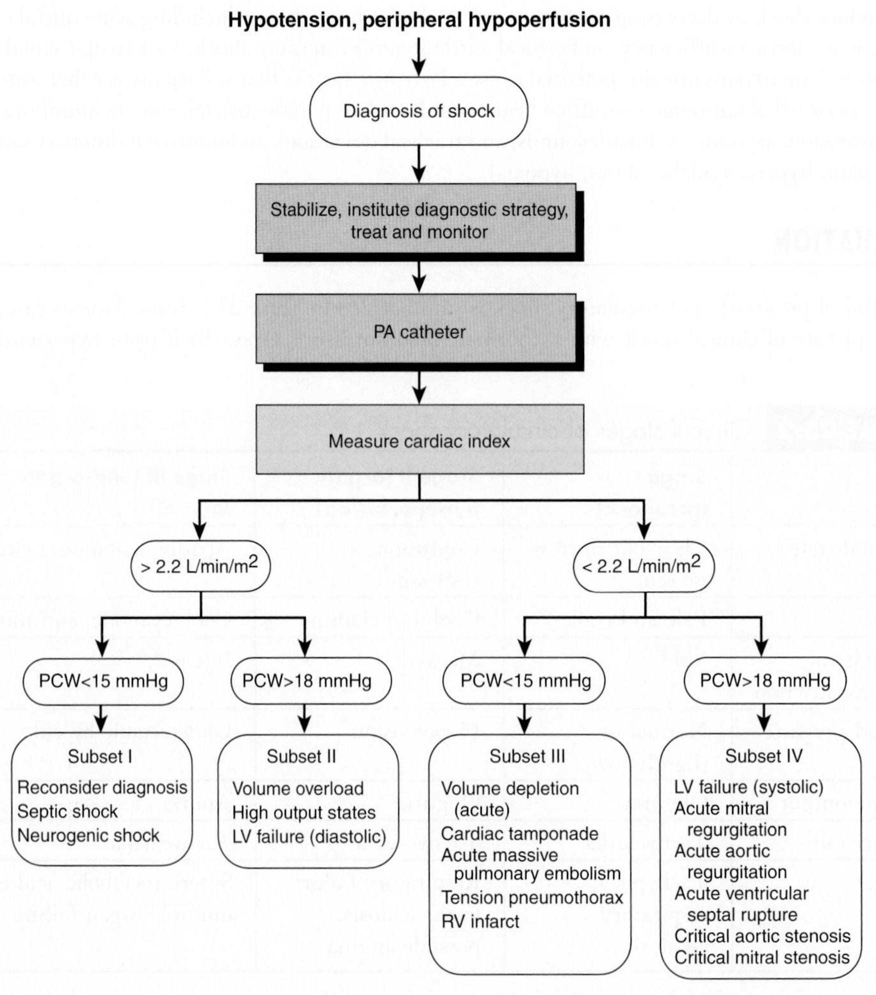

Figure 23.1 • Determination of hemodynamic subgroups in cardiogenic shock.

diseases, immunosuppressed states, and hypercoagulable conditions. Because tissue hypoxia is such an important part of the shock syndrome, early assessment of ventilation and oxygenation is needed. All patients should have a chest x-ray (CXR), which may be suggestive of congestive heart failure or infection, and arterial blood gas to evaluate for potential causes of shock and assess acid-base status. Following this assessment, further evaluation with laboratory and other testing should be performed. In many cases, the workup occurs in the intensive care unit and may take place while the patient is being prepared for pulmonary artery catheterization.

It is necessary to rule out hypovolemia in all patients presenting with symptoms of shock. The complete blood count will identify anemia and estimate the degree of blood loss in hemorrhagic shock. A comprehensive metabolic panel provides information about glucose, electrolytes, and renal function. Extreme hyperglycemia may point to hyperosmolar states that can cause polyuria. Electrolyte abnormalities including hypokalemia, hypo- or hypernatremia, and hypomagnesemia can be seen in patients with severe diarrhea and vomiting.

Sepsis is the most common cause of vasodilatory shock. Septic patients can present with either fever or hypothermia. All patients in whom sepsis is suspected should undergo a thorough investigation for infection including a CXR to rule out pneumonia. Urinalysis and urine cultures to identify urinary sources of infection should always be performed and sputum Gram stain and culture to identify respiratory pathogens should be attempted when sputum is available. Two sets of blood cultures on initial presentation prior to initiation of antibiotic therapy are needed to identify bacteremia and to help guide future therapy. Additional sets of blood cultures may be needed later depending on the clinical situation. Other laboratory testing including serum lactate, fibrinogen, and fibrin split products can identify patients likely to have sepsis related metabolic acidosis or disseminated intravascular coagulation. If adrenal crisis is suspected, serum cortisol measurement followed by functional assessment with a cosyntropin stimulation test may be needed. Measurement of serum amylase and lipase can identify acute pancreatitis. Computed tomography scanning of the abdomen to identify pancreatitis may or may not be helpful in the first few hours, but often is an important part of later management.

When indicated by the history and clinical presentation, early serum and urinary toxicology screening is important to exclude toxins; in particular situations, measurement of therapeutic drug levels to identify medication overdoses is warranted. Computed tomography and magnetic resonance imaging of the CNS including brain and spinal cord is needed in patients suspected to have neurogenic shock.

All patients presenting with shock should undergo an electrocardiogram to look for evidence of ischemia and acute infarction. This should be accompanied by measurement of serum cardiac enzymes. When an acute coronary syndrome is identified as the cause of shock, specialized management in a cardiac intensive care unit with a cardiac specialist is needed. Patients may require emergent cardiac catheterization and revascularization. Physical examination with attention to neck vein distention and findings associated with pulmonary edema is critical. CXR to look for evidence of cardiomegaly and pulmonary edema is very important. A two-dimensional echocardiogram can also help identify cardiomyopathic causes of cardiogenic shock that are ischemic and nonischemic. Mechanical causes of cardiogenic shock including valvular heart disease and obstructive causes such as cardiac tamponade are most easily assessed with echocardiography. All patients with shock should be placed on telemetry monitoring even if cardiogenic causes of shock are not suspected, because such monitoring increases the likelihood of detecting bradyarrhythmia and tachyarrhythmia. Tension pneumothorax should be suspected when the physical examination demonstrates asymmetric breath sounds, elevated jugular venous pressure (JVP), and hypotension. A CXR should be ordered and immediate intervention is required. Massive pulmonary embolism should be investigated when appropriate using either ventilation perfusion scanning, chest computed tomography with a pulmonary embolism protocol, and, in some cases, pulmonary angiogram.

CHAPTER 24

Syncope

Ann Maguire

Syncope is a sudden and brief loss of consciousness associated with a loss of postural tone. Recovery is usually spontaneous. Syncope is not a disease, but rather a symptom with causes ranging from benign to life-threatening. It is a common reason for emergency department evaluation and hospitalization; however, the etiology is often difficult to identify. The cause of syncope may be "unknown" in more than one third of cases. Because of the potential seriousness of this diagnosis and the high frequency of unknown etiology, it is helpful to approach the evaluation of patients with syncope in an organized fashion. The goal in evaluation of patients with syncope is to distinguish between benign and life-threatening causes of syncope so that hospitalization and invasive testing can be appropriately used in the care of those most at risk for adverse outcomes.

DIFFERENTIAL DIAGNOSIS

The causes of syncope can be broadly organized according to six major categories: neurally mediated syncope, cardiac syncope, orthostatic hypotension, neurologic disease, medications, and psychiatric disorders (Table 24.1).

Neurally Mediated Syncope

Neurally mediated syncope, also known as neurocardiogenic or reflex-mediated syncope, is the most common cause of syncope, particularly in younger patients without a history of organic heart disease. It includes three subtypes: vasovagal attacks or vasodepressor syncope, situational syncope, and carotid-sinus syncope or carotid sinus hypersensitivity. Individuals with neurally mediated syncope appear to be particularly susceptible to activities or exposures that stimulate the Bezold-Jarisch reflex. This reflex is activated via intracardiac vagal mechanoreceptors. Valsalva maneuver or prolonged standing may cause decreased cardiac venous return or venous pooling which leads to a drop in blood pressure and subsequent release of catecholamines. The catecholamine release triggers the Bezold-Jarisch reflex and results in a further increase in vagal tone causing simultaneous bradycardia and peripheral vasodilation. Hypotension and loss of consciousness may follow. This pathway explains vasovagal attacks and situational syncope quite well. In carotid sinus syncope, direct stimulation of the carotid artery can cause a cardioinhibitory (bradycardic) or vasodepressor response regardless of posture or adequacy of cardiac venous return.

Individuals with neurally mediated syncope often report a symptomatic prodrome that includes nausea, feelings of warmth, diaphoresis, and blurring or darkening of vision followed immediately by a brief loss of consciousness. Vasovagal attacks may occur after prolonged standing or intense emotional experiences such as unexpected pain, fear, or unpleasant sights, sounds, and smells. Patients may report syncope associated with throat or facial pain. Common causes of situational syncope include cough, defecation, micturition, or swallowing. Those with carotid-sinus syncope may experience syncope with head rotation or with pressure applied to the carotid sinus caused by shaving, tight collars, or tumors (Table 24.2).

TABLE 24.1 Causes of syncope

Cause	Mean prevalence (range)[a]
Neurally mediated syncope	
Vasovagal attack	18 (8–37)
Situational syncope	5 (1–8)
Carotid-sinus syncope	1 (0–4)
Psychiatric disorders	2 (1–7)
Orthostatic hypotension	8 (4–10)
Medications	3 (1–7)
Neurologic disease	10 (3–32)
Cardiac syncope	
Organic heart disease[b]	4 (1–8)
Arrhythmias	14 (4–38)
Unknown	34 (13–41)

[a]Percent of patients with syncope.
[b]Structural heart disease that causes syncope such as aortic stenosis, pulmonary hypertension, pulmonary embolism, or myocardial infarction.
Adapted from Figure 36.1 in Kochar 4th edition, p. 211 and Kapoor WN. Syncope. *N Engl J Med 2000*;343:1856–1862, with permission.

Cardiac Syncope

Cardiac causes of syncope can be categorized according to the presence or absence of organic heart disease and arrhythmia. Organic heart disease includes structural heart disease due to aortic stenosis, mitral stenosis, hypertrophic cardiomyopathy, and ischemic heart disease as well as vascular causes such as pulmonary embolus and pulmonary hypertension. Syncope in the setting of exertion is characteristic of patients who have severe aortic stenosis, hypertrophic cardiomyopathy, or ischemic heart disease. Syncope due to a sudden drop in cardiac output may also be a presenting symptom of life-threatening diseases such as aortic dissection and pericardial tamponade. Pulmonary embolism and pulmonary hypertension are uncommon vascular causes of syncope. Syncope in the setting of pulmonary embolism is caused by a massive thrombus formation leading to right ventricular failure, diminished right ventricular output, and consequent decreased left ventricular cardiac output.

Arrhythmias, either bradycardic or tachycardic, are more common cardiac causes of syncope. Bradyarrhythmias include sinus node disease, second- and third-degree heart block, and bradycardia associated with pacemaker malfunction. Medications causing bradycardia and syncope will be discussed separately. Tachyarrhythmias include ventricular tachycardia, torsades de pointes, ventricular fibrillation, and supraventricular tachycardia. A known history of ischemic heart disease or a dilated or hypertrophic cardiomyopathy makes arrhythmia more likely to be the cause of syncope. A family history of sudden cardiac death raises the possibility of ventricular fibrillation due to long QT syndrome or Brugada syndrome (pseudo right bundle branch block and persistent ST segment elevation in V1 to V3). Patients with bradycardia often experience sudden loss of consciousness without warning, whereas those with tachyarrhythmias are more likely to describe palpitations.

Orthostatic Hypotension

Syncope associated with changes in position is often due to orthostatic hypotension. When an individual assumes an upright posture, normal homeostatic mechanisms (arteriolar and venous constriction,

TABLE 24.2 Clinical features, electrocardiogram, and other key diagnostic testing related to common causes of syncope

Cause	Clinical features	Physical findings	Electrocardiogram	Testing
Vasovagal	Occurs after prolonged standing, associated nausea, diaphoresis, darkened vision	Normal	Normal	History may be diagnostic, tilt table testing
Situational	Occurs with cough, defecation, micturition, or swallowing	Normal	Normal	History may be diagnostic
Carotid sinus	Occurs with head rotation or carotid pressure	Sometimes carotid bruits	Normal	Carotid massage
Organic heart disease	Occurs with exertion, associated dyspnea	Normal exam, murmur	Evidence of ischemia or cardiomyopathy	Stress testing indicated
Arrhythmia	Palpitations prior to syncope	Normal exam or arrhythmia	Prolonged QT or other arrhythmia	Telemetry or Holter monitor
Orthostatic hypotension	Occurs upon standing	Characteristic rise in pulse and fall in blood pressure	Normal	Tilt table testing
Neurologic	Sudden onset, prolonged period of confusion or lethargy	Witnessed seizures, incontinence	Normal	Electroencephalogram
Medication-related	Multiple drugs, older age	Hypotension, bradycardia	Normal or prolonged QT	History may be diagnostic
Psychiatric	Frequent occurrence, young age, no injuries	Normal	Normal	History may be diagnostic

enhanced heart rate, and increased lower-extremity muscle tone) prevent a significant decrease in systolic blood pressure. Patients with orthostatic hypotension may have inadequate responses or impaired reflexes that cause postural symptoms. Symptomatic orthostatic hypotension may be related to inadequate volume due to dehydration or autonomic impairment caused by a primary autonomic neuropathy secondary to diabetes or other disorders. Medications known to cause orthostatic hypotension will be discussed separately. The hallmark of syncope due to orthostatic hypotension is that it usually occurs immediately upon standing. Vital signs demonstrate an increase in heart rate and a simultaneous drop in blood pressure with position changes from lying to sitting or standing.

Neurologic Disease

Neurologic disorders are an uncommon cause of syncope. Potential causes include migraine, transient ischemic attack (TIA), seizure, and subclavian steal syndrome. Seizures including unwitnessed grand mal seizures and temporal lobe epilepsy are by far the most common neurologic causes of syncope. TIA involving the vertebrobasilar artery can impair cerebellar circulation and lead to syncope. Basilar artery migraines are another reported cause of syncope. Symptoms that suggest a neurologic cause of syncope include witnessed seizure activity, headache, diplopia, and hemiparesis. Syncope due to cardiac and other causes may also result in brief spells of tonic-clonic activity or irregular muscle twitching making it difficult to distinguish these individuals from those with seizure as the underlying cause of syncope. The presence of incontinence or prolonged postictal lethargy and confusion make seizure activity more likely to be the primary cause.

Medications

Medications can lead to syncope by a variety of different mechanisms. Antihypertensives and antidepressant agents are the drug classes most likely to cause syncope. Diuretics are known to cause orthostatic hypotension. Vasodilating antihypertensives can increase the risk of vasovagal attacks and orthostatic hypotension. Beta blockers, clonidine, and cardioselective calcium channel blockers can lead to bradyarrhythmia and syncope. Tricyclic antidepressants and other drugs that cause QT prolongation can lead to ventricular fibrillation and syncope. Opiates, alcohol, and cocaine have been reported to cause syncope and seizures. Elderly patients in particular are at highest risk for medication-related syncope due to the increased prevalence of polypharmacy in this population, the increased risk for organic heart disease, and the greater prevalence of underlying autonomic impairment.

Psychiatric Disorders

A large proportion of patients with otherwise unexplained syncope have been diagnosed with a psychiatric disorder. Generalized anxiety disorder, panic disorder, major depression, and conversion disorders have all been reported to have an increased prevalence among patients who present with syncope. Psychiatric disorders should be considered as potential causes of syncope in young patients who faint frequently, those in whom syncope does not cause any injury, and in those who report many symptoms associated with their syncopal events.

EVALUATION

The most common causes of syncope are vasovagal attacks, organic heart disease, arrhythmias, orthostatic hypotension, and seizures. In many cases, it is possible to identify a potential cause of syncope using history and physical examination alone. Family members and other witnesses can be very helpful historians because they are in some cases better able to describe the events leading up to and following loss of consciousness. History taking should focus on postural symptoms (orthostatic or vasovagal syncope), exertional symptoms or a positive family history of syncope (cardiac syncope, prolonged QT syndromes), palpitations (tachyarrhythmias), postictal symptoms (neurologic syncope), situational symptoms (such as defecation and urination), use of medications, and history of organic heart disease (predisposing to arrhythmias or ischemia). Careful evaluation for the presence of physical findings including murmurs, carotid bruits, asymmetric pulses, and muffled heart sounds is important. Assessment of pulse and blood pressure while lying, sitting, and standing should be performed on all patients presenting with syncope during the initial examination. Every patient should also undergo electrocardiogram (ECG) testing to screen further for evidence of organic heart disease including ischemia, prolonged QT, and arrhythmia (Fig. 24.1).

Situations in which the history, physical examination, and ECG are often diagnostic in patients with syncope include vasovagal attacks, situational syncope, orthostatic hypotension, and polypharmacy. In other cases, the history, physical examination, and ECG may be highly suggestive. Examples include aortic stenosis, pulmonary embolism, seizure, and individuals in whom there is a strong family history of sudden cardiac death. These individuals should undergo further evaluation with specific testing that is dictated by the clinical scenario. Examples of appropriate testing include echocardiography to confirm valvular heart disease and cardiomyopathy, cardiac catheterization to look for evidence of acute coronary syndromes, ventilation-perfusion scanning or computed tomographic angiography to diagnose pulmonary embolism, electroencephalography to assess for seizures, or computed tomography scan of the brain to identify a focal neurologic lesion. Carotid or transcranial Doppler ultrasonography may be performed in the presence of bruits or when symptoms are suggestive of a neurovascular cause of syncope. Holter monitoring, Loop recorders, and electrophysiologic testing may be indicated when arrhythmia is suspected in individuals with a family history of sudden cardiac death. Routine use of basic laboratory tests is not recommended because of evidence that they rarely yield diagnostically useful information; however, these tests may be performed when they are indicated by the results of the history or physical examination.

Evaluation of Unexplained Syncope

After applying the algorithm (Fig. 24.1), a potential cause of syncope can be identified in nearly half of all patients. Before proceeding further, remaining patients with unexplained syncope should be stratified according to age and the likelihood that organic heart disease is present. In this way, it is possible to divide unexplained syncope into three branches.

BRANCH 1: HIGH LIKELIHOOD OF UNDERLYING ORGANIC HEART DISEASE

Patients likely to have organic heart disease are characterized by abnormal ECG, exertional symptoms, and sudden syncope without warning symptoms. All patients in this group should undergo echocardiography and cardiac stress testing. When these studies are abnormal, the next step is Holter monitoring or inpatient telemetry to identify arrhythmias. Those with evidence of ischemia will require appropriate revascularization procedures. Symptoms that increase the likelihood that syncope is related to an arrhythmia include: clustering of "spells," palpitations, sudden loss of consciousness, and use of certain medications. In appropriate cases, patients may require invasive electrophysiologic testing to make a diagnosis of tachyarrhythmia or bradyarrhythmia. If these studies fail to yield a diagnosis, tilt table testing and ultimately psychiatric evaluation is in order.

BRANCH 2: AGE >60 YEARS, WITHOUT LIKELY ORGANIC HEART DISEASE

Older individuals are at increased risk for carotid sinus syncope; therefore, this should be evaluated early. After examining the patient to verify the absence of carotid bruits, a carotid massage is diagnostically positive when more than 3 seconds of pressure results in asystole, hypertension, or both. Carotid massage can be performed at the bedside while the patient is monitored or during a tilt test. Following carotid massage, older patients should undergo echocardiography and cardiac stress testing. If there is evidence of organic heart disease, patients should undergo further evaluation as outlined in Branch 1. In the absence of organic heart disease, arrhythmia must be excluded. This can be investigated using

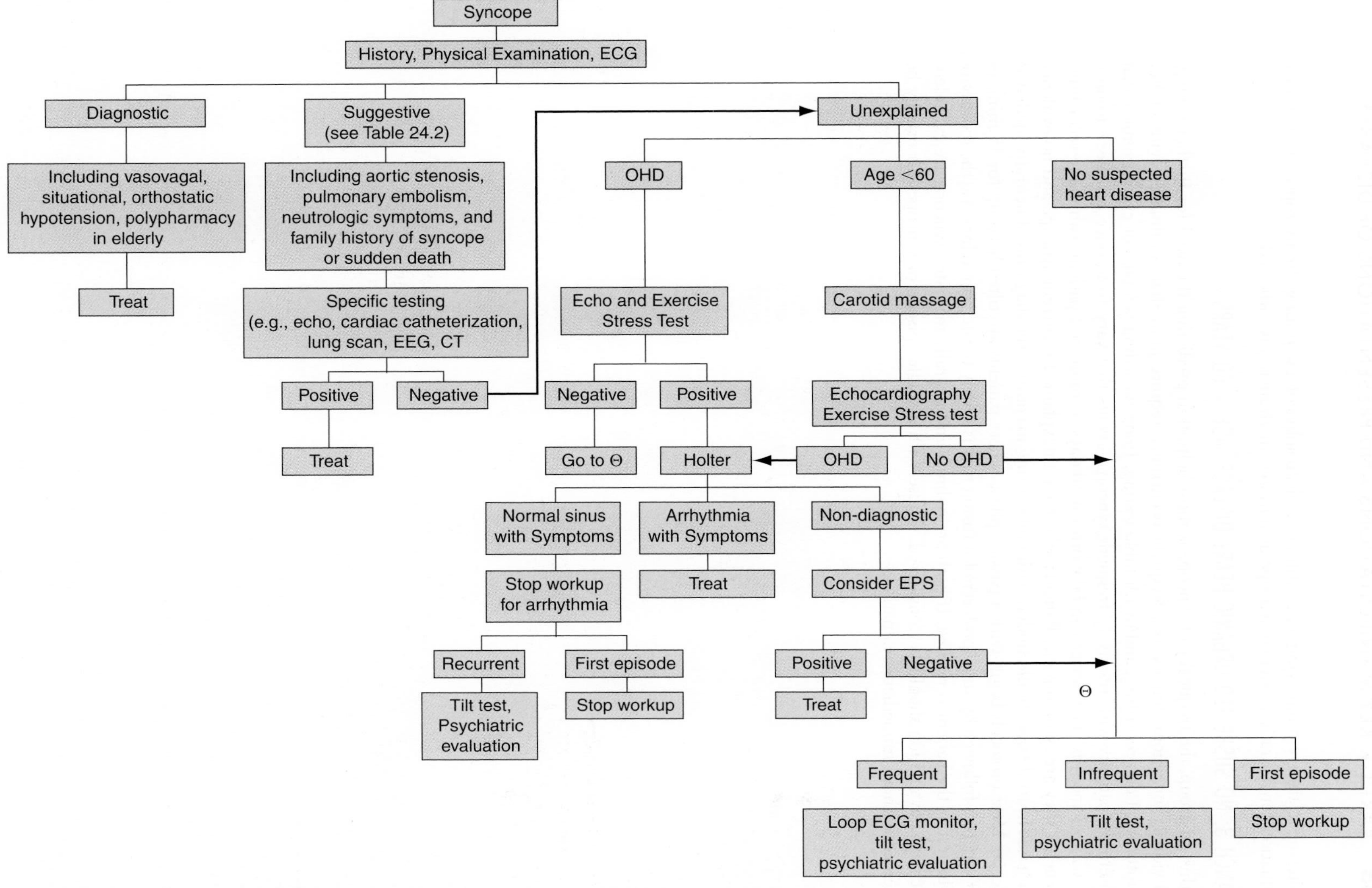

Figure 24.1 • Algorithm for diagnosing syncope. CT, computed tomography; ECG, electrocardiogram; EEG, electroencephalogram; EPS, electrophysiology study; OHD, organic heart disease. Adapted from Linzer M, Yang EH, Estes NA, et al. Diagnosing syncope, Part 1: value of history, physical examination, and electrocardiography. *Ann Intern Med* 1997;126:989–996.)

Holter or telemetry monitoring and ultimately electrophysiologic testing. In appropriate situations, evaluation for neurally mediated syncope as outlined in Branch 3 is indicated.

BRANCH 3: NO SUSPECTED ORGANIC HEART DISEASE, AGE <60 YEARS

In this subgroup, the frequency of syncope is most helpful in predicting the need for further testing. Individuals for whom syncope is a frequent occurrence require immediate evaluation with Holter monitoring, Loop recording, and/or tilt table testing. Loop recording is a type of event monitor that is useful in patients with relatively frequent syncopal events that vary from once per week to once every 2 to 3 months. The device can be worn for 30 days or more and patients can make recordings whenever they are symptomatic. Patients who have unexplained recurrent syncope and no evidence of organic heart disease should undergo tilt table testing to confirm the diagnosis of neurally mediated syncope. Most protocols begin with a passive phase where patients are tilted head up for 15 minutes at 60 degrees followed by an isoproterenol infusion that is slowly titrated up to increase the sensitivity of the test as the patient is retilted. If both arrhythmia and neurally mediated syncope are excluded, psychiatric evaluation should be considered. Those with a single episode of syncope can usually be observed without immediate evaluation.

CHAPTER 25

Thrombocytopenia

Gwen O'Keefe and Dario Torre

Thrombocytopenia is a platelet count usually less than 150,000/μL. Approximately 2.5% of the normal population may have platelet counts less then 150,000/μL. Low platelet counts are often found incidentally on complete blood counts obtained for other medical reasons, or when a patient presents with complaints of easy bruising or bleeding. Bleeding disturbances do not usually occur until the platelet count is below 50,000/μL, and spontaneous bleeding usually is not seen until the count is below 20,000/μL.

DIFFERENTIAL DIAGNOSIS

The differential diagnosis of thrombocytopenia is broad and can be grouped in four main categories characterized by different pathophysiologic mechanisms: pseudothrombocytopenia, decreased production, increased destruction, altered distribution (Table 25.1).

Pseudothrombocytopenia

It is important first to differentiate true thrombocytopenia from pseudothrombocytopenia. Spurious thrombocytopenia or pseudothrombocytopenia can be caused by platelet clumping seen in the peripheral smear. Clumps of platelets can be mistakenly counted or not properly differentiated from individual cells in the peripheral smear, resulting in a falsely low platelet count.

Decreased Production

Platelet production may be affected by bone marrow suppression. Viral agents (human immunodeficiency virus, Epstein-Barr virus, and hepatitis C virus), chemotherapy and radiation treatments, B12 deficiency, and folate deficiency can impair platelet production. Alcohol has toxic effect on bone marrow. Bone marrow infiltration by tumor or fibrosis can also decrease platelet production.

Increased Destruction

A number of conditions may cause thrombocytopenia by platelet destruction. In disseminated intravascular coagulation (DIC; Chapter 98), there is evidence of hemolysis, coagulation times are prolonged (prothrombin time [PT] and partial thromboplastin time [PTT]) d-dimer is elevated and fibrinogen is low. Thrombotic thrombocytopenic purpura (TTP) is characterized by the classic pentad: thrombocytopenia, microangiopathic hemolytic anemia, fever, renal failure, and change in mental status. TTP and hemolytic-uremic syndrome (HUS) will have schistocytes in the peripheral smear (Chapter 97). Immune thrombocytopenic purpura (ITP) may be idiopathic or secondary to autoimmune disease (systemic lupus erythematosus) or infections. It presents with petechiae, nonpalpable purpura, and a platelet count often <20,000/mL. In contrast with TTP or HUS, in ITP, renal failure and schistocytes on the peripheral smear are not present. ITP is often diagnosed after excluding other causes of thrombocytopenia such as TTP, HUS, or DIC.

Heparin-induced thrombocytopenia occurs approximately 5 to 10 days after initiation of heparin,

TABLE 25.1 Differential diagnosis of thrombocytopenia by pathophysiologic mechanism

Pseudothrombocytopenia
Platelet agglutination
Giant platelets
Decreased platelet production
Congenital lesions (Bernard Soulier)
Acquired states
Viral disease (human immunodeficiency virus, parvovirus, cytomegalovirus)
Nutritional deficiencies (vitamin B12)
Radio and chemotherapy
Aplastic anemia
Primary marrow disease
Metastatic disease
Leukemia
Drugs
Toxins
Alcohol
Altered distribution of platelets
Hypersplenism
Splenomegaly
Increased platelet destruction
Immune thrombocytopenic purpuras
Primary (autoimmune)
Secondary
Human immunodeficiency virus
Pregnancy
Drugs
—Heparin
—Quinine
—Gold
Disseminated intravascular coagulation Thrombotic thrombocytopenic purpura
Heparin-induced thrombocytopenia

or at times even after heparin has been discontinued. The most severe form (immune mediated) may present with arterial and venous thrombosis including deep venous thrombosis and pulmonary embolism, skin necrosis, and a platelet count that has fallen by 50% or more from the previous platelet count.

Altered Distribution or Pooling

Splenomegaly may cause pooling of platelets resulting in thrombocytopenia. Hypersplenism entails pooling coupled with platelet destruction. Causes of hypersplenism may include liver cirrhosis, congestive heart failure, and infiltrative disease such as leukemia and lymphomas. Massive transfusions may result in abnormal platelet distribution and low platelet counts.

EVALUATION

A complete history and physical examination can often provide clues to the cause of thrombocytopenia. A careful review of all medications taken by the patient should be done to investigate drug-induced thrombocytopenia. A family history of thrombocytopenia may point toward a congenital etiology such as Bernard Soulier, an autosomal recessive disease resulting in low platelet count. Poor nutritional status may suggest alcohol abuse as possible cause of low platelet count. Recent history of viral illnesses or a past history of hematologic diseases such as leukemias can provide clues to the diagnosis. A history of travel to endemic areas in a patient with fever and low platelet count may suggest malaria. Sepsis, vasculitis, DIC, and cardiac prosthetic valve can help determine the cause. Recent history of transfusions may indicate posttransfusion thrombocytopenia. Obtaining old values for comparison can help to determine if a slightly low value is the norm for that patient or date the onset of the thrombocytopenia.

On physical examination, most patients with chronic thrombocytopenia will have normal vital signs. The skin examination may show petechiae which are small flat red lesions usually located on feet and ankles. The confluence of numerous petechiae can result in purplish discoloration called purpura. Purpura in thrombocytopenic patients, as opposed to vasculitic purpura, is usually nonpalpable, not associated with burning or pain, and is usually located in dependent portions of the body

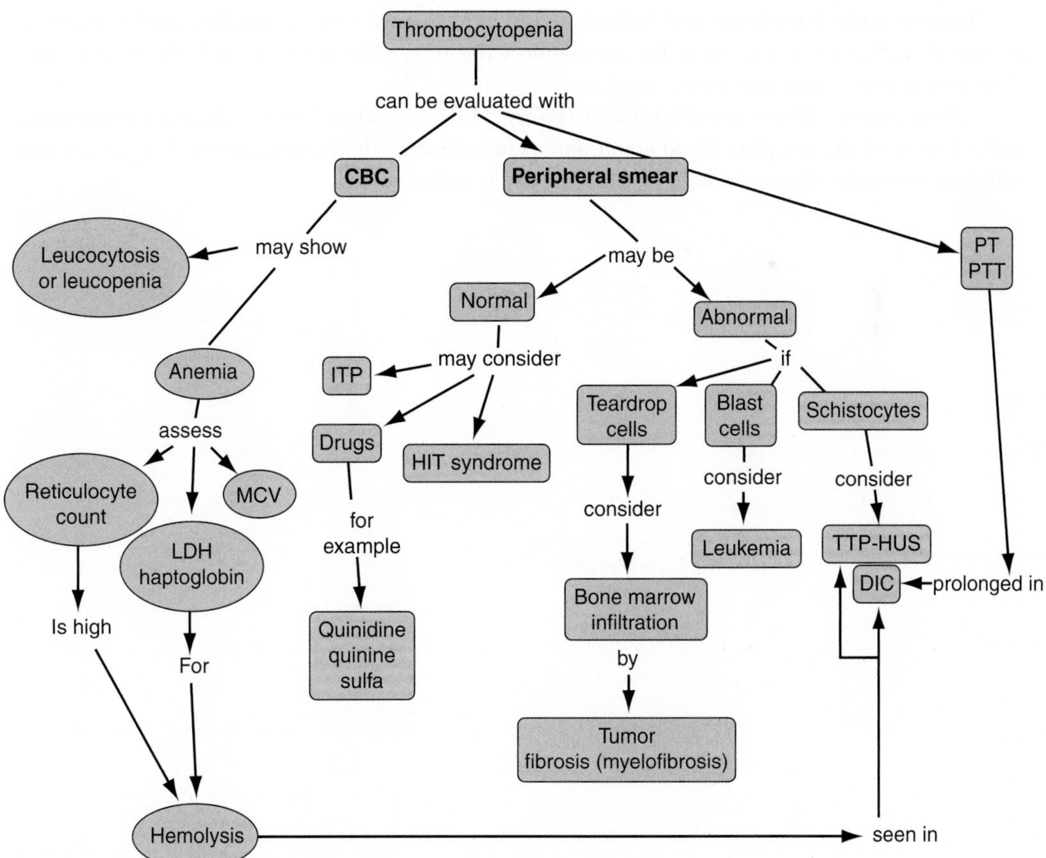

Figure 25.1 • Initial evaluation of thrombocytopenia. HIT, heparin-induced thrombocytopenia; ITP, immune thrombocytopenic purpura.

sparing the soles of the feet. Also the skin examination may reveal ecchymoses, small superficial lesions characterized by a red, purple, or orange discoloration, usually occurring in the absence of trauma. Mucosal bleeding manifesting as epistaxis or gingival bleeding may be present. A heart murmur can be a sign of high output secondary to an associated anemia. Splenomegaly may be the result of increased splenic sequestration of platelets (normally one third of platelets are sequestered in the spleen). Stigmata of chronic liver disease such as caput medusae, palmar erythema, nodular palpable liver, and jaundice may also indicate altered distribution or splenic sequestration as the cause of low platelets.

An initial laboratory evaluation should include a complete blood count (CBC) and a peripheral smear (Fig. 25.1).

A complete blood count should be obtained to measure the platelet count and assess the presence of concomitant anemia, leucocytosis, or leucopenia.

A peripheral smear is extremely helpful and a cost-effective test in the evaluation of thrombocytopenia. This is used to determine platelet clumping, platelet number, size, and morphology. It will also indicate abnormalities in other cell lines that can direct the diagnostic evaluation. The presence of schistocytes may suggest TTP, blast cells indicate leukemia, and large platelets may be seen in ITP. Teardrop cells may be found in myeloid metaplasia (fibrosis of the bone marrow) and Pelger-Huet anomaly in myelodysplasia. When the smear is normal, coagulation factors should be measured. Elevated D-dimer levels, PT, PTT, and low fibrinogen in the setting of sepsis or malignancy suggest DIC. Elevated lactate dehydrogenase and decreased haptoglobin indicate hemolysis.

The mean platelet volume will be increased in a destructive process and decreased in states of decreased production. If heparin-induced thrombocytopenic syndrome is suspected, the most specific diagnostic test is a serotonin release assay.

A bone marrow biopsy usually is not necessary. However, when history, physical examination, and a review of the complete blood count and examination of the peripheral blood smear are not sufficient to reach a diagnosis, bone marrow biopsy is indicated.

CHAPTER 26

Weight Loss

Marcos Montagnini

Clinically significant weight loss may be defined as the loss of 10 lbs (4.5 kg) or more than 5% of the usual body weight over a period of 6 to 12 months. Weight loss can be voluntary or involuntary. Involuntary weight loss is frequently encountered in clinical practice, is more common in the elderly, and is usually a sign of a serious medical condition or psychiatric disorder. Therefore, involuntary weight loss should always be investigated. Voluntary weight loss is of less concern, especially in an overweight patient who is trying to lose weight, but it can be a manifestation of an underlying eating disorder.

DIFFERENTIAL DIAGNOSIS

The most common causes of involuntary weight loss are outlined in Table 26.1. The differential diagnosis of weight loss can be separated into two broad categories: weight loss with normal or increased appetite, and weight loss with decreased appetite.

Weight Loss with Normal or Increased Appetite

Hyperthyroidism can present with heat intolerance, sweating, hair loss, palpitations, increased appetite, nervousness, insomnia, and amenorrhea or oligomenorrhea. Physical examination often reveals an anxious patient. Lid lag on downward gaze may be present. Skin is warm and moist, palms are erythematous, and hair is fine. Other findings include a fine tremor of the hands, tachycardia, a widened pulse pressure, systolic murmurs, atrial fibrillation, or supraventricular arrhythmias. In the elderly, both hypothyroidism and hyperthyroidism can present with weight loss and none of the classical signs or symptoms.

Diabetes mellitus (Chapter 64), when uncontrolled, presents with polyuria, polydipsia, and polyphagia. Physical examination reveals signs of dehydration such as decreased skin turgor, dry mucosa, hypotension, and tachycardia. Patients may complain of blurred vision and episodes of recurrent skin or mucosal infections. Patients with long-standing diabetes mellitus may present with anorexia and symptoms related to delayed gastric emptying such as nausea, vomiting, and abdominal distention. Many patients develop diarrhea accompanied by steatorrhea. Neuropathies, nephropathy, and retinopathy are also common in patients with long-standing disease.

Malabsorption commonly presents with weight loss, chronic malodorous diarrhea, and symptoms related to decreased absorption of proteins, fat, vitamins, and electrolytes. The patient may develop muscle wasting and edema (decreased protein absorption); paresthesias and tetany (decreased vitamin D and calcium absorption); bone pain (decreased calcium absorption); muscle cramps (excess potassium loss); easy bruisability, petechiae (decreased vitamin K absorption); hyperkeratosis, night blindness (decreased vitamin A absorption); pallor (decreased vitamin B12, folate, or iron absorption); glossitis, stomatitis, cheilosis (decreased vitamin B12 or iron absorption); and acrodermatitis (zinc deficiency).

Pheochromocytoma (Chapter 69) presents with hypertensive paroxysms accompanied by anxiety,

TABLE 26.1 Causes of involuntary weight loss

Causes of involuntary weight loss
Weight loss with increased appetite
Hyperthyroidism
Uncontrolled diabetes mellitus
Malabsorption
Pheochromocytoma
Weight loss with decreased appetite
Cancer
Chronic infections (tuberculosis, human immunodeficiency virus, parasites, subacute bacterial endocarditis, fungal)
Endocrinopathies (adrenal insufficiency, hypercalcemia, hyperthyroidism, diabetes mellitus)
Cardiovascular diseases (advanced congestive heart failure)
Pulmonary diseases (severe chronic obstructive pulmonary disease)
Renal diseases (end-stage renal disease)
Psychiatric disorders (depression, anxiety, schizophrenia, substance abuse)
Neurologic disorders (dementia, Parkinson's disease, brain tumors)
Connective tissue diseases
Drugs (antiepileptics, antidepressants, levodopa, digoxin, metformin, nonsteroidal anti-inflammatory drugs, chemotherapy agents)

headaches, palpitation, diaphoresis, and pallor. Some patients may have signs of hypermetabolism manifested as heat intolerance, sweating, and weight loss. Pheochromocytomas can also be asymptomatic and discovered incidentally.

Weight Loss with Decreased Appetite

Cancer usually manifests with symptoms that are nonspecific such as fatigue, weight loss, night sweats, low-grade fever, and decreased appetite. More specific signs or symptoms will depend on the primary location of the tumor. For example, gastrointestinal malignancies may present with nausea, vomiting, early satiety, abdominal pain, change in bowel function, melena, hematochezia, and palpable abdominal masses. Lung cancer frequently presents with cough, chest pain, sputum production, and hemoptysis. Bone cancer presents with localized or diffuse bone pain and pathological fractures. Metastatic bone cancer can lead to hypercalcemia, which causes fatigue, confusion, anorexia, nausea, constipation, polyuria, and dehydration.

Infections such as tuberculosis, fungal disease, parasite infections, subacute bacterial endocarditis, and human immunodeficiency virus can present with weight loss, fatigue, fever, night sweats, arthralgias, and decreased appetite. When infection is suspected, it is essential to ask about risk factors, including travel, occupation, living arrangements, lifestyle, and history of exposure. A thorough history and physical examination will elicit findings suggestive of the underlying disease.

Adrenal insufficiency (Chapter 69) manifests with anorexia, lethargy, weight loss, nausea, vomiting, muscle weakness, and diarrhea as a result of cortisol deficiency. Patients with primary adrenal insufficiency may have manifestations of aldosterone deficiency such as volume depletion, orthostatic blood pressure, and hyperpigmentation, particularly on the elbows, knees, buccal mucosa, and surgical scars. In females, loss of adrenal androgens leads to decreased pubic hair.

Advanced congestive heart failure (Chapter 28) presents with progressive fatigue and dyspnea at rest or with minimal exertion. Other symptoms include orthopnea, paroxysmal nocturnal dyspnea, and decreased appetite. Physical examination reveals tachypnea, jugular venous distention, S3 gallop, pulmonary congestion (rales, dullness over pleural effusion), peripheral edema, hepatomegaly, and ascites.

Advance lung disease presents with dyspnea at rest or with minimal exertion, cough, and sputum production. Patients with advanced lung disease frequently have an asthenic body build, tachypnea, prolonged expiration, hyperresonant chest, diminished breath sounds, wheezing, rales, clubbing, and cyanosis. Patients with long history of lung disease and pulmonary hypertension will develop signs right-sided heart failure.

Uremia often produces anorexia, nausea, and vomiting. Patients frequently report symptoms related to volume overload such as fatigue, dyspnea, and edema. Other uremic signs and symptoms include lethargy, seizures, myoclonus, asterixis, and peripheral neuropathies. Uremic pericarditis may manifest as chest pain, dyspnea, and a pericardial friction rub. Pruritus, anemia, and pallor are also common. Amenorrhea, impaired testicular function, and impotence are frequent in patients with end-stage renal disease.

Connective tissue diseases, especially rheumatoid arthritis (Chapter 47) and systemic lupus erythematosus (Chapter 48), also present with anorexia and weight loss. Common manifestations of connective tissue diseases include fatigue, fever, malaise, skin rashes, arthritis, myositis, mucosal lesions, alopecia, anemia, lymphadenopathy, splenomegaly, seizures, pleuritis, pericarditis, pneumonitis, nephritis, and vasculitis.

Psychiatric disorders should always be considered when an organic cause is not identified as the cause of weight loss. Weight loss and diminished appetite is found in 70% to 80% of patients with moderate to severe depression. Manic-depressive disorders, anxiety disorder, and schizophrenia may also be associated with anorexia and weight loss. Drug dependence, especially alcoholism, nicotine, opioids, cocaine, amphetamines, commonly result in anorexia and weight loss. Anorexia nervosa is always a consideration when a young woman has unexplained weight loss.

Neurologic conditions such as dementia (Chapter 144) and Parkinson's disease (Chapter 112) are often accompanied by decreased appetite and weight loss. Central nervous system tumors, especially those involving the hypothalamus, may present with anorexia and weight loss. Patients with dementia will present with progressive cognitive loss, personality changes, and the inability to care for themselves. Patients with Parkinson's disease will frequently report tremor, rigidity, slowness of movement, gait and posture abnormalities, falls, and deterioration in handwriting.

EVALUATION

Weight loss should be evaluated with a thorough history and physical examination with particular attention to diet and psychosocial factors. It is important to review medication use, as many drugs cause anorexia. Patients should also be screened for depression and anxiety. A cognitive screening test should be considered in an elderly patient with weight loss and anorexia to rule out dementia as a contributing factor. Appropriate tests should be ordered based on the history and physical findings.

An initial panel to assess unexplained weight loss include a complete blood count to look for infection, anemia, or lymphoproliferative disorder; chemistries (electrolytes, glucose, calcium, phosphorus) to look for evidence of diabetes mellitus, hypercalcemia, renal dysfunction, or other metabolic disorder; blood urea nitrogen and creatinine to screen for renal dysfunction; aspartate aminotransferase, alanine transferase, alkaline phosphatase, and bilirubin to assess for liver dysfunction; estimated sedimentation rate and C-reactive protein to look for connective tissue disease or chronic infection; and urinalysis to look for evidence of infection, renal disease, or dehydration.

A chest x-ray may be considered to evaluate the possibility of lung cancer, lung disease, congestive heart failure, tuberculosis, and lung abscess. A fecal occult blood test should be considered to rule out the gastrointestinal malignancy. Thyroid-stimulating hormone levels should be obtained to assess for hyperthyroidism or hypothyroidism. Additional tests may be ordered to detect specific conditions.

Pheochromocytoma is detected by measuring 24-hour urinary catecholamines, metanephrine, and creatinine. Once pheochromocytoma is confirmed biochemically, computed tomography scan, magnetic resonance imaging, and nuclear imaging should be performed to localize the lesion.

Fat malabsorption is suggested by stool fat determination by Sudan staining and confirmed by 72-hour fecal fat determination. More than 6 g of fat in a 72-hour collection stool sample is consistent with malabsorption. The D-xylose test is used to screen for diffuse small bowel mucosa disease. Small bowel biopsy is a valuable test in the differential diagnosis of malabsorptive disorders. Serum levels of calcium, albumin, iron, cholesterol, folate, and vitamin B12, serum-iron binding capacity, and prothrombin time can provide additional evidence of intestinal malabsorption.

Cancer of the gastrointestinal tract should be evaluated by colonoscopy and upper endoscopy. Abdominal ultrasound may be indicated to evaluate liver, kidney, and pancreatic masses. Imaging studies including computed tomography, magnetic resonance imaging, and positron emission tomography scans are utilized to diagnose solid tumor or metastatic lesions. Plain radiographs, bone surveys, and bone scan are utilized to diagnose metastatic bone disease. A bone marrow biopsy should be performed when a hematological malignancy is suspected.

The workup for infection should include an human immunodeficiency virus test in patients with risk factors; a purified protein derivative test and a chest x-ray should be considered in patients with suspected TB; blood cultures and echocardiogram should be done when there is a suspicion of endocarditis. Tests for fungal and diseases caused by parasites should be done when indicated.

Depressed ventricular function in congestive heart failure is confirmed by echocardiography, radionuclide ventriculography, or cardiac catheterization with angiography. Electrocardiogram abnormalities are frequently present in congestive heart failure and include arrhythmias, conduction delays, and nonspecific ST-T wave changes.

Chronic obstructive pulmonary disease is detected by pulmonary function test and arterial blood gases. Forced expiratory volume in 1 second is always reduced in chronic obstructive pulmonary disease. Total lung capacity, functional residual capacity, and residual volume may be increased. The carbon monoxide diffusion capacity is reduced in emphysema. Arterial blood gases demonstrate hypoxemia, hypercapnia, and metabolic compensation (increased serum bicarbonate) to maintain pH near normal.

If renal disease is detected in the initial elevation, further workup should include 24-hour urine collection for protein and creatinine determination. Imaging studies of the urinary tract such as ultrasound, pyelogram, and computed tomography scan should be performed to rule out urinary tract obstruction or tumor. An adrenocorticotropic hormone (ACTH) stimulation test should be done to screen for adrenal insufficiency. Further testing such as prolonged ACTH infusion test and insulin tolerance testing are indicated if the initial screening is abnormal.

The evaluation of connective tissue diseases include joint radiographs, synovial fluid analysis, rheumatoid factor (if rheumatoid arthritis is suspected), complement levels, serum immunoglobulins, antinuclear antibodies and subtypes (if systemic lupus erythematosus is suspected), Venereal Disease Research Laboratory test, prothrombin time, and partial thromboplastin time.

II

Diseases and Disorders

Cardiology

Geoffrey C. Lamb

CHAPTER 27

Coronary Artery Disease

James Kleczka

Coronary artery disease is defined by the development of atherosclerosis within the coronary vasculature, which often leads to impaired coronary blood flow. Although many advances have been made in the evaluation and treatment of coronary artery disease, it remains a significant burden both economically and clinically. The lifetime risk for coronary artery disease is 49% for men and 32% for women at age 40. Despite a significant decline in mortality related to cardiovascular disease over the past 50 years, coronary artery disease continues to be the leading cause of death in the United States.

The development of atherosclerosis is the primary etiology of coronary artery disease and may lead to chronic stable angina and ultimately acute coronary syndromes including unstable angina, myocardial infarction, and sudden cardiac death. It may also lead to the development of arrhythmias and congestive heart failure due to ischemic damage to the heart muscle. Atherosclerosis is the formation of plaque within the intima of large- and medium-sized blood vessels. Atherosclerotic plaque is comprised of multiple cell types including macrophages, foam cells (macrophages filled with cholesterol esters), smooth muscle cells, and lymphocytes. It also incorporates such substances as lipids, fibrous connective tissue, and minerals such as calcium. The development of atherosclerosis within the coronary arteries is a process that begins in childhood. This process is regulated by several environmental factors as well as the genetic makeup of an individual and the degree of endothelial dysfunction present.

The initial atherosclerotic lesions contain atherogenic lipoproteins, which release cytokines and cause an increase in macrophages and formation of foam cells. These most frequently develop at sites of focal thickening within the intima, which are present in everyone at birth. This thickening of the intima is an adaptation to local mechanical forces and is nonobstructive. These lesions progress to fatty streaks that consist of layers of foam cells and lipid-filled smooth muscles cells. Intermediate lesions may form after puberty and are the bridge between early and more advanced atherosclerosis. These lesions contain the same layers of foam cells and smooth muscle cells as fatty streaks. At this point, smooth muscle cells can divide and elaborate extracellular matrix, leading to the deposition of extracellular matrix and scattered accumulations of lipids within the evolving plaque. These scattered areas, once dense enough, can coalesce to form an extensive but well-defined lipid core. The lesion is now considered an atheroma. Atheromas are not typically obstructive and form in the third decade of life. They often are comprised of calcium and lymphocytes in addition to lipids. The lipid core can later begin to produce collagen which then forms a tough fibrous cap, which is then termed a fibroatheroma. Extensive calcification of the lipid core can also occur. Obstruction of coronary blood flow may accompany the development of these lesions and they may develop fissures, hematomas, or even thrombus. Once disruption of the fibrous cap occurs, they are classified as complicated lesions and are often the culprit of acute coronary syndromes (Fig. 27.1).

Traditional risk factors for development of atherosclerotic heart disease include smoking, diabetes mellitus, hyperlipidemia, hypertension, and family history of early coronary artery disease (males younger than 45 years, females younger than 55 years) (Table 27.1). Nearly 90% of patients with coronary artery disease have at least one of these major risk factors. More recently, additional risk

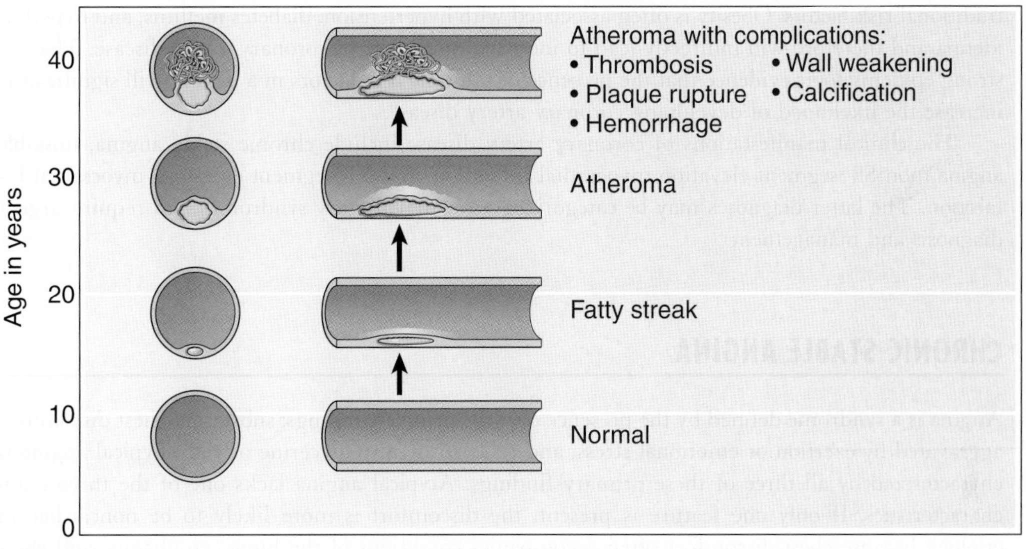

Figure 27.1 • Endothelial dysfunction.

factors have been taken into account including physical inactivity, obesity, dietary indiscretion, and psychosocial stress.

Cigarette smokers are two to four times more likely to develop coronary artery disease as compared to nonsmokers. They also have a two- to three-fold increased risk of dying as a result of their atherosclerotic heart disease. Smoking is also a strong independent predictor of sudden cardiac death in patients with a history of coronary disease. Diabetics have two to four times higher mortality related to coronary artery disease as compared to nondiabetics, and coronary disease is the leading cause of diabetes-related death. High levels of total cholesterol, low-density lipoprotein (LDL) cholesterol, and triglycerides have been found to accelerate atherosclerosis, as have low levels of high-density lipoprotein (HDL) cholesterol. HDL participates in reverse transportation of cholesterol from the tissues to the liver and therefore a high HDL will exert a protective effect. Nearly one in three adults in the United States has a history of hypertension, defined as systolic pressure above 140 mm Hg and diastolic pressure above 90 mm Hg. Approximately 69% of those presenting with a first heart attack have hypertension. The relative risk of developing coronary artery disease in patients with physical inactivity ranges from 1.5 to 2.4, which is comparable to that observed with the more

TABLE 27.1 Risk factors for coronary atherosclerosis

Modifiable	Nonmodifiable
Hypercholesterolemia	Age (men, >45 years; women, >55 years)
Cigarette smoking	Family history (men, <55 years; women, <65 years)
Hypertension Physical inactivity Low HDL-cholesterol (<35 mg/dL) Diabetes mellitus Truncal obesity	

traditional risk factors. Obesity is often associated with hypertension, diabetes mellitus, and hyperlipidemia and therefore will indirectly lead to increased incidence of coronary artery disease. There is strong epidemiologic evidence that the presence of multiple risk factors in a patient will significantly increase the likelihood of developing coronary artery disease.

The clinical manifestations of coronary artery disease include chronic stable angina, unstable angina, non-ST segment elevation myocardial infarction, and ST-segment elevation myocardial infarction. The latter diagnoses may be categorized as acute coronary syndromes and require urgent diagnosis and management.

CHRONIC STABLE ANGINA

Angina is a syndrome defined by the presence of three primary findings: substernal chest discomfort, aggravated by exertion or emotional stress, and relieved by nitroglycerine or rest. Typical angina is characterized by all three of these primary findings. Atypical angina lacks one of the three main characteristics. If only one feature is present, the discomfort is more likely to be noncardiac in etiology because chest discomfort often accompanies conditions of the lungs, esophagus, and chest wall. Chronic stable angina implies that the pattern of angina is predictable and unchanged.

Etiology

Typical angina is the result of cardiac ischemia caused by an imbalance in myocardial oxygen supply and demand. Increases in heart rate, chamber size, contractility, and blood pressure lead to increases in myocardial oxygen demand. At baseline, the myocardium will extract oxygen nearly maximally from coronary arterial blood. Therefore, the only way to increase supply to meet increased demand is to enhance coronary blood flow, the primary means of which is coronary arteriolar dilatation.

The most common etiology of ischemic chest pain is the presence of significant, obstructive atherosclerosis of at least one major epicardial blood vessel that impedes delivery of blood to the affected myocardium. In this setting, the vasculature distal to the obstruction has already maximally dilated in an attempt to increase coronary blood flow at rest. If myocardial oxygen demand increases, the vessels are unable to dilate further and cannot provide increased flow, leading to anginal symptoms. When coronary lesions become nearly completely obstructive, blood flow may be inadequate at baseline leading to rest angina.

Anginal symptoms and cardiac ischemia may also be caused by other entities that shift the delicate balance of supply and demand. Significant valvular heart disease, in particular severe aortic stenosis, can lead to ischemia. Severe coronary vasospasm can limit blood flow and cause ischemic chest pain and myocardial infarction. Severe left ventricular hypertrophy, arrhythmias such as ventricular or supraventricular tachycardia, hypertrophic cardiomyopathy, and conditions that significantly elevate intracardiac pressures such as uncontrolled hypertension may lead to an increase in myocardial oxygen demand and cause ischemic chest pain, even though obstructive coronary atherosclerosis may not be present.

Noncardiac causes of increased myocardial demand or reduced oxygen supply may produce angina in the setting of nonobstructive coronary artery disease. Examples of increased demand include the presence of hyperthermia, hyperthyroidism, sympathomimetic toxicity (cocaine), anxiety, and arteriovenous fistulae (cause high-output state). Reduced oxygen supply may be caused by severe hypoxemia, severe anemia, and hyperviscosity syndromes (polycythemia, thrombocytosis).

Clinical Manifestations

A detailed history is essential when a patient presents with complaints of chest pain. The history should focus on the quality of pain, location, duration, associated symptoms, and factors that aggravate or alleviate the pain. Anginal pain is often described as "tightness," "squeezing," "pressure," or "heaviness" in the chest. "Burning" pain is also frequently described and oftentimes mistaken for gastroesophageal reflux. Sharp pain is less likely to represent angina. Many patients will not classify their symptom as pain, but will rather call it "discomfort." The typical location is substernal, and the pain may radiate to the neck, jaw, shoulders, back, or arms. Chest pain may be absent in some cases with the pain located instead in the jaw, neck, arms, or epigastric region alone. It is also possible for a patient to have no complaints of pain and have a sole complaint of dyspnea. These "anginal equivalents" will worsen with exertion or emotional stress and improve with rest or nitroglycerine and may be the only indication of significant coronary disease. Isolated right- or left-sided chest pain, pleuritic pain, axillary pain, and abdominal or epigastric pain rarely represent true angina. Anginal chest pain usually lasts minutes. Pain lasting for many hours or continuous chest pain over a period of days is very unlikely to be anginal chest pain. Likewise, intermittent pain lasting seconds is more likely to be noncardiac. Anginal chest discomfort is often accompanied by shortness or breath, nausea, and diaphoresis. Angina can be graded based on duration and intensity using the Canadian Cardiovascular Society (CCS) classification system, which ranges from Class I (very strenuous work leads to symptoms) to Class IV (symptoms at rest) (Table 27.2).

The physical examination is often not helpful in patients with chronic stable angina because they are unlikely to have symptoms at the time of examination. Examination may reveal the presence of risk factors for coronary artery disease, such as elevated blood pressure or retinal changes to suggest hypertension. Careful examination of the peripheral vasculature may reveal diminished pulses or bruits consistent with peripheral atherosclerosis, which is often coexistent with coronary artery disease. The presence of xanthomas may indicate hyperlipidemia. The finding of chest discomfort that is reproduced by palpation might discourage the diagnosis of angina. Findings such as an S_3 or S_4 gallop, significant murmur, pericardial rub, or left ventricular heave indicate the presence of heart disease that may be secondary to ischemia.

Diagnosis

When a patient presents with a history of chest pain, one must consider not only obstructive coronary artery disease, but also other conditions that may cause or contribute to the development of angina.

TABLE 27.2 Grading of angina pectoris according to CCS classification

Class	Description of Stage
I	"Ordinary physical activity does not cause . . . angina," such as walking or climbing stairs. Angina occurs with strenuous, rapid, or prolonged exertion at work or receation.
II	"Slight limitation of ordinary activity." Angina occurs on walking or climbing stairs rapidly; walking uphill; walking or stair climbing after meals; in cold, in wind, or under emotional stress; or only during the few hours after awakening. Angina occurs on walking >2 blocks on the level and climbing >1 flight of ordinary stairs at a normal pace and under normal conditions.
III	"Marked limitations of ordinary physical activity." Angina occurs on walking 1 to 2 blocks on the level and climbing 1 flight of stairs under normal conditions and at a normal pace.
IV	"Inability to carry on any physical activity without discomfort—anginal symptoms may be present at rest."

CCS, Canadian Cardiovascular Society. Adapted from Campeau L. *Circulation* 1976;54:522–523, with permission.

These include conditions that may decrease myocardial oxygen supply and those that increase demand such as blood loss, hypoxia, or sepsis. Many of these conditions may lead to angina in the setting of otherwise nonobstructive coronary artery disease. In addition, there are many causes of noncardiac chest pain that one must keep in mind (Chapter 6). These include aortic dissection (Chapter 34), pulmonary embolism (Chapter 41), esophageal reflux (Chapter 71), costochondritis, and anxiety disorders, among others.

Based on the history taken, initial laboratory work might include thyroid function tests if hyperthyroidism is under consideration. If use of a sympathomimetic agent (cocaine) is suspected, a drug screen should be obtained. Checking the hemoglobin and hematocrit is essential to evaluate for anemia. A fasting lipid panel may be valuable in diagnosing hyperlipidemia, one of the major risk factors associated with the development of coronary artery disease.

In most cases of chronic stable angina, a chest x-ray will be normal and therefore routine use in the diagnosis of this entity is not suggested. This study is more helpful in patients with suspected aortic dissection or aneurysm, potential for significant pulmonary disease, evidence of congestive heart failure, or significant valvular heart disease in addition to chest pain. Enlargement of the mediastinum or cardiac silhouette may be seen in these cases.

ELECTROCARDIOGRAM

A resting 12-lead electrocardiogram should be obtained in all patients presenting with suspected anginal chest pain. In one half to two thirds of patients with chronic stable angina, the electrocardiogram will be normal, but this does not exclude the presence of significant obstructive coronary disease. Abnormal Q waves may be found indicating prior myocardial infarction. Electrocardiographic evidence of left ventricular hypertrophy or baseline ST-T wave changes can also be discovered which may suggest underlying coronary disease. A right or left bundle branch block will more frequently occur in patients with coronary artery disease as well. An electrocardiogram should be recorded in all patients with active chest pain. New abnormalities will be found in approximately 50% of patients with anginal chest pain and normal baseline electrocardiograms. The presence of dynamic ST segment elevation or depression, T-wave inversion, new left or right bundle branch block, or arrhythmia on electrocardiogram during an episode of chest pain are highly suggestive of ischemia and should expedite further workup.

STRESS TESTING

Stress testing is a valuable diagnostic tool when evaluating patients with suspected coronary artery disease. Many different modalities are available, including exercise stress testing; exercise stress test with nuclear imaging; pharmacologic (dipyridamole, dobutamine, adenosine) nuclear stress testing; and dobutamine, dipyridamole, or exercise/bicycle stress echocardiography.

Exercise stress testing is an important diagnostic and prognostic procedure in the assessment of patients with suspected or established coronary artery disease. It is widely available, costs little, and is generally safe, although both myocardial infarction and death have been reported (1 in 2,500 tests). These tests are performed frequently, do not always require a cardiologist, and are convenient for the patient as they can be done in the office or in the emergency department (Table 27.3).

Absolute contraindications to exercise stress testing include performing the test within 2 days of an acute myocardial infarction, in the presence of unstable angina not previously stabilized by medical therapy, uncontrolled cardiac arrhythmias, symptomatic severe aortic stenosis, decompensated heart failure, acute pulmonary embolism, pericarditis, and aortic dissection. Relative contraindications include the presence of left main stenosis, moderate stenotic valvular disease, electrolyte abnormalities, severe hypertension (systolic blood pressure >200 mm Hg, diastolic blood pressure >110 mm Hg), tachyarrhythmia or bradyarrhythmia, hypertrophic cardiomyopathy, high-degree atrioventricular nodal block, and inability to exercise adequately (Table 27.4).

Exercise can be performed utilizing a treadmill or a cycle ergometer device. The treadmill is

TABLE 27.3 Indications for exercise stress testing

Coronary artery disease (CAD)
A. Diagnosis Men with atypical angina Women with typical or atypical angina Asymptomatic men: • In special occupations (e.g., pilots, firemen, bus drivers, railroad engineers) • Two or more risk factors for atherosclerosis • Before entering exercise training programs
B. Prognosis (risk stratification) with establishing CAD diagnosis Stable angina Post myocardial infarction
C. Assessing treatment efficacy Medical Revascularization procedures (angioplasty, surgery)
Non-coronary artery disease
A. Evaluation and treatment efficacy of exercise-induced arrhythmias
B. Functional evaluation of Valvular heart disease
C. Functional evaluation in heart failure

TABLE 27.4 Contraindications to exercise stress testing

Cardiovascular
Acute myocardial infarction Recent in resting electrocardiogram Unstable angina Arrhythmias/conduction defects Uncontrolled life-threatening arrhythmias Second- or third-degree atrioventricular block Fixed-rate pacemaker Decompensated heart failure Critical aortic stenosis Severe obstructive hypertrophic cardiomyopathy Acute myocarditis, pericarditis, or endocarditis Uncontrolled hypertension (blood pressure >200/105 mm Hg)
Noncardiac
Severe pulmonary hypertension Acute pulmonary embolism or infarction Any acute, systemic illness

most commonly used in the United States. Results are given in terms of metabolic equivalents (METs). One MET is equal to 3.5 mL/kg/min, which is the standard basal oxygen uptake in a 70-kg, 40-year-old man. Reporting results in this fashion allows standardizing of workloads between different exercise protocols. Interpretation is based on several factors including ST-segment displacement (either depression or elevation), blood pressure response, pulse response, development of symptoms, and development of arrhythmias.

The sensitivity of an exercise stress test is estimated at 68%, while the specificity is estimated at 78%. The specificity is decreased in patients with electrocardiographic evidence of left ventricular hypertrophy, resting ST-segment depression, or patients on medical therapy with digoxin. When evaluating a patient with chest pain, one must take into account the pretest probability that the symptoms are due to coronary artery disease. This is accomplished by considering the age and sex of the patient in addition to the presence or absence of risk factors and the characteristics of the pain itself. For example, patients older than 50 years, in particular male patients, with typical anginal symptoms and multiple risk factors have a high probability of coronary artery disease. A positive test result would not provide any added benefit in the evaluation of such a patient, as coronary disease is already the suspected diagnosis. Likewise, a negative result would probably represent a false-negative test. Conversely, young female patients with no risk factors and atypical or noncardiac pain are very unlikely to have obstructive coronary disease as the cause of their symptoms, and a positive result would not be reliable. Exercise stress testing is most beneficial in those patients with intermediate pretest probability of disease.

NUCLEAR IMAGING

Nuclear imaging may be utilized with exercise stress testing to improve the sensitivity and specificity of the findings. This involves injection of nuclear isotopes at rest and peak exercise to produce images of myocardial regional uptake. This will allow localization of the area of ischemia and thus which artery is involved. Drugs such as thallium, sestamibi, and tetrofosmin have been used for this purpose. The use of nuclear perfusion scanning with exercise will increase both sensitivity (to ~90%) and specificity (60% to 90%). This modality is most beneficial in patients with abnormalities on resting electrocardiogram, which would reduce the sensitivity and specificity of a simple exercise stress test. These patients include those with baseline ST-segment depression, electrocardiographic changes of left ventricular hypertrophy, baseline left bundle branch block, paced rhythm, ventricular pre-excitation, and patients taking digoxin.

If patients are unable to exercise, pharmacologic nuclear stress testing can be performed. In this procedure, exercise as a stressor is replaced by vasodilators such as adenosine or dipyridamole, which will create a coronary steal phenomenon and, with injection of isotopes at rest and postvasodilator, produce images of myocardial regional uptake. Dobutamine has also been used to simulate the stress of exercise.

ECHOCARDIOGRAPHY

Echocardiography can also be performed during standard exercise stress testing or with pharmacologic stress to evaluate for ischemia. In this modality, there is no radiation exposure, results are available immediately, and the study is less costly as compared to nuclear scanning. Images are obtained at rest and with stress and are compared side by side to evaluate for regional wall motion changes. Sensitivity has been reported anywhere between 70% and 95%, with a specificity of 70% to 90%.

Echocardiography, the use of ultrasound to evaluate the heart, is not essential in the evaluation of angina or coronary artery disease, but it can provide useful information in various circumstances. An echocardiogram can assess for regional wall motion abnormalities suggestive of previous myocardial infarction. It can also be used as a tool to assess left ventricular systolic function and a variety of anatomical abnormalities that may lead to chest pain, such as severe aortic stenosis or hypertrophic cardiomyopathy. An echocardiogram can be quite valuable in the setting of active chest pain, as wall motion abnormalities would certainly be present if the pain were secondary to ischemia as a result of obstructive coronary artery disease.

CORONARY ANGIOGRAPHY

All previous diagnostic techniques discussed have been noninvasive studies performed with minimal risk to the patient. Selective coronary angiography is an invasive procedure wherein a catheter is advanced to the ostia of the left and right coronary arteries and contrast dye is injected. Digital images are taken and recorded in multiple views as the contrast is injected. This allows delineation of the coronary anatomy and will reveal significant coronary atherosclerosis. Coronary angiography remains the most accurate means of diagnosing clinically significant obstructive coronary artery disease. It will not provide information regarding the functional significance of lesions, nor can it predict which lesions will progress or lead to acute myocardial infarction. This procedure will provide a means of treating the underlying problem, as angioplasty and placement of coronary stents can be performed to relieve obstruction. Less than 0.5% of patients will experience a major complication such as death, myocardial infarction, and stroke. Patients presenting with classic anginal symptoms with a high pretest probability of coronary artery disease should directly undergo coronary angiography rather than noninvasive testing to evaluate their symptoms.

Newer noninvasive imaging modalities include cardiac magnetic resonance imaging (MRI) and computed tomography (CT) coronary angiography. MRI can be helpful in assessing myocardial perfusion but is not routinely performed in the assessment of coronary artery disease. CT coronary angiography is currently being studied in direct comparison to coronary angiography in the evaluation of anginal chest pain. Investigators are hopeful that this noninvasive imaging modality will compare favorably with coronary angiography in determining the extent and severity of coronary artery disease. Electron beam CT scanning can also be performed to evaluate the degree of coronary calcification present. This test has been shown to have prognostic significance depending upon the degree of calcification present, but is not helpful in determining the clinical significance or degree of obstructive coronary disease.

Treatment

The treatment of chronic stable angina consists of two major goals. The primary therapeutic goal is to prevent death and myocardial infarction. The secondary aim is to control symptoms and therefore episodes of ischemia. These objectives require a proper pharmaceutical regimen, interventions directed toward modifiable risk factors, and consideration of invasive or surgical procedures to deal with the presence of obstructive coronary artery disease. This section will deal primarily with pharmacologic management of chronic stable angina. Invasive and surgical interventions will be discussed later.

Antiplatelet agents are an important component of the treatment regimen. Aspirin inhibits cyclooxygenase and thromboxane A_2, which causes an antithrombotic effect. Its use has been shown to reduce the risk of adverse cardiovascular events by approximately 33% in those with chronic stable angina. Aspirin should be used on a routine basis in all patients with known coronary artery disease, whether stable or unstable. Clopidogrel irreversibly inhibits the glycoprotein IIb/IIIa receptors on platelets, thereby affecting platelet aggregation. Recent studies have shown that clopidogrel is likely as effective as aspirin in prevention of myocardial infarction and ischemic stroke in patients with known coronary artery disease. Clopidogrel is an acceptable substitute in the setting of allergy or intolerance to aspirin.

Studies of antithrombotic agents such as subcutaneous heparin and warfarin have failed to show any substantial benefit as compared to aspirin and therefore their use in patients with chronic stable angina is not recommended.

Multiple trials over the past decade have quite conclusively shown that lipid-lowering agents, in particular statins (simvastatin, atorvastatin), reduce the risk of major coronary events (fatal and nonfatal myocardial infarction) and overall mortality in patients with coronary artery disease, including chronic stable angina. There have also been studies showing some degree of coronary plaque regression with intensive lowering of LDL cholesterol. Given this data, aggressive lipid lowering with use of a statin (if tolerated) is recommended in all patients with coronary artery disease.

Blockade of beta-adrenergic receptors leads to reductions in heart rate and contractility, and therefore reduces myocardial oxygen demand. As a result, this class of medications is effective in treating anginal symptoms. These drugs have also been shown in multiple large trials to reduce mortality due to myocardial infarction and sudden cardiac death and to improve survival in those with previous myocardial infarct. They have also been shown to reduce the incidence of stroke and heart failure. Beta blockers are a first-line therapy in all patients with coronary artery disease unless contraindications to their use (severe bradycardia, decompensated heart failure) are present.

Inhibition of transmembrane calcium channels leads to vasodilation and a negative inotropic effect. Studies of calcium channel blockers directly compared to beta blockers have shown similar efficacy in relieving anginal symptoms. They are particularly effective in the treatment of coronary vasospasm. Recent studies indicate that short-acting dihydropyridine calcium channel antagonists enhance the risk of adverse events and should be avoided in patients with coronary artery disease. However, long-acting calcium channel blockers are effective at reducing angina and may be used in combination with or as a substitute for beta blockade. There is no significant long-term mortality benefit in patients with coronary disease. Their use is contraindicated in patients with decompensated heart failure and severe bradycardia.

Nitrates cause vasodilation, which can improve coronary perfusion and reduce myocardial oxygen requirements. They have also been shown to have antiplatelet effects in patients with chronic stable angina. This class of medication is effective in treating coronary vasospasm and leads to a reduction in anginal symptoms. Short-acting forms are commonly used for acute anginal attacks, whereas longer-acting forms are effective in prevention of recurrent angina. There is no mortality benefit afforded by nitrates. These drugs should not be used concomitantly with sildenafil and should be avoided in patients with hypertrophic obstructive cardiomyopathy and severe aortic stenosis. Nitrate tolerance can quickly develop with long-term use; therefore, a nitrate-free period each day is required.

Angiotensin-converting enzyme (ACE) inhibitors have been shown to reduce mortality due to cardiovascular death, myocardial infarction, and stroke. These drugs are especially effective in diabetics with coronary artery disease and in patients with left ventricular systolic dysfunction.

Overall, therapy for patients with chronic stable angina or asymptomatic coronary artery disease should include the addition of aspirin and beta blocker. Other antianginal therapy is added as needed. ACE inhibitors are started if left ventricular systolic dysfunction is noted and in the presence of diabetes. Aggressive modification of risk factors can positively affect outcomes. This includes lowering of LDL cholesterol with statins, if possible, tight control of blood glucose in diabetics, aggressive management of hypertension, and smoking cessation. Weight loss and exercise should be encouraged as well. Invasive evaluation with coronary angiography should be reserved for those with uncontrolled symptoms or evidence of ongoing ischemia.

ACUTE CORONARY SYNDROMES

Acute coronary syndromes include unstable angina, non–ST elevation myocardial infarction, and ST elevation myocardial infarction. These syndromes represent the clinical manifestations of acute myocardial ischemia, most likely due to obstructive coronary artery disease. All require early diagnosis and clinical management to minimize damage to the myocardium and potentially catastrophic complications, including death.

UNSTABLE ANGINA AND NON–ST SEGMENT MYOCARDIAL INFARCTION

Unstable angina and non–ST segment myocardial infarction (NSTEMI) are, in most cases, caused by significant atherosclerotic coronary disease. Disruption of atherosclerotic plaque leads to formation of thrombus and partial or transient occlusion of an epicardial coronary vessel. Both conditions are associated with considerable morbidity and mortality. Although each condition is similar in terms of etiology and clinical manifestations, NSTEMI is distinguished by the presence of myocardial injury.

Etiology

As noted in the previous discussion regarding chronic stable angina, the development of chest pain as a result of unstable angina or NSTEMI is due to an imbalance between myocardial oxygen supply and demand. The vast majority of cases are due to inadequate supply because of significant coronary atherosclerosis. Instead of a stable plaque altering blood flow, the plaque causing unstable angina has become disrupted leading to thrombus formation. In this setting, the thrombus is most often nonocclusive, although small platelet aggregates and parts of the plaque itself may embolize distally leading to evidence of myocardial injury and NSTEMI. Coronary vasospasm, severe atherosclerosis, and even nonobstructive coronary lesions may lead to NSTEMI in the setting of extrinsic stressors causing increased myocardial oxygen demand.

Clinical Manifestations

Unstable angina is distinguished from chronic stable angina in several ways. Although the symptoms are identical, it is their presentation that differs. Angina is considered to be unstable when it (a) occurs at rest and is prolonged, lasting greater than 20 minutes; (b) has been present in the past but has changed in frequency, severity, or threshold needed to bring on symptoms; and (c) new onset of anginal symptoms is at least CCS Class III. Patients with NSTEMI will present with resting symptoms, most commonly typical anginal chest pain. As with chronic stable angina, the patient's coronary disease may manifest as neck, jaw, arm, or epigastric pain, or even dyspnea; these symptoms should be considered an anginal equivalent if it appears it historically has been related to exertion or stress and relieved by rest or nitroglycerine.

Diagnosis

Given the significant degree of morbidity and mortality associated with both unstable angina and NSTEMI, a rapid diagnosis is essential so proper therapy may be instituted. When a patient presents with anginal symptoms, two decisions need to be made quickly. The provider needs to determine the likelihood that the symptoms represent an acute coronary syndrome. This assessment is based upon the history including presence of traditional risk factors for coronary artery disease, physical examination findings, electrocardiographic changes, and initial laboratory values. Next, the provider must determine the likelihood of an adverse outcome, such as death, myocardial infarction, or life-threatening arrhythmia. Consideration of the patient's history, character of the chest pain, clinical and electrocardiographic findings, and evaluation of blood work will aid in this assessment (Table 27.5). Patients determined to be at high risk of death or nonfatal cardiac events will require more intensive and invasive therapy acutely than a patient felt to be at low risk.

Once the likelihood of cardiac chest pain and adverse outcomes has been established, several initial tests should be performed. These include an evaluation of secondary causes of unstable angina and NSTEMI, which increase myocardial oxygen demand or decrease oxygen supply such as severe aortic valve stenosis, infection and fever, blood loss, tachycardia, hypoxemia, consideration of thyroid disease, and sympathomimetic use (e.g., cocaine).

TABLE 27.5 Risk stratification in unstable angina[a]

Feature	**High Likelihood** *Any of the following:*	**Intermediate Likelihood** *Absence of high-likelihood features and presence of any of the following:*	**Low Likelihood** *Absence of high- or intermediate-likelihood features but may have:*
History	Chest or left arm pain or discomfort as chief symptom reproducing prior documented angina Known history of CAD, including MI	Chest or left arm pain or discomfort as chief symptom Age >70 years Male sex Diabetes mellitus	Probable ischemic symptoms in absence of any of the intermediate likelihood characteristics Recent cocaine use
Examination	Transient MR, hypotension, diaphoresis, pulmonary edema, or rales	Extracardiac vascular disease	Chest discomfort reproduced by palpation
ECG	New, or presumably new, transient ST-segment deviation (≥0.05 mV) or T-wave inversion (≥0.2 mV) with symptoms	Fixed Q waves Abnormal ST segments or T waves not documented to be new	T-wave flattening or inversion in leads with dominant R waves Normal ECG
Cardiac markers	Elevated cardiac Tnl, TnT, or CK-MB	Normal	Normal

Feature	**High Risk** *At least 1 of the following features must be present:*	**Intermediate Risk** *No high-risk feature but must have 1 of the following:*	**Low Risk** *No high- or intermediate-risk feature but may have any of the following features:*
History	Accelerating tempo of ischemic symptoms in preceding 48 h	Prior MI, peripheral or cerebrovascular disease, or CABG, prior aspirin use	
Character of pain	Prolonged ongoing (>20 minutes) rest pain	Prolonged (>20 min) rest angina, now resolved, with moderate or high likelihood of CAD Rest angina (<20 min) or relieved with rest or sublingual NTG	New-onset or progressive CCS Class III or IV angina the past 2 weeks without prolonged (>20 min) rest pain but with moderate or high likelihood of CAD
Clinical findings	Pulmonary edema, most likely due to ischemia New or worsening MR murmur S_3 or new/worsening rales Hypotension, bradycardia, tachycardia Age >75 years	Age >70 years	
ECG	Angina at rest with transient ST-segment changes >0.05 mV Bundle-branch block, new or presumed new Sustained ventricular tachycardia	T-wave inversions >0.2 mV Pathological Q waves	Normal or unchanged ECG during an episode of chest discomfort
Cardiac markers	Elevated (e.g., TnT or Tnl >0.1 ng/mL)	Slightly elevated (e.g., TnT >0.01 but <0.1 ng/mL)	Normal

[a]Estimation of the short-term risks of death and nonfatal cardiac ischemic events in UA is a complex multivariable problem that cannot be fully specified in a table such as this; therefore, this table is meant to offer general guidance and illustration rather than rigid algorithms.

Braunwald E, Mark DB, Jones RH, et al. Unstable angina: diagnosis and management. Rockville, MD: Agency for Health Care Policy and Research and the National Heart, Lung, and Blood Institute, US Public Health Service, US Department of Health and Human Services; 1994; AHCPR Publication No. 94-0602.

Adapted from AHCPR Clinical Practice Guideline No. 10, Unstable Angina: Diagnosis and Management, May 1994. Braunwald E., Mark DB, Jones RH, et al. Unstable angina: diagnosis and management. Rockville, MD: Agency for Health Care Policy and Research and the National Heart, Lung, and Blood Institute, US Public Health Service, US Department of Health and Human Services; 1994; AHCPR Publication No. 94-0602.

ELECTROCARDIOGRAPHY

A 12-lead electrocardiogram should be obtained immediately, preferably when the patient is experiencing symptoms. Dynamic electrocardiographic changes, or changes that occur with symptoms and normalize once the symptoms are resolved, are highly predictive of the presence of significant obstructive coronary artery disease. Most commonly transient ST-segment depression or deep, symmetric T-wave inversion will occur during episodes of ischemic chest pain. These changes confer a poor prognosis (increased risk of death, nonfatal myocardial infarction, and need for urgent revascularization), especially when present in multiple leads.

BIOCHEMICAL MARKERS

Biochemical cardiac markers, or cardiac enzymes, are also quite useful for initial evaluation of patients with chest pain. These markers, when present in the bloodstream, indicate myocardial necrosis and therefore infarction. Multiple markers are routinely used for the purpose of detecting acute myocardial infarction.

Creatine kinase (CK) is released by muscle cells when damage occurs. CK-MB is an isoform of CK that is typically quite elevated with myocardial necrosis, but may also be elevated in severe skeletal muscle injury, so it lacks absolute specificity for cardiac muscle. Nonetheless, it has served as the principal serum marker of myocardial infarction for years. The test is rapid and cost efficient and levels begin to rise within 6 hours after the cell damage occurs. It will not detect very minor myocardial damage.

In recent years, levels of cardiac-specific troponin, troponin T and troponin I, have been utilized as the primary serum marker of myocardial necrosis. Cardiac troponin has greater sensitivity and specificity than CK-MB for detecting myocardial infarction and begins to rise within 6 hours of the initial event. Troponin remains elevated for up to 2 weeks after an infarct. If the troponin is elevated on presentation, the patient is no longer considered to have unstable angina but rather to have sustained an NSTEMI. Troponin can detect very small infarcts and at times is elevated even when the CK-MB is normal. In studies involving patients with chest pain, normal CK-MB, and no electrocardiographic changes, an elevated cardiac troponin has been found to be associated with a higher risk of death.

Serum myoglobin has also been utilized as a marker of acute myocardial necrosis because it can be elevated within 2 hours of the acute event. Myoglobin is released by both cardiac and skeletal muscle and therefore is not cardiac specific. Thus, a positive myoglobin is not helpful unless it is accompanied by elevation of other serum markers. A negative myoglobin, however, is helpful for ruling out an infarct due to its high sensitivity.

Treatment

Patients determined to have a low likelihood of cardiac chest pain or noncardiac chest pain are often discharged to home directly from the emergency room. Patients felt to have possible cardiac chest pain can often be managed as an outpatient or expedited through the emergency room. In the latter setting, the patient will be kept in the emergency department for 24 hours. Cardiac enzymes and 12-lead electrocardiograms will be checked at 6- to 12-hour intervals; if they remain normal, the patient will then undergo a stress test to further stratify their risk. If negative for ischemia, the presenting symptoms are not likely to be due to obstructive coronary artery disease and the patient is discharged to home. If the likelihood of cardiac chest pain is high, the stress test is positive, electrocardiograms or cardiac enzymes become abnormal, or if ongoing symptoms or hemodynamic instability are present, the patient should be admitted for further evaluation and management.

Once admitted, the patient's activity is generally restricted, especially if symptoms persist. If cyanosis or respiratory distress is present, oxygen should be placed on the patient. All patients admitted for chest pain should be placed on telemetry monitoring to evaluate for malignant arrhythmias associated with acute coronary syndromes.

Anti-ischemic medications can be used to control symptoms. Nitrates will reduce myocardial oxygen demand and increase delivery by reducing preload and afterload and promoting the dilation of epicardial coronary arteries and collateral circulation. Patients with ongoing cardiac chest pain are often started on intravenous nitroglycerine drips with titration of the dose until symptoms are relieved or hypotension develops. There have been no randomized controlled trials to demonstrate a mortality benefit of nitroglycerine in this setting. Morphine is recommended for pain relief in those with continued symptoms, as this drug can lead to venodilation and an increase in vagal tone, which can cause a reduction in heart rate (lowers myocardial oxygen demand). An adverse reaction to both of these drugs is hypotension; therefore, close monitoring of blood pressure is needed.

Beta blockers will lower heart rate and reduce contractility as well as blood pressure, leading to a decrease in myocardial oxygen demand. These drugs are contraindicated with hypotension, severe bradycardia, decompensated heart failure, or severe asthma. Intravenous metoprolol, esmolol, or propranolol can be used in unstable patients, whereas oral formulations can be given in lower risk settings. Many large studies have shown significant reduction in mortality and morbidity with the use of beta blockers and acute coronary syndromes or acute myocardial infarcts. Therefore, their use is recommended in all patients unless contraindicated. Calcium channel blockers are considered second- or third-line drugs in the setting of acute coronary syndromes, and dihydropyridines (nifedipine, among others) have been shown in some studies to be detrimental. Use of nondihydropyridines such as verapamil or diltiazem is recommended only when beta blockers are contraindicated.

ACE inhibitors have been found to be beneficial in those with left ventricular systolic dysfunction, diabetics, and patients with high-risk chronic coronary artery disease. They typically are added to the drug regimen of such patients presenting with a high likelihood of cardiac chest pain with high blood pressure despite the use of beta blockers and nitrates.

Given the underlying etiology of thrombus formation, patients with suspected acute coronary syndromes should be given adequate antiplatelet and antithrombotic therapy. Aspirin is essential in all patients with possible acute coronary syndromes, as studies have shown a significant benefit in terms of both morbidity and mortality when used in this patient population. If aspirin cannot be given due to allergy or intolerance, another antiplatelet agent such as clopidogrel should be given. Multiple studies have also shown mortality benefit when high-risk patients are given unfractionated or low molecular weight heparin. Long-term anticoagulation with warfarin has not been found to be useful and is therefore not recommended. Parenteral glycoprotein IIb/IIIa inhibitors (eptifibatide or tirofiban) are indicated in those with unstable angina or NSTEMI who have ongoing symptoms or other high-risk characteristics such as increasing cardiac enzymes or worsening electrocardiographic changes.

Lipid-lowering agents also should be started in patients with suspected acute coronary syndromes. Statins have been shown to reduce mortality in patients presenting with acute coronary syndromes, and patients with coronary artery disease require very tight control of lipids. If patients are intolerant to statins, other lipid-lowering agents should be instituted, such as niacin or fibrates.

Once this medical management is initiated, patients who have stabilized with resolution of symptoms and are considered to have possible ischemia are then monitored for at least 24 hours. Provided their cardiac enzymes show no evidence of acute myocardial infarction, they will then undergo risk stratification with stress testing, which was described previously.

Patients considered to have definite anginal symptoms or who have abnormal cardiac enzymes, persisting symptoms, or electrocardiographic changes undergo more invasive evaluation with coronary angiography (also described above). If significant obstructive coronary disease is found, therapeutic options include percutaneous coronary intervention and coronary artery bypass grafting.

PERCUTANEOUS CORONARY INTERVENTION

Percutaneous coronary intervention often involves performing angioplasty. This procedure entails maneuvering a small balloon to the site of significant stenosis within the coronary artery. The balloon is then inflated creating a dissection plane within the vessel. This will allow for increased blood flow. By itself, this procedure has historically been associated with restenosis rates of greater than 40%. Within the last 10 to 15 years, coronary stents have been introduced. These are small, wire, meshlike devices comprised of stainless steel, titanium, or cobalt that are mounted on a balloon. The stent is delivered to the area of significant plaque and deployed under high pressures. As a result, it will become embedded in the wall of the vessel, thereby increasing the luminal diameter. With stents, restenosis rates were initially reduced to 15% to 30%. The most recent innovation involves stents coated with immunomodulating agents such as sirolimus and paclitaxel, which prevent the growth of excess tissue within the stents. This has reduced restenosis rates to less than 5%. The metal stent that has been embedded in the arterial wall is thrombogenic, not only because it is a foreign body, but also because stent deployment leads to endothelial damage, which can set off a cascade leading to formation of a thrombus. Therefore, the patient should be maintained on antiplatelet therapy including aspirin and clopidogrel. These drugs will help maintain stent patency until the endothelium grows over the exposed metal stent, thereby eliminating any thrombogenic potential.

CORONARY ARTERY BYPASS GRAFTING

Coronary artery bypass grafting (CABG) involves the use of veins or arteries as conduits to supply blood to myocardium beyond significant stenoses within the coronary arteries. CABG is indicated in patients with significant left main coronary disease; patients with significant three-vessel coronary artery disease, especially those with diminished left ventricular systolic function; patients with diabetes; and significant two-vessel coronary disease wherein one of the lesions involves the proximal left anterior descending artery.

Once revascularization has been achieved, the patient is discharged home on much of the same medical regimen that was instituted in the hospital. This includes aspirin, beta blockers, and clopidogrel (if a stent was placed). Lipid-lowering therapy should be continued and ACE inhibitors should be used if there is evidence of left ventricular systolic dysfunction. Drugs required to control ischemic symptoms such as nitrates should be continued if needed. Continued modification of risk factors, including smoking cessation and strict glycemic control of diabetes, should be encouraged.

PRINZMETAL'S OR VARIANT ANGINA

Variant angina is a form of unstable angina that is caused by severe coronary vasospasm. This occurs spontaneously and is characterized by anginal chest pain occurring at rest and without any precipitating cause. Affected patients are usually younger, female, smokers, and without other significant risk factors for coronary artery disease. Patients often have manifestations of other vasospastic disorders such as migraine headaches and Raynaud's phenomenon. Most attacks resolve without progression to acute myocardial infarction, but infarction can happen in the setting of prolonged spasm. The spasm typically is focal and can occur at more than one site. When coronary angiography is performed, the arteries are often normal or show nonobstructive plaques. Treatment involves use of long-acting nitrates and calcium channel blockers. Prognosis is excellent in patients receiving proper medical therapy, especially when concomitant coronary disease is absent.

ST ELEVATION MYOCARDIAL INFARCTION

ST elevation myocardial infarction (STEMI) and its complications cause significant morbidity and mortality. Up to 45% of patients presenting with acute coronary syndromes are diagnosed with an acute STEMI. There are an estimated 500,000 ST elevation myocardial infarctions per year in the

United States alone, which signifies that this entity remains an important public health problem despite advances in therapy. The key to treating STEMI is early recognition and reperfusion therapy to re-establish blood flow. The faster the STEMI is diagnosed, the faster the infarct related blood vessel can be treated. This is of paramount importance as timely reperfusion will decrease the amount of myocardial necrosis and substantially reduce morbidity and mortality in a large number of patients.

Etiology

The pathophysiologic substrate of STEMI is called a vulnerable plaque. When the process of atherosclerosis leads to development of a lipid-laden fibrous plaque, the fibrous cap becomes prone to erosion or rupture. When this happens, it is often an abrupt process that exposes many prothrombotic substances to the blood. This leads to initiation of the clotting cascade and thus formation of what is many times an occlusive thrombus.

The vulnerable plaque is typically a nonobstructive lesion, often measuring 40% to 50% of the overall luminal diameter, and is therefore asymptomatic (and many times not recognized) prior to rupture. The majority are located at bifurcation points or acute bends in the arterial tree, points where sheer stress is greatest. Once a thrombus is formed it may completely occlude the vessel causing myocardial cell death. Myocardial cell death will lead to a process called ventricular remodeling, which involves changes in shape, size, and thickness of the ventricle. The myocardium affected by the infarct will thin and become dilated acutely, expanding into areas that are not damaged by myocardial necrosis. Areas of normal-functioning myocardium will attempt to compensate by muscle hypertrophy. This remodeling may lead to aneurysm and scar formation, which can serve as a nidus for malignant arrhythmia and significant reductions in left ventricular systolic function.

Clinical Manifestations

The patient suffering from STEMI may experience anginal chest pain of much the same quality as chronic stable angina but much more severe and unrelenting. It is acute in onset and may begin at rest or with exertion. The chest pain is often associated with difficulty breathing, nausea, emesis, and diaphoresis. Many times it will radiate to the neck, jaw, or arms. Almost 50% of all myocardial infarctions may be unrecognized due to a lack of chest pain based on data from the Framingham Study. Some patients will not experience any chest pain, but manifest only shortness of breath or pain located in other areas such as the neck, jaw, or epigastric region. These patients tend to be older, diabetic, and female. Because many expect dramatic chest pain to represent a myocardial infarction, the absence of chest pain will often cause patients to delay seeking medical care.

The initial history should target the patient's chest pain. The location, quality, time of onset, duration of the pain, and identification of where the pain radiates are all important aspects to investigate. The presence of previously diagnosed coronary disease and prior cardiac events or interventions (stents, CABG) should be determined. The presence or absence of risk factors is important to note, as is previously diagnosed peripheral vascular disease. One should also pay attention to problems that may interfere with antiplatelet or antithrombotic therapy such as active bleeding, history of bleeding disorders, recent surgical procedures, history of hemorrhagic stroke, and history of peptic ulcer disease. Associated symptoms should be noted including nausea, emesis, diaphoresis, and dyspnea.

The physical examination should focus on the stability of vital signs and clinical signs of hypoperfusion, evidence of heart failure (jugular venous distention, crackles on lung exam, left ventricular heave), assessment of heart murmurs or gallops, evidence of cerebrovascular disease (acute or chronic), and examination of peripheral pulses.

Diagnosis

Due to the implications of rapid diagnosis of acute STEMI and the potential reduction in morbidity and mortality once treatment has been initiated, it is imperative to efficiently evaluate the patient with a suspected acute coronary syndrome. The history, physical examination findings, and ancillary studies such as the electrocardiogram and cardiac enzymes must be accurately interpreted in a timely fashion.

A 12-lead electrocardiogram should be performed within 10 minutes of arrival, as this single study is most likely to influence therapy. Given this fact, many ambulances are now equipped to transmit a 12-lead electrocardiogram prior to the patient arriving at the hospital so therapy may be started sooner. If ST segment elevation is present, the patient will benefit from reperfusion therapy, as opposed to those with unstable angina and NSTEMI, in whom reperfusion therapy is generally not indicated. ST segment elevation should be seen in multiple contiguous leads to diagnose myocardial infarction. Mortality has been found to be higher in those with anterior ST elevation, left bundle branch block, and greater number of electrocardiogram leads involved.

Initial laboratory studies are drawn shortly after arrival but reperfusion therapy is generally not delayed until results are back. Cardiac enzymes should be obtained as well as a baseline complete blood count, basic metabolic panel, and coagulation panel. Although the diagnosis of STEMI will be made once the electrocardiogram has been obtained, cardiac biomarkers remain useful as they can provide prognostic information as well as allow estimation of infarct size. Recall that the most commonly used cardiac enzymes, namely CK-MB and cardiac troponin, begin to rise 3 to 6 hours after the initial infarct. Therefore, the initial set of cardiac enzymes will likely be normal if the patient as presented shortly after symptoms began. Troponin may stay elevated for several weeks after an infarct, whereas the CK-MB normalizes within days. Thus the CK-MB may be valuable in assessing recurrent chest pain after reperfusion if it begins to rise again (indicating reocclusion).

Treatment

Once the diagnosis of STEMI has been established, therapy to quickly and completely reestablish blood flow should be instituted. Most emergency departments have implemented protocols to deal with patients with suspected acute coronary syndromes to facilitate this process. Patients identified at high risk are immediately placed on telemetry and an electrocardiogram is performed within 10 minutes of arrival. If an acute STEMI is identified, a decision is made on reperfusion therapy within the next 10 minutes. Should cardiac catheterization and intervention be indicated, the goal to reperfusion is within 90 minutes of arrival to the emergency room. In hospitals where catheterization is not available, fibrinolytic agents are given. Should these methods fail, surgical intervention should be undertaken (CABG). Reperfusion of the infarct-related artery has been shown in multiple studies to be the main factor in determining both short- and long-term outcomes. It is now widely expected that fibrinolytic therapy will be instituted (door-to-needle time) within 30 minutes of presentation, and catheter-based intervention will lead to reperfusion (door-to-balloon time) within 90 minutes of presentation.

Fibrinolytic agents such as streptokinase or newer formulations such as alteplase, reteplase, and tenecteplase will lead to dissolution of thrombus at the site of plaque rupture, thereby reestablishing blood flow. Current recommendations state that these agents should be administered within 12 hours (ideally 3 hours) of symptom onset. They may also be given within 12 to 24 hours in the presence of continued symptoms and electrocardiographic changes. They should be utilized in settings where a catheterization lab is not readily available or a delay to catheterization is likely. Use of these agents has been shown to reduce relative mortality by up to 21%. Contraindications to fibrinolytic therapy include history of intracranial hemorrhage, significant closed head or facial trauma within the past 3 months, ischemic stroke within the past 3 months, patients with high risk for intracranial hemorrhage, or uncontrolled hypertension. The major complication of fibrinolytic therapy is life-threatening hemorrhage, in particular intracranial hemorrhage.

Percutaneous coronary intervention (angioplasty and stent placement) is a very effective reperfusion strategy for patients presenting with STEMI. This strategy will not only allow for intervention upon the infarct related artery, but will also identify patients who are better treated with coronary artery bypass grafting. A catheter-based invasive strategy will also reveal the occasional patient with STEMI who has vasospasm or spontaneous reperfusion and would not benefit from fibrinolytic therapy. Percutaneous coronary intervention will relieve obstruction by mechanically restoring luminal diameter with placement of a coronary stent within the lesion. At present, this procedure is preferred over fibrinolysis in several situations. If the proper facilities are immediately available and the patient is within 12 hours of symptom onset, the patient is in cardiogenic shock or severe heart failure, or symptoms persist within 24 hours of symptom onset, then primary percutaneous coronary intervention is the reperfusion therapy of choice. When directly compared with fibrinolysis, percutaneous intervention has demonstrated lower short-term mortality rates, lower incidence of nonfatal reinfarction, and less hemorrhagic stroke. Rates of major bleeding are higher with percutaneous intervention. Primary percutaneous intervention is not recommended in those who are greater than 12 hours out from onset of symptoms and are currently asymptomatic. Complications include arterial access site problems, allergies to contrast dye, and other technical complications such as coronary artery perforation.

Emergent coronary arterial bypass grafting should be performed in patients with failed percutaneous intervention, cardiogenic shock with left main disease, and life-threatening arrhythmias with significant left main or triple vessel coronary disease.

In terms of other medical therapy, hypertension should be immediately treated as high blood pressure will increase myocardial oxygen demand and worsen myocardial necrosis. Nitrates may be given for ongoing ischemic chest pain, uncontrolled hypertension, or evidence of congestive heart failure. Morphine may be given for additional pain relief. Aspirin at a dose of 162 to 325 mg should be given to all patients presenting with STEMI if the patient has not already taken it. Beta blockers should also be started upon presentation unless a contraindication exists. There is strong data to support a significant mortality benefit with both aspirin and beta blockade in the setting of STEMI. Unfractionated heparin has also been shown to reduce mortality in STEMI regardless of which reperfusion therapy is utilized. Clopidogrel may reduce mortality as well when given upon presentation. This drug may lead to excessive bleeding if surgical intervention is ultimately needed, and therefore should be withheld for at least 5 days prior to surgery. ACE inhibitors should be started in all patients with STEMI and anterior infarction, significant left ventricular systolic dysfunction, or pulmonary congestion. In patients who are intolerant of ACE inhibitors, angiotensin receptor blockers may be substituted. There is also evidence to support the use of ACE inhibitors in all patients with STEMI, although the magnitude of benefit is less than that noted in the above listed subgroups of patients. Calcium channel blockers may be used as a substitute for beta blockers if contraindications exist, but should not be utilized in patients with evidence of decompensated heart failure. Data also exists to support the use of statins upon admission for STEMI, regardless of initial lipid levels.

All acute STEMIs should be admitted to the cardiac intensive care unit for at least 24 hours of observation. Medications started on admission, such as beta blockers, aspirin, ACE inhibitors, and statins, are continued indefinitely unless they are not tolerated. Clopidogrel should be continued if percutaneous coronary intervention was performed. These medications should be continued upon discharge as well. Patients are then transferred to a stepdown unit where they continue to be monitored on continuous telemetry. The patient is typically discharged 72 hours after admission provided no complications have occurred. Of course, aggressive modification of cardiac risk factors should be undertaken upon discharge.

Complications

STEMI may be complicated by many life-threatening problems. If a significant amount of myocardial necrosis has occurred, hypotension, pulmonary vascular congestion, or cardiogenic shock may develop.

A low-output state may be present upon admission or it may develop over the first few days following presentation. Echocardiography can be performed to evaluate the contractility of both the left and right ventricles and the extent of myocardial damage, as well as assess for mechanical complications such as papillary muscle rupture with resultant mitral regurgitation, ventricular septal rupture, and left ventricular free wall rupture. If extensive remodeling has taken place, a left ventricular aneurysm may form which can lead to further reductions in left ventricular systolic function or rupture (Tables 27.6, 27.7, and 27.8).

Arrhythmias are also common after STEMI, particularly early after presentation. Ventricular fibrillation is most common in the first 4 hours after symptom onset and remains an important cause of mortality for at least the first 24 hours. Electrolyte abnormalities and acid-base disturbances will contribute to the development of ventricular fibrillation. Ventricular tachycardia is also a common

TABLE 27.6 Hemodynamic and other complications of myocardial infarction

Heart failure
With large MI that involves >28% of myocardial tissue With acute MR or large VSD
Cardiogenic shock
From a large MI causing heart failure and loss of cardiac output From acute MR (leading to severe heart failure and cardiogenic shock)
Postinfarction angina and infarct extension
Recurrent ischemic pain after relief of initial MI pain really represents unstable angina. Infarct extension indicates occurrence of another MI within 3 weeks of the preceding one.
Pericarditis
Complicates acute MI usually within the first 4 days
Thromboembolic complications
Mural thrombus may form often in anterior-wall MI (33%).
Left ventricular aneurysm
Usually follows an anterior Q-wave MI May cause congestive heart failure, and/or ventricular arrhythmias Persistent ST-segment elevation may be seen in leads showing Q waves.
Right ventricular infarction
Approximately 35% of patients with inferior or posterior LV infarction also sustain a RV infarction. ST elevation in right-sided lead V_4 on the ECG Hypotension, jugular venous distention, and low cardiac output
Dressler's syndrome (postmyocardial infarction syndrome)
About 3% of all cases of acute MI Occurs most often 2 weeks to several months after an MI Recurrent fever, chest pain, pericardial friction rub, leukocytosis, and bloody pericardial and/or pleural fluid.

ECG, electrocardiogram; LV, left ventricle; MI, myocardial infarction; MR, mitral regurgitation; RV, right ventricle; VSD, ventricular septal defect.

TABLE 27.7 Mechanical complications of myocardial infarction

Ventricular septal rupture with VSD
Occurs in 3% of cases of acute MI, usually in the first week after infarction Sudden, loud pansystolic murmur LLSB Severe CHF and/or cardiogenic shock
Acute MR
Due to a ruptured papillary muscle may lead to heart failure and/or cardiogenic shock
Rupture of LV free wall
Causes 10% of all deaths in acute MI Most patients die suddenly

CHF, congestive heart failure; LLSB, lower left sternal border; LV, left ventricle; MI, myocardial infarction; MR, mitral regurgitation; VSD, ventricular septal defect.

occurrence, usually within the first 48 hours. Most of these episodes are nonsustained (lasting less than 30 seconds). If nonsustained episodes are seen more than 4 days after STEMI, they may represent a higher risk of future cardiac arrest. Frequent premature ventricular contractions are not significant and should not be treated. Supraventricular tachycardia, in particular atrial fibrillation, occurs more commonly with large infarcts and in conjunction with other conditions like electrolyte abnormalities, heart failure, and pericarditis. Significant bradycardia is associated with inferior infarcts due to increased vagal tone. Heart block may develop as well depending upon the size of infarct. Bradycardias generally manifest early in the course of the infarct (Table 27.8).

Postinfarct pericarditis, or Dressler's syndrome, may occur in patients with large infarcts and appear several weeks following the initial event. ST segment elevation will again be apparent on the electrocardiogram and a pericardial rub may be heard on cardiac examination. Treatment is

TABLE 27.8 Arrhythmic complications of myocardial infarction

Sinus bradycardia
Common in early acute inferior-wall MI
Atrial tachycardia, atrial fibrillation
Due to left ventricle failure or atrial ischemia
Premature ventricular complexes
Occur in almost 90% of patients with acute MI, not treated unless symptomatic or sustained
Ventricular tachycardia, ventricular fibrillation (15% to 20%)
Primary within the first 48 hours of MI, usually do not recur Secondary ventricular tachycardia and fibrillation (later than 48 hours after MI) is recurrent, poor prognosis
AV blocks
More common in acute inferior wall MIs (because the right coronary artery supplies the inferior left ventricle wall, atrioventricular node, and His bundle)

MI, myocardial infarction.

with aspirin or other nonsteroidal anti-inflammatory drugs. Steroid use may cause further myocardial thinning at the site of infarct and may lead to rupture. Therefore, use of steroids with postinfarct pericarditis should be avoided if at all possible.

Acute stroke has been associated with anterior infarcts and diminished left ventricular systolic function and is usually embolic in nature. Risk of stroke is highest within the first month after the infarct and remains elevated for the first year.

CHAPTER 28

Heart Failure

Geoffrey C. Lamb

Heart failure is a general term referring to a constellation of disorders arising from problems with the pumping function of the heart. This dysfunction leads to a variety of systemic problems linked to disruption of the circulatory system, renal function, hormonal function, and neuroregulatory function. Such dysfunction can be asymptomatic or lead to symptoms ranging from simple fatigue to dyspnea and overt fluid congestion.

Heart failure is a common cause of morbidity and mortality affecting nearly 5 million people in the United States. It is predominantly a disease of aging, with approximately 2% of individuals between the ages of 40 to 59 years affected and nearly 10% of those over the age of 75 years. It is the most common cause of hospitalization in patients over 65 years, and more Medicare dollars are spent on the diagnosis and management heart failure than any other single diagnosis.

ETIOLOGY

In essence, heart failure occurs when the heart is unable to keep up with the metabolic demands of the body. Heart failure can be caused by *systolic dysfunction*, characterized by malfunction of the normal pumping capacity of the left ventricle, or *diastolic dysfunction*, which is characterized by normal systolic function and increased difficulty filling the left ventricle. It can also occur in the context of increased metabolic demand exceeding the normal capacity of the heart, or *high output failure. Right heart failure* can occur in the presence of increased pulmonary pressures or impairment of the right ventricular musculature (Table 28.1).

Typically the process of heart failure begins with an injury or disruption to the normal intricate balance of structures that contribute to normal heart functioning. This can include direct damage to the cardiac muscle (myocardial ischemia, myocarditis), obstruction to outflow (valvular disease, hypertension), or problems with filling (pulmonary hypertension, left ventricular hypertrophy). In response to this initial injury, there is active remodeling of cardiac muscle often with thickening or lengthening of the myocardial muscle. This is accompanied by infiltration of inflammatory cells and deposition of fibrin. Systemically, the changes in perfusion pressures and hemodynamics lead to a host of hormonal responses, including activation of the renal angiotensin-aldosterone system and the sympathetic nervous system

Systolic dysfunction usually is characterized by a decline in the *ejection fraction* of the left ventricle, the proportion of blood in the left ventricular chamber that is pumped out with each stroke. The most common cause of systolic dysfunction is ischemic cardiomyopathy secondary to coronary artery disease. Myocardial infarction or stunned myocardium leads to areas of poor contractility and inefficient ventricular output. The next most common cause is cardiomyopathy, disease in which there is global loss of contractility in the ventricle. Fully 50% of cases of cardiomyopathy are idiopathic with the remainder due to myocarditis, viral infections, infiltrative diseases, hypertension, substance abuse, and toxins (Table 28.1). Systolic dysfunction can also be triggered by pressure overload, volume overload or a chronic high output state. *Pressure overload* or increased afterload can be caused by

TABLE 28.1 Etiology of congestive heart failure

Predominantly systolic dysfunction	Predominantly diastolic dysfunction
Conditions causing pressure overload: Hypertension Aortic stenosis Coarctation of aorta Pulmonary hypertension Pulmonary thromboembolic disease	Marked left ventricular hypertrophy Hypertrophic cardiomyopathy Hypertension Severe myocardial ischemia Mitral stenosis Left atrial myxoma Infiltrative cardiomyopathies (amyloidosis, hemochromatosis)
Conditions causing volume overload: Aortic incompetence Mitral incompetence Ventricular septal defect Atrial septal defect	
Myocardial contractile failure: Myocardial infarction Dilated cardiomyopathies	

obstruction of the ventricular outflow tract as in aortic stenosis and coarctation of the aorta or by increased vascular pressure as in systemic hypertension. Left ventricular hypertrophy develops to compensate for the increased workload, but over years this leads to failure of the contraction and dilation of the cardiac muscle in the ventricle. *Volume overload* can occur due to disorders such as aortic regurgitation, patent ductus and ventricular septal defect. In contrast to pressure overload, the ventricle dilates early and undergoes hypertrophy over years.

Diastolic dysfunction is caused by disruption of the normal filling of the left ventricle. It is characterized by the development of congestive heart failure (CHF) in the presence of a normal ejection fraction. Most commonly, diastolic dysfunction is caused by left ventricular hypertrophy. As the ventricle gets thicker and stiffer, it becomes more difficult to fill. The contractile force needed to fill a stiff ventricle leads to an increase in left atrial pressure, which in turn can lead to dilation of the thin walled left atrium. If atrial fibrillation develops, it can exacerbate the situation by further delaying filling and decreasing the filling pressure. Triggers can include anything that leads to left ventricular hypertrophy including hypertension, hypertrophic cardiomyopathy, or aortic stenosis. Diastolic dysfunction can also be triggered by disorders that interfere with the flow into the ventricle such as mitral stenosis or atrial myxoma.

High output failure often occurs in the setting of an intrinsically unhealthy heart. Systemic disease that forces the ventricle to operate at its highest output over several years (such as anemia, hyperthyroidism and direct arterial-venous shunts) can lead to muscle fatigue. The ventricle dilates leading to a chronic volume overload and further dilation.

Right heart failure is characterized by a decrease in the right ventricle pumping function. Most cases of right heart failure stem from a disorder that leads to pulmonary hypertension, which in turn creates a pressure load on the ventricle. Examples of disorders leading to isolated right ventricular failure include mitral stenosis, pulmonary embolism, and chronic lung disease. However, the most common cause of right ventricular failure is left ventricular failure. As the left ventricle fails and pulmonary arterial pressure rises, the pressure load on the right ventricle is increased. Ultimately dilation of the right ventricle occurs, leading to failure. This in turn leads to an increase in systemic venous pressures. Rarely, disease affecting the right ventricle alone, such as a right ventricular infarction, can lead to right ventricular failure in the absence of pulmonary hypertension.

CLINICAL MANIFESTATION

The classic manifestation of left heart failure is dyspnea. This typically is caused by a combination of diminished compliance of the lungs in the presence of pulmonary venous congestion and ventilation-perfusion mismatch due to edema within the lung tissue. Early in the disease, dyspnea is seen primarily on exertion. However, as the disease progresses, pulmonary congestion is increased in the supine position leading to *orthopnea* and *paroxysmal nocturnal dyspnea.* Orthopnea is the sensation of shortness of breath when lying flat and relieved on sitting up. Paroxysmal nocturnal dyspnea is the sudden onset of severe shortness of breath while lying down sleeping, forcing the patient to sit or stand to get relief.

At the extreme, the patient may develop pulmonary edema. This is manifested by marked shortness of breath even when upright. Associated symptoms may include a sense of chest tightness, anxiety, diaphoresis, and pallor. Pulmonary edema may also trigger a cough. This can be accompanied by production of frothy sputum that may be blood tinged.

In the presence of increasing venous congestion and right heart failure, patients often notice dependent edema, especially in the distal extremities. Passive congestion of the liver can cause right upper quadrant discomfort and a sense of abdominal bloating, nausea, and loss of appetite. Patients may also notice daytime oliguria and increasing nocturia.

Strikingly, in patients with biventricular failure or left ventricular failure in the face of progressive right sided failure, pulmonary congestion may actually diminish due to the reduction of right ventricular perfusion pressure. Such patients may have minimal dyspnea or orthopnea despite advanced disease. In patients for whom the dominant manifestation is inadequate perfusion as opposed to congestion, symptoms may simply consist of fatigue, lethargy, and poor exercise tolerance.

Regardless of the specific symptom complex, severity is commonly gauged using the New York Heart Association (NYHA) Functional Classification of Congestive Heart Failure (Table 28.2).

On examination, physical signs are largely related to the manifestations of venous congestion and ventricular dysfunction. On inspection, patients in pulmonary edema typically are sitting upright and are in visible respiratory distress. Tachypnea and tachycardia frequently are seen. An irregularly irregular pulse suggests atrial fibrillation. Hypertension at the time of presentation is unusual if there is significant systolic dysfunction because of the inability of the ventricle to generate high pressures. Accordingly, the presence of hypertension at the time of initial evaluation is associated with the presence of diastolic dysfunction as the etiology in close to two thirds of patients.

Inspection of the neck can reveal jugular venous distension, a manifestation of right-sided failure. Elevation of the jugular venous pulse to greater than 3 cm above the sternal angle has a 60% sensitivity

TABLE 28.2 New York Heart Association functional classification of congestive heart failure

Class	Description
I	Symptoms with greater than ordinary activity (i.e., no impairment)
II	Symptoms with ordinary activity (i.e., mild impairment)
III	Symptoms with minimal activity, asymptomatic at rest (i.e., significant impairment)
IV	Symptoms at rest (i.e., severe impairment)

and near 80% specificity for increased atrial filling pressure. A positive *hepatojugular reflux*, persistent elevation of the jugular venous pulse with firm pressure over the liver, is more specific (94%) for the presence for congestive heart failure. Lung examination may reveal basilar rales, rhonchi, and dullness at the bases in the presence of left ventricular failure.

Palpation of the heart can reveal the sustained left ventricular heave of left ventricular hypertrophy, the slight tapping sensation of the ventricle in the presence of mitral stenosis or the diffuse, displaced Part of Maximal Impulse (PMI) of a dilated left ventricle. Careful auscultation of the heart can reveal characteristic heart sounds and murmurs. An S3 over the apex is a sign of a dilated, poorly contractile left ventricle and is highly predictive of the presence of heart failure, but is only present in half of patients. An S4 is associated with a noncompliant left ventricle and may suggest left ventricular hypertrophy but is not reliable for distinguishing diastolic from systolic dysfunction. A crescendo-decrescendo systolic murmur, especially located along the left upper sternal border, should lead to consideration of occult aortic stenosis. A blowing systolic murmur radiating from the apex toward the axilla suggests mitral regurgitation. This may be a cause of CHF or occur as the left ventricle dilates and enlarges the mitral ring. Dilation of the right ventricle can lead to the development of tricuspid regurgitation manifested as a holosystolic murmur along the left lower sternal border and a prominent jugular venous pulse that peaks during systole (v-wave).

In the presence of right-sided heart failure, hepatomegaly can develop. Typically this is mildly tender to palpation. In the presence of tricuspid regurgitation, pulsations can be felt. Pitting edema is common in the presence of heart failure. This generally is located in the dependent areas of the body such as the ankles and feet; however, in patients who are bedbound, it may best be identified over the sacrum.

DIAGNOSIS

The goals of the diagnostic workup are to confirm the diagnosis of heart failure, assess the severity of the disorder, and identify the underlying etiology.

In addition to the characteristic symptoms of heart failure identified earlier, the history is an important tool in determining the underlying cause of the heart failure. It is important to inquire about drug consumption, alcohol use, and illicit substance use. A number of prescription drugs have side effects that can manifest as heart failure (Table 28.3). Alcohol is a myocardial suppressant and a number of illicit drugs (cocaine, heroin) can cause myocardial toxicity. The physical examination can also provide clues to etiology including valve disorders, rhythm problems, and metabolic disorders such as hyperthyroidism.

Chest radiography is the first diagnostic test of choice. Typical findings suggestive of heart failure include cardiomegaly, interstitial edema, and vascular redistribution (cephalization) of the pulmonary veins. Cardiomegaly is seen in approximately 80% of patients with heart failure but is not very specific (80%). Findings of interstitial edema such as Kerley B lines, peribronchial cuffing, and perihilar haziness—especially in combination with cephalization—are found in less than half of cases but when present are much more specific (98%) (Fig. 28.1).

Initial laboratory work should include urinalysis, creatinine, electrolytes, albumin, and liver function tests to look for renal failure, nephrotic syndrome, and liver disease as alternate causes of fluid retention as well as to identify end-organ disease such as renal failure and electrolyte disturbances. If the clinical examination suggests high-output failure or atrial fibrillation, or if the patient is older than 65 years, thyroid testing should also be obtained (including a free T4 and thyroid-stimulating hormone) and a complete blood count should be obtained to look for anemia.

B-type natriuretic protein (BNP) is also helpful in diagnosing CHF. BNP is a peptide released from the ventricle when myocytes are subjected to increased stretch. A BNP >100 pg/mL has a

TABLE 28.3 Prescription drugs known to cause or exacerbate heart failure

Drug type	Specific examples
Amphetamines	
Antiarrhythmic agents	Disopyramide Amiodarone
Beta-adrenergic blockers	Propranolol
Calcium channel blockers	Verapamil Diltiazem
Nonsteroidal anti-inflammatory drugs	Ibuprofen Indomethacin
Thiazolidinediones	Rosiglitazone Pioglitazone
Chemotherapeutic drugs	Doxorubicin

90% sensitivity and a 75% specificity for heart failure. In a low probability patient, a BNP level <100 pg/mL can rule out heart failure.

An electrocardiogram should be obtained routinely. It is often nonspecific but it is almost always abnormal in the presence of substantial left ventricular dysfunction. It can be useful to detect ischemia, infarction, arrhythmias, or left ventricular hypertrophy.

When the patient is stabilized, some method of assessing left ventricular function should be

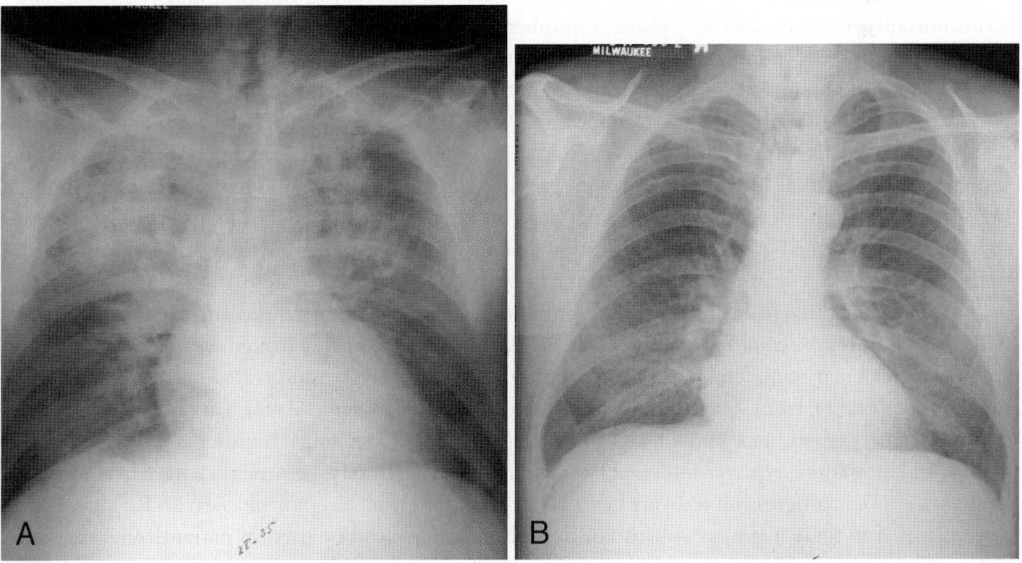

Figure 28.1 • **A.** Chest radiograph in acute cardiogenic pulmonary edema showing bilateral confluent opacities ("bat-wing"). **B.** Follow-up x-ray a few days later, showing significant clearing, although some mild congestive changes remain.

obtained to confirm the diagnosis and guide therapy. An echocardiogram is particularly useful because it is noninvasive and can be used to estimate left ventricular ejection fraction and ventricular dimensions thus distinguishing diastolic from systolic dysfunction. It can also identify structural abnormalities such as valve disease and septal defects. Other alternatives for estimating ejection fraction include radionuclide techniques such as multiple-gated acquisition scanning (MUGA) or contrast ventriculography performed during cardiac catheterization. Cardiac stress testing should be considered when reversible ischemia is suspected. It is indicated whenever congestive heart failure occurs in the context of prior myocardial infarction or prior history of ischemia. Depending on the stability of the patient and the clinical context, either stress testing or coronary artery catheterization should be considered when CHF is associated with angina or electrocardiographic changes. Cardiac catheterization is not routinely required unless the diagnosis is in question or there is strong evidence that the proximal cause of heart failure is acute ischemia. When performed, catheterization reveals high pulmonary capillary wedge and left ventricular end-diastolic pressures and abnormally wide arteriovenous oxygen differences.

TREATMENT

The treatment of acute congestive heart failure focuses on symptom relief and stabilization of the patient. Patients should be allowed to sit in the upright position. Oxygen supplementation is useful to decrease the workload of the heart and relieve some dyspnea. Loop diuretics, such as furosemide, are the mainstay of treatment and typically are administered intravenously, either intermittently or continuously. Morphine sulfate given intravenously can help relieve the sensation of dyspnea and associated anxiety. The subsequent reduction in adrenergic stimuli can also lead to vasodilation. Nitrates can be useful to increase venous dilation. They are particularly useful in the setting of heart failure exacerbated by ischemic heart disease. Nitroprusside may be employed if the heart failure occurs in the context of severe hypertension. Inotropic agents such as digoxin, dobutamine, and milrinone are not routinely used but can be helpful in refractory cases.

The management of chronic heart failure focuses on improving function and reducing long-term mortality. Over the last few years, a number of drugs have been demonstrated to prolong life expectancy and improve function by reducing afterload, promoting ventricular remodeling, reducing adrenergic stimulation, and modulating the angiotensin–aldosterone system. The American College of Cardiology and American Heart Association (ACC/AHA) have established guidelines for the treatment of heart failure based on a staging system created in 2001 (see Fig. 28.2) This staging system emphasizes that heart failure is a progressive disease and that intervention in individuals at high risk prior to the development of symptoms can have significant benefit. This staging system is complementary to the New York classification system which serves as a method of classifying symptom severity and can be used in conjunction the ACC/AHA staging system.

Angiotensin-converting enzyme (ACE) inhibitors should be the first-line drug used in all patients with heart failure. ACE inhibitors modulate the renin-angiotensin system, reduce afterload, and can facilitate ventricular remodeling. Most importantly, they have been demonstrated in controlled studies to reduce mortality from heart failure. They are indicated in stage A for patients with diabetes mellitus, hypertension, and known atherosclerotic disease and in stage B patients with a previous myocardial infarction, hypertension, and left ventricular hypertrophy, because they have been demonstrated to prevent progression to overt heart failure. Angiotensin-receptor blockers (ARB) have been demonstrated to serve a similar role as ACE inhibitors. They can be used in patients who meet the criteria for ACE inhibitor use in those who are ACE intolerant. There is little evidence of added benefit to using an ACE inhibitor and an ARB together.

Beta blockers—specifically bisoprolol, carvedilol, and metoprolol succinate—have been also demonstrated to reduce mortality in heart failure. Beta blockade reduces the workload of the heart,

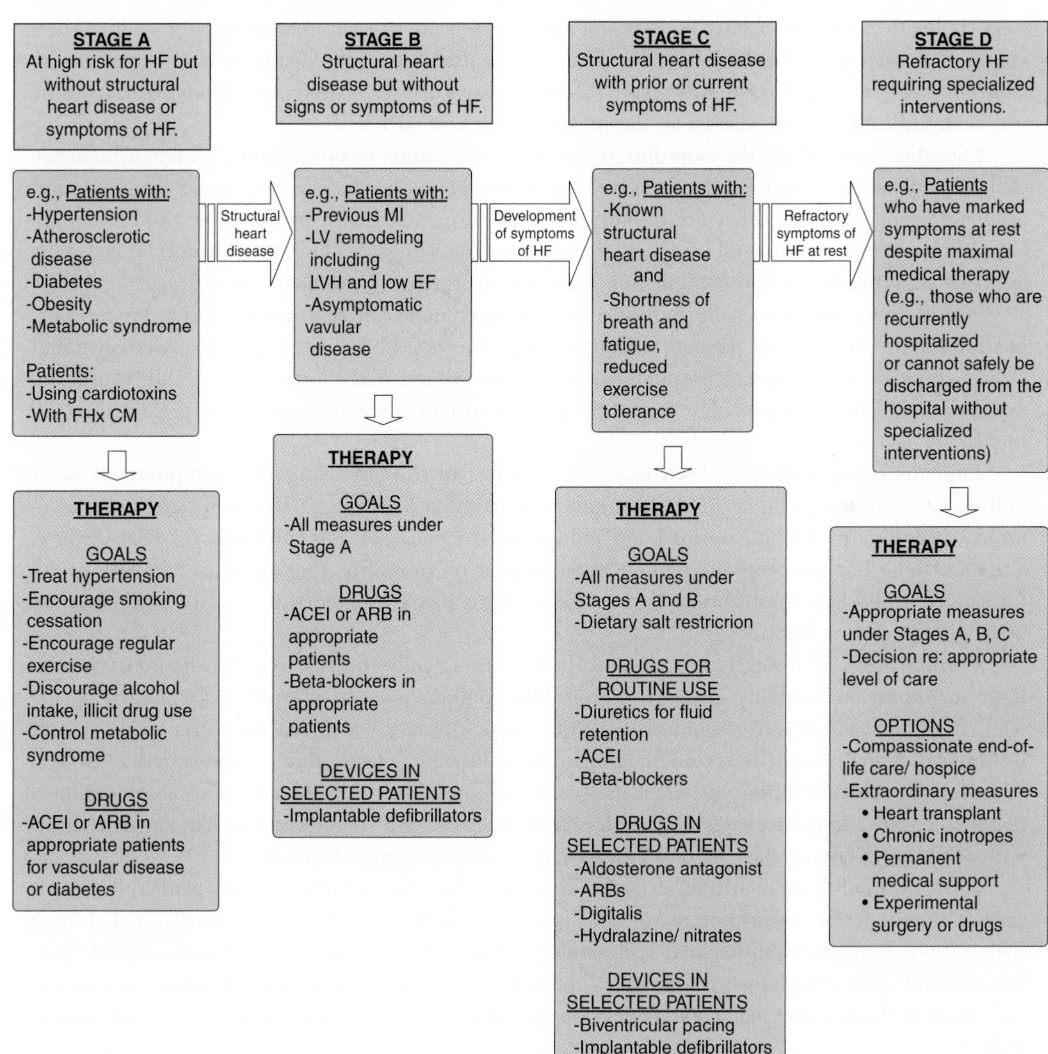

Figure 28.2 • Stages in the development of heart failure/recommended therapy by stage. ACEI, angiotensin-converting enzyme inhibitor; ARB, angiotensin-receptor blocker; FHx CM, family history of cardiomyopathy. (Reproduced from Hunt SA, Abraham WT, Chin MH. ACC/AHA 2005 Guideline Update for the Diagnosis and Management of Chronic Heart Failure in the Adult—Summary Article: A Report of the American College of Cardiology/American Heart Association Task Force on Practice Guidelines [Writing Committee to Update the 2001 Guidelines for the Evaluation and Management of Heart Failure]. *Circulation* 2005;112:1825–1852, with permission.)

decreases the impact of sympathetic nervous system stimulation, and reduces blood pressure. They serve as an important component of management in all patients with symptomatic heart failure, stages B, C, or D. Even in the absence of symptoms, beta blockers should be used in patients with stage B heart failure who have underlying structural heart disease, remodeling, or reduced left ventricular ejection fraction (LVEF). They can also be useful in stage A patients with hypertension. Contraindications include primarily severe reactive airways disease, symptomatic bradycardia, cocaine use, or significant valvular disease in the presence of a normal LVEF.

Diuretics, particularly the loop diuretics such as furosemide or bumetanide, remain a mainstay of therapy. They have not been shown to prolong life but are quite effective in reducing symptoms and reducing hospitalizations. They are recommended for all patients with symptomatic fluid retention. Current guidelines recommend using weight and symptoms to guide dosing of diuretics. It is important that diuretics be used in combination with sodium restriction to maximize efficacy.

Aldosterone inhibition using spironolactone or eplerenone can be a useful adjunct in late-stage heart failure in symptomatic patients resistant to loop diuretics. These agents have been demonstrated to reduce death and recurrent hospitalization in these groups. They must be used with caution to avoid hyperkalemia and probably should be avoided in patients with a creatinine greater than 2.0 mg/dL.

Digitalis compounds have been used for centuries to treat the congestive symptoms of heart failure. Currently, digoxin is the safest digitalis preparation available. It has been demonstrated to improve symptoms of fluid overload and reduce the frequency of hospitalization for heart failure, although there has not been any demonstrated impact on mortality. Digoxin is particularly useful for rate control when atrial fibrillation is present. Digoxin is associated with toxicity and should be used with caution at high doses.

Combinations of hydralazine and isosorbide were actually the first regimen demonstrated to have an impact on mortality in heart failure. This combination was ultimately supplanted by the ACE inhibitors which were demonstrated to be more effective. However, there has been a recent resurgence of hydralazine/isosorbide combinations following a study that demonstrated a survival advantage in African Americans when used as an adjunct to existing therapy. This combination is reasonable to use in patients who are intolerant of ACE or ARB therapy and in African Americans with NYHA functional class III or VI heart failure despite standard therapy.

Lifestyle modification to reduce factors that exacerbate heart failure or independently impair cardiac function play an important role in disease management. Concomitant cardiac risk factors such as hypertension, dyslipidemia, and smoking should be managed using standard guidelines. Alcohol and other drugs known to impair cardiac function should be avoided. Regular exercise can maximize performance. Once patients develop symptoms, sodium restriction becomes important as well.

Ultimately, heart transplantation can be an option for patients with end-stage heart failure. It is reserved for patients with intractable functional Class III or IV CHF who have little likelihood of survival during the next 6 to 12 months. The ideal patients are relatively young (60 years) and without multiorgan disease. In such patients, the chances of improved quality of life and return to employment are high. Significant pulmonary hypertension (pulmonary vascular resistance >6 Wood units), collagen vascular disease, positive human immunodeficiency virus status, and severe, complicated diabetes mellitus are the major contraindications.

COMPLICATIONS

One of the common causes of death in patients with impaired ventricular function is ventricular arrhythmia and sudden death. Implantable cardioverter- defibrillator devices have been clearly shown to prolong life in those heart failure patients with a low LVEF and documented ventricular arrhythmias, prior cardiac arrest, or syncope of unclear etiology. Several trials have also demonstrated reduced mortality from cardiac arrhythmias in asymptomatic patients with a low LVEF. However routine placement of an implantable cardioverter-defibrillator device in all patients with a low LVEF remains controversial. It is not clear that such devices reduce total mortality and in some patients placement of an implantable cardioverter-defibrillator can reduce quality of life.

Heart failure remains a disease with high mortality. For patients hospitalized with a first episode of heart failure, the 1-year mortality averages approximately 33%. Mortality rates range from 7.6% at 1 year for women younger than 50 years with no comorbidities to more than 60% for men older than 75 years with three or more comorbidities. To date, only the use of ACE inhibitors/ARBs and beta blockers at the time of discharge have been shown to have any effect on these numbers.

CHAPTER 29

Cardiomyopathies / Myocarditis

Tayyab Mohyuddin

The cardiomyopathies are a group of diseases that primarily affect myocardial muscle structure and function in the absence of a secondary cause such as coronary artery disease, hypertension, or valvular dysfunction. Cardiomyopathies can be categorized into three clinical subgroups: dilated, hypertrophic, and restrictive. Dilated cardiomyopathies primarily exhibit systolic dysfunction, whereas hypertrophic and restrictive cardiomyopathies primarily exhibit diastolic dysfunction.

DILATED CARDIOMYOPATHY

Dilated cardiomyopathy (DCM) is a common cause of heart failure with an estimated prevalence of 36.5 per 100,000 persons in the United States. African American males are more commonly affected than other ethnic groups. Left and/or right ventricular dilatation with impaired contractile function is characteristic of this disorder. Nonspecific histomorphological changes include interstitial and perivascular fibrosis as well as myocyte hypertrophy and atrophy.

Etiology

Although the etiology is unknown in most cases, DCM is likely the sequela of infectious, metabolic, or toxic insults (Table 29.1). Toxic exposures include alcohol, cocaine, antineoplastic agents, and thyroid disease.

Alcoholic cardiomyopathy usually results from heavy alcohol consumption over years. A genetic predisposition may play a role in certain individuals. Left ventricular (LV) dysfunction appears to be dose dependent. Specific toxins, ethanol itself, and a metabolic product, acetaldehyde, have been shown to impair cardiac excitation-contraction coupling resulting in oxidative damage. Cessation of alcohol intake before the development of clinical heart failure usually can reverse the LV dysfunction.

Peripartum cardiomyopathy generally occurs in the last month of pregnancy or early after delivery. Numerous mechanistic etiologies (infectious, immunologic, and nutritional) have been suggested but the true cause remains unclear. Most patients have recovery of ventricular function following delivery but the risk of recurrence with subsequent pregnancy is nearly 50% and the risk of irreversible cardiac damage increases with subsequent pregnancies.

Familial cardiomyopathy is seen in 20% to 40% of patients with DCM with various patterns of inheritance including autosomal dominant, X-linked, autosomal recessive, and mitochondrial inheritance. Mutations may be present in genes encoding for the myocyte cytoskeleton (dystrophin and desmin), the sarcomere (beta-myosin heavy chain, troponin, cardiac alpha-actin, alpha-tropomyosin), or other proteins.

Arrhythmogenic right ventricular cardiomyopathy (ARVC) is characterized by replacement of right ventricular myocardium by fatty or fibrofatty tissue. ARVC is genetically heterogeneous.

Clinical Manifestations

Exertional intolerance due to dyspnea or fatigue is the most common presentation, although the first manifestation may be overt congestive heart failure with orthopnea, paroxysmal nocturnal dyspnea,

TABLE 29.1 Known causes of dilated cardiomyopathy

Toxins	Inflammatory or infectious causes
Ethanol[a] Chemotherapeutic agents: doxorubicin, bleomycin Cobalt[a] Antiretroviral agents: zidovudine[a], didanosine[a], zalcitabine[a] Phenothiazine[a] Carbon monoxide[a] Lead[a] Mercury[a] Cocaine[a]	Infectious Viral: Coxsacki virus, cytomegalovirus[a], human immunodeficiency virus Rickettsial Bacterial: diphtheria Mycobacterial Fungal Parasitic Toxoplasmosis[a] Trichinosis, Chagas' disease Collagen vascular disorders Systemic lupus erythematosus, progressive systemic sclerosis, dermatomyositis Hypersensitivity myocarditis[a] sarcoidosis[a], peripartum dysfunction[a]
Metabolic abnormalities	**Neuromuscular causes**
Nutritional deficiencies Thiamine[a], selenium[a], carnitine[a] Endocrinologic disorders Diabetes mellitus, hypothyroidism[a], thyrotoxicosis[a], Cushing's disease, acromegaly[a], pheochromocytoma[a] Electrolyte disturbances: Hypocalcemia[a], hypophosphatemia[a]	Duchenne's muscular dystrophy Fascioscapulohumeral muscular dystrophy Erb's limb girdle dystrophy Myotonic dystrophy Fredreich's ataxia
Familial cardiomyopathies	

[a]Potentially reversible either spontaneously or with treatment.
From Dec GW, Fuster V. Idiopathic dilated cardiomyopathy. *N Engl J Med* 1994;331:1564–1575, with permission.

and volume overload (Chapter 28). Despite normal coronary arteries, up to one third of patients report angina-like chest pain. Syncope is usually secondary to an arrhythmia. ARVC patients in particular can present with chest pain, palpitations, or sudden cardiac death. Symptoms in these patients are often secondary to ventricular tachycardia with a left bundle branch block morphology.

The physical examination varies with the extent of ventricular dilatation, dysfunction, and neurologic compensation. Sinus tachycardia is common. Systolic blood pressure is often low, typically with a narrow pulse pressure. Jugular venous distension is present with a prominent V wave when tricuspid regurgitation is present. The apical impulse is often diffuse and laterally displaced. Atrial (S4) and ventricular (S3) gallops and systolic murmurs are common. Systolic murmurs can result from mitral or tricuspid regurgitation due to annular dilatation and chordal geometric distortion. The lung exam can have bilateral end inspiratory crackles. Asymmetric dullness to lung percussion is often secondary to a pleural effusion. Ascites, hepatomegaly, and bilateral pedal edema are seen when venous pressures are high.

Diagnosis

Blood tests are of limited value. The brain natriuretic peptide level is typically elevated, which can be useful to suggest a cardiac cause in patients who present primarily with dyspnea. The electrocardiogram is nonspecific. Common findings include sinus tachycardia or atrial fibrillation, left atrial enlargement, repolarization changes, and intraventricular conduction delays. The chest radiograph can demonstrate cardiomegaly, pulmonary vascular congestion, or pleural effusions.

Echocardiography is the most useful test. The echocardiogram shows ventricular dilatation, with normal, minimally thickened or thinned walls and decreased systolic function. Coronary angiography, performed to exclude coronary artery disease, is by definition without flow-limiting obstructions. In selected patients such as those with suspected ARVC, other diagnostic studies include cardiac magnetic resonance imaging (MRI) and right ventricular angiography.

Treatment

Treatment focuses on the management of the heart failure (Chapter 28). Nonpharmacologic therapies include salt restriction, exercise, alcohol cessation, smoking cessation, and weight reduction. Drug therapy for heart failure with renin-angiotensin axis inhibitors (angiotensin-converting enzyme receptor blockers or angiotensin receptor blockers) and beta-adrenergic blockade improves symptoms and prolongs survival. Most patients require loop diuretics to relieve symptoms of volume overload such as edema. Aldosterone antagonists are used in patients with New York Heart Association class III/IV symptoms.

Patients with atrial fibrillation, a mural thrombus or prior thromboembolism should receive chronic anticoagulation. Patients with left bundle branch block and LV systolic dysfunction have been shown to benefit from resynchronization therapy. Implantable cardioverter defibrillators have been shown to reduce mortality in patients with an ejection fraction of less than 35%. Cardiac transplantation is an option for refractory cases.

HYPERTROPHIC CARDIOMYOPATHY

Hypertrophic cardiomyopathy (HCM) is a disorder characterized by myocyte hypertrophy and disarray, in the absence of hemodynamic stress capable of producing hypertrophy (e.g., hypertension, obesity, exercise). When outflow tract obstruction is present, the entity is called hypertrophic obstructive cardiomyopathy (HOCM).

The prevalence is 1 in 500 in the U.S. population. The approximate annual mortality is 1 % in patients with HCM and 2% in patients with HOCM. Hypertrophic cardiomyopathy is the most common cause of death among high school athletes in the United States.

Etiology

Hypertrophic cardiomyopathy is a genetic disorder. Most patients have a positive family history consistent with an autosomal dominant pattern of inheritance. Missense mutations of genes that encode the cardiac sarcomeric proteins (beta-myosin heavy chain, cardiac troponin T, myosin-binding protein C, alpha-tropomyosin, and beta-myosin light chains) are present.

The pathophysiology of HOCM is complex and involves various mechanisms. The pattern of hypertrophy is asymmetric, affecting the interventricular septum more than the posterolateral segments of the left ventricle. An apical or concentric distribution may be present. Initial contraction of the ventricle is usually normal however as outflow from the left ventricle progresses and the ventricle contracts outflow obstruction can occur. Outflow tract obstruction is dynamic and changes with preload, afterload and contractility. Conditions that decrease the preload (hypovolemia, diuretics, Valsalva), decrease the afterload (vasodilators), and increase the contractility (exercise, sympathomimetics) can increase the pressure gradient and the outflow obstruction. Systolic anterior motion of the mitral valve (SAM) is the apposition of the anterior mitral valve leaflet against the hypertrophied septum during systole. The obstruction increases diastolic filling pressures leading to decrease in cardiac output and myocardial ischemia. Secondary mitral regurgitation can occur in patients with SAM.

Clinical Manifestations

Most patients with HCM are asymptomatic. When symptoms occur they can be highly variable. Exertional dyspnea, fatigue, chest pain, palpitations, dizziness, exertional syncope, and sudden cardiac death have been noted.

The physical examination classically reveals a fast rising arterial pulse, pulsus bisferiens (a pulse with double peaks), double apical precordial impulse, and a fourth heart sound. The double impulse represents the initial normal outflow, obstruction as systole progresses, then a second rise in flow as the ventricle relaxes. On auscultation the hallmark finding is a harsh, diamond-shaped systolic murmur best heard at the base. Maneuvers that decrease the LV cavity size (Valsalva, standing) augment the murmur and maneuvers, which increase venous return, and ventricular volume (passive leg raising) decreases the murmur.

Diagnosis

The electrocardiogram typically shows LVH and prominent septal Q waves in the precordial leads (pseudoinfarct pattern). This phenomenon can be confused with myocardial ischemia or infarction. The chest radiograph may show cardiomegaly but is often normal.

Echocardiography remains the definitive diagnostic test, showing asymmetric septal hypertrophy (septal thickness >1.5 times that of posterior wall or an interventricular septal thickness >15 mm). SAM is seen in about one half of the cases and is quite specific for LV outflow tract obstruction. Maneuvers like Valsalva can provoke latent obstruction. Cardiac catheterization shows an elevated left ventricular diastolic pressure and allows measurement of the pressure gradient between the left ventricle cavity and the left ventricle outflow tract.

All first-degree relatives should have a screening echocardiogram every 5 years and for adolescents every year until they are 18 years of age. Genetic testing for diagnosis and screening likely will become commercially available.

Treatment

The goal of therapy is relief of symptoms and prevention of sudden cardiac death. Initial therapy should incorporate a beta blocker which can decrease the outflow gradient, improve diastolic filling, and reduce myocardial ischemia by slowing the heart rate. Calcium channel blockers and disopyramide have been used but are not recommended as first-line therapy. Vasodilators such as nitroglycerin should be avoided in patients with HOCM. Patients should be advised to avoid dehydration and strenuous exercise.

Surgical treatment, myectomy for HOCM, usually resolves the gradient and improves symptoms. Symptomatic patients with a resting gradient greater than 30 mm Hg are the best candidates for myomectomy. The operative mortality in experienced centers is 1% to 3%. A potentially less invasive approach to reduce the size of the obstruction is percutaneous septal ablation. Alcohol is infused in a septal perforator artery with a resulting controlled infarction of the hypertrophied septum. The appropriate septal perforator is identified by contrast echocardiography to target myocardial damage. Known complications include heart block, inappropriate infarction, and cardiac perforation. Long-term follow-up data on these patients is limited to case reports only.

Dual chamber pacing has been advocated as an alternative therapeutic approach. This derives from the recognition that initiating contraction in the right ventricle instead of the left alters septal movement during systole and results in the reduction of the gradient. Long-term data are controversial and do not support pacing as first-line therapy.

Patients with major risk factors (prior cardiac arrest, sustained ventricular tachycardia, massive hypertrophy, or a family history of sudden death) are candidates for an implantable cardioverter defibrillator. Outflow obstruction or mitral regurgitation mandates endocarditis prophylaxis.

RESTRICTIVE CARDIOMYOPATHY

Restrictive cardiomyopathy (RCM) is the least common form of cardiomyopathy. Impaired ventricular filling due to high ventricular pressures results in diastolic dysfunction. Systolic function is often preserved.

Etiology

The major causes of RCM are shown in Table 29.2. In cardiac amyloidosis, deposition of insoluble amyloid protein fibrils occurs in the interstitium. On histology, amyloid deposits are stained red with Congo red, showing green birefringence under polarized light.

In endomyocardial fibrosis, fibrosis of the endomyocardium occurs in one or both ventricles and the atrioventricular valves. Mural thrombi can result in partial cavity obliteration. Two types of endomyocardial fibrosis have been described. Löffler's endocarditis is associated with a hypereosinophilic state (Churg-Strauss syndrome, idiopathic hypereosinophilia). Cardiac damage results from intracytoplasmic granular content of activated eosinophils. The second type of endomyocardial fibrosis is endemic to parts of Africa, Asia, South America, and Central America. The etiology is unknown.

In cardiac sarcoidosis, granulomas can involve the pericardium, myocardium, or endocardium. Conduction abnormalities and fatal arrhythmias can occur. African Americans are afflicted more than other ethnic groups.

In hemochromatosis, iron deposition is secondary to a hereditary state (autosomal recessive), multiple transfusions, or a hemoglobinopathy.

TABLE 29.2 Causes of restrictive cardiomyopathy

Myocardial	**Endomyocardial**
Noninfiltrative	Endomyocardial fibrosis[a]
Idiopathic[a]	Hypereosinophilic syndrome
Familial	Carcinoid heart disease
Diabetic	Metastatic cancers
Infiltrative	Radiation[a]
Amyloidosis[a]	Anthracycline toxicity[a]
Sarcoidosis[a]	Drug-related fibrous endocarditis
Fatty infiltration	Serotonin
Gaucher's disease	Methysergide
Storage diseases	Ergotamine
Hemochromatosis	Mercurial agents
Fabry's disease	Busulfan
Glycogen storage disease	

[a]More frequent than the others in clinical practice.

Clinical Manifestations

High filling pressures result in a decreased cardiac output. The typical presentation is dyspnea on exertion. The jugular venous pressure is elevated and may rise with inspiration (Kussmaul's sign). RCM may mimic constrictive pericarditis clinically. Compared to constrictive pericarditis, the apical impulse is usually palpable, mitral regurgitation is more common, and pulmonary pressures are higher.

Diagnosis

The electrocardiogram often shows sinus tachycardia, low voltage in the limb leads, nonspecific ST-T changes, and a left bundle branch block. Chest radiography can show cardiomegaly and pulmonary venous congestion. On echocardiography, the valves are normal; the LV is thickened and is not dilated. A computed tomographic scan can be useful to exclude pericardial thickening and constrictive pericarditis. Contrast-enhanced magnetic resonance imaging and positron emission tomography scan are most sensitive for the diagnosis of sarcoidosis. Cardiac catheterization shows elevated right and left ventricular end diastolic pressures. Endomyocardial biopsy is useful in the diagnosis of amyloidosis, hemochromatosis, and endomyocardial fibrosis.

Treatment

Treatment is aimed toward the underlying clinical condition causing RCM and the relief of heart failure symptoms. For hemochromatosis, specific treatments include deferoxamine and phlebotomy. For amyloidosis, chemotherapy, autologous stem cell transplantation, and cardiac transplantation improve survival in certain cases but the overall prognosis remains poor. In endomyocardial fibrosis, surgical excision of fibrotic endocardium is an option. In cardiac sarcoidosis, corticosteroids may slow the progression but the incidence of ventricular tachycardia is unaffected. An implantable cardioverter defibrillator should be placed in sarcoidosis patients with nonsustained ventricular tachycardia or syncope. Diuretics and vasodilators should be used with caution in all forms of RCM so that LV preload is not compromised.

MYOCARDITIS

Myocarditis is an inflammation of the myocardium, with infection as the most common cause. The true incidence of myocarditis is difficult to estimate because of variable clinical presentations and diagnostic criteria.

Etiology

The causes of myocarditis are listed in Table 29.3. Multiple infectious etiologies have been implicated, the most common being enterovirus coxsackie B. Recent data also show that geographical variations exist in viral etiology. Parvovirus B19 has been identified in German patients and hepatitis C virus in Japanese patients. Pathogenesis involves direct viral infection and/or the ensuing host immune response.

Human immunodeficiency virus patients develop myocarditis and left ventricular dysfunction secondary to involvement by virus, medications, or other opportunistic infections. Lyme carditis is caused by *Borrelia burgdorferi* and is typically manifested as arrhythmias or heart block.

Chagas disease is caused by *Trypanosoma cruzi*, commonly in Central and South America. Rarely, patients develop an acute myocarditis, but approximately 30% of patients develop a chronic cardiomyopathy. Various mechanisms such as persistent parasitemia and oxidative stress have been implicated in the pathogenesis. Dilatation of cardiac chambers, conduction abnormalities, and arrhythmias are characteristic. Cases are now found in the United States with immigration from these countries.

TABLE 29.3 Causes of myocarditis

Infectious	
Bacterial	Diphtheria (toxin), infective endocarditis, Lyme disease (Borrelia burgdorferi)
Fungal	Aspergillus
Mycoplasma	
Parasitic	Toxoplasmosis, trypanosomiasis (Chagas' disease), trichinosis
Rickettsial	Rocky Mountain spotted fever
Viral	Adenovirus, Coxsackie groups A and B, cytomegalovirus, ECHO viruses, hepatitis B, human immunodeficiency virus (may be opportunistic infections or drug effects), influenza, poliomyelitis, rubella, rubeola
Inflammatory	
Idiopathic giant cell	Myocarditis, rheumatic fever, sarcoidosis
Connective tissue diseases	Systemic lupus erythematosus, rheumatoid arthritis
Vasculitis	Polyarteritis nodosa, Churg-Strauss vasculitis
Hypereosinophilic syndrome	
Toxic	
Drugs	Aerosol propellants, daunorubicin, emetine, phenothiazine, tricyclic antidepressants
Physical agents	
Radiation	

Medications including penicillin, sulfonamides, tricyclics, and clozapine can cause myocarditis by a hypersensitivity reaction. Autoimmune states including systemic lupus erythematosus, rheumatoid arthritis, and systemic sclerosis have been associated with myocarditis.

Clinical Manifestations

Myocarditis shows highly variable clinical features. Patients can present with a viral prodrome, chest pain, or congestive heart failure. Fulminant myocarditis presents with hemodynamic instability. The physical examination in most patients has no specific findings. Some patients may present with signs of heart failure (Chapter 28).

Diagnosis

The sedimentation rate is commonly elevated as are other markers of myocardial injury such as creatine kinase-MB, aspartate aminotransferase, and lactate dehydrogenase. Troponin T has been shown to be a useful marker for myocarditis as well. If myocarditis is confirmed, serology for suspected triggering agents such as Lyme titers is warranted.

The electrocardiogram shows tachycardia, low voltage, and nonspecific ST-T changes. Atrial and ventricular extrasystoles and atrioventricular block are common, especially in Lyme carditis. The chest radiograph may be normal or show signs of heart failure.

Echocardiography may show depressed LV systolic function or a pericardial effusion. Nuclear scan with indium-111 or gallium-67 labeled antimyosin antibodies, which bind to cardiac myocytes with disrupted sarcolemmal membranes, can quantify myocardial inflammation and necrosis. Contrast magnetic resonance imaging shows focal myocardial enhancement as well as wall motion abnormalities strongly suggestive of myocarditis.

Treatment

The usual treatment is supportive care. Patients with fulminant myocarditis require hemodynamic support and may require mechanical circulatory support as a bridge to recovery.

Most patients recover ventricular function (LVEF) within weeks. Immunosuppression is not effective, although several new immune-modulating therapies are under investigation.

CHAPTER 30

Valvular Heart Disease

Geoffrey C. Lamb

The heart is an intricate structure of contracting chambers and valves that serve to maintain forward flow of blood and a careful balance of perfusion pressures with the various structures of the body. Disruption of that balance can lead to interference with flow and increased pressure behind the "pump." The four major valves of the heart—aortic, mitral, pulmonic, and tricuspid—can each have disorders leading to leakage across the valve, regurgitation, or narrowing leading to obstruction and stenosis. Of these, the disorders involving the left-sided valves are most clinically significant, although tricuspid lesions can have hemodynamic impact as well.

AORTIC STENOSIS

Aortic stenosis (AS) is a narrowing of the aortic valve structure in the left ventricular (LV) outflow tract leading to obstruction to flow through the valve. The normal valve size ranges from 3 to 4 cm^2. In general it must be narrowed to less than 25% of its normal size before there is any impact on the circulation. It is one of the most common valve disorders, accounting for one quarter of all patients with valve disease.

Etiology

The most common cause of AS in this country is senile calcification of the valves. This accounts for nearly two thirds of cases. Calcification affects the degenerating valve from the base of the cusp and progresses toward the free edge. The cusps become increasingly less mobile and may fuse. Risk factors for this process seem to parallel coronary artery disease risk. A total of 10% to 35% of cases are attributable to rheumatic fever. Inflammation leads to injury of the valve and ultimately leads to calcification of the valve, typically from the free edge of the valve and progressing toward the base. Most cases also involve some degree of aortic regurgitation. Mitral valve involvement is also present in 80% of cases. In case series, congenital bicuspid aortic valve lesions account for 5% to 30% of cases. Bicuspid aortic valvular disease is the most common congenital heart disorder and occurs in 1 to 2 per 1,000 births. In general, aortic stenosis becomes more common as individuals age. In screening studies, 2.5% of patients aged 75 years have AS, whereas fully 8% of those aged 85 years will have AS. Individuals with rheumatic fever and bicuspid valves tend to become symptomatic at younger age, often between ages 30 and 50 years, whereas those with senile degeneration of the valves are more likely to have problems between ages 50 and 80 years.

Regardless of cause, AS has a consistent course. Turbulent blood flow across an abnormal valve can lead to accelerated fibrosis and degenerative changes in the valve due to mechanical stress. Calcium can develop along with the fibrosis, causing increasing rigidity of valve leaflets and immobility of the cusps. This obstruction leads to increased LV wall stress and filling pressures, LV hypertrophy, and finally, chronic LV pressure overload. These changes impair epicardial to endocardial blood flow, while at the same time increasing myocardial O_2 demands and contributing to an abnormal relaxation response of a stiff, hypertrophied ventricle. For many years, most patients are asymptomatic, although valve area may be decreasing and the pressure gradient across the valve increasing. However, LV dilatation, systolic or diastolic dysfunction, and clinical deterioration eventually supervene.

Clinical Manifestations

Once AS becomes symptomatic, patients may manifest with angina, dyspnea on exertion, exertional syncope, or heart failure. Prior to that point, patients may have very subtle impairments in exercise tolerance that may just be attributed to being "out of shape" or "old age." The development of symptoms signal a poor prognosis if left untreated, with an average survival of 2 to 3 years.

On physical examination, there can be several clues to the presence of significant AS. The classic murmur is a coarse crescendo-decrescendo murmur heard in mid to late systole, radiating to the carotid artery (Chapter 16). Markers of severe disease on physical examination include a delay felt in the upstroke of the pulse in the carotid artery, a sustained left ventricular heave when feeling for the point of maximum impulse, a soft A2 portion of the second heart sound, and delay of the murmur to late systole. The absence of radiation of the murmur to the carotid is a strong argument against the presence of AS.

Diagnosis

When AS is suspected, initial workup should include an electrocardiogram (ECG), a chest x-ray, and an echocardiogram. The ECG should show left ventricular hypertrophy. There may be a left ventricular strain pattern or a left bundle branch block. Occasionally, as left atrial pressures increase, atrial fibrillation may be seen. The chest x-ray can give information about the cardiac silhouette and may demonstrate early heart failure. On occasion, calcification in the area of the aortic valve can be seen.

The echocardiogram is the mainstay of diagnosis. The two-dimensional echocardiogram is useful for visualizing the valve itself and confirming the presence of disease and allows one to determine left ventricular function. Doppler echocardiography allows measurement of the outflow velocity across the valve so that a mean transvalvular pressure gradient and valve area can be estimated. Severe AS typically has a valve area less than 1.0 cm^2 and a gradient >50 mm Hg. It is also helpful to detect concomitant regurgitation or other valvular abnormalities.

Exercise stress testing can be useful in asymptomatic patients. It can identify patients with a limited exercise tolerance or an abnormal exercise response such as a drop in blood pressure. Exercise testing should only be performed under close supervision with careful monitoring of blood pressure and the ECG. In patients who are symptomatic, exercise testing offers little additional value and is potentially dangerous; as such, it should not be performed.

Cardiac catheterization and coronary angiography are indicated when valve replacement is being considered. Coronary artery disease is present in greater than 33% of patients with AS and greater than 50% of those over 70 years of age. Revascularization performed at the same time as valve replacement has no increased mortality over valve replacement alone. Catheterization is also indicated if there is a substantial discrepancy between the echocardiogram and the clinical presentation.

Treatment

The only effective treatment for severe AS is valve replacement. The American College of Cardiology and American Heart Association (ACC/AHA) have published guidelines as to when valve replacement should be considered. In essence, valve replacement is recommended in any patient who is symptomatic, anyone with moderate to severe stenosis undergoing open heart surgery for another reason, or in anyone who is asymptomatic with severe AS who has LV dysfunction or exercise-induced hypotension.

Balloon valvotomy is recommended for children, adolescents, and young adults in whom a stenosed valve is likely congenital with fused cusps and extensive calcification has not occurred. These individuals have a high success rate with good long-term palliation and little complication.

Valvotomy does not work well in older adults, especially when there is a large amount of calcification contributing to the stenosis.

Patients who are asymptomatic, have good LV function, and good exercise tolerance should be monitored on a regular basis but do not require surgery. They should receive prophylaxis for endocarditis when undergoing potentially contaminated invasive procedures such as dental work. There is no medical therapy that has been shown to be helpful.

AORTIC REGURGITATION

Aortic regurgitation occurs when blood leaks backward through the aortic valve into the left ventricle during diastole. This can occur due to dilation of the aorta or the aortic ring or due to disease of the valve leaflets themselves. The prevalence is about 5 per 10,000 people. Men between the ages of 30 and 60 years are most commonly affected.

Etiology

The most common cause of chronic aortic regurgitation is an idiopathic dilation of the aortic root. Although the etiology remains unclear, it appears to be related to medial degeneration and is highly associated with hypertension and progressive age. Other causes of a dilated aortic root and valve ring include connective tissue diseases (e.g., Marfan's syndrome), aortic dissection, autoimmune diseases (e.g., ankylosing spondylitis), aortitis (giant cell arteritis), mediastinal irradiation, and syphilis. The next most common cause is a congenital bicuspid valve. With progressive calcification and rigidity of the valves, incomplete closure is common. Other triggers of intrinsic valve disease are trauma to the valve itself and inflammatory processes such as endocarditis and rheumatic fever. Drugs have also been associated with development of aortic insufficiency, including dexfenfluramine and pergolide (Table 30.1).

In chronic aortic regurgitation, there is a combined volume and pressure overload due to the reflux of blood back into the ventricle. The ventricle adapts by dilating and developing hypertrophy over time, allowing the heart to maintain a normal ejection fraction for many years. The rapid drop in aortic filling due to the regurgitation leads to a very low diastolic blood pressure. Concomitantly, the increased left ventricular volume leads commonly to elevated systolic pressures and a very wide pulse pressure. Normalization of systolic blood pressure can be a marker of left ventricular decompensation. As the disease progresses, the ability of the left ventricle to compensate with exercise declines, which is often the first sign of systolic dysfunction. During the early stages of ventricular decompensation, repair of the valve will lead to normalization of systolic function. If the left ventricle becomes too dilated, however, recovery becomes incomplete and life expectancy may be limited even with repair.

Acute aortic regurgitation usually occurs in response to an acute event such as aortic dissection, valve destruction from endocarditis, or chest wall trauma. A sudden volume load is created on the left ventricle. Because the ventricle cannot expand as quickly as the volume load, left ventricular end diastolic pressure increases rapidly, which can lead to a rapid decline in cardiac output and cardiogenic shock.

Clinical Manifestations

Chronic aortic regurgitation is most commonly identified as an incidental finding on clinical examination. Symptom onset usually is insidious and manifests as dyspnea on exertion. Patients may attribute the symptoms to "old age" or being out of condition. Occasionally, if the disease has progressed to severe systolic dysfunction, patients may complain of palpitations due to the rapid heart rate and distended ventricle. Angina can occur both due to insufficiency in the coronary arteries and/or

TABLE 30.1 Causes of aortic regurgitation

Intrinsic Valve disease (46%)	Aortic dilation (54%)
Congenital (25%) Endocarditis (18%) Rheumatic (3%)	Idiopathic (33%) Dissection (10%) Marfan's (5%) Aortitis (4%)
Miscellaneous (1%)	
Congenital valve Ventricular septal defect Supra- and subvalvular stenosis Aneurysm sinus of Valsalva	
Connective tissue Osteogenesis imperfecta Ehlers-Danlos	
Autoimmune disease Ankylosing spondylitis Rheumatoid arthritis Systemic lupus erythematosus	
Aortitis Giant cell arteritis Takayasu's disease	
Syphilis	
Drugs Dexfenfluramine Pergolide	
Chest trauma	
Mediastinal irradiation	

From Roberts WC, Ko JM, Moore TR, et al. Causes of pure aortic regurgitation in patients having isolated aortic valve replacement at a single US tertiary hospital (1993 to 2005). *Circulation* 2006;114:422–429.

partial ostial occlusion. Physical examination can reveal a number of clues to the presence of aortic regurgitation. The blood pressure typically has a very large pulse pressure with diastolic pressures frequently below 50 mm Hg and occasionally down to 0 mm Hg. The wide pulse pressure has lead to a number of physical signs, many of which have acquired eponyms (Table 30.2). Auscultation reveals an early diastolic decrescendo murmur best heard with the bell along the left sternal border. S1 is typically soft and S2 is often single because of incomplete closure of the aortic valve. Palpation reveals a dynamic left ventricular heave that may rock the chest.

Acute aortic insufficiency often presents in dramatic fashion with pulmonary edema or cardiogenic shock. The large pulse pressures seen in chronic regurgitation usually are not seen due to the rapid decompensation of the left ventricle.

Diagnosis

Oftentimes, the diagnosis of aortic regurgitation can be made on the basis of physical examination alone. Initial evaluation of the patient presenting with suspected aortic regurgitation should begin

TABLE 30.2 Physical signs of aortic regurgitation

Finding	Sign
Bobbing of the head with heart beat	de Musset's sign
Pistol shot sound over femoral artery	Traube's sign
Murmur over femoral artery when compressed Compressed proximally: systolic Compressed distally: diastolic	Duroziez's sign
Capillary pulsations in nail bed	Quincke's pulse
Rapid rise and collapse of pulse	Corrigan's pulse
Double impulse of arterial pulse	Bisferiens pulse

with an ECG, chest x-ray, and an echocardiogram. The ECG typically will show left ventricular hypertrophy and left atrial enlargement due to the volume overload. A left bundle branch block may be present. Atrial fibrillation is uncommon. The chest x-ray will show an enlarged left ventricle and occasionally left atrial enlargement. It is useful to look for pulmonary venous congestion. On occasion, calcification in the area of the aortic valve can be seen.

The echocardiogram is indicated to confirm the diagnosis of aortic regurgitation and assess the severity of the disease. Findings include coarse diastolic fluttering of anterior mitral leaflet, left ventricular hypertrophy and aortic (and left ventricular) dilatation. Doppler will show retrograde flow across the valve during diastole. The echocardiogram is useful to identify the nature of the underlying lesion, LV dimension, and systolic function.

Further testing is often not necessary in patients who are asymptomatic and have good exercise tolerance. In patients for whom exercise tolerance is equivocal or who are sedentary, exercise echocardiography testing can be useful to assess the functional capacity of the ventricle and evaluate the hemodynamic impact of exercise. A decline in systolic function with exercise is an early sign of systolic dysfunction. If patients are symptomatic, cardiac catheterization and angiography are indicated.

Treatment

Medical management is directed toward reducing the volume of regurgitant blood flow and improving the amount of blood directed forward into the aorta, largely by reducing afterload. Studies demonstrating effectiveness of this approach are limited. To date, only the vasodilators hydralazine and nifedipine have been shown to have some modest benefit. Digoxin is not effective. In general, medical management is indicated only for chronic therapy in patients who are symptomatic or have systolic dysfunction and have a contraindication to surgery, for asymptomatic patients who have severe regurgitation and a dilated LV but normal systolic function, or in patients who have hypertension.

Surgery with replacement of the aortic valve is the treatment of choice for aortic regurgitation. If performed early in the process of LV decline, LV function can be restored. Surgery should be reserved for patients with severe aortic regurgitation. Patients with severe aortic regurgitation are considered candidates for surgery if they have New York Heart Association (NYHA) Class III or IV symptoms (Table 28.2), NYHA class II symptoms with progressive LV dilation, or a declining ejection fraction on serial testing; have angina; or have an EF <0.50 even if asymptomatic. There is no survival advantage for surgery in patients who are asymptomatic and have a normal ejection fraction or who have LV end diastolic dilation less than 70 mm. Surgery is also reasonable in patients with severe aortic regurgitation who are undergoing open heart surgery for another reason. In patients with aortic root disease, it may also be necessary to perform an aortic root repair.

In patients with mild to moderate disease or who are asymptomatic, serial follow-up is important. Yearly clinical follow-up is usually adequate with repeat echocardiography every 2 to 3 years. If the aortic regurgitation is severe but does not meet criteria for surgery, follow-up echocardiograms every 6 months may be necessary.

Complications

As with all patients with pathologic valve disease, patients with aortic regurgitation are at risk for endocarditis. Antibiotic prophylaxis should be provided for all dental procedures and procedures that carry a risk of bacterial contamination. If left untreated while progressing, aortic regurgitation can lead to irreversible LV dysfunction. Untreated disease often progresses to overt congestive heart failure with a low ejection fraction.

MITRAL STENOSIS

Mitral stenosis is an obstruction to flow from the left atrium into the left ventricle caused by a problem with the mitral valve. The normal mitral valve area is generally between 4 to 5.0 cm^2. Symptoms almost never occur unless the valve narrows to less than 2.5 cm^2. It is relatively uncommon, with a prevalence of 0.1% in the United States.

Etiology

Mitral stenosis is almost always due to rheumatic heart disease. The injury is triggered by repeated episodes of carditis with healing and fibrosis. The commissures between leaflets fuse, contracting, thickening, and potentially calcifying. In developed countries, the process is very slowly progressive, often taking 20 to 40 years to become symptomatic. Other causes of mitral stenosis are rare but can include infective endocarditis, malignant carcinoid syndrome, systemic lupus erythematosus, left atrial myxoma, endomyocardial fibroelastosis (a congenital "parachute" deformity of the valve), and massive mitral valvular calcification.

When flow across the valve decreases, left atrial pressures increase leading to dilation and hypertrophy. Pulmonary venous and ultimately pulmonary arterial pressures increase leading to right ventricular hypertrophy. Flow across the mitral valve occurs only during diastole and thus is very rate dependent. Tachycardia impairs left ventricular filling and thus cardiac output is compromised with increasing heart rate.

Clinical Manifestations

Although most cases of mitral stenosis follow rheumatic fever, 60% of patients with rheumatic heart disease never recall having had rheumatic fever or any of the classic symptoms. Most patients remain relatively asymptomatic for more than 20 years. Onset of symptoms can be very subtle. Typically the first manifestation is increasing dyspnea on exertion. As the obstruction progresses, the shortness of breath comes on with less and less exertion. It is often a full 10 years from onset of symptoms until they become disabling. When the stenosis becomes severe, however, patients notice orthopnea and paroxysmal nocturnal dyspnea. Pulmonary fluid overload can occur rapidly, so-called flash pulmonary edema. Palpitations from premature atrial contractions and atrial fibrillation become common as the left atrium dilates. Atrial fibrillation is present in 30% to 40% of patients with symptomatic mitral stenosis.

Early in the disease, the only manifestation on physical examination may be the characteristic murmur and accompanying heart sounds. S1 is loud. The characteristic diastolic rumbling murmur is best heard with the patient lying in the left lateral decubitus position using the bell of the stethoscope positioned at the apex. An opening snap can sometimes be heard with the diaphragm midway between the apex and the left sternal border. As the disease progresses, findings of pulmonary hypertension and right-sided heart failure may be observed. Other valves are frequently involved so ausculatory findings of aortic or tricuspid valve disease may be noted as well.

Diagnosis

Initial evaluation of the patient with suspected mitral stenosis should incorporate a chest x-ray, an ECG, and two-dimensional and Doppler echocardiogram. The ECG will show changes of atrial enlargement including a prolonged biphasic or notched P wave, P mitrale. Atrial arrhythmias, especially atrial fibrillation, are common. A right-sided strain pattern with right axis deviation and right ventricular hypertrophy may develop later in the disease. Chest x-ray will show left atrial enlargement. Pulmonary vascular congestion may be seen in the presence of a small or normal left ventricular silhouette. Calcification of the mitral valve may be seen on occasion.

The diagnostic test of choice, however, remains the echocardiogram. The two-dimensional echocardiogram can reveal the status of the valve leaflets, chamber size, and function. The Doppler echocardiogram can reveal the gradient across the valve and an estimated valve area can be calculated. It can also be helpful in estimating the pulmonary artery pressures.

In patients who are not physically active, stress testing with echocardiography may be helpful. Limitations in exercise with a rise of a transmitral gradient over 15 mm Hg and pulmonary artery hypertension with systolic pressure >60 mm Hg are indicators for further evaluation. Catheterization should be performed for anyone for whom valvotomy or surgery is being considered.

Treatment

Medical treatment for mitral stenosis focuses primarily on slowing the heart rate and preventing complications of the disease. Drugs such as beta blockers or calcium channel blockers can slow the heart rate allowing better left ventricular filling. Digoxin has not been shown to be helpful. Because most patients have had rheumatic fever, it is important to prophylax against recurrent rheumatic fever. Patients should also be treated as high risk for endocarditis.

The initial intervention of choice is percutaneous mitral balloon valvotomy. Any symptomatic patient with a valve area <1.5 cm^2 or pulmonary hypertension should be evaluated for valvotomy. Mitral valve repair is an option if balloon valvotomy is not available. Mitral valve replacement works well and is the accepted approach if a patient has severe disease and is not considered a candidate for balloon valvotomy or repair.

Complications

If untreated, the mortality for patients with mitral stenosis is extremely high. If limiting symptoms develop, the 10-year mortality rate is 0% to 15%. Causes of death are heart failure in 60% to 70%, systemic embolism in 20% to 30%, pulmonary embolism in 10%, and infection in 1% to 5%.

As noted previously, atrial fibrillation develops in 30% to 40% of patients. Anticoagulation is warranted unless there is a direct contraindication. Other indications for anticoagulating include a prior episode of systemic embolism or left atrial diameter ≥55 mm.

MITRAL REGURGITATION

Mitral valve regurgitation (MVR) is the retrograde flow of blood from the left ventricle into the left atrium as a result of failure of the mitral valve to fully close. The prevalence of MVR in the United States is roughly 2%. The prevalence increases significantly with age, with only 0.5% of those under 45 years and more than 9% of those older than 75 years affected. Mitral valve prolapse (MVP) is somewhat of a special case. MVP with and without regurgitation is quite common and has been estimated to be present in up to 2.5% of the population.

Etiology

The mitral valve apparatus is a complicated structure involving intricate coordination of the leaflets, chordae tendineae, papillary muscles, the annulus, and the supporting left ventricular wall structures. Abnormalities in any of the components can lead to incompetence and leakage across the valve. Historically, the most common cause of mitral regurgitation was rheumatic fever. However, as the incidence of this disease has declined in the developed world, mitral valve prolapse and idiopathic causes have become more common causes (Table 30.3). Acute mitral regurgitation is most commonly caused by infective endocarditis, trauma, or acute myocardial ischemia leading to papillary muscle dysfunction or rupture.

Mitral valve prolapse is characterized by excessively large leaflets or chordae tendineae. With systole, they are displaced superiorly at least 2 mm when viewed echocardiographically. It is typically seen in patients who are relatively lean. It can be acquired in individuals with severe starvation as in anorexia nervosa.

In the presence of mitral valve regurgitation, the increased volume load in the left atrium leads to an increase in left ventricular preload. In chronic disease, the increase in end-diastolic volume leads to an increase in stroke volume. Afterload is effectively reduced because of the regurgitation back into the atrium unloading the pressure on the ventricle. As such, the ventricle remains compensated despite the volume load and the patient remains asymptomatic. Over time, however, the chronic volume load can lead to dysfunction of the left ventricular muscle and further dilation of the ventricle.

TABLE 30.3 Causes of mitral valve regurgitation
Abnormal leaflets and commissures
Postinflammatory (rheumatic heart disease)
Infective endocarditis
Mitral valve prolapse
Trauma
Methysergide
Abnormal tensor apparatus
Ruptured papillary muscle or chordae tendinea
Papillary muscle dysfunction usually due to ischemic heart disease (myocardial infarction)
Abnormal left ventricular cavity and/or annulus
Left ventricular enlargement (myocarditis, hypertrophic cardiomyopathy, congestive cardiomyopathy)
Calcification of mitral ring
Aneurysm of left ventricle involving mitral annulus
Idiopathic myxomatous degeneration, myxoma
Marfan's syndrome
Ehlers-Danlos syndrome
Pseudoxanthoma elasticum
Autoimmune
Systemic lupus erythematosus
Scleroderma
Takayasu's arteritis
Ankylosing spondylitis

Pulmonary congestion can occur. In acute onset MVR, the volume load occurs too rapidly to allow the ventricle to adapt to the volume load and pulmonary congestion can occur quickly.

Clinical Manifestations

As with mitral stenosis, patients can be asymptomatic for many years. The first signs of decompensation are relatively subtle. Patients become limited by dyspnea on exertion and fatigue. Over time symptoms are more consistent with right heart failure and tricuspid insufficiency as pulmonary congestion and hypertension develop. Palpitations are common due to the volume load on the atrium and atrial fibrillation occurs in up to 57% of patients.

On physical examination, the apical impulse is enlarged and deviated laterally consistent with the volume overload on the left ventricle. Auscultation in severe mitral regurgitation often reveals a third heart sound and a blowing systolic murmur heard best over the apex and radiating to the axilla. The presence of a midsystolic click and a late systolic murmur suggests mitral valve prolapse. In the presence of acute rupture of a chordae, the murmur may radiate along the left sternal border instead. In advanced disease, there may be signs of right-sided failure including jugular venous dilation with a dominant V wave, a right ventricular heave, and the blowing respirophasic murmur of tricuspid regurgitation.

Diagnosis

As with other valve disorders, initial evaluation should incorporate an ECG, chest x-ray, and an echocardiogram. An ECG may show enlargement of the left atrium and, in advanced cases, right ventricular strain. It is most useful to assess the underlying rhythm. Chest x-ray is similarly nonspecific. It may reveal left ventricular hypertrophy and pulmonary congestion.

The echocardiogram is necessary to estimate the left ventricular and atrial volumes, the left ventricular ejection fraction (LVEF), and the severity of the regurgitation. Visualization of the valve can also give clues as to the etiology, clarifying whether the disease is due to dilation of the annulus, abnormality in the valve leaflets or a problem with the tensor apparatus. Patients who are asymptomatic should be followed annually to watch for a decline in the LVEF. Exercise testing is useful only for patients for whom an exercise history is unreliable. Catheterization is only useful when surgery is planned or when coronary artery disease is suspected.

Treatment

Medical treatment is useful only for patients with acute mitral regurgitation as a temporizing measure until surgery is feasible. Vasodilator therapy can serve to reduce afterload and increase forward flow in this setting. In chronic mitral regurgitation, the decrease in afterload is not helpful and may be dangerous.

Surgical repair of the valve is the treatment of choice when conditions are suitable. Indications for repair include symptomatic mitral regurgitation, asymptomatic mitral regurgitation with ejection fraction <0.6 and an end diastolic volume of >45 mm, and asymptomatic patients with an end diastolic volume >50 mm. Repair may also be useful in asymptomatic patients with atrial fibrillation or pulmonary hypertension. Valve replacement with preservation of the mitral apparatus should be considered if repair is not feasible, typically in patients with significant damage from rheumatic fever, ischemia, or calcification of the leaflets.

TRICUSPID REGURGITATION

Tricuspid regurgitation is the presence of retrograde flow from the right ventricle into the right atrium during systole across an incompetent tricuspid valve. Clinically significant primary tricuspid regurgitation is uncommon. It is commonly seen with dilation of the right ventricle and the annulus.

Etiology

Tricuspid regurgitation may exist with or without underlying pulmonary hypertension. When pulmonary hypertension is present, secondary tricuspid regurgitation develops as a result of right ventricular failure and dilatation, which stretch the tricuspid annulus. This type of "functional" tricuspid regurgitation commonly follows LV failure, mitral stenosis, and cor pulmonale due to chronic obstructive pulmonary disease. In the absence of pulmonary hypertension, acquired TR follows infective endocarditis (intravenous drug abuse), carcinoid syndrome, and right ventricular dysfunction due to right ventricular infarction. Tricuspid valve prolapse, Ebstein's anomaly, and atrial septal defect (ostium primum) are congenital lesions associated with tricuspid regurgitation.

The pathophysiologic consequences of tricuspid regurgitation include elevation of right atrial pressures, right ventricular volume overload, and the development of signs and symptoms of systemic venous congestion.

Clinical Manifestations

Symptoms of tricuspid regurgitation are primarily those of right-sided heart failure and the underlying disease process responsible for tricuspid regurgitation. Physical examination shows jugular venous distension, prominent *v* wave with a rapid *y* descent and hyperdynamic parasternal impulse (right ventricular lift), a holosystolic murmur along the lower left sternal border that waxes and wanes with respiration, an enlarged pulsatile liver, and peripheral edema.

Diagnosis

The ECG may show right atrial enlargement and right ventricular hypertrophy. Atrial fibrillation and right bundle branch block are common. Transthoracic echocardiography may define the etiology of tricuspid regurgitation (prolapse, ruptured chordae, or vegetations). Doppler echocardiography, by measuring RV systolic and peak pulmonary artery pressures, can help assess its severity.

Treatment

Except for endocarditis prophylaxis and the possible need for diuretics to manage peripheral edema, no specific treatment is indicated for mild to moderate tricuspid regurgitation. Tricuspid valve repair or annuloplasty may be performed in conjunction with mitral valve repair for severe tricuspid regurgitation due to mitral valve disease. In tricuspid valve endocarditis, excision of the tricuspid valve may be called for, especially for native valve infection due to *Staphylococcus aureus* or a fungal organism.

TRICUSPID STENOSIS

Tricuspid stenosis (TS) is a narrowing or constriction of the tricuspid valve orifice that leads to obstruction to RV inflow. Pathophysiologic sequelae of this obstruction include the development of right atrial hypertension and hypertrophy and decreased cardiac output due to decreased ventricular filling.

Etiology

Tricuspid stenosis is rarely an isolated valvular lesion. In adults, it is almost always due to rheumatic valvulitis, for which the pathology is similar to mitral stenosis. Other causes of tricuspid stenosis include carcinoid syndrome, congenital heart disease, and fibroelastosis. Right atrial myxoma occasionally mimics tricuspid stenosis.

Clinical Manifestations

Because rheumatic heart disease causes the majority cases, most patients with tricuspid stenosis are women. Patients may report easy fatigability, which may be due to the associated mitral stenosis.

Physical findings are a large *a* wave in the jugular venous pulse with a slow *y* descent, a loud S_1, and a low-pitched diastolic rumble along the left sternal border. This murmur typically increases with inspiration and often has a presystolic accentuation. Hepatomegaly, jaundice, presystolic liver pulsation, ascites, and pedal edema may also occur.

Diagnosis

ECG and chest x-ray show evidence of right atrial enlargement. Chest x-ray may also show a distended superior vena cava. Transthoracic echocardiography confirms the diagnosis and may identify other associated valvular lesions.

Treatment

Valve repair or replacement is required for symptomatic patients with tricuspid stenosis.

CHAPTER 31

Pericardial Disease

Vishal Ratkalkar

The pericardium is a thin layer of tissue that covers the outer surface of the heart. This tissue helps to anchor the heart in place and prevents excessive movement of the heart within the chest. A number of diseases can affect the pericardium and its function including inflammation (pericarditis), accumulation of fluid between the layers (pericardial effusion and tamponade), and thickening (constrictive pericarditis).

PERICARDITIS

Pericarditis, with its diverse causes, refers to the acute or chronic inflammation of the visceral and parietal pericardium. Pericarditis causes a characteristic chest pain that is often the reason for seeking medical attention. Pericarditis is more common in males than in females, and has a predilection for adolescents and young adults.

Etiology

The inflammation of pericarditis can be caused by both infectious and noninfectious etiologies (Table 31.1). Infiltration of inflammatory cells and the triggering of the inflammatory process lead to fibrin deposition in the pericardium. This in turn causes fluid exudation which may lead to the development of a pericardial effusion. The nature of the effusion—serous, bloody, or purulent—will depend on the nature of the underlying cause.

Clinical Manifestations

The most common symptom of pericarditis is chest pain. The onset may be insidious or abrupt. It typically presents as a sharp pain behind the sternum worsened by supine posture, coughing, or deep breathing, and relieved by sitting up and leaning forward. Presumably such posturing reduces local pressure on inflamed pericardial surfaces. However, the pain may vary in quality, location, and radiation, and may be associated with dyspnea. At times, there may be an intense, steady, crushing, substernal discomfort that radiates to the shoulder, neck, or nape of the neck, mimicking an acute myocardial infarction. A history of recent infections (especially flu-like infections), a history of myocardial infarction, presence of cancer, and medication history may provide clues to the etiology.

Fever, tachycardia, and pericardial friction rub are classic findings. The physical examination focuses on careful listening with a stethoscope for the pericardial rub, which is a scratchy sound produced by the heart muscle rubbing against the inflamed pericardium. This finding strongly suggests the diagnosis of pericarditis. Other findings, such as distended veins in the neck and swollen ankles and feet, can suggest impaired venous return due to a pericardial effusion, which often accompanies pericarditis.

Diagnosis

The initial evaluation consists of a medical history, physical examination, and an electrocardiogram (ECG). Pericarditis frequently produces characteristic findings on the ECG, usually elevated ST

TABLE 31.1 Frequent causes of pericarditis

Cause	Comment
Idiopathic infections	No unique features but resembles viral pericarditis
Viral	Most cases are viral. Commonly due to Coxsackie B virus in young adults. Pneumonia and pleuritis usually associated.
Bacterial	Uncommon cause, but important in immunocompromised hosts.
Tuberculosis	Pleural and/or systemic disease commonly associated. Eventually constrictive pericarditis may follow.
Purulent pericarditis	Follows pericardial "seeding" during bacteremia; extension of contiguous infection; or penetrating chest wounds and esophageal perforation (Boerhaave's syndrome)
Rheumatic fever[a]	Pericarditis associated with valvulitis or myocarditis
Noninfectious	
Uremia	Chronic end-stage renal disease generally present. Exuberant fibrinous pericardial reaction, often with hemorrhagic fluid. Reversible with dialysis.
Connective tissue diseases	Pericarditis part of pan serositis in systemic lupus erythematosus (SLE), rheumatoid arthritis (RA), and progressive systemic sclerosis. Pericarditis and/or effusion develop sometime in the course of SLE and 30% of RA. May precede pancarditis in SLE.
Trauma	May follow significant closed chest trauma. Myocardial contusions and transient myopericarditis associated.
Post-MI	"Early" form commonly follows 10% to 15% of transmural MI in first few days, due to pericardial extension of epicardial inflammation directly from the injured myocardium. May be confused with recurrent ischemic pain and/or reinfarction. "Late" form (Dressler's syndrome) follows MI by 2 weeks to 2 years; may be recurrent. Autoimmune basis. Associated hemorrhagic pleural effusion, high fever.
Postpericardiotomy syndrome	Follows open-heart surgery or procedures involving opening the pericardium. Features similar to Dressler's syndrome.
Postirradiation	May follow radiation to the chest for lung cancer, lymphoma, or breast cancer

MI, myocardial infarction.

segments in most leads (Fig. 31.1). These findings in conjunction with the characteristic pain and/or pericardial rub are usually sufficient for a physician to make a presumptive diagnosis of pericarditis. The ECG can also suggest other causes of chest pain, such as a recent or past myocardial infarction (Table 31.2).

ECG changes occur in about 90% of cases. Nearly one half of these changes evolve through three phases. In phase I, the PR segment is depressed, the ST segment is diffusely elevated with an upward concavity, and the T waves are upright. The PR depression is an insensitive but specific ECG sign. Seen in two thirds of all cases, it may be the sole ECG change in some patients. In several

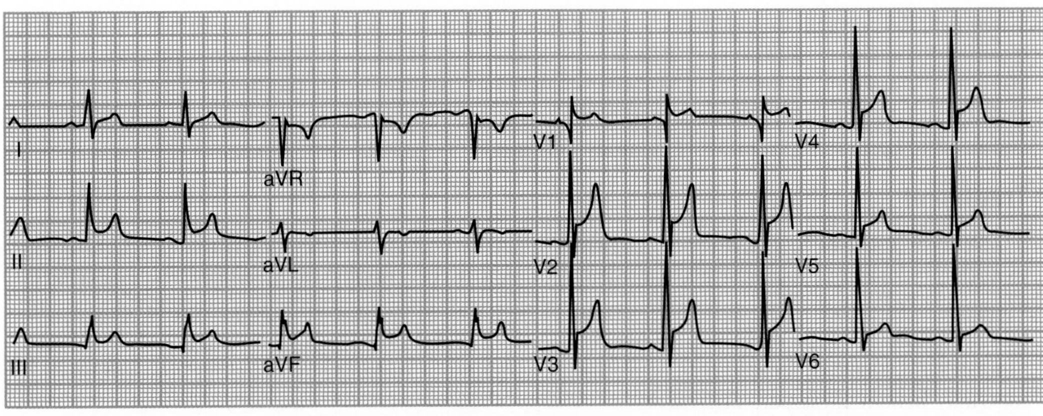

Figure 31.1 • Electrocardiogram changes in acute pericarditis.

days, phase II follows, with isoelectric ST segments and flattened T waves. In phase III T waves are inverted, often with low-voltage QRS complexes. Although atrial extra systoles and atrial fibrillation may occur, ventricular arrhythmias are uncommon.

Blood tests and chest radiographs may be helpful but are often nonspecific. Pericarditis is often associated with leukocytosis and an elevated sedimentation rate. Elevation of a creatinine kinase–MB fraction can be indicative of concomitant myocarditis. If the etiology is not apparent, serologies for typical infectious agents and connective tissue diseases, as well as screening for renal, metabolic, and liver disease, may guide further management. The chest radiograph is commonly abnormal. Cardiomegaly is present in 97% to 100% of cases due to either left ventricular hypertrophy or pericardial effusion.

An echocardiogram should be obtained in the presence of suspected pericardial disease. The

TABLE 31.2 ECG differentiation of acute pericarditis and acute myocardial infarction

	Pericarditis	Acute myocardial infarction
ECG leads involved	Usually diffuse; spares aVR, V_1	Regional changes that correspond to distribution of coronary blood flow; may see reciprocal changes in other leads
PR segment	Usually depressed early	Normal
ST segments	Concave upward	Convex upward
Persistence of ST-segment changes	Days	Hours to days
Time course of T-wave changes	T waves invert after ST returns to baseline	T waves invert within hours while ST segment is still elevated
Q waves	Absent	Present unless non–Q wave infarct pattern
R-wave amplitude	Never lost	May be lost

echocardiogram is usually unable to visualize the thin pericardium well enough to see the presence of inflammation. It is, however, very useful for determining if pericardial effusion is present. It helps estimate the amount of fluid that has accumulated and assess whether the fluid is compressing the chambers of the heart. Large-sized pericardial effusions can lead to incipient tamponade or shock and need to be drained to improve hemodynamics.

Treatment

The specific medical management of pericarditis has two goals: to provide symptom relief and to treat the underlying process, if needed. Symptomatic patients usually are given bed rest and aspirin or another nonsteroidal anti-inflammatory agent such as ibuprofen. Although pericarditis has a self-limited course in most cases, nearly one fourth, especially those with immunologically mediated processes, may have prolonged pain or recurrent symptoms. Colchicine and tapering doses of prednisone may benefit these patients.

PERICARDIAL EFFUSION AND CARDIAC TAMPONADE

A pericardial effusion is a fluid collection that develops between the visceral and parietal layers of the pericardium. With larger amounts, pericardial pressure rises sharply and intracardiac and pulmonary diastolic pressures rise. Chamber pressures equalize, leading to a decline in ventricular filling and eventually cardiac output. Ultimately, systemic blood pressure falls and shock supervenes. This condition is known as cardiac tamponade.

Etiology

The causes of pleural effusion are similar to those that cause pericarditis, although not all causes of pericarditis are equally likely to lead to severe effusion or tamponade. Malignancy is the most common cause of pericardial tamponade (54%). Metabolic disorders such as chronic renal failure or myxedema are the next most common (14%). Vascular causes such as acute myocardial infarction or perioperative bleeding cause 6%, whereas infections lead to about 5% of cases. Approximately 14% are ultimately labeled as idiopathic (Table 31.3).

Clinical Manifestations

Patients may present with shortness of breath, chest pain, pressure, discomfort, light-headedness, syncope, palpitations, cough, dyspnea, hoarseness, anxiety, and confusion (Table 31.4). Patients with rapid accumulation of fluid may show classic signs of cardiac tamponade. Hypotension, jugular venous distension, and diminished heart sounds constitute the classic Beck's triad, present in 10% to 40% of cases of tamponade. Physical examination may also reveal pulsus paradoxus, tachycardia, and hepatojugular reflux. *Pulsus paradoxus* (a fall in systolic blood pressure on inspiration by more than 10 mm Hg) is seen in almost 75% of these cases. Normally, inspiration augments venous return to the right ventricle (RV) and its end-diastolic volume. RV filling displaces the interventricular septum towards the left ventricle (LV), thereby slightly decreasing LV end-diastolic volume. In pulsus paradoxus, the inspiratory RV expansion is exaggerated and RV filling occurs at the expense of LV filling. Although pulsus paradoxus is an important bedside clue, it is neither sensitive nor specific. Many of the findings may be absent or attenuated in patients with hypovolemia who experience "low-pressure tamponade." A pericardial friction rub can also be observed in some patients. It is best heard in the supine position, at end exhalation, with the diaphragm of the stethoscope.

Diagnosis

Chest x-ray may show a globular heart or "water bottle" heart (Fig. 31.2). Transthoracic echocardiography is the most sensitive and specific test in suspected pericardial effusion. Small effusions (less

TABLE 31.3 Causes of pericardial effusion

Infectious
Viral (e.g., human immunodeficency virus)
Tuberclulosis
Fungi
Parasites
Syphilis
Bacterial
Noninfectious pericarditis
Acute myocardial infarction
Uremia
Malignancy both primary and secondary
Benign tumors
Hypothyroidism
Trauma
Severe chronic anemia
Post radiotherapy
Post cardiac surgery
Autoimmune diseases (e.g., systemic lupus erythematosus, scleroderma, rheumatoid arthritis)
Drug induced (e.g., hydralazine)
Idiopathic

TABLE 31.4 Classic signs of cardiac tamponade

Sign
Dyspnea Anxiety ("sense of impending doom")
Tachycardia
Signs of low cardiac output Fatigue, weakness, and confusion Tachycardia Hypotension (systolic blood pressure often <100 mm Hg) Narrow pulse pressure
Marked neck vein distension (prominent *x* and absent *y* descents)
Pulsus paradoxus
Muffled heart sounds
Signs of compression of adjacent organs

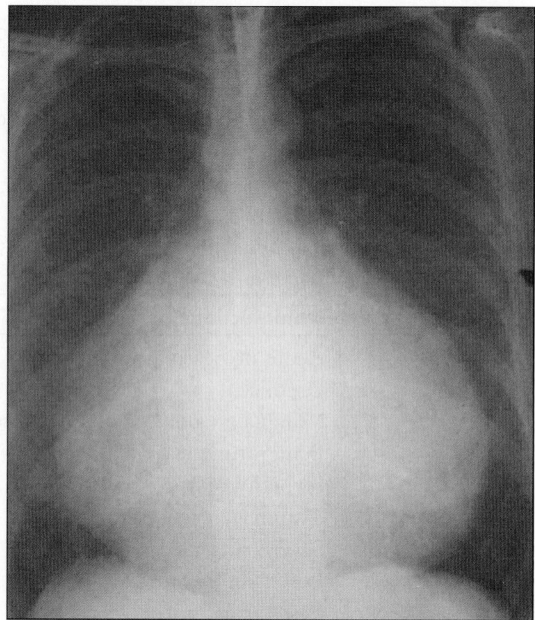

Figure 31.2 • "Water bottle" heart.

than 300 mL) may appear on the subxiphoid view as an echo-free space between the posterior cardiac wall and parietal pericardium. Larger effusions may be seen both anteriorly and posteriorly. Right atrial compression and RV diastolic collapse are sensitive and specific echocardiographic signs of early tamponade. These findings may be seen when the cardiac output is only modestly decreased, before systemic hypotension and pulsus paradoxus occur, and thus foretell impending clinical cardiac tamponade with hemodynamic collapse.

Right-heart catheterization may detect coexistent conditions, such as LV failure or effusive-constrictive disease, and document hemodynamic improvement after pericardial drainage. Right-sided systolic pressures and the pulmonary capillary wedge pressure are moderately high. In tamponade, right atrial, RV, and LV end-diastolic pressures are all equal (diastolic equalization of chamber pressures).

Treatment

Treatment of pericardial effusion depends on the presence or absence of cardiac tamponade. Tamponade is a medical emergency and symptoms such as cyanosis, shock, or a change in mental status require urgent drainage of the fluid. This drainage is accomplished with a procedure called pericardiocentesis, in which a needle or catheter is inserted through the chest wall to aspirate the fluid. Pericardiocentesis is also indicated if a purulent effusion is suspected. In the absence of these indications, pericardial effusions usually are managed by treating the underlying cause.

CONSTRICTIVE PERICARDITIS

Constrictive pericarditis is a disorder caused by inflammation of the pericardium with subsequent thickening, scarring, and contracture of the pericardium. The pericardial space is partially or completely obliterated by fibrous adhesions formed during a previous bout of acute pericarditis. The diagnosis requires evidence of systemic venous congestion without myocardial dysfunction or other causes of congestion.

Etiology

The most common causes of constrictive pericarditis are conditions that induce chronic inflammation of the pericardium: tuberculosis, radiation to the chest, and cardiac surgery. Less frequent causes are mesothelioma of the pericardium or from incomplete drainage of abnormal fluid accumulating in the pericardial sac, which can occur in purulent pericarditis or in postsurgery hemopericardium. Constrictive pericarditis may also develop without an apparent cause (idiopathic).

Clinical Manifestations

Symptoms may include atypical or typical chest pain, chest heaviness or pressure, fatigability, or peripheral edema. Patients may report dyspnea on exertion in severe cases. Many patients are asymptomatic until the advanced stages of disease. Specific etiologies of effusive-constrictive pericarditis may have characteristic antecedent histories that suggest pericardial disease (e.g., tuberculosis, renal failure, malignancy, radiation therapy, and cardiovascular surgery).

Common findings may include pulsus paradoxus, jugular venous distension, tachycardia, tachypnea, hepatomegaly, ascites, peripheral edema, pleural effusion (in the absence of left-sided congestive signs), or auscultation of a pericardial friction rub.

Percussible cardiac dullness at the apex can be present. Heart sounds can be muffled. Occasionally there is a characteristic pericardial knock after the second heart sound that occurs when the expansion of the ventricle is suddenly stopped by the immobile constrictive pericardium.

Diagnosis

Chest radiographs may show extensive pericardial calcification in about one half of cases, but calcification alone is not pathognomonic of constriction. The ECG may show low-voltage QRS complexes and nonspecific ST-T changes. In severe cases, electrical alternans may occur. Atrial arrhythmias are common, and atrial fibrillation occurs in about 50% of patients.

Echocardiography is used to establish normal LV function and to rule out cardiac tamponade and other causes of right-sided heart failure. Cardiac catheterization sometimes may be necessary to assess hemodynamics. Computed tomography or magnetic resonance scans of the chest can document pericardial thickening and thus distinguish constrictive pericarditis from restrictive cardiomyopathy.

Treatment

Medical therapy is primarily supportive. Depending on the etiology, steroids, nonsteroidal anti-inflammatory agents, or antibiotics may be needed. The most effective therapy for effusive-constrictive pericarditis is pericardiectomy, with complete removal of the parietal and visceral membranes. The perioperative mortality rate with this procedure can be high. In patients who may have a high mortality rate with thoracotomy and have a significant chance of effusion recurrence with needle drainage alone, a pericardial-peritoneal window is an effective treatment for recurrent pericardial effusions.

CHAPTER 32

Arrhythmias

Lee Biblo

Under normal circumstances, the cardiac electrical system is controlled by the sinus node. The sinus node is the dominant cardiac pacemaker directing atrial depolarization across the atria from right to left and top to bottom. Electrical activity spreads to the ventricles via the atrioventricular (AV) node and the bundle of His, and then through the right and left bundles generating a narrow QRS complex. An arrhythmia is in essence a disruption of this activity, leading to an abnormal electrical pattern.

ETIOLOGY

Arrhythmias are classified as either supraventricular or ventricular based on their site of origin. Figure 32.1 documents some common supraventricular arrhythmias. Arrhythmias are also classified according to mechanism: automatic, triggered, or re-entrant.

Automatic arrhythmias include abnormal rates of discharge of the normal cardiac pacemaker, the sinus node (e.g., sinus bradycardia or tachycardia), or of an ectopic pacemaker that can be in the atria (automatic atrial tachycardia), AV node (junctional tachycardia), or ventricle (accelerated idioventricular rhythm).

Triggered activity may occur singly or in salvos and is caused by afterdepolarizations that affect the action potential of myocardial cells. Torsades de pointes, a "twisting" polymorphic ventricular tachycardia, is a specific type of triggered arrhythmia that is observed in situations where the QT interval has been prolonged. The QT interval is calculated from the electrocardiogram (ECG); a standardized

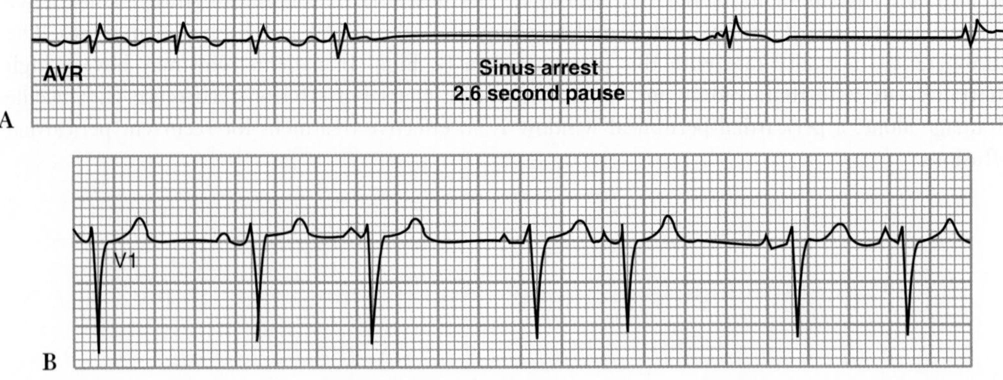

Figure 32.1 • **A.** Sinus arrest. Following a run of supraventricular tachycardia at a rate of 110 beats/min, sinus arrest occurs, resulting in a 2.6-sec pause, followed by a slow junctional escape rhythm at a rate of 30 beats/min. This type of alteration, between a tachyarrhythmia and a bradyarrhythmia, is a characteristic of the sick-sinus syndrome. **B.** Premature atrial complexes. In this strip, premature atrial complexes are conducted without aberration.

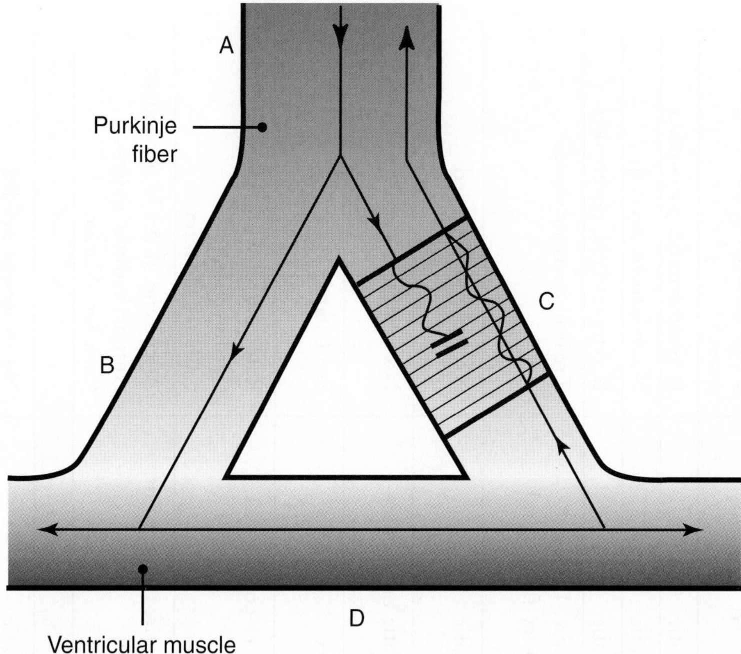

Figure 32.2 • Mechanism of re-entry in a branched terminal of the Purkinje system contacting ventricular muscle. An impulse traveling antegrade in Purkinje fiber A exhibits a unidirectional block in Purkinje fiber C. However, the initial impulse from fiber A is able to conduct normally through Purkinje fiber B via ventricular muscle back to Purkinje fiber C. The additional time allows this impulse to travel retrograde to the distal branch of fiber C (which has not yet been depolarized) and through the previous site of the unidirectional block to again reach fiber A. If retrograde conduction is slow enough for the cells of fiber A to have regained excitability, then a self-perpetuating circuit or re-entrant loop is formed. In this example, ventricular tachycardia would result.

QT interval relative to heart rate is called the QTc interval. Numerous clinical (e.g., abrupt bradycardia, ischemia, or electrolyte disturbances [hypokalemia, hypomagnesemia, hypocalcemia]) or drug-induced (e.g., specific antiarrhythmic, antibiotic, antipsychotic, or gastrointestinal drugs) states can prolong the QT interval and precipitate this arrhythmia. The common theme in most prolonged QT states is delay in the potassium current that underlies phase 3 of the myocardial action potential.

Re-entry is the most common mechanism underlying pathologic arrhythmias. Re-entry requires an area of slow conduction, unidirectional block, and two pathways (Fig. 32.2). Re-entrant arrhythmias can involve the atria (atrial fibrillation, re-entrant atrial tachycardia, or atrial flutter), the AV node (AV nodal re-entrant tachycardia), the ventricles (ventricular tachycardia), or both the atria and ventricle when a bypass tract crosses the fibrous atrioventricular annulus (AV reentrant tachycardia). Any factor that can alter conduction velocity and/or refractoriness may contribute to the substrate needed for re-entrant arrhythmias. Ventricular re-entrant arrhythmias are almost always associated with structural heart disease.

CLINICAL MANIFESTATIONS

The clinical presentation of patients with arrhythmias is quite variable. Palpitation, lightheadedness, and syncope are common symptoms. A nonspecific presentation may include fatigue, dyspnea, or exertional intolerance. Table 32.1 lists the most common arrhythmias organized by site of origin.

TABLE 32.1 Types of arrhythmias

Type	Characteristic	Mechanism	Treatment
Atrial			
Sinus tachycardia	Sinus rate >100 bpm	Automatic	Treat underlying physiologic stress
Sinus bradycardia	Sinus rate <60 bpm	Automatic	If symptomatic: pacemaker
Sinus arrhythmia	Varying sinus rate, usually respirophasic	Automatic	No treatment needed
Sinus arrest (Fig. 32.1A)	Pause in rhythm without P wave	Automatic	If symptomatic: pacemaker
Multifocal atrial tachycardia (Fig. 32.3A)	Rate >100 bpm with at least 3 distinct P wave morphologies	Automatic. Linked to respiratory failure and hypoxia	Treat underlying disease
Wandering atrial pacemaker	Rate <100 bpm, with at least 3 distinct P wave morphologies	Automatic	No treatment needed
Premature atrial complexes (Fig. 32.1B)	Early, non-sinus P wave morphology	Automatic or re-entry	No treatment needed
Atrial fibrillation (Chapter 33)	Irregularly irregular ventricular response without distinct P waves	Re-entry	See Chapter 33
Atrial flutter (Fig. 32.4)	Saw tooth-like flutter waves with rate of ~300 bpm	Macro–re-entry	Rate control with AVN blockers Cardioversion Catheter ablation
Atrial tachycardia (Fig. 32.3B)	Rapid atrial rhythm P wave preceeds QRS	Automatic, triggered or re-entry	Adenosine, if AVN dependent Anti-arrhythmic drugs Catheter ablation
Junctional			
Premature junctional beats	Early beat with normal QRS; retrograde P wave	Automatic	No treatment needed
Junctional escape rhythm (Fig. 32.5A)	Slow (40–60 bpm) regular beats with normal QRS. Retrograde P wave only	Automatic (failure of sinus node)	If no reversible cause: pacemaker

AV junctional tachycardia (Fig. 32.5B)	AV node rate > sinus rate and >100 bpm	Automatic. Associated with myocardial infarction, myocarditis, or digoxin toxicity	Treat underlying cause
AV nodal reentry tachycardia (Fig. 32.6)	Narrow complex tachycardia with rate 150–250, P wave is usually buried within QRS	Re-entry	Catheter ablation
Concealed bypass tract tachycardia (Fig. 32.7)	Narrow complex tachycardia with retrograde P wave. No delta wave present in sinus rhythm.	Re-entry	Adenosine for acute termination Catheter ablation
Nonconcealed bypass tract tachycardia	Narrow complex tachycardia with retrograde P wave. Delta wave present in sinus rhythm (Fig. 32.8).	Re-entry	Adenosine for acute termination Catheter ablation
Ventricular			
Premature ventricular complexes (Fig. 32.9)	Premature wide complex QRS	Automatic or re-entry	Treat underlying disease
Ventricular tachycardia (Fig. 32.10)	Wide complex QRS tachycardia	Automatic, triggered or re-entry	Anti-arrhythmic drugs Cardioversion Implantable cardioverter defibrillator (ICD)
Torsades de pointes (Fig. 32.11)	Ventricular tachycardia with oscillating QRS complexes, associated with a prolonged QT interval	Triggered	Correct underlying cause
Ventricular escape beats	Wide complex rhythm at 20–40 bpm	Automatic or re-entry	Pacemaker if symptomatic
Accelerated idioventricular rhythm (Fig. 32.12)	Wide complex rhythm at 60–100 bpm	Automatic, associated with coronary reperfusion	No treatment needed
Ventricular fibrillation (Fig. 32.13)	Absence of distinct ventricular activity	Re-entry	Defibrillation ICD

A
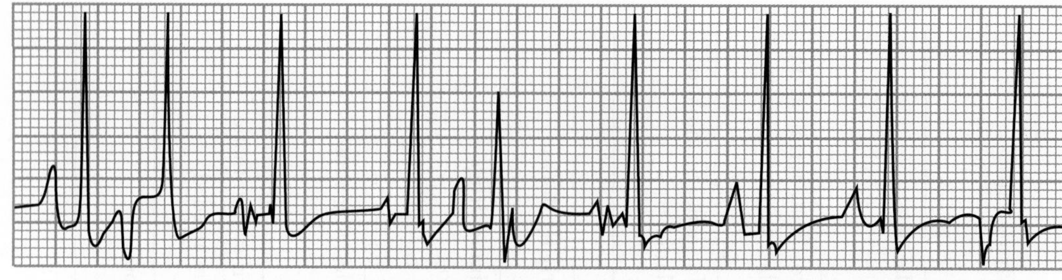

B
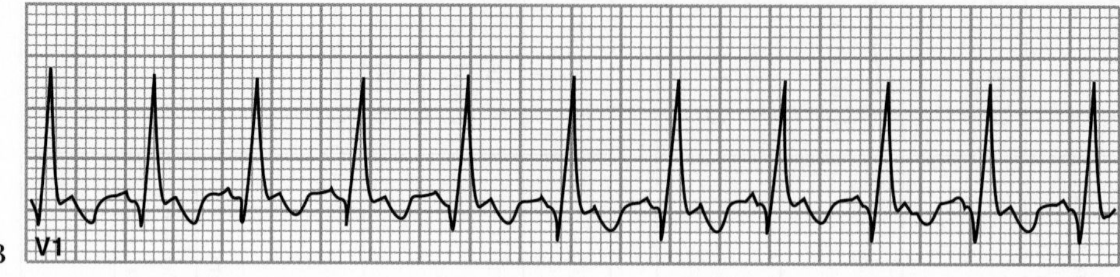

Figure 32.3 • **A.** Multifocal atrial tachycardia, more than three different P-wave morphologies are evident. **B.** Paroxysmal atrial tachycardia with 2:1 AV conduction. The P waves occur at 250 beats/min, resulting in a ventricular rate of 125 beats/min. Paroxysmal atrial tachycardia with AV conduction block is associated with by digitalis intoxication.

DIAGNOSIS

The 12-lead electrocardiogram, 24-hour ambulatory ECG monitor, and ECG event recording can establish the diagnosis. Twelve-lead ECG tracings, rather than single-lead tracings, are preferable for the analysis of an arrhythmia.

Vagal maneuvers can help in the differential diagnosis of tachyarrhythmias. By increasing vagal tone, a slight transient decrease of rate will occur in sinus tachycardia; but abrupt termination of AV nodal re-entrant tachycardia (AVNRT) or orthodromic-AV re-entrant tachycardia (O-AVRT) occurs if AV block is induced.

Adenosine can produce AV node block, which will terminate transient AVNRT or O-AVRT. Adenosine can "unmask" atrial fibrillation, atrial flutter, or atrial tachycardia when AVN block occurs making diagnosis definitive.

Electrophysiologic (EP) studies can be important diagnostic tools, particularly with the emergence of effective nonpharmacologic therapies. The ability to trace specific pathways and map conduction has allowed increasingly more precise diagnosis and treatment using ablative techniques.

TREATMENT

First-line therapy for a tachyarrhythmia is often an antiarrhythmic drug. The Vaughan-Williams classification (Table 32.2) places antiarrhythmic drugs into classes. This classification scheme logically groups these drugs, but with significant variations in the electrophysiological, hemodynamic, or myocardial depressant effects even within a given class. The safe use of any antiarrhythmic drug depends on a thorough knowledge of the pharmacology, dose range, metabolism, drug interactions, and side-effect profile. Most often during an acute supraventricular arrhythmia, adenosine is tried initially. If not successful, the next option usually is a beta-blocker or a short-acting calcium channel

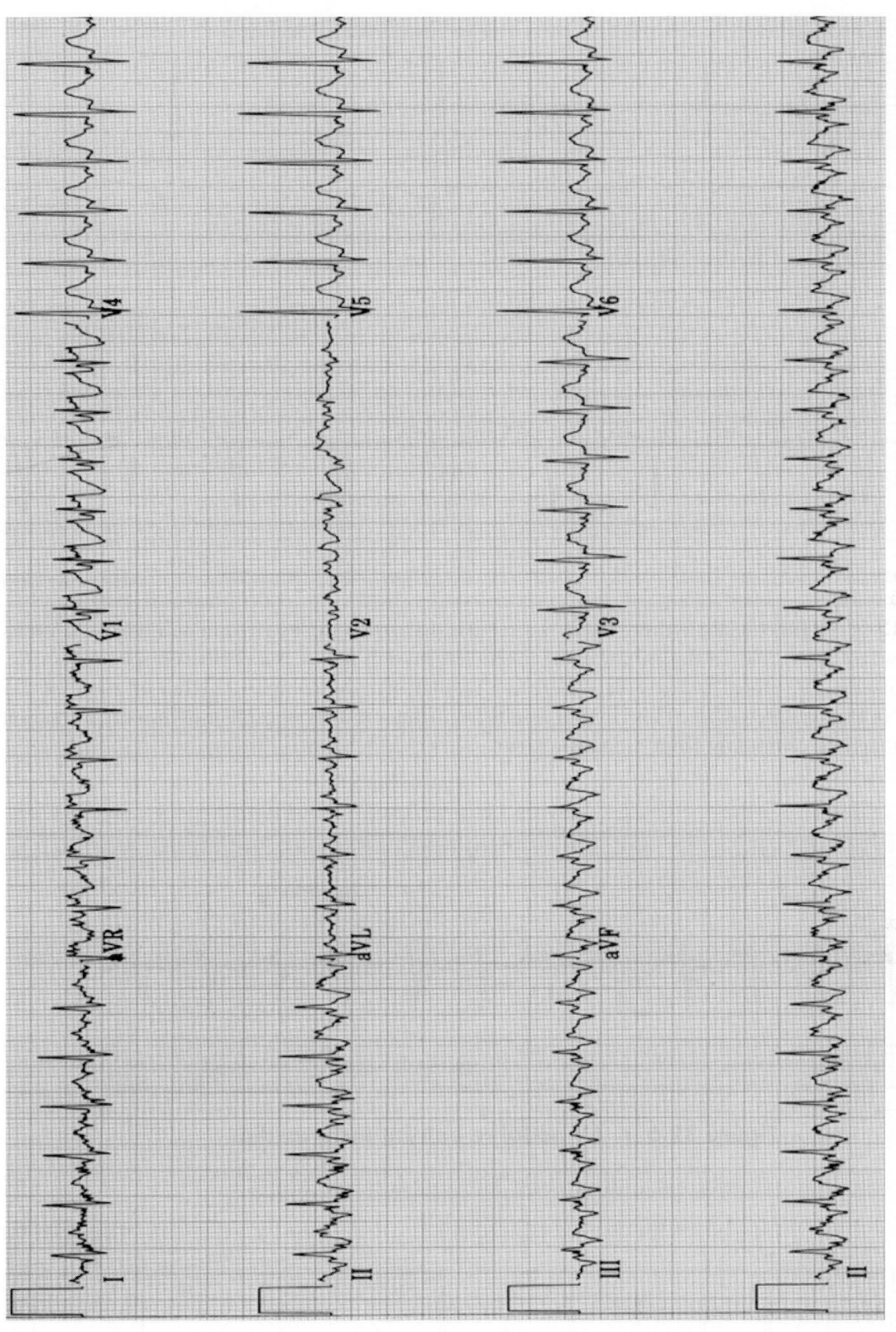

Figure 32.4 • This 12-lead electrocardiogram demonstrates atrial flutter with an atrial rate of 300 bpm with 2/1 AV conduction resulting in a ventricular rate of 150 bpm. The classic "saw tooth" pattern is best seen in lead III in this electrogram.

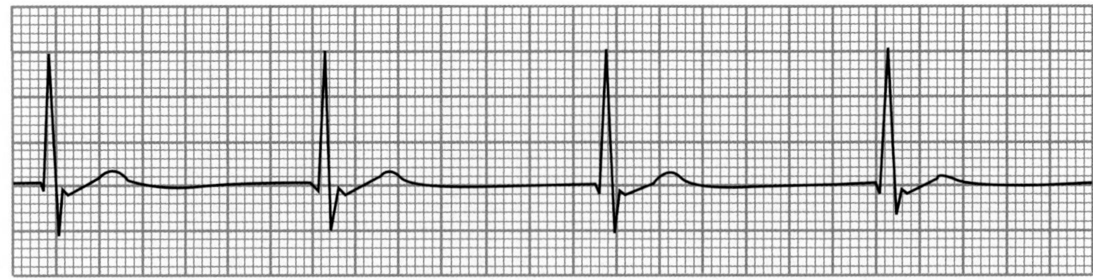

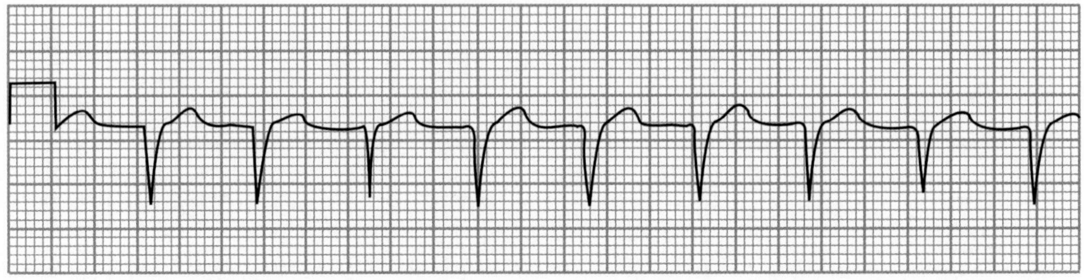

Figure 32.5 • **A.** Junctional rhythm. There is a regular, narrow-complex rhythm at a rate of 52 beats/min. No P waves are visible. In this instance, the junctional rhythm serves as a passive escape mechanism. **B.** Nonparoxysmal junctional tachycardia. There is a regular, narrow complex rhythm at a rate of 125 beats/min. No P waves are visible. This rhythm results from abnormal enhancement of impulse formation at the AV junction, commonly from digitalis toxicity.

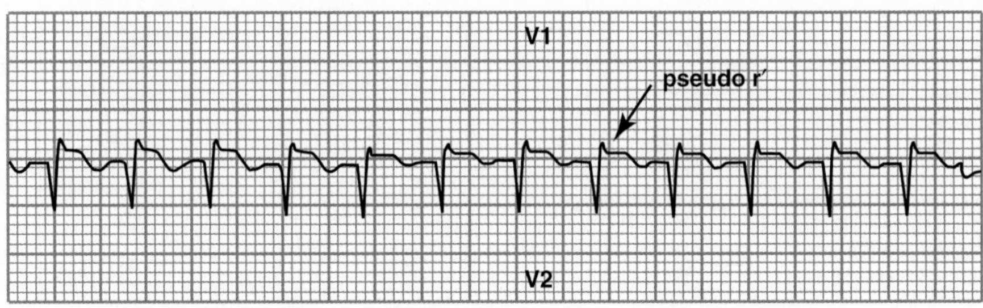

Figure 32.6 • **AV nodal re-entrant tachycardia.**

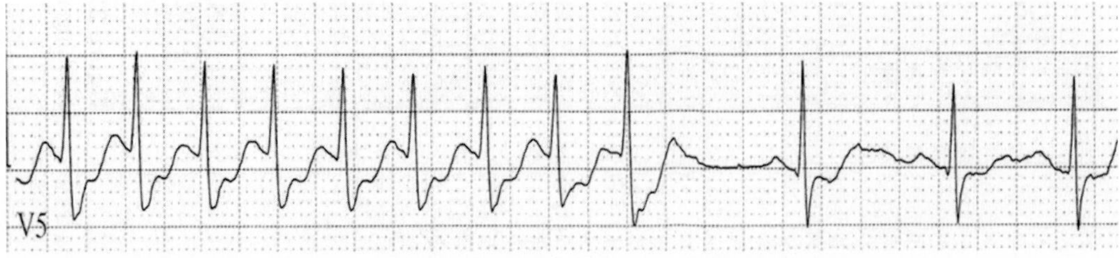

Figure 32.7 • **This electrocardiogram tracing shows termination of orthodromic AV re-entrant tachycardia after the administration of intravenous adenosine.** Retrograde P waves are likely seen after the QRS and are designated by arrows. No delta wave is apparent in sinus rhythm, thus this bypass tract is concealed and can only conduct in a retrograde fashion.

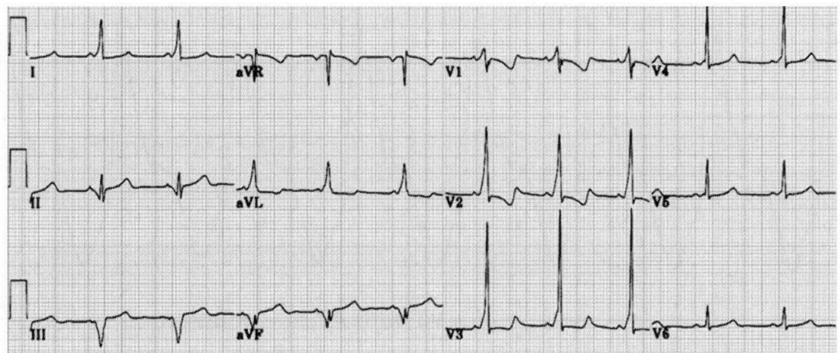

Figure 32.8 • This 12-lead ECG demonstrates ventricular pre-excitation. The initial portion of the QRS is slurred (delta wave) representing slow cell to cell ventricular depolarization via the bypass tract. This is best seen in lead V2.

blocker. Vagal maneuvers or intravenous (IV) adenosine can terminate AVNRT and O-AVRT as these arrhythmias are AV-node dependent.

Radiofrequency catheter ablation is emerging as the treatment of choice for supraventricular tachycardias. In AVNRT, ablation of the slow pathway in the AV node is the preferred treatment. Catheter ablation of the bypass tract has become the first-line therapy for all forms of O-AVRT.

Cardioversion is useful for treatment of atrial flutter and occasionally atrial fibrillation. Patients with hemodynamic compromise during atrial fibrillation (AF) require immediate cardioversion.

In a patient who presents with the acute onset of ventricular tachycardia, IV lidocaine or IV amiodarone are usually the initial agents of choice. If the patient is hemodynamically unstable, prompt restoration of sinus rhythm by electrical cardioversion is necessary. Patients with the potential for recurrent sustained ventricular tachycardia often require an implantable cardioverter defibrillator (ICD) for rescue therapy. Underlying cardiac conditions must always be optimized. The risk of ventricular tachycardia or ventricular fibrillation in patients is predicted by the extent of left ventricular (LV) dysfunction. Primary prevention with an ICD is now advocated in those patients with LV dysfunction with an ejection fraction less than 35%.

A permanent pacemaker consists of an electrode lead (or leads) and a pulse generator. In most circumstances, two electrode leads are inserted transvenously, one into the right atrial appendage and one into the right ventricular apex. The generator is placed in a subcutaneous pocket below the clavicle. The power source is a lithium battery with a life expectancy of 5 to 10 years.

A letter code designation is used to describe the complex function of pacemakers. The first letter indicates the chamber paced; the second letter, the sensed chamber; the third, the mode of the pacemaker response to a spontaneous cardiac impulse; and the fourth letter indicates that the pace-

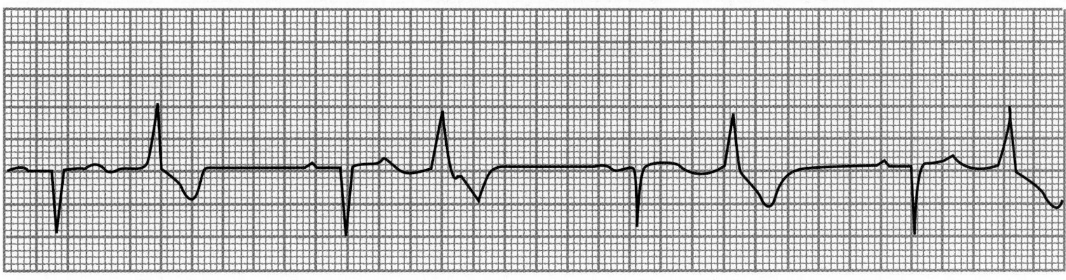

Figure 32.9 • Bigeminy. Every other QRS represents a premature ventricular complex (PVC).

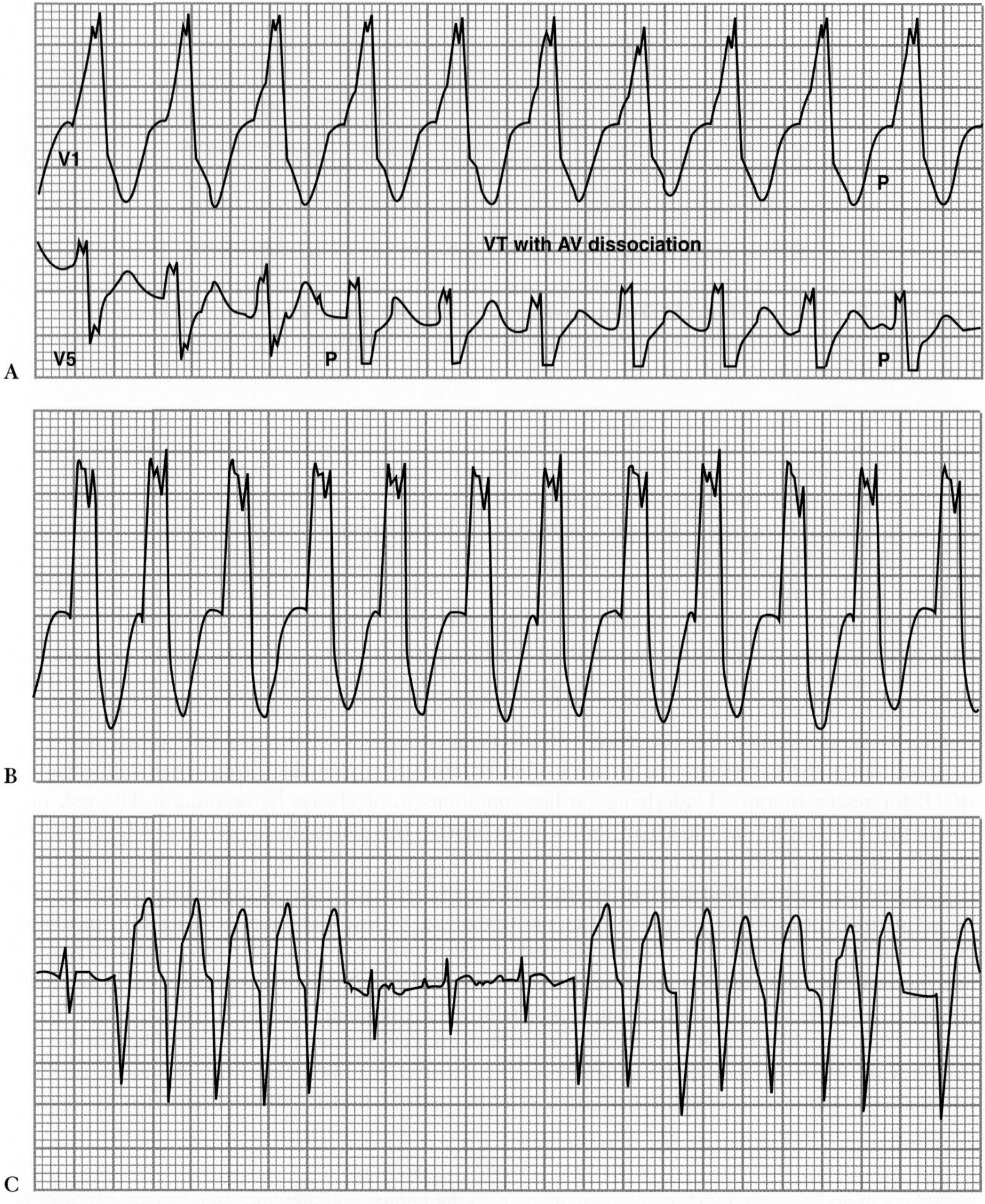

Figure 32.10 • Ventricular tachycardias (VT). **A.** VT with AV dissociation. This strip demonstrates VT at 130 beats/min with evidence of dissociated P waves (P). AV dissociation during a wide QRS tachycardia defines the tachycardia as ventricular in origin. **B.** Monomorphic VT. This contrasts with the pattern of polymorphic VT (Fig. 32.11). **C.** Nonsustained VT. These five- and eight-beat runs demonstrate that VT is often absolutely regular.

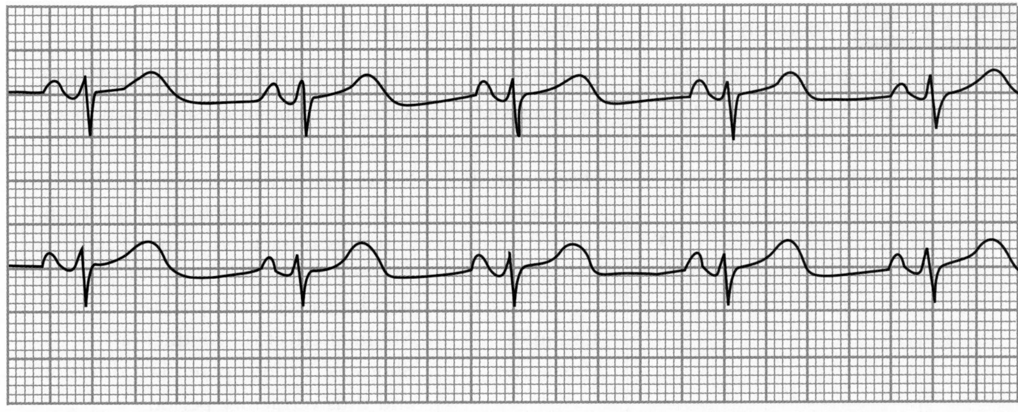

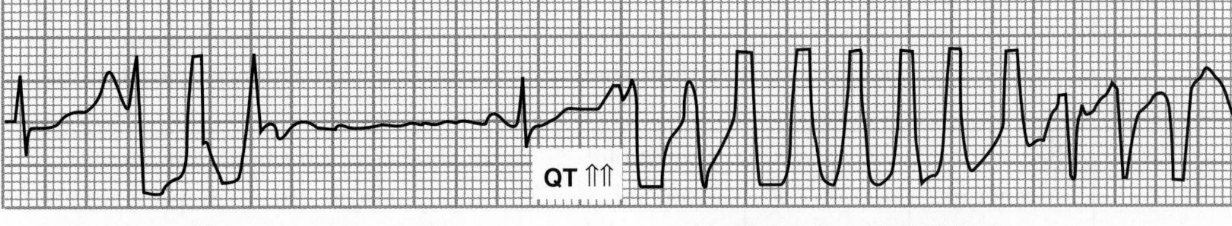

Figure 32.11 • Torsades de pointes. The upper strip demonstrates sinus bradycardia with a mildly prolonged Q-T interval. The lower strip demonstrates the twisting pattern of Torsades de pointes.

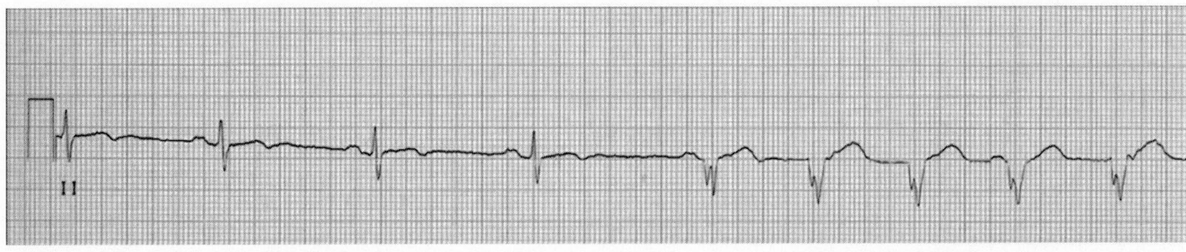

Figure 32.12 • This electrocardiogram tracing demonstrates sinus rhythm with the onset of an accelerated idioventricular rhythm. AV dissociation is demonstrated by the dissociation between the wide bents and P waves in the second half of the tracing.

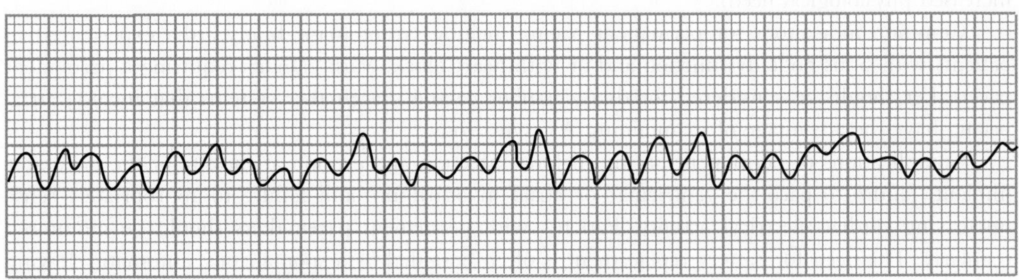

Figure 32.13 • No discrete QRS complexes are present.

TABLE 32.2 Vaughan Williams classification of antiarrhythmic drugs

Class	Category	Subclass	Agent(s)	Primary Electrophysiological Effects
I	Sodium-channel blockers	A	Procainamide	Moderate inhibition of phase 0 depolarization
			Disopyramid	Slows conduction
			Quinidine	Prolongs action potential duration, and thus refractory period
		B	Lidocaine	Mild/moderate inhibition of phase 0 depolarization
			Tocainide	Minimal effect on conduction
			Mexiletine	Shortens action potential duration and thus refractory period
		C	Flecainide	Marked inhibition of phase 0 depolarization
			Propafenone	Marked slowing of conduction
			Ethmozine	Little effect on action potential duration
II	Beta-adrenergic receptor blockers	—	Propanolol Atenolol Metoprolol Others	In absence of catecholamines, no electrophysiologic effect; in presence of catecholamines, slows SA nodal discharge rate and slows conduction through AV node
III	Potassium-channel blockers	—	Amiodarone Bretylium Dofetilide Ibutilide Sotalol	Prolongs repolarization
IV	Calcium-channel blockers	—	Verapamil Dilitiazem	Activates in slow-response cells Slows SA nodal discharge rate; slows conduction and increases refractory period of AV node

maker has the property of rate modulation (i.e., the unit can increase its pacing rate in response to increased physiological need).

Common indications for permanent pacing include symptomatic bradycardia experienced in patients with sinus node dysfunction and or with heart block. Most patients requiring a permanent pacemaker should be considered for dual-chamber pacing. Pacemaker systems that include atrial pacing have the advantage of maintaining AV synchrony.

Complications of permanent pacing include infection and erosion at the site of the generator implant, failure to pace the ventricular or atrial myocardium, and failure to appropriately sense underlying cardiac electrical activity. Patients with permanent pacemakers should be monitored regularly. The need for battery replacement is often heralded by a spontaneous, automatic slowing of the pacing rate, a property built into the pacemaker to alert the physician to the need for battery replacement.

SUMMARY

Cardiac arrhythmias are ubiquitous and range in clinical spectrum from benign to lethal. Characterization of the arrhythmia prior to treatment is important to a successful outcome. Initial characterization via electrocardiography is preferred. Clinical risk stratification is often accomplished by examining the underlying cardiac substrate. With LV dysfunction, cardiac arrhythmias carry a more ominous prognosis.

CHAPTER 33

Atrial Fibrillation

Lee Biblo

Atrial fibrillation is found in 2% to 4% of the population in the United States. In the young adult, atrial fibrillation is uncommon; however, the incidence doubles each decade of life, such that atrial fibrillation is found in 13% to 15% of those over age 80 years. Atrial fibrillation is associated with a high incidence of stroke, estimated at 5% to 6% per year. In addition, atrial fibrillation appears to convey a mortality risk independent of other factors.

ETIOLOGY

Until the mid-1990s, re-entry was felt to form the mechanistic framework for the maintenance of atrial fibrillation. Several re-entrant wave fronts simultaneously circulated in both atria. The wave fronts activate the atria randomly, disappear and reform, and once established, follow pathways of excitation largely guided by differences in atrial tissue refractoriness.

Contemporary studies suggest that rapidly firing foci originating in one or more of the pulmonary veins underlies atrial fibrillation. These rapidly firing foci can enter the left atrium, initiate, and then maintain the multiple wave fronts necessary for sustained atrial fibrillation. The atria of most patients with atrial fibrillation have structural abnormalities, ranging from fibrosis to dilatation. Common cardiac syndromes like hypertension, valve disorders, coronary disease, and ventricular dysfunction enhance changes in atrial tissue refractoriness that support atrial fibrillation. Patients with a structurally abnormal atrial tissue likely require fewer rapidly firing foci to enter the left atrium to maintain atrial fibrillation.

In addition to the above noted cardiac conditions, several noncardiac conditions are associated with atrial fibrillation. Hyperthyroidism leads to a hyperadrenergic state. Holiday heart refers to atrial fibrillation that occurs 24 hours after an episode of binge drinking. Both hyperthyroidism and alcohol withdrawal seen in the holiday heart syndrome appear to shorten atrial refractoriness and may allow triggers from the pulmonary veins to enter the left atrium that previously were blocked by atrial tissue refractoriness.

Underlying pulmonary diseases including pneumonia, pulmonary emboli, chronic lung diseases, and acute respiratory failure can lead to atrial fibrillation. Hypoxia can also lead to changes in atrial tissue refractoriness that may facilitate atrial fibrillation.

CLINICAL MANIFESTATIONS

Patients with atrial fibrillation can present with a variety of symptoms, although many patients are asymptomatic or minimally symptomatic. Likewise, in a single patient with paroxysmal atrial fibrillation, approximately two thirds of the episodes are asymptomatic.

The usual presentation is palpitation or a sense of cardiac awareness. Patients can feel an uneasiness or irregularity in their heartbeat. The ventricular response or heart rate can be normal or near normal at rest. However, with minimal exertion, the heart rate can abruptly increase to high rates, creating a sense of breathlessness. As atrioventricular nodal (AV) conduction is catecholamine dependent, a rapid ventricular response during effort leads to exertional intolerance.

During atrial fibrillation, stasis can lead to thrombus formation in the left atrial appendage. The stroke risk in nonvalvular atrial fibrillation is about 6% per year. Recurrent cerebral emboli may also manifest as a progressive "unexplained" deterioration in cognitive function.

A persistent rapid ventricular response can lead to a tachycardia-mediated cardiomyopathy. This may be the most common cause of a reversible nonischemic cardiomyopathy.

The loss of the atrial contraction can lead to a variety of hemodynamic issues, particularly in those patients with diastolic heart disease. Patients with diastolic heart disease (e.g., left ventricular hypertrophy, aortic stenosis, cardiac amyloid) decompensate with the onset of atrial fibrillation because these conditions are very preload dependent.

DIAGNOSIS

All patients with atrial fibrillation require a thorough history and physical examination. Classically, the heartbeat is irregularly irregular. The pulse will vary in intensity due to the changes in preload and in the diastolic interval. An electrocardiogram documents no discrete atrial electrical activity.

An echocardiogram can determine the presence of valvular disease or left ventricular dysfunction. A stress test will characterize the patient's functional ability and look for signs of coronary ischemia.

Laboratory work should include a thyroid-stimulating hormone to exclude hyperthyroidism.

TREATMENT

General Management

The management of patients with atrial fibrillation requires the diagnosis and subsequent treatment of underlying cardiac and noncardiac disorders. If hyperthyroidism exists, return to the euthyroid state usually will return the patient to sinus rhythm. Binge alcohol ingestion or sympathomimetic drugs may precipitate atrial fibrillation and, obviously, should be addressed with the patient. Underlying abnormal pulmonary disorders should be treated when present.

Associated cardiac conditions such as valvular heart disease, coronary artery disease, hypertension, or congestive heart failure must be optimized. Despite optimal medical treatment of all noncardiac issues and the underlying cardiac milieu, atrial fibrillation often persists.

In 10% of patients with atrial fibrillation, no associated cardiac or noncardiac abnormality is present. These patients are classified as having "lone" atrial fibrillation.

ACUTE TREATMENT

The acute treatment of atrial fibrillation is dictated by the clinical condition of the patient. The loss of atrial systole and the shortening of the diastole can lead to a decrease in cardiac output. If the patient is hemodynamically unstable, acute cardioversion is often necessary. In the absence of acute hemodynamic compromise, control of the rapid ventricular response is initially indicated. This strategy is called rate control.

Administration of an intravenous (IV) calcium channel blocker is commonly used for the acute control of the rapid ventricular response during atrial fibrillation. IV diltiazem often successfully controls the ventricular response in atrial fibrillation. The average time to a therapeutic response is less than 7 minutes from the beginning of the IV infusion. Diltiazem may be associated with hypotension;

however, usually blood pressure improves with the control of the rapid ventricular response. Esmolol, an ultrafast-acting beta-blocker, has also been used to acutely control the rapid ventricular response.

Classically, digoxin has been used acutely to control the rapid ventricular response. However, the therapeutic use of digoxin is inconsistent and often ineffective. The median time until adequate control of the ventricular response is 11.6 hours. Thus, the use of digoxin for the acute control of ventricular response in atrial fibrillation has been relegated to a secondary position. Digoxin may have a role as an adjunct to other AV node blocking agents, especially in patients with concomitant congestive heart failure.

LONG-TERM TREATMENT

Rhythm Control

When the patient's rapid ventricular response has been controlled, a decision must be made regarding the restoration of sinus rhythm versus simply continuing to control the ventricular response. The decision whether or not to cardiovert a patient with atrial fibrillation is complicated. If the onset of atrial fibrillation can be estimated at less than 48 hours, the usual clinical practice is to perform the cardioversion independent of the state of anticoagulation. This recommendation is based on the assumption that a thrombus usually takes more than 48 hours to form.

In patients with paroxysmal atrial fibrillation, asymptomatic episodes occur more frequently than symptomatic episodes. Thus, determining the onset of atrial fibrillation by using the patient's appreciation of symptoms may be hazardous. If the onset of atrial fibrillation cannot be determined or is greater than 48 hours, there are two strategies for attempting cardioversion to sinus rhythm. The first strategy requires systemic anticoagulation for a 3-week period prior to elective electrical or pharmacologic cardioversion. This period of anticoagulation reduces the risk of embolization after cardioversion from 5% to 1%.

The second strategy permits cardioversion without an antecedent 3-week period of systemic anticoagulation if an atrial thrombus is not documented by transesophageal echocardiography. Atrial stunning (evidence of sinus rhythm electrically but without effective mechanical contraction) can exist for several weeks after a cardioversion and predisposes to blood stasis in the atria. Therefore, systemic anticoagulation with heparin transitioning to warfarin must begin with and continue after the cardioversion for at least 4 weeks, although long term anticoagulation is often required.

In the second strategy, if an atrial thrombus is documented by transesophageal echocardiography, systemic anticoagulation should occur for 3 weeks prior to cardioversion. Cardioversion is then safe and the patient is treated for at least 4 more weeks after cardioversion with systemic anticoagulation therapy, although long term anticoagulation is often required.

A high rate of recurrence occurs in patients cardioverted without antiarrhythmic drug therapy. By 3 months, only 30% of patients who have undergone successful cardioversion remained in sinus rhythm. Thus, antiarrhythmic agents are usually initiated just prior to or just after cardioversion in most patients.

The decision to use antiarrhythmic drug therapy is complex. The benefits of sinus rhythm with the restoration of atrial-ventricular synchrony, improved cardiac output, and physiologic heart rate control are clear. These benefits must be weighed against the risks of antiarrhythmic drug therapy. Class IA, Class IC, and Class III agents have been used to maintain sinus rhythm. Several studies have demonstrated an increase in mortality in patients who received antiarrhythmic drugs, presumably due to proarrhythmia. Seemingly paradoxical, the greatest risk of proarrhythmia appears immediately after cardioversion when sinus rhythm emerges. Drugs like quinidine and sotalol prolong repolarization to a greater extent at slower heart rates, thereby enhancing the possibility of Q-T interval prolongation and a ventricular arrhythmia. In contrast, amiodarone, a Class III agent, has an extremely low proarrhythmic risk and remains the antiarrhythmic agent of choice in patients with structural heart disease. In patients without structural heart disease, the risk of proarrhythmia is low and the antiarrhythmic agent of choice is usually flecainide.

Enthusiasm for maintaining sinus rhythm must be tempered not only by the risk of proarrhythmia, but also by the high rate of recurrence. Class IA agents (quinidine, procainamide, disopyramide), Class IC agents (flecainide, propafenone), and Class III agents (sotalol, amiodarone) appear to have similar efficacy at preventing atrial fibrillation recurrences. At 6 months to 1 year, approximately 50% of the antiarrhythmic drug–treated patients will have had a recurrence, as opposed to approximately 80% of these patients treated with placebo. If atrial fibrillation recurs from time to time, cardioversion may be an acceptable therapeutic strategy in an effort to maintain sinus rhythm.

In many patients with atrial fibrillation, attempts at maintaining sinus rhythm are difficult if not futile. Frequent recurrences of atrial fibrillation, concerns related to antiarrhythmic drug toxicity, or other adverse effects (both cardiac and noncardiac) may mitigate against further attempts to maintain sinus rhythm. In such instances, a rate control strategy is reasonable.

It has been demonstrated that rate control is equivalent to rhythm control as a long-term strategy. Beta-blockers are the preferred AV nodal blocking agent.

ANTICOAGULATION

A meta-analysis of clinical anticoagulation trials showed a 68% risk reduction in stroke when comparing warfarin adjusted to an International Normalized Ratio between 2 and 3 versus placebo ($p <$ 0.001). The benefits of aspirin compared to placebo were marginal. Risk stratification on the basis of this meta-analysis showed that patients with a history of hypertension, recent congestive heart failure, or previous thromboembolism were at the greatest risk for stroke. The incidence of stroke was highest (17.6% per year) if a patient had two or three risk factors. If only one of those risk factors was present, the risk was 7.3% per year. The low-risk group comprised those patients less than 60 years in age and without any risk factors. These patients likely do not require systemic anticoagulation.

ENDOCARDIAL ELECTRICAL ISOLATION

Recently, several groups of investigators have developed catheter-based methods to cure atrial fibrillation. Endocardial electrical isolation of the pulmonary veins from the left atrium effectively prevents the rapidly firing foci from entering the left atrium. These foci appear necessary to regenerate the many re-entrant wavelets necessary to sustain atrial fibrillation. Cure rates approaching 80% have been reported with catheter-based procedures. A stroke risk of ~ 1% appears to limit frontline use of this procedure. This method is currently only being used in those patients who remain symptomatic despite optimal therapy. Endocardial electrical isolation of the pulmonary veins if successful (as judged by the absence of episodes of atrial fibrillation for 1 year after the procedure) would then obviate the need for systemic anticoagulation.

Currently, either a rhythm- or a rate-control strategy directed at the atrial fibrillation is acceptable. Anticoagulation with warfarin is usually necessary. With further advances, ablative procedures will likely evolve to first-line therapy.

COMPLICATIONS

The major complications of atrial fibrillation bear repeating. The stroke risk in nonvalvular atrial fibrillation is about 6% per year. Recurrent cerebral emboli may also manifest as a progressive "unexplained" deterioration in cognitive function.

A persistent rapid ventricular response can lead to a tachycardia-mediated cardiomyopathy. This may be the most common cause of a reversible nonischemic cardiomyopathy.

The loss of the atrial contraction can lead to a variety of adverse hemodynamic events, particularly in those patients with diastolic heart disease. Patients with diastolic heart disease (e.g., left ventricular hypertrophy, aortic stenosis, cardiac amyloid) are very preload dependent and can decompensate with the loss of atrial contraction.

CHAPTER 34

Aortic Dissection

James Kleczka

Aortic dissection is a very serious, potentially fatal disease of the aorta caused by a tear of the intima that allows blood to dissect into the vessel wall. It is one of the most common causes of aortic rupture and therefore must be identified quickly so therapy—medical or surgical—can be instituted.

ETIOLOGY

Aortic dissection results from a tear in the intima that allows creation of a false lumen, which is propagated by pulsatile aortic flow. The initial insult is thought to be damage to the media of the aortic wall with subsequent hemorrhage into the media. This can dissect into and disrupt the intimal layer. A tear in the intima, usually transverse, often occurs near the proximal end of the hematoma, which allows blood to extend the area of hemorrhage within the aortic wall and enlarge the false lumen. The false lumen often occupies 50% of the circumference of the aorta. When a dissection plane begins in the ascending aorta, it will usually extend along the greater curvature into the arch. When involving the descending aorta, the dissection plane is most often located laterally but may propagate in a spiral fashion. A second tear may occur distally, allowing blood to flow from the false lumen back into the true lumen.

There are two commonly used systems to classify aortic dissections. The Stanford classification system divides dissections into Type A and Type B. Type A dissections are proximal and involve the ascending aorta, whereas Type B dissections are distal (usually beyond the left subclavian artery) and involve the transverse or descending aorta. The DeBakey classification system specifies three types of dissection. Type I dissections originate in the ascending aorta and propagate into the descending aorta. Type II dissections are limited to the ascending aorta. Type III dissections originate in the descending aorta and propagate distally. In the majority of cases, the intimal tear occurs in the ascending aorta just above the aortic valve, with the false lumen extending to the aortoiliac bifurcation. Less frequently, the dissection is limited to the descending aorta.

Dissections found in the descending aorta most commonly arise from penetrating aortic ulcers associated with large ulcerated atherosclerotic plaques. These ulcers can disrupt the media, forming a hematoma and thereby provide a site prone to dissection. Patients with Marfan's syndrome are predisposed to cystic medial necrosis, which can lead to intramural hematoma, most commonly in the aortic root and ascending aorta, and are also sites that are prone to dissection.

Predisposing factors include systemic hypertension, which is found in 70% to 80% of patients with aortic dissection. As noted above, those with Marfan's syndrome and cystic medial necrosis are at higher risk of dissection, and aortic dissection is a major cause of morbidity and mortality in this patient population. There is also an increased frequency of dissection in patients with bicuspid aortic valve and coarctation of the aorta. Traumatic dissection may occur as a result of major mechanical trauma, such as a motor vehicle accident, or iatrogenic trauma, perhaps caused by intraaortic plaque

TABLE 34.1 Predisposing factors for aortic dissection

Acquired
Long-standing hypertension (most common)
Atherosclerosis
Trauma to chest wall
Syphilis
Giant cell arteritis
Congenital
Marfan's syndrome
Bicuspid aortic valve

disruption during a cardiac catheterization. Aortic dissection is twice as common in men than women and usually manifests between the ages of 40 and 70 years (Table 34.1).

CLINICAL MANIFESTATIONS

Patients will present with sudden onset of severe pain, many times described as a "tearing" sensation. The pain is most commonly located in the chest but has also been described in the back between the scapulae. As the dissection propagates further, it may extend into the epigastric and lumbar regions. The pain does not typically wax and wane, but rather remains severe throughout its course. Patients may also present with syncope if the dissection has extended into the cerebral or spinal circulation.

An expanding dissection may compress adjacent structures and lead to symptoms that may not be attributed to aortic dissection. If the airways are compromised, the patient may appear in significant respiratory distress. Dysphagia may be present if the esophagus is compressed. Other findings may include hoarse voice, Horner's syndrome, or even superior vena cava obstruction. If dissection extends into the aortic root, it may compromise blood flow through the right coronary artery and patients may present with an acute inferior myocardial infarction. It may also interfere with the integrity of the aortic valve leading to significant aortic regurgitation and acute pulmonary edema. This occurs in approximately 50% of patients with proximal dissections. Other physical findings of severe aortic regurgitation can be found on examination as well, including a loud diastolic murmur and bounding pulses. Extension into the pericardium can occur, in which case the patient may present with evidence of pericardial tamponade such as hypotension, jugular venous distention, and diminished heart sounds. Dissection can also extend into major aortic branches such as the innominate and subclavian arteries, or distally into the iliac arteries. This may lead to diminished pulses and possibly evidence of circulatory compromise.

When a patient presents with symptoms consistent with aortic dissection, the physical examination should focus on potential related findings such as the presence of aortic regurgitation, asymmetric or absent peripheral pulses, or findings consistent with a longstanding history of hypertension. Neurological deficits including hemiplegia may be present if dissection has propagated into the cerebral vasculature (Table 34.2).

DIAGNOSIS

Patients presenting with hypotension may have already ruptured their aorta and therefore a rapid diagnosis is essential. Routine diagnostic studies should include a plain chest x-ray. This study will

TABLE 34.2 Clinical features of aortic dissection by type and location

Clinical features	More frequent	Comments
Chest or back pain	DD	May radiate to any area of the thorax or abdomen
		Described as tearing
Abrupt onset	DD	Described as sharp May occur in two thirds of cases
Hypertension	DD	Two thirds of cases at presentation
Acute aortic insufficiency	AD	May lead to acute heart failure Dissection through the aortic valve
Cardiac tamponade	AD	Due to rupture of the aorta into the pericardial space
Stroke	AD	Due to dissection extending into the carotid arteries or decreased cardiac output
Hemothorax	AD	Due to rupture of the aorta into the pleural space
Blood pressure differential	AD	Difference ≥20 mm Hg between arms
Acute myocardial ischemia or myocardial infarction	AD	Due to coronary occlusion
Syncope	AD	Associated with poor outcome

AD, ascending dissection; DD, descending dissection.

be abnormal in most patients with aortic dissection, revealing a widened mediastinum in most cases. Aortic intimal calcification may be separated from the adventitial border by more than 1 cm. A "double lumen" due to a less radiopaque false lumen and left-sided pleural effusions may also be seen.

The 12-lead electrocardiogram will in most cases be unrevealing. If the dissection has extended into the ostia of either coronary artery, ST elevation may be seen, simulating a true acute myocardial infarction.

Further imaging is usually required to confirm the diagnosis of aortic dissection. Computed tomography and magnetic resonance imaging are both very sensitive and specific for diagnosing dissection and defining the extent of damage but are somewhat time consuming. Echocardiography, in particular transesophageal echocardiography, can also be utilized to assess the size and extent of dissection in the ascending and descending aorta with high sensitivity and specificity, but is not as accurate in imaging the aortic arch. Aortic angiography, an invasive study performed using peripherally inserted catheters, has historically been the gold standard in the diagnosis of aortic dissection. This will allow for imaging of coronary arteries, as well preparation for surgical repair of the dissection.

TREATMENT

When untreated, mortality due to aortic dissection is greater than 90% at 1 year. Up to 35% will die within the first 24 hours and 50% within the first 48 hours. Patients presenting with hypotension have a much worse prognosis, as this typically indicates rupture of the aorta. The prognosis is also worse in proximal as opposed to distal dissection. With prompt therapy, survival can exceed 80%.

Given the extreme mortality risk, it is imperative that medical management begin as soon as the diagnosis of aortic dissection is entertained. Goals include stopping propagation of the dissection and minimizing risk of rupture. The patient should always be admitted to a critical care unit with constant hemodynamic monitoring. Most patients admitted with aortic dissection are hypertensive, which will increase the shear stress on the aortic wall. Therefore, medications to lower systemic pressure and decrease cardiac contractility, which will in turn decrease the probability of continued propagation of the dissection plane, should be started. Intravenous beta-blockers such as esmolol or metoprolol are often used as first-line medical therapies. In cases of more severe hypertension, intravenous nitroprusside can be employed. Goals should be a heart rate in the 60s with systolic blood pressures between 100 and 120 mm Hg. Some drugs that cause arterial vasodilation, such as hydralazine or minoxidil, may cause a reflex increase in heart rate, thus increasing shear stress, and should be avoided. If arterial hypotension is present, aortic rupture must be considered, which will require emergency surgical repair.

Surgical repair should be considered in all cases. Patients presenting with proximal dissection should undergo surgical repair as soon as possible. The patient should be stabilized medically prior to the operation because emergency repair carries an extremely high risk. If symptoms persist, however, surgery should be performed regardless of stability. Patients with uncomplicated distal aortic dissections should be treated medically, as there has been no benefit shown to be associated with early surgical intervention in this group. If distal aortic dissections involve major branches including the renal or mesenteric circulation, or if there is continued pain suggesting propagation or a high likelihood of rupture, surgical repair should be pursued. Some patients are clearly not candidates for an operation of this magnitude due to comorbid illnesses. Those patients must be treated with maximal medical therapy, converting intravenous therapies to oral therapy to maintain systolic blood pressure between 100 and 120 mm Hg.

Long-term therapy will involve continued blood pressure control, regardless of whether or not surgical repair was performed. Beta-blockers are highly beneficial and should be continued, with additional antihypertensive agents being added when needed.

COMPLICATIONS

Perioperative complications leading to increased morbidity and mortality include myocardial infarction, cardiac tamponade, sepsis, spinal ischemia leading to hemiplegia, and renal failure. Many other complications of dissection are found upon the initial presentation and are described above.

Pulmonary

Ralph Schapira

CHAPTER 35

Bronchial Asthma

Linus Santo Tomas

Asthma is chronic inflammatory disease of the airways characterized by airway hyperresponsiveness and episodic obstruction to expiratory airflow (airway obstruction). Patients may present with cough, wheezing, or shortness of breath.

ETIOLOGY

The airway inflammation in asthma is mediated mainly by mast cells, eosinophils, and TH2 lymphocytes. Neutrophilic inflammation is less characteristic but has been described in sudden-onset and fatal asthma exacerbations. Cytokines and proinflammatory substances released by these cells contribute to hyperresponsiveness of the airway and lead to bronchoconstriction, airway edema, mucus hypersecretion, and denudation of the airway epithelium. Early in its course, the airway obstruction in asthma is almost always fully reversible with treatment, but undertreatment and poor control can lead to airway remodeling, which can evolve into persistent (fixed) airway obstruction.

The exact mechanism by which asthma develops has not yet been fully elucidated. However, a number of host and environmental factors have been identified. Atopy, typified by exuberant immunoglobulin E–mediated immune response to allergens, is a strong risk factor for developing asthma. There may be a genetic component to this since atopy may have a familial predisposition. Obesity has also been implicated as a risk factor for the development of asthma. Environmental factors that have been identified as possible factors in the development of asthma include exposure to allergens, certain infections, inhaled substances at the workplace, and diet in early childhood. Although tobacco smoke and air pollution are known to be associated with exacerbations of asthma, their role in the initial development of the disease is unclear.

CLINICAL MANIFESTATIONS

Individuals with asthma usually present with episodes of chest tightness, wheezing, cough, and breathing difficulties. These symptoms may be precipitated by inhaled irritant substances or allergens and may worsen with other comorbidities or exposures (Table 35.1). Some patients may be predictably worse during certain seasons, and a diurnal variation with symptoms being worse at night or early morning is characteristic of asthma. There may be family history of asthma or atopic disease.

Physical examination may be normal in the absence of an exacerbation of asthma. Findings that may assist in diagnosis include use of accessory respiratory muscle groups, hyperexpansion of the thorax, prolonged expiratory time, decreased breath sounds, and wheezing on auscultation. Due to markedly decreased air flow, wheezing may be absent with a very severe exacerbation. Other clues to predisposing risk factors for asthma include the presence of nasal polyps and skin manifestations of atopic dermatitis or eczema.

TABLE 35.1 Exposures or factors that can worsen asthma symptoms
Pollen
Inhaled chemicals or dusts
Upper respiratory infection
Animal dander
Dust mites (can be in beddings or carpeting)
Mold
Smoke (tobacco, wood)
Changes in weather
Extreme emotions
Exercise
Gastroesophageal reflux disease
Postnasal drip
Menses
Medication allergies
Beta-blockers

DIAGNOSIS

In patients who refer classic symptoms of asthma (wheezing, dyspnea) triggered by typical allergens that readily and completely resolve with the administration of asthmatic treatment, a clinical diagnosis of asthma may be made. In other patients whose symptoms and clinical course are not so typical, additional testing is needed.

Pulmonary Function Tests

Pulmonary function tests include peak expiratory flow rates (PEFR) and spirometry. A decreased PEFR has a low specificity and can be seen with other pulmonary processes. Peak flow measurements are dependent on patient effort and may be reduced in both obstructive and restrictive diseases, hence reducing their diagnostic utility. Monitoring diurnal variation in peak expiratory flows (PEFs) can be mostly helpful in monitoring disease activity outside the pulmonary function laboratory.

The clinical suspicion of asthma should be confirmed with spirometry in patients who are able to perform this. Performance of the test maneuver may not be satisfactory in children under 7 years old but can be considered for patients over 4 years of age. Spirometry done before and after an inhaled short-acting β2-agonist bronchodilator can help confirm whether a patient has airways obstruction and determine whether there is significant improvement in pulmonary function after an inhaled bronchodilator is given (a significant bronchodilator response). The criterion standard for the diagnosis of airway obstruction is a decrease in the ratio of the forced expiratory volume in 1 second (FEV1) to forced vital capacity (FVC) below that predicted for the subject. The normal FEV1/FVC varies from about 85% in young adults to about 65% in the oldest adults. A significant bronchodilator response is defined by a 12% and 200 mL increase in the FEV1 or FVC compared to baseline. Importantly, a FEV1/FVC that normalizes after the administration of an inhaled bronchodilator—demonstrating reversible airway obstruction—supports the diagnosis of asthma. If the baseline and postbronchodilator spirometry do not demonstrate airway obstruction, a methacholine challenge test may be indicated to confirm asthma. Bronchoprovocation with inhaled methacholine

TABLE 35.2 Differential diagnoses for asthma

Other pulmonary or cardiovascular diseases
Chronic bronchitis or emphysema
Cystic fibrosis
Bronchiectasis
Infectious bronchiolitis
Bronchiolitis obliterans
Nonasthma eosinophilic lung diseases
Congestive heart failure
Pulmonary embolism
Upper and large airway diseases
Vocal cord dysfunction
Foreign body aspiration
Laryngeal, tracheal, and other large airway tumors
Tracheomalacia
Tracheal and bronchial stenosis
Common nonasthma causes of chronic cough
Postnasal drip
Gastroesophageal disease

should trigger a reduction in FEV1 of at least 20%. Spirometric findings of airway obstruction that significantly improve to normal or near normal values after a bronchodilator should be correlated with clinical features to make a more accurate diagnosis of asthma. For suspected exercise-induced asthma, spirometry can be taken before and after a supervised exercise activity.

Other lung function tests such as lung volume measurements and diffusing capacity of carbon monoxide may assist in distinguishing asthma from emphysema or other lung diseases.

Chest Radiograph

A chest x-ray is not necessary to make a diagnosis of asthma and it is almost always normal. However, it may be helpful in excluding other diseases that can present similarly (e.g., congestive heart failure) as well as recognize comorbid conditions. The chest radiograph during an acute exacerbation may reveal hyperinflation and subsegmental atelectasis from mucous plugging. In the presence of fever, chest pain, and wheezing, a chest x-ray may be warranted to exclude the presence of pneumonia. Furthermore, differential diagnoses that may present with similar symptoms should be considered and ruled out (Table 35.2).

MANAGEMENT

Asthma management requires an integrated approach that entails involving patients in their care, identifying and avoiding risk factors, and periodic evaluation of disease control to optimize further treatment. Patient education that teaches the recognition of exacerbating factors and symptoms of worsening disease control should be an integral part of management.

TABLE 35.3 Classification of asthma severity by clinical features before treatment

Severity	Controller treatment
Intermittent	
Symptoms <2 days/week Nocturnal dyspnea ≤ twice a month FEV1 ≥80% predicted	Short-acting β2-agonist as needed
Mild persistent	
Symptoms >2 days/week but not daily Exacerbations may affect activity and sleep Nocturnal symptoms 3-4 times a month FEV1 ≥80% predicted	Low-dose inhaled corticosteroid Leukotriene modifiers Mast-cell stabilizers (Cromolyn/Nedocromil) Theophylline (not preferred)
Moderate persistent	
Symptoms daily Nocturnal symptoms once/week but not nightly Daily use of inhaled short-acting β2-agonist FEV1 >60% but <80% predicted	Low-dose inhaled corticosteroid + long-acting inhaled β_2-agonists Medium-dose inhaled corticosteroid alone Low-dose inhaled corticosteroid + leukotriene modifier Low-dose inhaled corticosteroid + sustained release theophylline
Severe persistent	
Symptoms daily Frequent exacerbations Nocturnal symptoms often nightly Limitation of physical activity FEV1 ≤60% predicted	High-dose inhaled corticosteroid + long-acting β_2-agonist Addition of a leukotriene modifier and/or a sustained release theophylline can be considered Addition of oral corticosteroid may be needed Anti-immunoglobulin E antibody treatment can be considered

Rapid-acting inhaled β2-agonists can be used for any severity to relieve acute symptoms.

The management of asthma involves aiming for long-term control as well as treatment of acute exacerbations. An assessment of a patient's severity of disease, based on clinical symptoms, lung function variability, and the type of medications needed to control symptoms, is vital to instituting appropriate therapy and management modification (Table 35.3). A stepwise approach to treatment is recommended depending on the severity of asthma, with the goal of maintaining disease control with the least amount of medications. Periodic assessment of asthma control is needed because the disease can have a variable clinical course and response to treatment. Pharmacologic therapy can be broadly classified into reliever and controller medications. Reliever medication usually consists of an inhaled short-acting β_2-agonist that works by effecting bronchodilation through bronchial smooth muscle relaxation. Controller medications are given with the aim of reducing inflammation in the airways as well as targeting longer durations of bronchodilation.

TABLE 35.4 Hospitalization criteria for acute exacerbation of asthma

FEV1 <50%
O_2 satuation <91% on room air (<95% if pregnant)
Respiratory rate >30/min
Pulse rate >120/min
If patient has any of the following: • Breathlessness at rest • Difficulty speaking phrases • Decreased alertness due to respiratory symptoms • Uses accessory muscles • Evidence of poor air movement • Not subjectively halfway back to baseline

Acute exacerbations of asthma can be precipitated by identified triggers but may also occur without a clear heralding event. They are characterized by worsening shortness of breath, wheezing, and significant reduction in the FEV1 or PEF when compared to the patient's best values.

Mild exacerbations, with PEF reduction of less than 20% from baseline, can usually be treated as an outpatient. However, some exacerbations are best managed in the hospital and very severe exacerbations should be admitted to an intensive care unit (Table 35.4). Treatment primarily involves increasing the frequency of inhaled rapid-acting bronchodilators and giving systemic corticosteroids.

TABLE 35.5 Treatment of severe asthma exacerbation

Oxygen
Aim for oxygen saturation >90% Aim for oxygen saturation >95% if pregnant or has heart disease Monitor until response is stable
Inhaled short-acting β_2-agonist
Repetitive or continuous administration is most effective way of reversing airflow obstruction Selective β_2-agonists: albuterol, terbutaline, pirbuterol, bitolterol High-dose metered-dose inhaler (MDI) w/spacer = nebulization Nebulize if unable to coordinate
Inhaled anticholinergic
Should be considered in severe exacerbations Ipratropium bromide + β_2-agonist Provides additional bronchodilation
Systemic corticosteroid
Prednisone, methylprednisolone, prednisolone 120–180 mg/day in 3 or 4 divided doses for 48 hours Then 60–80 mg/day until PEFR ≥70% Oral route is as effective as intravenous if absorption is not a concern

Inhaled bronchodilators, such as a short-acting β_2-agonist or its combination with an inhaled short-acting anticholinergic, can be given every 20 to 30 minutes with acute severe asthma (Table 35.5). Systemic corticosteroids can be given orally or intravenously. Adequate oxyhemoglobin saturation ($\geq$90%) should also be ensured by supplementation if necessary. Worsening oxygenation, hypercapnia, lethargy, and worsening sensorium are usually indicators of impending respiratory arrest. Vigilance should be maintained in identifying patients who continue to worsen and may need mechanical ventilation.

CHAPTER 36

Chronic Obstructive Pulmonary Disease

Linus Santo Tomas

Chronic obstructive pulmonary disease (COPD) is a group of pulmonary disorders characterized by permanent (irreversible) obstruction to expiratory airflow (airway obstruction). Chronic inflammation, in response to inhaled tobacco smoke, noxious gases, and dusts, damages the airways and lung parenchyma. COPD has traditionally been classified into subtypes of chronic bronchitis and emphysema, although many patients have both. Chronic bronchitis is defined as a chronic productive cough for more than 2 years and emphysema is characterized by destruction of alveolar walls that lead to an abnormal increase in the size of the distal airspaces.

The distinction of COPD from asthma is important as asthma is characterized by intermittent airway obstruction and the management of asthma is different from that of COPD. Bronchial hyperresponsiveness (defined as periodic changes in forced expiratory volume in 1 second [FEV1]), although usually of lesser magnitude than in asthma, may be observed in COPD. The important distinction is that asthma is characterized by reversible airway obstruction, whereas COPD is characterized by permanent airway obstruction. Studies indicate that chronic poor asthma control can eventually lead to structural changes and airway obstruction that is persistent—asthma that evolves into COPD in the absence of smoking. Nevertheless, there are some differentiating features of asthma and COPD (Table 36.1).

ETIOLOGY

Inflammation is a key element in the pathogenesis of COPD. Inhalation of tobacco smoke or of other noxious gases activates macrophages and epithelial cells to release chemotactic factors that recruit more macrophages and neutrophils. In turn, macrophages and neutrophils release proteases that destroy structural elements in the lungs. Proteases can be counteracted by endogenous antiproteases but an imbalance between these, with predominance of protease activity, predisposes to the development of COPD. The generation of highly reactive oxygen species such as superoxide, hydroxyl free radical, and hydrogen peroxide has also been identified as a contributing factor in the pathogenesis because these substances can increase destruction of proteases.

The chronic inflammation leads to bronchial wall epithelial metaplasia, mucous hypersecretion, increased smooth muscle mass, and fibrosis. There is also ciliary dysfunction of the epithelium, impairing clearance of the already increased mucous production. Clinically, this is what manifests as chronic bronchitis, typified as a chronic productive cough. In the lung parenchyma, protease-mediated breakdown of structural elements leads to emphysema. Loss of alveolar attachments results in reduced elastic recoil of the lung and dynamic airway collapse due to removal of the tethering support in smaller noncartilaginous airways. All these processes result in a mostly fixed airway obstruction and other physiologic features that are characteristic of COPD (Table 36.2).

Airway obstruction produces unventilated or under ventilated alveoli; continued perfusion of these alveoli leads to hypoxemia (low PaO_2) from mismatching of ventilation and blood flow (V/Q mismatch). Ventilation of unperfused or poorly perfused alveoli increases dead space (V_d), causing

TABLE 36.1 Comparative features of COPD and asthma

	COPD	Asthma
Clinical history	Onset usually older age Tobacco smoking exposure No family history of atopy Diurnal variation is not that prominent	Onset usually younger age Allergen exposure Family history of asthma or atopy Nocturnal and early morning worsening is characteristic
Diagnostic tests		
Spirometry	Obstruction is not fully reversible	Obstruction is fully reversible
Diffusing capacity	Reduced (with emphysema)	Usually normal
Chest radiograph	Hyperinflation is more persistent, bullous disease may be evident	Hyperinflation during exacerbation, but may otherwise be normal
Pathology	Mucous gland metaplasia Loss of alveolar tissue (emphysema)	Mucous gland hyperplasia Intact alveolar structure
Inflammation	Macrophages and neutrophils predominate CD8+ Lymphocytes	Mast cells and eosinophils predominate CD4+ Lymphocytes
Treatment		
Inhaled corticosteroids	For moderate to severe disease	For mild to severe persistent disease
Leukotriene modifier	Not recommended	Used as controller medication
Inhaled anticholinergic	Used for maintenance and during exacerbations	Used for exacerbations; not indicated for maintenance

TABLE 36.2 Pathogenesis of COPD

Pathogenic mechanisms	Pathologic changes	Physiologic consequences
Inflammation Proteinase vs. antiproteinase Oxidative stress	Central airways Peripheral airways Lung parenchyma Pulmonary vasculature	Mucous hypersecretion Ciliary dysfunction Airflow limitation and hyperinflation Gas exchange abnormality Pulmonary hypertension Systemic effects

inefficient CO_2 removal. Hyperventilation normally compensates for this, thus producing a normal $PaCO_2$. However, hyperventilation, which further increases the work required to overcome the already increased airway resistance, ultimately fails, resulting in CO_2 retention (hypercapnia) in some patients with advanced COPD.

Risk Factors for COPD

Tobacco smoking is currently the primary risk factor for COPD in developed countries. A total of 85% to 90% of patients with COPD have previous or current history of tobacco smoking. On the other hand, only about 15% of smokers develop COPD, indicating that there likely are other constitutional or genetic factors that determine the risk of developing airway obstruction. Alpha-1-antitrypsin deficiency is the only genetically linked risk factor that we know of at present, but the propensity of COPD to occur in certain families indicates that there are other hereditary factors yet to be identified. Indoor and outdoor pollution as well occupational exposure to dusts and gases have been associated with development of COPD. Other risk factors that have been implicated include the presence of bronchial hyperresponsiveness, lower birth weight, impaired fetal lung growth, and lower socioeconomic status.

CLINICAL MANIFESTATIONS

The cardinal symptoms of established COPD are cough and expectoration, which tend to be maximal in the morning and reflect pooling of secretions overnight. A productive cough, intermittent at first, becomes almost a daily occurrence with time. Sputum is clear and mucoid, but may become thick, tenacious, and yellow, and even blood-streaked during intercurrent bacterial respiratory infections. Wheezing is generally present, especially during respiratory infections.

Exertional dyspnea develops as the disease progresses. With advanced disease, dyspnea may occur with minimal activity and even at rest as gas exchange abnormalities worsen. With moderate to severe disease, physical examination may reveal decreased breath sounds, prolonged expiration, rhonchi, and hyperresonance to percussion. Because advanced disease may be complicated by pulmonary hypertension and cor pulmonale, signs of right-sided heart failure (including jugular venous distension, hepatomegaly, and lower extremity edema) may also be seen. Clubbing of the digits is not a feature of COPD and when present should arouse suspicion of another disorder, especially bronchogenic carcinoma.

DIAGNOSIS

A complete history and detailed physical examination are important in establishing a diagnosis of COPD. However, pulmonary function testing is necessary for the diagnosis.

Pulmonary Function Tests

The diagnosis of COPD is supported by finding of persistent airway obstruction on a postbronchodilator spirometry (defined by a FEV1/forced vital capacity [FVC] less than predicted for the subject). Lung volume measurements may reveal an increased residual volume and total lung capacity though the diagnosis of airway obstruction is only made by demonstrating an abnormality in the FEV1/FVC. The diffusing capacity for carbon monoxide is usually reduced with emphysema but preserved in patients with chronic bronchitis.

Pulmonary function generally declines progressively, and although less accurately predictable in a given patient, the average yearly loss in FEV1 is 50 to 100 mL. The loss of FEV1 is accelerated in patients who continue to smoke. Activity is markedly limited when the FEV1 is about 1.0 L. The postbronchodilator FEV1, performance on a 6-minute walk, level of dyspnea, and body mass index have been identified as predictors of survival.

Chest Radiograph and Other Tests

The chest radiograph (CXR) may reveal lung hyperinflation, flat diaphragms, a narrow heart shadow, and bullous disease on a frontal view and an increased retrosternal air space on a lateral projection. However, the chest radiograph may be normal in the early stages of the disease and is not a sensitive test for the diagnosis of COPD. Emphysematous changes are more easily seen on a computed tomography scan of the chest but this is not a cost-effective or recommended modality for screening COPD. Nonetheless, although imaging can suggest the presence of COPD, only spirometry is the criterion standard for the diagnosis of airway obstruction.

Arterial blood gas measurement is recommended when the FEV1 is below 40% of predicted for the subject, with evidence of cor pulmonale and during severe acute exacerbations to assess not just oxygenation but also possible hypercapnia.

Testing for alpha-1-antitrypsin is recommended for patients who are diagnosed to have COPD at a young age (<45 years old) or have strong familial history of obstructive lung disease.

MANAGEMENT

Recent management consensus guidelines have used the severity of COPD, based on the FEV1, to guide therapy (Fig. 36.1). The only interventions that have so far been proven to improve survival are smoking cessation and long-term oxygen therapy (LTOT) for those who have significant hypo-

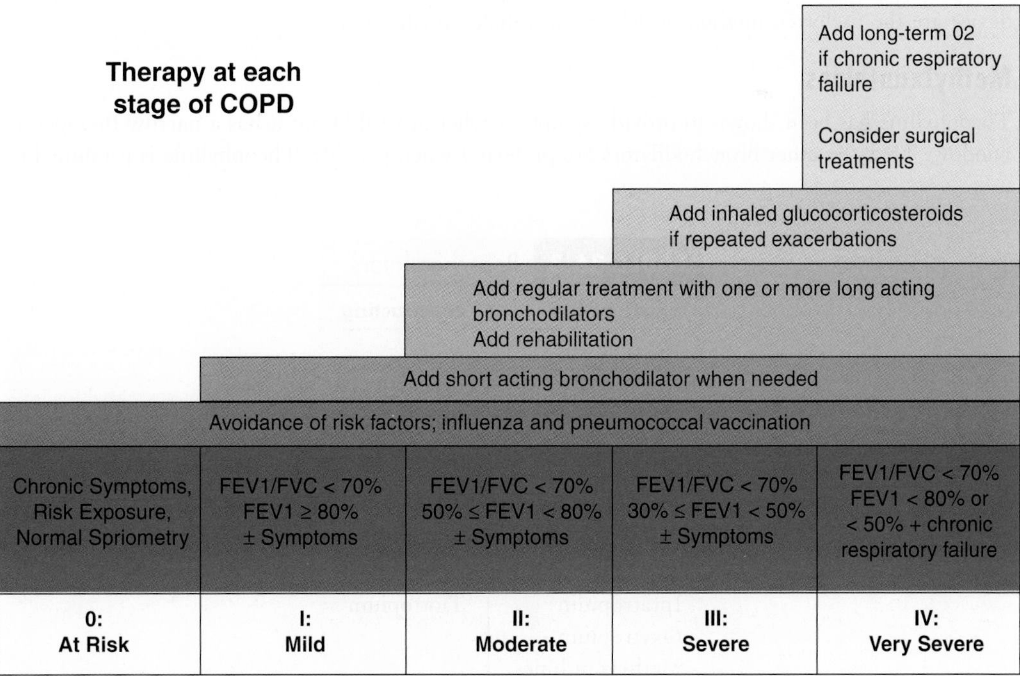

Figure 36.1 • Severity classification of COPD and therapeutic options. (Adapted from the Global Strategy for the Diagnosis, Management and Prevention of COPD, Global Initiative for Chronic Obstructive Lung Disease (GOLD) 2006. Available from: http://www.goldcopd.org, with permission).

xemia at rest. Thus, all patients with COPD should be encouraged to stop smoking. Nonsmokers who develop COPD should also be encouraged to avoid occupational or environmental exposures that may be contributing factors in their disease. Vaccination against influenza should be given yearly, generally in early autumn. Pneumococcal vaccine is recommended; immunity wanes after about 5 years and revaccination may be required in patients at high risk of serious pneumococcal infection.

Bronchodilators

Bronchodilators can be classified as short-acting and long-acting agents and fall into three main pharmacologic classes (Table 36.3). Short-acting bronchodilators may be the only medication needed to relieve symptoms in patients with mild disease. With increasing severity of COPD, the long-acting bronchodilators may offer symptomatic benefit for longer periods. All symptomatic patients with the diagnosis of COPD should be given a trial of inhaled bronchodilators, regardless of whether spirometry shows a significant bronchodilator response.

Anticholinergics can be used as a first-line treatment in COPD. Ipratropium bromide is a short-acting anticholinergic that is poorly absorbed from the airways when given as an aerosol and has little effect on mucociliary clearance. Tiotropium is a long-acting anticholinergic that has been shown to sustain higher FEV1 troughs. Anticholinergics are not as effective in the maintenance pharmacotherapy of asthma as in COPD.

β_2-agonists presumably cause bronchodilation by stimulating adenyl cyclase and increasing intracellular cyclic adenosine monophosphate (cAMP). β_2-agonists may be administered in combination with anticholinergics to optimize bronchodilatory effects.

Bronchodilators can be delivered with a metered-dose inhaler (MDI) using a spacer device or as a dry-powder inhaler (DPI), providing fixed-dose, targeted delivery into the airway and thus minimizing systemic effects. Nebulizers deliver a larger dose, involve bulky equipment, and require skills in equipment care and medication dispensing. Thus, properly used MDIs attached to a spacer device are the preferred method of delivery of inhaled medications.

Methylxanthines

Theophylline has been shown to provide symptom relief in COPD but it has a narrow therapeutic window. Thus the other bronchodilators are preferred when possible. Theophylline is presumed to

TABLE 36.3 Bronchodilators

Short-acting	Long-acting
β_2-agonists	
Albuterol Fenoterol Metaproterenol Pirbuterol Terbutaline	Formoterol Salmeterol
Anticholinergic	
Ipratropium Oxytropium Methylxanthines Aminophylline Theophylline	Tiotropium

TABLE 36.4 Indications for continuous long-term oxygen therapy

Resting arterial partial pressure of oxygen ≤55 mm Hg or arterial oxygen saturation 88%
Resting arterial partial pressure of oxygen 56 to 59 mm Hg or arterial oxygen saturation 89% with the following conditions:

a. Electrocardiographic evidence of cor pulmonale, or
b. Erythrocythemia with hematocrit >56%, or
c. Edema due to congestive heart failure

provide benefit by phosphodiesterase inhibition and increase in the levels of cAMP. It is also thought to augment diaphragmatic contractility by enhancing diaphragmatic blood flow. This beneficial effect on diaphragmatic function may help minimize or prevent diaphragm fatigue or respiratory failure in advanced COPD. Periodic drug level monitoring and the use of slow-release preparations are recommended.

Corticosteroids

Inhaled corticosteroids should be considered in severe to very severe COPD (FEV1 <50% predicted especially those with recurrent exacerbations. Systemic corticosteroids, oral or intravenous, are used in the management of acute exacerbations. Systemic corticosteroids are given for up to 2 weeks with acute exacerbations requiring hospitalization; longer treatment is not recommended because no further benefit is achieved and there is increased incidence of side effects. Although corticosteroids are part of the armamentarium in the treatment of COPD its effects are not as dramatic as in asthma.

Pulmonary Rehabilitation

When customized for the patient with COPD (or other debilitating respiratory disorders), a comprehensive program in pulmonary rehabilitation can improve exercise capacity, psychosocial functioning, and overall health-related quality of life. These programs do not improve longevity or pulmonary function, but they have been shown to reduce hospitalizations.

Long-Term Oxygen Therapy

Oxygen is an inhaled medication and LTOT can prolong life and improve quality of life in selected patients with COPD (Tables 36.4 and 36.5). The criteria to prescribe oxygen are not based on dyspnea but rather on the result of standardized testing for hypoxemia at rest and with exertion done in a pulmonary function laboratory. Dyspnea does not necessarily correlated with hypoxemia; many dyspneic patients are not hypoxemic and many patients who are hypoxemia are not dyspneic. There

TABLE 36.5 Indications for long-term oxygen therapy during exercise and sleep[a]

1. Arterial partial pressure of oxygen ≤55 mm Hg or arterial oxygen saturation 88% during exercise or low-level activity
2. Arterial partial pressure of oxygen ≤55 mm Hg or arterial oxygen saturation 88% during sleep

[a]The need for long-term oxygen therapy during exercise or sleep is usually determined by a minute walk test or sleep study respectively.

are universally recognized criteria as to which patients with COPD should receive LTOT, based on the level of hypoxemia. It should be used for at least 15 hours per day to provide survival benefit. It is usually delivered with a nasal cannula attached to an oxygen source. There are very portable oxygen units and there are devices that can help conserve oxygen delivery.

Surgical Options

Bullectomy, lung volume reduction surgery, and lung transplantation are surgical options that can be considered in patients with very severe COPD. Referral to a specialist in a specialized center is indicated to further evaluate appropriateness of these procedures.

Treatment of Exacerbations

Generally, exacerbations occur more frequently as the FEV1 decreases. Most are precipitated by respiratory infections that are likely viral but may also be due to bacterial flora that are commonly found in the upper respiratory tract. Moderate to severe exacerbations characterized by worsening dyspnea, cough, and increased sputum production and purulence benefit from antibiotic treatment that covers for *Haemophilus influenzae*, pneumococci, and *Moraxella catarrhalis*. *Pseudomonas aeruginosa* coverage needs to be considered in patients who have had three or more exacerbations in the past year. Oral or intravenous corticosteroids are used in severe exacerbations as mentioned above. Noninvasive positive pressure mechanical ventilation should be considered because it may help prevent invasive mechanical ventilation (requiring intubation) in some patients.

CHAPTER 37

Interstitial Lung Disease

Linus Santo Tomas

Interstitial lung diseases (ILDs) include a wide array of disorders that primarily, but not exclusively, affect the lung compartment that lies between the epithelial cells of the alveoli and the endothelial cells of the capillaries—the lung interstitium.

ETIOLOGY

Some ILDs are attributed to inhalational exposure or are associated with nonpulmonary or other systemic disease (Table 37.1). Others have no clear cause that has yet been identified, such as sarcoidosis, but have been well recognized for decades. On the other hand, the idiopathic interstitial pneumonias (IIP) have only more recently been characterized as a number of distinct clinicopathologic entities with various prognosis and response to treatment.

Regardless of etiology, interstitial lung diseases share some common clinical features. An initial alveolar epithelial injury leads to an alveolitis; inflammation in the lung interstitium and collagen deposition by mesenchymal cells follow. Fibrosis and destruction of the alveolar capillary units culminate in "end-stage lung disease" and chronic respiratory failure. In any tissue injury, a balance ordinarily prevails between inflammation and repair. This balance is disturbed in ILD and the inflammation is perpetuated. The type, route, and duration of the injury, the genetic predisposition of the host, and comorbid factors all determine the severity and rate of progression of the lung disease.

Idiopathic pulmonary fibrosis (IPF) is the most common form of idiopathic interstitial pneumonias (IIP) (Table 37.1). IPF is a progressive disease of unknown etiology. Its pathogenesis includes inflammation and fibrosis of the pulmonary interstitium leading to destruction of the alveolar capillary units. Despite its distinct clinical, histologic, and roentgenographic aspects, it is diagnosed only after excluding other forms of ILD. There are a number of hypothesis on how IPF develops, but the predominant thought at present is that injury to the epithelial cells initiates a dysregulation of inflammation, which eventually leads to abnormal healing with formation of abundant scar tissue.

Usual interstitial pneumonia (UIP) is the characteristic feature of IPF on histology. UIP is denoted by the presence of temporal heterogeneity of fibrotic changes when lung tissue sections are viewed under the microscope. This means various stages are seen, from normal lungs to active fibrosis and end-stage honeycombing. Not all lung areas are involved in earlier stages of the disease, such that basal and peripheral lung areas tend to be more severely involved. There are other end-stage interstitial lung diseases that may have a UIP pattern on histology. Thus, other causes of ILD have to be ruled out to make the clinical diagnosis of IPF.

CLINICAL MANIFESTATIONS

The clinical manifestations of an ILD may vary according to the etiology. Because ILD is often associated with a systemic disorder, the manifestations of the primary disease may be more prominent

TABLE 37.1 Etiologic classification of interstitial lung diseases

Connective tissue diseases
Ankylosing spondylitis, polymyositis-dermatomyositis, rheumatoid arthritis, Sjögren's syndrome, systemic lupus erythematosus, systemic sclerosis
Complications of treatment
Drug-related: amiodarone, nitrofurantoin, chemotherapeutic agents
Hematopoietic stem cell transplantation: idiopathic pneumonia syndrome
Radiation pneumonitis
Environmental and occupational
Hypersensitivity pneumonitis
Inorganic dusts, asbestosis, coal-workers pneumoconiosis, silicosis
Gastrointestinal and liver disease
Inflammatory bowel disease
Primary biliary cirrhosis
Hereditary disorders
Tuberous sclerosis
Neurofibromatosis
Metabolic storage disorders
Neoplastic
Lymphangitic carcinomatosis
Pulmonary Langerhans cell histiocytosis
Granulomatous idiopathic disease
Sarcoidosis
Idiopathic interstitial pneumonias
Idiopathic pulmonary fibrosis
Nonspecific pulmonary fibrosis
Cryptogenic organizing pneumonia
Acute interstitial pneumonia
Lymphocytic interstitial pneumonia
Desquamative interstitial pneumonia
Respiratory-bronchiolitis interstitial lung disease

than the pulmonary symptoms. Symptoms of ILD are often chronic, but an acute onset with rapid progression is well known. The usual symptoms are gradually progressive dyspnea, dry cough, and chest pain, which may be pleuritic. Hemoptysis may follow severe cough or signify pulmonary hemorrhage syndromes that manifest as ILD. Pulmonary histiocytosis X and lymphangioleiomyomatosis may present with recurrent pneumothoraces.

In diagnosing occupational pneumoconioses, hypersensitivity pneumonitis (HP), and drug-induced ILD, it is critical to obtain a history of exposure to possible offending agents (e.g., silica, asbestos, inorganic dusts, or cytotoxic drugs). Although smokers do not seem to develop HP, they are at risk for eosinophilic granuloma and Goodpasture's syndrome.

Tachypnea is an early and constant feature of ILD. Finger clubbing is seen in 50% of patients especially in the presence of hypoxia. End-inspiratory rales vary, depending on the disease entity. Rales (crackles) can be heard on auscultation in idiopathic pulmonary fibrosis and asbestosis, but are less commonly heard in granulomatous ILD (sarcoidosis, HP, silicosis, and eosinophilic granuloma).

Diagnosis

A clinical assessment with focused history and physical examination is the first step. Specific inquiries should be made about symptoms, their progression, and impact on daily activities. Determine exposure to tobacco smoke, noxious agents, or respirable substances in the workplace and/or through hobbies, and the temporal relationship of such exposure to symptoms. An inquiry should be made on medication use and other treatments, including radiation. Family history can also be helpful, such as with familial pulmonary fibrosis and sarcoidosis.

Chest x-rays are abnormal in 90% of ILD cases. Besides the features of the primary disease, other findings include low lung volumes or diffuse interstitial (nodular, reticular, or reticulonodular) abnormalities. High-resolution computed tomography has a high sensitivity in diagnosing ILD but is less specific in determining the underlying process.

In patients with other signs and symptoms of connective tissue disease, directed diagnostic testing for the characteristic laboratory abnormalities may help confirm the etiologic diagnosis: for example, elevated creatinine kinase in polymyositis, specific antinuclear antibody patterns in scleroderma and lupus erythematosus, or rheumatoid factor in rheumatoid arthritis. ILD occurring in these settings may be attributed to these specific disorders without resorting to lung biopsy.

Pulmonary function studies usually show a restrictive impairment in ILD (characterized by a decrease in total lung capacity). The DL_{CO} is typically reduced. The PaO_2 and $PaCO_2$ are low. The PaO_2 declines further with exercise compared to the value at rest.

For some ILDs, like occupational diseases such as silicosis and asbestosis, an appropriate history and characteristic radiologic features may be enough to make the diagnosis. A fiberoptic bronchoscopic biopsy may suffice to confirm certain diseases such as sarcoidosis or hypersensitivity pneumonitis. More commonly, a video-assisted thoracoscopic surgical biopsy or an open thoracoscopic lung biopsy is needed. Most disorders that cause ILD, including idiopathic pulmonary fibrosis, will ultimately require a surgical biopsy to establish a specific diagnosis and determine the prognosis.

In IPF, the erythrocyte sedimentation rate may be high. Immunologic abnormalities including cryoglobulins, rheumatoid factor, antinuclear antibodies, and elevated serum immunoglobulins are frequent. Arterial hypoxemia can be present at rest or on exercise, and is mostly due to ventilation-perfusion mismatching. Pulmonary function studies show a restrictive ventilatory impairment. The DL_{CO} is reduced. Chest roentgenograms may reveal low lung volumes, ground glass opacities, or reticular, reticulonodular, or nodular infiltrates. A high-resolution computed tomography scan of the chest is recommended for better definition of abnormalities. Honeycombing signifies advanced disease.

MANAGEMENT

There is no uniformly successful or satisfactory therapy for ILD that is diagnosed at an advanced stage. If an offending agent (especially medication or inhaled organic antigens) is identified, removal might stop further progression and even result in some improvement. Treatment also depends on the type of ILD diagnosed. Corticosteroids and other immune-modulating drugs have been used in various ILDs but response depends on the underlying cause. Evaluation of response to treatment usually includes assessment of symptoms, pulmonary function tests, and chest imaging studies (x-ray or computed tomography scan).

Optimal pharmacotherapy in IPF is controversial. A trial of corticosteroids can be made but objective evidence of improvement after a few months, based on physiologic and pulmonary function or radiologic studies, must be sought to justify continuing treatment. Other treatments that may be considered are acetylcysteine, azathioprine, and other immune-modulating drugs. Newer treatment options are continuing to be studied.

In all forms of interstitial lung diseases, pulmonary rehabilitation should be offered and oxygen supplementation should be prescribed when patients become hypoxemic on room air. Referral for possible lung transplantation should also be considered for those whose function continues to decline precipitously despite a trial of medical management.

CHAPTER 38

Pleural Effusions

Siddhartha Singh

The pleura is a serous membrane that surrounds the lung and lines the inside of the chest cavity. It has two layers: parietal (adjacent to the chest wall) and visceral (adjacent to the lung). These two layers essentially adhere to each other, with the pleural space between them normally containing only a tiny amount of low-protein fluid. A pleural effusion is said to be present when there is an accumulation of fluid in this pleural space.

ETIOLOGY

An accumulation of fluid in the pleural space is caused by an imbalance between fluid production and resorption. The resorptive capacity of the pleural drainage system is large; hence, most often pleural effusions represent overproduction. This overproduction may be caused by two pathogenetic mechanisms.

First, systemic factors alter hydrostatic or oncotic pressures without altering the pleural permeability; the pleura are intrinsically normal. Such effusions are called *transudative* effusions. The most common causes of transudative effusions are left-sided heart failure, cirrhosis, and the nephrotic syndrome. Treatment of the underlying cause in turns treats the pleural effusion.

Second, factors (inflammation, infection, or invasion by malignant cells) lead to an increased production of pleural fluid by increasing the permeability of the pleura; the pleura are intrinsically abnormal. These effusions are called *exudative* effusions. The most common causes are malignancy (metastatic to the pleural space, such as lung cancer), tuberculosis (tuberculous pleuritis), parapneumonic effusion (an effusion ipsilateral to pneumonia), collagen vascular diseases (such as rheumatoid arthritis), and pancreatitis. These factors cause intrinsic damage to the pleura, resulting in the formation of a pleural effusion.

The increased permeability of the pleura in exudative effusions leads to the presence of large molecules like proteins in the pleural fluid. Markers of inflammation are usually present in higher concentrations in exudative effusions compared to a transudate. Common causes of exudative and transudative effusions are listed in Table 38.1.

CLINICAL MANIFESTATIONS

The symptoms associated with pleural effusions are those of the underlying process. If pleural inflammation is the cause, then pleuritic chest pain (chest pain worse on deep inspiration) may be present. A mid- to large-sized pleural effusion can cause dyspnea by displacing lung tissue, leading to atelectasis and ventilation-perfusion mismatch.

On chest examination, pleural effusion is characterized by dullness to percussion and decreased breath sounds to auscultation within the area of dullness. On occasion, bronchial breath sounds can

TABLE 38.1 Common causes of pleural effusion by type

Type of effusion[a]	Most common causes
Transudative (caused by abnormalities of oncotic or hydrostatic forces with a normal pleura)	Congestive heart failure Nephrotic syndrome Cirrhosis with ascites (movement of ascites into the pleural space)
Exudative (caused by intrinsic damage to the pleura with alterations in pleural permeability)	Pneumonia Cancer (malignant effusion) Pulmonary embolism Tuberculosis Pancreatitis

[a]Based on measurement of lactate dehydrogenase and total protein or serum and pleural fluid.

be heard just above the effusion when atelectasis is present. Lung examination findings differentiating plural effusion from pneumothorax are listed in Table 38.2.

DIAGNOSIS

Pleural effusion is in most cases detected using a posterior-anterior (PA) and lateral chest x-ray. Pleural fluid is radiodense and usually accumulates at the most dependent part of the thoracic cavity, causing blunting of the costophrenic angle and formation of a meniscus.

A lateral decubitus chest x-ray (with the side of the pleural effusion down or dependent) is helpful to check if fluid is free flowing or restricted to certain areas of the pleural space by loculations and to more adequately visualize the underlying lung parenchyma. Transudates tend to be free flowing. A chest computed tomography scan can further characterize the effusion and visualize associated abnormalities, such as a lung mass or adenopathy in the chest.

Pleural fluid analysis is the cornerstone of diagnosing the cause of a pleural effusion. In the setting of frank congestive heart failure, watching for the resolution of an effusion with treatment of heart failure can suffice. However, if the cause of a pleural effusion is unknown, a thoracentesis is indicated to characterize the effusion.

Thoracocentesis

Characterization of the pleural fluid as a transudate or an exudate is an important step in diagnosis. This requires removal of a sample of pleural fluid by thoracentesis, performed percutaneously using

TABLE 38.2 Lung examination findings in pleural effusion, pneumonia, and pneumothorax

Diagnosis	Percussion	Breath sounds	Vocal fremitus
Pleural effusion	Stony dull	Decreased	Decreased
Pneumonia	Dull	Bronchial	Increased
Pneumothorax	Resonant	Decreased	Decreased

TABLE 38.3 Diagnostic pleural fluid values suggestive of specific disorders

Test	Utility
Glucose	Low glucose in parapneumonic effusion may indicate need for drainage. Low glucose is also present in malignancy and rheumatoid arthritis.
pH	Low pH (<7.10) in parapneumonic effusions may indicate need for drainage; low pH may also indicate esophageal rupture.
Cytology	Useful for identifying tumor cells.
Gram stain	Correlates well with the organism causing the pneumonia. If positive, the effusion needs drainage.
Culture	Positive culture correlates with organism infecting the pleural space and the associated pneumonia; requires chest tube drainage.
Pus	Gross pus on pleural fluid exam indicates need for chest tube drainage.
Amylase	High levels suggest malignancy, esophageal rupture, or pancreatitis.

a local anesthetic. Differentiation of a transudate from an exudate is based on Light's criteria, which require simultaneous measurement of lactate dehydrogenase (LDH) and total protein from the serum and pleural effusion. If any of the three criteria are present, then the pleural fluid is an exudate:

1. Ratio of pleural fluid to serum protein >0.5
2. Ratio of pleural fluid to serum LDH >0.6
3. Pleural fluid LDH level more than two thirds the upper limit of normal for serum

A transudate is said to be present when none of these criteria are met.

Transudates require no further analysis of the pleural fluid and treatment of the underlying cause (i.e., heart failure). Further testing on the pleural fluid is indicated if an exudate is detected. The exact battery of tests to be ordered depends on the clinical scenario thought to be causing the exudative effusion. Table 38.3 lists examples of the tests that can be ordered and their utility.

If the cause of an exudative effusion remains unclear, consideration should be given to tests such as thoracoscopy, needle biopsy of the pleura, or open pleural biopsy.

THERAPY

Treatment of transudative pleural effusions is directed at the underlying cause of the effusion, usually congestive heart failure or cirrhosis. With control of these underlying conditions, the effusion will usually diminish in size or completely resolve.

Treatment of exudative effusions is usually more complex and specific to the cause of the exudate. A few need special mention.

A pleural effusion ipsilateral to pneumonia is termed a *parapneumonic effusion*. *Uncomplicated* parapneumonic effusions are free-flowing pleural effusions associated with a pneumonia not requiring chest tube drainage and treated with antibiotics alone. These effusions are exudates but do not require drainage; rather continued treatment of the underlying pneumonia and observation by chest radiograph to assure resolution is indicated.

Complicated parapneumonic effusions are caused by intense inflammation in the pleural space. They are characterized by any of the following: a pleural fluid appearance of gross pus (empyema), pH <7.20, organisms on culture or Gram stain, a pleural fluid glucose <60 mg/dL or LDH >1,000 U/L. These effusions typically do not respond well to antibiotics alone and may require chest tube or open surgical drainage. *Malignant effusions* (caused by direct invasion of the pleural space by malignant cells) can be the initial presentation of a malignancy and are usually diagnosed by pleural fluid cytology, which shows malignant cells. Treatment options are typically limited and prognosis is poor.

Tuberculosis pleuritis is characterized by a lymphocyte-predominant exudative effusion; diagnosis is made by pleural fluid cultures and acid fast bacilli (AFB) smears along with percutaneous pleural biopsy sent for culture and AFB stain. When done together, these tests typically make the diagnosis in about 90% of cases. Pleural fluid analysis alone has a very low likelihood of making a diagnosis. *Pulmonary embolism* is associated with the development of pleural effusions, which are usually exudated; consideration should always be given to pulmonary embolism if the cause of an effusion is not clear, particularly in a patient at risk for pulmonary embolism.

CHAPTER 39

Pneumothorax

Siddhartha Singh

A pneumothorax is the presence of gas in the pleural space and is classified as spontaneous, traumatic, or iatrogenic (Fig. 39.1). Primary spontaneous pneumothorax occurs in persons without clinically known lung disease—most commonly in young, tall men—and is unrelated to trauma or any precipitating factor. Secondary spontaneous pneumothorax is a complication of pre-existing lung disease such as emphysema with rupture of a bleb into the pleural space. Iatrogenic pneumothorax results from a complication of a diagnostic or therapeutic intervention, typically a thoracentesis. Traumatic pneumothorax is most commonly caused by penetrating or blunt trauma to the chest, with air entering the pleural space from the atmosphere through the chest wall. A tension pneumothorax is usually associated with positive pressure mechanical ventilation and causes the progressive accumulation of air in the pleural space, culminating in compression of mediastinal structures and cardiovascular collapse.

ETIOLOGY

The pleural space usually contains a small amount of fluid and no gas. This space is at a negative pressure as compared with the atmospheric pressure and the pressure in the alveoli. Any connection between the pleural space and the atmosphere (penetrating trauma) or the underlying lung (rupture of a bleb) will lead to air being sucked into the pleural space. This gas in the pleural space causes lung collapse and shortness of breath, and is associated with impaired gas exchange. In individuals with compromised lung function, a pneumothorax can causes life-threatening hypoxemia. A tension pneumothorax is usually associated with diminished venous return and hypotension due to distortion and pressure on the vena cava.

CLINICAL MANIFESTATIONS

Virtually all individuals with a pneumothorax present with ipsilateral pleuritic chest pain or the onset of acute dyspnea. Chest pain ranges from minimal to severe and, at onset, can be described as "sharp" and later as a "steady ache." Tachycardia is a common physical finding. In patients with a larger pneumothorax (usually defined as ≥15% of the hemithorax), the findings on examination may include decreased movement of the chest wall, a hyperresonant percussion note, diminished fremitus, and decreased or absent breath sounds on the affected side.

EVALUATION

Any patient with sudden onset of shortness of breath should be evaluated for pneumothorax by a chest radiograph to assess the possibility of a pneumothorax. On the chest x-ray, gas in the pleural

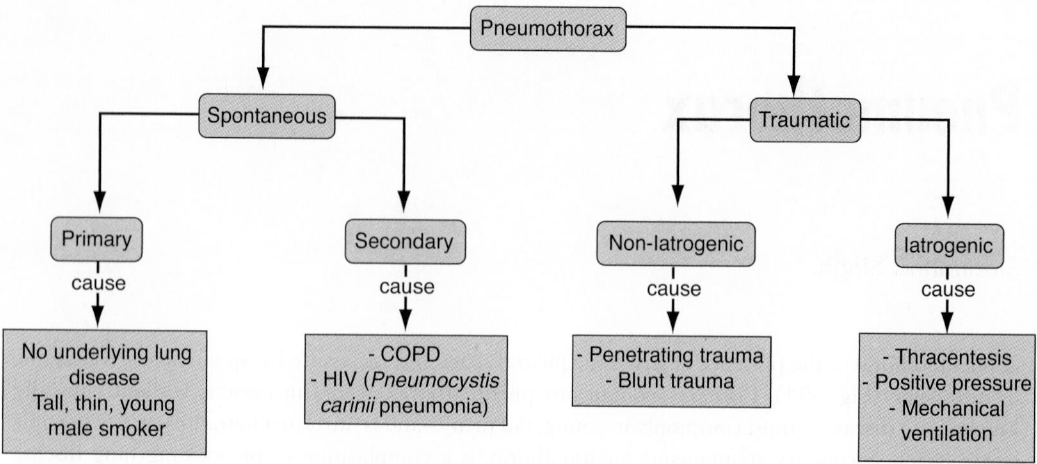

Figure 39.1 • Differential diagnosis of pneumothorax.

space is radiolucent and causes separation of the visceral pleura from the chest wall. This intervening area is free of lung or vascular markings. An outwardly convex white visceral pleural line is visible along the lung margin. A bulla may mimic a pneumothorax but it is concave toward the chest wall and completely surrounded by visceral pleura. A skinfold mimics the visceral pleural line but is usually seen crossing the chest cavity. A computed tomography scan of the chest may be required to definitively differentiate a bulla from a pneumothorax.

Arterial blood gas measurement is useful to assess the degree of hypoxia and any ventilatory compromise. The results typically indicate an increase in the alveolar–arterial oxygen gradient and acute respiratory alkalosis.

TREATMENT

The goals of treating a pneumothorax are to remove of the air from the pleural space and prevent recurrence of pneumothorax. Options to remove the pleural air include: (a) observation alone with administration of supplemental oxygen to hasten reabsorption of the pneumothorax, (b) aspiration of the area with a catheter that is then immediately removed, and (c) insertion of a chest tube attached to a water-seal device followed by hospitalization (Fig. 39.2). Generally, chest tube insertion is required for a large primary spontaneous pneumothorax or a secondary spontaneous pneumothorax. Complications of chest-tube drainage include pain, the introduction of skin flora into the pleural space resulting in infection, incorrect placement of the chest tube, and hemorrhage into the pleural space.

Intervention to prevent recurrence is often required in patients with a secondary spontaneous pneumothorax because these patients often have limited cardiopulmonary reserve. Also, patients with more than one primary spontaneous pneumothorax or a persistent pneumothorax complicating the initial episode should be considered for interventions aimed at preventing recurrence. This is commonly done by *pleurodesis*, a procedure consisting of instillation of a sclerosing agent into the pleural space through a chest tube to cause adherence of the visceral and parietal pleura. In the presence of ruptured bullae, thoracoscopy or surgery may be required to resect the bullae in order to prevent recurrences.

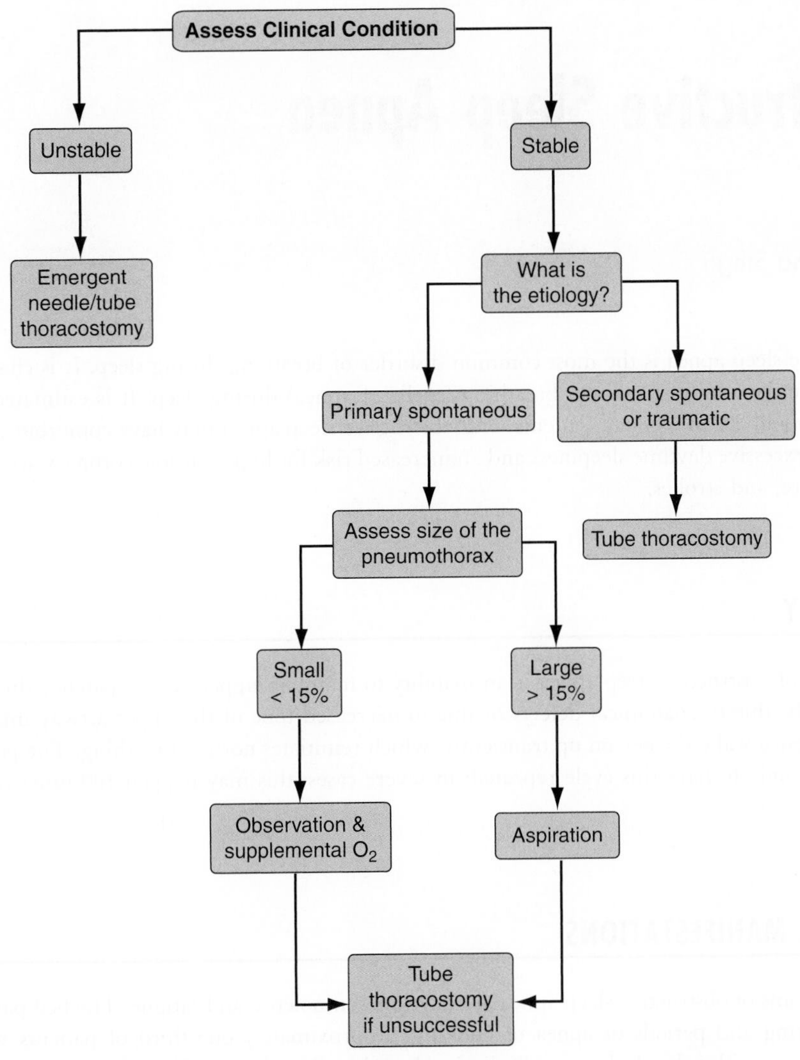

Figure 39.2 • Assessment and management of pneumothorax.

COMPLICATIONS

Tension pneumothorax (TP) may occur in patients on mechanical ventilation or as a complication of a spontaneous pneumothorax. It is a medical emergency and a high clinical suspicion is important because often there is often no time to obtain a chest radiograph to confirm the diagnosis. Patients present with tachycardia, hypotension, jugular venous distension, and absent breath sounds in the affected hemithorax.

In a patient suspected of having a TP, a large needle should be inserted immediately in the second intercostal space of the affected pleural space. A tube thoracostomy should be then immediately performed.

CHAPTER 40

Obstructive Sleep Apnea

Siddhartha Singh

Obstructive sleep apnea is the most common disorder of breathing during sleep. It is characterized by multiple episodes of pauses in breathing (spells of apnea) during sleep. It is estimated to affect 4% of men and 2% of women. Patients with obstructive sleep apnea may have comorbid conditions, including excessive daytime sleepiness and an increased risk for hypertension, coronary artery disease, heart failure, and strokes.

ETIOLOGY

The cause of obstructive sleep apnea is an inability to maintain upper airway patency during sleep. This may be due to anatomical defects or due to decreased tone of the upper airway musculature. Spells of apnea wake the person up transiently, which reinitiates normal breathing. The person then falls asleep only to have this cycle repeated; in severe cases, this may happen 100 times in an hour of sleep.

CLINICAL MANIFESTATIONS

The symptoms of obstructive sleep apnea are daytime somnolence and fatigue. The bed partner may report snoring and periods of apnea or choking. Approximately one third of patients with sleep apnea awaken with a headache, usually lasting less than 30 minutes. There is higher incidence of motor vehicle accidents in patients suffering from obstructive sleep apnea.

On physical examination, the patients are usually obese, hypertensive, and have a large neck circumference. In severe cases, it is not uncommon for a patient to fall asleep during the examination. Inspection of the oropharynx can reveal an elongated soft palate, tonsillar hypertrophy, an enlarged tongue, or a poorly visualized posterior pharynx. Edema is common. Findings of pulmonary hypertension and cor pulmonale (right-sided heart failure) may be present in severe cases (Chapter 28) (Table 40.1).

DIAGNOSIS

Any patient suspected of suffering from obstructive sleep apnea should undergo a multichannel sleep study or polysomnography. Patients are monitored during sleep with an electroencephalogram, flow monitors over the airway, pulse oximetry, and chest wall monitors, which detect periods of apnea or hypopnea during sleep and determine the severity of apnea. These episodes of apnea expressed

TABLE 40.1 Signs and symptoms OSA
Signs of upper airway obstruction during sleep (snoring, gasping, witnessed apneas)
Insomnia
Daytime sleepiness
Obesity

per hour of sleep give us the apnea-hypopnea index (AHI). If the AHI is 5 or greater, a diagnosis of obstructive sleep apnea is made (Table 40.2).

TREATMENT

The decision to treat and the choice of treatment modality do not depend solely on the AHI. The threshold to treat is lower and the intensity of treatment is higher in patients who have severe daytime symptoms, who are at a high risk for motor vehicle accident, and those with significant comorbidities such as coronary artery disease.

Conservative treatment is acceptable for patients with mild daytime symptoms. It consists of advocating that the patients sleep on their side rather than back, weight loss, and avoiding the use of sedatives such as benzodiazepines and alcohol.

More severe cases often benefit from continuous positive airway pressure (CPAP), which involves the application of continuous positive pressure to the airways during sleep using a device (CPAP machine) that delivers positive airway pressure through a face mask or nasal pillows. This provides pneumatic splinting of the upper airways and prevents collapse and consequent obstruction and apnea. Polysomnography is usually performed with a patient fitted with CPAP in order to assess the benefits of CPAP in reducing the AHI.

Other treatment modalities may be used if CPAP is not tolerated or is ineffective. These consist of oral devices for mandibular or tongue repositioning during sleep and surgery such as uvulopalatopharyngoplasty, tonsillectomy, or tracheostomy. Tracheostomy is curative because it bypasses the airway obstruction. However, it is reserved for severe cases of obstructive sleep apnea that cannot be treated by more conservative measures.

TABLE 40.2 Differential diagnosis of obstructive sleep apnea
Poor sleep hygiene
Sleep deprivation
Narcolepsy
Periodic limb movement disorder, circadian rhythm disturbance

CHAPTER 41

Venous Thromboembolic Disease

Siddhartha Singh

Venous thromboembolism (VTE) is a disease process characterized by the formation of a blood clot in the venous system (deep venous thrombosis [DVT]) and the subsequent dislodgement (embolization) of the clot to the lungs by way of the pulmonary arteries (pulmonary embolism [PE]). PE and DVT are clinical representations of the same pathogenetic mechanism and share the same basic therapeutic approaches.

More than 500,000 patients are diagnosed with a VTE in the United States yearly and 200,000 patients die every year as a result of PE. The mortality of untreated VTE is high (30%), and it is a major preventable cause of death in hospitalized patients. Indeed, DVT prophylaxis is an important and often overlooked intervention.

ETIOLOGY

The initial event in VTE is the formation of a clot in the venous system. Clots most commonly form in the proximal deep veins of the lower extremity (iliofemoral venous system). Clots can also form in the distal veins of the lower extremity (calf and popliteal veins) and in 10% of cases can develop in the veins of the upper extremity (axillosubclavian veins). Virchow proposed a triad of local trauma, hypercoagulability, and venous stasis as causes of thrombosis; the triad holds true to this day. The risk factors for DVT are listed in Table 41.1. Upper extremity DVT has become an important complication of the placement of subclavian catheters.

The risk factors associated with PE are the same as that for the initial thrombotic event. Other than inadequate treatment of DVT, there is no known risk factor that predicts patients who will have embolization of the established thrombus. Most pulmonary emboli come from the deep venous system of the lower extremities, although upper extremity DVTs are as likely to embolize to the lungs as are lower extremity DVTs. Calf vein thrombi rarely embolize. Death due to PE is caused by the inability of the heart to overcome the resistance of a large clot obstructing the pulmonary arteries, resulting in acute right ventricular failure and death. PE can produce hypoxia and tachypnea through a complex interplay of physiological responses (shunt, V/Q mismatch, and an increase in dead space). The pleuritic chest pain sometimes associated with PE is due to pulmonary infarction and irritation of the visceral pleura. Only about 10% of PEs cause pulmonary infarction distal to the part of the lung supplied by the occluded pulmonary artery.

CLINICAL MANIFESTATIONS

VTE may present with clinical features of PE or DVT or both. The diagnosis of PE and DVT can be difficult as the physical examination and laboratory findings are very nonspecific and insensitive. It is important to recognize the clinical features that might predispose an individual to a DVT and

TABLE 41.1 Risk factors for thrombosis classified per Virchow's triad

Trauma to the veins
Central or femoral venous catheter placement
History of deep venous thrombosis or pulmonary embolism
Hypercoagulability
Cancer
Oral contraceptive use
Thrombophilia (inherited: factor V Leiden mutation)
Pregnancy
Stasis
Recent surgery (risk of DVT/PE varies by type of surgery)
Obesity
Congestive heart failure
Stroke
Varicose veins
Pregnancy
Long-distance travel with prolonged immobility
Miscellaneous
Hypertension
Cigarette smoking

subsequent PE (Table 41.1). Understanding these risk factors can help one develop a pretest probability of VTE and assess the need for further evaluation.

The presentation of a PE may range in severity from asymptomatic (occult PE) to sudden cardiac death from right ventricular failure. Most commonly, patients diagnosed with PE have symptoms that include dyspnea, pleuritic chest pain, cough, and hemoptysis (Table 41.2). On physical examination, the patient may have a fever, tachypnea, tachycardia, an S4, and loud P2 component of the second heart sound. Some patients can present with chronic, occult PE demonstrated by the insidious onset of right-sided heart failure.

A DVT presents as an acute to subacute onset of pain, swelling, and redness of an extremity, usually a lower extremity. On physical examination, the patient may have fever. The extremity may be found to be swollen, erythematous, tender, and warm. Homan's sign (pain on dorsiflexion of the foot) may be present.

DIAGNOSIS

History and physical examination are extremely important to establish the pretest likelihood of PE, which is essential to assess the need for further testing and their interpretation (Table 41.3).

Laboratory Tests

Routine laboratory tests are nonspecific and not very helpful. If pulmonary embolism is suspected, the initial diagnostic tests should be an arterial blood gas and a D-dimer. The classic blood gas pattern associated with PE is decreased PaO_2, decreased $PaCO_2$, and an increased alveolar to arterial

TABLE 41.2 Symptoms and signs of pulmonary embolism

Symptom/sign	Incidence (%)
Pleuritic pain	74
Dyspnea	85
Apprehension	59
Cough	53
Hemoptysis	30
Chest pain	14
Syncope	13
Tachypnea	92
Rales	58
Increased P_2	53
Tachycardia	44
Fever	43
Diaphoresis	33
Gallop	34
Phlebitis	32
Edema	24
Cyanosis	19

From Bell WR, Simon TL, DeMets DL. The clinical features of submassive and massive pulmonary emboli. *Am J Med* 1977;62:355–360, with permission.

TABLE 41.3 Estimating the pretest probability of pulmonary embolism

Criteria	Points
Clinical signs/symptoms for deep venous thrombosis (objectively measured leg swelling and pain on palpation in the deep vein region)	3.0
Heart rate >100/min	1.5
Immobilization (bedrest, except to access the bathroom for 3 or more consecutive days) or surgery in the previous 4 weeks	1.5
Previous objectively diagnosed deep venous thrombosis or pulmonary embolism	1.5
Hemoptysis	1.0
Malignancy (cancer under therapy or palliative care, or treatment stopped within the past 6 months)	1.0
Pulmonary embolism as likely or more likely than an alternative diagnosis (using clinical information, chest x-ray, and necessary blood tests)	3.0

Total score <2, low probability; 2 to 6, intermediate probability; >6, high probability.
Adapted from Wells PS, Anderson DR, Rodger M, et al. Excluding pulmonary embolism at the bedside without diagnostic imaging: management of patients with suspected pulmonary embolism presenting to the emergency department by using a simple clinical model and d-dimer. *Ann Intern Med* 2001;135:99, with permission.

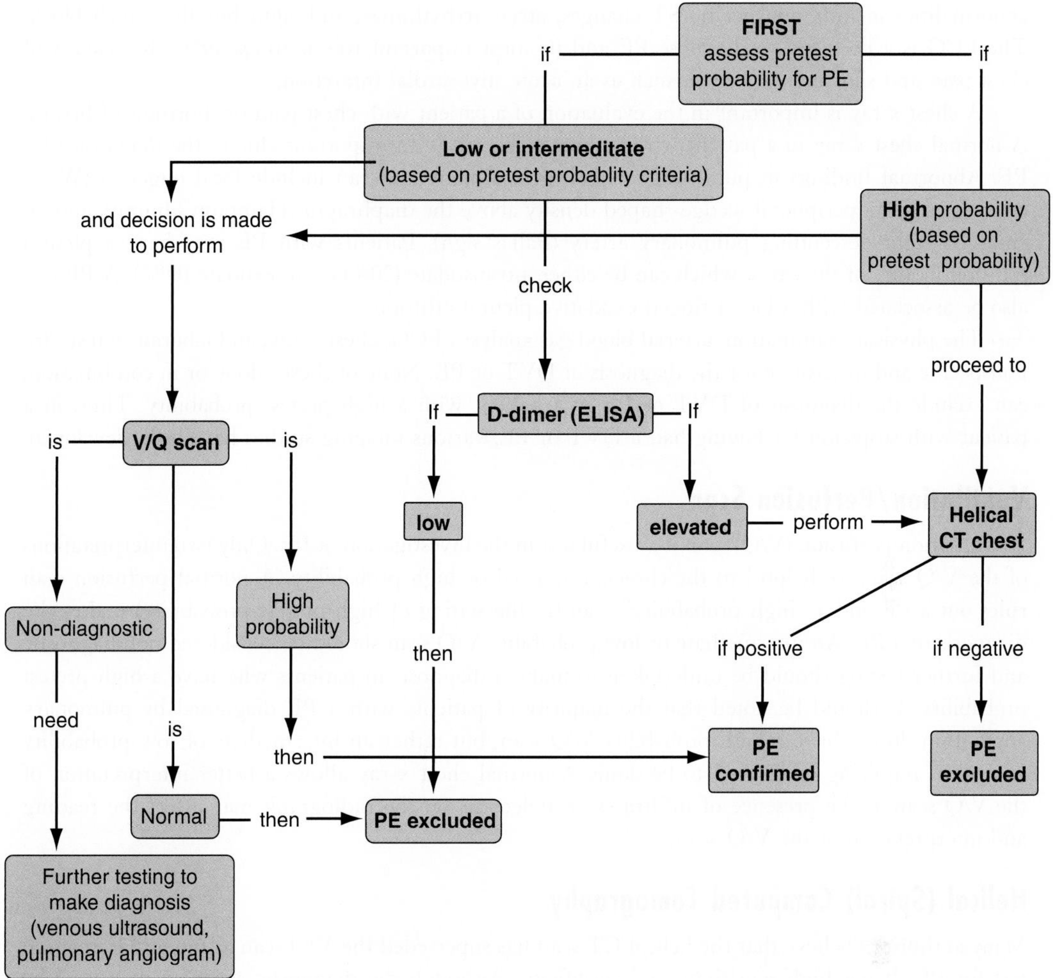

Figure 41.1 • Diagnostic approach to the diagnosis of patients with suspected pulmonary embolism.

gradient (A-a gradient). However, this pattern is seen in a variety of conditions other than PE (panic attacks, infection) and hypoxemia may not be present in 10% to 15% of PE cases.

D-dimer

The D-dimer is an important blood assay in the workup of a suspected DVT or PE. Because a negative D-dimer assay has a high negative predictive value for VTE, in the setting of low clinical suspicion or pretest probability it may exclude the diagnosis of VTE or PE. However, more recently it was found that in patients with low or intermediate probability for PE and a D-dimer ≥500 μg/L (elevated), PE was diagnosed by helical computed tomography (CT) in about 25% of cases (Fig. 41.1)

Electrocardiogram and Chest Radiograph

On electrocardiogram (ECG), the most common abnormality detected is sinus tachycardia. The classic pattern is an S wave in lead I and a Q wave in lead III, but this is uncommon. Other abnormalities include nonspecific ST changes, atrial arrhythmias, and right bundle branch block. The ECG is a poor test to diagnose PE and its most important role is to exclude other causes of chest pain and shortness of breath such as an acute myocardial infarction.

A chest x-ray is important in the evaluation of a patient with chest pain or shortness of breath. A normal chest x-ray in a patient who is short of breath is an important clue to the diagnosis of a PE. Abnormal findings in pulmonary embolism are many and can include focal oligemia (Westermark's sign), a peripheral wedge-shaped density above the diaphragm (Hampton's hump), and an enlarged right descending pulmonary artery (Pallas sign). Patients with PE may have a pleural effusion in 40% of the cases, which can be either a transudate (20%) or an exudate (80%). A PE can also be associated with a blood-tinged exudative pleural effusion.

The physical examination, arterial blood gas analysis, ECG, chest x-ray, and laboratory tests are nonspecific and insensitive for the diagnosis of DVT or PE. None of these, alone or in combination, can exclude the diagnosis of DVT or PE in a patient with a high pretest probability. Thus, in a patient with suspicion for having had a DVT or PE, various imaging studies have been developed.

Ventilation/Perfusion Scan

A ventilation/perfusion (V/Q) scan is a useful test in the investigation of PE. Only two interpretations of the V/Q scan are helpful to the clinician: normal or high probability. A normal perfusion scan rules out a PE and a "high probability" scan (in the setting of high pretest probability) makes the diagnosis of a PE. An intermediate or low probability V/Q scan should be considered nondiagnostic and further testing should be undertaken to make a diagnosis in patients who have a high pretest probability. It should be noted that the majority of patients with a PE diagnosed by pulmonary angiogram do not have a high probability V/Q scan, but rather an intermediate or low probability scan, thus requiring other tests to be done. A normal chest x-ray allows a better interpretation of the V/Q scan as the presence of infiltrates or atelectasis on the radiograph may affect the reading and interpretation of the V/Q scan.

Helical (Spiral) Computed Tomography

Many authorities believe that the helical CT scan has superseded the V/Q scan as the initial imaging test for PE. It has high sensitivity and specificity. Although the diagnostic accuracy may vary by hospital and reader's expertise, helical CT has a particularly high specificity in the setting of a high or intermediate clinical suspicion (96% and 92%, respectively). Thus assessment of the clinical suspicion is extremely important because it may increase the accuracy (sensitivity, specificity, and predictive value) of the test. It has the advantages of being quick, having the ability to evaluate the pulmonary parenchyma in addition to the pulmonary vasculature, and it can assess for DVT of the lower extremities. It has the disadvantages of requiring significant radiocontrast dye exposure and a significant dose of radiation.

Pulmonary Angiogram and Magnetic Resonance Angiography

Pulmonary angiogram has long been considered the definitive diagnostic test for PE. This may not be true for long as rapid advances in helical CT scanning are poised to make the helical CT equally effective at diagnosing PE without the mechanical risks of central vein catheterization.

Risks may include reaction to contrast, respiratory failure, or cardiac arrhythmia (such as complete heart block in patients with pre-existing right bundle branch block).

At present, magnetic resonance angiography is not a part of the usual battery of tests for PE, but with further technological advances may become a useful test. It has the potential advantage of avoiding nephrotoxic radiocontrast exposure. Magnetic resonance imaging is an excellent test to diagnose lower extremity DVT.

Lower Extremity Venous Ultrasound

In patients with clinical features of DVT, lower extremity compression ultrasonography (DUS) of the deep venous system should be considered a first-line imaging test. DUS is noninvasive and simple to perform. When proximal DVT is suspected, DUS has a 97% positive predictive value and a 98% negative predictive value. In patients with a suspected PE, the diagnosis of DVT by DUS can negate the need for further invasive testing (such as helical CT) because the treatment of DVT and PE is the same. Nonetheless, the absence of DVT does not rule out PE; in about 50% of patients, the entire DVT will have embolized. In the setting of clinical suspicion, a normal DUS must be followed-up by further testing to exclude the possibility of PE.

Echocardiogram

An echocardiogram may aid in the diagnosis of PE, especially massive PE. A pattern of regional right ventricular dysfunction or failure can suggest a massive PE. Some experts contend that an echocardiography can identify patients that may benefit from thrombolytic therapy. However, the use of echocardiography in the diagnosis of PE remains limited.

A number of multimodality algorithms are available based on the above principles and can be used to guide the diagnostic work-up of PE (Fig. 41.1).

Once the diagnosis of a VTE is confirmed in a patient with no obvious precipitating risk factors, the presence of a hypercoagulable state should be considered. The evaluation should include factor V Leiden mutation (the most common hypercoagulable state), homocysteine levels, and antiphospholipid antibodies. Protein C, protein S, and antithrombin 3 levels should not be part of the routine workup at the time of initial presentation because their levels are decreased in the acute thrombotic state and by therapy of VTE with anticoagulation.

TREATMENT

The mainstay of management DVT and PE is anticoagulation with heparin and warfarin unless there is a contraindication to such therapy. The use of anticoagulants is to prevent propagation of the DVT and to prevent further episodes of PE. The body's natural fibrinolytic system dissolves the DVT and PE. Initially patients should be treated with heparin (either unfractionated heparin or low molecular weight heparin [LMWH]). LMWH may be used for its ease of administration, lack of required monitoring, and lower rate of thrombocytopenia. Unfractionated intravenous heparin may be a better choice in patient with poor renal function or those who are obese. In such patients, LMWH cannot be accurately dosed without monitoring of levels. Warfarin is usually started on the day of starting heparin and can be used as the sole agent after 3 to 5 days of overlap with heparin and after the prothrombin time (expressed as the international normalized ratio) is within therapeutic range (2.0 to 3.0) for at least 24 hours. Increasingly, with the availability of low molecular weight heparins, the treatment of DVT and PE is as an outpatient in patients who are clinically stable.

The optimal duration of anticoagulation remains controversial. In general a shorter duration (3 to 6 months) of therapy should be considered in patients with a transient predisposing factor for PE, such as short-term immobility due to orthopedic surgery. Lifelong therapy is indicated for patients with nonmodifiable and persistent risk factors (e.g., antiphospholipid antibody syndrome).

In patients for whom anticoagulation is not feasible, an alternative is inferior vena cava interruption using a filter. These are not commonly employed because they induce stasis and a prothrombotic state, lack significant efficacy, and carry the risk of filter migrating through the vessel wall. The indications for insertion of a venacaval filters include: (a) short-term contraindication to anticoagulation, such as an immediate postsurgical state or concurrent hemorrhage; (b) recurrent DVT or PE

TABLE 41.4 Indications for inferior vena caval interruption
Recurrent pulmonary embolism despite adequate anticoagulation
Documented venous thromboembolism with any of the following: Contraindication to anticoagulation Necessity for premature discontinuation of anticoagulation
Chronic, recurrent pulmonary embolism in the setting of pulmonary hypertension and cor pulmonale
During pulmonary embolectomy
Septic pelvic thrombophlebitis
Paradoxical embolism
Residual, large, free-flowing ileofemoral thrombus in the setting of massive pulmonary embolism

while on anticoagulation; or (c) a patient with right-sided heart failure from an initial PE in whom the risk of a subsequent PE causing death is large (Table 41.4).

Systemic thrombolytic therapy may be lifesaving in patients with PE and acute right-sided heart failure resulting in cardiogenic shock. Thrombolytic agents include tissue plasminogen activator, streptokinase, and urokinase. Thrombolytic therapy has replaced thrombectomy (surgical embolectomy) in patients with life-threatening PE. However, the use of thrombolytic therapy has to be weighted against the risk of significant hemorrhage.

Prophylactic therapy for patients at risk for DVT and PE is an important consideration for all patients admitted to the hospital. Regimens consisting of subcutaneous standard heparin or LMWH are recommended. For patients that have a contraindication to heparin, the use of mechanical devices such as lower extremity sequential compression devices can be effective.

COMPLICATIONS

The most feared complication of DVT is sudden death from acute right-sided heart failure. Early diagnosis and initiation of anticoagulation therapy can decrease the risk of PE. Patients with occult, chronic PE can present with evidence of pulmonary arterial hypertension and chronic right-sided heart failure. DVT can result in the postphlebitic syndrome characterized by chronic venous stasis in the affected extremity.

CHAPTER 42

Asbestosis

Ralph Schapira

Pulmonary fibrosis caused by asbestos inhalation is called asbestosis. Asbestosis is one of several pleuropulmonary diseases caused by asbestos exposure (in addition to calcified and noncalcified pleural plaques, pleural effusion, rounded atelectasis, malignant mesothelioma, and bronchogenic carcinoma).

Asbestos describes a group of heat-resistant fibrous minerals. Chrysotile, crocidolite, amosite, and anthophyllite are four of the more important forms. Because asbestos has thousands of industrial uses, occupational asbestos exposure is common. Examples of professions potentially at risk include boiler makers, brake lining makers or workers, construction workers, dock workers, filter workers, insulation workers, gasket makers, pipe coverers or cutters, plumbers, rock miners, ship builders, and steam fitters. The use of asbestos has been banned in the United States because of the adverse health effects of exposure.

A latent period of 20 years or more usually follows exposure before clinical or x-ray manifestations appear. Because the development of asbestosis is dose dependent, this latent period may be shorter with more intense exposure.

ETIOLOGY

Chemoattractants are released when the inhaled asbestos activates both macrophages and dual complement pathways. Chemoattractants recruit neutrophils, which interact with asbestos to produce oxygen radicals (superoxide anion, hydrogen peroxide, and hydroxy radicals) that damage proteins and lipid membranes. Lipid peroxides may autocatalyze and perpetuate damage even without further asbestos exposure. Pathologic findings include both diffuse interstitial fibrosis and asbestos bodies (asbestos fibers coated with protein and iron). The respiratory bronchioles are thickened with connective tissue and fibrosis proceeds centrifugally.

Macrophages accumulate, but granuloma or nodules (similar to silicosis) are absent. In advanced asbestosis, extensive fibrosis causes airspace distortion and a honeycomb pattern with cystlike spaces.

CLINICAL MANIFESTATIONS

Dyspnea on exertion is the most common symptom, usually manifesting after 20 or more years of asbestos exposure. Cough, usually dry, may also be present. Tightness or pain in the chest may be reported, especially in advanced cases. Basilar rales and finger clubbing are the most important findings.

DIAGNOSIS

Pulmonary function testing shows a restrictive impairment, with reduced DL_{CO}; hypoxemia is present at rest or on exercise. Chest x-rays show interstitial, predominantly lower-zone infiltrates. Pleural thickening and hyaline pleural plaques may be present along the lateral chest wall and calcified pleural plaques may involve the pleura of the diaphragm. Hilar node enlargement or calcification is rare.

Diagnosis depends on obtaining a history of significant occupational exposure, clinical features, typical x-ray findings, and the restrictive abnormality. A clinical diagnosis is usually sufficient and lung biopsy is only occasionally needed. Both asbestos bodies and interstitial fibrosis, the hallmarks of asbestosis, are essential if a pathologic diagnosis is needed.

MANAGEMENT

No specific treatment exists for asbestosis. Asbestosis may progress even in the absence of continued exposure. Besides efforts directed at prevention (i.e., avoiding exposure to asbestos), prompt treatment of respiratory infections is necessary because infections may accelerate the fibrosis.

COMPLICATIONS

Complications of asbestosis are progressive fibrosis leading to cor pulmonale and respiratory failure. The risk of bronchogenic carcinoma of all cell types may be higher in persons exposed to asbestos in the absence of cigarette smoking. Clearly, asbestos-exposed smokers are at particularly higher risk, as smoking and asbestos are synergistic cocarcinogens.

CHAPTER 43

Tuberculosis

Kesavan Kutty

Over one third of the world's population is infected by *Mycobacterium tuberculosis*, the causative agent of tuberculosis. In United States, there were 14,517 cases (4.9 active cases per 100,000 persons) in 2004, most often afflicting racial and ethnic minorities (Asians, Native Hawaiians and other Pacific Islanders, non-Hispanic blacks, Hispanics, American Indians, and Alaskan natives, in that order) and foreign-born persons.

ETIOLOGY

Primary tuberculosis infection consists of the following sequence: infection with *M. tuberculosis (*ssp. *hominis, africanum, and bovis)* through droplets from an active case of pulmonary tuberculosis, phagocytosis by alveolar macrophages, bacterial replication, development of a silent pneumonitis, and associated lymphadenopathy (together called the primary [Ghon] focus), lymphohematogenous bacillary spread, and generation of secondary (Simon) foci. Both Ghon and Simon foci resolve and heal; the host's cell-mediated immunity kills most of the bacilli in these foci. These clinically silent events of the primary infection generally manifest only a positive tuberculin skin test (purified protein derivative [PPD]). After containment of initial infection by caseation, residual mycobacteria become dormant and linger in these foci (latent infection).

Simon foci involving upper lobes of the lung, growing ends of bones, and renal cortices might reactivate after some latency, or occasionally progress immediately. Most clinical tuberculosis cases follow such endogenous reactivation, in which host hypersensitivity to tuberculoprotein evokes tissue liquefaction, cavitation, and bacterial replication. However, exogenous reinfection can also produce disease. Almost 10% of infected patients will develop subsequent disease, 5% within 2 years of infection and another 5% in the years following. Many conditions enhance this risk (Table 43.1).

Reactivation tuberculosis primarily occurs in the lung (84%); a less common site is pleura (tuberculosis pleuritis). The resulting pleural effusion usually resolves spontaneously, but frank cavitary pulmonary tuberculosis develops in over 65% of patients within 2 years. A cavity might erode a blood vessel with resulting systemic hematogenous dissemination (military tuberculosis).

Tuberculosis and Human Immunodeficiency Virus Coinfection

Worldwide, a large proportion of newly diagnosed cases of tuberculosis has human immunodeficiency virus (HIV) coinfection, with one increasing the proliferation of the other. HIV coinfection strongly enhances risk of reactivation of latent tuberculosis infection. Persons with the dual infection have twice the mortality of persons with HIV alone. Often, HIV-positive patients with tuberculosis demonstrate little or no response (anergy) to tuberculin skin test. Granulomas form poorly and cavitation seldom occurs. Chest radiographs may be deceptively normal or minimally abnormal. However, the unfettered bacterial replication in these persons creates abundant bacilli in these persons, rendering them highly infectious.

TABLE 43.1 Tuberculosis: selected factors that favor development of active disease following latent infection
Age (extremes of age, childhood)
Race (see text)
Impaired integrity of the cellular immune mechanisms
Human immunodeficiency virus infection/acquired immune deficiency syndrome
Corticosteroid, cytotoxic or other immunosuppressive therapy (including therapy with anti-tumor necrosis factor [e.g., infliximab] agents)
End-stage renal disease
Malnutrition
Hematological and reticuloendothelial malignancies
Associated diseases
Diabetes mellitus
Silicosis
Prior gastrectomy
Infection with measles virus
Alcoholism/drug addiction
Being underweight (≥10% below ideal body weight)

CLINICAL MANIFESTATIONS

Primary tuberculosis, often asymptomatic, occurs most often in childhood and youth, and in about 15% of the elderly Americans. In all forms of tuberculosis, symptoms lag until the disease is moderately advanced. Weight loss, night sweats, and fever are general symptoms. Chest pain, cough, sputum, and hemoptysis (occasionally massive and life-threatening) are ascribed to pulmonary tuberculosis, which might mimic an acute bacterial pneumonia or cause catastrophic respiratory failure. An infrequent but deceptive presentation in the elderly is a chronic, unresolving, or slowly resolving pneumonia. Physical findings include fever and signs of inanition, and (in pulmonary tuberculosis), signs of cavitation, consolidation, and/or pleural effusion. Extrapulmonary tuberculosis often involves the kidneys, bones, and meninges. Fever (sometimes fever of unknown origin), weight loss, progressive respiratory insufficiency, and prostration characterize miliary tuberculosis; meningitis is frequent.

DIAGNOSIS

Anemia and hyponatremia are common. Abnormal liver function tests may signify hepatic involvement. Acid-fast stains of sputum may be positive, depending on the bacillary load and the extent of cavitation. The cerebrospinal fluid (CSF) in tuberculous meningitis is characteristically clear, with high protein and low glucose (about 45 mg/dL) and a high cell count that is neutrophilic initially and lymphocytic later. Although the organism may be detected in the CSF—especially through polymerase chain reaction (PCR)—associated pulmonary or other extracranial disease is key to suspecting tuberculous meningitis.

The slow growth of *M. tuberculosis* delays diagnosis. The BACTEC-TB system can detect mycobacterial growth in culture. Nucleic acid probes with PCR hasten detection and speciation of the organism. Nucleic acid tests cannot supplant traditional culture techniques because only the latter can provide drug susceptibility information.

Primary infection usually appears as a hazy, uncavitated, unilateral, peripheral, middle or lower lung infiltrate, with hilar lymphadenopathy. In reactivation tuberculosis, the infiltrates are generally bilateral, often symmetrical, and typically involve the apical and/or posterior segments of upper lobes. Cavitation and fibrosis are common, but hilar adenopathy is not. HIV coinfection often evokes atypical x-ray patterns. Most importantly, with HIV infection, no pulmonary infiltration might accompany pulmonary tuberculosis.

A tuberculin skin test (PPD), chest x-ray, and sputum acid-fast (AFB) smears should be done when pulmonary tuberculosis is suspected. PPD is positive in most cases (>85%) of active tuberculosis. A positive sputum smear does not necessarily mean tuberculosis, but suffices to initiate infection control (isolation) precautions and drug therapy if the clinical picture is compatible. When smears are negative, transbronchoscopic biopsy of the affected lung can rapidly and reliably provide a diagnosis, if caseating granulomas are seen. Bronchial brushing and lavage or transthoracic needle aspiration biopsy of pulmonary nodules may also provide material for microbiologic studies. Antimicrobial sensitivity testing should follow the identification of any positive cultures. Culture is positive in most (75%) cases. Extrapulmonary tuberculosis is diagnosed by processing pathologic material obtained from infected sites as described above.

TREATMENT

Isolation, mask, and negative flow ventilation help prevent droplet spread. Recent outbreaks of multidrug-resistant (MDR-TB, which is resistant to at least two first-line drugs) and extensive drug-resistant tuberculosis (XDR-TB, which is MDR-TB that is also resistant to at least three second-line drugs) have necessitated several initial drug regimens (Table 43.2). Baseline liver function studies are obtained before treatment. Treatment rapidly renders patients noninfectious, probably in about 2 weeks. Patients should be advised to avoid alcohol during treatment. Isoniazid (INH), rifampin (RFN), pyrazinamide (PZA), ethambutol (EMB), and streptomycin (SM), where available, are considered first-line drugs. Directly observed therapy is proven to ensure compliance. Common side effects of antituberculous drugs are abnormal liver tests, hepatitis (INH, RFN, PZA), peripheral neuropathy (INH), orange discoloration of secretions and urine (RFN), hyperuricemia (PZA), vestibular toxicity and nephrotoxicity (SM), and optic neuritis (EMB). INH is given with pyridoxine (50 mg daily) to prevent neurotoxicity. The same treatment principles underlie HIV coinfection, but a minimum of 9 months is needed. Immediate contacts should be identified and given PPD testing and, if positive, a chest x-ray examination; all are treated with INH and pyridoxine for latent tuberculosis infection. With positive PPD, therapy is given for 6 months; those with negative PPD are retested 3 months later and, if the PPD is unchanged, therapy is stopped. Indications for tuberculin skin testing and treatment of latent infections appear in Table 43.3.

When clinical suspicion of tuberculosis complicating HIV is high and the sputum AFB smear is positive, RNA or DNA probes for confirmation render no additional benefit. The same is true when clinical suspicion of tuberculosis is low and the sputum AFB smear is negative in a HIV-positive person. Concurrent therapy with rifampin and protease inhibitors and/or nonnucleoside reverse transcriptase inhibitors lead to subtherapeutic levels of these antiretroviral agents; these agents in turn inhibit metabolism of rifampin, leading to toxic levels of rifampin. Thus, rifampin is not used with these agents. Rifabutin, the alternative, can be used with these agents, except for ritonavir (unless dose is significantly reduced) and delavirdine.

TABLE 43.2 Treatment regimens for active tuberculosis, incorporating HIV status

Drug resistance	HIV status		Concurrent antiretroviral therapy
	Negative	Positive	
None	INH, RFN, PZA, and EMB for 2 months; then INH and RFN for 4 months	INH, RFN, PZA, and EMB for 2 months; then INH and RFN for 7 months **OR** INH, PZA, and EMB for 2 months; then INH and RFBN for 7 months	No PI or NNRTI with RFN. RFBN may be used with indinavir or nelfinavir but not with saquinavir, ritonavir, or NNRTIs
Isoniazid	RFN, PZA, and EMB for 6 months	RFN, PZA, and EMB for 9 months **OR** PZA, EMB, and RFBN for 9 months	No PI or NNRTI with RFN RFBN may be used with indinavir or nelfinavir but not with saquinavir, ritonavir, or NNRTIs
Rifampin	INH, PZA, and EMB for 18 to 24 months	INH, PZA, and EMB for 18 to 24 months **OR**	All may be used
		INH, PZA, SM, and EMB for 2 months; then INH, PZA, and SM for 7 to 10 months	All may be used

Adapted from Havlir DV, Barnes PF. *N Engl J Med* 1999;340:369; Bass JB Jr., Farer LS, Hopewell PC, et al. Treatment of tuberculosis and tuberculosis infection in adults and children. *Am J Respir Crit Care Med* 1994;149:1359–1374; and *MMWR Morb Mortal Wkly Rep* October 30, 1998;47:1–57, with permission.
EMB, ethambutol; INH, isoniazid; NNRTI, nonnucleoside reverse transcriptase inhibitors; PI, protease inhibitors; PZA, pyrazinamide; RFBN, rifabutin; RFN, rifampin; SM, streptomycin.

Targeted tuberculin skin testing using PPD, correct interpretation of the PPD skin test, and administration of pharmacological therapy to treat latent tuberculosis infection (LTBI) are the key public health efforts to decrease the incidence of active tuberculosis. LTBI HIV-infected persons is treated with daily or twice-weekly INH and pyridoxine for 9 months, or by daily PZA and RFN for 2 months. An emerging diagnostic serological assay that detects interferon-gamma producing T cells is being actively studied and may complement or replace PPD skin testing in the future. Until that time, the PPD skin test is the best available screening test for LTBI.

TABLE 43.3 Indications for tuberculin (PPD) skin testing

1. Suspected active tuberculosis
2. Targeted tuberculin testing[a]
   a. Close contacts (within 1 to 2 years) of active cases
   b. Associated medical or other conditions that increase risk of tuberculosis (human immunodeficiency virus, silicosis, chronic renal failure, diabetes mellitus, or persons significantly underweight ≥5%, immunosuppression [daily prednisone dose of 20 mg or more] or solid organ transplantation, injection drug users, cancer of head or neck, homeless persons, long-term institutional residence [nursing home, prisons, psychiatric institutions]
   c. Persons whose chest radiographs are consistent with prior tuberculosis
   d. Health care workers with high risk of infection
   e. Recent immigrants from countries with a high prevalence of tuberculosis

[a]PPD testing aims to detect latent tuberculosis infection. It is targeted to persons at high risk for latent tuberculosis infection or high risk to develop active disease. Latent tuberculosis infection indicated by a positive skin test is treated regardless of age if risk factors exist such as HIV infection, close contacts, skin test conversion within a 2-year period, chest radiographs consistent with prior tuberculosis, intravenous drug use, or predisposing medical conditions as indicated above. Otherwise, treatment should be considered for those with a positive skin test only if less than 35 years of age. (See *Am J Resp Crit Care Med* 2000;161(Suppl):S221–S247 for details.)
PPD, purified protein derivative.

CHAPTER 44

Sarcoidosis

Linus Santo Tomas

Sarcoidosis is a systemic disease of unknown etiology. Its essential features are a compatible clinical picture along with noncaseating epithelioid cell granulomas in several affected organs and tissues that either resolve or become featureless hyaline connective tissue. Ninety percent of the patients with sarcoidosis are between 20 and 40 years of age with a higher prevalence in the United States among African Americans and women. The predilection for race, certain human leukocyte antigen types, and family clustering indicates a genetic basis.

ETIOLOGY

The noncaseating granuloma, which is a reaction against an unidentified antigenic stimulus, contains epithelioid cells, giant cells, lymphocytes, and plasma cells with variable fibrosis and hyalinization. The CD_4 T-cells are increased in all affected tissues and decreased in the peripheral blood, which indicates their redistribution. Mononuclear phagocytes, epithelioid cells, and giant cells are transformed monocytes, which are attracted into the lung by monocyte chemotaxis, initiated by sarcoid lung T-lymphocytes. Proliferation of all these cells perpetuates the granuloma.

CLINICAL FEATURES

Sarcoidosis is often detected incidentally by an abnormal chest x-ray, obtained generally while evaluating another illness or, less commonly, during a pre-employment physical examination. Symptoms of sarcoidosis arise from the granulomatous involvement of various organs. The lungs are affected in more than 90% of patients with sarcoidosis; thus, pulmonary symptoms predominate. Cough is generally dry; sputum and hemoptysis are infrequent. Physical examination findings of rales over the lung fields and clubbing of fingers are rarely noted.

Extrapulmonary involvement is suggested by signs and symptoms of respective organ dysfunction (Table 44.1).

DIAGNOSIS

A chest radiograph should always be performed. The chest radiograph patterns of sarcoidosis are shown in Table 44.2. Differentiation is mainly from lymphomas and other causes of mediastinal adenopathy such as mycobacterial and fungal infections, toxoplasmosis, berylliosis, and metastatic renal cell carcinoma.

Tissue confirmation is recommended in all cases. Transbronchoscopic lung biopsy is the recommended initial procedure. It is a simple, safe, low-morbidity procedure with a high diagnostic yield.

TABLE 44.1 Extrapulmonary manifestations of sarcoidosis

Dermatological (20%)
Erythema nodosum Pyoderma gangrenosum Subcutaneous nodules Lupus pernio
Opthalmologic (20%)
Anterior or posterior uveitis Keratoconjunctivis Cardiac (10%) Cardiomyopathy Conduction abnormalities (complete heart block)
Musculoskeletal (5% to 10%)
Acute polyarthritis or chronic arthritis
Metabolic/renal
Hypercalcemia (15%) with hypercalciuria (50%) Nephrocalcinosis
Systemic
Generalized lymphadenopathy (35% to 40%) Hepatomegaly
Central nervous system (1% to 5%)
Facial palsy Central diabetes insipidus (hypernatremia) Basilar meningitis

TABLE 44.2 Chest radiograph classification and prognosis

Stage	Radiographic findings	Spontaneous remission rate
0	Normal	
I	Bilateral hilar lymphadenopathy	55% to 90%
II	Bilateral hilar lymphadenopathy with pulmonary infiltrates	40% to 70%
III	Pulmonary infiltrates without bilateral hilar lymphadenopathy	10% to 20%
IV	Pulmonary fibrosis	None

The yield depends on the stage of the disease and the experience of the operator; it is more than 90% in stage 2 and 3 disease when at least four lung biopsies are done. Even in stage 1 disease, the yield is good (40% to 90%), reflecting microscopic lung involvement despite normal lung fields on chest x-ray.

Other possible biopsy sites are skin or palpable lymph nodes. Biopsy of erythema nodosum is not recommended as they do not show granulomas. Liver biopsy is not indicated even in the presence of hepatomegaly and abnormal liver function tests. Mediastinoscopy may be needed in some instances when bronchoscopic biopsy is nondiagnostic. Thoracoscopic or open lung biopsy is seldom indicated.

Laboratory Features

Laboratory testing is not useful in the diagnostic evaluation of sarcoid; however, there are a number of characteristic laboratory findings. Cutaneous anergy and leukopenia reflect T-cell kinetics, and serum immunoglobulins rise due to the B-cell overactivity. Hypercalcemia is from calcitriol (1,25 dihydroxycholecalciferol), one of the many biologically active agents secreted by activated macrophages. Other important anomalies are hypercalciuria, hyperuricemia, elevated serum angiotensin-converting enzyme (ACE), and lysozyme. ACE is elevated in nearly 80% of sarcoidosis patients. Elevated ACE may be seen in many other diseases, but elevations greater than two times the upper limits of normal are less common and seen in tuberculosis, other granulomatous diseases, Gaucher's disease, and hyperthyroidism.

Management

Spontaneous resolution is so frequent in stage 1 that all that is needed is observation until resolution unless it transforms into another stage. Corticosteroids are the major drugs available for treatment of sarcoidosis. Vital organ involvement (e.g., eye, heart, kidney), hypercalcemia and disfiguring skin lesions, and progressive pulmonary disease (best indicated by worsening pulmonary function tests) are indications for corticosteroid treatment. Treatment with prednisone can be initiated at 20 to 40 mg daily or its equivalent on alternate days for 8 to 12 weeks. Higher doses of steroids should be considered with neurologic or cardiac involvement. If improvement follows or if worsening has been halted, then the dose is tapered by 5 to 10 mg every 8 to 12 weeks with clinical, physiologic, and x-ray monitoring. The minimum steroid dose needed to maintain the improvement is then given every other day. Therapy is discontinued after 2 years; observation is continued for possible relapse.

For patients with skin lesions, uveitis, and nasal polyps, topical corticosteroid may be used. Nonsteroidal anti-inflammatory drugs are useful in treating musculoskeletal pain and erythema nodosum. In selected patients, including those refractory to prednisone cytotoxic agents such as methotrexate, azathioprine and cyclophosphamide can be used. Chloroquine and hydroxychloroquine have also been used to treat pulmonary sarcoidosis, skin lesions, and hypercalcemia.

CHAPTER 45

The Solitary Pulmonary Nodule

Linus Santo Tomas

Solitary pulmonary nodule (SPN), a roentgenographic diagnosis, is a single, well-circumscribed (surrounded by aerated lung tissue), spherical pulmonary density. By convention, it is 3.0 cm or less in diameter (>3.0 cm in diameter are designated as "masses"). SPNs are not accompanied by chest x-ray evidence of atelectasis, pleural effusion, or hilar or mediastinal adenopathy. SPNs may be either calcified or uncalcified. Although many are benign, some SPNs represent a potentially curable stage of lung cancer. Thus, it is essential to estimate the probability of malignancy of an SPN in order to decide on an appropriate approach.

ETIOLOGY

A significant proportion of SPNs are malignant, from 10% to 68% depending on the series and patient population. Bronchogenic carcinoma tops the list of malignant SPNs. The incidence of bronchogenic cancer varies with advancing age and smoking history. The majority of benign SPNs are infectious granulomas of mycotic or mycobacterial etiology. Other benign causes include hamartomas, noninfectious inflammatory disease such as sarcoidosis and rheumatoid nodules, intrapulmonary lymph nodes, and even pulmonary infarcts.

DIAGNOSIS AND MANAGEMENT

Because lung cancer presenting as an SPN has a highly favorable prognosis (5-year survival rate of 50% to 80%), an organized and rapid approach to assessment and management of all SPNs is essential. "Watchful waiting" of a SPN in a patient with risk factors for lung cancer is unacceptable and a diagnostic evaluation in those patients must be undertaken immediately. Computed tomography (CT) imaging and the application of probabilistic reasoning (a high pretest probability of a lesion being benign or malignant) are important components of the decision-making process. The essentials in decision-making include a thorough clinical history, physical examination, and review of current and old roentgenograms. Age, history of smoking, presence of coexistent lung disease, and roentgenographic (CT if available) appearances of the nodule are important considerations. A SPN that has been stable on comparison with old chest radiographs for 2 years or more is highly unlikely to be malignant. Thus, an effort should always be made to obtain previous chest radiographs for comparison—potentially the easiest way to establish a benign diagnosis.

Nonsurgical aids to diagnosis include CT densitometry, positron-emission tomography (PET), transthoracic fine-needle aspiration biopsy (FNAB), and bronchoscopy. A *diffusely* calcified lesion or

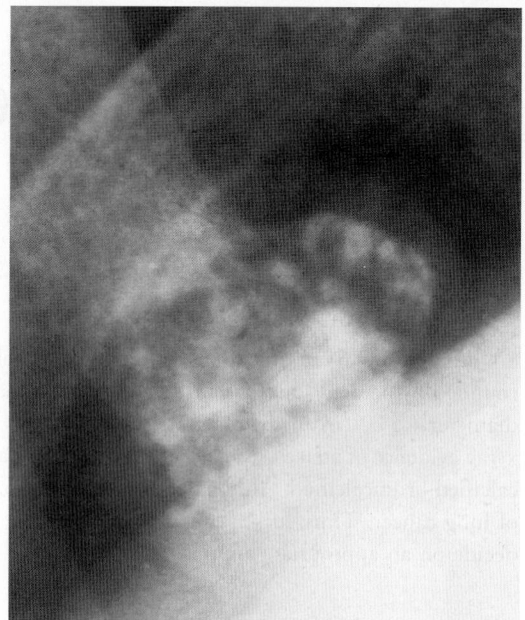

Figure 45.1 • Solitary pulmonary nodule: "popcorn" calcification in a benign long nodule.

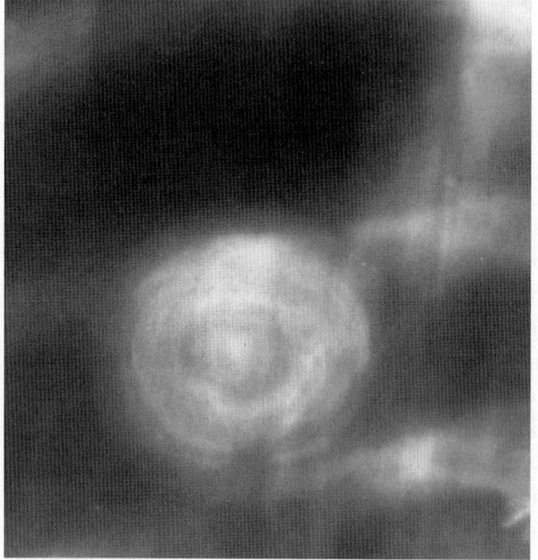

Figure 45.2 • Solitary pulmonary nodule: benign concentric calcification in a histoplasmoma.

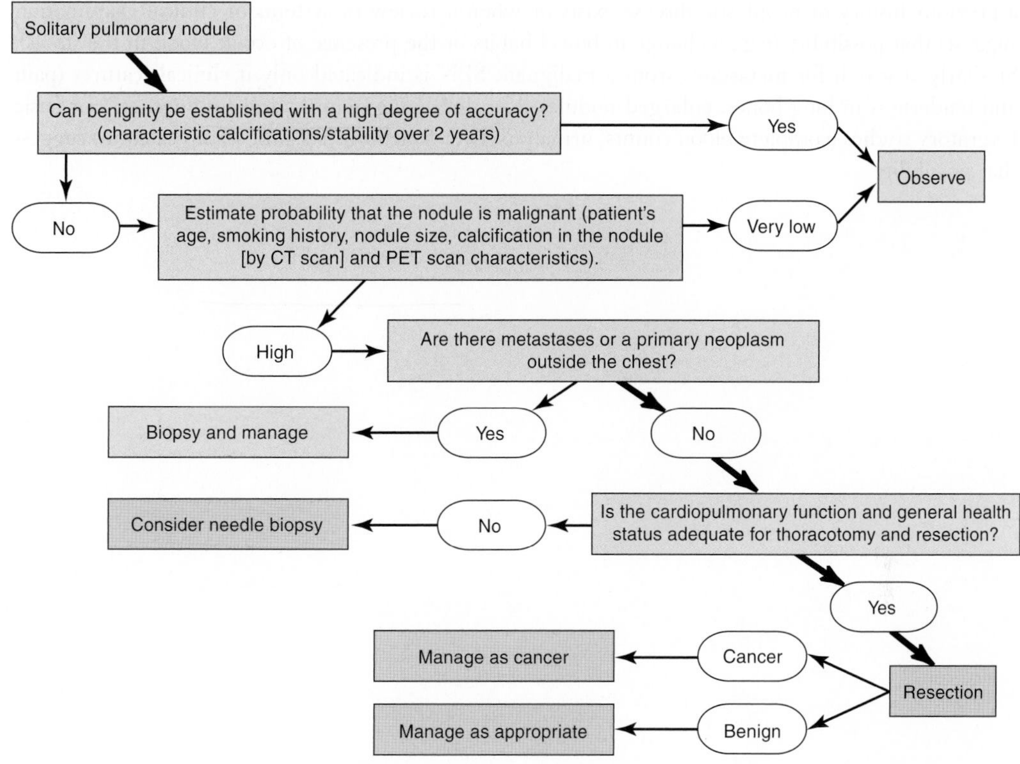

Figure 45.3 • Suggested approach to managing solitary pulmonary nodule.

a lesion that has a *specific* benign pattern of calcification (i.e., "onion skin" in the case of a histoplasmoma) is conclusive of a benign SPN. PET has up to 97% sensitivity but lower specificity for malignancy in lesions that are at least 1 cm in diameter. Bronchoscopic biopsy and brushings is of limited value in small and peripheral lesions, but may have better diagnostic yield (40% to 70%) for centrally located lesions that are 2 to 3 cm in diameter and have a bronchus leading to the SPN on CT imaging. FNAB of SPN yields a positive result for malignancy in up to 90% of the cases when the nodule is malignant. These results vary widely. However, the diagnosis of a specific benign disease is definitively made by FNAB much less frequently (30% to 40%) and unless a specific benign diagnosis is made, the SPN can not be assumed to be benign. FNAB is indicated when resection is not feasible and a preoperative diagnosis is essential. Other possible indications include a patient with borderline pulmonary function, in whom a definitive diagnosis of malignancy could lead to surgical resection.

Unless a specific benign lesion can be established with a high degree of accuracy, surgical resection of the SPN is indicated. Two generally accepted criteria of benignity are: (a) radiographic stability of the lesion, with no change in size for at least 2 years; and (b) characteristic patterns of calcification (usually requiring CT), which include "popcorn" (Fig. 45.1), concentric (Fig. 45.2), or central bull's-eye patterns. Younger age (<35 years) and an absence of smoking history also support a benign etiology. The management of SPN is outlined in Figure 45.3. Watchful waiting of a lesion that might be malignant is not acceptable medical practice. Video-assisted thoracoscopic surgery and open thoracotomy are utilized to make a definitive diagnosis and for complete resection.

The search for an extrapulmonary neoplasm producing a metastatic SPN is indicated only when a previous history of neoplastic disease exists or when a review of systems or clinical examination suggests that possibility (e.g., a change in bowel habits or the presence of occult blood in the stools). Similarly, a search for metastases from a malignant SPN is indicated only if clinical features (pain and tenderness in long bones, enlarged nodular liver, localizing neurological findings, etc.) or basic laboratory studies (complete blood counts, urinalysis, liver function tests, and serum calcium) suggest that possibility.

Rheumatology

Deidre Faust, Paul Halverson, and Steven Denson

CHAPTER 46

Osteoarthritis

Steven Denson and Paul Halverson

Osteoarthritis (OA), also known as degenerative joint disease (DJD), is the most common form of arthritis, appearing in the majority of people over the age of 60 years with either clinical or radiographic evidence of the disease. It is characterized by the slow, insidious, and progressive breakdown and fragmentation of articular cartilage.

ETIOLOGY

OA initially develops in joints where the cartilage has lost a significant amount of its glycosaminoglycan content. Gradually worsening fissures develop in the cartilage surface, with subsequent fragmentation and eventual total loss of cartilage, leaving bare bone. At the same time, underlying bone becomes sclerotic and abnormal bone growth develops at the margins of the joint (osteophyte formation). The result is an asymmetric loss of cartilage along the lines of greatest force within a joint, with findings of bare, dense, ivory-like bone where the joint cartilage used to be—a process called eburnation, or bone sclerosis.

There are two types of OA: primary and secondary. Primary OA has no clear etiology but is thought to have a genetic predisposition. It is diagnosed by exclusion of secondary OA causes. Secondary OA is linked to specific conditions known to cause damage to cartilage. Although the pathogenesis is not well understood, the commonly recognized risk factors include obesity (with involvement of the weightbearing joints); injury from trauma, prior inflammation, infection, or surgery involving the joint; repetitive trauma from work or sports; or other medical conditions such as metabolic (e.g., hemochromatosis) or congenital (e.g., epiphyseal disease, collagen gene mutations, or Perthes disease) illnesses (Table 46.1).

CLINICAL MANIFESTATIONS

The joints most commonly involved are the proximal and distal interphalangeal joints and the first carpometacarpal joints of the hands, the first metatarsophalangeal joints in the feet, the hips, knees, and apophyseal joints of the spine. Symptoms consist of the gradual onset of joint pain. Typically, pain occurs after use of the joint (relieved with rest) and after periods of prolonged inactivity (such as after sitting, a condition called "gelling"). Morning stiffness can occur and is usually less than 30 minutes duration. Involvement of the knees and spine is typically worsened with activity and improved with rest. Signs include bony enlargement, decreased range of motion, and coarse crepitus. Generally, there is minimal or no inflammation of the affected joints.

TABLE 46.1 Conditions predisposing to osteoarthritis
Mechanical trauma
Weightbearing joints in obese persons
Prior joint trauma
Excessive joint use (occupational)
Previous inflammatory arthritis
Congenital joint dysplasias
Avascular necrosis of bone
Metabolic diseases affecting cartilage
Hemochromatosis
Ochronosis
Calcium pyrophosphate crystal deposition
Neurologic disorders
Diminished pain perception

Classic examination findings include Heberden's nodes in the distal interphalangeal joints, or Bouchard's nodes of the proximal interphalangeal joints (Fig. 46.1). Other characteristic joint deformities in OA include squaring (shelf sign) of the first carpometacarpal joint, bunion (hallux valgus abduction of the great toe relative to medial deviation of the first metatarsophalangeal joint), bow legs (genu varus of the medial), and knock knees (genu valgus of the lateral) in the

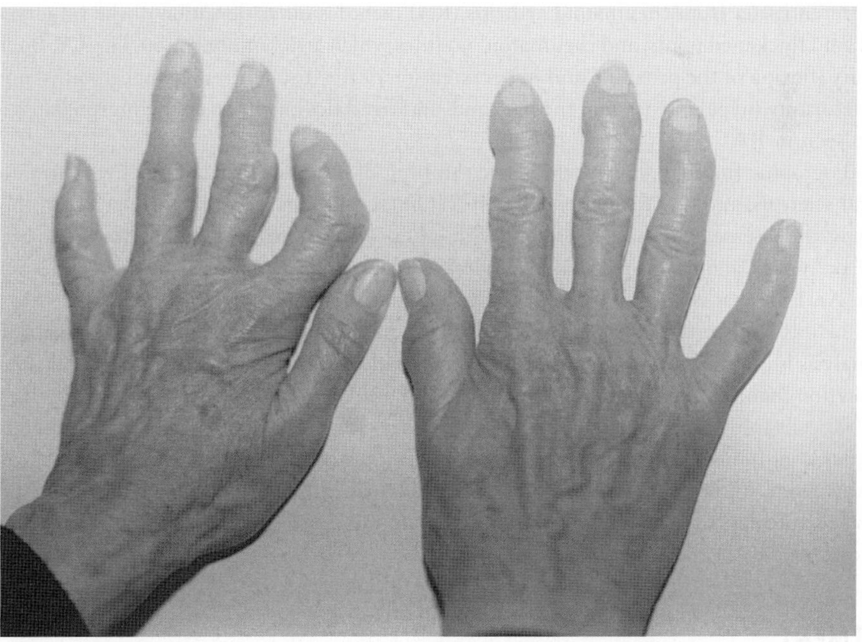

Figure 46.1 • Hands of an elderly woman with osteoarthritis showing osteophytic enlargement of the proximal interphalangeal joint (Bouchard's nodes) and distal interphalangeal joints (Heberden's nodes), as well as angulation deformity in some joints.

TABLE 46.2 Common deformities in osteoarthritis

Joint	Deformity
Distal interphalangeal	Heberden's node
Proximal interphalangeal	Bouchard's node
First carpometacarpal	Squaring (shelf sign)
First metatarsophalangeal	Hallux valgus (bunion)
Knee: medial femorotibial compartment	Genu varus (bow legs)
Knee: lateral femorotibial compartment	Genu valgus (knock knees)

femorotibial compartments (Table 46.2). This may be present along with crepitus, pain, and bony ridges.

DIAGNOSIS

Diagnosis is usually made clinically and by exclusion of other arthritides. OA can be differentiated by absent or minimal inflammation, the absence of systemic findings, and the involvement of weightbearing and high-use joints. Spinal arthritis must be differentiated from more serious diseases such as metastatic disease, multiple myeloma, osteoporosis, infection, and other bone diseases.

OA joint pain can also be differentiated from periarticular soft tissue injury by the frequent finding in OA of pain with any direction of movement, whereas periarticular injury elicits pain when the ligament or soft tissue is strained. OA of the hips can be differentiated from greater trochanteric bursitis, which is more lateral and does not limit movement.

Differentiation from rheumatoid arthritis (RA) includes ulnar deviation of the fingers; swollen, painful, and thickened joints; and rheumatoid nodules which are commonly noted in RA. Boutonnière deformity (flexion of the proximal and hyperextension of the distal interphalangeal joints) and "swan neck" deformity (hyperextension of the proximal and fixed flexion of the distal interphalangeal joints) are also seen in RA.

Radiographic findings show asymmetric thinning of the joint space, osteophyte formation, subchondral sclerosis, and cyst formation (Fig. 46.2). These findings may not correlate with the clinical severity of the disease, and may be present with other forms of arthritis. Laboratory tests are usually normal or mildly abnormal, particularly the erythrocyte sedimentation rate (ESR) and C-reactive protein. An ESR that is normal (between 30 and 80 mm/hour) is more consistent with OA, whereas an ESR of >100 suggests a more serious condition such as infection or rheumatoid arthritis. Synovial fluid analysis is most useful for excluding other arthritides. The fluid typically has <1,500 leukocytes/mm^3, predominantly monocytes, as compared to inflammatory arthritis, which typically has a count of >2,000 cells/mm^3 with a neutrophil predominance. Joint fluid tends to be more viscous in OA than other conditions. There are several biomarkers currently being researched for OA, but none are mainstream studies yet. Pathology often reveals calcium pyrophosphate dihydrate or apatite crystals (calcium crystals are the most common type in OA), and subchondral bone trabecular microfractures.

TREATMENT

Management of OA is aimed at preserving function (strength, motion, and alignment) and minimizing pain. The first line of therapy for OA is acetaminophen to the maximum safe dose (4 g/day

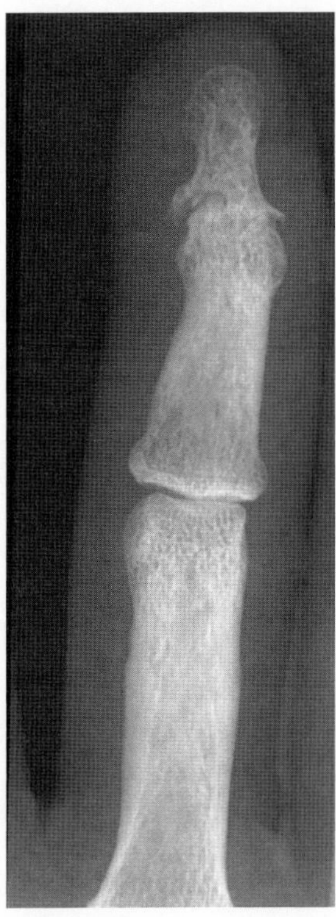

Figure 46.2 • Radiograph of the third digit of a patient with osteoarthritis (erosive type) showing osteophyte formation, joint erosion, and mild sclerosis.

in nonalcohol-consuming patients). Additional treatment includes nonacetylated salicylates such as salsalate. The next line includes nonsteroidal anti-inflammatory agents (NSAIDS), although these should be limited due to side effects such as renal insufficiency, gastrointestinal bleeds, and hypertension. Drugs with a stronger cyclooxygenase 2 (COX2) inhibitory effect (e.g., ibuprofen) or selective COX2 effect are recommended, although several COX2 inhibitors have recently been linked to myocardial infarction and subsequently withdrawn from the market. Opioid analgesics are of limited value and are usually restricted to the management of acute pain, or to scenarios where NSAIDS are contraindicated (as with renal disease, congestive heart failure, hypertension, peptic ulcer disease, or NSAID or aspirin hypersensitivity). There is no general utility to oral or parenteral corticosteroids. Intra-articular corticosteroid injections are occasionally helpful in relieving the low-grade chronic inflammation often found in OA, but have limitations on frequency and total amount that can be administered. Hyaluronate injections, designed to improve synovial fluid viscoelastic properties and/or decrease intra-articular inflammation, have inconsistent efficacy and require 3 to 5 repeated injections to complete a series.

Nutritional supplements are of debated utility as well, but commonly used supplements include glucosamine sulfate, chondroitin sulfate, and S-adenosylmethionine (SAM). These agents are thought to either limit or reverse the cartilage loss. Controlled studies have suggested benefit from glucosamine sulfate comparable to that seen in NSAID use but studies of other agents show either conflicting or inconsistent benefit from their use. Topical agents such as capsaicin or lidocaine will occasionally provide symptomatic relief at localized areas. Capsaicin may take several weeks to reach its maximum potency.

Physical therapy is helpful in maintaining strength and joint mobility, and often helps to reduce the level of pain on a particular joint. Assistive devices may also help in decreasing the pressure and weight on an affected joint; for instance, a walker will decrease the weight on a knee by up to 50%, a cane by 25% to 30%. Assistive devices should be prescribed and taught by a qualified health professional. Weight loss in overweight or obese individuals is also advised, as this will reduce the forces acting on a joint and both decrease the pain and slow further injury.

Surgery is a treatment of last resort. Arthroscopic surgery to the knees is of questionable benefit in typical OA without underlying injury. Joint replacement surgery is utilized for moderate to severe OA refractory to more conservative treatment. Knee replacement or grafting has been shown to have good efficacy for improving pain and mobility. Hip and shoulder replacements are done primarily for pain control because they can be associated with decreased range of motion in the joint.

CHAPTER 47

Rheumatoid Arthritis

Deidre Faust and Paul Halverson

Rheumatoid arthritis (RA) is a systemic disorder of unknown etiology characterized by a destructive arthropathy that cannot be cured and can result in severely reduced functional capacity and shortened lifespan. It afflicts approximately 1% of the population, predominantly females who outnumber males 3:1.

ETIOLOGY

The underlying mechanism is that of an autoimmune process. In RA, the synovium is infiltrated with T lymphocytes, plasma cells, and macrophages. Antigen-expressing CD4+ T cells stimulate synovial fibroblasts, monocytes, and macrophages to produce interleukins 1, 6, and tumor necrosis factor–alpha. These cause the active inflammation and joint destruction in RA. Within the synovium, immunoglobulins (including Rheumatoid factor [RF] are actively synthesized.

Neutrophils predominate in RA joint fluid. As they phagocytize immune complexes, they release lysosomal enzymes locally and generate reactive oxygen species. Both these enzymes and the reactive oxygen species may cause cartilage destruction. Prostaglandins are elevated in such joint fluids. Cytokines—including interleukins 1 and 6, tumor necrosis factor, and probably other growth factors—activate synovial fibroblasts and possibly chondrocytes. Unchecked, rheumatoid synovitis causes sustained inflammation with eventual thinning of cartilage, erosion of bone, and weakening of ligamentous structures, resulting in joint instability and deformity. The same cytokines involved in joint inflammation with RA ultimately lead to a reduced lifespan partially related to the increased cardiovascular morbidity in patients with RA.

Although the exact etiology of RA is unknown, predisposing factors include obesity, smoking, prior blood transfusion, adverse outcome of pregnancy, and increased red meat consumption.

CLINICAL MANIFESTATIONS

Rheumatoid arthritis has a variable natural history. Most patients experience recurrent and protracted exacerbations with gradual, cumulative, and irreversible tissue destruction. Less commonly, a single episode may be followed by lasting remission. Rare patients have progressive unremitting systemic disease, causing crippling disability and death.

Joint swelling and pain are the most common and predominant manifestations of rheumatoid arthritis. Joint swelling is often accompanied by more systemic manifestations such as malaise, fatigue, and weight loss. It may also be accompanied by chest pain, shortness of breath, dry eyes, and skin changes. The onset of systemic and musculoskeletal symptoms is insidious over weeks to months in most patients, but more rapid (and sometimes acute) in the remainder. Because of the multiple systems that RA can affect, it is of utmost importance that a thorough review of systems and physical is completed.

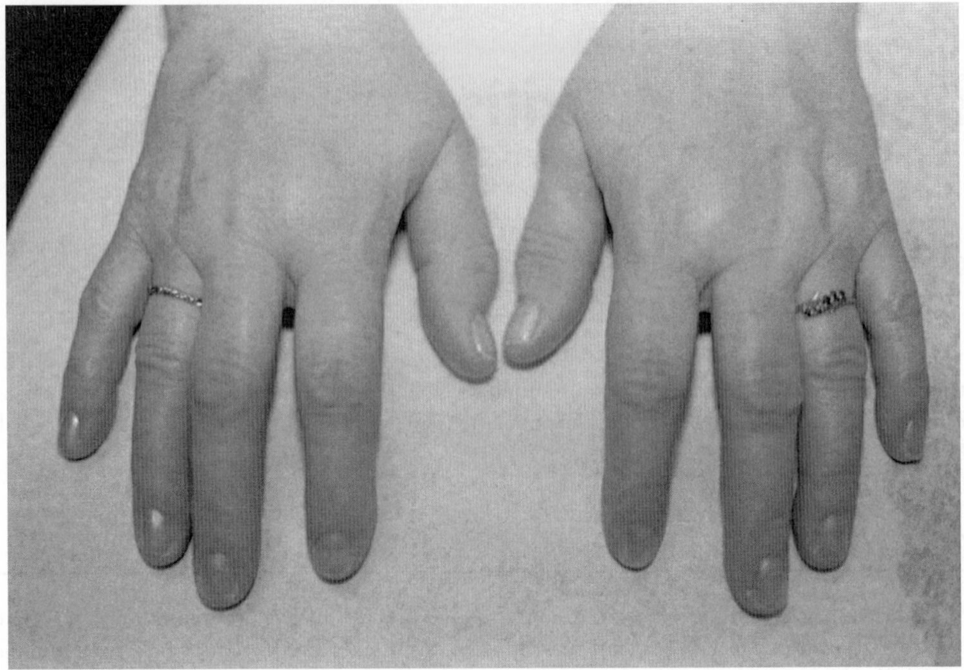

Figure 47.1 • Hands of a woman with early rheumatoid arthritis showing synovial thickening of the metacarpophalangeal and proximal interphalangeal joints.

Virtually any diarthrodial (synovial) joint may be involved, including the cricoarytenoid. Symmetric involvement is more common, but even if the initial presentation is asymmetric, with time, symmetry usually prevails. Morning stiffness may last for 1 hour or longer. Muscle atrophy may occur around involved joints, so that activities of daily living (e.g., household and self-care activities) become difficult. In some patients, there may be severe flares in one or a few joints or periarticular structures that last only a few days (palindromic rheumatism).

The joints most commonly involved are the proximal interphalangeal (PIP), metacarpophalangeal (MCP), and wrist, followed by the knee, ankle, metatarsophalangeal (MTP), shoulder, and elbow. Joint enlargement results from soft tissue swelling (synovitis) or synovial fluid accumulation (Fig. 47.1). Synovitis is usually detected as a "bogginess" of the joint on palpation while an effusion is noted as fluctuance in the tissue surrounding the joint. Affected joints may be warmer than nonaffected joints, but significant heat and erythema are not classic findings. Tendons may also develop synovitis, which is manifested on examination as thickening of the tendon sheath.

Chronic synovitis and tenosynovitis result in characteristic joint deformities classic for chronic rheumatoid arthritis. Patients may have swan neck deformities, Boutonnière's sign, ulnar deviation, cock-up toes, or hammer toes. Chronic tenosynovitis may result in decrease mobility of the fingers or trigger finger (Figs. 47.2 and 47.3, Table 47.1).

Rheumatoid nodules are a pathognomic finding in RA. Although these nodules are only present in 20% of patients with RA, when found, they are very specific for it. Virtually all patients with rheumatoid nodules are seropositive for RF. These nodules can occur in any organ, but the most common are (in diminishing order) subcutaneous, pulmonary (Fig. 47.4), and myopericardial. Rheumatoid nodules that are located subcutaneously are not attached to underlying structures such as tendons or bones and commonly occur in areas of pressure. Rheumatoid nodules tend to mirror disease activity. A common time to get rheumatoid nodules is at the onset of treatment with methotrexate.

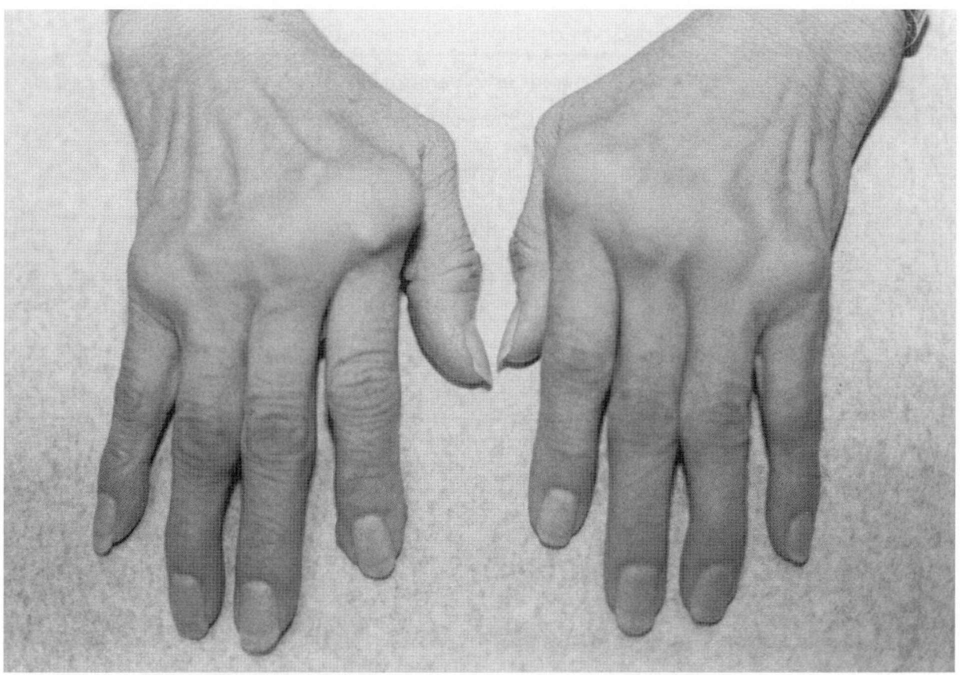

Figure 47.2 • Hands of a woman with chronic rheumatoid arthritis showing ulnar deviation, metacarpophalangeal subluxation, and swan neck deformities.

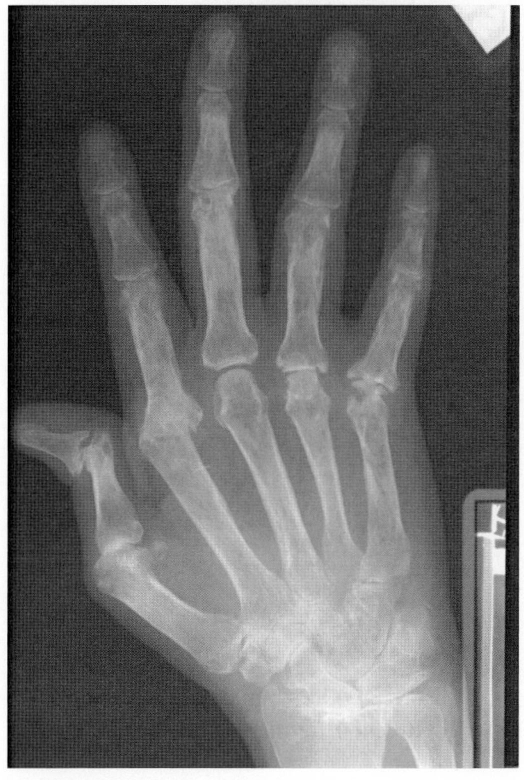

Figure 47.3 • Radiograph of the right hand of a woman with chronic rheumatoid arthritis. Joint erosions are present in the carpal bones and second metacarpophalangeal joint. Joint space narrowing and subluxation also are present.

TABLE 47.1 Common joint deformities in rheumatoid arthritis

Deformity	Joint involvement
Swan neck	Hyperextension of proximal interphalangeal and flexion of distal interphalangeal
Boutonnière	Flexion of proximal interphalangeal and extension of distal interphalangeal
Ulnar deviation of fingers	Radial deviation of carpal bones
Cock-up toes	Metatarsal head subluxation
Hammer toes	Metatarsal head subluxation leading to pressure necrosis of dorsal proximal interphalangeals
Bunion (hallux valgus)	First metatarsophalangeal

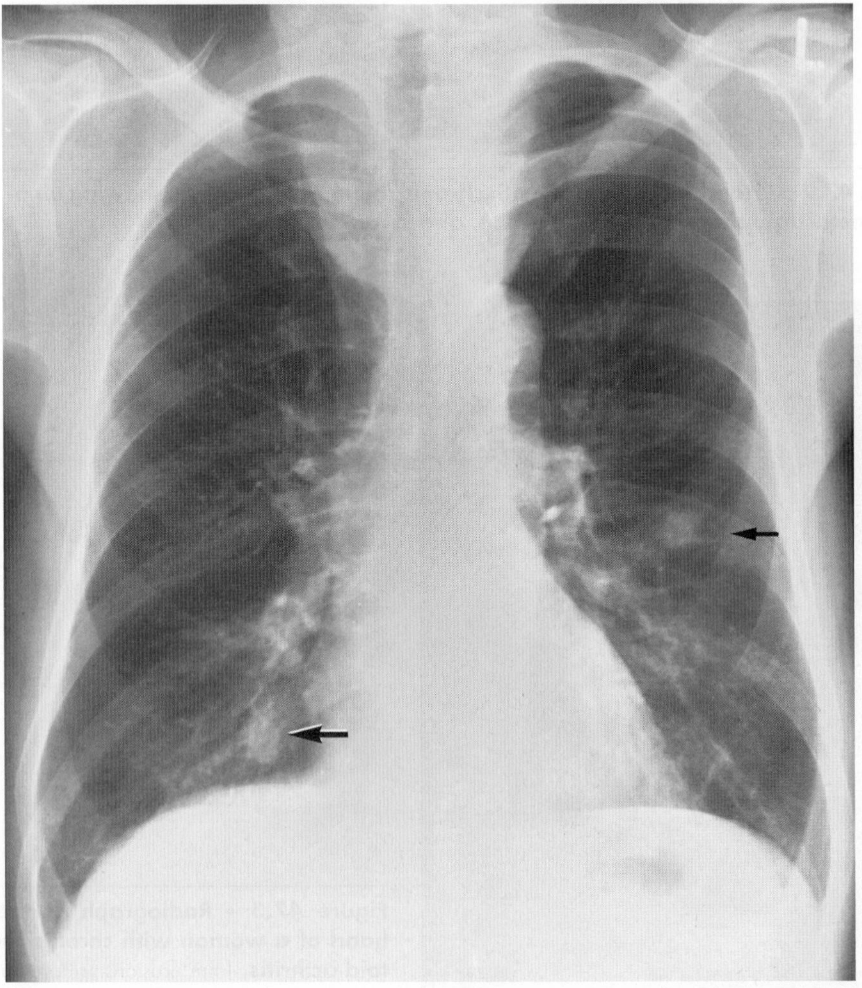

Figure 47.4 • Chest radiograph of a patient with chronic rheumatoid arthritis showing rheumatoid lung nodules.

TABLE 47.2 Revised American College of Rheumatology criteria for rheumatoid arthritis (1987)

1. Morning stiffness for at least one hour and present for at least 6 weeks
2. Swelling of three or more joints for at least 6 weeks
3. Swelling of wrist, metacarpophalangeal, or proximal interphalangeal joints for 6 or more weeks
4. Symmetric joint swelling
5. Hand roentgenogram changes typical of rheumatoid arthritis that must include erosion or unequivocal bony decalcification
6. Rheumatoid nodules
7. Serum rheumatoid factor by a method that yields positive results in less than 5% of normals

With exclusion of other joint disorders and fulfillment of four or more criteria, the diagnosis of RA is likely.
Reprinted from Arnett FC, Edworthy SM, Bloch DA, et al. The American Rheumatism Association 1987 revised criteria for the classification of rheumatoid arthritis. *Arthritis Rheum* 1988;31:315–324, with permission.

In summary, examination findings classic of RA include symmetric joint swelling with synovial bogginess most commonly involving the MCPs, PIPs, and MTP joints. Other examination findings helpful in making the diagnosis (if present) include rheumatoid nodules, joint effusions, and tenosynovitis.

DIAGNOSIS

A committee of the American College of Rheumatology developed a set of seven clinical criteria for epidemiologic and demographic use. These criteria, because they are nonspecific, usually indicate only that an inflammatory arthritis is present (Table 47.2).

Laboratory evaluation in patients who have physical examination findings of RA include rheumatoid factor and antibodies to citrulline containing proteins (anti-CCP). Almost 80% of patients with RA are seropositive for RF; however, 5% of the general population is positive for RF as well. Anti-CCP has a sensitivity of 60% and carries a specificity of >95%. Other serologic markers that are not specific but are helpful in making the diagnosis include the erythrocyte sedimentation rate and C-reactive protein. These are helpful in indicating that an inflammatory process is present when elevated and they are even more helpful in monitoring disease response. Thrombocytosis and anemia of chronic disease are also indicative of active inflammation.

Radiographs are usually not helpful in very early rheumatoid arthritis. Initially, radiographs may show only soft-tissue swelling. Classically, periarticular demineralization, symmetric joint space narrowing, and marginal articular erosions are seen as the disease progresses. In severe cases, marked bony destruction due to bony resorption and malalignment due to weakened capsular, tendinous, and ligamentous structures may occur (see Fig. 47.3). Joint ankylosis is unusual in RA.

TREATMENT

Therapy for RA is directed at reducing inflammation, controlling pain, halting progressive joint erosion, interrupting visceral involvement, and maintaining muscle strength, joint alignment, and joint mobility while awaiting remission. Because the disease course varies widely, medical therapy should be tailored to suppress synovitis or extra-articular manifestations of RA, if feasible, without exposing the patient to excessive risks of drug therapy. Early aggressive treatment is warranted, given the serious disability and premature mortality due to RA. Success of treatment usually is measured both clinically and in studies by following patients' reports of pain and physical disability, and by measuring levels of acute phase reactants such as erythrocyte sedimentation rate and C-reactive protein. All therapies are aimed at treatment of symptoms as no cure is available.

Therapy is begun with a full dose of nonsteroidal anti-inflammatory drugs (NSAIDs). Response is graded in terms of relief of pain, morning stiffness, and joint swelling and tenderness. Patients also should be questioned regarding potential side effects of NSAIDs including headache, rash, weight gain, dyspepsia, abdominal pain, or any other gastrointestinal symptoms. Many RA patients report some response to NSAIDs but continue to have pain, morning stiffness, and joint swelling. If NSAIDs fail to control pain and joint swelling adequately after 2 months, second-line drug therapy should be initiated.

The second-line agents, sometimes called disease-modifying antirheumatic drugs (DMARDs), include methotrexate hydroxychloroquine, minocycline, auranofin (oral gold), sulfasalazine, azathioprine, intramuscular gold, and penicillamine. Of these, methotrexate is typically the first and the most commonly used. Gold and penicillamine are rarely used. Single drugs may be adequate in milder cases, but combinations of drugs are being prescribed increasingly, usually with methotrexate, which has been referred to as an "anchor drug." Methotrexate is typically very well tolerated with its most common side effects being gastrointestinal upset or oral ulcers. One drawback of these drugs is their delayed onset of action. Cyclophosphamide and other alkylating agents clearly suppress RA as well, although an increased risk of malignancy relegates them to use only for serious complications of RA, such as rheumatoid vasculitis. Each of these agents has its own unique, and in some cases potentially severe, toxicity that requires monitoring.

Fortunately, significant progress has been made in the last several years for the treatment of RA. New DMARDs specific to mediators of inflammation such as tumor necrosis factor have provided more potent treatments that have significantly altered the treatment of rheumatoid arthritis Table 47.3. The newer agents have demonstrated promising results in reducing joint destruction and improving patient's perception of physical disability.

TABLE 47.3 Newer disease modifying anti-rheumatic drugs (DMARDs)

Agent	Mechanism
Leflunomide	Pyrimidine pathway antagonist
Etanercept, Infliximab	Anti-tumor necrosis factor
Anakinra	Anti-interleukin-1 receptor antagonist
Adalimumab	Monoclonal antibody and an inhibitor of tumor necrosis factor
Rituxan	Monoclonal antibody
Abatacept	Costtimulatory signal modulator. Inhibits T cell production and cytokines

Systemic corticosteroid therapy has an immediate ameliorative effect on inflammation. However, the long- and short-term side effects of high, or even moderate, doses of steroids argue against their use except in limited situations, including life-threatening visceral disease (e.g., pericardial tamponade, systemic vasculitis). Low-dose steroids, usually prednisone (5 mg/day), sometimes are used in patients with more severe RA who are beginning a remittive regimen in order to maintain function and employability while awaiting a therapeutic response. The long-term goal is always to discontinue steroids, although a few patients with the most severe RA may require low-dose treatment for years.

Intra-articular steroids are of value when the clinical picture is dominated by one or two joints, and this approach may control the local inflammatory response for months. It is inadvisable to inject a given joint any more than 3 or 4 times per year, because excess exposure to intra-articular steroids has been reported to result in a Charcot-like arthropathy.

COMPLICATIONS

Complications of rheumatoid arthritis are numerous because of the multitude of associated systemic symptoms. RA affects nearly every organ system including the cardiovascular system, skin, eyes, lungs, nervous system, and blood. Interestingly, the kidneys are almost never affected (Table 47.4).

Tenosynovitis at the wrist may produce carpal tunnel syndrome or cystic enlargement around the extensor tendons. Prolonged tenosynovitis may cause attrition and eventually rupture of extensor tendons, usually the fourth and fifth, resulting in inability to actively extend those digits. At the knee, expansion of the gastrocnemius-semimembranosus bursa by one-way flow of synovial fluid may produce a Baker's cyst in the popliteal space. This cyst usually is asymptomatic but may cause pain behind the knee or may rupture into the calf, simulating a deep vein thrombosis (pseudothrombophlebitis).

Neck pain in a patient with long-standing RA should prompt an evaluation of the cervical spine for C1-C2 subluxation, an incomplete dislocation. Cervical spine radiographs in flexion and extension may reveal widening of the space between the odontoid process and anterior arch of C1, suggesting laxity of supporting ligaments. This type of cervical instability as well as vertical subluxation of the odontoid into the foramen magnum may cause impingement on the spinal cord, with paralysis and respiratory failure. (It is important for an anesthesiologist to be aware of any cervical spine abnormalities prior to any contemplated surgery and intubation.)

Serious forms of pulmonary disease include interstitial pneumonitis producing restrictive lung disease and bronchiolitis obliterans. Again, pulmonary nodules can also be seen and may result in a restrictive lung disease or Caplan's syndrome.

Cardiovascular complications include an increased risk for coronary artery disease and pericarditis. Coronary artery disease is responsible for approximately 45% of deaths in patients with rheumatic arthritis. The exact mechanism causing this increase has not been elicited; however, it is thought that the same cytokines and inflammatory markers responsible for joint destruction are also responsible for endothelial dysfunction, plaque formation, and rupture. Patients with RA have an inherently increased risk for coronary artery disease; however, treatment for RA (especially steroids) can also increase cardiovascular mortality. Furthermore, disability and joint pain limit patients' ability to exercise, further increasing risk for cardiovascular disease. In addition to coronary artery disease, patients with rheumatoid arthritis can develop pericarditis. It is often asymptomatic but can result in constrictive pericarditis and heart failure.

Sjögren's syndrome (sicca complex) is found in RA, systemic lupus erythematosus, other connective tissue diseases, or by itself without another associated disease. Lymphocytic infiltration of lacrimal and salivary glands produces dysfunction and damage, followed by reduced formation of tears and saliva. Prominent symptoms include dry eyes (sicca syndrome) as well as burning, matter formation,

TABLE 47.4 Extra-articular manifestations of rheumatoid arthritis

Skin
Rheumatoid nodules
Vasculitis lesions
Mucous membranes
Sjögren's syndrome (20%)
Eyes
Sjögren's syndrome
Episcleritis
Scleromalacia perforans
Heart
Pericarditis
Lungs
Pleurisy
Pulmonary rheumatoid nodules
Interstitial pneumonitis
Bronchiolitis obliterans
Pneumoconiosis (Caplan's syndrome)
Nervous system
Compression neuropathy
Median nerve
Posterior interosseus syndrome
Peripheral neuropathy
Mononeuritis multiplex (in vasculitis)
Cervical cord compression (C1-2 subluxation)
Hematologic
Anemia
Leukopenia
Felty's syndrome
Leukocytosis
Thrombocytosis
Vascular
Rheumatoid vasculitis

and dryness of the mouth. Patients require frequent instillation of artificial tears or gels to prevent symptoms and corneal ulcers. Cholinergic agents (e.g., oral pilocarpine, cevimeline) or artificial saliva may reduce mouth dryness. In some patients, lymphocytic infiltration of lungs, kidneys, or other sites may evoke organ dysfunction. Hematologic complications of RA include anemia of chronic disease, Felty's syndrome, and an increased risk for malignancy.

Felty's syndrome, affecting 1% of patients, is a triad of RA, splenomegaly, and cytopenia, usually leukopenia. Nearly all such patients are seropositive for RF in high titers, with more erosive, destruc-

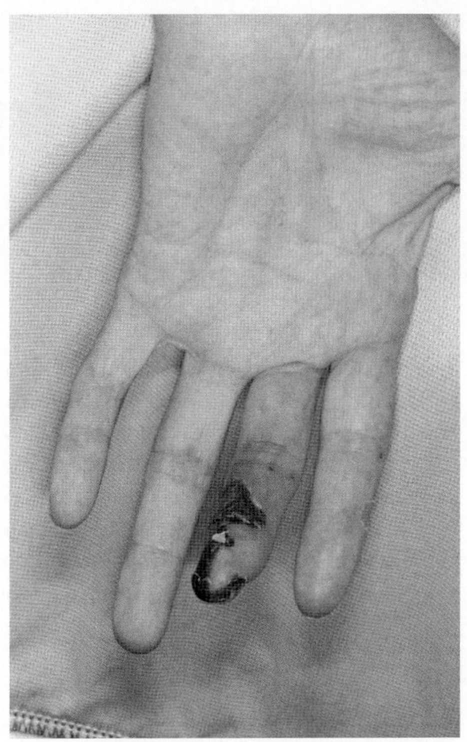

Figure 47.5 • Digital gangrene of the middle finger in a patient with systemic vasculitis related to rheumatoid arthritis.

tive arthritis than the average patient with RA. Such patients are at high risk for life-threatening pyogenic infections, although the actual peripheral blood leukocyte count and risk for infection are poorly correlated. Many RA patients have significant leukopenia without splenomegaly.

Signs of vasculitis occur in 8% of RA patients. In most, this includes minor digital infarcts (brown spots). In 1% of patients, nearly all of whom are RF-seropositive in high titers, a severe systemic vasculitic syndrome occurs, with fever, skin ulcers, digital gangrene (Fig. 47.5), and organ infarction.

CHAPTER 48

Systemic Lupus Erythematosus

Deidre Faust and Paul Halverson

Systemic lupus erythematosus (SLE) is an autoimmune disease most commonly manifesting as a polyarthritis. The term lupus erythematosus was first used to describe the nodular red ulcerating lesions of the skin. It was Sir William Osler who first characterized it as a systemic disease in a 1904 paper, "On the visceral manifestations of the erythema group of skin diseases." SLE can have varying presentations ranging from a superficial skin rash and mild arthralgias to a severe life-threatening systemic illness with multiorgan involvement. It afflicts about 0.1% of the general population but appears to be slightly more common and more severe in nonwhites. It is much more common in women (90%) and usually begins between the ages of 15 and 40 years.

ETIOLOGY

The underlying cause of SLE is unknown. The disease is characterized by an increased frequency of human leukocyte antigen (HLA)-B8, HLA-DR2, and HLA-DR3; along with the concordant occurrence of disease in monozygotic but not dizygotic twins, this strongly suggests a genetic predisposition. The predilection for women suggests the influence of estrogen on the immunologic abnormalities. Environmental factors, such as exposure to ultraviolet light, may activate both the skin disease and the systemic disease.

SLE is characterized by antibodies to the nuclei of cells, known as antinuclear antibodies (ANA), although a wide range of immunologic effects can be present. The presence of elevated immunoglobulin levels reflects B-cell stimulation. Specific autoantibodies are present, which cause disease by direct reaction with a target tissue (e.g., immune thrombocytopenia) or by tissue deposition of the resulting immune complex (e.g., SLE nephritis, immune complex vasculitis). These immune complexes are poorly cleared by the reticuloendothelial system, perhaps due to a concomitant inherited deficiency of one of several complement components.

Some drugs can induce ANA and, occasionally, overt clinical symptoms of SLE (drug-induced lupus). Procainamide, hydralazine, isoniazid, diphenylhydantoin, and penicillamine are the most common offenders. Over 60% of patients taking procainamide develop a positive ANA titer with time, but only 5% of these develop symptoms of SLE. Most often, such patients have only fever, serositis, and arthritis. Cessation of the drug usually leads to alleviation of symptoms over several weeks to months, although the serologic changes may persist for years.

CLINICAL MANIFESTATIONS

Systemic lupus erythematosus potentially involves every body system (Table 48.1). However, not all systems are affected in any given case and they may not all be present at initial presentation in some cases. Oftentimes, the diagnosis is made based on the evolution of symptoms and signs over time.

TABLE 48.1 Revised American College of Rheumatology criteria for the diagnosis of systemic lupus erythematosus (1982)

Criterion	Comment
Malar (butterfly) rash	Spares nasolabial folds
Discoid skin lesions	Atrophic scarring may occur in older lesions
Photosensitivity	Unusual reaction to sunlight
Oral ulcers	Usually painless; may be nasopharyngeal
Nonerosive arthritis	Involves >2 peripheral joints
Serositis	Pleuritis (pleurisy, pleural rub, or effusion) or pericarditis (abnormal electrocardiogram, rub, or pericardial effusion)
Renal disorder	Persistent proteinuria >0.5 g per 24 hours, or >3% proteinuria on dipstick, or cellular casts
Neurological disorder	Seizures or psychosis in the absence of offending drugs or metabolic derangements
Hematologic disorder	Cytopenias on >2 occasions: hemolytic anemia with reticulocytosis, leucopenia <4,000/mm^3, or lymphopenia <1,500/mm^3, or thrombocytopenia <100,000/mm^3
Immunologic disorder	Antinative DNA or anti-Smith antibodies or positive anticardiolipin antibody, or false-positive VDRL
Antinuclear antibody	Abnormal ANA titer in the absence of drugs associated with drug-induced lupus

For the purposes of case definition, diagnosis of SLE requires the presence of 4 of these 11 criteria, either serially or simultaneously.

Adapted from Tan EM, Cohen AS, Fries JF, et al. The 1982 revised criteria for the classification of systemic lupus erythematosus. *Arthritis Rheum* 1982;25:1271–1277. Hochberg MC. Updating the American College of Rheumatology revised criteria for the classification of systemic lupus erythematosus. *Arthritis Rheum* 1997;40:1725, with permission.

The integument is commonly affected in SLE. A faint, relatively nonspecific malar rash is seen in 25% of patients. A butterfly rash over the cheeks is considered classic, but is seen in only about 5% of cases. Discoid lesions occur in about 10%. Other skin lesions include photosensitive skin eruptions, urticaria, macular or papular eruptions, bullae, and panniculitis. Livedo reticularis, Raynaud's phenomenon, nail-bed telangiectasia, splinter hemorrhages, and Osler's nodes (tender, erythematous thickenings in the finger pads) reflect the underlying vasculitis. Oral mucosal or nasal septal ulcerations are common but are painless and therefore frequently missed. Patchy alopecia or brittle hair ("lupus hair") is seen in about 15% of cases and reflects involvement of the skin appendages.

Joint pain and swelling together represent the most frequent manifestation of SLE, and are seen in 95% of patients. Typically, the arthritis is nondeforming and nonerosive, unlike that in rheumatoid arthritis. However, a minority of patients can develop rheumatoid arthritis-like ulnar deviation and swan-neck deformities secondary to periarticular soft-tissue changes (Fig. 48.1) Aseptic necrosis of bone, most often involving the femoral or humeral heads, can follow steroid therapy or vasculitis.

Serositis may occur as pericarditis, pleuritis, or peritoneal inflammation. Pericarditis occurs in 25% of patients with SLE but rarely causes cardiac malfunction (Fig. 48.2) Angina or myocardial infarction can result from vasculitis of the small coronary vessels or from coronary atherosclerosis as a result of corticosteroid therapy. Aortic or mitral valve insufficiency is seen in the rare patient with valvulitis. A form of aseptic endocarditis has been described (Libman-Sacks). It typically is asymptomatic but may predispose to bacterial endocarditis.

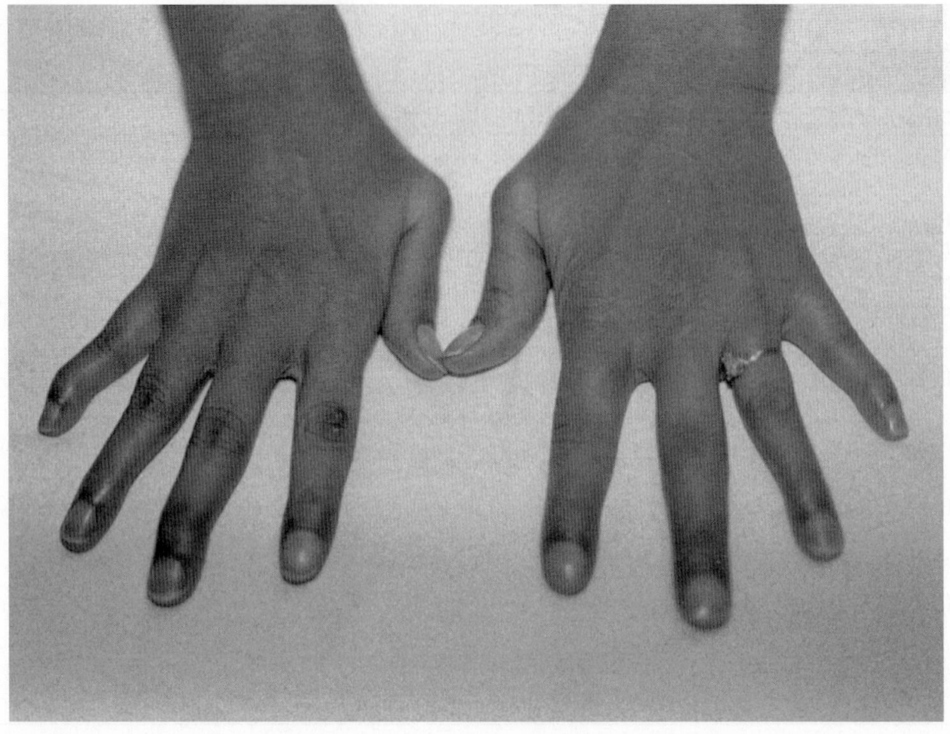

Figure 48.1 • Hands of a woman with systemic lupus erythematosus, showing synovitis in several proximal interphalangeal joints and swan-neck deformities.

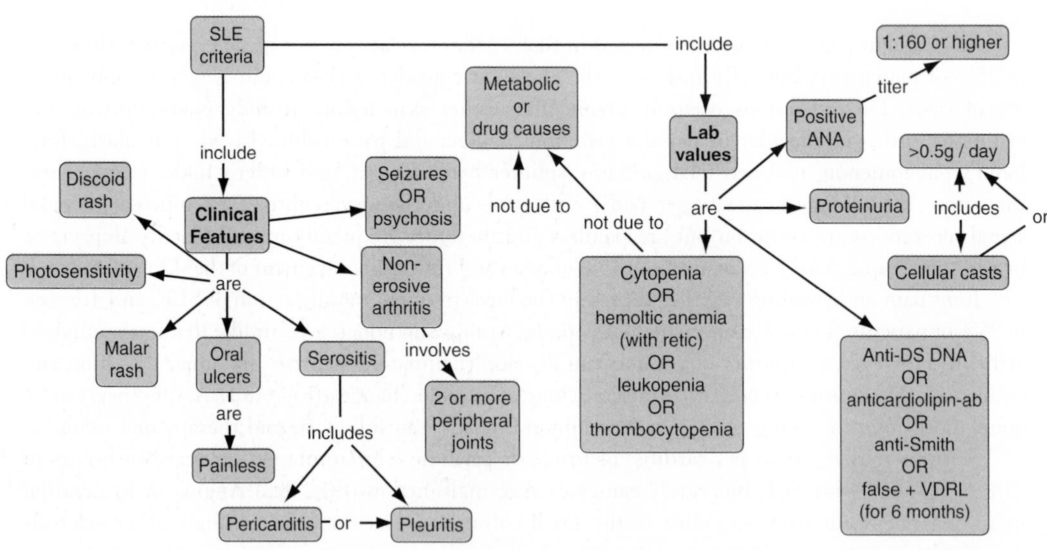

Figure 48.2 • Systemic lupus erythematosus criteria. Anti-DS DNA, anti–double-stranded DNA.

Pleuritis, the most common pleuropulmonary manifestation, is seen in 30% of cases. Lupus pneumonitis is uncommon. Thus, a pulmonary infiltrate in SLE is more apt to be infectious than a result of the underlying pulmonary disease.

About 25% of patients exhibit some form of neurologic involvement. Virtually any central or peripheral neurologic structure can be affected, although seizures, cerebrovascular accidents, and organic mental syndromes predominate. Lupus cerebritis leading to diffuse cortical atrophy, irreversible dementia, and organic brain syndrome is especially ominous.

Another pathogenetic mechanism for central nervous system lupus is vaso-occlusive stroke. These patients usually present with physical signs of one or more specific ablative neurologic defects, which may be detectable on computed tomography, magnetic resonance imaging, or arteriography. Vascular occlusion in these patients is due to vasculitis or thromboembolism, the latter of which is related to hypercoagulability from antiphospholipid antibodies or lupus anticoagulant.

Proximal muscle weakness may reflect myositis with elevation of muscle enzymes and other features of myositis (Chapter 49).

About one half of patients with SLE develop clinically apparent renal disease suggested by hematuria or proteinuria (Chapter 81). Renal biopsies usually reveal some form of glomerulonephritis. In general, the more diffuse the involvement, the worse the prognosis. Patients with minimal or focal change on light microscopy have a generally benign prognosis, and those with pure membranous change have an intermediate prognosis. About one third of patients with focal or membranous change, however, can progress in time to diffuse lupus glomerulonephritis. Evidence also suggests that a higher degree of chronic change on biopsy (e.g., scarring, crescents) identifies patients who do less well over several years. Thus, it is likely that every patient with clinically apparent renal involvement warrants treatment.

Most patients with SLE have anemia of chronic disease. In 5% or less, the anemia is an autoimmune hemolytic type. Granulocytopenia or lymphopenia also can occur. Although mild thrombocytopenia occurs in one third of patients, severe autoimmune thrombocytopenia develops in only 5%.

DIAGNOSIS

The diagnosis of SLE is based on clinical and laboratory findings based on criteria established by the American College of Rheumatology (Table 48.1). For the purpose of clinical studies, the case definition requires that four or more criteria be met serially or simultaneously for an unequivocal diagnosis of SLE. Many patients with SLE acquire four criteria only after some years.

ANA, anti-DNA, and the variety of other autoantibodies possible in SLE are listed in Table 48.2. The presence of anti-Smith or high titers of antinative DNA antibodies are virtually diagnostic, but they are only present in 40% to 50% of cases. Conversely, a negative ANA virtually excludes SLE, except in the unusual subgroup of "subacute cutaneous lupus," in which the ANA is negative but anti-Ro (SSA) antibodies are present. This subgroup of SLE patients features primarily photosensitivity, causing annular skin lesions and arthritis.

Depressions of serum hemolytic complement correlate with immune complex nephritis or, alternatively, may reflect congenital absence of one of the complement components (C2 deficiency is the most common). The latter patients are significantly more likely than the general population to develop SLE, polymyositis, or another autoimmune disease.

Twenty percent of SLE patients have a false-positive Venereal Disease Research Laboratory (VDRL) test, which may antedate full-fledged SLE by decades. Among these, 5% have a prolonged partial thromboplastin time, attributable to an antibody against the platelet factor III–factor X–factor V complex (lupus anticoagulant) or anticardiolipin antibody.

Up to 50% of patients may have anticardiolipin antibodies, lupus anticoagulant, or both. Hemorrhagic problems are rare in such patients. Instead, about one third are at risk for thromboembolic

TABLE 48.2 Antinuclear antibodies: frequency of positive finding in various rheumatic diseases (%)

Antibody	Systemic lupus erythematosus	Diffuse scleroderma	CREST	Polymyositis/ dermatomyositis	Rheumatoid arthritis	Drug-induced lupus	Mixed connective tissue disease	Sjögren's syndrome
Antinuclear antibody	>95	95	95	20–50	15–35	>95	>95	75
Antinative DNA	50							
Smith	40							
Ribonucleoprotein	40	15	10	15			>95	15
Centromere			50					
Histones	30				20	>95		
Scl-70		40	15					
SS-A/Ro	25[a]			10	10[b]			50
SS-B/La	15							25
PM-1				30–50				

[a]Positive in subacute cutaneous lupus, in which ANA may be negative.
[b]SS-A/Ro positive patients usually have secondary Sjögren's syndrome.
CREST, calcinosis, Raynard syndrome, esophageal dysmotility, sclerodactyly, telangiectasia.

disease, which may take the form of venous thromboembolism, stroke, or other vascular occlusive syndromes. Anticardiolipin antibody also identifies a group with recurrent spontaneous abortions, some of whom have no evidence of SLE.

The antiphospholipid syndrome should be considered in women with recurrent spontaneous abortions or persons with a hypercoagulable state (younger persons or those with recurrent thrombotic episodes without other risk factors). A prolonged partial thromboplastin time or thrombocytopenia may be the tip off.

Synovial analysis in active arthritis typically reveals 2,000 to 5,000 leukocytes/mm^3. In patients with renal disease, a nephritic picture (microscopic hematuria or red cell casts), serum creatinine, blood pressure, serologic changes, and the degree of proteinuria can predict quite accurately the changes on biopsy. The closest correlate of lupus glomerulonephritis is a low serum complement, and the second is a high level of antinative DNA.

TREATMENT

Treatment of SLE is based on its severity. Rapid onset and the presence of both anti-DNA antibodies and low serum complement suggest more severe disease. Arthritis and, often, serositis respond to aspirin or other NSAIDs. Both arthritis and dermatologic manifestations can be treated with antimalarial agents, but ophthalmologic monitoring is required to detect early toxicity.

Indications for high-dose corticosteroid therapy (prednisone, 60 to 100 mg/day or equivalent, in divided doses) include severe multisystem disease, serositis unresponsive to NSAIDs, central or peripheral nervous system disease, vasculitis, hemolytic anemia, immune thrombocytopenia, and glomerulonephritis. Controlling blood pressure in hypertensive lupus patients is critical to prevent further renal deterioration. If an excessive dose of corticosteroid is required to suppress disease activity, azathioprine, mycophenolate mofetil, or methotrexate may affect disease control and be steroid-sparing. Cytotoxic drugs (e.g., cyclophosphamide) are indicated primarily for active renal disease.

Drug-induced lupus is treated by withdrawal of the offending agent, which leads to the gradual disappearance of symptoms and eventually of the ANA.

The prognosis for SLE patients has improved over the years. Since the introduction of corticosteroids, 5-year survival rates of 93% to 94% are reported. The use of cytotoxic agents delays the onset of renal failure requiring dialysis. Infection is the most common cause of death, and those with renal and central nervous system disease have the worst 5-year survival rate.

CHAPTER 49

Polymyositis and Scleroderma

Steven Denson and Paul Halverson

POLYMYOSITIS

Polymyositis (PM) is an idiopathic systemic inflammatory myopathy that is often grouped alongside of dermatomyositis (DM), rhabdomyositis, and inclusion body myositis that share the common feature of inflammation of skeletal muscle. PM and DM are also seen in other rheumatologic conditions. Peak incidence of myositis disorders is in the fifth and sixth decades of life, but can occur at any time. Women are affected twice as often as men, and blacks are more commonly affected than whites. Myositis, usually DM, develops alongside of a malignancy in 25% of cases.

Etiology

Polymyositis and dermatomyositis appear to be mediated by unknown autoimmune processes. Triggers may be environmental or viral in patients who are susceptible. Staining of pathologic material indicates that CD8-positive T cells predominate in polymyositis, whereas in dermatomyositis CD4-positive T cells and B cells predominate. Perivascular infiltration of lymphocytes and histiocytes is seen. Both polymyositis and dermatomyositis are associated with human leukocyte antigen (HLA)-B8, HLA-DR3, and DRW52 phenotypes, suggesting some degree of genetic susceptibility.

Clinical Manifestations

The most common (70% to 95%) presenting complaints include difficulty in standing from seated or lying positions, difficulty climbing or descending stairs, difficulty kneeling, and difficulty raising the arms. Proximal muscle groups are affected more than distal muscles, which are involved in only 20% of cases. Joint and muscle aches can develop in a quarter of cases, along with stiffness, swelling, and induration of the muscles. Oropharyngeal skeletal muscles found in the pharynx and upper third of the esophagus can develop weakness and atrophy, leading to dysphagia and possible aspiration. Respiration can be affected by involvement of the intercostal muscles.

Physical examination findings of a heliotrope (reddish purple) periorbital and eyelid rash with some associated edema differentiate DM from PM. A second rash can include deep red popular plaques on extensor surfaces of the knuckles, elbows, knees, and medial malleoli (Gottron's sign), and can also involve the neck, shoulders, and upper torso. There can be whitish scaling and dilated nailfold capillaries with hyperemia. The presence of cutaneous vasculitis with tender nodules, periungual infarctions, and digital ulcerations is more common with a concurrent neoplasm.

Diagnosis

Laboratory studies often show increased creatinine kinase, erythrocyte sedimentation rates, lactate dehydrogenase, aldolase, and aspartate transaminase levels. Antinuclear antibody levels are elevated in more than half of cases. Imaging studies such as a fluoroscopic swallowing study demonstrate dysphagia in 15% of cases in the pharynx and upper one third of the esophagus, and distal hypomotility of questionable significance in the esophagus in 50% of cases. Electrocardiograms are often abnormal, showing conduction delays in 50% of patients.

Muscle biopsies, ideally of the weakened but not atrophied deltoid or femoral muscles, demonstrate lymphocytic infiltrate between muscle fibers and around blood vessels, patchy areas of necrosis with phagocytic invasion, destruction and regeneration of muscle fibers, and inflammatory infiltrates.

The common diagnostic criteria for inflammatory myopathies in general include:

1. Bilaterally symmetric muscle weakness, usually in proximal muscle groups.
2. Rash characteristics of DM including Grotton's papules and a heliotrope rash.
3. Elevated muscle enzymes.
4. Myopathic changes noted on electromyelograph.
5. Muscle biopsy findings that exclude other myopathies.

Other medical problems that resemble polymyositis need to be excluded from the diagnosis. Thyroid disorders (both hypo- and hyperthyroidism), drug reactions (steroids, hydroxychloroquine, tryptophan, statins, zidovudine, and clofibrate among others), other rheumatologic disorders (systemic lupus erythematosus or sarcoidosis) and nervous system disorders (myasthenia gravis, multiple sclerosis, chronic inflammatory polyneuropathy) need to be excluded. An alternative form of myositis, called inclusion body myositis, can occur typically in older white men, has a more insidious onset and course, and is often resistant to treatment for polymyositis. The diagnosis is made by the presence of basophilic-rimmed vacuoles on light microscopy and filamentous nuclear or cytoplasmic masses on electron microscopy.

Treatment

Treatment is usually with corticosteroids, initiated at high doses of 40 to 60 mg/day and maintained at these high doses for 1 to 3 months. The creatinine kinase level is monitored as a gauge of therapy, and corticosteroids are adjusted downward based on a drop in this marker. Methotrexate and azathioprine are used as steroid-sparing agents. Most patients will eventually come off steroids, but there is a high risk of relapse. Oral hydroxychloroquine and topical steroids are used for the treatment of rashes associated with dermatomyositis. Prognosis is usually fair, with three quarters of patients surviving more than 8 years, and half having a full recovery. Approximately one third have residual weakness and one fifth have persistent active disease requiring long-term steroid management. Malignancy and comorbid conditions have a poorer prognosis, and in most cases death is due to either the malignancy or to infection.

SYSTEMIC SCLEROSIS SCLERODERMA

Progressive systemic sclerosis (PSS) is a disease characterized by thickening and fibrosis of the skin and internal organs. Although the skin manifestations are one of the most evident manifestations of this disease, it is the internal organ involvement that most often affects the morbidity and mortality of this disorder. It is relatively uncommon, with an incidence of 10 to 20 per million persons per year.

Etiology

The exact cause of systemic sclerosis is unknown. It appears to be autoimmune mediated largely through lymphocytes. Recent theories have invoked serum matrix metalloproteinases, antibody activation of platelet derived growth factor, and transforming growth factor–beta. Regardless of trigger, the process seems to evolve through four stages. Early in the disorder, it is characterized by proliferative vascular lesions that lead to obliterative microvascular disease. Ultimately ischemia develops leading to atrophy and fibrosis.

Clinical Manifestations

SKIN INVOLVEMENT

Skin involvement is characterized by thickening and hardening of the skin. The fingers (sclerodactyly), hands, and face are generally involved earlier in the disease.

VASCULAR ABNORMALITIES

Vascular abnormalities are generally diffuse but are more prominent in the distal extremities. Raynaud's phenomenon, defined as sequential color changes (white, blue, and red) in the digits precipitated by cold, stress, or even change in temperatures, is present in more 90% of patients.

INTERNAL ORGAN INVOLVEMENT

Extracutaneous organ involvement includes the gastrointestinal tract, lungs, kidneys, and heart. Gastrointestinal manifestations include gastroesophageal reflux, with subsequent chronic esophagitis and stricture formation, and abnormal motility. Pseudo-obstruction and bacterial small bowel overgrowth with malabsorption may also be present. However, half of these patients may be asymptomatic.

Pulmonary involvement is found in over 70% of patients with systemic sclerosis. The two most frequent clinical manifestations of lung involvement are interstitial lung disease (pulmonary fibrosis) and pulmonary hypertension, which results in exertional dyspnea with exertion and diminished exercise tolerance. Patients with systemic sclerosis have also an increased risk of lung cancer.

Renal impairment is present in 60% to 80% of patients. Patients can develop proteinuria, a mild elevation in plasma creatinine concentration, and/or hypertension. Scleroderma renal crisis may occur with sudden onset of renal failure and malignant hypertension.

Cardiac disease may manifest with pericarditis, pericardial effusion, and heart failure, as well as conduction disturbances and arrhythmias. Peripheral and central nervous system involvement may reveal peripheral neuropathies, myopathy, headache, seizures, and stroke.

One variant of systemic sclerosis is known as CREST (**C**alcinosis, **R**aynaud's phenomenon, **E**sophageal dysmotility, **S**clerodactyly [tight skin below metacarpal phalangeal (MCP) or on face], and **T**elangiectasia [hands and face]) syndrome. CREST seems to have a better prognosis than progressive systemic sclerosis. The skin disease is limited to the distal extremities and there is less lung and kidney involvement. Pulmonary hypertension can occur late in the disease despite relatively limited lung parenchymal disease.

Diagnosis

The diagnosis of systemic sclerosis is a clinical diagnosis. Typical skin thickening (sclerosis), Raynaud's phenomenon, signs and symptoms of multiple organ involvement coupled with the detection of characteristic autoantibodies are highly suggestive of systemic sclerosis.

Laboratory and imaging tests may be helpful to suggest extracutaneous organ involvement. Urinalysis may reveals mild proteinuria with few cells or casts; a chest radiograph or computed tomography of the chest may show evidence of interstitial lung disease or pulmonary fibrosis. An echocardiogram may show decreased left ventricular function suggestive of cardiomyopathy. An electrocardiogram may reveal conduction abnormalities or evidence of pericarditis.

Antitopoisomerase I (Scl-70) antibodies and anticentromere antibody can be diagnostically useful. Antitopoisomerase is positive in 20% to 40% of patients with scleroderma and in greater than 70% of those with PSS. Anticentromere antibody is only present in up to 10% of those with PSS but is present in up to 90% of those with CREST. A skin biopsy may be needed to confirm the diagnosis.

Treatment

The treatment of scleroderma is complex. In general, the treatment is supportive. The nature and distribution of organ involvement may dictate the specific therapy needed. All patients should be treated with gastric acid suppression and antireflux measures to reduce the likelihood of esophageal stricture. Skin should be protected with lubricating creams. Symptomatic gastroparesis can be treated with metoclopramide. Periodic treatment for bacterial overgrowth in the gut may be helpful.

In patients with aggressive lung involvement, immunomodulators and other agents such as cyclophosphamide, glucocorticoids, or cyclosporine can be used and may help stabilize the progression off the disease. A renal crisis in patients with scleroderma can be life threatening and should be treated immediately by controlling blood pressure. The drug of choice is an angiotensin-converting enzyme inhibitor.

CHAPTER 50

Sjögren's Syndrome

Steven Denson and Paul Halverson

Sjögren's syndrome (also known as sicca syndrome) is a chronic, progressive inflammatory process of the exocrine glands. Although the disease can present at all ages, the mean age of onset is 50 years and the incidence increases with age. Ninety percent of cases are female.

ETIOLOGY

The underlying cause is unknown, but there is evidence to suggest an autoimmune process with lymphocyte infiltration of the exocrine glands, and autoantibodies to ribonucleoproteins Ro and La (SS-A and SS-B, respectively). Half of cases are primary. The other half have related rheumatologic (rheumatoid arthritis, systemic lupus erythematosus) or connective tissue disorders associated with the syndrome. As with many rheumatologic conditions, there is likely a genetic predisposition with an environmental or pathological trigger.

CLINICAL MANIFESTATIONS

The usual presenting symptoms involve the mouth and eyes, but exocrine glands of the respiratory, vaginal, and gastrointestinal tracts are also involved. The most common presenting complaints are of a dry mouth with difficulty chewing and swallowing foods, and of burning, itching, and dry "gritty" eyes. Twenty percent of patients will also have symptoms of Raynaud's syndrome (paroxysmal bilateral cyanosis of the fingers and toes due to arterial contraction caused by cold, emotion, or other triggers). Dry skin is also a common complaint.

On examination, the findings of dry, erythematous mucous membranes with severe dental caries, a firm parotid gland, or gland enlargement are notable on oral examination and can be found in some cases. The eyes will also reveal dry mucous membranes and decreased tearing (keratoconjunctivitis), fluorescein staining can reveal ulceration, and a positive Schirmer's test (diminished flow of tears down a strip of filter paper) is a notable finding.

DIAGNOSIS

General laboratory tests show a normocytic-normochromic anemia, elevations in erythrocyte sedimentation rate and C-reactive protein, and occasionally leukopenia. Immunological tests reveal anti-Ro (SS-A) and anti-La (SS-B) antibodies in about 70% of cases, and an elevated rheumatoid factor is also seen. There are no useful imaging studies, although positive findings of decreased flow on parotid and salivary scintigraphy support the diagnosis. Biopsy of the lips for labial exocrine gland involvement is done when the diagnosis is in question.

TREATMENT

The majority of Sjögren's cases are limited in the scope of the disease and have a relatively benign prognosis; treatment is supportive. Oral symptoms are managed by careful oral hygiene, the use of artificial saliva preparations, and salivary gland stimulants (such as oral pilocarpine or cevimeline). Artificial tears and protection of the eyes from ultraviolet radiation control ocular manifestations. Skin and vaginal dryness is managed with moisturizing creams. In the small percentage of cases with lymphoma or life-threatening complications, corticosteroids and immunosuppressives may be necessary.

COMPLICATIONS

Ten percent of cases also have lymphocyte infiltration of the lungs, kidneys, muscles, and lymph nodes. Twenty percent have associated vasculitis symptoms. There is also a significant association with neurological deficits, both central and peripheral; this includes sensory neuropathy in both peripheral and cranial nerves, neurogenic bladder, stroke, seizure, and progressive transverse myelopathy. Lymphoma is also an associated complication of late Sjögren's, and presents most often as a low-grade B-cell extranodal lymphoma.

CHAPTER 51

Seronegative Spondyloarthropathies

Steven Denson and Paul Halverson

The seronegative spondyloarthropathies are a group of disorders that are negative for rheumatoid factor, and have involvement of the back, inflammation at ligamentous or tendon insertions into bone, or involve peripheral arthritis (Table 51.1). There is a tendency for the human leukocyte antigen (HLA) B27 to be positive in many of these disorders, but due to its prevalence in healthy individuals, it is felt to be neither sensitive nor specific. Some patients may present with a pattern of arthritis characteristic of a spondyloarthropathy but without evidence of ankylosing spondylitis, psoriatic arthritis, reactive arthritis, or inflammatory bowel disease. These cases are referred to as undifferentiated spondyloarthritis.

ANKYLOSING SPONDYLITIS

Ankylosing spondylitis (AS) is a chronic progressive joint inflammation of axial skeleton, with prevalence in the United States of 0.1% to 0.5%. The disease often manifests with pain and stiffness in the spine, often beginning in the teen years and early 20s. White males are the most commonly affected group by a 9:1 ratio.

Clinical Manifestations

The presenting symptom is often intermittent back pain, usually lumbar, that may radiate down into the thighs. It is worse on arising and often associated with morning stiffness but improves with exercise. The disease progresses gradually with ascending spinal inflammation and a loss of back motion due to ankylosis. There may also be buttock pain from sacroiliac involvement. One third of all cases progress to involve the shoulders and hips. Costovertebral joint involvement may cause chest pain and restricted chest expansion. There are otherwise few specific systemic symptoms to the disease; fatigue and malaise may accompany the condition.

The clinical examination can reveal (in progressed disease) loss of lumbar lordosis, which fails to reverse with forward flexion thoracic kyphosis, flexion of the neck, all leading to a stooped posture.

Diagnosis

Laboratory evaluation is limited. There is an elevation of the erythrocyte sedimentation rate in up to 85% of cases with characteristically negative rheumatoid factor serology. There is an association with HLA-B27 antigen, but this is neither sensitive nor specific given its prevalence in the healthy white population. Imaging with plain radiographs may progress from normal studies to sacroiliitis, squaring of the vertebral bodies, and eventual ligamentous ossification and joint fusion with the characteristic "bamboo spine" pattern.

Treatment

Treatment of AS involves anti-inflammatory medications, initially with aspirin or nonsteroidal anti-inflammatories, and later with anticytokine agents such as anti–tumor necrosis factor (TNF) agents.

TABLE 51.1 Features of spondyloarthropathies

	Sacroiliitis	Spine	Peripheral arthritis	Iritis	Aortitis	Cutaneous	Gastrointestinal	Genitourinary
Ankylosing spondylitis	+ + +[a]	+ + +[b]	+	+	+ +	–	–	–
Reiter's syndrome	+ + +[c]	+ + +[d]	+ + +[e]	+ +[f]	+	+ + +	+ +	+ + +
Psoriatic arthritis	+ +[c]	+ +[c]	+	+	+	+ + +	–	–
Inflammatory bowel disease	+ + +[a]	+ + +[b]		+	+	–	+ + + +	–

[a] Bilateral involvement.
[b] Ascending pattern.
[c] Can be asymmetric (i.e., unilateral syndesmophyte or one side larger than the other).
[d] Tendency toward "skip pattern" (i.e., skips vertebral segments).
[e] Usually in lower extremity.
[f] Conjunctivitis is the first manifestation in most patients.

There is little evidence that immunomodulatory agents such as methotrexate and sulfasalazine benefit axial disease. There is generally little use for systemic corticosteroids.

Physical therapy and exercise help maintain range of motion and limit symptoms. Surgery is limited to hip replacement in affected individuals, or cervical spinal fusion with atlantoaxial subluxation.

Complications

The long-term course of AS is of gradual progression of disease over the course of decades, with very little impact on overall mortality. Small percentages go on to develop fibrosis of the cauda equina with associated radicular symptoms—the "cauda equina syndrome." Atlantoaxial subluxation can cause spinal cord compression. Nonarticular symptoms include anterior uveitis in up to one quarter of patients, and inflammation of the aortic root causing aortic insufficiency or atrioventricular conduction disturbances. The rarer manifestations include renal disease with immunoglobulin A nephropathy or amyloidosis, bowel mucosal ulceration, osteopenia, restricted chest expansion, and apical lung infiltrates that may cavitate.

REITER'S SYNDROME AND REACTIVE ARTHRITIS

Reiter's syndrome and reactive arthritis are characterized by sterile joint inflammation following infections at nonarticular sites, often related to sexually transmitted infections (most commonly with *Chlamydia trachomatis*) or postdysentery (when infected with *Shigella*, *Salmonella*, *Yersinia*, *Campylobacter*, or *Clostridium difficile*). Reiter's syndrome complicates up to 2% of nongonococcal infections, and up to 1.5% of dysentery (formally termed "reactive arthritis" in these cases).

Clinical Manifestations

Reiter's syndrome features the classic triad of arthritis, conjunctivitis, and nongonococcal urethritis. The arthritis tends to be oligoarticular and involving lower extremity joints more than upper extremity. Enthesitis (inflammation of the tendons or tendon-bone insertions) is commonly noted at the insertion sites of the plantar fascia and the Achilles tendon. Other features include spondylitis, mucocutaneous lesions (painless ulcers on the tongue, palate, and glans of the penis), keratoderma blenorrhagicum (a characteristic hyperkeratotic rash on the soles or palms), urogenital involvement (including prostatitis, urethritis, circinate balanitis, and occasionally cystitis), and remote system involvement (such as pericarditis, peripheral neuropathy, or constitutional symptoms of fever, weight loss, and malaise).

Symptoms will often develop 1 to 2 weeks after sexual exposure, or within the timespan for the foodborne infection, and can last for several months. Ninety-five percent of cases will resolve within 6 months, although half will have a recurrence over the next several years with a risk of approximately 10% per year. A minority of cases will develop persistent arthritis.

Diagnosis

Diagnosis is based on the constellation of symptoms and clinical features; it requires the presence of the arthritis with urethritis or cervicitis, and at least one of the extra-articular features. Half of patients will have evidence of *Chlamydia* infection with antichlamydial antibodies, antigens, or organism fragments on biopsy, or positive cultures. Sedimentation rates and white blood counts will typically be elevated, and there may be a concurrent normochromic anemia.

Treatment

Treatment is directed at the offending bacteria, with doxycycline (100 mg twice daily for 7 to 14 days) for *Chlamydia* infections, and ciprofloxacin (500 mg twice daily for 7 to 28 days, depending on the risk of a carrier state) for the *Salmonella*, *Shigella*, *Yersinia*, and *Campylobacter* infections. Other treatments are symptomatic, such as nonsteroidal anti-inflammatory medications for the treatment of the arthritis. Refractory arthritis can also be treated with methotrexate, sulfasalazine, or azathioprine. The mucocutaneous lesions and conjunctivitis are also treated symptomatically, except for uveitis, which may require intraocular steroids.

PSORIATIC ARTHRITIS

Psoriatic arthritis is an inflammatory condition affecting the peripheral or spinal joints that occurs in approximately 6% of cases of psoriasis. Psoriasis itself involves approximately 1% to 2% of the population. Psoriatic arthritis is thought to have a strong—albeit complex—genetic predisposition, with HLA and non-HLA loci identified. It is more common in women and more often develops in early to middle adulthood.

Clinical Manifestations

Seventy percent of cases are asymmetric oligoarthritides; 5% to 15% of cases involve only the distal interphalangeal joints; 15% are symmetric and can mimic rheumatoid arthritis. In 5% of cases, the most destructive form of psoriatic arthritis, termed "arthritis mutilans," can occur with severe osteolysis and telescoping of fingers ("opera-glass hands") and spinal involvement. In most cases (75%), the skin lesions precede joint inflammation, in 15% the arthritis comes first, and in the remaining 10% the two develop concurrently. The severity of the dermatitis does not correlate well with the arthritis.

Other features common to the other seronegative spondyloarthropathies include enthesitis of the Achilles tendon, pelvic bones, and plantar fascia; tenosynovitis of the hand flexor tendons; and dactylitis ("sausage" finger or toe). Nail lesions (pits, transverse depressions, subungual hyperkeratosis, and onycholysis) are frequently seen.

Diagnosis

Laboratory tests are helpful in excluding other diseases, and rheumatoid factor and antinuclear antibody tests are usually (although not always) negative. Elevations can be seen in the erythrocyte sedimentation rate and C-reactive protein, and there may be a concurrent anemia and hyperuricemia. In severe psoriatic arthritis, radiographs show a whittling of the distal phalanges causing the "pencil in cup" (acro-osteolysis) appearance that is common in psoriatic arthritis. Erosions and effusions in the absence of osteopenia are also commonly found, as are the fluffy changes of periostitis.

Treatment

Treatment is similar to rheumatoid arthritis, with steroid-sparing agents as the first line—acetaminophen and nonsteroidal anti-inflammatory agents. In more severe, progressive, or refractory cases, methotrexate, azathioprine, and sulfasalazine may be effective. Antimalarials such as hydroxychloroquine may help with the arthritis, but can precipitate a dermatitis flare. Psoralen ultraviolet A, when used for psoriatic dermatitis, may improve symptoms in peripheral joints as well. Anti-TNF agents have proved to be valuable additions to the treatment of both skin and joint disease in patients not responding to conventional therapies.

ARTHRITIS AND INFLAMMATORY BOWEL DISEASE

Inflammatory bowel disease (IBD) can present with multiple extraintestinal manifestations, the most common of which is anemia, and the second most common is arthritis. This affects 20% of patients with IBD, and occurs more often with Crohn's disease (20%) than with ulcerative colitis (12%).

Clinical Manifestations

Two types of arthritis tend to develop in IBD. The first involves peripheral joint arthritis, usually of the large joints; this tends to be an asymmetric oligoarthritis that parallels flairs of the IBD. The second is a spondylitis very similar to ankylosing spondylitis and is independent of the intestinal flares.

Diagnosis

The diagnosis of arthritis associated with inflammatory bowel disease is made largely on clinical grounds. Pattern of presentation and the finding of joint involvement on physical examination in the context of inflammatory bowel disease meet the criteria for diagnosis.

Laboratory tests often reveal a mild anemia. Sedimentation rate and C-reactive protein are often elevated. Antinuclear antibodies and rheumatoid factor generally are negative. pANCA is positive in 60% of patients with ulcerative colitis and somewhat less often in patients with Crohn's disease. If spondylitis is suspected, x-rays of the sacroiliac joints may reveal sacroiliitis.

Treatment

Treatment is more limited, because nonsteroidal agents used in other arthritides are not safe for use in IBD for fear of precipitating bowel ischemia, or of precipitating a flare-up of the intestinal disease. When appropriate, treatment should be directed at the bowel disease. The spine disease is treated similarly to ankylosing spondylitis, with physical therapy.

The peripheral disease is treated similarly to psoriatic arthritis, and methotrexate, sulfasalazine, and azathioprine are helpful. Infliximab may be helpful, but runs the risks of severe side effects, particularly in patients not receiving treatment on a continuing basis.

CHAPTER 52

Wegener's, Polyarteritis Nodosa, Polymyalgia Rheumatica, and Temporal Arteritis

Steven Denson and Paul Halverson

Vasculitis is a broad, heterogenous group of disorders commonly linked by the presence of inflammation (as manifested by the presence of leukocytes), ischemia, and necrosis in blood vessel walls, as well as more generalized tissue ischemia in the surrounding tissues or affected organs. A common classification system divides vasculitides based on the size of vessels involved (small, medium, and large), but often the grouped conditions have little clinical, histological, or serologic similarity. This classification is shown in Table 52.1.

Polyarteritis nodosa (PAN) is a systemic necrotizing vasculitis involving primarily the medium size and occasionally the small muscular arteries. It has a mean age of onset of about 50 years, and the incidence increases with age. PAN affects men more than twice as often as women. *Wegener's granulomatosis* is a multisystem vasculitis occurring in small to medium arteries as well as involvement of arterioles and venules. Men and women are equally affected, and the mean age of onset is 40 years, although it can occur at any age. *Giant cell arteritis,* often referred to as temporal arteritis, is a granulomatous arteritis of predominantly large vessels, but may also affect medium-sized arteries. The most affected vessels are the cranial vessels, but the aorta and some of its branches can also be affected. Women are twice as likely as men to develop this. It is extremely unlikely in patients younger than 50 years of age. *Polymyalgia rheumatica* (PMR) is a syndrome, closely related to giant cell arteritis, featuring neck, shoulder, and hip girdle pain and stiffness in the morning. It is thought to be part of a continuum of giant cell arteritis that also includes temporal arteritis. Like giant cell arteritis, PMR is rare before the age of 50 years, with a mean age of onset of 70 years, and women are twice as likely as men to be affected. The cause is unknown.

ETIOLOGY

The mechanisms are not well understood, but thought to include immune complex–mediated damage and a secondary inflammatory response in the vessels. Cell-mediated immunity is the likely cause in most forms of vasculitis. Vasculitides are broadly characterized as primary (arising without a clear predisposing factor) or secondary (related to another condition, such as systemic lupus erythematosus, rheumatoid arthritis, or an infection). In general the underlying causes remain unknown, although there are likely genetic and environmental components to the process.

PAN is thought to be immune complex–mediated. Thirty to 50% of cases have an associated hepatitis B antigenemia, and hepatitis B antigen, immunoglobulin, and complement in the vessel walls. Histology of the vessels reveals segmental transmural inflammation with areas of necrosis with damage to the internal and external elastic lamina. Also notable is the absence of venous involvement and of granulomatous inflammation. Wegener's granulomatosis also is mediated by immune complex deposition and an autoimmune response, although the triggers are less well defined. Pathology usually reveals granulomatous arteritis of all sizes of vessels.

TABLE 52.1 Types of features of vasculitis based on blood vessel size

Medium to large arteries	
Temporal arteritis	Giant cell arteritis, affects mostly cranial arteries in the elderly
Takayasu arteritis	Aortic arch involvement in young, usually Asian women
Small to medium arteries	
Polyarteritis group Polyarteritis nodosa	Necrotizing vasculitis with renal, abdominal, coronary, central nervous system and peripheral nerve involvement
Churg-Strauss vasculitis	Similar to above with pulmonary involvement and eosinophilia
Overlap syndrome	Features of several types of vasculitis
Small to medium arteries, veins	
Wegener's granulomatosis	Granulomatous vasculitis, involves upper and/or lower respiratory tract, eyes, ears, kidneys, skin
Arterioles, capillaries, venules	
Hypersensitivity vasculitis	Leukocytoclastic vasculitis (often with "palpable" purpura)
Rheumatoid vasculitis Lupus vasculitis Drug-induced vasculitis Essential mixed cryoglobulinemia Malignancy Henoch-Schönlein purpura	Purpura, joint pain, abdominal pain, glomerulitis

CLINICAL MANIFESTATIONS

Polyarteritis Nodosa

PAN tends to involve the kidney, gastrointestinal tract, skin, muscles, joints, genitourinary and reproductive systems, nervous system (both central and peripheral), and heart. It questionably affects the lungs, reflecting a difficulty in clinically distinguishing PAN from allergic granulomatosis (Churg-Strauss syndrome), which has a frequent background of asthma and eosinophilia.

Presenting symptoms are often nonspecific but reflect multisystem involvement including fever, weakness, weight loss, malaise, livedo reticularis, and abdominal pain. Other symptoms relate to the organ system affected by the vascular involvement. For example, mesenteric arteritis can cause abdominal pain (and can cause an acute abdomen), cholecystitis, nausea, vomiting, and bleeding. Renal arteritis can cause progressive renal failure, hypertension (particularly new-onset diastolic hypertension), hematuria, and proteinuria. Nervous system involvement can cause seizures, stroke, headache, and mononeuropathy multiplex (nontraumatic involvement of two or more portions of the peripheral nervous system in different areas of the body).

Other characteristic symptoms involve the skin, particularly erythematous subcutaneous nodules, persistent livedo reticularis, and purpura. Muscle weakness, myalgia, and arthralgia are common, as is myocardial ischemia. There are no pathognomonic findings but physical examination is useful to help define the extent of the disease.

Wegener's Granulomatosis

The classic triad of organ system involvement includes the kidney, upper, and lower respiratory tract involvement. Upper airway involvement usually includes otitis, mucositis, and sinusitis. There can also be involvement of the peripheral and central nervous systems, skin, eyes, gastrointestinal tract, and joints with either granulomatous disease or vasculitis, or both.

Symptoms of arthralgia, fever, cough, and nasal complaints (drainage, bleeding, sinus pain) are the most common presenting complaints. Pulmonary infiltrates are found in approximately three quarters of patients, sinusitis in approximately two thirds, and arthralgias in slightly less than one half. Fevers and cough occur in only one third of patients. The eyes are involved in half of patients, ranging from conjunctivitis to uveitis, and should be evaluated in any patients with a suspected diagnosis. Likewise, skin lesions such as papules, ulcers, or subcutaneous nodules are also found in approximately half of patients. Disease complications can include saddle nose deformities from septal necrosis, deafness from refractory otitis, interstitial lung disease, and skin ulcers or gangrene.

Giant Cell Arteritis

Visual disturbances are very common, and transient blindness (amaurosis fugax) without any evidence of disease to the eye itself should increase the index of suspicion. Other symptoms include tenderness and claudication of the jaw or tongue particularly with chewing, neurological symptoms (usually transient ischemic attack or strokelike symptoms), a sore throat and cough, or a low-grade fever. More generalized arthralgias, myalgias, or arthritis can also develop. Physical examination may reveal palpable temporal arteries with tenderness.

Polymyalgia Rheumatica

Typical manifestations include neck, shoulder, and hip girdle pain, associated with myalgia, and malaise, fatigue, and weight loss. Stiffness is a prominent symptom, especially in the morning and after prolonged inactivity (gelling). Physical examination is relatively nonspecific but tenderness should be limited to muscles and not involve the joints themselves.

DIAGNOSIS

Polyarteritis Nodosa

Diagnosis is clinically based on history with corroborating physical findings. The American College of Rheumatology has established 10 criteria for diagnosis:

1. Unexplained weight loss of more than 4 kg
2. Myalgias weakness or polyneuropathy
3. New-onset hypertension of greater than 90 mm Hg
4. Neuropathy (either mononeuropathy or polyneuropathy)
5. Livedo reticularis
6. Testicular pain or tenderness
7. Serologic evidence of current or prior hepatitis B infection
8. Elevated serum blood urea nitrogen or creatinine levels
9. Arteriographic abnormalities not otherwise explained
10. Biopsy evidence of neutrophils in small- to medium-sized arteries

There are no diagnostic laboratory tests, and abnormalities tend to reflect the organ systems involved. There tends to be an elevation in the erythrocyte sedimentation rate (ESR), C-reactive protein, rheumatoid factor, and leukocyte count (specifically neutrophil count). Positive hepatitis B or C serology increases suspicion. Cryoglobulinemia or low complement levels (C3 or C4) occur in about one quarter of cases. Urinalysis showing abnormal sedimentation suggests renal involvement, and elevated creatinine kinase (CK) levels suggest muscle involvement, blood urea nitrogen, and creatinine. An elevated antineutrophil cytoplasmic antibody (ANCA) level argues against PAN but does not necessarily rule it out. Imaging can show aneurysm formation related to the damaged vessel walls (i.e., mesenteric, renal, or hepatic artery aneurysms), and would support the diagnosis. Ideally a tissue biopsy of an affected area's arteries shows the necrotizing inflammation at varying stages described above, whereas affected organs may show thrombosis or infarction.

Wegener's Granulomatosis

Laboratory evaluation of Wegener's includes a markedly elevated ESR and ANCA (particularly c-ANCA, which is reasonably specific; p-ANCA is nonspecific but also elevated) levels, low to moderate elevations of rheumatoid factor, leukocytosis, thrombocytosis, and anemia on complete blood count, and evidence of renal involvement either with elevated creatinine levels or a urinalysis showing hematuria, cellular casts, and proteinuria. Radiographic evaluation includes chest x-rays showing multiple bilateral nodular cavitary infiltrates and densities. Sinus films and computed tomography scans can show evidence of bony erosion. Diagnosis is based on biopsies with a compatible clinical presentation. Biopsies should be taken from involved tissues, and should demonstrate granulomatous inflammation of an artery.

Giant Cell Arteritis

The American College of Rheumatology requires three of five criteria to support the diagnosis of giant cell arteritis:

1. Disease onset after the age of 50 years
2. New headache localized to the scalp area or to one temple
3. Tenderness of the temporal artery or decreased pulsation
4. Elevated erythrocyte sedimentation rate (ESR) levels of greater than 50 mm/hr
5. Arterial biopsy (usually of a temporal artery) showing either a necrotizing arteritis with a predominance of mononuclear cells or a granulomatous process with multinucleated giant cells in the intima or media of large vessels

Alternative criteria include tenderness and claudication of the jaw or tongue, particularly with chewing, if the ESR is not elevated (may occur in 10% of patients).

Laboratory evaluation focuses on the ESR, and on excluding other diseases. It is common to see mild normocytic normochromic anemia, and increased acute phase reactants (elevated white blood cell and platelet counts). Imaging with cranial arteriography may help with the diagnosis if areas of smooth-walled constriction can be seen, although this is not often done in clinical situations. The formal diagnosis is usually based on biopsy. Typically a 2- to 6-cm portion of temporal artery on the affected side is taken because there tends to be skip lesions. A contralateral biopsy can be performed if the initial one is negative.

Polymyalgia Rheumatica

Laboratory analysis is generally non specific and not diagnostic. There is typically a very high ESR along with other acute phase reactants such as C-reactive protein, fibrinogen, complement, and platelet counts. Serum creatinine kinase and muscle enzyme levels are usually normal, as are other muscle evaluations such as electromyelogram and muscle biopsy. There are no imaging tests to help confirm the diagnosis, although they help to rule out other conditions.

TREATMENT

Polyarteritis Nodosa

Management of PAN is dependent on the stage of the disease, and on the organ systems involved. Initial therapy with corticosteroids is usually beneficial, and monotherapy will induce disease remission in half of the cases. Intravenous therapy can be started in severe cases. Cyclophosphamide is added to the regimen in the refractory half, and methotrexate can be added as a steroid-sparing agent to help maintain response. Azathioprine is also used in certain settings as an adjunctive treatment. Therapy is maintained for 6 to 12 months to decrease the chance of relapse. Angiotensin-converting enzyme inhibitors are effective in treating hypertension. Other treatments depend on and are specific to the organ systems involved. Five-year survival with treatment is approximately 80%, with most deaths occurring within the first 18 months of the disease. Untreated PAN has a 13% 5-year survival.

Wegener's Granulomatosis

Treatment is initiated with prednisone at high doses, with cyclophosphamide added either to critically ill patients, or to maintain remission. Azathioprine has been used as an alternative to cyclophosphamide in patients who cannot tolerate it. Methotrexate is also used to maintain remission. Trimethoprim-sulfamethoxazole has been occasionally used either as single therapy in limited disease, or to augment the prednisone and cyclophosphamide. Treatment is usually 3 to 6 months to induce remission, then for 1 to 2 years to maintain remission before considering tapering. Untreated, Wegener's is nearly always fatal, usually from progressive renal failure.

Giant Cell Arteritis

Prednisone is the first line of treatment, and confirmed disease requires on average 2 to 4 years of treatment to induce remission. Initial high dose (60 mg/day) steroids can be tapered after 1 to 2 months slowly to a maintenance dose of 10 to 15 mg, and then adjusted by symptoms and ESR level. Methotrexate is used when there is a contraindication to steroids (such as brittle diabetes, heart failure, and osteoporosis).

Blindness is a significant risk if temporal arteritis develops (up to 20% depending on studies), and other complications can develop when active arteritis is present, such as stroke. When the diagnosis is strongly suspected, steroids should be started even before a biopsy is done although ideally a biopsy should be performed within 4 days of starting steroids.

Polymyalgia Rheumatica

Treatment is usually with prednisone at low doses of 15 mg/day, and the response is often dramatic and rapid. Symptoms improve or resolve within 1 to 2 days of initiation. This response is also used to presumptively confirm the diagnosis. Prednisone is usually continued at a very slow taper over 24 to 36 months, and the average length of the disease is 3 years. Relapses are common, although the general prognosis with treatment is good.

CHAPTER 53

Gout and Other Crystal-Induced Synovitis

Diedre Faust and Paul Halverson

Crystals associated with synovial inflammation include monosodium urate (gout), calcium pyrophosphate dihydrate (pseudogout), and, less often, hydroxyapatite, oxalate, and adrenocorticosteroid esters. Cholesterol crystals are occasionally found in chronic joint effusions but probably are inert. Acute crystal-induced arthritis is rapid in onset and self-limited. Differences in crystal morphology and clinical features are helpful in diagnosis.

The pathophysiology of crystal-induced synovitis is incompletely understood. Although crystals certainly are causative in acute gouty arthritis and pseudogout, crystals occasionally may be seen in quiescent joints as well. The precise inciting event in vivo is unknown but may involve crystal shedding from preformed cartilaginous or synovial deposits. Crystal phagocytosis by neutrophils in vitro induces release of lysosomal enzymes, humoral mediators, and chemotactic factors associated with acute inflammation.

Gout is the most common cause of crystal-induced synovitis and probably the best understood.

GOUT

Gout is a metabolic disease in which hyperuricemia and arthritis are variably expressed. Gout is caused by the deposition of monosodium urate crystals in the synovium. It occurs primarily in men, with onset usually in the fourth through sixth decades; in women, it is more likely to follow menopause.

Etiology

Gout is linked to high levels of uric acid; however, there is not an absolute association between hyperuricemia and gout. Hyperuricemia is a biochemical abnormality defined solely by the serum urate concentration that results from increased production of urate, decreased excretion, or both (Table 53.1). Acute gout may be triggered by trauma, alcohol ingestion (particularly beer), acute medical illness, surgical procedures, and certain drugs (Table 53.1). Dietary factors also seem to play a role. Increased meat ingestion seems to be correlated with gouty attacks, but starvation has also been associated. Colder temperatures and poorly perfused distal joints also make gouty attacks more likely. Not all factors responsible for the precipitation of urate crystals are known, however, because hyperuricemia does occur without urolithiasis or gout.

Clinical Manifestations

Three possible stages of gout exist: acute gouty arthritis, intercritical gout, and tophaceous gout.

Acute gout features acute inflammatory arthritis, which usually is monoarticular and most often involves lower extremity joints. An acute gouty attack is very painful. In 60% of cases, the first attack involves the first metatarsophalangeal (MTP) joint (podagra) or other joints in the foot. Acute gout also may occur in the ankle, the prepatellar or olecranon bursae, and midfoot, in which location it may resemble cellulitis (gouty cellulitis). Within a few hours, the affected joint becomes red, swollen,

TABLE 53.1 Conditions associated with hyperuricemia

Urate Overproduction	Urate Renal Underexcretion
Idiopathic (primary) gout	Idiopathic (primary) gout
Inherited enzymatic defects	Clinical disorders
Polycythemia vera	Hypertension
Paget's disease	Dehydration
Hemolytic diseases	Obesity
Psoriasis	Sarcoidosis
Obesity	Renal insufficiency
Myelo- and lymphoproliferative diseases	Lead toxicity
Drugs Cytotoxic agents High-dose salicylates Ethanol Warfarin	Drugs Ethanol Diuretics Low-dose salicylates Cyclosporine Levodopa
	Starvation Acidosis Toxemia of pregnancy Salt restriction

warm, and tender, but usually the attack resolves on its own within a few days to a few weeks without leaving apparent sequelae. Fever may be present. In a minority, the initial episode may be polyarticular. Tophi (discussed later in this chapter) usually follow years of gout; they are rare in conjunction with the first attack.

As the acute gouty attack subsides, the patient becomes asymptomatic (intercritical gout). In most patients, a second attack occurs within 6 months to 2 years. Ensuing attacks may become polyarticular and may last longer, yielding a different clinical picture from early gout. In this later phase, gout is suggested by prior hyperuricemia, a history of gout, palpable tophi, and episodes of acute arthritis.

If recurrent gout is untreated, nodules (tophi) can develop on the extensor surfaces of the elbows, in joints, and in surrounding tissues, especially the interphalangeal joints of the hands or feet and the helix of the ear. Tophi usually are firm and, when aspirated, yield a chalky white material containing monosodium urate crystals.

Chronic tophaceous gout may mimic rheumatoid arthritis, with arthralgias, progressive stiffness, nodules, joint swelling, and deformity (Fig. 53.1), and even a high erythrocyte sedimentation rate and positive rheumatoid factor. Acute attacks manifest only soft-tissue swelling on radiographs, but chronic gout manifests punched-out erosions at the ends of phalanges, most commonly at the medial aspects of the head of the first MTP joint. These are highly typical of tophaceous gout.

Diagnosis

The diagnosis of gout is made by clinical findings and also aspiration of monosodium urate crystals from the synovium. Patients with gout will have clinical symptoms as above. Symptoms that are specifically helpful in making the diagnosis of gout are rapid development of severe pain, erythema,

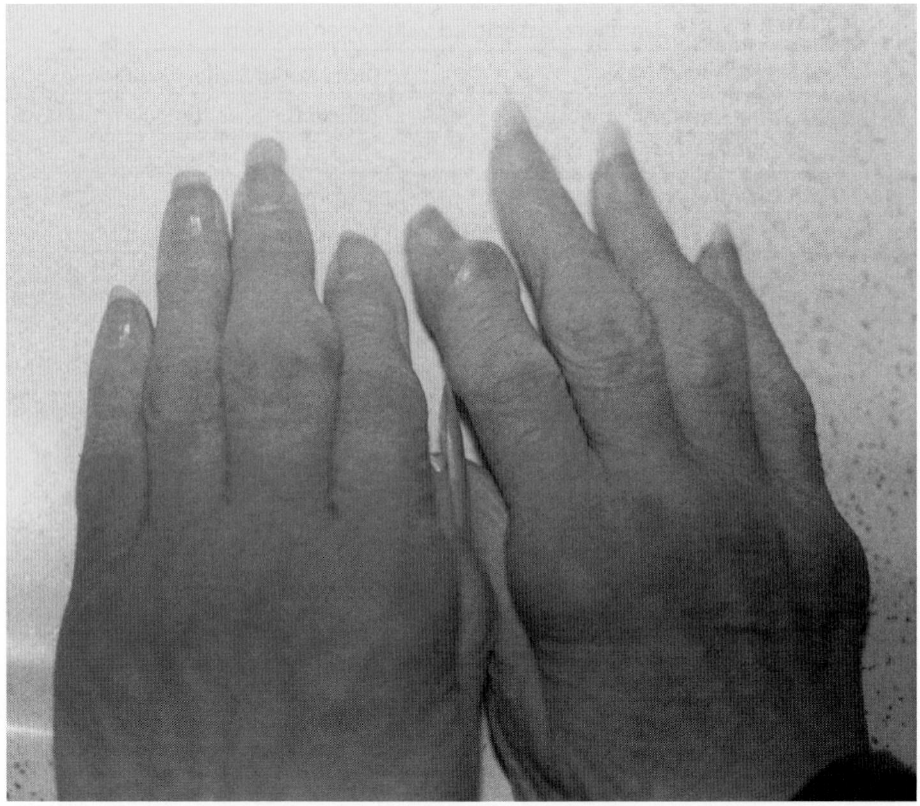

Figure 53.1 • Hands of an elderly woman with chronic tophaceous gout. Some of the tophi appear to have formed in joints with previous osteoarthritic changes.

swelling, and involvement of the first metatarsal. Hyperuricemia is characteristic of gout; however, normal serum urate values may be seen during the acute attack. Plain radiographs may be helpful in chronic gout; indeed, tophi may be detected first on radiographs before they are clinically recognized. However, radiographs are not helpful in diagnosing early-onset gout or acute gouty attacks. A clinical response to empiric treatment with colchicine is very suggestive.

Definitive diagnosis requires identification of monosodium urate crystals aspirated from the affected joint, a tophus, or even from an asymptomatic (e.g., seemingly unaffected) first MTP joint. Synovial effusions in acute gout typically are inflammatory (5,000 to 50,000 leukocytes/mm^3, mostly neutrophils). Characteristic needle-shaped, strongly negatively birefringent crystals of monosodium urate crystals are seen either intra- or extracellularly on synovial fluid examination with a compensated polarizing microscope.

Treatment

ACUTE MANAGEMENT

Nonsteroidal anti-inflammatory drugs (NSAIDs) or colchicine are the usual first lines of treatment for acute gout. Oral colchicine is given in doses of 0.6 mg every 1 to 2 hours until either gout improves, gastrointestinal side effects (nausea, vomiting, or diarrhea) occur, or a total of 3.0 to 4.0 mg has been given. Intravenous colchicine, 1 to 2 mg, one or two doses, avoids gastrointestinal side effects. Colchicine should be used in lesser doses or not at all in elderly persons or patients with impaired renal function because of the increased risks of bone marrow suppression. A clinical response is not specific for gout because other crystal arthropathies, such as acute pseudogout or calcific tendinitis, also may respond.

Indomethacin, up to 200 mg/day in divided doses, usually for 4 to 5 days, is effective and more convenient than colchicine, but the maximal dosage often produces central nervous system and gastrointestinal side effects. Other NSAIDs may be similarly effective but have been used less commonly in acute gout. Oral steroids are particularly useful in patients with polyarticular gout who do not respond to initial therapies or for those who have contraindications to NSAIDs and colchicine. Intra-articular steroids are helpful for patients with monoarticular gout and those who cannot take oral medications. Other alternatives when oral therapy is not possible include intravenous (IV) methylprednisolone (20 to 50 mg/day), adrenocorticotropic hormone (40 to 80 U/day), or IV colchicine.

PROPHYLAXIS

Small doses of colchicine (0.6 mg once or twice daily) or another NSAID may be prescribed as prophylaxis against recurrent attacks, but this prophylaxis does not prevent crystal deposition and possible joint destruction. Instead, after acute gout resolves, chronic hypouricemic therapy should be initiated. Such therapy is indicated in patients with frequent recurrent attacks, tophi (clinically or radiographically manifest), or nephrolithiasis. Achieving a serum urate concentration <6.0 mg/dL prevents further monosodium urate crystal deposition (although some patients may require even further lowering of the serum urate).

Decreased uric acid excretion accounts for hyperuricemia in at least 90% of cases with the remainder being overproducers. A 24-hour urinary uric acid estimation should differentiate the overproducer from the underexcretor. The uricosuric drug probenecid may be used if the daily uric acid excretion is <800 mg per 24 hours on a regular diet or when allergy to allopurinol is present. It is contraindicated with creatinine clearance below 60 mL/min or nephrolithiasis.

Allopurinol and its metabolite oxypurinol inhibit xanthine oxidase to decrease uric acid synthesis. It is used in patients who excrete in excess of 800 mg uric acid per 24 hours on a regular diet and in those with severe tophaceous gout, chronic renal insufficiency, or allergy to uricosurics. Probenecid should be avoided in the overproducer because of the risk of nephrolithiasis. In contrast, allopurinol is commonly used in underexcretors because of its ease of administration (once-daily dosing).

The newest treatment available for gout is febuxostat. Febuxostat is a nonpurine xanthine oxidase inhibitor similar to allopurinol; however, it is not excreted by the kidneys and therefore may be safe in patients with mild to moderate renal failure

Complications

Recurrent gout attacks can lead to joint destruction, deformity, loss of function, and chronic pain. Chronic tophaceous gout can also lead to deformity and disability related to tophi deposition. Uncontrolled hyperuricemia is associated with several renal diseases: renal stones, urate nephropathy, and uric acid nephropathy. Uric acid renal stones occur in 10% to 25% of patients with gout but actually occur more often without gout or hyperuricemia. Urate nephropathy results from deposition of sodium urate crystals in the renal tubular epithelium and adjacent interstitium. It is rare in the absence of gout and is a late event in the natural history of gout, with very high serum urate levels.

CHAPTER 54

Infectious Arthritis

Steven Denson and Paul Halverson

Infectious arthritis is defined as bacterial, fungal, or viral infection of a joint and the tissues surrounding it. There are approximately 20,000 cases annually, with a slight male over female predominance. The type of infection varies with age, and we will address the most common adult causes here. (Please also see Chapter 61.)

ETIOLOGY

Bacterial

Bacterial arthritis accounts for most cases of septic arthritis, with half being caused by *Neisseria gonorrhea*, and a significant percentage of adult septic arthritis also caused by staphylococcal species, streptococcal species, and other gram-negative rods. Three million gonococcal infections occur annually in the United States, with 1% developing bacteremia and arthritis as a manifestation of disseminated gonococcal infection. Tuberculosis is a rare but important cause of infectious arthritis; it occurs in 1% to 3% of patients with tuberculosis. Staphylococcal infections, particularly *Staphylococcal aureus*, become more common with advancing age as compared to neisserial infections. These bacteria are able to bind to certain glycoproteins in joint spaces; therefore, they are more apt to cause septic arthritis and are the most common pathogens in postoperative joint infections. Most bacterial joint infections are monoarticular, but up to 10% can be polyarticular. Tuberculous joint infections can be polyarticular in up to 10% of cases, and Lyme disease tends to be polyarticular or to have migrating arthritis.

Bacterial infections tend to be spread hematogenously, or in rare occasions by direct inoculation of the joint through trauma or surgery. Those joints with prior injury from gout, other arthritides, the presences of a prosthesis or foreign body, or penetrating trauma are more likely to develop an infection. Although any joint can become infected, large joints such as the knees, hips, shoulders, or ankles are particularly vulnerable. Joint damage occurs as a result of proteolytic enzymes released by neutrophils in response to the infection, which then go on to damage the articular surface ground substance and erode the joint cartilage. Additional mediators and endotoxins from the bacteria themselves may further damage the joint cartilage. Individuals at risk of developing septic arthritis include the immunosuppressed (either through human immunodeficiency virus [HIV], medications, or illnesses that cause immunosuppression such as diabetes, malignancy, liver diseases, or congenital immunosuppression), intravenous (IV) drug abusers, those with other arthritis conditions, concurrently infected individuals, those with prosthetic joints, or those either undergoing joint surgery or with direct or penetrating trauma to a joint. IV drug users have a higher incidence of involvement in the sacroiliac or sternoclavicular joints. In patients with *Neisseria gonorrhea,* spread is usually hematogenous from the site of infection in the genital, rectal, or oral mucosa to the joints. Most vulnerable are the knees, hips, wrists, and ankles. In mycobacteria tuberculosis, spread is also usually hematogenous, but can also be from an adjacent osseous focus. Other mycobacterial organisms can cause infections, but this is usually limited to immunosuppressed individuals.

Fungal

Fungal infections are relatively uncommon and unusual causes of monarticular arthritis. Infection usually occurs from either hematogenous spread, or from direct inoculation with injury or surgery. Sporotrichosis (*Sporothrix schenckii*) can develop in gardeners or persons who work with contaminated soil. *Coccidioides immitis*, *Histoplasma capsulatum*, *Blastomyces dermatitidis*, *Pseudallescheria boydii*, *Cryptococcus neoformans*, *Candida*, and *Aspergillus* can be hematogenously spread in immunocompromised individuals, those with debilitating illnesses (such as diabetes or renal disease), intravenous drug users, or those with disseminated disease. *Candida* species have been identified in postoperative wound infections or in prosthetic joint infections.

Viral

Viral arthritis has a variety of common pathogens, with HIV, rubella, mumps paramyxovirus, human parvovirus B19, enteroviruses (Coxsackie and echovirus), hepatitis B and C viruses, and herpesvirus (mostly Epstein-Barr and varicella) being the most common pathogens. Various endemic areas have viral infections that cause arthritides, dependent on locale, such as alphavirus variants in Africa and Asia. Viruses can cause arthritis via direct synovial tissue infection, or as part of the immune response.

CLINICAL MANIFESTATIONS

Common presenting complaints usually include pain and tenderness in the affected joint, with limitation or loss of motion, tenosynovitis (inflammation of the tendon and its sheath), and effusion. Symptoms such as fevers, chills, and malaise may be present, but are unreliable because many other arthritic conditions can cause these as well. Up to 90% of patients will develop fevers at some point in the infection.

In patients with gonococcal arthritis, 10% of cases may be polyarticular, and there may be a distinctive dermatitis-arthritis-tenosynovitis (inflammation of the tendon and its surrounding sheath) picture. The typical dermatitis lesions occurring in neisserial infections are tender, petechial, or necrotic pustular nodules on an erythematous base. It is notable that monoarthritis in disseminated infection may also be present in 40% without skin lesions or tenosynovitis. Arthritis may also develop without genitourinary symptoms (although cultures will be positive in these areas).

With tubercular arthritis, half of all cases occur in the thoracic or lumbar spine as Pott's disease with possible paraspinous abscess formation. The remaining half are comprised of the weightbearing joints of the hips and knees (15% of cases) and the ankles and wrists (each 5% to 10%). Small joints are rarely involved. Diagnosis is often delayed because symptoms are usually less severe and more indolent. Often, early complaints of back pain and muscle spasms gradually progress into localized tenderness, nerve root compression with referred pain, and kyphosis in Pott's disease. In nonaxial joints, the early symptoms may only be of localized soft tissue swelling. Pulmonary symptoms of tuberculosis are unusual in skeletal tuberculosis.

Joint disease and arthritis related to *Borrelia burgdorferi* infection is usually a manifestation of late Lyme disease, although polyarticular migrating arthralgias and erythema migrans can be seen in early disease as well. The symptoms rarely reach the level of pain and inflammation seen in other infectious arthritides, and their presence should raise suspicion for other causes of arthritis.

In viral-induced arthritis, the pattern of infection is different for each type of virus, but ranges from monoarticular to symmetric polyarticular involvement and can be accompanied by systemic symptoms.

HIV presents with arthritis that can be caused both by the primary viral infection, and also as a bacterial infection related to the immunocompromised state. HIV can cause a severe form of Reiter's syndrome, with widespread joint involvement usually in the lower extremities and a rash resembling pustular psoriasis. Most joint infections in HIV are due to *Staphylococcus aureus*, *Streptococcus*, and *Salmonella*. Bacterial infection must be excluded before attributing the arthritis to the HIV virus.

DIAGNOSIS

Joint infections must be evaluated with arthrocentesis whenever the suspicion arises, preferably within 12 hours of suspicion, unless there is an overlying infection. Infected synovial fluid is usually cloudy, with low viscosity and poor mucin clot formation (a test evaluating clot formation when synovial fluid is mixed with 5% acetic acid in equal amounts) when compared to noninfected synovial fluid, which has a clear yellow color, high viscosity, good mucin clot formation, and low white blood cell (WBC) count with few neutrophils. The infected fluid cell count is usually greater than 50,000 WBC, but may range from 5,000 to 250,000 leukocytes/mm^3. A neutrophil predominance is common. Glucose levels in the fluid are usually less than 50% of concurrent serum samples. A Gram stain and culture of the fluid will reveal an organism in two thirds of cases. An exception is gonococcal arthritis, in which synovial analysis will not usually yield a gonococcal organism and cultures of the fluid are often negative. If gonococcal arthritis is suspected, rectal, urethral, and cervical cultures should be done. *Neiserria gonorrhea* and *Hemophilus influenza* should be grown on chocolate agar in addition to the blood agar plates. Additional cultures should also be obtained for fungal, mycobacterial, and anaerobic bacteria if there is clinical suspicion for these as infecting agents.

Diagnosis of tubercular disease is dependent on clinical suspicion and culture. Synovial fluid from these joints is usually positive on acid-fast stain in only 30% of cases, although cultures are positive in 80% and cultures from biopsied tissues are positive in 90%. Biopsy remains the quickest and most reliable diagnostic tool.

Most patients with Lyme disease who develop chronic symptoms are positive on enzyme-linked immunosorbent assay and Western blot testing, but this does not necessarily mean the arthritis is *Borrelia* related. Immunologic studies of the synovial fluid are recommended to confirm the presence of Lyme arthritis.

Any fungal organisms in a properly collected synovial specimen should be considered pathogenic. Diagnosis is usually dependent on biopsy and culture, which in turn defines the antifungal antibiotic choices.

In patients with septic arthritis, peripheral blood laboratory analysis will usually show elevated white blood count and acute phase reactants, such as elevated erythrocyte sedimentation rate (ESR) and markedly elevated C-reactive protein. Of note, ESR may be in a normal range in 20% of cases. Blood cultures should be drawn and, if positive, repeated while on antibiotic treatment until negative.

X-ray evaluation of the joint will often show only soft tissue swelling early in the course of the infection, but may start to show joint space loss in as early as 1 week due to damage and loss of cartilage, and thinning of the subchondral bone in as little as 2 days. Radiolucent areas can develop from gas-forming bacteria, but may also be a vacuum phenomenon in normal bone and joints. Tagged white blood cell scans will nonspecifically reveal inflammation and infection. Computed tomography and magnetic resonance imaging scans will also help determine if concurrent osteomyelitis is present by showing the extent of bone involvement or destruction, and may help define the extent of joint, cartilage, and tendon involvement. There are no unique radiographic findings for mycobacteria tuberculosis; chest radiography is normal in more than 50% of cases; however, the index of suspicion is higher in patients with active or old evidence of tuberculosis on chest radiograph with concurrent back or joint pain.

Diagnosis of viral arthritis is usually made through correlating clinical history and serologic tests. ESR is elevated and the synovial fluid is inflammatory (high neutrophil count, but not always as high as with bacterial; low viscosity; poor mucin clot formation) but gram-stain negative.

TABLE 54.1 Intravenous antibiotic therapy based on culture results

Organism	Antibiotic	Alternate
Staphylococcus	Nafcillin	Vancomycin
Streptococcus	Penicillin G	Vancomycin, cefazolin, clindamycin
Neisseria gonorrhoeae	Ceftriaxone	Spectinomycin
Haemophilus	Third-generation cephalosporin	Chloramphenicol
Enterobacteriaceae		
Escherichia coli, Salmonella, Klebsiella, Enterobacter, Proteus	Gentamicin	Tobramycin, amikacin
Pseudomonas	Antipseudomonal penicillin, plus gentamicin	

TREATMENT

The American College of Rheumatologists suggests that any inflammatory joint fluid in a febrile patient be considered infectious until excluded by culture. Antibiotics usually are initiated empirically after arthrocentesis and cultures are drawn, and are based on clinical suspicion (Tables 54.1 and 54.2). Unless gonococcal infection is suspected, parenteral antibiotics are started with a cephalosporin-based antibiotic plus vancomycin for gram-positive cocci. For gram-negative organisms, a third-generation cephalosporin should be started. An aminoglycoside should be added if *Pseudomonas*

TABLE 54.2 Initial antibiotic therapy for suspected septic arthritis with a negative Gram stain, based on patient's age

Age	Suggested regimen	Alternate	Coverage
<3 months	Penicillinase-resistant penicillin, third-generation cephalosporin		Gram-positive cocci, coliforms
3 months to 14 years	Penicillinase-resistant penicillin, third-generation cephalosporin	Vancomycin	Staphylococci, Streptococci, *H. influenzae*
15 to 40 years	Third-generation cephalosporin	Nafcillin (if Gram stain shows gram-positive cocci in clusters)	*Neisseria gonorrhoeae,* Staphylococci
>40 years	Penicillinase-resistant penicillin, third-generation cephalosporin	Vancomycin, percent third-generation cephalosporin	Staphylococci, coliforms

aeruginosa is suspected. If *Staphylococcus aureus* or gram-negative organisms are found, 3 to 4 weeks of parenteral antibiotics followed by 2 weeks of oral antibiotics are recommended. If anaerobic bacteria are suspected, then clindamycin is added. Management of gonococcal infections are with ceftriaxone 1 g IV or IM daily for at least 14 days or 7 days after symptoms resolve, or with spectinomycin 2 g IM every 12 hours for 10 days. Antibiotic therapy is tailored to culture and sensitivity results when available. Treatment for viral infections is supportive.

Treatment for mycobacteria tuberculosis–associated septic arthritis is the same as for pulmonary tuberculosis, namely isoniazid, rifampin, pyrazinamide, and ethambutol. A minimum 6-month course of therapy is recommended by the Centers for Disease Control and Prevention, with longer courses recommended in patients who are slow to respond or immunosuppressed. Surgical intervention is recommended in patients with spinal involvement and neurological deficits, severe kyphosis greater than 40 degrees, or progression of deficits despite therapy.

If Lyme disease is suspected, treatment is usually with oral penicillin or doxycycline for 4 to 6 weeks as the first line. Parenteral antibiotics might be helpful in refractory cases.

If fungal elements are identified, the nature of the organism dictates the antifungal drug selection. Surgical lavage of the infected joints is often necessary.

Pain should be treated initially by immobilization of the joint, with passive range of motion reintroduced gradually to prevent contractures and decreased joint motion. Anti-inflammatory pain medications should be avoided to prevent confusion over the therapeutic response. Effusions should be drained as often as necessary. A surgical consult should be obtained if the joint cannot be drained with arthrocentesis, the hip is infected, pus is loculated, or the arthritis is not responding to treatment within 3 to 4 days. In these cases, the joint may need to be irrigated and cleaned with an arthroscopy or arthrotomy, depending on the joint.

Infectious Diseases

Michael Frank

CHAPTER 55

Pneumonia

Jasna Jevtic

Despite great strides in infectious disease over the past century, pneumonia is still a common cause of morbidity and mortality among adults, particularly those with underlying diseases. It is the number one cause of death among infectious diseases in the United States and the seventh leading cause of death overall. There are approximately 5 million cases of pneumonia in the United States each year, with the majority of patients being treated as an outpatient. Over 1 million cases are still hospitalized annually.

Pneumonias are divided into two categories: community-acquired pneumonia (CAP) and nosocomial pneumonia which will be discussed here. Nosocomial pneumonia is defined as pneumonia developing after a patient has been hospitalized, usually for an unrelated condition.

The spectrum of nosocomial pneumonia can include hospital-associated pneumonia (HAP), health care–associated pneumonia (HCAP), and ventilator-associated pneumonia (VAP). HCAP includes any patient who was hospitalized in an acute care hospital for more than 2 days within 90 days of the infection; resided in a long-term care facility; received recent intravenous antibiotics, chemotherapy, or wound care within the past 30 days of the current infection; or attended a hospital or hemodialysis clinic. These categories are meant to provide a framework for the initial evaluation and management of the immunocompetent host with bacterial causes of pneumonia.

ETIOLOGY

The causative organisms for pneumonia vary with age, comorbidities, severity of disease, clinical setting (i.e., category), and geographic location.

Community-Acquired Pneumonia

Although *Sreptococcus pneumoniae* remains an important cause of CAP, its relative role has declined in recent years as newer pathogens have emerged. A specific etiology is identified in only about one half of cases of CAP. A few agents cause most cases, including: *S. pneumoniae, Haemophilus influenzae, Mycoplasma pneumoniae, Chlamydia pneumoniae, Legionella pneumophila,* or viruses. A longer list of encountered pathogens in the immunocompetent host is shown in Table 55.1.

Pneumonia occurs by three possible routes: inhalation or aspiration of organisms (most common), hematogenous spread, or contiguous spread of organisms (from peritonsillar abscess or pharyngeal infection).

Reasons contributing to the difficulty in isolating an organism are multifold. They include the initiation of empiric antibiotics prior to culture, the inability to expectorate an adequate sputum sample, and the difficulty in isolating organisms such as pneumococci even with an adequate sputum sample (i.e., containing abundant neutrophils).

Nosocomial Pneumonia

Pneumonia is the leading cause of death from nosocomial infection and ranks second to urinary tract infections for all causes of hospital-acquired infection, accounting for up to 15%. The most

TABLE 55.1 Causative agents in community-acquired pneumonia

Bacteria	Viruses
Streptococcus pneumoniae	Influenza
Haemophilus influenzae	Adenovirus
Legionella pneumophila	Respiratory syncytial virus
Mycoplasma pneumoniae	Severe acute respiratory syndrome
Chlamydia pneumoniae	Avian influenza
Anaerobes (oral)	**Fungi**
Moraxella catarrhalis	*Histoplasma capsulatum*
Staphylococcus aureus	*Coccidioides immitis*
Chlamydia psittaci	*Blastomyces dermatitidis*
Mycobacterium tuberculosis	*Cryptococcus neoformans*

common microbial causes are listed in Table 55.2. Pneumonia that develops in the hospital setting is due to either aspiration of oropharyngeal flora or bacteremia, with aspiration being the most frequent mechanism. Oropharyngeal colonization typically occurs within 2 days after hospitalization, with offending organisms such as *Pseudomonas aeruginosa*, enteric pathogens, and other gram-negative aerobic bacilli. Daily monitoring of cultures from various sites has shown that the enteric gram-negative organisms are primarily derived from the patient's own flora, whereas *P. aeruginosa* appears to be from the environment. Predisposing factors for nosocomial pneumonia are listed in Table 55.3.

Pneumonia in the Immunocompromised Host

Common causes of pneumonia as associated with specific defects in immune defenses are outlined in Table 55.4. Pneumonias in these patients may be acquired either at home or in the hospital, and

TABLE 55.2 Common causative microbes in nosocomial pneumonia

Agent	Approximate frequency (%)
Pseudomonas aeruginosa	17
Staphylococcus aureus	15
Klebsiella spp.	7
Escherichia coli	6
Haemophilus influenzae	6
Serratia marcescens *Proteus mirabilis* *Enterobacter spp.* *Acinetobacter spp.* *Legionella pneumophila*	5
Streptococcus pneumoniae	<3

TABLE 55.3 Predisposing factors associated with nosocomial pneumonia

Predisposing factor	Comment
Intubation, mechanical ventilation	Disruption of cough mechanism; damage to respiratory epithelium, equipment colonized by bacteria
Respiratory (aerosol-generating) equipment	Equipment colonized by bacteria; frequent handling of tubes
Advanced age	Poor cough, impaired local defenses
Underlying disease	Debilitation, increased aspiration risk
Prior antibiotics	Selection
Recent surgery	Aspiration
Antacids, H_2 blockers	Increased stomach colonization and subsequent aspiration
Poor infection control precautions (e.g., hand washing)	Enhanced risk of transmission of gram-negative organisms from patient to patient within the same units

TABLE 55.4 Pneumonia in the immunocompromised host

Immune defect (clinical examples)	Common microbes causing pneumonia	Common chest radiographic patterns
Neutropenia		
Cancer chemotherapy	Gram-negative bacilli	No infiltrate/lobar
	Staphylococcus aureus	No infiltrate/lobar
	Aspergillus spp.	Cavitary/diffuse
γ-Globulin deficiency/dysfunction		
Multiple myeloma	*Streptococcus pneumoniae*	Lobar
Acquired immune deficiency syndrome Common variable hypogammaglobulinemia Lymphoma	*Haemophilus influenzae*	
Cell-mediated deficiency		
Acquired immune deficiency syndrome	*Pneumocystis carinii*	Diffuse
Transplant	*Cryptococcus neoformans*	Nodular/cavitary/diffuse
Corticosteroid therapy	*Aspergillus spp.*	Nodular/cavitary/diffuse
	Mycobacterium spp.	Diffuse
	Legionella spp.	Lobar/diffuse
	Herpes viruses	Diffuse

the clinician must be aware of the possibility of one of these immune defects when taking the patient's history. The clinical features and diagnosis of pneumonia in the immunocompromised host will be discussed separately in the appropriate chapters (Chapters 63, 101, and E7).

CLINICAL MANIFESTATIONS

Community-Acquired Pneumonia

Given the many etiologies in CAP, clues from the medical history, environmental history, and host factors (i.e., underlying disease) may be helpful in suggesting the causative organism (Table 55.5). Symptoms of pneumonia include fever, chills, pleuritic chest pain, and cough, which may or may not be productive. Confusion, gastrointestinal symptoms, and hepatic dysfunction, once felt to be specific to *Legionella* pneumonia, are no longer considered unique to it.

Pulmonary examination is important; however, a normal lung examination does not exclude the presence of pneumonia. On palpation, if typical consolidation is present, tactile fremitus is increased in the affected area and dullness to percussion is also found. On auscultation rales, crackles or bronchial breath sounds may be heard. In addition, egophony (E to A change), bronchophony, and whispered pectoriqui may be detected upon auscultation. These maneuvers are an important component of the evaluation of patients suspected to have CAP; however, clinical features and physical examination findings may vary or be lacking in the elderly or debilitated patient.

The etiology for pneumonia cannot be reliably determined from the clinical presentation alone. Furthermore, the belief and the importance that pneumonias could be separated based on their presentation into "typical" and "atypical" types may have been overestimated. Typical pneumonias resemble the classical presentation of pneumococcal pneumonia: acute onset, high fever, rigors, pleuritic chest pain, and productive cough. Atypical pneumonias present with a more subacute onset, nonproductive cough, and less ill-appearing patient, as exemplified by pneumonias due to *Mycoplasma pneumoniae*, *Legionella pneumophila*, and *Chlamydia pneumoniae*. Nonetheless, these distinctions are now less important than previously emphasized.

Nosocomial Pneumonia

The combination of fever, productive cough, elevated white blood cell count, hypoxemia, and a new infiltrate on chest radiographs in a hospitalized patient strongly suggest nosocomial pneumonia. The diagnosis is not always straightforward as fever and cough may not always be present. Alternatively, fever and a high white blood cell count may be explained by other entities, such as possible catheter-associated infections or antibiotic-associated colitis. Other disease states that may also cause a chest infiltrate and hypoxemia include pulmonary embolus, pleural effusion, tumor, pulmonary hemorrhage, a mucus plug with atelectasis, and aspirated tube feeding.

DIAGNOSIS

Diagnostic evaluation beyond the history and physical examination includes a chest radiograph, analysis of pulmonary secretions (i.e., sputum), blood cultures, and other ancillary tests.

Chest Radiograph

The chest radiograph is the gold standard for diagnosing pneumonia. It must be interpreted with clinical findings in mind because its appearance will not accurately predict the etiology. Other conditions such as pulmonary edema or hemorrhage, malignancy, and some connective tissue diseases are often indistinguishable from pneumonia on radiography. Common radiographic patterns in pneumo-

TABLE 55.5 Environmental and host factors suggesting a microbial etiology of community-acquired pneumonia

Clinical feature	Potential etiology
Environmental factors	
Residence in or travel to:	
Southwestern United States	*Coccidioides immitis*
Mississippi, Ohio River Valleys	*Histoplasma capsulatum* *Blastomyces dermatitidis*
Exposure to bat caves	*Histoplasma capsulatum*
Exposure to psittacine birds, turkeys	*Chlamydia psittaci*
Exposure to contaminated air-conditioning system	*Legionella pneumophila*
Prison, homeless shelter residence	*Streptococcus pneumoniae* *Mycobacterium tuberculosis*
Outbreak in winter season	Influenza virus
Cluster cases	*Mycoplasma pneumoniae* Influenza virus
Host factors Human immunodeficiency virus/acquired immune deficiency syndrome Transplant status	*Streptococcus pneumoniae* *Pneumocystic carinii* *Cryptococcus neoformans* *Aspergillus spp.*
Chronic obstructive lung disease	*Streptococcus pneumoniae* *Haemophilus influenzae* *Moraxella catarrhalis*
Diabetes mellitus	*Streptococcus pneumoniae* *Staphylococcus aureus*
Alcoholism	*Streptococcus pneumoniae* *Staphylococcus aureus* *Klebsiella pneumoniae* Oral anaerobes
Elderly age	*Streptococcus pneumoniae* Influenza virus
Young, healthy adult	*Mycoplasma pneumoniae* *Streptococcus pneumoniae* *Chlamydia*

nias by different etiologic agents are shown in Table 55.6. Lobar consolidation is classically due to bacterial pathogens such as *S. pneumoniae*, whereas interstitial infiltrates are more likely seen with viruses, *M. pneumoniae*, or *Pneumocystis carinii*. *P. carinii* may present initially with interstitial infiltrates and without a prior diagnosis of human immunodeficiency virus, thus generating diagnostic confusion with pneumonias due to other pathogens. Cavitation features are found prominently in anaerobic, gram-negative, or tuberculous causes of pneumonia.

Radiographic evaluation for the presence of a concomitant pleural effusion is also important.

TABLE 55.6 Radiologic patterns of community-acquired pneumonia

Community-acquired pneumonia	Chest x-ray patterns
Lobar consolidation	Interstitial
Streptococcus pneumoniae	Viruses
Haemophilus influenzae	*Pneumocystis carinii*
Moraxella catarrhalis	*Mycoplasma pneumoniae*
Mycoplasma pneumoniae	*Chlamydia psittaci*
Legionella pneumophila	Cavitation
Chlamydia pneumoniae	Mixed aerobes/anaerobes
Multifocal opacities *Streptococcus pneumoniae* *Legionella pneumophila* *Staphylococcus aureus*	Aerobic gram-negative bacilli *Mycobacterium tuberculosis*

Nearly 50% of patients with pneumococcal pneumonia show pleural effusions (frank empyema in only 1% to 5%).

Sputum Gram-stain and Culture

Pulmonary secretions can usually be analyzed noninvasively by examining expectorated sputum. Sputum Gram stain and culture pose many problems, despite their traditional role in the diagnosis of pneumonia. Up to 40% of patients may produce a poor sputum sample or none at all. Cultures take time and are therefore not helpful initially. Although *S. pneumoniae* and *H. influenzae* often can be pathogens, their presence on culture may reflect only oropharyngeal colonization. The sputum Gram stain is more specific than sputum cultures.

Sputum Gram stains are most predictive when one adheres to strict criteria of acceptability. Only samples with less than 10 epithelial cells and over 25 neutrophils per low-power field are acceptable for analysis. On such samples, the finding of a positive Gram stain is highly predictive of a subsequent positive sputum culture result and validates the culture finding. However, finding none or a few mixed organisms on Gram stain may also alert one to the presence of a not easily identifiable organism (i.e., *M. pneumoniae*, *L. pneumophila*, *Mycobacterium tuberculosis*). Pretreatment culture of expectorated sputum should be performed only if a good-quality specimen can be obtained taking into account collection method, transport, and processing of samples.

Although the routine use of sputum cultures in the initial management of CAP has been questioned, pretreatment cultures are recommended in patients with severe disease, those intubated or likely to be infected with unusual pathogens (including *S. aureus*, *P. aeruginosa*, or other gram-negative bacilli) and if antibiotic sensitivity needs to be determined.

When sputum is not obtainable by expectoration or after induction, respiratory secretions may be obtained by invasive methods, such as by fiberoptic bronchoscopy using bronchoalveolar lavage (BAL). BAL, which has not been fully evaluated in CAP, is an expensive method and may be potentially compromised by contamination with oral flora.

Blood Cultures

Patients with severe CAP requiring hospitalization should routinely have blood cultures (two sets) performed, as well as assessment of arterial oxygen saturation. Despite the low yield of blood cultures,

5% to 15% in a large series of patients hospitalized with CAP, the impact of a positive blood culture on antibiotic management should not be underestimated. Therefore, blood cultures are recommended for all patients with severe CAP, as well as hosts with impaired immunity such as patients with asplenia, complement deficiencies, chronic liver disease, and leukopenia.

Other Studies

Other potentially helpful diagnostic tests include a complete blood count, blood chemistries, cold agglutinins, and antibody titers. Tests for *Legionella* involve a direct fluorescent antibody assay, which can be done on sputum, pleural fluid, or other pulmonary secretions. *Legionella* and pneumococcal antigen assay may also be performed on urine in select laboratories. Although none of these tests is recommended in the initial outpatient management of patients with low severity CAP, complete blood count, electrolytes, and renal function tests can be helpful in assessing prognosis and need for hospitalization.

TREATMENT

Only occasionally do all the pieces of the diagnostic puzzle fit together easily to yield an etiology of CAP; hence, therapy is empiric most of the time. For empiric outpatient therapy, a macrolide alone is appropriate.

The initial evaluation also entails determining the need for hospitalization by calculating the Pneumonia Severity Index. A significant abnormality in vital signs (i.e., hyperthermia, tachycardia, hypotension, extreme tachypnea), changes in mentation, respiratory failure, inability to take medications at home, or other risk factors for complications (i.e., renal insufficiency) are indications for hospitalization. A combination of a macrolide and a beta-lactam agent (such as ceftriaxone and azithromycin) is the preferred empiric therapy. A respiratory fluoroquinolone (such as moxifloxacin) is an alternative for the patient with a beta-lactam allergy.

Treatment of nosocomial pneumonia is also usually empiric with most pathogens requiring 10 to 14 days of therapy. Special attention should be paid to underlying host factors that may predispose to specific pathogens, prior antibiotic use, and pathogens unique to specific institutions or units. Infections due to gram-negative organisms in the appropriate setting (i.e., necrotizing pneumonia) should be treated for 21 days.

Traditionally, broad-spectrum antibiotic combinations (i.e., antipseudomonal penicillin or cephalosporin, with or without an aminoglycoside) are used to cover the common gram-negative pathogens such as *K. pneumoniae*, *Pseudomonas aeruginosa*, and *Serratia marcescens*. Vancomycin or linezolid should be used in the setting of methicillin-resistant strains of *Staphylococcus aureus*.

COMPLICATIONS

Once the patient's therapy is underway, attention must be focused on possible complications. A resurgence of fever after an initial period of defervescence is a frequent clue to a complication.

Poor coughing can lead to an accumulation of secretions or a mucus plug can obstruct an airway, leading to partial collapse of a segment or lobe of a lung with resulting atelectasis. Chest percussion, chest gravity drainage, and/or endotracheal suction to remove secretions and help re-expand the atelectatic segment should be tried before resorting to bronchoscopy.

In severely ill patients or those who do not respond promptly to treatment, radiography should be repeated because a severe and rapidly progressive pneumonia may evolve into pleural effusion or empyema. The development of a loculated pleural effusion or empyema requires thoracentesis and possible chest tube drainage (Chapter 38). Failure of the pneumonia to respond to therapy or a history of multiple recurrent pneumonias may also require sputum cytologies and bronchoscopy to inquire about the presence of a partial obstructing airway lesion or an endobronchial tumor.

Lung abscesses form as a complication of a localized area of pneumonia or when a neoplasm becomes necrotic and contains purulent material. *S. aureus*, gram-negative organisms, and anaerobes may be the infecting organisms. Lung abscess may present with an indolent course, accompanied by fever, weight loss, chronic purulent cough, and an air fluid level on chest radiograph. A chest computed tomography or a bronchoscopy may be necessary to confirm the diagnosis.

CHAPTER 56

Urinary Tract Infection

Jasna Jevtic

Approximately 50% of adult women report having had a urinary tract infection (UTI) at some point in their lifetime. Ten percent of adult women in the United States have at least one UTI each year. This lifelong higher incidence of UTIs in women peaks between ages 16 to 35 years due to sexual activity and diaphragm use. The prevalence of UTI by age groups in women and men is shown in Table 56.1. Infections of the urinary tract entail a broad terminology (Table 56.2).

Asymptomatic bacteriuria refers to the presence of a positive urine culture in an asymptomatic person. Symptomatic individuals may be further divided into those with infection in the lower (cystitis) or upper urinary tract (pyelonephritis). Acute cystitis is an infection of the bladder that can result in pyelonephritis if ascending to the upper urinary tract.

UTIs may be complicated or uncomplicated. A complicated UTI is defined as a urinary infection associated with factors listed in Table 56.2. Also, UTIs may be isolated or recurrent. Recurrent UTIs may be further categorized into relapsing infections or reinfections. Relapsing infections that occur within 2 weeks of completion of treatment are caused by the same organism. In contrast, reinfection is defined as a recurrent infection where each episode is caused by a different microorganism. Urethritis is discussed in Chapter 139.

ETIOLOGY

UTIs are caused by a subset of fecal microbes that invade the genitourinary tract. Some strains of bacteria are especially uropathogenic, and some hosts are especially susceptible to these strains (i.e., women).

Establishing whether a UTI is uncomplicated or complicated early may help to determine the uropathogen (Table 56.3). Most uncomplicated episodes of either cystitis or pyelonephritis (>80%) are due to certain strains of *Escherichia coli.* Approximately 10% of cases of uncomplicated cystitis result from a coagulase-negative staphylococci, *Staphylococcus saprophyticus,* which is not the case with pyelonephritis. Complicated UTIs, on the contrary, arise from a wider range of organisms. Most are gram-negative, but gram-positive organisms and fungi are also frequent. Enteric gram-negative organisms and enterococcal species predominate as the leading cause of prostatitis.

Cystitis usually occurs by the ascent of pathogenic microorganisms from the urethra to the bladder. Pyelonephritis can result from further ascent of these microbes; hematogenous spread from a different focus of infection to the kidney may occur. As mentioned, acute, uncomplicated cystitis usually is caused by a few uropathogenic *E. coli* strains that normally colonize the bowel. Predisposing factors in women include the close proximity of the female genitourinary tract to the anus with subsequent colonization of the vagina and the urethral meatus. After such colonization, the shorter female urethra permits an easier ascent of organisms to the bladder, a process that is facilitated by sexual activity.

The increased incidence in older men is primarily due to prostatic hypertrophy, incontinence, and long-term urinary catheterization.

TABLE 56.1 Epidemiology of urinary tract infections by age

Age group	Prevalence (%)	
	Women	Men
<1 year	1	1
1 to 5 years	4–5	0.5
6 to 15 years	4–5	0.5
16 to 35 years	20	0.5
36 to 65 years	35	20
>65 years	40	35

Adapted and reprinted with permission from Stamm WE. In: Gorbach SL, Bartlett JG, Blacklow NR, eds. *Infectious diseases*. Philadelphia: WB Saunders; 1992:788–798.

CLINICAL MANIFESTATIONS

Acute cystitis is characterized by frequency, urgency, and (less commonly) hematuria. The presence of fever, nausea, vomiting, flank pain, and costovertebral tenderness suggest the diagnosis of pyelonephritis. The common "classic" symptoms of acute cystitis and pyelonephritis, as seen in young women, are shown in Table 56.4.

Catheterized patients may have either nonspecific symptoms or no symptoms at all except fever. Whereas suprapubic tenderness and gross hematuria are seen in only 10% and 30% of cystitis cases,

TABLE 56.2 Urinary tract infections: a glossary of terms

Bacteriuria	Bacteria in the urine (usually $>10^5$ bacteria/mL)
Cystitis	Infection of the lower urinary tract
Pyelonephritis	Infection of the upper urinary tract
Acute urethral syndrome	Symptoms of UTI with $>10^5$ bacteria/mL
Complicated UTI	UTI in the presence of: • a structural anatomic abnormality • diabetes mellitus • elderly age • immunosuppressive states • recent urologic instrumentation • antibiotic resistance • pregnancy
Recurrent UTI	Repeated UTI that may be either a relapse or reinfection

UTI, urinary tract infection.

TABLE 56.3 Common microbes causing uncomplicated and complicated urinary tract infections

Uncomplicated	Complicated
Escherichia coli	*Escherichia coli*
Staphylococcus saprophyticus	*Klebsiella spp.*
	Enterobacter spp.
	Proteus spp.
	Pseudomonas spp.
	Enterococcus spp.
	Staphylococcus epidermidis
	Yeast (*Candida spp.*)

respectively, they are fairly specific findings for cystitis. As many as one third of patients who have only symptoms of cystitis have unrecognized pyelonephritis.

In evaluating patients with urinary catheters, one must realize that bacteriuria is common and that most catheter-associated urinary tract infections are asymptomatic. When symptoms are present, they may range from fever or flank pain to sepsis or septic shock. Asymptomatic bacteriuria is a fairly common finding in elderly patients without catheters and is usually an incidental finding on routine urinalysis.

DIAGNOSIS

Urine Dipstick

Leukocyte esterase, which can be detected by a dipstick method, is indicative for the presence of pyuria; however, it is somewhat less sensitive than a urine microscopic examination. Nitrite can also be identified by dipstick and indicates the presence of micro-organisms such as *Enterobacteriaceae*, which convert urinary nitrate to nitrite.

TABLE 56.4 Differentiating clinical features of cystitis and pyelonephritis

Cystitis	Pyelonephritis
Dysuria	Dysuria and frequency
Urinary frequency	Fever
Urgency	Flank pain
Suprapubic tenderness (10%)	Nausea and vomiting
Gross hematuria (30%)	Malaise

When UTI is clinically suspected, a urine sample for microscopic analysis should be obtained for confirmation.

Urinalysis

A clean, midstream voided sample is preferred in most patients, although urine can be obtained from a urethral catheter in those who are already catheterized.

Inflammatory cells (pyuria) and erythrocytes (hematuria) in a clean-catch urine sample support the diagnosis of a UTI. Pyuria (defined as more than 5 to 10 white blood cells per high-power field on a centrifuged specimen of urine) is a common finding present in clinically significant UTI (95% sensitivity); however, because it can also occur in other conditions such as gonococcal urethritis, its specificity is reduced (71% specificity). The presence or number of white blood cells does not differentiate a lower from an upper UTI (for example, pyelonephritis), but the presence of white blood cell casts is a hallmark of pyelonephritis.

Erythrocytes (hematuria) are not as commonly seen in UTI as white blood cells. Hematuria may suggest the possibility of urinary stones or tumor, and decrease the likelihood of urethritis, which is not normally associated with hematuria. Gram-stain findings may help guide initial therapy in a complicated case (i.e., recurrent UTIs).

Urine Culture

A urine culture growing $>10^5$ colony forming units of an organism per milliliter of urine is considered to be a positive finding. Urine culture before treatment is generally not necessary in women with uncomplicated cystitis because the typical treatment usually covers the narrow spectrum of causative organisms. However, the increasing emergence of antibiotic resistance, recurrence less than 1 month after treatment, and the presence of features of complicated infection may warrant pretreatment urine cultures. Also, any patient with suspected pyelonephritis, complicated UTI, or a history of resistant organisms should have a urine culture.

In men with uncomplicated cystitis, a pretreatment urine culture should be obtained. Recurrent infection and the absence of obvious factors leading to a UTI (for example, the presence of urinary catheter) may warrant urologic and imaging evaluation. Urethritis and prostatitis should also be considered in men with urethral discharge and no pyuria on urinalysis.

Individuals with symptoms of cystitis who show no growth or nonsignificant bacterial growth on urine culture often require inspection of the genitalia for urethral discharge. Evidence of urethritis and urethral discharge on examination requires gram staining and cultures to aid in diagnosis and management.

TREATMENT

Successful management of a UTI is based on a clinical estimation of the site of infection, coupled with knowledge of likely pathogens and pharmacokinetics of antibiotics in the urine. The standard management of an acute uncomplicated UTI in an otherwise healthy, nonpregnant woman requires only a short (3-day) course of a first-line antimicrobial agent such as trimethoprim/sulfamethoxazole or a fluoroquinolone. The choice of first-line agents may need to be changed, however, in situations where antimicrobial resistance is suspected. Prolonged therapy should be given to those with symptoms lasting for 7 days or more, diabetes, immunosuppression, elderly, pregnancy, or an anatomic urinary tract abnormality because this indicates a complicated UTI (Table 56.5).

Initial management of patients with pyelonephritis is based on the need for hospitalization and intravenous therapy. Some patients, particularly younger individuals, can be given outpatient oral therapy, whereas more symptomatic patients should be given parenteral agents. With clinical improvement, one can substitute a suitable oral agent for a total of a 14-day course.

TABLE 56.5 Suggested antibiotic regimens for urinary tract infections

Cystitis	Pyelonephritis
Trimethoprim/sulfamethoxazole[a]	Trimethoprim/sulfamethoxazole[a]
Trimethoprim[a]	Third-generation cephalosporin
Quinolone	Quinolone
Amoxicillin or amoxicillin clavulanic acid	Aminoglycoside plus antipseudomonal penicillin
Cephalexin	

[a]Although all drugs carry some fetal risk, these agents should be used with caution in early pregnancy.

In evaluating patients with urinary catheters, one must remember that bacteriuria is common and that most catheter-associated UTIs are asymptomatic. Only symptomatic patients should be treated; treatment includes removal or replacement of the catheter and initiation of parenteral antibiotics. Antibiotic selection is similar to that for complicated pyelonephritis with special attention to the institutional nosocomial flora.

In general, treatment of asymptomatic bacteriuria is not recommended in catheterized or noncatheterized adults. Those populations in which asymptomatic bacteriuria should be treated, however, include children, pregnant women, and prior to any invasive urologic procedure.

COMPLICATIONS

Patients with multiple episodes of UTIs, impaired renal function, pyuria with white cell casts, bacteriuria, and an IVP showing an abnormal renal pelvis (i.e., calcium deposits and cortical scars) can be diagnosed as having chronic pyelonephritis. Resulting renal disease may progress slowly and silently to the point of renal insufficiency.

Individuals with vascular disease of the kidney or with urinary tract obstruction who develop severe pyelonephritis are at risk for renal papillary necrosis. Hematuria, flank or abdominal pain, and chills and fever are the most common presenting symptoms. Acute renal failure with oliguria or anuria sometimes occurs.

An uncommon complication of acute pyelonephritis includes medullary abscesses when foci of cellular material coalesce to form a single or multiple distinct cavities in the interstitium of the kidney. The onset of renal abscess is abrupt with chills and fever, followed by costovertebral pain and tenderness. Medullary abscesses are usually accompanied by pyuria and transient hematuria may occur at the onset. Early in the disease, the diagnoses of ureteral stones or acute hydronephrosis should be entertained. Computed tomography scans usually demonstrate the abscess as a fluid-filled defect. Treatment consists of a more prolonged duration of antibiotics, adequate fluids, and analgesia, usually resulting in prompt recovery. Persistent fever following adequate treatment indicates incorrect diagnosis or need for surgical drainage.

CHAPTER 57

Cellulitis

Susan Davids

Cellulitis is defined as an infection of the dermis with extension into the subcutaneous tissue. It can occur in any part of the body, but is most often seen in the extremities. Cellulitis is an infection seen in both the outpatient and inpatient settings. The true prevalence and incidence of cellulitis is not known, but it is accepted as a common problem.

Erysipelas is a superficial cellulitis that does not extend into the subcutaneous tissue. This infection is characterized by swelling and erythema of the skin with well-demarcated borders.

ETIOLOGY

Cellulitis is most often caused by *Streptococcus pyogenes* and *Staphylococcus aureus.* However, depending on the predisposing factor for bacterial invasion, a number of bacteria could be involved (Table 57.1).

There are many predisposing factors to the development of cellulitis, but the most common causes are a prior history of cellulitis and anything that disrupts the dermis layer including surgery, trauma (including radiation), leg ulcers, and dermatoses, particularly tinea pedis. Venous insufficiency and lymphatic disruption are also important predisposing factors, especially for recurrent cellulitis.

Depending upon the predisposing factors, the bacterial cause is narrowed down to guide treatment choices. However, the exact bacterial cause is not known in most cases.

Bite wounds are common from dogs, cats, and humans, and the likelihood of infection at the site depends on the degree of tissue injury and delay in obtaining appropriate wound care. Although there is usually a localized cellulitis, there may be a deeper soft-tissue infection (including abscesses), septic arthritis, or osteomyelitis or metastatic foci from bacteremia. The normal flora of the animal and human skin are the common organisms that cause infection (Table 57.2).

Erysipelas is usually caused by group A β-hemolytic streptococci. Other rarely isolated organisms are groups B, C, or G streptococci. The pathogen enters through an abrasion, surgical incision, puncture wound, ulcer, injury, or fissure in the nose, ears, or perineum. Any draining site may serve as a source of infection, but sometimes no portal of entry is apparent.

CLINICAL MANIFESTATIONS

Cellulitis presents as an acute spreading area of erythema, with tenderness, warmth, and swelling. Unlike erysipelas, the borders of the lesions lack distinct boundaries and are not elevated. Tender regional adenopathy is common and lymphangitis may be present.

TABLE 57.1 Causes of cellulitis and associated conditions

Etiologic agents	Predisposing conditions	Antimicrobial agents
Streptococcus pyogenes (and other streptococci)	Trauma, puncture wound, tinea pedis	Penicillin, macrolide, clindamycin
Staphylococcus aureus	Trauma, puncture wound, tinea pedis	Methicillin-susceptible *S. aureus*– • Penicillins (dicloxacillin PO, nafcillin IV) • First-generation cephalosporin • Clindamycin • Tetracycline • TMP-SMZ Methicillin-resistant *S. aureus* • Vancomycin • Linezolid • TMP-SMZ • Clindamycin • Daptomycin • Tetracyline
Gram-negative bacteria (e.g., Enterobacteriaceae, *Serratia*, *Pseudomonas*, *Proteus* spp.)	Granulocytopenia	Third-generation cephalosporins, extended spectrum penicillins, quinolones, aminoglycosides
Vibrio spp. (e.g., *Vibrio vulnificus, Vibrio parahaemolyticus*)	Traumatic wound in salt water or brackish inland water	Doxycycline plus third-generation cephalosporin
Aeromonas hydrophila	Traumatic wound in freshwater	Ciprofloxacin or third-generation cephalosporins plus aminoglycosides
Erysipelothrix rhusiopathiae	Abrasion from handling saltwater fish, poultry, meat, hides	Penicillin, ciprofloxacin, or cefotaxime
Clostridium perfringens	Contaminated traumatic or surgical wound	Penicillin, clindamycin, chloramphenicol
Nonclostridial anaerobic cellulitis (*Bacteroides*, *Peptostreptococcus*, *Peptococcus*, aerobic streptococci, gram-negative bacilli)	Diabetes mellitus, local trauma	Broad-spectrum therapy to cover the range of pathogens

TMP-SMZ, Trimethoprim-sulfamethoxazole

TABLE 57.2 Bite wound infections

Type of bite	Usual	Antimicrobial therapy
Dog or cat	*Pasteurella multocida* and other *Pasterella* spp. *Staphylococcus aureus, Streptococcus* spp. Capnocytophaga canimorsus *Prevotella* spp., *Fusobacterium* spp. *Bacteriodes* spp, *Prophyromonas* spp. *Peptostreptococcus* spp.	Amoxicillin-clavulanic acid
Human	*Streptococcus* spp. (especially *S. viridans*), *Staphylococcus aureus, Eikenella corrodens,* *Prevotella* spp., *Peptostreptococcus* spp. *Fusobacterium* spp., *Bacteroides* spp.	Amoxicillin-clavulanic acid

Although most patients have mild systemic manifestations, patients can present with fever, chills, myalgias, and mental status changes, which commonly precede the skin eruption. Laboratory abnormalities are usually seen only in severe cases.

Classically, erysipelas is a sharply circumscribed, red, tender or painful plaque (See Color Plate 10). The skin can appear finely dimpled, resembling an orange peel. The lesions progress rapidly by peripheral extension of the raised indurated borders. In severe cases, the warm edematous plaques become blisters or bleeding into the skin (purpura) may occur. The most common site was previously the face, but now the lower extremities are more frequently affected. Fever, chills, headache, and malaise precede and accompany the onset of the skin eruption, and the patient appears toxic. Some report gastrointestinal symptoms, arthralgias, and changes in mental status. Leukocytosis is common and often exceeds 20,000/ mm^3.

DIAGNOSIS

The diagnosis of soft tissue infections is primarily clinical. The etiology is often difficult to determine and in mild cases is usually unnecessary. In more severe cases and with certain exposures, it may be necessary to isolate the infecting organism. Blood cultures are positive in less than 5% of the cases and should be reserved for febrile patients with severe disease. Aspirating the leading edge of the cellulitis yields an etiologic diagnosis in about only 25% of cases. Culture of a punch biopsy has a slightly higher yield. Needle aspiration or a punch biopsy should only be performed in those patients where typical treatment fails, or in those with risk factors for recurrent cellulitis.

In assessing clinical severity several algorithms have been proposed; however, most have been developed with retrospective studies or expert opinion.

Methicillin-resistant *Staphylococcus aureus* (MRSA) always needs to be considered as a cause of cellulitis, especially in those who fail standard treatment for cellulitis. A careful history should be taken to identify risk factors for community-acquired MRSA, including: history of MRSA infection, being from a community with a high prevalence of MRSA, recurrent skin disease, living in crowded conditions (i.e., homeless shelter, military barracks, jail), participation in contact sports, injection drug use, male with a history of having sex with men, or a member of a Native American, Pacific Island, or Alaskan Native population.

Because the diagnosis of cellulitis is largely clinical, the differential diagnosis may include contact dermatitis, insect bite, acute gout, deep venous thrombosis, fixed-drug reaction, or lymphedema. Less common diagnoses to be considered include pyoderma gangrenosa, Sweet's syndrome, lupus, sarcoid, urticaria, and hematologic malignancies.

When erysipelas presents in its classic form (bright red, indurated facial plaque with distinct borders), there is little diagnostic difficulty. Sometimes the lesions may resemble allergic contact dermatitis, urticaria, scarlet fever, systemic lupus erythematosus, tuberculoid leprosy, or relapsing polychondritis. Culture of this closed infection is difficult to obtain and rarely of use in initial management.

Radiographic evaluation of cellulitis is rarely necessary and is done only when considering osteomyelitis or necrotizing fasciitis. Misdiagnosis of cellulitis could delay the diagnosis of necrotizing fasciitis, a rapidly progressive, life-threatening deep tissue infection.

TREATMENT

The treatment of cellulitis continues to change with the emergence of resistant organisms, making the treatment decisions more complex. MRSA, an emerging pathogen, can either be hospital acquired (HA-MRSA) or community acquired (CA-MRSA). CA-MRSA more commonly causes skin and soft tissue infections than HA-MRSA, and can be more virulent.

Nonetheless, treatment should be directed at the most likely organism depending on the risk factors present (Tables 57.1 and 57.2). In most cases, cellulitis is due to *Streptococcus pyogenes* or *Staphylococcus aureus*; both are covered by penicillinase-resistant penicillin (dicloxacillin, nafcillin). Parenteral therapy may be necessary when a systemic response is prominent or the patient has clinically significant comorbid conditions (diabetes, neutropenia, cirrhosis, cardiac failure, renal insufficiency, or asplenia) until clinical improvement occurs. Most patients are treated as outpatients with oral therapy. If CA-MRSA or HA-MRSA is suspected, vancomycin would be the treatment of choice in the inpatient setting, and TMP-SMX or tetracyclines could be used for outpatients. Certain types of cellulitis with tissue necrosis (e.g., clostridial anaerobic cellulitis) require both antibiotics and surgical debridement.

Penicillin is the drug of choice for erysipelas. Improvement is rapid and dramatic. Penicillin-allergic patients are given erythromycin or clindamycin. A semisynthetic penicillin or cephalosporin is used when *S. aureus* is a potential second pathogen. Cool compresses provide symptom relief for tender, warm, blistered plaques, and swelling is controlled with immobilization and elevation. With chronic or recurrent infection, a bacterial reservoir and a possible portal of entry (e.g., macerated skin of tinea pedis) should be determined. Treatment for predisposing factors for cellulitis or erysipelas should be initiated.

COMPLICATIONS

Cellulitis can lead to complications such as osteomyelitis, particularly in the setting of patients with diabetic ulcers and necrotizing fascitis. Complications of erysipelas are rare but can include infections distant to the site of erysipelas or cellulitis via bloodstream spread (including infective endocarditis), osteomyelitis, septic arthritis, poststreptococcal glomerulonephritis, venous sinus, thrombosis, and streptococcal toxic shock syndrome (rare).

CHAPTER 58

Meningitis and Encephalitis

Michael Frank

Meningitis is defined as inflammation of the meninges covering the brain and is identified clinically by the demonstration of white blood cells in the cerebrospinal fluid (CSF).

Encephalitis involves inflammation of the brain itself, but it is more accurate to think of these as processes on a continuum rather than as distinct entities, and many infections may cause meningoencephalitis. Encephalitis typically has altered mental status early in the illness without meningeal signs, whereas meningitis has meningeal signs usually without focal signs early. Meningitis can be further subdivided into acute versus chronic; chronic is defined as being present for longer than 4 weeks.

Acute meningitis usually is divided into bacterial versus aseptic meningitis. Aseptic meningitis usually is viral but can be caused by other infectious agents or even be noninfectious. Acute bacterial meningitis has an incidence of 4 to 6 cases per 100,000 people; even today, it remains as one of the bacterial infections that will kill previously healthy persons without appropriate therapy. Acute bacterial meningitis is a medical emergency requiring immediate attention and prompt initiation of therapy to avoid mortality.

ETIOLOGY

Acute meningitis has a variety of causes (Table 58.1). Two organisms together cause 80% of all cases of community-acquired bacterial meningitis in adults: *Streptococcus pneumoniae* (pneumococcus) and *Neisseria meningitidis* (meningococcus). *Haemophilus influenzae* used to be a common cause in children before widespread adoption of the *H. influenzae* type b (Hib) vaccine. Meningococcal meningitis may occur in young adults sporadically or during epidemics.

Pneumococcus is seen in all ages, but is the most common organism in the adult. Predisposing factors for pneumococcal meningitis include otitis media or mastoiditis (30%), pneumonia (20%), and head trauma (10%). The number of sporadic bacterial meningitis cases increases in the autumn and winter months and declines during the spring, reaching a nadir during summer when, in contrast, enteroviral aseptic meningitis peaks.

Enteric gram-negative bacillary meningitis is seen primarily in trauma, neurosurgical, or hospitalized patients. Whereas coagulase-negative staphylococcus is seen in patients with CNS shunts, *S. aureus* usually is related to trauma or endocarditis. Among adults, *Listeria* meningitis may occur in the elderly, alcoholics, or those with defective cell-mediated (T-cell) immunity.

Aseptic meningitis is a misnomer because it denotes culture-negative meningitis (usually with lymphocytic predominance in the CSF), even though infectious agents are usually the cause. In particular, viral agents are the most common cause, with enteroviruses leading the list (Coxsackie and echo viruses).

The classic definition of subacute or chronic meningitis is meningitis exceeding 4-weeks duration.

TABLE 58.1 Causes of acute meningitis

Infectious		Noninfectious
Typical "bacterial" CSF	"Aseptic" CSF findings	
Streptococcus pneumoniae	Enteroviruses	Medications
Neisseria meningitidis	Human immunodeficiency virus	Connective tissue diseases
Haemophilus influenzae	Herpes simplex	Lymphoma or other malignancy
Listeria monocytogenes	*Treponema pallidum*	Neurosarcoidosis
Streptococcus agalactiae	*Borrelia burgdorferi*	
Staphylococci	Rickettsiae	
Gram-negative bacilli		

CSF, cerebrospinal fluid.

The diagnosis can further be classified into lymphocytic or neutrophilic meningitis; causes of each are listed in Table 58.2.

Encephalitis may be epidemic or nonepidemic. Epidemic forms include mosquito-borne arbovirus encephalitides including St. Louis, La Crosse, West Nile, and eastern and western equine encephalitis in the United States; Japanese encephalitis is common in Southeast Asia. Rarely, enteroviruses or measles virus may cause encephalitis. The nonepidemic form is most commonly due to herpes simplex virus. Rabies remains rare in the United States.

CLINICAL MANIFESTATIONS

The acuteness of presentation and findings vary according to the process. Fulminant symptoms with fever, lethargy, and nuchal rigidity make bacterial meningitis likely, which calls for immediate lumbar puncture (LP) and antibiotic therapy within 1 hour. A subacute history over weeks or months,

TABLE 58.2 Causes of chronic meningitis by cerebrospinal fluid cell predominance

Lymphocytic	Neutrophilic
Tuberculosis	Actinomycosis
Syphilis	*Nocardia*
Lyme disease	*Brucella*
Fungal (*Cryptococcus, Coccidiodes, Histoplasma*)	*Candida*
Sarcoidosis	Aspergillosis
Vasculitis	Medications
Behcet syndrome	
Tumor	
Parameningeal focus of infection	

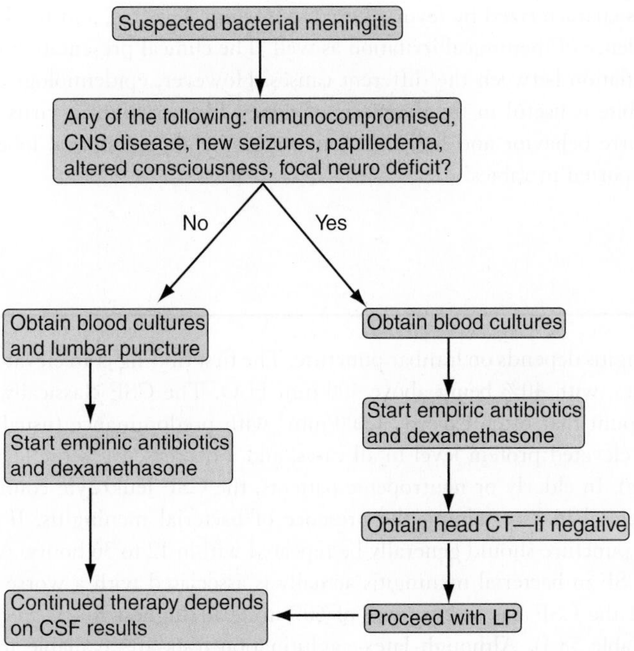

Figure 58.1 • Algorithm for the management of suspected bacterial meningitis.

especially with focal signs and symptoms, implies a mass effect; computed tomography (CT) scan is indicated first because lumbar puncture may be risky. When these distinctions are blurred and meningitis is still a consideration, blood cultures are drawn, antibiotics are given, and lumbar puncture is deferred until the CT scan is completed. See Figure 58.1 for an algorithm of the management of suspected bacterial meningitis in adults.

One fourth of patients with bacterial meningitis have a rapid onset with headache, lethargy, and confusion within 24 hours (Table 58.3). In the others, symptoms evolve over 1 to 7 days. In some patients, the features of meningitis may develop as an aftermath of or in continuity with a pneumonic process. Fever, neck stiffness, and altered mental status are considered the "classic triad" of acute bacterial meningitis, but all three are present in only 44% of patients. However, almost all patients will have at least two of the following four symptoms: fever, headache, neck stiffness, and altered mental status. Focal findings, mostly consisting of cranial nerve deficits (especially cranial nerves 3, 6, and 8), may be noted in 10% to 20% of patients. Papilledema is rare. Petechial or purpuric rash is a clue to meningococcal infection and indicates meningococcemia.

The classic clinical presentation of aseptic meningitis includes headache, fever, and neck pain and stiffness (meningismus) in children or young adults during the summer months.

TABLE 58.3 Clinical features of bacterial meningitis

Very common	Less common
Fever	Kernig and Brudzinski signs
Headache	Seizures
Neck stiffness (meningismus)	Vomiting
Confusion	Focal neurologic deficits

Encephalitis is characterized by fever, altered sensorium, seizures, and focal neurologic deficits. There may be evidence of meningeal irritation as well. The clinical presentation of encephalitis does not allow differentiation between the different causes. However, epidemiologic clues are useful. A history of animal bite is useful in the diagnosis of rabies. Herpes simplex virus (HSV) encephalitis classically has bizarre behavior and hallucinations suggestive of a temporal lobe focus. There may be hydrophobia reported in rabies.

DIAGNOSIS

Diagnosis of meningitis depends on lumbar puncture. The first finding is an elevated opening pressure in virtually all cases, with 40% being above 400 mm H_2O. The CSF classically shows an elevated white blood cell count that often exceeds 1,000/mm^3 with predominance (usually more than 80%) of neutrophils, an elevated protein level in all cases, and a decreased glucose level below 40 mg/dL (hypoglycorrhachia). In elderly or neutropenic patients, the CSF leukocyte count may not be high; Gram stain is essential in ascertaining the presence of bacterial meningitis. If the diagnosis is in doubt, the lumbar puncture should generally be repeated within 12 to 36 hours. A lower white blood cell count in the CSF in bacterial meningitis actually is associated with a worse prognosis.

Gram stain of the CSF has a sensitivity of 60% to 90% (highest for *S. pneumoniae*) and has a 97% specificity (Table 58.4). Although latex agglutination tests are available for *H. influenzae, S. pneumoniae,* and *N. meningitidis,* they do not contribute to diagnosis beyond Gram stain. CSF cultures are reportedly positive in 80%, with blood cultures being positive in 40% to 80%. It is crucial to obtain blood cultures before starting antibiotics, even if lumbar puncture is delayed by the need to obtain a head CT and empiric antibiotic coverage will be started. Starting antibiotics before obtaining the CSF may decrease the yield of the CSF Gram stain and culture, but the CSF cell counts, glucose, and protein will still be reliable, as will blood cultures obtained first.

The CSF in aseptic meningitis may be neutrophilic in two thirds of patients (usually less than 200 cells/mm^3) initially, changing to mononuclear predominance in 6 to 24 hours. The CSF glucose level is usually normal and protein is less than 100 mg/dL. Viral cultures of CSF and throat swabs may be positive. Occasionally, viral meningitis can resemble a bacterial process, with neutrophil counts as high as 500/mm^3. Usually, on repeat lumbar puncture within 12 to 36 hours, the cellular response becomes mononuclear.

Routine laboratory evaluation of the CSF for chronic meningitis may include the following tests: cryptococcal antigen, VDRL, Lyme serology, cytology, fungal cultures, and mycobacterial cultures.

TABLE 58.4 Laboratory abnormalities in bacterial meningitis

Test	Frequency
CSF opening pressure elevated	Always
CSF protein elevated	Always
CSF Gram stain positive for bacteria	60% to 90%
CSF culture positive	80%
Blood cultures positive	40% to 80%
CSF glucose:serum glucose ratio <0.40	80%

CSF, cerebrospinal fluid.

High-volume lumbar punctures with multiple cultures may be necessary. If no diagnosis is made and clinical status is worsening, then treatment for tuberculosis should be initiated.

Specific microbiological diagnosis is difficult in encephalitis. The CSF response is nonspecific and may be normal in 5% of cases due to HSV. Magnetic resonance imaging and electroencephalography may be suggestive of HSV, but their specificity is unknown. Polymerase chain reaction of the CSF has become the best tool for diagnosing HSV, short of brain biopsy.

TREATMENT

Important general principles in the treatment of acute bacterial meningitis include the imperative need to start treatment immediately and the need to use very high doses of antimicrobials. Any delay in initiation of appropriate therapy is associated with increased morbidity and mortality. Very high dosing regimens are needed to ensure adequate levels of antibiotic in the CSF.

The initial treatment approach to the patient with meningitis is outlined in Table 58.5. Increasing antibiotic resistance among pneumococci has prompted changes in empiric antibiotics used in adults. Presently, a third-generation cephalosporin is recommended for initial community-acquired bacterial meningitis, along with vancomycin until penicillin susceptibility is known; ampicillin should be added for individuals at risk for *Listeria* infection (elderly, alcoholic, or immunosuppressed patients).

In general, 7 days of therapy is necessary for meningococci, 7 to 10 days for *H. influenzae,* 10 to 14 days for pneumococci, and 21 days for *Listeria* or gram-negative rods. Data now support the use of adjunctive corticosteroids, to lessen the complications resulting from inflammation, in children with *H. influenzae* meningitis and in adults with pneumococcal meningitis. The adjunctive steroids (high-dose dexamethasone) must be started at the same time as the empiric antibiotics and so should be started presumptively in all cases of suspected bacterial meningitis; therapy can later be modified depending on results of Gram stain and culture.

Management of encephalitis is complicated by the nonspecific clinical picture for individual causative agents. The difficulty in making a specific microbiological diagnosis, the difficulty in ruling out HSV, and the clinician's reluctance to perform a brain biopsy for HSV further compound the management dilemma. Because of these factors and because HSV is the only treatable cause, acyclovir is usually given at 10 mg/kg every 8 hours for 14 to 21 days whenever HSV is a possible cause. Patients whose conditions progress despite treatment should undergo brain biopsy.

COMPLICATIONS

Complications of meningitis can be separated into those that are more immediate at the time of the infection and those that are more permanent resulting from the inflammation and tissue damage.

TABLE 58.5 Choice of empiric antibiotic therapy for bacterial meningitis in adults

Predisposing factor	Likely pathogens	Empiric antibiotics
Age 16 to 50 years, otherwise healthy	*S. pneumoniae, N. meningitidis*	Vancomycin + ceftriaxone
Age 50 or older	*S. pneumoniae, N. meningitidis, Listeria monocytogenes*, aerobic gram-negative bacilli	Vancomycin + ceftriaxone + ampicillin
Immunocompromised or alcohol abuse	*S. pneumoniae, Listeria, H. influenzae*	Vancomycin + ceftriaxone + ampicillin

Infectious complications include subdural empyema, brain abscess, bacteremia, and septic shock. Repeat lumbar puncture is indicated if there is not clinical improvement within 48 hours; CSF gram stain and culture should be negative. Immediate noninfectious complications include disseminated intravascular coagulation, syndrome of inappropriate antidiuretic hormone, and hyponatremia. Several serious neurologic complications can be seen, including development of hydrocephalus (in 3% to 8%), cerebral edema (6% to 10%), or even transtentorial herniation of the brain. Seizures occur in 15% to 23% of adults with bacterial meningitis, and infarcts can result from inflammation occluding the basilar arteries.

Acute bacterial meningitis results in death in 19% to 37% of cases, depending on the particular organism; higher mortality is seen in pneumococcal infections. Other permanent complications include residual neurological deficits, mostly cranial nerve palsies in about 14%. Up to 27% of survivors may have residual cognitive impairment, usually slowed mentation, and a small percentage may have aphasia or hemiparesis. Prompt use of adjunctive dexamethasone may lower the rate of complications.

Finally, it is important to mention the prevention of bacterial meningitis. Patients suspected of having meningococcal meningitis should be placed in isolation. Close contacts of patients with meningococcal meningitis should receive antimicrobial prophylaxis. There are effective vaccines against all three of the most common causes of bacterial meningitis: the polyvalent pneumococcal conjugate and polysaccharide vaccines for infants and older adults, the meningococcal polysaccharide vaccine for young adults, and the Hib vaccine for infants.

CHAPTER 59

Sepsis Syndrome

Jasna Jevtic

The concept of sepsis encompasses a diverse group of disorders that are grouped under one name because they share the common properties of both an infection and a resultant systemic inflammatory response. Occasionally patients with established bacteremia do not mount a septic response. The terminology of sepsis (Table 59.1) provides a simple and practical framework for identifying these disorders.

Stepwise increases in mortality occur with progression from systemic inflammatory response syndrome to sepsis to severe sepsis to septic shock. Approximately 750,000 cases of severe sepsis occur in the United States each year with more than 100,000 deaths per year.

Bacteremia is defined as the invasion of blood by bacteria, as detected by blood cultures. Because blood circulates in a closed system, bacteremia always presupposes an infectious focus elsewhere in the body (the source), from which the blood becomes seeded. For any infection, bacterial or otherwise, the development of bloodstream invasion implies a worse prognosis and a major threat to life. Bacteremic and/or septic patients have a higher rate of complications, longer hospital stay, and higher mortality with rates ranging from 20% to 50%. The epidemiology of bacteremia differs depending on whether it is community-acquired or nosocomial.

Community-acquired bacteremia traditionally refers to infections detected within 72 hours of hospitalization (unless the patient was a resident of a long-term care facility). Although the use of 72 hours may seem arbitrary, the separation of bacteremias into community-acquired and nosocomial has implications in terms of the organism(s) involved, source of the bacteremia, complication rate, and mortality.

ETIOLOGY

Community-acquired bacteremia is more frequent among the elderly. The most frequent sources and most common organisms are listed in Table 59.2. In some cases, more than one organism may be detected in blood cultures. Once contamination has been excluded, polymicrobial bacteremia suggests the biliary tract, intra-abdominal sepsis, or a urinary tract infection as a source.

Some organisms tend to be associated with specific underlying infections (e.g., pneumococcal bacteremia with pneumonia). It is also important to note that in some cases, the source may remain elusive after a diligent search, a feature most likely to occur with *Escherichia coli*, *Enterococcus*, *Pseudomonas*, *Bacteroides*, and some polymicrobial bacteremias.

Nosocomial bacteremias may be primary or secondary. A source is identifiable in the secondary and absent in the primary types. However, bacteremia occurring from an intravascular device in the absence of local purulent infection at the infusion site is also considered primary nosocomial bacteremia.

Risk factors for nosocomial bacteremia are summarized in Table 59.3. Most nosocomial bacteremias arise from skin (i.e., postoperative wound or intravenous catheter infections), intra-abdominal, urinary tract, pulmonary (pneumonias), or other focal infections. The most common organisms

TABLE 59.1 Definitions of systemic inflammatory response syndrome, sepsis, severe sepsis, and septic shock

Term	Definition
Systemic inflammatory response syndrome	Evidence of two or more of the following: • Temperature >38°C (100.4°F) or <36°C (96.8°F) • Heart rate >90/minute • Respiratory rate >20/min or $PaCO_2$ <32 mm Hg • White blood cell count >12,000/mm^3 or <4,000/mm^3 or 10% immature band forms
Sepsis	Systemic inflammatory response syndrome in response to a confirmed infectious process
Severe sepsis	Sepsis associated with organ dysfunction, hypoperfusion, or hypotension; perfusion abnormalities may include but are not limited to lactic acidosis, oliguria, or altered mental status
Septic shock	Sepsis-induced hypotension and perfusion abnormalities despite adequate fluid resuscitation, plus above criteria for severe sepsis

Adapted from American College of Chest Physicians/Society of Critical Care Medicine. Consensus conference: definitions for sepsis and organ failure and guidelines for the use of innovative therapies in sepsis. *Crit Care Med* 1992;20:864, with permission.

TABLE 59.2 Community-acquired bacteremia: most frequent source(s) and common organisms

Organism	Most likely primary infectious process/source	Next most likely source
Escherichia coli	Urinary tract infection	Biliary tract (unknown in some cases)
Streptococcus pneumoniae	Pneumonia	Meningitis
Klebsiella species	Biliary tract	Urinary tract/lower respiratory tract
Staphylococcus aureus	Lower respiratory tract	Endocarditis
Enterococcus species	Urinary tract	
Proteus mirabilis	Urinary tract	
Pseudomonas Aeruginosa	Urinary tract	
Streptococcus bovis	Endocarditis	
Streptococcus viridans	Endocarditis	

Data from Esposito AL, Gleckman RA, Cram S, et al. Community-acquired bacteremia in the elderly: analysis of one hundred consecutive episodes. *J Am Geriatr Soc* 1980;28:315–319, with permission.

TABLE 59.3 Risk factors for nosocomial bacteremia

Host factors
Elderly patient
Systemic antimicrobial therapy
Multiple trauma or burns
Life-threatening underlying illness
Granulocytopenia
Immunosuppression (corticosteroids or cytotoxic agents)
Environmental factors
Intensive care unit
Vascular or nonvascular invasive device
Hemodialysis
Infusion of large volume of parenteral fluids or blood products

Adapted from Maki DG. Nosocomial bacteremia. An epidemiologic review. *Am J Med* 1981;70:724, with permission.

causing nosocomial bacteremias are *Staphylococcus aureus*, *Staphylococcus epidermidis*, *Klebsiella*, group D streptococcus, *Sreptococcus pneumoniae*, and *Escherichia coli*.

The systemic inflammatory response syndrome (SIRS) represents physiological derangements that are nonspecific but are expected to be present in patients with sepsis. However, some patients with clinically overt sepsis do not fulfill the definition for SIRS; hence, the definitions are only valid for practical purposes. The innate immune response to infection involves a rapid inflammatory reaction that is activated over minutes to days and provides an immediate defense against pathogens until one's own immunity develops. The complex interactions among microbial signal molecules, leukocytes, humoral factors, and the vascular endothelium can result in sepsis, but the exact molecular pathogenesis of sepsis syndrome is unknown.

CLINICAL MANIFESTATIONS

In general medical wards, bacteremia is much more prevalent among the elderly and those with diabetes mellitus, chronic renal failure, cerebrovascular accidents, or underlying neoplastic disease.

Features of bacteremia are listed in Table 59.4. Classic symptoms are fever and shaking chills, but rigors may be absent in the debilitated patient. In a significant number of patients, the fever and chills are preceded by hyperventilation and changes in mental status. Although fever is the general rule, bacteremia without fever has been well-documented. The elderly, especially those with associated renal failure or hypoalbuminemia, seem to exhibit this feature more frequently. Bacteremia may be detected incidentally in these persons from the blood cultures performed to elucidate some other problem. Although the lack of fever is a poor prognostic sign, the development of hypothermia is even more ominous.

SIRS is an inflammatory response to an infection or disease that is recognized by the presence of two or more of the following criteria listed in Table 59.1. When the clinical signs of SIRS are present together in the setting of a documented infection, sepsis has ensued.

In severe sepsis, organ dysfunction or hypoperfusion are present. Thus mental status changes, especially lethargy, and rarely agitation may occur. Further findings may include decreased urine output, metabolic acidosis, hypotension, hypoxemia, and hepatic dysfunction.

TABLE 59.4 Manifestations of bacteremia
Fever
Confusion, drowsiness, delirium
Lethargy
Tachycardia
Hyperventilation
Chills/rigors
Hypotension
Nausea/vomiting
Hypotension
Diarrhea
Falls
Incontinence from altered mentation

Multiorgan failure and hypotension refractory to prolonged fluid resuscitation are key manifestations of septic shock. Septic shock affects the major organs by shunting blood away from noncritical tissue (i.e., skin) to maintain perfusion to critical organs (i.e., brain, liver, and kidney). Signs of impaired organ perfusion that occur in shock include cool, vasoconstricted skin (due to redirection of blood flow to core organs). Obtundation or restlessness may indicate central nervous system involvement or liver failure (i.e., hepatic encephalopathy). Urine output must be closely monitored as oliguria or anuria indicates renal impairment. Hypoperfusion ultimately results in anaerobic metabolism, lactic acidosis, and death. Multiple organ dysfunction correlates with poor outcomes in adult patients and also identifies a spectrum of severity in patients with sepsis.

DIAGNOSIS

A complete history is a key component of the clinical evaluation. Attention to underlying diseases, travel, exposures, and other factors is essential. Signs and symptoms pointing to a source should be sought (i.e., headache, joint pain, or diarrhea may suggest the site of focal infection). Careful, thorough physical examination should be completed because in immunosuppressed hosts, disease manifestations may be absent or blunted. Patients with gram-positive bacteremias may show diffuse reddening of the skin (erythroderma), and those with *Pseudomonas bacteremias* may show a central vescicular lesion surrounded by a halo of erythema and induration, which becomes ulcerated (ecthyma gangrenosum). Patients who manifest symptoms or signs suspicious for bacteremia should have two sets of blood culture performed.

Further testing is dictated by the clinical setting. Usually, complete blood counts, liver function tests, and coagulation studies are performed. If there is no apparent source, a urinalysis and chest radiograph should be done. Abdominal pain may prompt computed tomographic (CT) imaging. Obstructing hydronephrosis should be excluded if a urinary tract infection is the focus. As well, one should always entertain diseases that require immediate surgical consultation and/or intervention.

Major problems related to blood cultures are the occurrence of false-positive (positive blood culture with no bacteremia) and false-negative cultures. The frequency of false-positive blood cultures varies widely; most are related to contamination from the skin flora. Clues for recognizing false-positive cultures are listed in Table 59.5. False-negative cultures may be due to an inadequate volume

TABLE 59.5 Clues to false-positive blood culture results
Isolation of the following organisms:
• Diphtheroids
• Staphylococcus epidermidis
• Bacillus species[a]
Inability to isolate same organisms in subsequent cultures
Isolation of multiple organisms in the same culture
Isolation of organism after delayed bacterial growth (broth only)
Same species, but with varying antibiotic sensitivity patterns
Lack of correlation with clinical course
No identifiable primary infection by the same organism
Lack of identifiable predisposing factors, such as:
• Prosthetic devices
• Intravenous drug abuse
• Recent hospitalization
• Immunosuppression
Lack of leukocytosis or left shift

[a]Isolation of enteric gram-negative aerobic organisms, *Streptococcus pyogenes*, or *Streptococcus pneumoniae* is seldom false-positive.
Adapted from Aronson MD, Bor DH. Blood cultures. *Ann Intern Med* 1987;106: 246–253, with permission.

of blood sampled (<15 mL/culture), an inadequate number of blood cultures obtained, improper technique, or the low prevalence of the bacteremia in a given condition (low pretest probability).

TREATMENT

Successful management of sepsis requires urgent measures to treat the local site of infection, to provide hemodynamic and respiratory support, and to eliminate the offending pathogen.

Appropriate antibiotic selection is extremely important in the early phases of sepsis, because mortality is reduced as much as 50% when antibiotics are chosen properly. Because microbiological data are not available for 1 to 2 days, initial antibiotic selection should be empiric and broad spectrum, directed against both gram-positive and gram-negative bacteria. Few guidelines exist for the initial selection of empiric antibiotics in sepsis syndrome. Risk factors for nosocomial infections (i.e., catheter-related infection) and the clinical setting (i.e., neutropenia, nonneutropenia) must be considered. The hospital's antibiogram (antibiotic resistance patterns) should be available with recommendations varying for individual institutions. Once blood culture results become available, antibiotic coverage should be narrowed.

Beyond antimicrobial therapy, "source control" is an important strategy for certain types of sepsis patients. This is particularly important for patients with abscesses or other localized sources of infection where drainage and debridement are the mainstay of treatment. Patients with empyema, sinusitis, chest and/or mediastinal infections, and occasionally skin or soft-tissue infection may also benefit from this approach.

The other major cornerstone to sepsis therapy is fluid resuscitation. This is a common theme for patients with both severe sepsis and septic shock, typically requiring 4 to 8 liters of crystalloid fluid resuscitation. Vasopressors are useful in patients who remain hypotensive despite adequate fluid resuscitation or who develop cardiogenic pulmonary edema. There is no definitive evidence of the superiority of one vasopressor over another.

The development of recombinant human activated protein C (rhAPC), has emerged as a specific therapy for patients with severe sepsis. Administration of rhAPC has been associated with reduced overall risk of death in patients with severe sepsis in recent large clinical trials. Guidelines for determining which patients should receive activated protein C are still evolving. In patients with septic shock and apparent insufficient adrenal reserve, corticosteroid therapy has been shown to improve hemodynamics and survival. Adequate nutritional support is essential for optimal immune function and appears to be beneficial in the treatment of sepsis.

COMPLICATIONS

Septic patients carry an overall mortality of 30%, which is influenced by several factors such as the source, identity, and virulence of the organism on one hand, and a number of host factors on the other, including the status of the specific defenses, functional status, underlying diseases, and the presence or absence of complications. Mortality rates increase with increasing age and with hospital-acquired bacteremia.

A well-known complication in septic shock is sepsis-related acute respiratory distress syndrome (ARDS or "shock lung"). Pulmonary dysfunction typically develops within 24 to 48 hours of the initial event. Patients develop rapidly worsening tachypnea, dyspnea, and hypoxemia requiring high concentrations of supplemental oxygen. Dry cough and chest pain may also be present. The physical examination usually reveals cyanosis, tachycardia, tachypnea, and diffuse rales in the chest. Patients almost always require mechanical ventilation, which may contribute to complications of barotrauma and nosocomial pneumonia. Long-term survivors of ARDS have shown only mild abnormalities in pulmonary function and are often asymptomatic.

Other complications of sepsis syndrome include deep venous thrombosis, gastrointestinal bleeding, malnutrition, negative effects from sedative and neuromuscular blocking medications, and catheter-related infections.

CHAPTER 60

Endocarditis

Jasna Jevtic

Endocarditis, an inflammation of the endocardium, may be infective or nonbacterial. Infective endocarditis (IE) is caused by bacterial or fungal infections of the endocardium. In nonbacterial thrombotic endocarditis, there is an absence of infection. IE may be classified into native-valve or prosthetic-valve IE (bioprosthesis or mechanical) or that related to intravenous (IV) drug abuse, each with its unique list of causative organisms.

Native-valve endocarditis is most common in men aged over 50 years, especially elderly diabetic men. Predisposing valvular lesions are mitral valve prolapse (30% to 50%), rheumatic heart disease (30%), and congenital heart disease (10% to 20%) with a bicuspid aortic valve, pulmonic stenosis, ventricular septal defect, aortic stenosis, IHSS, or patent ductus arteriosus. Degenerative disease of the aortic and mitral valves is responsible in some elderly patients. In rare cases, no predisposing valve lesion is found. Endocarditis may be responsible for 5% to 10% of hospital admissions for febrile intravenous drug abusers (IVDA), generally affecting younger men with a predilection for right-sided valves, notably the tricuspid valve.

Prosthetic valve endocarditis accounts for 10% to 20% of endocarditis cases, typically occurring in males over age 60 years. Aortic valve prostheses are much more likely to be involved than mitral valve prostheses. Because of differences in pathogenesis and pathogens in prosthetic valve endocarditis (PVE), classification into early or late onset is important. Early-onset PVE occurs within 60 days of surgery; with late-onset endocarditis, symptoms are noted after 60 days.

ETIOLOGY

Pathogenesis

The characteristic lesions of infective endocarditis are vegetations on valves. Vegetations can also form on the endocardial surfaces of cardiac chambers or vessels, such as right ventricle in ventricular septal defect, pulmonary artery in patent ductus arteriosus, or left ventricular outflow tract in hypertrophic cardiomyopathy. In the setting of infective endocarditis, the vegetations consist of aggregates of platelets, fibrin, bacteria, and rarely neutrophils. Clots or shreds of fibrin form on an ulcerated valve surface in nonbacterial thrombotic endocarditis.

The evolution of IE requires two processes: an abnormal valve surface and transient bacteremia (Fig. 60.1). Endocarditis tends to occur in high-pressure areas (left side of heart) and downstream from where blood flows through a narrow opening at a high velocity from a high- to low-pressure chamber. The disease usually arises secondary to localization of micro-organisms on sterile vegetations composed of platelets and fibrin. During brief bacteremias, this sterile "vegetation" becomes a source where bacteria adhere. With bacterial colonization and further deposition of platelets and fibrin, valvular infection progresses to damage the valvular architecture. Progressive destructive changes cause or worsen valvular insufficiency. When infection extends into the valve annulus, abscesses and

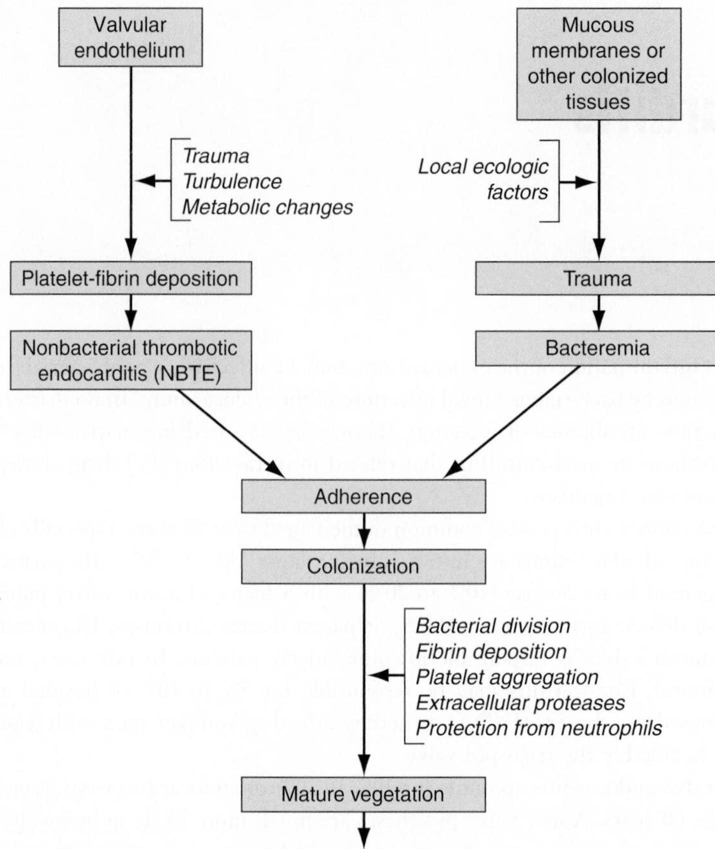

Figure 60.1 • Pathogenesis of infective endocarditis. (Adapted from Bayer AS, Scheld WM. Endocarditis and intravascular infections. In: Mandell GL, Benett JE, Dolin R, eds. *Mandell, Douglas, and Bennett's Principles and Practice of Infectious Diseases.* Philadelphia: Churchill & Livingstone, 2000:859, with permission.)

conduction disturbances result. Vegetations may detach and embolize systemically, involving the skin, brain, kidneys, and lung (in right-sided endocarditis).

Characteristics of the Micro-organisms

Staphylococcus aureus, *Staphylococcus epidermidis*, *viridans streptococci*, and *enterococci* are common causes of IE, because of both the relatively high rate at which they cause transient bacteremia and their avid adherence to normal and abnormal valve surfaces.

Over half of the cases of culture-proven native-valve endocarditis are due to streptococci, typically the *Streptococcus viridians*. Streptococci are normal inhabitants of the mouth and gingiva; hence, minor dental trauma can evoke transient bacteremia and endocarditis. Enterococcal endocarditis often has a subacute course in older (>60 years) men but when seen in young women, it occurs at <40 years of age. Genitourinary disorders or manipulations (i.e., cystoscopy, prostatectomy, urinary catheterization, pregnancy or Cesarean section) are frequent precipitating events. *Streptococcus bovis* bacteremia characteristically occurs with colonic polyps or colon cancer.

S. aureus causes up to 25% of all cases of culture-proven IE. Fungal IE should be considered in IV drug abusers and those with recent cardiovascular surgery or prolonged IV antibiotic therapy. Recent antibiotic use and infections with slow-growing (HACEK group: *Haemophilus parainfluenzae,*

Actinobacillus actinomycetemcomitans, Cardiobacterium hominis, Eikenella species, and *Kingella* species) or fastidious (nutritionally deficient streptococci, fungi, brucellae, chlamydiae, psittacosis, and Q fever) microbes may result in negative cultures in nearly 5% of cases of IE.

CLINICAL MANIFESTATIONS

IE affects persons of all age groups, but mostly older men. The clinical features of IE may be constitutional, cardiac, embolic, and immunologic (Table 60.1).

Constitutional symptoms, being nonspecific, may delay diagnosis of IE. The most common cardiac symptom of IE is dyspnea, which is usually related to congestive heart failure. Major emboli complicate one third of cases, causing protean manifestations with involvement of different organs (skin, abdominal viscera, brain). Thus, sudden neurologic events in young patients should arouse suspicion of IE.

The virulence of the organism and its ability to adhere to the valve also influence the clinical picture. Thus, *S. aureus* endocarditis presents as an acute, fulminant illness with high hectic fever, predominant cardiovascular signs, and scant peripheral stigmata of endocarditis. Rapid valve destruction, hemodynamic instability, and extracardiac metastatic abscesses are its other features. Continuous, community-acquired *S. aureus* bacteremia should always be treated as endocarditis, especially if a primary source is not apparent. Endocarditis due to the viridans streptococci has an insidious onset with a low-grade fever and frequent extracardiac manifestations. A tendency for systemic emboli, ostensibly from large bulky vegetations, is typical of fungal endocarditis.

Fever and heart murmur are characteristic but not uniformly seen. Fever may be absent in

TABLE 60.1 Clinical features of infective endocarditis

Type	Common	Less common
Constitutional	Fever (80%), chills, weakness (40%), sweats, anorexia, weight loss, malaise (each 25%)	Nausea, vomiting, abdominal pain, myalgias/arthralgias, back pain, headache
Cardiac	Dyspnea, which may be acute or insidious (40%); cardiac murmur (>85%)	Chest pain in 15%; myocardial infarctions due to emboli to coronary arteries from valvular vegetations; a new murmur/ changing murmur very infrequent
Embolic	Major emboli (>35%) to different organs (e.g., abdominal pain due to splenic or mesenteric infarction; focal neurologic symptoms)	Janeway lesions (nontender, hemorrhagic, macules on the palmar and plantar surfaces) seen in about 10%
Immunologic	Splenomegaly and clubbing (each in up to 50% of cases)	Conjunctival, oral mucosal, and lower-extremity petechiae; splinter hemorrhages in about 15% (very nonspecific); Osler nodes (multiple, 2–5 mm, tender, nodular lesions on the fingers or toes, seen in 15% (nonspecific)

elderly patients and those with heart failure, malnutrition, or in renal failure (urea has antipyretic properties). In many patients, particularly the elderly, the cardiac auscultatory findings of endocarditis are often inseparable from signs of prior valvular disease and high output (fever, anemia).

IE in IVDAs often presents with pleuritic chest pain and cough. In over half the cases, the responsible microorganism is *S. aureus* (50%), followed by streptococci in 20%, gram-negative bacilli (esp. *Pseudomonas aeruginosa*) in 20%, and fungi (esp. *Candida* sp.) in 10% of cases. The geographical location (eastern versus western United States) may affect the microbial etiology. A murmur is common, but the classical triad of tricuspid regurgitation, a pulsatile liver, and the waxing-waning systolic murmur occurs in one third of cases. The mitral and aortic valves also may be involved.

DIAGNOSIS

Blood cultures are positive in over 95% of cases, being the key diagnostic test for IE. No more than three sets of cultures are routinely necessary in the first 24 hours unless antibiotics have been given in the preceding 2 weeks. The laboratory should be notified of the clinical suspicion of IE, so as to enable prolonged incubation and subculture techniques. When the bacteremia is continuous all sets of blood cultures will be positive in most patients. Persistent bacteremia without an identifiable source (i.e., an infected IV line) should arouse the suspicion of IE. Minimum inhibitory concentration (MIC) should be measured to guide the choice and dose of antimicrobials.

A normochromic, normocytic anemia is very common. In subacute cases, the white blood cell count may be normal or modestly high. The erythrocyte sedimentation rate (ESR) is almost always high, but a normal ESR does not exclude IE. Positive VDRL and rheumatoid factor may be present. Proteinuria, occasionally in the nephrotic range, and microscopic hematuria are generally noted. Gross hematuria may follow renal emboli or infarcts. Red and white blood cell casts reflect an immune-complex-mediated glomerulonephritis when present on urine microscopy.

Chest x-rays may show septic pulmonary emboli and/or pneumonia in about 50% of patients. Septic pulmonary emboli (i.e., bilateral, multiple, small patchy infiltrates that may cavitate) are typical of right-sided endocarditis. The chest x-ray may also show heart failure. In suspected prosthetic valve endocarditis, fluoroscopy typically shows abnormal valve motion or "rocking" by a loose prosthesis.

The electrocardiogram may show signs of myocardial infarction and ST-T changes in the setting of coronary artery emboli and myocarditis. The electrocardiogram should also be monitored for conduction defects such as complete heart block, which may be the result of a valvular abscess extending into the septum.

Echocardiography has a critical role in the diagnosis and management of IE (Fig. 60.2). Findings highly predictive of IE include characteristic vegetations, abscesses, new prosthetic valve dehiscence, or new valvular regurgitation. Although echocardiography should be performed in all cases of suspected IE, it is not an appropriate screen for IE in clinical situations where fever or bacteremia is unlikely to be caused by IE. Transthoracic echocardiography (TTE), with a sensitivity of about 70% for large (>5 mm) vegetations and few false-positive results, can assess the severity of valvular incompetence and detect vegetations and local complications (i.e., perforated leaflet, chordal rupture, myocardial ring abscesses). Nearly 80% of infected, native, left-sided valve vegetations may be detected. A normal study does not exclude IE as small vegetations may be missed. Keep in mind that adequate imaging may not be achieved in patients with obesity, chronic obstructive lung disease, and chest wall abnormalities.

Transesophageal echocardiography (TEE), with a sensitivity of over 90% for detecting vegetations, can detect smaller vegetations and identify periannular abscesses, mycotic aneurysms, and pulmonic valve vegetations. Because TEE is more sensitive both for the diagnosis of IE and for detecting complications, TEE should be performed in essentially all cases of suspected endocarditis.

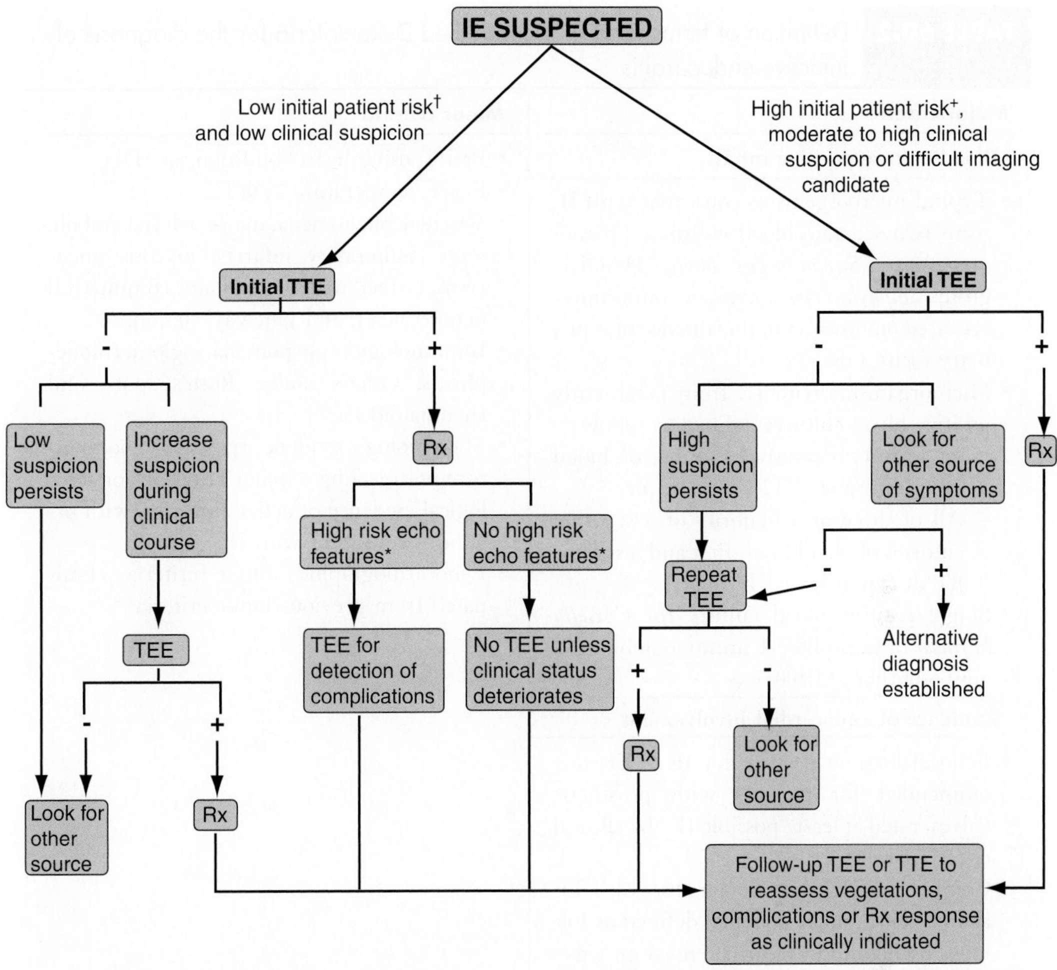

Figure 60.2 • An approach to the diagnostic use of echocardiography. *High-risk echocardiographic features include large and/or mobile vegetations, valvular insufficiency, suggestion of perivalvular extension, or secondary ventricular dysfunction (see text). †For example, a patient with fever and a previously known heart murmur and no other stigmata of IE. + High initial patient risks include prosthetic heart valves, many congenital heart diseases, previous endocarditis, new murmur, heart failure, or other stigmata of endocarditis. Rx, antibiotic treatment for endocarditis. (Reproduced from Bayer AS, Bolger AF, Taubert KA, et al. Diagnosis and management of infective endocarditis and its complications. *Circulation*. 1998;98:2936–2948, with permission.)

Modified Duke criteria for diagnosing IE incorporate pathologic and clinical aspects, which includes both major and minor criteria (Table 60.2). The approach to the patient with suspected IE is outlined in Figure 60.2.

TREATMENT

General principles of treating infective endocarditis include the use of bactericidal rather than bacteriostatic antibiotics as failure to sterilize the vegetations increases the risk of relapse, the use of IV

TABLE 60.2 Definition of terms used in the modified Duke criteria for the diagnosis of infective endocarditis

Major criteria	Minor criteria
Blood culture positive for IE • Typical microorganisms consistent with IE from two separate blood cultures: *Viridans streptococci, Streptococcus bovis*, HACEK group, *Staphylococcus aureus*, or community-acquired enterococci in the absence of a primary focus; OR • Microorganisms with IE from persistently positive blood cultures defined as follows: At least two positive cultures of blood samples drawn >12 hrs apart, **or** All of three or a majority of 4 separate cultures of blood (with first and last sample drawn at least 1 hr apart) • Single positive blood culture for *Coxiella burnetii* or anti-phase 1 immunoglobulin G antibody titer >1:800	• Predisposing heart condition, or IDU • Fever, temperature >38°C • Vascular phenomena, major arterial emboli, septic pulmonary infarcts, mycotic aneurysm, intracranial hemorrhage, conjunctival hemorrhages, and Janeway's lesions • Immunologic phenomena: glomerulonephritis, Osler's nodes, Roth's spots, and rheumatoid factor • Microbiologic evidence: positive blood culture not meeting a major criterion[a] or serological evidence of active infection with organism consistent with IE • Echocardiographic minor criteria eliminated from previous Duke criteria
Evidence of endocardial involvement • Echocardiogram positive for IE (TEE recommended for patients with prosthetic valves, rated at least "possible IE" by clinical criteria, **or** • Complicated IE [paravalvular abscess]; TTE as first test in other patients) defined as follows: oscillating intracardiac mass on valve or supporting structures, in the path of regurgitant jets, or on implanted material in the absence of an alternative anatomic explanation, **or** • Abscess, **or** • New partial dehiscence or prosthetic valve; new Valvular regurgitation (worsening or changing or pre-existing murmur not sufficient)	
Definite diagnosis of infective endocarditis: • 2 major criteria; **or** • 1 major criterion and 3 minor criteria; **or** • 5 minor criteria	

[a]Excludes single positive cultures for coagulase-negative staphylococci and organisms that do not cause endocarditis.
TEE, transesophageal echocardiography; TTE, transthoracic echocardiography.

TABLE 60.3 Endocarditis treatment table

Organism	Valve	Drug(s) and duration
Staphylococci, methicillin-susceptible	Native	Nafcillin × 6 weeks
	Prosthetic	Nafcillin × 6 weeks + Rifampin × 6 weeks + Gentamicin × 2 weeks
Staphylococci, methicillin-resistant	Native	Vancomycin × 6 weeks
	Prosthetic	Vancomycin × 6 weeks + Rifampin × 6 weeks + Gentamicin × 2 weeks
Streptococci, penicillin-susceptible (MIC <0.12)	Native	Penicillin × 4 weeks
	Prosthetic	Penicillin × 6 weeks
Streptococci, relatively penicillin resistant (MIC >0.12)	Native	Penicillin × 4 weeks + Gentamicin × 2 weeks
	Prosthetic	Penicillin × 6 weeks + Gentamicin × 6 weeks
Enterococci, penicillin-susceptible	Native	Ampicillin × 4–6 weeks + Gentamicin × 4–6 weeks
	Prosthetic	Ampicillin × 6 weeks + Gentamicin × 6 weeks

MIC, minimum inhibitory concentration.
Adapted from Baddour LM, et al. Infective endocarditis: diagnosis, antimicrobial therapy, and management of complications. *Circulation* 2005;105:394–434, with permission.)

antimicrobial therapy, and ensuring high antibiotic concentrations for prolonged periods so as to eradicate slow-growing organisms.

Empiric antibiotics may be given to patients with suspected IE, especially those who are acutely toxic or in heart failure. Streptococci, staphylococci, and enterococci pose special problems, given the recent emergence of drug-resistant strains. Once blood culture results are available, regimens should be tailored to the specific organism and its in vitro sensitivities (Table 60.3). With optimal treatment, most patients (>90%) with native-valve endocarditis attain a microbiologic cure.

Positive blood cultures are the cornerstone of diagnosis of IVDA-related IE; hence, patients with fever and IVDA should be observed closely until blood cultures are reported sterile. The cure rate in right-sided *S. aureus* endocarditis exceeds 90% if promptly and appropriately treated. Persistent fever and septic emboli are not indications for surgical intervention; hence, valve excision or debridement is usually reserved for those with persistent uncontrolled bacteremia.

Because of differences in pathogenesis and pathogens in early-onset versus late-onset prosthetic valve endocarditis (PVE), classification is important. *Staphylococcus epidermidis* is the most frequent organism in early PVE supporting the role of intraoperative contamination. Causative organisms in late disease resemble those of native-valve endocarditis. Suggested treatment of early PVE due to *S. epidermidis* takes into account the resistance patterns of this organism. Both early and late PVE often need reoperation for valve replacement.

Valve surgery is required in about 25% of cases of IE. Common indications (discussed in the next section) are congestive heart failure (>70% of cases), hemodynamic compromise, persistent infection, periannular extension of infection, systemic emboli, splenic abscess, and mycotic aneurysms as discussed below.

COMPLICATIONS

The patient's age, comorbid conditions, the valve affected, virulence of the organism, and complications of treatment all influence the prognosis. Recurrent fever may reflect local complications (i.e., myocardial or valve ring abscess, metastatic abscesses), drug fever, or progression to sepsis.

Patients at high risk of complications are those with special issues determined by clinical factors (those with prolonged symptoms or poor response to therapy), predisposition (IE superimposed on prosthetic cardiac valves, cyanotic heart disease, previous endocarditis or systemic shunts), site of lesion (left-sided IE), or causative organisms (staphylococci and fungi). Complications of IE include congestive heart failure (CHF), systemic embolization, perivalvular and splenic abscesses, and mycotic aneurism.

Congestive Heart Failure

Among all the complications of IE, CHF has the greatest impact on prognosis. In native valve IE, acute CHF occurs more frequently in aortic valve infections (29%) than with mitral (20%) or tricuspid disease (8%). CHF may develop acutely from perforation of a native or bioprosthetic valve leaflet, rupture of infected mitral chordae, valve obstruction by bulky vegetations, or sudden intracardiac shunts from fistulous tracts or prosthetic dehiscence. Heart failure also may develop more insidiously despite administration of appropriate antibiotics as a result of progressive worsening of valvular insufficiency and ventricular dysfunction. The degree of tolerance of CHF is valve dependent, with acute aortic regurgitation being least tolerant and acute tricuspid regurgitation most tolerant.

Risk of Embolization

Systemic embolization occurs in 22% to 50% of cases of IE. Emboli often involve major arterial beds, including the lungs, coronary arteries, spleen, bowel, and extremities. Up to 65% of embolic events involve the central nervous system the majority lodging in the distribution of the middle cerebral artery. The highest incidence of embolic complications is seen with vegetations >10 mm in diameter occurring on the anterior mitral leaflet and in IE caused by *S. aureus*, *Candida*, HACEK, and *Abiotrophia* organisms. Most emboli occur within the first 2 to 4 weeks of antimicrobial therapy. Prediction of individual patient risk for embolization is extremely difficult.

Periannular Extension of Infection

Extension of IE beyond the valve annulus predicts a higher mortality rate, more frequent development of CHF, and more frequent cardiac surgery. Perivalvular abscesses are particularly common with prosthetic valves because the annulus, rather than the leaflet, is the usual primary site of infection. Clinical parameters for the diagnosis of perivalvular extension of IE are inadequate. Persistent bacteremia or fever, recurrent emboli, heart block, CHF, or a new pathological murmur in a patient with IE on appropriate antibiotics may suggest extension. Drainage of abscess cavities, excision of necrotic tissue, and closure of fistulous tracts often accompany valve replacement surgery.

Splenic Abscess

Splenic abscess is a well-described but rare complication of IE. In contrast, splenic infarction is a common complication of left-sided IE (40% of cases). Clinical splenomegaly, which is present in up to 30% of cases of IE, is not a reliable sign of splenic infarction or abscess. Pain in the left upper quadrant, back, left flank, or generalized abdominal tenderness may be associated with either splenic infarction or abscess. Persistent or recurrent bacteremia, persistent fever, or other signs of sepsis are suggestive of splenic abscess, and patients with these findings should be further evaluated.

Mycotic Aneurysms

Mycotic aneurysms (MAs) are uncommon complications of IE that result from septic embolization of vegetations to the arteries or the intraluminal space occurring most frequently in the intracranial arteries, followed by the visceral arteries and the arteries of the upper and lower extremities.

The clinical presentation of patients with intracranial MAs is highly variable. Patients may develop severe headache, altered sensorium, or focal neurological deficits (i.e., hemianopsia or cranial neuropathies). In some patients, there are no clinically recognized findings before sudden subarachnoid or intraventricular hemorrhage.

Intrathoracic or intra-abdominal MAs often are asymptomatic until leakage or rupture occurs. The appearance of a tender, pulsatile mass in a patient with IE should suggest an extracranial MA. Hematemesis, hematobilia, and jaundice suggest rupture of a hepatic artery MA; arterial hypertension and hematuria suggest rupture of a renal MA; and massive bloody diarrhea suggests the rupture small or large bowel MA. Most extracranial MAs will rupture if not excised.

CHAPTER 61

Osteomyelitis

Susan Davids

Osteomyelitis, or bone infection, is an inflammatory process caused by a pyogenic organism, which can be difficult to diagnose and treat. There are three types of osteomyelitis based on the initial mechanism of infection: (a) spread from a contiguous infection following trauma, bone surgery or joint replacement, or local spread from a soft-tissue focus of infection; (b) vascular insufficiency, primarily foot soft tissue infections that spread to the bone (e.g., infected diabetic foot ulcers); or (c) hematogenous spread. Osteomyelitis can be also be characterized as an acute, subacute, or chronic infection. Acute osteomyelitis develops after several days to weeks (usually from hematogenous spread), subacute may develop after several weeks to a month (usually from spread from contiguous infection), and chronic begins after a few months (usually from vascular insufficiency).

ETIOLOGY

The bone is highly resistant to infection and is only infected with trauma, a foreign body, or a very large inocula of an organism. Bone infection is associated with tissue edema and destruction of bone trabeculae and matrix. Vascular occlusion also occurs and results in bony necrosis, called sequestra.

The etiology of infection depends on the type of osteomyelitis (Table 61.1).

Hematogenous Osteomyelitis

Hematogenous osteomyelitis occurs predominantly in children and affects the long bones. Adults are rarely affected, but if they are, they are generally over the age of 50 years. The most common sites involved are thoracic or lumber vertebrae. Hematogenous osteomyelitis can also occur in younger adults, but is primarily seen in intravenous drug users or those with sickle cell disease. The bacteria involved are usually based upon the age and risk factors of the patient. For adults, the most common organism is *Staphylococcus aureus*, followed by gram-negative bacilli; however fungi and *Mycobacterium tuberculosis* also needs to be considered.

Patients with sickle cell disease are 10 times more likely to be infected with *Salmonella spp*. than any other bacteria.

Risk factors for hematogenous osteomyelitis include central lines, urinary catheters, dialysis, urinary tract infections, or endocarditis.

Spread from a Contiguous Infection

This type of infection involves prosthetic joint replacements or other implants (pins/screws), trauma (open fracture), bone surgery or local sites of infection (decubitus ulcers). *S. aureus* and *Staphylococcus epidermidis* are the most common organisms. The organism responsible for posttraumatic osteomyelitis includes many possibilities depending on the exposure at the time of the injury (i.e., soil, water), which could include gram-negative bacilli, anaerobic organisms, or endemic organisms to the community, including fungi.

TABLE 61.1 Categories and etiology of osteomyelitis

Underlying disease	Typical organisms
Hematogenous spread Endocarditis, infected intravascular catheter, urinary tract infection, intravenous drug use	*Staphylococcus aureus, Pseudomonas aeruginosa* (and other gram-negative bacilli), *Candida* spp.
Sickle cell disease	*Salmonella* spp., *S. aureus*
Secondary to a contiguous focus	
Without vascular insufficiency	*S. aureus,* gram-negative bacilli, anaerobes
Contamination from surgery or trauma, local soft-tissue infection (e.g., decubitus ulcer) Prosthetic joint	 *Streptococcus epidermidis*
With vascular insufficiency	
Lower-extremity soft-tissue injury in a patient with diabetic neuropathy and vascular insufficiency	Staphylococci, streptococci, enterococci, gram-negative bacilli, anaerobes

Orthopaedic prosthetic devices can have an infection rate up to 15%. Infection, usually initiated at the bone cement interface, occurs by local introduction of organisms or, less commonly, hematogenously. Staphylococci (both coagulase-negative and positive) are the most frequent pathogens, followed by streptococci and gram-negative bacilli.

Due to Vascular Insufficiency

Patients with diabetes or vascular insufficiency develop this type of osteomyelitis, which is usually a chronic and generally affects the feet. The infection originates from a break in the skin or an ulcer. There are a variety of organisms that can cause osteomyelitis due to vascular insufficiency, including staphylococci, streptococci, enterococci, gram-negative bacilli, and anaerobes.

CLINICAL MANIFESTATIONS

The clinical manifestations may vary by type of osteomyelitis.

Hematogenous Osteomyelitis

Hematogenous osteomyelitis has features of systemic illness, including chills, fever, malaise, and pain. There can also be local swelling at area of local infection especially when the infection originated from an infected intravenous catheter, or from intravenous drug use. In patients with vertebral involvement, the patient may present with back pain, similar to pain from other musculoskeletal diseases; however, most patients will have pain and tenderness over the involved vertebrae.

Spread from a Contiguous Infection

Osteomyelitis after an orthopedic implant (prosthetic joint or other implant) can occur less than 3 months (acute) and up to 24 months or greater after the implant. If acute, the patients will have acute joint pain, effusion, erythema, warmth at the implant site, and fever. Those presenting later usually have a more mild presentation, such are persistent joint pain or implant loosening. Those with a very late presentation usually are infected by hematogenous spread and not from contiguous spread.

The features of a posttraumatic osteomyelitis or post bone surgery include poor wound or bone healing. Patients may also have local signs of infection including pain, warmth, erythema, swelling, and drainage from the wound site. Fever may be present, but is more likely to be low grade if the infection is chronic.

Osteomyelitis due to infected pressure ulcers occurs in 17% to 32% of patients. The diagnosis is difficult to establish, but poor wound healing with or without systemic symptoms can be present. There are no proven signs or symptoms that correlate with osteomyelitis, including fever, bone exposure, duration of ulcer, or purulent drainage.

Due to Vascular Insufficiency

Generally patients will have a soft-tissue infection or ulcer in the feet for greater than 1 week, particularly over bony prominences. Usually, the patient is afebrile. Pain may be present and can be severe; however, there can be an absence of pain in patients with diabetic neuropathy. The ability to advance a sterile probe to bone confirms the diagnosis. In cases of early osteomyelitis, clinical presentation and exam can be negative.

DIAGNOSIS

A careful history and physical should always be performed. A radiographic evaluation should be done in all types of osteomyelitis and is essential in the follow-up of the patient.

Plain radiographs that reveal typical periosteal elevation and soft tissue swelling, narrowing or widening of joint spaces, or bone destruction are diagnostic of osteomyelitis and warrant initiation of treatment. However, because these changes may take up to 3 weeks from the onset of the disease to develop, a negative radiographic film does not exclude the diagnosis of osteomyelitis (plain radiographs have low sensitivity but high specificity in the diagnosis of osteomyelitis).

Radionuclide studies can detect early osteomyelitis, but can have false positives can occur with diabetic arthropathy, gout, trauma, and surgery. Radionuclide studies are useful when osteomyelitis is suspected but no obvious site of infection is detected.

Both computed tomography (CT) and magnetic resonance imaging (MRI) can detect edema and periosteal reaction, articular damaged, and soft tissue swelling early. The accuracy of the CT can be degraded due to artifacts caused by bone or metal including titanium, which is commonly used in orthopedic procedures.

MRI is the imaging modality of choice for the diagnosis of osteomyelitis, particularly in diabetic patients. MRI reveals early bone edema, even prior to radionuclide studies. However, there is a lag of resolution of edema after full antimicrobial eradication, so may not be helpful in guiding the response to therapy.

Positron emission tomography (PET) is also being considered as an imaging modality for osteomyelitis.

Definitive diagnosis of osteomyelitis, however, is achieved by culturing a biopsy or aspirate of affected bone.

Special diagnostic considerations are discussed based on mechanism of infection.

Hematogenous Osteomyelitis

Bone tenderness can be present in these patients; therefore, a thorough bone evaluation should be done. If febrile, blood cultures should be done, but they are frequently negative. If the blood cultures are negative and the imaging studies reveal osteomyelitis, a needle biopsy with multiple specimens should be performed because many organisms can cause this disease, including bacteria, fungi, and mycobacteria. If the first biopsy is negative, it should be repeated; if it is again nondiagnostic, the options include an open surgical procedure or empirical therapy.

Spread from a Contiguous Infection

If an infected prosthetic is diagnosed by one of the imaging tests, joint fluid should be sampled to isolate the pathogen. When the diagnosis is in question, more than one arthrocentesis should be performed to confirm the pathogen. If a pathogen is not isolated, a bone biopsy should be done. Sinus tract cultures are usually not helpful, unless *S. aureus* is isolated.

In those patients with decubitus ulcers, clinical judgment is very poor at making the diagnosis. Those patients with nonhealing or progressive ulcers should have imaging and bone biopsy.

Due to Vascular Insufficiency

In this type of osteomyelitis, when bone is exposed in the ulcer bed or a sterile probe can reach bone, the diagnosis of osteomyelitis is confirmed. However, imaging is always performed as noted above, and microbial diagnosis is best made by bone biopsy.

TREATMENT

Treatment depends upon many factors and particularly the type of osteomyelitis. However, early antibiotic treatment produces the best results.

Osteomyelitis is treated using an antibiotic appropriate for the pathogen. Antibiotics are traditionally given parenterally for 4 to 6 weeks, although long-term oral antibiotics are appropriate in certain settings (e.g., oral quinolones for sensitive gram-negative organisms).

Antimicrobial therapy is usually sufficient therapy; surgical debridement may be integral to successful therapy in selected cases, especially in chronic osteomyelitis, in which necrotic bone precludes proper penetration of antibiotics. Inadequate debridement is one of the causes of high recurrence rates. With pre-existing ulcers or prior debridement, tissue flaps may be necessary.

Surgery for vertebral osteomyelitis is usually limited to relieve compression of the spinal cord or to drain epidural or paravertebral abscesses.

In diabetic or vascular insufficiency infections, surgery to improve blood flow should be done. Amputation may be necessary if there is no response to revascularization and antibiotics.

In patients with a prosthetic infection, successful treatment usually involves removal of the prosthesis, followed by a 6-week course of appropriate antibiotics and then reimplantation.

COMPLICATIONS

Complications can include sepsis, amputation, or recurrent infection. In vertebral osteomyelitis, potential complications include soft-tissue extension of the infection, paraspinal abscess, and spinal cord compression.

CHAPTER 62

Syphilis

Susan Davids

Syphilis is a sexually transmitted disease with both cutaneous and visceral manifestations caused by *Treponema pallidum*. First described 500 years ago, syphilis has been called the "great imitator" due to its variety of clinical presentations. After the introduction of penicillin in the 1940s, the rate of syphilis in the United States fell dramatically to a nadir in the late 1950s. But, in 1990 the United States suffered a miniepidemic thought to be due to human immunodeficiency virus (HIV). Although by 2000, the incidence had declined to the lowest rates, the incidence of syphilis since has risen; in 2004, primary and secondary cases reported to the Centers for Disease Control and Prevention increased 11%. The increase was seen primarily in men who have sex with men. However, for the first time in many years, the rate of syphilis did not decrease in women and increased in almost all racial and ethnic groups, most notably in black men. In the United States, the southeast and urban areas are most affected. Outside of the United States and other developed countries, syphilis remains a very significant problem with approximately 3 to 4 million new cases of syphilis each year in the following areas: Latin American and the Caribbean, south and southeast Asia, and sub-Saharan Africa.

ETIOLOGY

Syphilis is caused by the spirochete *T. pallidum*. It is a very small (less than 20 μm in length), slender, coiled organism that replicates slowly (estimated dividing time of 30 hours) and cannot grow in vitro. Syphilis is spread person-to-person with the primary route of transmission through sexual contact. Spirochetes migrate through minute fissures in mucous membranes or skin in adults via direct contact with the syphilitic ulcerative lesion called a chancre (primary stage) or condylomata lata (flat, wartlike plaques that occur in the secondary stage). Vertical transmission may also occur because the spirochete can cross the placenta to infect a fetus. Very rarely, it is transmitted by accidental inoculation or blood transfusion.

Transmission occurs early in the disease in the either primary or secondary stages of syphilis. *T. pallidum* enters the lymphatics and bloodstream, disseminating to almost any organ in the body. The incubation period is nearly 3 weeks, but can vary from a few days to 3 months depending on the size of the inoculum.

Other sexually transmitted diseases (STDs) such as HIV, chlamydia, and gonorrhea may coexist with syphilis; the diagnosis of any one of these should prompt a search for the others.

CLINICAL MANIFESTATIONS

Syphilis is classified into the four categories of *primary, secondary, latent,* and *tertiary phases,* which differ in their clinical manifestations and treatment. It may also be divided into the two broad categories of *early* and *late* syphilis. Early syphilis is defined as the first 2 years of disease and encompasses primary syphilis, secondary syphilis, and early latent syphilis. Late syphilis includes late latent and tertiary syphilis.

Primary Syphilis

The chancre is the hallmark of primary syphilis. The chancre develops 3 to 4 weeks after exposure to the *T. pallidum* at the site of contact. The lesion begins as a single red papule and evolves into a painless ulcer. The chancre is accompanied by bilateral, nontender regional adenopathy and resolves in about 6 weeks.

Although usually solitary and localized to the genitals, chancres may be multiple (especially in HIV patients) and involve oral mucosa, rectum, face, axilla, breasts, or distal extremities. In women, a chancre may be overlooked because it may occur on the cervix. It can occur as a mixed infection with chancroid (*Hemophilius ducreyi*) or become superinfected.

Secondary Syphilis

Secondary syphilis, indicating acute dissemination, usually occurs 2 to 8 weeks after the chancre appears. Some patients may have no history of a chancre, as the primary infection may have been asymptomatic or unrecognized. Secondary syphilis can cause a wide variety of signs and symptoms.

Cutaneous findings are the most prominent feature in the secondary stage, occurring in 90% of cases. The most characteristic cutaneous finding is a nonpruritic, nonpainful, symmetrical rash of reddish-brown macules and papules, which may scale and follow the lines of cleavage in the skin. The rash involves the entire trunk and extremities including the characteristic involvement of the palms and soles. Even in nontreated patients, the rash eventually resolves; however, it can occur again.

Other cutaneous lesions observed at this stage are mucous patches, condyloma lata, syphilitic pharyngitis, and patchy "moth-eaten" alopecia. Characteristically, none of these lesions are pruritic as well. Mucous patches are white, eroded papules that arise on the tongue; tonsils; gingival, buccal, and labial mucosa; cervix; vagina; labia minora; glans; and corona of the penis. Condyloma lata, which occur in moist intertriginous areas, are pink exophytic papules that are very infectious, and should be distinguished from condyloma acuminate (human papillomavirus).

Systemic features include fever, headache, anorexia, arthralgias, fatigue, sore throat, and generalized lymphadenopathy. The gastrointestinal tract, kidneys, liver, central nervous system, prostate, lungs, and bones may also be infected. Anemia, leukocytosis, significantly elevated alkaline phosphatase, and a high erythrocyte sedimentation rate are the notable laboratory findings.

Without treatment, resolution can occur within 10 weeks and lesions heal with pigmentary changes. However, any of the above symptoms can occur again.

Latent and Tertiary Stages

Latent syphilis occurs when there is a positive test for syphilis without any manifestations of disease. The latent stage is classified as early or late latent. Early latent refers to disease acquired during the preceding 12 months. Early and late latent must be distinguished as treatment differs.

Tertiary syphilis comprises three types: neurosyphilis, cardiovascular syphilis, and late benign (i.e., gummatous) syphilis. Tertiary syphilis can occur 1 to 25 years after the initial infection; however, it is now extremely rare in the United States due to early treatment.

Neurosyphilis is divided into two categories: (a) early involvement of the central nervous system limited to the meninges, and (b) parenchymal involvement. The majority of infected people with neurosyphilis are asymptomatic, but they can present with a wide variety of neurological signs and symptoms including but not limited to: stroke, personality changes, ataxia, ophthalmic symptoms (Chorioretinitis), dementia, and sensory involvement. Tabes dorsalis, now rare, was once the most common form of neurosyphilis, affecting the posterior columns.

Cardiovascular syphilis refers medial necrosis of the aorta (aoritis) causing aortic aneurysms mainly of the ascending aorta, which causes aortic insufficiency. Coronary stenosis also may occur.

Late benign syphilis, gummatous, is a form of granulomatous disease and can occur anywhere. On the skin, gummas can be raised lesions or appear ulcerative. Gummas can also appear to be mass lesions and mimic malignancies when in the central nervous system or other organs. Gumma rarely affects the vital organs and quickly responds to treatment; therefore, they are labeled benign.

DIAGNOSIS

Syphilis is diagnosed by correlation of the clinical findings and the results of serological tests for syphilis, because *T. pallidum* cannot be grown in vitro. A thorough history and physical must first be done, concentrating on the sexual history, syphilis history, and a very thorough examination of the oral mucosa, skin, genital and perianal area, and a detailed neurological assessment.

In patients with a chancre of primary syphilis or the condylomata lata of secondary syphilis, dark-field examination allows direct visualization of the spirochete and should be performed. A scraping of the lesion is placed on a slide and viewed with a phase-contrast microscope. However, the necessary expertise may not be available in all facilities.

Serologic tests for syphilis include nontreponemal tests and a specific antitreponemal antibody test. The former tests are nonspecific and include the Venereal Disease Research Laboratory (VDRL) or the rapid plasma reagin (RPR). These tests measure immunoglobulin (Ig) M and IgG antibodies directed against a lipid antigen formed by interaction of *T. pallidum* and the host, and are used for screening or following up disease activity. A fourfold change (two dilutions) is considered significant.

Because of frequent false-positive results (Table 62.1), a confirmatory test is usually done using treponemal tests, such as the fluorescent treponemal antibody absorption (FTA-ABS) or the microhemagglutination assay (MHA-TP) for antibody to *T. pallidum*. All patients with syphilis should be evaluated for HIV infection.

TREATMENT

Penicillin remains the drug of choice for all stages of syphilis (Table 62.2). The type of penicillin used, the dosage, and the duration of treatment depend on the stage of disease. For penicillin-allergic patients, oral doxycycline or erythromycin may be used, except in neurosyphilis because these drugs

TABLE 62.1 Causes of false-positive results in serologic tests for syphilis

Infectious causes	Noninfectious causes
Other spirochetes	Narcotic addicts
Tuberculosis	Connective tissue disorder
Leprosy	Pregnancy
Endocarditis	Old age
Mycoplasma infection	Chronic liver disease
Rickettsial infection	Laboratory error
Hepatitis	
Infectious Mononucleosis	

TABLE 62.2 Treatment of primary, secondary, and late syphilis

Stage	Treatment regimen	Comments
Primary, secondary, and early latent	Benzathine penicillin 2.4 MU intramuscularly (IM) in a single dose	If penicillin allergic, doxycycline 100 mg orally twice daily or tetracycline 500 mg orally four times daily for 28 days for all stages; desensitize for syphilis complicating pregnancy
Late latent or unknown duration	Benzathine penicillin 7.2 MU total, administered as 2.4 MU weekly IM doses for 3 weeks	
Tertiary syphilis (excluding neurosyphilis)	Benzathine penicillin 7.2 MU total, administered as 2.4 MU weekly IM doses for 3 weeks	
Neurosyphilis	Aqueous crystalline penicillin G 18–24 MU per day, administered as 3–4 MU IV every 4 hours or continuous infusion, for 10–14 days	If compliance can be ensured, could use procaine penicillin 2.4 MU IM once daily PLUS probenecid 500 mg orally four times a day, both for 10–14 days

do not penetrate the cerebrospinal fluid. Penicillin desensitization should be strongly considered for penicillin-allergic patients with neurosyphilis and in penicillin-allergic women regardless of the stage. A clinical and serological reexamination should occur 6 and 12 month after treatment. A patient is considered to have either failed treatment or have been reinfected if they have persistent or recurrent signs and symptoms and/or have sustained elevated nontreponemal titers. If treatment failure is suspected, the individual should have a repeat HIV test as well as cerebrospinal fluid analysis. In patients with reinfection or treatment failure, retreatment consists of weekly penicillin G 2.4 million units IM for 3 weeks, unless neurosyphilis is present.

Management of syphilis in patients with HIV is similar to that for the non-HIV patient, and close follow-up is necessary with serological examination at 1, 2, 3, 6, 9, and 12 months. Penicillin-allergic patients should be desensitized.

Sexual partners need to be evaluated clinically and serologically to direct their treatment regimen.

COMPLICATIONS

Patients treated adequately for early syphilis should have complete resolution of their disease. However, in untreated patients with late-stage syphilis, both cardiac and neurosyphilis may have nonreversible components.

CHAPTER 63

HIV Infection

Michael Frank

In 1981, a publication in *Morbidity and Mortality Weekly Report* about clusters of cases of *Pneumocystis* pneumonia and Kaposi's sarcoma in previously healthy gay men led to the recognition of a new disease that became known as acquired immunodeficiency syndrome (AIDS). In 1983, a virus was isolated from lymph tissue of patients with the new disease, and a serologic test for infection with the virus was developed by 1985. This newly identified virus eventually was named human immunodeficiency virus (HIV) type 1. It is now known that HIV evolved from genetically similar simian immunodeficiency virus (SIV), which infects chimpanzees in central Africa, and that introduction into the human species likely occurred decades before its identification. By that point, HIV infection had spread around the world.

The Joint United Nations Programme on HIV/AIDS estimated in 2005 that globally 38.6 million people were living with HIV infection. While the majority of cases were still in subSaharan Africa, the countries of Asia had the fastest growing rates of new infections. By the end of 2004, a cumulative total of 529,113 people had died of AIDS in the United States. As of 2004, an estimated 1.2 million people in the United States were living with HIV infection, with an estimated one fourth of them unaware of their infection. Although new infections continued to rise in all categories, the rates were increasing fastest in minorities and women, most of whom acquired the disease through heterosexual contact. The development of successful treatment for HIV infection has led to dramatic reductions in the death rate due to AIDS in the United States and the developed world, although the prevalence has continued to increase (Figure 63.1).

ETIOLOGY

HIV-1 is a member of the retrovirus family, with two copies of single-stranded RNA in each virion. This family also includes several animal lentiviruses, human T-cell lymphotropic viruses I and II, and HIV-2. HIV-2 is genetically very similar to certain SIVs that infect monkeys, and in humans causes a more indolent, slowly progressive or nonprogressive infection. HIV-1 is now universally accepted as the cause of AIDS and has numerous different subtypes. The clinical relevance of different subtypes for the most part results from some viral load assays being less able to detect the less common subtypes. HIV serologic testing usually detects antibodies to all HIV-1 subtypes. HIV-1, like all retroviruses, contains an enzyme, reverse transcriptase, which transcribes the viral RNA into double-stranded DNA to be integrated into the host cell genome. The life cycle of HIV is pictured in Figure 63.2.

The most common mode of transmission of HIV is through sexual contact. It can also be spread through blood or blood products, or from mother to child in utero, during delivery, or through breastfeeding. HIV is found in semen and vaginal secretions. Transmission rates per sexual encounter are highest for anal intercourse; for vaginal intercourse, transmission is more likely from an infected

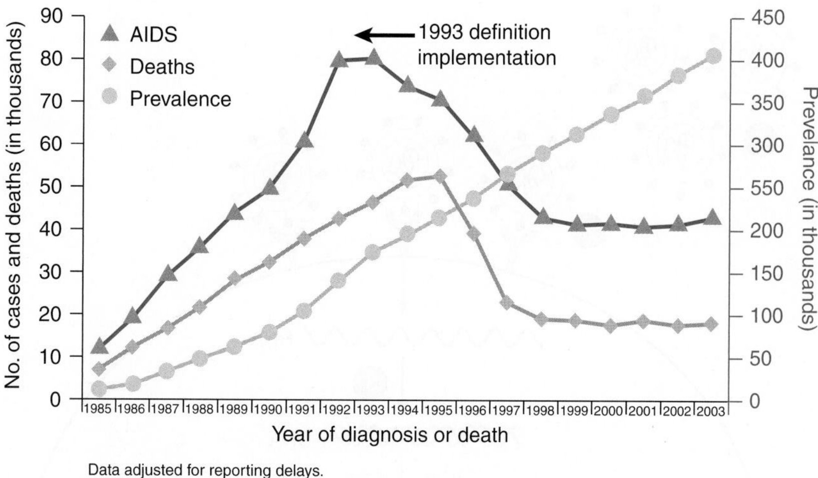

Figure 63.1 • Estimated number of AIDS cases, deaths, and persons living with AIDS, 1985–2003, United States.

male to an uninfected female than vice versa. The sexual transmission of HIV can be significantly reduced by the use of condoms. The transmission of HIV by contaminated needles has been significantly reduced in areas where clean needle exchange programs have been implemented, and the transmission of HIV during pregnancy and labor can be all but eliminated by the appropriate use of antiretroviral therapy.

The primary target of HIV infection is the CD4+ T-lymphocyte, although HIV can be taken up by other cells with these receptors and certain chemokine receptors, such as macrophages, dendritic cells, and microglial cells. Within days of infection, HIV rapidly disseminates throughout the lymphoid system and the central nervous system. Infection with HIV is a very dynamic process: even during the long asymptomatic period of infection, viral turnover is actually on the order of a billion new virions a day. Besides these actively infected cells with rapid turnover, there exist a much smaller number of long-lived latently infected T-cells with integrated HIV. These are "invisible" to the immune system and antiretroviral therapy, and present a major obstacle to strategies for curing HIV infection.

CLINICAL MANIFESTATIONS

The natural course of HIV infection is shown schematically in Figure 63.3. Within a few weeks of primary infection with HIV, most newly infected persons go through an initial symptomatic illness known as the acute retroviral syndrome. Although most of these acutely infected persons do seek medical attention for their illness, the correct diagnosis is not usually made, and the symptoms usually resolve spontaneously over a few week period. Typical presenting symptoms of acute HIV infection are listed in Table 63.1. This illness is similar in many ways to the presentation of infectious mononucleosis. It can be distinguished from colds and influenza by the lack of any nasal congestion, cough, or other respiratory symptoms. If present, the rash is usually an erythematous maculopapular rash, most prominent on the trunk and face, and may include ulcerations of the oropharynx and genitals. Neurologic manifestations of acute HIV infection are most often related to aseptic meningitis, but may also be due to a peripheral neuropathy, radiculopathy, or facial nerve palsy.

Whether or not HIV infection is diagnosed during the acute stage, it then moves into an

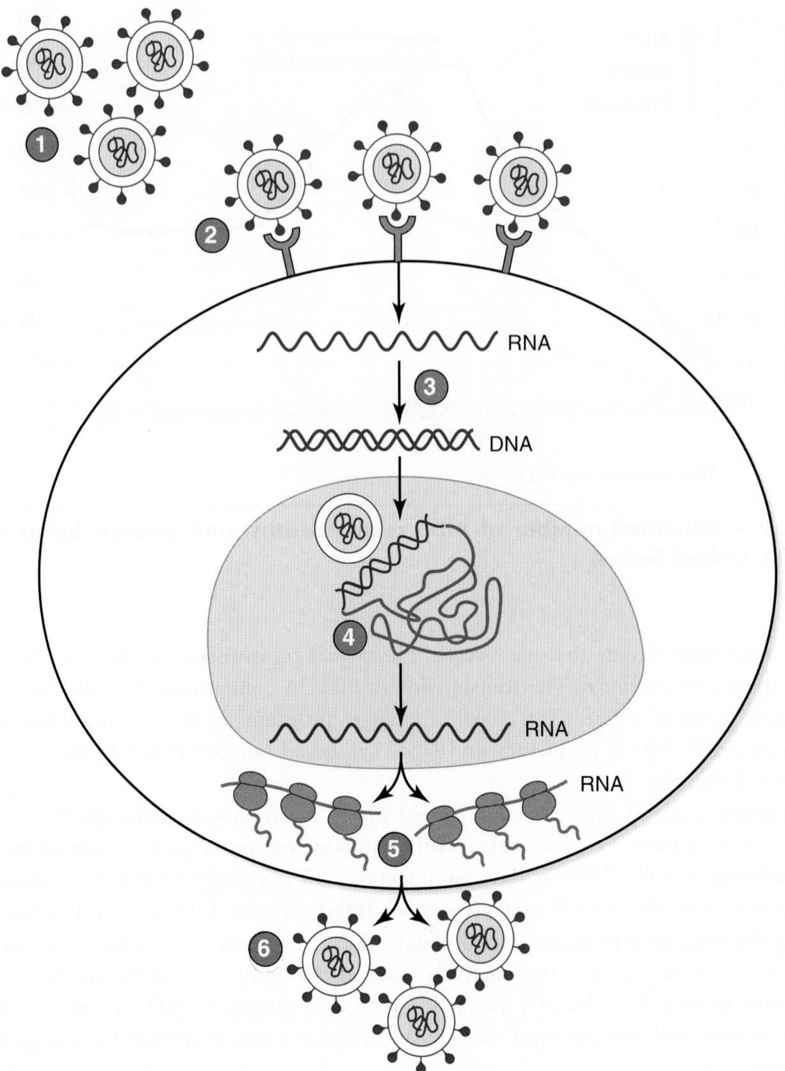

Figure 63.2 • Life cycle of HIV virus. 1, virions; 2, attachment to CD4 receptor; 3, reverse transcriptase; 4, incorporation of provirus into the host genome; 5, protein coating; 6, mature viral particle.

asymptomatic stage that usually lasts several years. During this time, HIV-infected persons may look and feel well. Some manifestations of chronic HIV infection may occur, however, especially over time as the disease progresses and the CD4+ T-cell count falls (Table 63.2). These symptoms are nonspecific and may be the only manifestation of HIV infection during this time, so any such complaint without other known explanation should prompt HIV testing. Persistent generalized lymphadenopathy is an especially important finding. The CD4 count at which common opportunistic infections occur is shown in Figure 63.4.

In addition, during this stage of mild immunosuppression, patients may present with common infections that do not qualify as opportunistic infections (because they do occur in normal hosts) but that are more severe or prolonged in HIV infection. Examples of these include severe or recurrent episodes of vaginal candidiasis, orolabial or genital herpes simplex, pneumococcal pneumonia, and

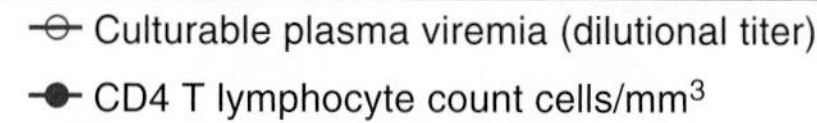

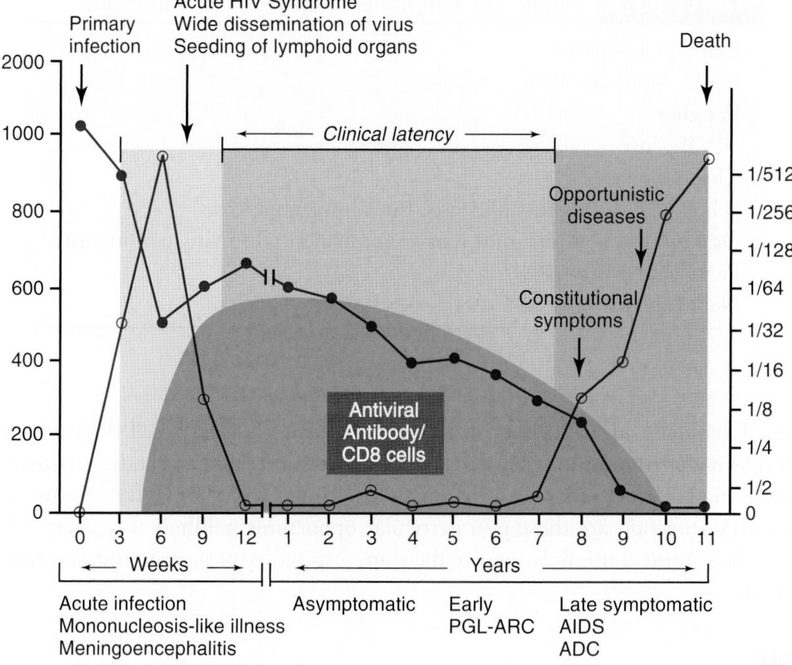

Figure 63.3 • Time course of typical HIV infection. Widespread viral dissemination occurs early in the primary infection and encompasses an abrupt decline in peripheral blood CD4+ T-cell number. The ensuing immune response is accompanied by a decrease in plasma viremia (culturable virus) and a lengthy period of clinical latency. However, the CD4+ T-cell count continues to decline during this period until a critical level is reached, where the risk of opportunistic infections is markedly increased. ADC, AIDS dementia complex; ARC, AIDS-related complex; PGL, persistent generalized lymphadenopathy.

TABLE 63.1 Signs and symptoms of the acute retroviral syndrome

Sign/symptom	Frequency (%)
Fever	96
Lymphadenopathy	74
Pharyngitis	70
Rash	70
Myalgias/arthralgias	54
Diarrhea	32
Headache	32
Nausea/vomiting	27
Hepatosplenomegaly	14
Weight loss	13
Thrush	12
Neurologic symptoms	12

TABLE 63.2 Signs and symptoms of chronic HIV infection
Lymphadenopathy
Fever, night sweats
Fatigue
Weight loss
Chronic diarrhea
Seborrheic dermatitis, psoriasis, tinea, onychomycosis
Oral aphthous ulcers, oral hairy leukoplakia, gingivitis/periodontitis
Peripheral neuropathy
Nephropathy

herpes zoster. Eventually HIV infection leads to significant CD4+ T-cell depletion, compromise primarily of cell-mediated immunity (and to a lesser degree decreased antibody responses and phagocytic responses), and increased risk for opportunistic infections (see below). Often, the initial presenting symptoms of HIV infection are those of a particular opportunistic illness that is an AIDS-defining complication. These most commonly involve the skin, respiratory or gastrointestinal tracts, or central nervous system.

DIAGNOSIS

The preferred means of diagnosing HIV infection is through serologic testing. It is now recognized that targeted testing of only those individuals in traditional "high-risk" groups, or those with oppor-

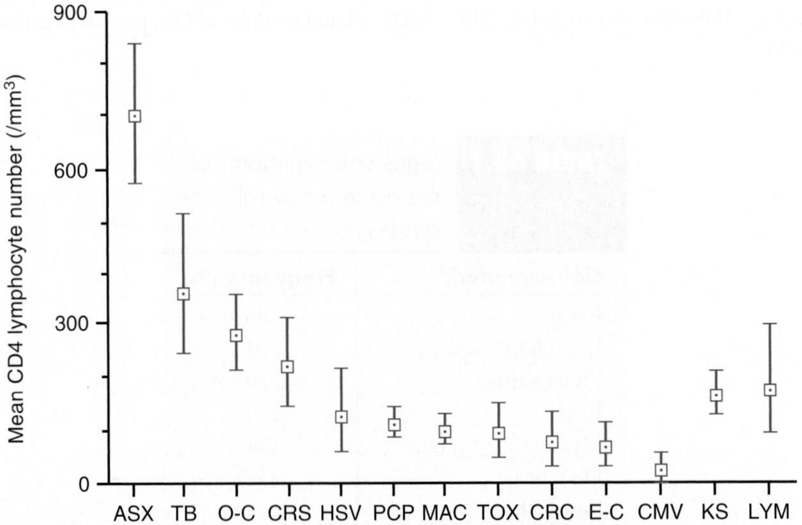

Figure 63.4 • Mean CD4 cell levels with standard deviations (boxes) and 95% confidence intervals (bars) in 222 HIV-infected patients with opportunistic diseases and HIV-infected asymptomatic controls. ASX, asymptomatic; CMV, cytomegalovirus retinitis; CRC, cryptococcal meningitis; CRS, cryptosporidiosis; EC, esophageal candidiasis; HSV, recurrent herpes simplex virus; KS, Kaposi's sarcoma; LYM, lymphoma; MAC, *Mycobacterium avium* complex; OC, oral candidiasis; PCP, *Pneumocystis carinii* pneumonia; TB, tuberculosis; TOX, toxoplasmosis.

TABLE 63.3 Indications for HIV testing

Symptoms/signs of acute retroviral syndrome
Symptoms/signs of chronic HIV infection
Opportunistic infection
Severe, recurrent, or persistent infection that does not qualify as opportunistic
Presence of tuberculosis, hepatitis B, hepatitis C, other sexually transmitted diseases, hemophilia
History of at-risk behavior (multiple sex partners, men who have sex with men, injection drug use)
Sexual partner of someone who engages in at-risk behavior
Adults in population areas with high (>1%) prevalence
Known or suspected exposure to HIV
Victim of sexual assault
Patient request
All pregnant women
Child born to HIV-infected mother
Occupational exposure to blood/body fluid (both source patient and exposed worker)
Blood/semen/organ donor

tunistic infections, misses the majority of those with HIV infection, and thus misses the best opportunity to intervene before progression as well as to interrupt further transmission. The Centers for Disease Control and Prevention now advocates widespread routine HIV testing. Accepted indications for HIV testing are listed in Table 63.3.

Serologic testing for HIV infection is a two-stage procedure. Initially an enzyme-linked immunosorbent assay (ELISA) is performed. If this is negative, then the test is negative. If the first ELISA is positive, then it is repeated. Only samples repeatedly positive on ELISA undergo confirmatory testing. The confirmatory test is a Western blot (WB). The ELISA is a more sensitive test but the WB is more specific. The combination of ELISA and confirmatory WB testing is extremely sensitive (99.5%) and specific (99.99%). The WB test has three possible outcomes: positive (confirming HIV infection), negative (indicating the positive ELISA was a false-positive), or indeterminate (if there are one or more bands present but not enough to meet criteria for positive). In high-risk individuals, an indeterminate WB result most often occurs during the process of seroconversion, and repeat testing and/or polymerase chain reaction (PCR) testing can be helpful. Patients with multiple, repeated, persistently indeterminate WB results are very unlikely to have HIV infection.

Rapid HIV tests are now available to be performed on either blood or saliva; the kits can be used in an office or clinic and will give results in 10 to 20 minutes. This makes them especially useful in settings such as emergency rooms, primary care clinics, and STD clinics. Because the rapid test is only an ELISA, any positive result must be confirmed with standard HIV testing including a Western blot.

False-negative antibody tests for HIV can occur during the "window" period of the first few weeks of acute infection, before the infected person has mounted an antibody response. Thus, during the acute retroviral syndrome, testing for HIV should include a viral test such as a quantitative HIV RNA PCR in addition to HIV antibody testing. During acute HIV infection, the level of viremia is very high, so the quantitative PCR (viral load) is usually in the tens of thousands or hundreds of thousands of copies per milliliter. A viral load level of only a few hundred is more likely to be a false positive in this setting. Because of problems with false positives and false negatives, HIV nucleic acid testing such as PCR is less reliable than antibody testing and should not be used to diagnose HIV infection, except in two situations: (a) possible acute infection where the antibody may not yet have turned positive, as just described; and (b) for testing in newborns born to HIV-infected mothers. In this setting, the infant's HIV antibody test will always be unreliable because the mother's HIV antibody has crossed the placenta, and a virus-specific test such as DNA PCR is needed to diagnose HIV infection in the infant.

T-lymphocyte subset testing to determine the CD4+ count should never be used as a surrogate for HIV testing to try to make a diagnosis of HIV infection. CD4+ T-cell quantification is neither sensitive nor specific for HIV infection, because most people with HIV infection go through a long period of time with normal CD4+ counts and because many other illnesses can affect the CD4+ T-cell count.

TREATMENT

Treatment of HIV infection has become more complicated and more successful as more treatment options have become available. Selection and management of specific antiretroviral medication regimens should only be undertaken by physicians who have expertise in the area. The general principles of HIV therapy, however, are straightforward and important to understand. Remember that the goal of HIV treatment is to restore and maintain immunologic function so as to prevent opportunistic infections and death. Treatment should be started for symptomatic infection, or in asymptomatic infection when CD4+ T-cell counts have begun to fall but well before they have reached a high-risk AIDS-defining level (<200). Most experts recommend initiating treatment at CD4+ counts around 350. Today's regimens, if prescribed and taken correctly, can be very successful at restoring CD4+ T-cell levels to normal, with consequent elimination of the previous risk of opportunistic infections. When CD4+ counts are low, however, opportunistic infection prophylaxis is crucial; prophylactic agents and indications are shown in Table 63.4.

The most important principle in treating HIV infection is to maximally suppress viral replication. Treatment is monitored by viral load level testing. Viral load should fall markedly within the first few weeks after starting therapy, reach undetectable levels after a few months, and stay undetectable thereafter. Any consistently detectable level of viral load indicates ongoing viral replication, and allowing the virus to replicate in the presence of any drug will inevitably select for resistance to that drug. Therefore, regimens involving multiple drugs from multiple classes (typically two nucleoside analogue reverse transcriptase inhibitors plus either a nonnucleoside reverse transcriptase inhibitor

TABLE 63.4 Prophylaxis for opportunistic infections in AIDS

Opportunistic infection	Indication	Preferred drug
Pneumocystis carinii (jiroveci)	CD4 <200	TMP/SMX DS daily or 3 times/week
Toxoplasmosis	CD4 <100 and positive serology	TMP/SMX DS daily
Mycobacterium avium complex	CD4 <50	Azithromycin 1,200 mg/week
Tuberculosis	PPD >5 mm	INH 300 mg/day for 9 months

Also recommended are the 23-valent polysaccharide pneumococcal vaccine, influenza vaccine annually, hepatitis B vaccine in susceptible individuals, and hepatitis A vaccine for high-risk patients.
INH, isoniazid; PPD, purified protein derivative; TMP/SMX, trimesnoprim/Sulfamethoxazole.

or a protease inhibitor) are used to totally suppress viral replication and prevent the development of resistance. Resistance testing, either genotypic or phenotypic, is routinely used to guide choices of specific active drugs for the regimen.

Because any missed doses of the medications allows the drug level to fall, which favors the selection of drug resistant virus, strict adherence to the regimen is absolutely crucial and must be maintained at all times—considerable patient education and counseling must be devoted to this end for treatment to be successful in the long run. Because the patients being treated are usually asymptomatic before starting therapy, counseling about and trying to minimize or avoid adverse drug effects is important. Likewise, because the patients will need to be continued on the regimens for many years, minimizing long-term toxicity is vital. The major long-term toxicity concerns of present regimens have to do with metabolic side effects, such as hyperlipidemia, insulin resistance, lipodystrophy (fat redistribution), and mitochondrial toxicity. Finally, many of the antiretroviral agents, especially the nonnucleosides and protease inhibitors, have important interactions with each other and with numerous other medications that can significantly raise or lower drug levels. Possible interactions must always be considered whenever any medication is prescribed, and either the dosing adjusted or an alternative agent used if necessary.

COMPLICATIONS

The major complication of HIV infection is progressive immune system dysfunction with the development of AIDS, defined as a CD4+ T-cell count of below 200 or the onset of an AIDS-defining opportunistic infection or malignancy. The most common and significant complications are listed in Table 63.5 and can be divided into infections, malignancies, and immunologic or metabolic syndromes. The incidence of these has been dramatically reduced by appropriate use of antiretroviral therapy.

Pneumocystis carinii pneumonia (PCP) has historically been the most common AIDS-defining opportunistic infection. Occurring in patients with CD4+ counts less than 200 who are not on

TABLE 63.5 Most common or significant complications of HIV/AIDS

Pneumocystis carinii (jiroveci) pneumonia
CNS toxoplasmosis
Mucocutaneous candidiasis, especially oral and esophageal
Cryptococcal meningitis
Disseminated histoplasmosis
Tuberculosis, especially extrapulmonary
Disseminated *Mycobacterium avium* complex
Cytomegalovirus, especially retinitis, less often gastrointestinal or CNS
Herpes simplex virus
Varicella zoster virus
Progressive multifocal leukoencephalopathy
Kaposi's sarcoma
Non-Hodgkin's lymphoma, including primary CNS lymphoma
HIV encephalopathy/dementia
Wasting syndrome
Lipodystrophy syndrome

CNS, central nervous system.

prophylaxis, it usually presents with the subacute onset of dyspnea, dry cough, and fever. While a variety of chest x-ray findings are possible, the typical pattern seen is diffuse bilateral interstitial infiltrates; the presence of a pleural effusion or hilar/mediastinal lymphadenopathy argues strongly against a diagnosis of PCP. Definitive diagnosis requires demonstration of the organism in sputum or bronchoalveolar lavage, but treatment is often empiric in the appropriate setting. Because PCP is readily treatable (and preventable), it needs to be a prime consideration in any patient with a CD4 count possibly less than 200 who is not on prophylaxis and who presents with a lower respiratory infection. Toxoplasmosis is a protozoan infection, usually of the brain, in patients not on prophylaxis with CD4+ counts under 100. Presentation is most commonly subacute with focal neurologic deficits or seizures, and brain magnetic resonance imaging shows multiple ring-enhancing lesions.

Candida infections are very common in AIDS and are usually of skin or gastrointestinal/genital mucosal surfaces, rather than invasive. Although vaginal or cutaneous candidiasis can occur at any CD4+ count, oral or esophageal candidiasis usually indicates a CD4+ count less than 250. Oral thrush most commonly presents as painless whitish plaques that can be scraped off the oral mucosa; esophageal involvement should be considered with any dysphagia or retrosternal pain, and is an important distinction because it requires more intensive treatment. *Cryptococcus neoformans* infection can present as pulmonary or disseminated disease but usually is identified as subacute meningitis presenting as indolent progressive headache, fever, and sometimes mental status changes. Focal deficits and seizures are less common. Diagnosis of cryptococcal meningitis is made by lumbar puncture with fungal culture or cryptococcal antigen testing of the cerebrospinal fluid. Histoplasmosis is a fungal infection found mostly in a geographic area following the Mississippi and Ohio River valleys, and in AIDS patients usually presents as disseminated disease involving the lungs, liver/spleen and gastrointestinal tract, skin, and bone marrow.

Tuberculosis is much more common in patients with HIV, even at higher CD4+ counts, and is also much more likely to present as extrapulmonary or even disseminated disease. Treatment of concomitant tuberculosis and HIV infection is complicated by drug interactions and is different from standard regimens used in HIV-negative patients. Testing for HIV should be done in all persons diagnosed with tuberculosis, and purified protein derivative testing (with >5 mm induration indicating a positive reaction) should be performed in all persons with HIV infection. *Mycobacterium avium* complex infection usually presents as disseminated disease in patients with CD4+ counts less than 50, manifested by fevers, sweats, weight loss, lymphadenopathy, hepatosplenomegaly, and bone marrow involvement. Diagnosis can be made by acid-fast bacilli culture of blood, bone marrow, lymph node, or liver.

Cytomegalovirus (CMV) disease in AIDS is most often retinitis, presenting with floaters or fixed visual field deficits in patients with CD4+ counts usually less than 50, and progressing to blindness if not treated. Funduscopic examination by an experienced ophthalmologist can make the diagnosis. CMV may also cause colitis, esophagitis, encephalitis, or polyradiculitis. Orolabial, genital, or perianal herpes simplex disease episodes can in HIV become much more severe, persistent, or frequent, even at high CD4+ counts, and may be the initial manifestation of HIV infection. Likewise, an episode of herpes zoster may be the initial indication of HIV even with high CD4+ counts. At lower CD4+ levels, herpes zoster can present as disseminated disease. Progressive multifocal leukoencephalopathy is caused by JC virus, a polyomavirus, and presents with insidious mental status changes and slowly progressive focal neurological deficits.

Kaposi's sarcoma has been the most common malignancy in HIV/AIDS, and is now known to be caused by human herpes virus type 8. Often multifocal, lesions are typically reddish, violaceous, or brownish, painless initially, and may be macules, papules, plaques, or nodules. Noncutaneous involvement is more worrisome, and can include oral, pulmonary, or gastrointestinal lesions. Non-Hodgkin's lymphoma, usually associated with Epstein-Barr virus, is as much as 600 times more common in AIDS than in HIV-negative controls, and is more often associated with "B" symptoms (fevers, night sweats, weight loss) and extranodal involvement, including primary central nervous system (CNS) lymphoma.

HIV-associated dementia is a chronic encephalopathy due to CNS infection and immune activation by HIV. It presents usually in CD4+ counts less than 200, with apathy, memory loss, cognitive slowing, and psychomotor retardation. Wasting syndrome is defined as involuntary loss of >10% of body weight, and is more commonly seen at CD4+ counts under 200. An increasingly more common metabolic complication of HIV and its treatment is lipodystrophy. Although its cause is not yet clear, it appears to be correlated with duration and severity of HIV infection, and also with duration of and specific agents used for HIV therapy. Lipodystrophy consists of two processes which may coexist to varying degrees: (a) visceral fat accumulation, which, as in HIV-negative persons, is associated with insulin resistance and the metabolic syndrome; and (b) subcutaneous fat atrophy, especially of face and extremities. Like the development of lactic acidosis (seen in about 1% of patients on long-term antiretroviral therapy, and potentially life-threatening), the lipoatrophy is believed to be a manifestation of chronic mitochondrial toxicity. Elevated triglycerides and low high-density lipoprotein cholesterol are a common metabolic consequence of HIV infection. Treatment of HIV often adds the adverse effect of raising total and low-density lipoprotein cholesterol, further increasing the risk for future cardiovascular disease.

Endocrinology

Irene O'Shaughnessy and Albert Jochen

CHAPTER 64

Diabetes Mellitus and Hypoglycemia

Jennifer Zebrack

DIABETES MELLITUS

Diabetes mellitus is a syndrome of altered carbohydrate, fat, and protein metabolism resulting from an absolute or relative deficiency of insulin resulting in hyperglycemia. Diabetes mellitus affects approximately 6% of the U.S. population and often coexists with the metabolic syndrome. Longstanding diabetes is commonly associated with chronic complications of retinopathy, nephropathy, neuropathy, and accelerated atherosclerosis.

Etiology

Diabetes mellitus is a heterogeneous disorder with two subtypes. Type 1 diabetes mellitus, caused by autoimmune destruction of the pancreatic beta cells, accounts for less than 10% of cases. It is typically characterized by severe insulin deficiency, sudden onset of symptoms, and risk for diabetic ketoacidosis (DKA). It usually occurs in young patients, but a late-onset form may occur in adults. These patients require insulin therapy for survival.

Type 2 diabetes mellitus, formally called adult-onset diabetes, is the most common type and accounts for over 90% of all cases of diabetes. Both genetic and environmental factors (e.g., obesity) contribute to its development. Type 2 diabetes is characterized by insulin resistance, relative insulin deficiency, and a more gradual onset of hyperglycemia. Peripheral tissues, such as muscle, fat, and liver, are abnormally resistant to the effects of insulin, resulting in decreased glucose uptake and inappropriate hepatic gluconeogenesis. Insulin secretion is usually sufficient to prevent ketoacidosis, but DKA may occur during severe illness or stress in these patients. These patients may require insulin to control blood glucose levels.

Impaired fasting glucose (IFG) and impaired glucose tolerance (IGT) are intermediate states between normal blood glucose and diabetes mellitus (previously termed "borderline" diabetes). These states are associated with insulin resistance and are risk factors for type 2 diabetes. Gestational diabetes mellitus (GDM) is defined as glucose intolerance diagnosed during pregnancy and complicates between 3% and 4% of all pregnancies in the United States. Gestational diabetes occurs as a result of insulin resistance, and these women are also at risk for developing type 2 diabetes.

In other types of diabetes, entities such as pancreatic insufficiency (e.g., chronic pancreatitis, hemochromatosis, pancreatectomy), Cushing's syndrome, and acromegaly are the underlying cause. Drugs, including glucocorticoids and nicotinic acid, can produce hyperglycemia in patients predisposed to type 2 diabetes.

Clinical Manifestations

The classic triad of polyuria, polydipsia, and polyphagia (excessive eating) arises from hyperglycemia, which leads to glycosuria upon exceeding the renal threshold. Glucose acts as an osmotic diuretic, leading to polyuria and, hence, polydipsia. Loss of calories evokes a sensation of excess hunger and

TABLE 64.1 Diagnosis of diabetes mellitus in nonpregnant adults

Random glucose >200 mg/dL with symptoms of hyperglycemia
or
Fasting venous plasma glucose ≥126 mg/dL on two or more occasions
or
Oral glucose (75 g) tolerance test showing a 2-hour glucose level of ≥200 mg/dL

polyphagia. Patients may also complain of blurred vision and weight loss despite excess food intake. Skin infections, vulvovaginitis (inflammation of the vulva and the vagina), and balanitis (inflammation of the glans penis) may cause the patient to seek medical care. Diabetic ketoacidosis may also be the initial manifestation of type 1 diabetes. Type 2 diabetes often is detected by screening examinations. Peripheral neuropathy is often present when type 2 diabetes is diagnosed and may be the presenting feature. Less commonly, type 2 diabetes presents with vascular complications, such as myocardial infarction, peripheral vascular disease, or chronic kidney disease.

Diagnosis

Table 64.1 shows the accepted criteria for the diagnosis of diabetes in an adult. Commonly, type 1 diabetic patients are diagnosed by the first criterion; type 2 diabetes patients are diagnosed by the second. Oral glucose tolerance testing (OGTT) is reserved for individuals with potential symptoms of diabetes or its complications as well as fasting plasma glucose below 126 mg/dL. IFG is defined as fasting plasma glucose between 100 and 125 mg/dL, and IGT is defined as plasma glucose between 140 and 199 mg/dL, after a 2-hour OGTT.

Treatment

PATIENT EDUCATION AND MONITORING

All diabetic patients should be educated about the goals of therapy, glucose monitoring, dietary changes and physical activity, sick day management, and chronic complications of diabetes. All diabetic patients should wear a medical bracelet or necklace at all times. Diabetic education should be reinforced at every opportunity, whether in the outpatient or inpatient setting. If available, utilizing a team approach (e.g., diabetic nurse educators, dieticians) is preferred.

Self-monitoring of capillary blood glucose (e.g., fingersticks or alternate site testing) is recommended for all patients with diabetes; frequency of testing is individualized and depends on the diabetic therapy being used and the degree of glucose control. The American Diabetes Association recommends fasting and premeal glucose levels of 90 to 130 mg/dL with postprandial glucose levels (1 to 2 hours after the beginning of a meal) less than 180 mg/dL. Diabetic patients should be monitored for urine ketones (e.g., diabetic ketoacidosis) during illness (i.e., fever, nausea, vomiting, abdominal pain) or if blood glucoses persist above 300 mg/dL.

Glycosylated hemoglobin (HbA_{1c}) is a covalent modification of hemoglobin by glucose, and its amount is proportional to the mean blood glucose level. HbA_{1c} provides an average and objective measurement of blood glucose over the past 2 to 3 months. The correlations between HBA_{1c} and mean blood glucose level are listed in Table 64.2. HbA_{1c} levels should be maintained below 7%. All patients with diabetes should receive HbA_{1c} testing at least every 6 months if blood glucoses are well controlled and approximately every 3 months if blood glucoses are uncontrolled or changes in therapy have been made.

The prevention of the chronic complications of diabetes is an important part of diabetic care. Screening for early diabetic nephropathy with a urine microalbumin and maintaining blood pressure

TABLE 64.2 Correlation between HBA_{1c} and mean plasma glucose level

HbA_{1c} (%)	Mean blood glucose level (mg/dL)
6	135
7	170
8	205
9	240
10	275
11	310
12	345

below 130/80 mm Hg is recommended. A lipid profile should also be checked annually. Foot and eye examinations are important in the prevention of foot ulcers, infections, and diabetic retinopathy. The timing and frequency of these screening recommendations are discussed below.

NONPHARMACOLOGIC TREATMENT

Diet and physical activity are essential components of diabetes therapy. The daily caloric intake usually is prescribed as three major meals with two or three snacks during a 24-hour period. Carbohydrates should provide 45% to 65% of total calories, protein should account for 15% to 20%, and total fat should make up 25% to 35% (saturated fat limited to <7% and minimize trans fat intake). Patients should strive to maintain an ideal body weight. Patients with type 2 diabetes are usually obese and should be encouraged to lose weight by prescribing lower-calorie diets and physical activity for most days of the week.

PHARMACOLOGIC TREATMENT

Insulin

Insulin Preparations and Delivery In 1982, human insulin, produced by recombinant molecular technology, became available and has replaced animal sources of insulin. Insulin preparations are listed in Table 64.3. Regular insulin is unmodified and acts rapidly. Newer rapid-acting insulin (lispro, aspart, glulisine) contain amino acid substitutions that enable them to act even faster than regular insulin. Intermediate- and long-acting insulin has been modified to prolong the insulin action. Insulin is typically given subcutaneously via syringe, pen, or insulin pump. Preferred inject sites include the abdomen, thighs, and arms. In severe hyperglycemia and diabetic ketoacidosis, intravenous administration of regular insulin is usually required.

Principles of Insulin Therapy Insulin is typically prescribed in such a way that it roughly approximates the idealized profile of insulin secretion in a nondiabetic person (Fig. 64.1). This profile arises from both basal insulin secretion (occurring in the absence of eating) and nutrient-stimulated insulin secretion with meals. For instance, short-acting insulin is typically given before two or three meals to mimic nutrient-stimulated insulin secretion and to promote metabolism of the ingested calories. Intermediate- or long-acting insulin is given once or twice daily to mimic basal insulin secretion. Most diabetics require a dose of intermediate- or long-acting insulin in the evening in order to suppress nocturnal hepatic gluconeogenesis, which can lead to prebreakfast hyperglycemia.

Starting Insulin Therapy In general, the initial starting insulin dose for a nonobese patient is approximately 0.5 to 1.0 units/kg/day given subcutaneous in divided doses. Common insulin regimens

TABLE 64.3 Insulin preparations

Type of insulin	Onset (hours)	Peak (hours)	Duration (hours)
Rapid			
Regular	0.5–1	2–4	6–8
Lispro	0.25–0.5	0.5–1.5	3–5
Aspart	0.2–0.3	1–3	3–5
Glulisine	0.3–0.4	1	4–5
Intermediate-acting			
Lente	3–4	6–12	16–20+
NPH	2–4	6–10	14–18+
Long-acting			
Ultralente	4–6	10–16	24–36
Glargine	1–2	Flat	24
Detemir	—	Peakless	Up to 23

are listed in Table 64-4). The standard regimen (also known as the "split-mixed" regimen) is a mixture of intermediate-acting and rapid-acting insulin given before breakfast and before the evening meal. Traditionally, approximately two thirds of the total daily dose of insulin is given in the morning and one third before supper; two thirds of each injection consists of intermediate-acting insulin and one third consists of rapid-acting insulin (the "rule of thirds"). Premixed insulin preparations are available that consist of fixed ratios of two different insulin types. These preparations can be used to simplify insulin administration in some patients.

Adjusting Insulin Therapy Insulin adjustments are made prospectively based on the patient's glucose levels. For intermediate-acting insulin, the prebreakfast glucose levels reflect the adequacy

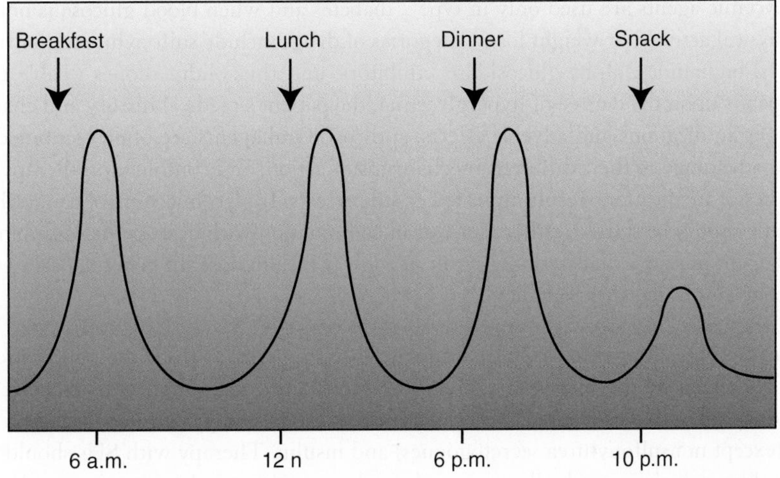

Figure 64.1 • Idealized profile of a 24-hour insulin secretion pattern in a nondiabetic individual.

TABLE 64.4 Common insulin regimens

Prebreakfast	Prelunch	Presupper (p.m.)	Bedtime (h.s.)
NPH/Reg	—	NPH/Reg	—
NPH/Reg (or lispro or aspart)	—	Reg (lispro or aspart)	NPH
Reg (or lispro or aspart)	Reg (or lispro or aspart)	Reg (or lispro or aspart)	Reg (or lispro or aspart)
Lispro or aspart	Lispro or aspart	Lispro or aspart	Insulin glargine

of the p.m. (or bedtime [h.s.]) dosage, and the presupper levels reflect the adequacy of the a.m. dosage. For rapid-acting insulin, the prelunch glucose levels can help adjust the a.m. dosage, just as the h.s. level can help adjust the p.m. dosage.

In some patients, the presupper intermediate-acting insulin (NPH, lente) peaks between 2 and 4 a.m., causing overnight reactions. These reactions can be avoided by giving the NPH (or lente) at bedtime. By also adding a dose of rapid-acting insulin prelunch, the morning intermediate-acting insulin can be eliminated in many patients.

For a select group of patients, continuous insulin infusion via an insulin pump can provide intensive glucose control. The pump provides a basal rate of insulin, and preprandial boluses are patient-directed, based on the carbohydrate content of each meal.

Complications of Insulin Therapy The most common complication of insulin therapy is hypoglycemia. Unfortunately, many insulin-dependent diabetics with long-standing diabetes have hypoglycemic unawareness; as a result, the first symptom of hypoglycemia may be cognitive impairment or seizures. Weight gain is common with insulin therapy. Insulin allergy and lipoatrophy have decreased in frequency with improved, highly purified insulin preparations.

Oral Hypoglycemic Agents

Oral hypoglycemic agents are used only in type 2 diabetes and when blood glucose is not controlled with diet, physical activity, or weight loss. Categories of drugs include sulfonylureas, nonsulfonylurea secretogogues, biguanides, alpha-glucosidase inhibitors, and thiazolidinediones (Table 64.5). Drug selection depends upon the degree of hyperglycemia, the patient's medical history and characteristics, the drug's contraindications and adverse effects, and cost. Oral agents are often combined with each other to take advantage of their different mechanisms of action, and combination therapy may allow for lower doses of medications resulting in fewer side effects. If glycemic control cannot be attained, insulin therapy should be started, either alone or in combination with oral agents. Combining insulin with an oral agent in type 2 diabetes may result in a lower insulin dose. In general, oral hypoglycemic agents are contraindicated in pregnancy.

Sulfonylureas The sulfonylureas (SUs) stimulate insulin secretion from the pancreatic beta cells. Most are metabolized by the liver and excreted by the kidney, so caution with advanced forms of liver and kidney disease is warranted. SUs can be use as monotherapy or in combination with other oral agents (except nonsulfonylurea secretogogues) and insulin. Therapy with SUs should begin with the smallest dose, which is gradually increased until optimal control or maximum dose has been reached. Common adverse effects include weight gain and hypoglycemia, which can be severe and prolonged, especially when there is impaired kidney function or no oral intake.

TABLE 64.5 Oral hypoglycemic agents

Class	Primary mechanism of action	Products	Mean HbA_{1c} reduction
Sulfonylureas	Increase insulin secretion by pancreatic beta cells	Gliclazide Glimepiride Glipizide Glyburide	1% to 2%
Non-SU secretagogues	Increase insulin secretion by pancreatic beta cells	Nateglinide	0.5% to 1%
		Repaglinide	1% to 2%
Biguanides	Inhibit hepatic gluconeogenesis	Metformin	1% to 2%
Thiazolidinediones	Increase peripheral glucose uptake	Pioglitazone Rosiglitazone	1.5%
Alpha-glucosidase inhibitors	Decrease carbohydrate absorption by small intestine	Acarbose Miglitol	0.5% to 1%

Nonsulfonylurea Secretogogues Like the sulfonylureas, two newer nonsulfonylurea secretagogues, repaglinide and nateglinide, stimulate the release of insulin from pancreatic beta cells. Compared to the SUs, they have a more rapid onset, shorter half-life, and are administered three times per day before each meal (targeting postprandial glucose). Like the SUs, adverse effects include weight gain and hypoglycemia, but theses effects are probably less frequent with non-SU secretogogue use. Like SUs, they are also metabolized by the liver and cleared by the kidney, so caution with liver and kidney disease is warranted. They can be used as monotherapy or with a biguanide (i.e., metformin). Efficacy of repaglinide is similar to SUs, while nateglinide is slightly less effective. Dosing of non-SU secretagogues is less convenient, but they may be preferred in someone with irregular meals. They are also more expensive than SUs.

Biguanides Metformin is the only member of a class of drugs called biguanides that is approved for use in the United States. Biguanides decrease glucose levels primarily through inhibition of hepatic gluconeogenesis. In addition, metformin is sometimes used in patients with impaired glucose tolerance to prevent progression to type 2 diabetes. Weight gain is not a side effect of metformin, and patients may actually lose weight while taking it. Hypoglycemia also does not occur with metformin monotherapy. For these reasons, metformin is usually the preferred first-line choice in an obese patient who does not have any contraindications to its use. Metformin can be used alone or in combination with either insulin or other oral agents, such as sulfonylureas, nonsulfonylurea secretogogues, and thiazolidinediones. The side effects of metformin are primarily gastrointestinal (i.e., nausea, diarrhea, abdominal pain) and can be minimized if the dose is started low, increased gradually, and taken with food. Lactic acidosis, sometimes fatal, has been reported. Metformin-associated lactic acidosis occurs primarily, if not solely, in patients with renal failure (baseline creatinine ≥1.5 for men and ≥1.4 for women), hepatic dysfunction, or congestive heart failure. Others at risk for metformin-associated lactic acidosis include alcoholics and those patients who are dehydrated or acutely ill (e.g., sepsis). For this reason, use of the drug is contraindicated in these patients. Metformin should be held before patients undergo radiographic contrast studies and restarted only after creatinine retesting.

Thiazolidinediones Although the mechanism of action is not clearly understood, thiazolidinediones (TZDs) are insulin-sensitizing agents that decrease insulin resistance in peripheral tissues. TZDs bind to the nuclear receptor known as peroxisome proliferator-activated receptor gamma. This activation results in the transcription of genes that improve insulin sensitivity and glucose uptake, especially by skeletal muscle cells. The first TZD, troglitazone, was removed from the market in 1998 because of hepatic necrosis as a rare but lethal idiosyncratic adverse effect. Other TZDs, rosiglitazone and pioglitazone, are currently available; they are used as monotherapy or in combination with insulin (pioglitazone only), sulfonylureas, or metformin. Hypoglycemia does not occur with TZD monotherapy. TZDs are similar in efficacy to SUs and metformin, with a mean decrease in HbA_{1c} of approximately 1.5%. However, the TZDs are the most expensive of the oral diabetic agents and are associated with weight gain and edema. They are contraindicated in patients with New York Heart Association class III or class IV heart failure or hepatic dysfunction. Liver transaminases should be checked prior to starting a TZD and monitored periodically thereafter.

Alpha-Glucosidase Inhibitors Alpha-glucosidase is an enzyme of the brush border of the small intestine that breaks down carbohydrates. Alpha-glucosidase inhibitors delay the absorption of carbohydrates from the gastrointestinal tract and primarily reduce postprandial hyperglycemia. These agents are nonsystemic, and hypoglycemia and weight gain do not occur with monotherapy. However, because they are less efficacious, alpha-glucosidase inhibitors are rarely used as monotherapy. They are often used in combination with sulfonylureas; if hypoglycemia occurs with combination therapy (i.e., sulfonylurea + alpha-glucosidase inhibitor), glucose must be ingested to reverse low blood glucose (not complex carbohydrates). Adverse effects include abdominal pain, flatulence, and loose stools.

Complications

The major morbidity and mortality due to diabetes result from chronic complications, which consist of macrovascular disease (accelerated atherosclerosis) and microvascular disease (retinopathy, nephropathy, and neuropathy). Suboptimal glucose control is directly related to the risk of developing long-term complications, particularly of the microvasculature. A major emphasis in the treatment of diabetes is the prevention or delay of complications by modifying risk factors.

MACROVASCULAR DISEASE

Coronary Artery Disease and Stroke

Myocardial infarction and stroke occur more frequently, at an earlier age, and with greater severity in diabetic men and women than in nondiabetic persons. Even patients with impaired glucose tolerance are at a greater risk for the development of atherosclerosis. Coronary artery disease is the leading cause of mortality in people with diabetes. Because of autonomic neuropathy, myocardial ischemia or frank infarction in diabetes may be asymptomatic; it may present as diabetic ketoacidosis or be diagnosed incidentally by a routine electrocardiogram. Therefore, tobacco cessation is strongly recommended and dyslipidemia is treated aggressively. Lipid screening should occur at least annually and more often if needed to reach goals. The goal low-density lipoprotein cholesterol is <70 mg/dL in diabetics with cardiovascular disease and <100 mg/dL in those without. Triglycerides should be <150 mg/dL, and high-density lipoprotein >40 mg/dL in men and >50 mg/dLin women. The goal blood pressure in diabetic patients is 130/80 mm Hg. Obesity and inactivity increase the risk for macrovascular disease; maintaining ideal body weight and physical activity should be strongly encouraged. Aspirin should be recommended for those with documented cardiovascular disease and considered for those diabetics over the age of 40 years who have risk factors.

Peripheral Vascular Disease

Involvement of large or medium-sized blood vessels in the lower limbs is a common complication of diabetes. A diagnosis of arterial insufficiency is suggested by a history of claudication. Physical examination reveals absent or weak peripheral pulses. Noninvasive vascular testing is used to confirm the diagnosis. Patients with peripheral vascular disease often cannot supply the increased blood flow needed to heal foot infections, such as cellulitis and ulcerations. The inability to heal these infections leads to osteomyelitis, gangrene, and amputations.

MICROVASCULAR DISEASE

Diabetic Retinopathy

Diabetic retinopathy is a leading cause of blindness in the United States. However, with yearly ophthalmologic examinations and preventive eye care, significant vision loss is prevented in all but a small fraction of patients. Type 2 diabetic patients should have an annual examination beginning after diagnosis, while type 1 diabetics should have their initial annual exam within 3 to 5 years after onset of the disease. Less frequent examinations (every 2 to 3 years) may be considered in those diabetics with normal eye exams. Diabetic retinopathy has two stages: background retinopathy and proliferative retinopathy. Background retinopathy may progress to the proliferative stage and cause vitreous hemorrhage, retinal detachment, and vision loss. In addition to retinopathy, cataracts and glaucoma are more prevalent in the diabetic population.

Diabetic Nephropathy

Diabetic nephropathy is often present along with retinopathy, and occurs in approximately one third of patients. The specific lesion of diabetic nephropathy is nodular sclerosis (Kimmelstiel-Wilson lesion), visible on light microscopy as a rounded hyaline mass at the center of the glomerular lobules. More common, but less specific, is diffuse glomerulosclerosis with thickening of the glomerular basement membrane and an increased mesangial matrix. Microalbuminuria (20 to 300 mg per 24 hours) heralds future development of gross proteinuria and should be checked annually in all type 2 diabetics starting at diagnosis and all type 1 diabetics who have had diabetes for 5 or more years. Progressive nephropathy results in heavy proteinuria and the development of nephrotic syndrome, which typically progresses to renal failure and the need for hemodialysis within 5 years.

The treatment of diabetic nephropathy should be aimed at strict control of hypertension (goal blood pressure <130/80 mm Hg) in addition to good glycemic control. Uncontrolled hypertension exacerbates worsening of renal function. Microalbuminuria and nephrotic syndrome should be treated with an angiotensin-converting enzyme (ACE) inhibitor (or angiotensin-receptor blocker if an ACE inhibitor is contraindicated or not tolerated). A decrease in protein intake may slow the progression of nephropathy. Hemodialysis, peritoneal dialysis, and renal transplantation are used to manage end-stage chronic kidney disease.

Diabetic Neuropathy

Diabetic neuropathy affects both the peripheral and the autonomic nervous systems. Distal, symmetric polyneuropathy is the most common form of diabetic peripheral neuropathy. It usually occurs in a stocking-glove distribution with numbness, tingling, burning, and/or pain in the feet and lower legs. Tendon reflexes and response to sensory stimuli, particularly vibration, are decreased. Patients with peripheral neuropathy are at risk for long-term complications of infection and amputation, especially if peripheral vascular disease coexists. All diabetic patients should receive an annual foot examination, including visual inspection, peripheral pulses, and sensation. The monofilament examination is currently the best screening test to detect clinically significant neuropathy. Patient education regarding foot care and daily monitoring for skin breakdown is essential.

Therapy of uncomfortable peripheral neuropathy involves the use of drugs such as gabapentin, tricyclic antidepressants, and anticonvulsants. Topical agents (e.g., capsaicin) are effective at times.

Focal peripheral neuropathies include mononeuropathies and entrapment syndromes. Examples of focal neuropathies are femoral and cranial nerve palsies, especially the third nerve. Carpal tunnel syndrome is an example of an entrapment syndrome and is more common in diabetic patients.

Autonomic neuropathies can affect nearly all organs, more notably the skin, the cardiovascular, gastrointestinal, and genitourinary systems. Diminished sweating (anhidrosis) of the feet can result in drying, cracking, and ulcer formation. Diabetic patients with autonomic neuropathy may present with postural hypotension (without compensatory tachycardia). Gastroparesis presents as early satiety, vomiting after meals, and increasing frequency of hypoglycemic episodes. Patients may also experience alternating bouts of diarrhea and constipation (enteropathy). Bacterial overgrowth secondary to stasis may contribute to diarrhea. Impotence, with preserved libido, is a common manifestation of diabetic autonomic neuropathy and affects 75% of diabetic men 60 to 65 years old. Neurogenic bladder may also occur.

DIABETIC KETOACIDOSIS AND NONKETOTIC HYPEROSMOLAR COMA

Diabetic ketoacidosis and nonketotic hyperosmolar coma are potentially fatal complications of diabetes. The distinction between ketoacidosis and nonketotic diabetic coma is not absolute; mild ketonemia may be present in patients with a hyperosmolar state. DKA is more common in type 1 diabetes and occurs in up to 5% of type 1 diabetes patients per year. However, nonketotic hyperosmolar coma occurs only in type 2 diabetes and is less common.

DIABETIC KETOACIDOSIS

Etiology

DKA evolves as a consequence of insulin deficiency, which is further complicated by an excess of counterregulatory hormones (i.e., catecholamines, growth hormone, glucocorticoids, and glucagon). A precipitating event such as infection, injury, myocardial infarction, pregnancy, or noncompliance with insulin is usually present. In the setting of stress or illness, patients often intentionally or unintentionally discontinue insulin, which can rapidly cause DKA. Without insulin, increased lipolysis makes increased amounts of free fatty acids available to the liver; they are oxidized, and ketone bodies (acetoacetate and β-hydroxybutyrate) are formed as byproducts. Ketone bodies release hydrogen ions into the body fluids, causing the pH to fall (metabolic acidosis).

Clinical Manifestations

The onset of DKA is characterized by an increase in symptoms of hyperglycemia, such as polyuria and polydipsia, but symptoms may be nonspecific. Patients with previously undiagnosed diabetes may give a history of weight loss. Nausea, vomiting, and vague abdominal pain are common. Lethargy may be present. On physical examination, signs of volume depletion are usually evident (e.g., dry skin/tongue, orthostasis, hypotension). Increasing H^+ ion concentration leads to an increased rate and depth of respiration (Kussmaul respiration) and "fruity" breath (secondary to ketosis) may be present. Electrolyte abnormalities (e.g., hyponatremia, hyperkalemia, metabolic acidosis, azotemia) are usually present. Respiratory distress and shock can occur.

Diagnosis

The hallmark features of DKA are marked hyperglycemia, anion gap metabolic acidosis, and ketonemia. Blood glucose generally ranges between 400 and 800 mg/dL, but may be as low as 250 mg/dL. The concentration of serum ketone bodies can be obtained, but this test is sensitive to acetoacetate only (not to β-hydroxybutyrate). Measurement of electrolytes and pH reveals a high anion gap metabolic acidosis. Normal anion gap ($[Na^+] - [Cl^- + HCO_3^-]$) is below 12 mEq/L; in general, the higher the level above 16 mEq/L, the greater the severity of ketoacidosis.

Treatment

DKA is a life-threatening situation. Management requires close observation, preferably in an intensive care unit. The essentials of treatment are replacement of fluid and electrolyte replacement, the reversal of ketogenesis (and resulting metabolic acidosis), insulin administration, and management of precipitating events. Hyperglycemia, if significant, can easily be corrected; it is the acidosis that is far more difficult to treat.

The fluid losses in DKA range between 4 and 10 L. Fluid therapy should be started with normal saline (0.9%) so as to achieve a prompt re-expansion of the circulating blood volume. In the first hour, 1 L of normal saline should be administered rapidly, followed by a liter of normal or half-normal saline (0.45%) in the next hour. The remainder of the fluids can be given more slowly until the patient's volume status is restored. Patients with congestive heart failure may require more gradual fluid replacement.

Insulin therapy is required to eliminate ketogenesis and metabolic acidosis. Following an initial intravenous bolus of 10 to 15 units (U) of regular insulin, regular insulin should be administered as a continuous IV infusion with an initial rate of 0.1 U/kg/hour (or 5 to 10 U per hour). Plasma glucose should be monitored hourly. An appropriate decrease in glucose is 50 to 75 mg/dL/hour; decreases of more than 100 mg/dL per hour should be avoided. When plasma glucose reaches approximately 250 mg/dL, the intravenous fluid should be changed from normal saline to 5% glucose in half-normal saline with the insulin drip decreased to 0.05 U/kg/hr. It is imperative to avoid hypoglycemia because it may predispose to cerebral edema and brain damage. In addition, rebound ketoacidosis may occur if the insulin is stopped prematurely before ketogenesis has resolved.

Electrolyte abnormalities are common and should be monitored every 1 to 2 hours. Total body potassium is depleted, despite the deceptively normal or even high serum levels that appear initially. Hyperkalemia occurs when acidosis shifts potassium to the extracellular compartment. Insulin administration and correction of acidosis will reverse this shift; therefore, hypokalemia should be anticipated. Consequently, it is necessary to begin potassium administration at initiation of therapy, unless hyperkalemia, oliguria, or renal failure is present. The amount of potassium added to the intravenous fluids is typically 10 to 30 mEq per hour, but may be higher if hypokalemia is present initially. Hypophosphatemia is common during therapy for ketoacidosis; because it reverses with refeeding, however, phosphate administration is not generally required. Return of the anion gap to normal is a reliable marker of resolution of the metabolic acidosis. Most cases do not require administration of sodium bicarbonate, but it should be administered if the pH is below 7.1.

A diligent search for precipitating causes should follow. If a bacterial infection is detected, appropriate antibiotics are required. It is necessary to rule out silent myocardial infarction by serial electrocardiography and appropriate blood tests.

HYPEROSMOLAR HYPERGLYCEMIC NONKETOTIC COMA (HYPEROSMOLAR COMA)

Etiology

Hyperosmolar coma is much less common than diabetic ketoacidosis (DKA) and usually occurs in older patients with type 2 diabetes. Conceptually, these patients usually have enough insulin to prevent ketosis and acidosis, but not enough to prevent hyperglycemia.

Clinical Manifestations

The evolution of the hyperglycemia, glycosuria, dehydration, and shock is similar but usually more insidious than DKA. Patients usually present with a history of polyuria, polydipsia, and progressive fatigue of several days' or weeks' duration. The condition typically is precipitated by an associated illness, such as infection, myocardial infarction, stroke, hip fracture, or exacerbation of an underlying chronic illness. Decreased oral intake over a period of time is also typical. Physical examination reveals evidence of severe dehydration and impaired mentation, although frank coma is unusual despite the name. Focal neurologic signs, although often seen, usually resolve with treatment.

Diagnosis

Severe hyperglycemia is present with blood glucose usually ranging from 600 to 1,300 mg/dL. The serum osmolarity is greatly increased (>320 mOsm/L), as measured directly or estimated by the following formula: serum osmolarity = 2 (Na × K) + glucose/18 + blood urea nitrogen/2.8. Plasma ketones usually are absent or, if present, occur in very small amounts. In contrast to DKA, a significant metabolic acidosis is usually not evident, with the pH greater than 7.3 and bicarbonate over 20 mEq/L. Azotemia and other electrolyte abnormalities are common.

Treatment

The principles of treatment are similar to those of DKA (i.e., fluid replacement, intravenous insulin therapy, electrolyte replacement, and search for precipitating cause), although the volume depletion usually is more profound than in DKA. Thus, whereas insulin therapy is a key component of the management of DKA, fluid replacement is the cornerstone of treatment of hyperosmolar coma. Often, the hyperglycemia can be corrected with fluids alone. If neurologic impairments are present, repeated neurologic evaluations are recommended.

HYPOGLYCEMIA

Hypoglycemia, a deficiency of glucose concentration in the blood, can occur in diabetic (usually iatrogenic) and nondiabetic individuals. Recurrent episodes of hypoglycemia result in a reduced ability to recognize these symptoms (hypoglycemic unawareness).

Etiology

Hypoglycemia has numerous causes and can be classified as one of two types (based on the temporal relationship between ingestion of a meal and the onset of clinically relevant symptoms). Fasting hypoglycemia is not seen until several hours after a meal has been fully digested and absorbed, whereas postprandial hypoglycemia often occurs within the first few hours after food intake (Table 64.6).

Fasting hypoglycemia is far more prevalent than the postprandial type, and most cases are drug induced (iatrogenic hypoglycemia). Insulin and the sulfonylureas cause most episodes. It is seen often in patients with type 1 diabetes attempting to maintain tight control with insulin. It also is seen in patients with type 2 diabetes taking oral hypoglycemic agents. Ethanol potentiates the hypoglycemic effects of both of these agents; it can also induce hypoglycemia alone by directly inhibiting gluconeogenesis. Factitious hypoglycemia has also been observed in nondiabetic psychiatric patients who have access to syringes and insulin or diabetic oral agents. Other causes include severe renal and hepatic failure, adrenal insufficiency, and insulinomas. Insulinomas are rare pancreatic β-cell tumors; most of these tumors are benign and small.

The best documented form of postprandial hypoglycemia in adults is alimentary hypoglycemia caused by surgical procedures leading to the rapid movement of ingested food into the small intestine (e.g., pyloroplasty, gastric bypass, gastrectomy). An idiopathic (functional) form of reactive hypoglycemia remains debatable; it often is erroneously diagnosed by both physicians and patients. These persons tend to be thin, anxious, and emotionally labile, with somatic features of autonomic hyperactivity such as gastric hypermotility and irritable bowel syndrome. Early type 2 diabetes is occasionally seen with postprandial hypoglycemia.

TABLE 64.6 Causes of hypoglycemia

Fasting	Postprandial
Insulin	Alimentary
Oral sulfonylurea agents	Idiopathic
Ethanol	Early type 2 diabetes mellitus
Medications:	
Pentamidine	
Salicylates	
Propranolol	
Sulfamethoxazole	
Disopyramide	
Tumor hypoglycemia	
Insulinomas	
Adrenal insufficiency	
Prolonged starvation	
Liver failure	
Uremia	

Clinical Manifestations

Hypoglycemia manifests clinically by symptoms of catecholamine release and/or neuroglycopenia (Table 64.7). Catecholamine release-related symptoms predominate when the blood glucose falls precipitously and include tremors, sweating, palpitations, and hunger. With a more gradual decrease in glucose or in patients with hypoglycemic unawareness, the initial symptoms are often those involving the central nervous system (neuroglycopenia), such as headache, irritability, confusion, seizures, or coma.

Diagnosis

Although hypoglycemic symptoms often develop when blood glucose drops below 45 mg/dL, many healthy adults are asymptomatic at this level, thus making it difficult to define clinically significant hypoglycemia. Rather, definitive diagnosis depends on the presence of Whipple's triad: adrenergic or neuroglycopenic symptoms consistent with hypoglycemia, low blood glucose level, and relief of the symptoms when blood glucose is restored to normal.

Definitive diagnosis may require hospital admission with serial blood glucose, insulin, and C-peptide monitoring during a supervised fast. C-peptide, an inactive cleavage fragment of proinsulin, is released in the body in amounts equal to insulin. Insulinoma is suspected when there are inappro-

TABLE 64.7 Symptoms of hypoglycemia

Adrenergic	Neuroglycopenic
Sweating	Headache
Tremors	Irritability
Palpitations	Confusion
Pallor	Seizure
Hunger	Coma

priately high levels of insulin and C-peptide during a fast. In factitious hypoglycemia with insulin use, the presence of insulin antibodies, an inappropriately low C-peptide level, and high levels of circulating insulin is often diagnostic. A urine screen for sulfonylureas can help with the diagnosis if a prescription error or factitious use of a sulfonylurea is suspected.

Treatment

The treatment of hypoglycemia depends on the cause and severity. Mild hypoglycemia can be treated with sugar-containing food or beverages for rapid effect. Intravenous dextrose is indicated for more severe hypoglycemia or in those unable to take oral intake. Hypoglycemia from sulfonylureas can be insidious and protracted. Patients who develop severe hypoglycemia due to these drugs should be hospitalized and given intravenous glucose with close observation. Patients with known hypoglycemic unawareness should monitor blood glucose frequently. Postprandial hypoglycemia is usually managed with small, frequent meals and reassurance. If an insulinoma is diagnosed, surgical excision is usually curative. For those patients with symptoms suggestive of idiopathic (functional) hypoglycemia, evaluation for impaired glucose tolerance may be indicated.

CHAPTER 65

Disorders of Parathyroid, Calcium, Vitamin D, and Metabolic Bone Diseases

Jennifer Zebrack

Calcium has two major physiologic functions: (a) calcium salts provide the rigidity and strength of the skeleton, and (b) ionized calcium plays critical roles in blood clotting, neuromuscular and membrane physiology, and signal transduction. Calcium kinetics are shown in Figure 65.1. Despite the high variability in dietary calcium intake, overall calcium balance is maintained principally by efficient regulation of intestinal calcium absorption. Circulating serum calcium takes three forms: free (ionized), albumin-bound, or complexed to citrate or phosphate. Only the ionized calcium is hormonally regulated and biologically active. Changes in the serum albumin affect the total serum calcium level, but not the biologically active ionized calcium. When the albumin level is abnormal, the total serum calcium can be calculated by adding 0.8 mg/dL to the serum calcium for each 1 g/dL the serum albumin level is below 4 g/dL. Alternatively, ionized calcium can be measured directly.

The parathyroid gland secretes parathyroid hormone (PTH), an 84-amino acid polypeptide, in close and inverse relation to the serum calcium level. PTH maintains serum calcium levels in three ways: by stimulating osteoclast activity thereby causing bone resorption and the release of calcium into the circulation; increasing the distal tubular reabsorption of calcium in the kidney; and stimulating renal 1α-hydroxylase. PTH also increases urinary phosphate excretion.

The active form of vitamin D, 1,25-dihydroxyvitamin D, increases absorption of dietary calcium in the small intestine and maintains calcification of the bone matrix. Its two precursors are ergocalciferol (synthetically derived from vegetable sterols) and the naturally occurring 7-dehydrocholesterol, both of which are activated sequentially in the skin, liver, and kidneys (Fig. 65.1). The major storage form of vitamin D is 25-hydroxyvitamin D; its production is not homeostatically regulated. The conversion of 25-hydroxyvitamin D to 1,25-dihydroxyvitamin D is accomplished by 1α- hydroxylase in the kidney, which is regulated primarily by PTH.

HYPERCALCEMIA

Hypercalcemia exists when the serum calcium level exceeds 10.2 mg/dL (2.55 mmol/L) or when the ionized calcium exceeds 5.28 mg/dL (1.32 mmol/L).

Etiology

Primary hyperparathyroidism and hyperkalemia of malignancy account for 90% to 95% of hypercalcemia cases. Causes of hypercalcemia are shown in Table 65.1. Primary hyperparathyroidism is seen more often in women than in men, and its peak incidence is around the sixth decade. Primary hyperparathyroidism results from one of three pathologic conditions: a single benign parathyroid adenoma that produces excessive PTH (85%); diffuse hyperplasia of all four glands, accounting for most of the remaining 15% and often occurring in the setting of the multiple endocrine neoplasia (MEN) syndromes; and parathyroid carcinoma, accounting for less than 1% of cases.

Malignancies are commonly associated with disorders of calcium metabolism. Neoplasms may secrete PTH-related protein (PTHrP), causing the so-called humoral hypercalcemia of malignancy.

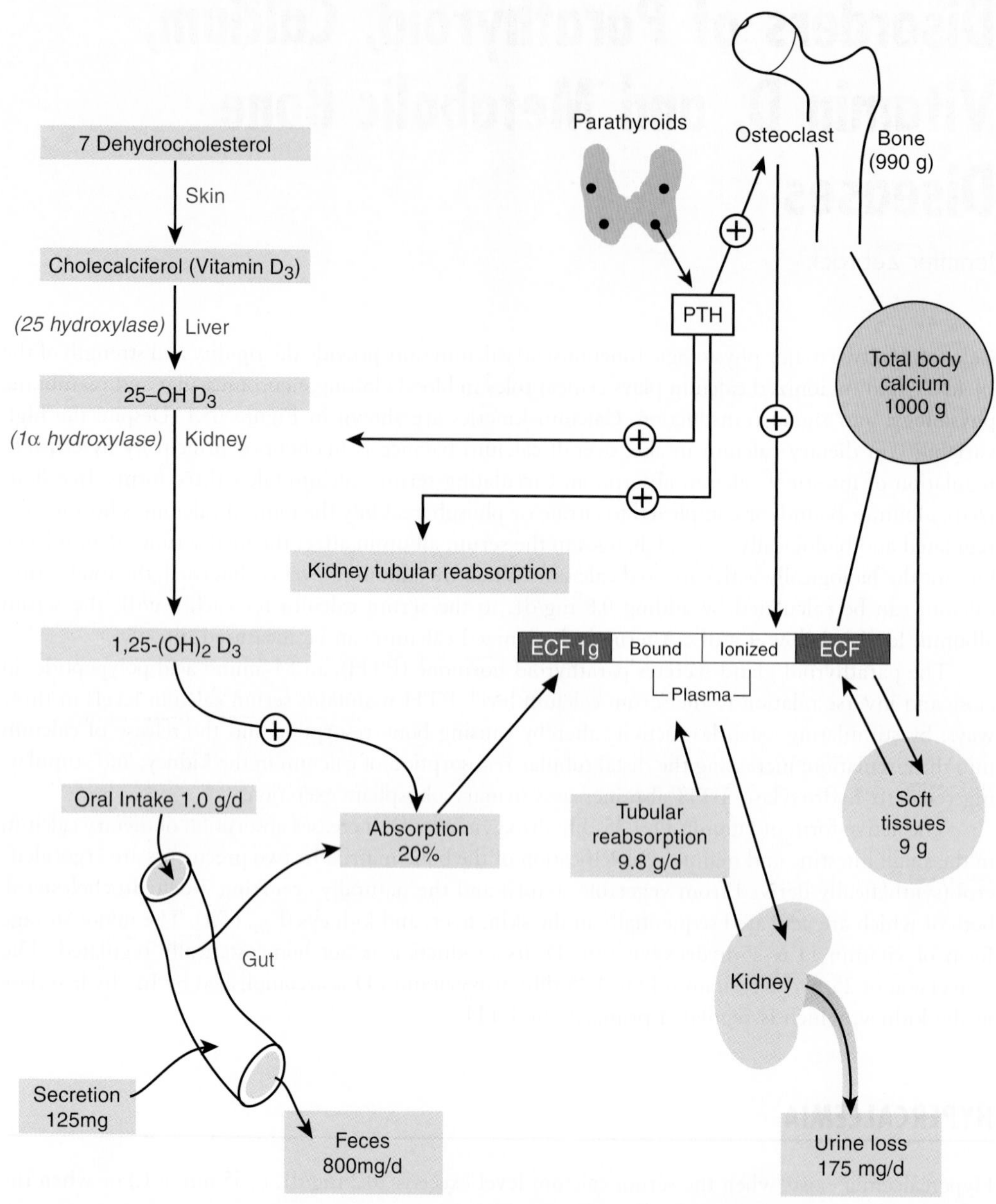

Figure 65.1 • Calcium balance on an average diet.

PTHrP, although distinct from PTH, has amino-terminal homology with PTH and can mimic its effects on PTH receptors. PTHrP is produced most commonly by squamous cell cancers (head, neck, lung, and esophagus), renal cell carcinoma, and breast cancer. Metastases with extensive localized bone destruction constitute the second most common mechanism of tumor-related hypercalcemia, called osteolytic hypercalcemia. Hematologic neoplasms (e.g., multiple myeloma and lymphoma) cause hypercalcemia by releasing osteoclast-activating cytokines and, occasionally (in lymphomas), 1,25-dihydroxyvitamin D.

TABLE 65.1 Causes of hypercalcemia

Common	Less common	Factitious
• Primary hyperparathyroidism • Malignancy	• Medications (lithium, thiazides) • Vitamin D intoxication • Familial hypocalciuria hypercalcemia • Sarcoidosis • Acute immobilization • Renal failure • Hyperthyroidism • Milk-alkali syndrome	• Increased calcium-binding proteins (e.g., hypergammaglobulinemia)

Clinical Manifestations

Hypercalcemia can evoke a variety of systemic signs (Table 65.2); however, symptoms usually occur only if the serum calcium is greater than 12 mg/dL. Hypercalcemia that is acute and/or severe (greater than 14 mg/dL) usually causes more symptoms such as weakness, anorexia, nausea, vomiting, dehydration, renal failure, confusion, or coma (hypercalcemic crisis).

In primary hyperparathyroidism, the serum calcium level typically ranges from 10.5 to 13 mg/dL; occasionally it is severely elevated. Patients may be completely asymptomatic, present with symptoms of hypercalcemia, or experience organ damage from the hypercalcemia. Nephrolithiasis is common and is the harbinger in many patients. Severe, chronic hypercalciuria can lead to nephrocalcinosis and renal failure. Increased bone resorption causes demineralization and osteopenia. Advanced disease may classically, but rarely, lead to osteitis fibrosa cystica, with bone cysts, pathological fractures, and brown tumors.

Most cancer-related hypercalcemia complicates an already diagnosed advanced malignancy and is associated with a poor prognosis. The features of advanced cancer usually dominate the presentation with weight loss, anorexia, fatigue, and pain from bone metastases. Hypercalcemia of malignancy is more likely than primary hyperparathyroidism to cause a hypercalcemic crisis.

Diagnosis

The recognition of hypercalcemia has increased markedly in recent decades with routine laboratory testing. The most likely causes, primary hyperparathyroidism and hypercalcemia of malignancy, can usually be differentiated by the clinical presentations. Most patients with primary hyperparathyroidism have mild hypercalcemia (<13 mg/dL) and either are asymptomatic or manifest a complication of chronic hypercalcemia, such as nephrolithiasis. Patients with malignancy, however, typically present with advanced cancer and manifest more acute, severe hypercalcemia. On laboratory evaluation (Table 65.3), patients with primary hyperparathyroidism usually have a significantly elevated intact PTH level; it is low-normal or nondetectable in patients with hypercalcemia of malignancy. Measurement of urinary calcium excretion may be useful to (a) exclude familial hypocalciuric hypercalcemia when clinical and laboratory features suggest mild primary hyperparathyroidism, and (b) determine the long-term risk for nephrolithiasis and nephrocalcinosis in patients with mild hyperparathyroidism.

Treatment

The definitive treatment of single adenomas is surgical removal. In cases of four-gland hyperplasia, three of the glands usually are removed. A portion of the remaining gland is either left in place or

TABLE 65.2 Clinical manifestations of hypercalcemia

Renal
Nephrolithiasis
Impaired concentrating ability (polyuria, polydipsia, and dehydration)
Renal tubular defects (natriuresis)
Interstitial nephritis
Nephrocalcinosis
Renal failure
Gastrointestinal
Constipation
Anorexia
Nausea
Peptic ulcer
Pancreatitis
Neuromuscular
Muscle weakness
Lethargy
Somnolence
Coma
Hyporeflexia
Psychiatric
Apathy
Depression
Psychosis
Cardiovascular
Pruritus (calcium deposition within the skin)
Band keratopathy (calcium deposition within the cornea)
Ectopic calcification
Shortened QT interval on electrocardiogram (characteristic)
Increased sensitivity to digoxin

TABLE 65.3 Laboratory evaluation of hypercalcemia

Initial work-up
Serum calcium, albumin, phosphate, and creatinine
Parathyroid hormone level
Urine calcium excretion (24-hour urine collection)
Additional tests sometimes useful
Ionized calcium
SPEP, UPEP
Chest radiograph
Computed tomography, magnetic resonance imaging of chest and abdomen

SPEP, serum protein electrophoresis; UPEP, urine protein electrophoresis

TABLE 65.4 Medical therapy of hypercalcemic crisis

Step I:	Intravenous normal saline to reverse dehydration and establish brisk urine output
Step II:	Cautious use of furosemide (e.g., 20 mg twice daily) to promote further urine calcium excretion Note: Furosemide should be started only after adequate hydration has been established
Step III:	Individualized use of calcitonin or pamidronate Less commonly indicated are plicamycin, glucocorticoids, oral phosphate, indomethacin, dialysis, or gallium

transplanted to the forearm to foster access if hypercalcemia persists and reoperation is needed. Serum calcium falls postoperatively within several hours of successful surgery. Transient postoperative hypocalcemia may occur after removal of an adenoma because of suppression of the remaining normal glands. Permanent hypoparathyroidism can follow if all four glands are removed surgically. Observation for postoperative hypocalcemia is critical.

Some advocate deferring surgery in asymptomatic patients with mild hypercalcemia (<11 mg/dL), especially those who are elderly or frail and poorly suited for general anesthesia. If medical management without surgical intervention is selected, bone mass and renal function should be closely monitored.

When malignancy is the cause, treatment is directed toward the primary tumor. Hypercalcemic crisis is treated medically (Table 65.4). In many patients with terminal cancer, one may elect not to treat the hypercalcemia but to provide only palliative and supportive care because the hypercalcemia of malignancy is usually associated with advanced and untreatable cancer.

HYPOCALCEMIA

Hypocalcemia can be due to a decrease in either the albumin-bound or ionized (free) fraction of the serum calcium. It is defined as a corrected serum calcium less than 8.4 mg/dL (2.1 mmol/L) or ionized calcium less than 4.65 mg/dL (1.16 mmol/L).

Etiology

Hypocalcemia is usually due to a deficiency in the production, secretion, or action of PTH or of 1,25-dihydroxyvitamin D. Because PTH decreases renal tubular phosphate reabsorption, hypocalcemia due to PTH deficiency or resistance is associated with hyperphosphatemia (Table 65.5). In contrast, 1,25-dihydroxyvitamin D normally increases renal tubular phosphate reabsorption. Thus, hypocalcemia due to a deficiency of or resistance to vitamin D is associated with hypophosphatemia.

Causes of hypoparathyroidism include surgical removal of the parathyroid glands, autoimmune disorders, and infiltrative diseases. Hypomagnesemia can decrease PTH secretion and cause renal and skeletal resistance to PTH; hypocalcemia does not usually develop until the serum magnesium falls below 1.0 mg/dL. Rarely, hypocalcemia is from PTH resistance from a hereditary condition of pseudohypoparathyroidism (PHP).

Renal failure is the most common cause of hypocalcemia. As the glomerular filtration rate falls below 30 mL per minute, PTH can no longer produce phosphaturia, resulting in hyperphosphatemia and subsequent hypocalcemia. PTH levels are elevated in this setting (secondary hyperparathyroidism). Other contributing factors in renal failure include the reduced production of 1,25-dihydroxyvita-

TABLE 65.5 Causes of hypocalcemia as integrated with serum phosphate level

Hyperphosphatemia	Hypophosphatemia
Parathyroid hormone-related	**Vitamin D-related**
PTH deficiency Congenital Acquired Postsurgical Autoimmune Infiltrative Chronic hypomagnesemia (may cause PTH resistance also) Idiopathic PTH resistance Pseudohypoparathyroidism	Deficient vitamin D Poor diet/no sun exposure Malabsorption Impaired 1-hydroxylation of 25-hydroxyvitamin D Resistance to vitamin D Vitamin D-dependent rickets, types 1 and 2
Parathyroid hormone-unrelated	
Endogenous Renal failure Hemolysis Rhabdomyolysis Tumor lysis syndrome Exogenous phosphate load Laxatives and enemas	

min D by the kidney and skeletal resistance to the actions of PTH. Hyperphosphatemia from conditions such as rhabdomyolysis, tumor lysis syndrome, and excessive phosphate administration can also result in hypocalcemia.

Vitamin D deficiency from decreased dietary intake, lack of sunlight, or malabsorption can cause hypocalcemia. Because the liver is the site of 25-hydroxylation, liver disease impairs this stage of vitamin D metabolism. Rarely, hypocalcemia can result from vitamin D resistance (vitamin D–dependent rickets).

Pancreatic lipase, which is released in acute pancreatitis, liberates free fatty acids from the surrounding retroperitoneal and omental fat. These free fatty acids chelate calcium ions, resulting in hypocalcemia (a poor prognostic sign). The hungry bone syndrome occurs when calcium and phosphate are acutely deposited into bones, causing hypocalcemia; it is typically seen within hours after a parathyroidectomy (excision of a parathyroid gland) for primary hyperparathyroidism.

Several medications can also cause hypocalcemia. Phenytoin, phenobarbital, and glutethimide impair 25-α hydroxylation of vitamin D; foscarnet may chelate circulating calcium; and cholestyramine may interfere with vitamin D absorption. Finally, cisplatin and pentamidine may produce urinary magnesium wasting.

Clinical Manifestations

The clinical manifestations depend on the degree, rate of development, and duration of hypocalcemia (Table 65.6), but often there are no symptoms. The hallmark of severe hypocalcemia is tetany, caused

TABLE 65.6 Clinical manifestations of hypocalcemia

Clinical manifestations of hypocalcemia
Cardiac
Decreased myocardial contractility
Congestive heart failure
Prolonged QT interval
Dental
Hypoplasia of teeth/enamel
Dental caries
Delayed eruption of teeth
Neurologic
Paresthesias (toes, fingers, and perioral regions)
Muscle cramps/fasciculations
Chvostek's sign (Fig. 65.2A)
Trousseau's sign (Fig. 65.2B)
Tetany
Seizures
Basal ganglia calcifications
Mental status changes
Ophthalmologic
Cataracts
Optic neuritis
Papilledema

by spontaneous sensory and motor discharges in peripheral nerves and featuring muscular twitching, spasms, or seizure. A prolonged QT interval on electrocardiogram is also a classic manifestation of hypocalcemia. Chvostek's sign may be elicited by tapping the facial nerve approximately 2 cm in front of the ear lobe and just below the zygomatic arch (Fig. 65.2A). A positive response is a twitching of the lip at the angle of the mouth. Trousseau's sign is tested by inflating a blood pressure cuff 10

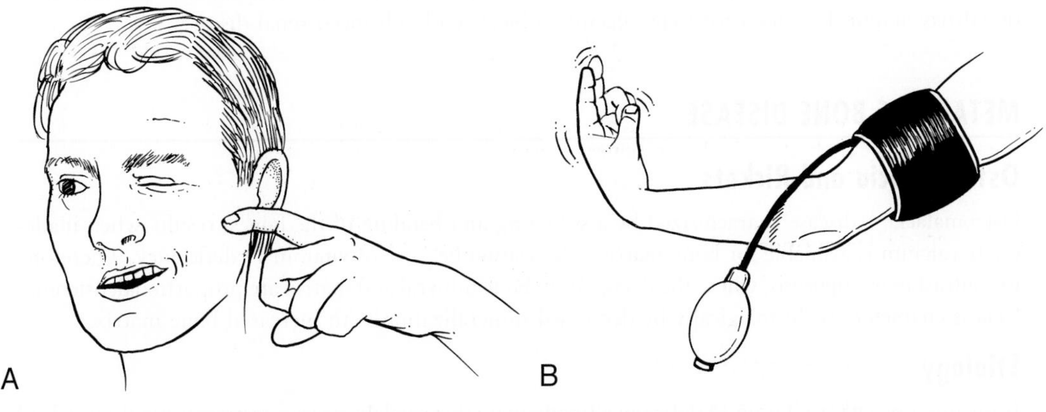

Figure 65.2 • Positive Chvostek's sign and Trousseau's sign.

TABLE 65.7 Laboratory values of hypoparathyroidism, vitamin D deficiency, and pseudohypoparathyroidism

	Hypoparathyroid	Vitamin D deficiency	Pseudohypoparathyroidism
PTH	↓	↑	↑
Calcium	↓	↓	↓
Phosphate	↑	↓	↑

to 20 mm Hg above the patient's systolic blood pressure for 3 to 5 minutes, thus reducing the blood supply to the ulnar nerve. In hypocalcemia, this maneuver causes the classic "obstetrician's hand" (Fig. 65.2B). Whereas Chvostek's sign is positive in 10% to 20% of normal persons, Trousseau's sign is rarely present normally.

Diagnosis

Once hypocalcemia has been found, checking a PTH level will aid in diagnosis. Generally, PTH is low and phosphate levels are high in PTH deficiency, while PTH is high and phosphate levels are low in disorders of vitamin D (Table 65.7). Chronic renal failure usually exhibits elevated PTH and due to secondary hyperparathyroidism and hyperphosphatemia secondary to uremia. In states of PTH resistance, such as pseudohypoparathyroidism, PTH and phosphate levels are also elevated. Pseudohyperparathyroidism is associated with Albright hereditary osteodystrophy. This syndrome is characterized by short stature, obesity, *café au lait* spots, mental retardation, and shortened fourth and fifth metacarpophalangeal and metatarsal (MTT) joints. When vitamin D deficiency is suspected, it usually is necessary to measure only the metabolite 25-hydroxyvitamin D because it is consistently low in states of vitamin D deficiency. Circulating 1,25-dihydroxyvitamin D levels are less consistently depressed.

Treatment

Acute hypocalcemia is treated by intravenous calcium gluconate or calcium chloride (Table 65.8). Vitamin D and calcium supplements are therapeutic mainstays of all forms of parathyroid hormone and vitamin D deficiencies. If possible, the pharmacotherapy of vitamin D should allow for regulated production of 1,25-dihydroxyvitamin D. For example, if a hypocalcemic patient has normal renal function, a simple vegetable-derived vitamin D preparation should be used. Alternatively, 25-hydroxyvitamin D is used to treat patients with normal kidney function and liver disease, whereas 1,25-dihydroxyvitamin D is used for hypocalcemic subjects with advanced renal disease.

METABOLIC BONE DISEASE

Osteomalacia and Rickets

Osteomalacia, a disease characterized by a softening and bending of the bones, results when inadequate calcium is available for bone matrix calcification because of vitamin D deficiency. Therefore, in contrast to osteoporosis, where the decreases in bone mineral and matrix are proportional, osteomalacia is characterized histologically by decreased mineralization with increased bone matrix.

Etiology

It is caused by either vitamin D deficiency (inadequate diet, malabsorptive gastrointestinal disorders) or diseases or other factors that impair conversion of vitamin D to 1,25-dihydroxyvitamin D (liver

TABLE 65.8 Therapy for hypocalcemia

Acute symptomatic hypocalcemia (tetany)

1. Ten percent calcium gluconate (90 mg of elemental Ca^{2+}/10 mL ampule)
   a. Dilute 2 × 10 mL ampules of calcium gluconate in 50 to 100 mL of D^5 solution. Infuse 2 mg/kg body weight over 5 to 10 minutes; or 10% calcium chloride (272 mg of elemental calcium/10 mL ampule)
   b. Dilute 1 × 10 mL ampule in 50 to 100 mL of D^5 solution. Infuse 2 mg/kg over 5 to 10 minutes
2. Continue IV calcium until over tetany is controlled
   This rapid infusion may ameliorate symptoms for 15 minutes to several hours
   a. Follow rapid loading infusion by a slower infusion of 15 mg/kg of calcium gluconate mixed with D^5 infused over 6 to 12 hours

Chronic hypocalcemia

1. Mild vitamin D deficiency
   Multivitamin containing 400 IU of vitamin D daily
   Oral calcium, 800 to 1,200 mg daily
2. Hypoparathyroidism
   Oral elemental calcium 1 to 2 g in 3 divided doses
   1, 25-dihydroxyvitamin D: 0.25 to 2.0 μg/day
   Vitamin D: 25,000 to 100,000 IU/day

disease, renal disease, or anticonvulsant therapy). The decreased intestinal absorption of calcium reduces its availability to mineralize bone matrix. A compensatory increase in parathyroid hormone levels leads to increased bone mineral resorption by osteoclasts.

Clinical Manifestations

Clinical features vary depending on the age at onset, the precipitating causes, and the presence or absence of concomitant hypocalcemia. Rickets is osteomalacia occurring in children prior to epiphyseal closure. Children with rickets have bowing of long bones, growth retardation, bone pain, and delayed dentition. Adults with osteomalacia present with bone pain and pathological fractures. Associated hypocalcemia leads to hypotonia, muscle weakness, and tetany.

Diagnosis

Imaging studies show diffuse demineralization (osteopenia), increased trabecular markings, and pseudofractures. Serum calcium and phosphate often are low, and alkaline phosphatase is high. PTH levels are elevated (secondary hyperparathyroidism).

Treatment

Therapy of osteomalacia includes administration of vitamin D or its active metabolite, 1,25-dihydroxyvitamin D, and, where possible, identification and treatment of the underlying disease or diseases.

Paget's Disease of Bone

The hallmark of Paget's disease (osteitis deformans) is disordered bone remodeling with an increase in the rate of bone turnover. Although it usually is focal, Paget's disease may be widespread. The pelvic bones are most commonly involved, followed by skull, femur, lumbosacral spine, clavicles, ribs, and tibia. Excessive bone resorption results in areas of radiolucency on radiographs (osteoporosis circumscripta). The normal marrow is replaced by fibrovascular connective tissue. Excessive osteoblastic activity replaces resorbed bone, but new bone is organized haphazardly, with multiple, irregular cement lines; histologically, it has a characteristic mosaic pattern.

Etiology

The etiology of Paget's disease is unknown, but it may be caused by a slow-activating viral infection in genetically susceptible individuals. Up to 20% to 30% of those affected have a family history.

Clinical Manifestations

Paget's disease is rare before middle age, but estimates suggest that it may be present in 3% of persons over age 40 years. Because most patients are asymptomatic, the disease usually is discovered incidentally on radiographs or by an isolated, otherwise unexplained rise in alkaline phosphatase. Serum calcium and phosphate usually are normal. However, hypercalcemia can follow immobilization in patients with Paget's disease. It can also present with swelling, deformity, or pain in a long bone. Skull enlargement may cause an increase in hat size over the years. Temporal bone involvement may cause hearing loss, and Pagetic bone growth and basal skull compression may evoke other neurologic symptoms. Vertebral and long-bone fractures may result from structural bone abnormalities; these fractures and deformities together may cause loss of height. With widespread disease, the high skeletal blood flow raises cardiac output, thus leading to heart failure. Osteogenic sarcoma occurs in less than 1% of cases. Although the coarse, dense Pagetic bone appears abnormally dense on radiographs, its strength is not enhanced; the irregular structure makes it weaker than normal bone, thus causing fractures and deformities.

Diagnosis

Plain skeletal radiographs, especially of the pelvis, skull, femur and lower spine, are useful in diagnosis. Bone scans, which are more sensitive than radiographs, can define the extent of Paget's disease, but the findings are nonspecific and overlap with degenerative arthritis and metastatic cancer. Bone turnover in Paget's disease is focally increased. Therefore, markers of osteoblast activity (serum alkaline phosphatase) and of osteoclast activity (urine hydroxyproline) usually are high in active disease; observing changes in their levels can be helpful in monitoring response to therapy.

Treatment

The major goals of drug therapy are to reduce pain, limit the development of further deformities, and prevent neurologic complications. Aspirin or nonsteroidal anti-inflammatory agents can help relieve pain. If symptoms are clearly attributable to Paget's disease, more specific therapy can be given, but it can be difficult to judge whether back pain in a patient with Paget's disease is due to Paget's disease or to coexisting degenerative disc disease. The use of a bisphosphonate or calcitonin may suppress disease activity. Oral bisphosphonates, such as etidronate, alendronate, or risedronate, are typically given cyclically; pamidronate is given in a series of intravenous infusions to produce a prolonged remission in symptoms. Mithramycin is less useful because of its hepatic, renal, and hematologic toxicity. Disease activity should be monitored during therapy.

CHAPTER 66

Thyroid Diseases

Ty Carroll

The thyroid gland is the largest of the solely endocrine glands of the human body. The normal adult gland weighs 20 g, but pathologic growth, known as goiter, can produce a gland weighing over several hundred grams. The thyroid is shaped much like a butterfly and is located inferiorly and laterally to the thyroid cartilage. It consists of a right and left lobe connected by a small isthmus, which lies over the second or third cartilaginous ring of the trachea (Fig. 66.1). In more than 60% of the population, a small pyramidal lobe extends superiorly from the isthmus along the tract of the thyroglossal duct.

The follicle is the structural unit of thyroid tissue. The follicle consists of a single layer of cuboidal follicular cells enclosing a cavity filled with colloid, a gel-like material that serves as a reservoir of thyroid hormone. The thyroid also contains a small number of parafollicular cells (C cells) that secrete calcitonin and are unrelated to thyroid hormone metabolism. The gland receives its rich blood supply from superior and inferior thyroidal arteries.

THYROID HORMONE SYNTHESIS

Thyroxine (T_4) and triiodothyronine (T_3) are the two major hormones produced in the thyroid (Fig. 66.2). Their production begins as iodide is actively transported via the Na+/I into the follicular cell. Once in the cell, the iodide is organified in a reaction catalyzed by thyroid peroxidase. The organification creates monoiodotyrosine (MIT) and diiodotyrosine (DIT) bound to thyroglobulin.

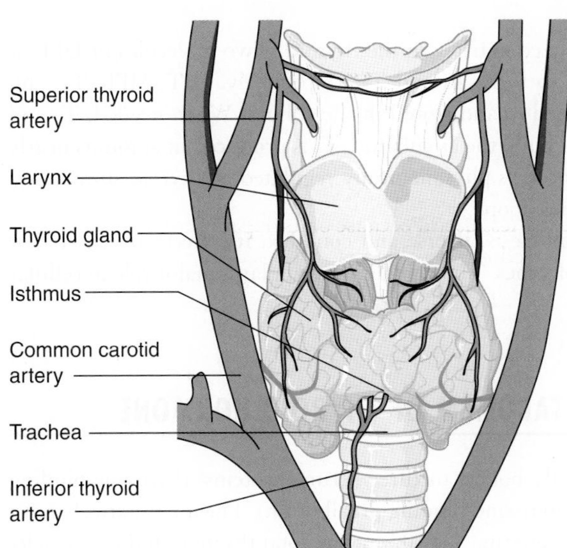

Figure 66.1 • Anatomy of the thyroid gland.

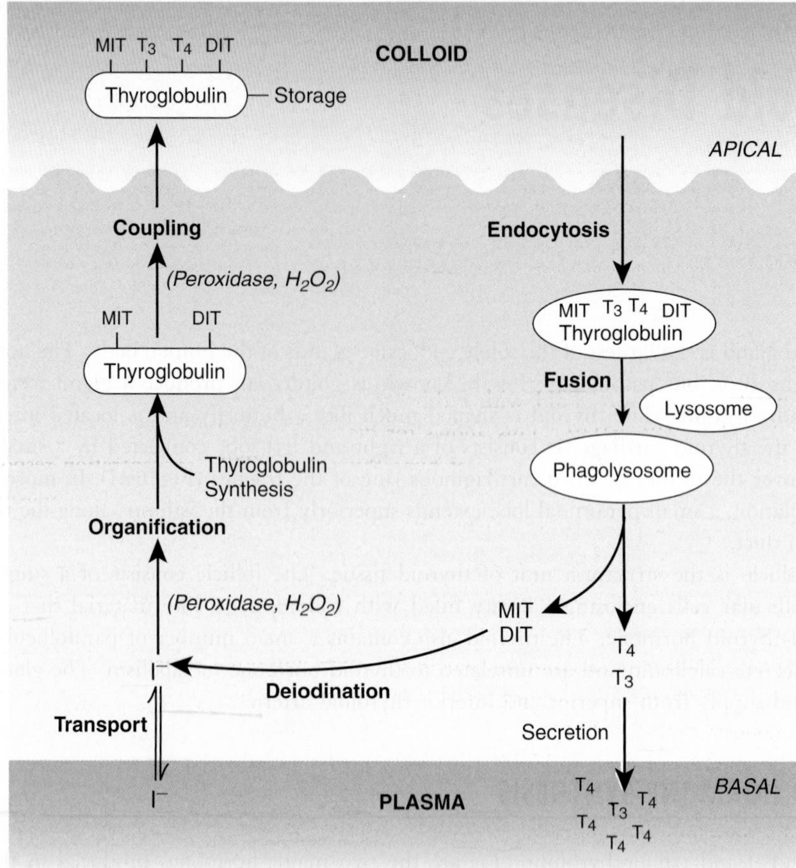

Figure 66.2 • Pathway of biosynthesis of thyroid hormones. (From West JB [ed]. *Best and Taylor's Physiological Basis of Medical Practice,* 12th ed. Baltimore: Williams & Wilkins; 1991:813, with permission.)

Thyroglobulin is a protein produced and utilized entirely in the thyroid. Two molecules of DIT or one molecule of each DIT and MIT couple to form T_4 and T_3, respectively. DIT, MIT, T_3, and T_4 bound to thyroglobulin are then transported to and stored in the colloid. When needed, T_3 and T_4 are cleaved from thyroglobulin and secreted into the circulation. T_4 is produced in amounts nearly 10-fold greater than T_3. Each step of this process is physiologically regulated by thyroid stimulating hormone (TSH) via a classic negative feedback loop.

The function of circulating thyroid hormone is diverse and complex. Its effects are exerted at the nuclear level by increasing transcription of genes. These genes in turn play a major role in cellular growth, development, and metabolism.

PERIPHERAL CIRCULATION AND METABOLISM OF THYROID HORMONE

T_3 and T_4 circulate in the bloodstream tightly bound to three serum proteins: thyroxine-binding globulin (TBG), albumin, and transthyretin (thyroxine-binding prealbumin). The quantitatively most important of the binding proteins is TBG, accounting for 70% of the total thyroid-binding capacity of the serum. More than 99% of both T_3 and T_4 are protein bound. Although T_4 is more abundant than T_3, T_3 interacts with intranuclear receptors at a higher affinity and is more important in producing the biological effects of thyroid hormone. T_4 is converted to T_3 intracellularly in its target cells by the action of 5′-deiodinase. T_4 also may be metabolized to metabolically inactive reverse T_3 by 5-deiodinase.

LABORATORY TESTS OF THE THYROID

Numerous laboratory measurement of thyroid function currently exist; however, measurement of serum TSH, free T_4 (fT_4), and occasionally total T_3 (tT_3) have the most diagnostic utility.

Most laboratories measure TSH with a third-generation immunometric assay that can detect serum levels less than 0.01 mIU/L. This allows for discrimination between suppressed and absent TSH, which is important in the diagnosis of hyperthyroidism. TSH concentration responds logarithmically to changes in T_3 and T_4. This logarithmic response together with very sensitive assays makes TSH the single best test of thyroid function in most circumstances.

As such, TSH is the best arbiter of thyroid function, except in cases of: (a) secondary hypothyroidism, when the pituitary fails to secrete adequate TSH in response to hypothyroidism; (b) in acute illness, where the TSH may be transiently elevated or suppressed without true thyroidal pathology; and (c) in recovery from hyperthyroidism, where the TSH will often remain suppressed for several months as thyroid hormone levels return to normal. In these circumstances, fT_4 and tT_3 should be measured in concert with the TSH.

Because thyroid hormones are highly protein bound, any change in binding protein concentrations leads to changes in the total hormone levels. Measurement of non–protein bound or free hormone rather than total hormone eliminates confounding caused by fluctuations in binding protein concentrations and allows one to assess the biologically active level of hormone. Accurate assays to measure fT_4 are widely available and should be used in place of total T_4 measurements. Likewise, fT_3 assays are available; however, they may not achieve the level of accuracy of the fT_4 assay.

IMAGING TESTS OF THE THYROID

Radionuclide uptake and scanning, ultrasound, computed tomography (CT), and magnetic resonance imaging (MRI) are all available to image the thyroid. Each has its own inherent advantages and disadvantages, and no imaging modality can definitively diagnose or rule out malignancy. There are two distinct radionuclide imaging tests used in evaluation of the thyroid. Radionuclide uptake measurement produces no images of the thyroid but produces functional information. In radionuclide uptake measurement, patients are given ^{131}I, ^{123}I, or ^{99m}Tc pertechnetate, which is then concentrated by the thyroid gland. The total amount of radionuclide uptake is then measured. Increased uptake signifies hyperactivity of the gland and low uptake indicates hypofunction or damage of the thyroid. Radionuclide scanning is similar to uptake measurement but produces images of the thyroid that show areas of increased and decrease uptake. Ultrasound gives excellent anatomical information including whether nodules are cystic or solid. In addition, it can detect many nodules not palpable on physical examination. As a result, ultrasound is used as a supplement to physical examination in the characterization of thyroid nodules and to follow nodule growth over time. CT and MRI are not routinely used for thyroid imaging due to cost and relatively small advantage over ultrasound.

THYROID DISEASE

The thyroid has three cardinal disease states: overproduction of hormone, underproduction of hormone, and abnormal growth which includes thyroid cancer.

HYPERTHYROIDISM

Hyperthyroidism affects <1% of the U.S. population. It is characterized by an excessive amount of circulating thyroid hormone, which causes a hypermetabolic state.

A list of signs and symptoms of hyperthyroidism can be found in Table 66.1. All causes of hyperthyroidism have similar clinical manifestations; however, subtleties in presentation can help differentiate the underlying cause. For example, Graves' disease often has an abrupt onset with severe symptoms, whereas thyroiditis is a transient and often milder form of hyperthyroidism, and in toxic multinodular goiter the onset of symptoms is insidious. This being said, the patient's age at onset and coexisting medical conditions are often as important as the underlying cause in determining the presentation of hyperthyroidism. Younger patients are more likely to present with classic symptoms of nervousness, hyperhidrosis, palpitations, and tachycardia. Older individuals usually have more subtle complaints and can manifest apathetic hyperthyroidism with weight loss, depression, and atrial fibrillation.

There are many causes of hyperthyroidism but Graves' disease, toxic multinodular goiter, and thyroiditis account for a large majority of all cases of hyperthyroidism.

Thyroid crisis (thyroid storm) is a rare life-threatening complication of hyperthyroidism. In most

TABLE 66.1 Clinical manifestations of hyperthyroidism

Symptoms	Frequency (%)	Signs	Frequency (%)
Nervousness	99	Tachycardia	100
Increased sweating	91	Goiter	100
Heat intolerance	89	Skin changes	97
Palpitations	89	Bruit over thyroid	77
Fatigue	88	Eye signs[a]	71
Weight loss	85	Atrial fibrillation	10
Tachycardia	82	Splenomegaly[a]	10
Dyspnea	75	Gynomastia	10
Weakness	70		
Increased appetite	65		
Eye complaints[a]	54		
Swelling of the legs	35		
Hyperdefecation (without diarrhea)	33		
Diarrhea	23		
Anorexia	9		
Constipation	4		
Weight gain	3		

[a]Much more common in Graves' disease.
Adapted from Williams RH. Thiouracil treatment of thyrotoxicosis. *J Clin Endocrinol* 1946:6:1–22, with permission.

instances, thyroid storm is ushered in by a precipitating event in patients with previously untreated Graves' disease and severe hyperthyroidism. Precipitating events include infections, surgery, and trauma. The features of this condition include fever, which may be high, restlessness, confusion, and, occasionally, frank psychosis. Cardiac arrhythmias are common and cardiovascular collapse may supervene. Treatment includes propylthiouracil (800 to 1,200 mg) given orally or by nasogastric tube. Iodide is given to block thyroid hormone synthesis and peripheral T_4 to T_3 conversion. Antithyroid drugs must precede the iodide because iodide also is a substrate for thyroid hormone synthesis. β-blockers are a critical component of the therapy. Glucocorticoids are administered to offset a relative adrenal insufficiency. Both propranolol and corticosteroids also lower the peripheral conversion of T_4 to T_3. A precipitating event should be searched for carefully and, if found, appropriately treated.

Graves' Disease

Graves' disease is the most common cause of hyperthyroidism and accounts for 60% to 90% of all cases of hyperthyroidism. The exact trigger of Graves' disease is still unclear; however, the pathophysiology is created by autoantibodies to the TSH receptor that stimulate the thyroid to produce increased amounts of thyroid hormone.

CLINICAL FEATURES

Graves' disease presents similar to other causes of hyperthyroidism with nervousness, palpitation, tachycardia, and increased sweating. In this condition, the thyroid is diffusely enlarged, firm, and nontender (Fig. 66.3), and a bruit is audible over the gland in 75% of patients. Graves' disease is also associated with several distinct and more specific nonthyroidal entities, ophthalmopathy, and dermopathy.

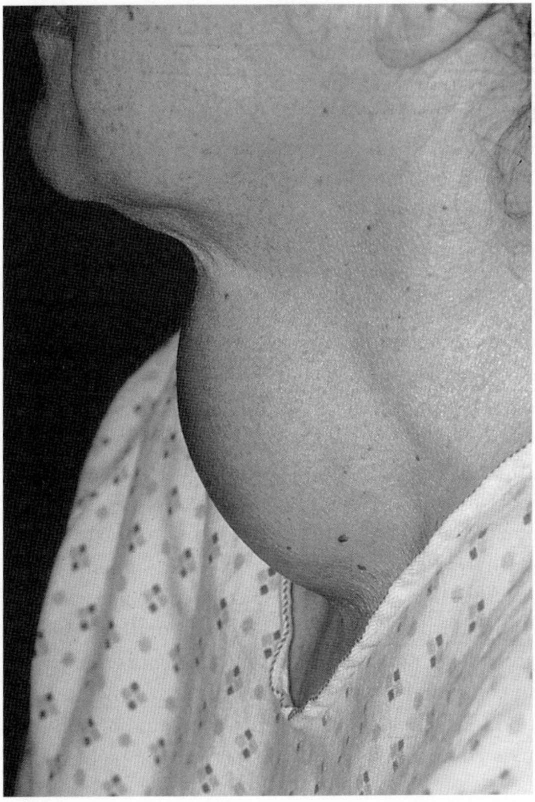

Figure 66.3 • A large, diffuse goiter as seen in Graves' disease.

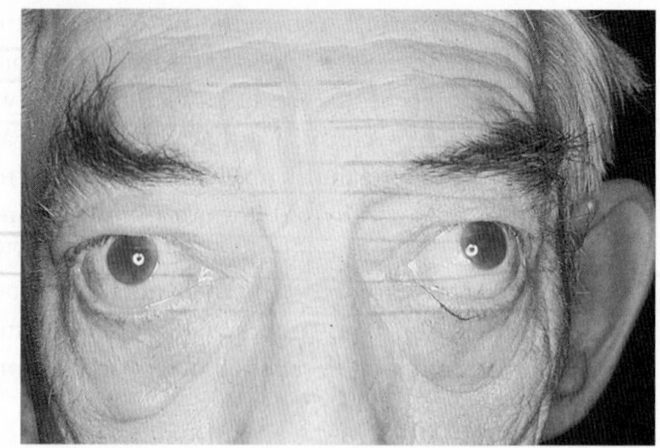

Figure 66.4 • Graves' ophthalmopathy. (Photograph courtesy of James M. Cerletty, MD, Department of Medicine, The Medical College of Wisconsin, Milwaukee, WI.)

Ophthalmopathy (Fig. 66.4) is present in 25% of patients with Graves' disease and generally manifests at the time of diagnosis of hyperthyroidism but can occur prior to or after the appearance of hyperthyroidism. It results from inflammation of the eye and orbital tissues and can range from eye irritation to proptosis and ophthalmoplegia (Fig. 66.5). Dermopathy is rare and results from mucopolysaccharide deposition in the dermis. It is characterized by thick, firm, elevated patches of skin (Fig. 66.5).

DIAGNOSIS

Graves' disease is a diagnosis made on both biochemical and clinical grounds. As in any case of suspected hyperthyroidism, thyroid function tests should be ordered. The TSH will be suppressed in patients with true hyperthyroidism. The fT_4 and tT_3 will be elevated, confirming the diagnosis and assessing the degree of hyperthyroidism. Total T_3 is necessary in the rare case of T_3 thyrotoxicosis where the fT_4 is normal despite hyperthyroidism with a suppressed TSH. In this situation, the tT_3 will be elevated confirming the diagnosis of hyperthyroidism (Table 66.2).

Individuals with thyroid function tests indicating hyperthyroidism and either ophthalmopathy or dermopathy are diagnosed with Graves' disease. Individuals with suspected Graves' disease but without ophthalmopathy or dermopathy often undergo radionuclide uptake measurement to assist in the diagnosis. An elevated uptake confirms the diagnosis of Graves' disease.

THERAPY

The natural history of Graves' is generally one of persistent disease, but individuals may have remission and relapse, therefore predicting the course of an individual patient is difficult. As such, all patients should undergo therapy with antithyroid medication, ^{131}I, or rarely surgery. One of these three modalities can be used to effectively treat essentially all patients with Graves' disease. In addition, β-blockers alleviate many of the adrenergic manifestation of hyperthyroidism including tachycardia, tremor, and excessive sweating. The traditional β-blocker used is propranolol, but newer agents are also effective.

The thioureas, propylthiouracil and methimazole, are the two medication used to treat Graves' disease in the United States. Both agents decrease thyroid hormone levels by blocking organification of iodide. They require at least 4 weeks to achieve full effect. Their side effects include nausea, rash, and agranulocytosis. ^{131}I is highly effective in treating Graves' disease. ^{131}I is given orally and taken up and concentrated in the thyroid where it exerts a local radiation effect over the course of several months. Most individuals develop permanent hypothyroidism within 6 months after therapy and require lifelong thyroid hormone supplementation. Surgery is the selected therapeutic option only in selected cases when thyroid enlargement causes compressive symptoms or because of physician and patient preference.

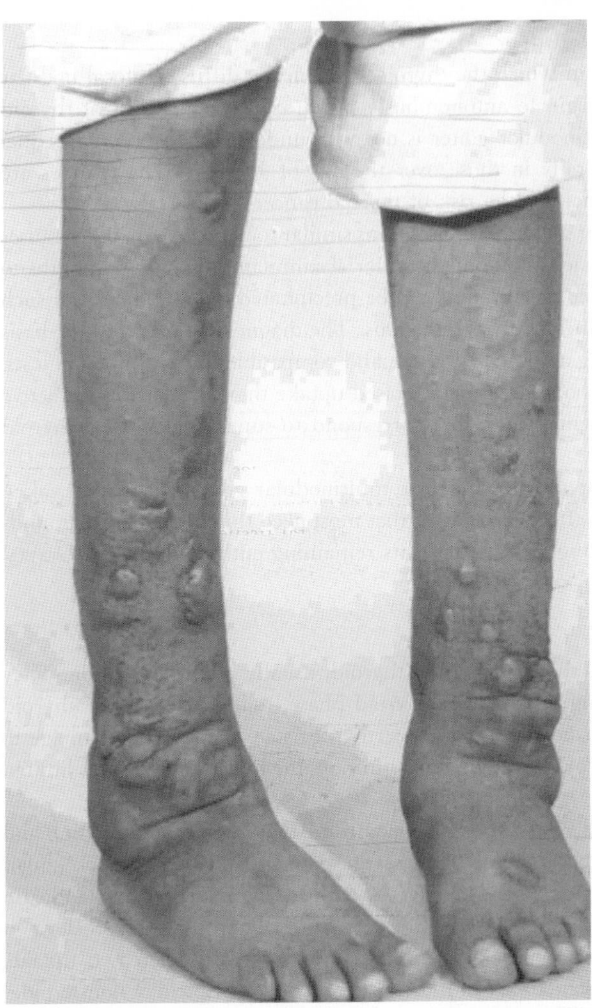

Figure 66.5 • Graves' dermopathy. (Photograph courtesy of James M. Cerletty, MD, Department of Medicine, The Medical College of Wisconsin, Milwaukee, WI.)

TABLE 66.2 Evaluation of hyperthyroidism

	Euthyroid	**Graves' disease**	**Toxic multinodular goiter**	**Thyroiditis**
Thyroid stimulating hormone	Normal	Low	Low	Low
Total T3	Normal	High	High	High
Free T4	Normal	High	High	High
Radionuclide Scanning	Normal	Increased uptake	Focal increase	Decreased uptake

Toxic Multinodular Goiter

Toxic multinodular goiter is a condition in which the thyroid gland has a diffuse or focal nodular enlargement. These nodules grow and begin to autonomously produce excess amounts of thyroid hormone. The pathogenesis of toxic multinodular goiter is not well understood. It occurs in equal frequency in men and women and generally in those over the age of 40 years. The nodules are generally benign adenomas and do not increase the risk of thyroid cancer.

Again, patient with toxic multinodular goiter have symptoms similar to patients with other causes of hyperthyroidism. The symptoms of toxic multinodular goiter accumulate slowly over months to years as the nodules continue to grow. Acute symptoms can be precipitated by an iodine load such as intravenous contrast dye or by acute illness such as infections. The diagnosis is made on the basis of history, a thyroid examination revealing a nodular thyroid, and compatible thyroid function tests. If radionuclide scanning is performed it shows areas of increased uptake that correlate to overactive or "hot" nodules, as well as areas of absent uptake that correspond to suppressed normal thyroid tissue.

^{131}I is the treatment of choice in individuals with toxic multinodular goiter. The ^{131}I is taken up avidly by the hot nodules and exerts its effect at the areas that most need therapy. Often surrounding normal thyroid tissue is spared resulting in more patients remaining euthyroid than in Graves' disease after therapy.

Thyroiditis

Thyroiditis refers to a group of disorders that damage the thyroid, usually by inflammation. They share a common natural history beginning with a hyperthyroid phase, followed by a hypothyroid phase, then usually a return to the euthyroid state. The hyperthyroid state is caused by damage to the follicle and unregulated release of thyroid hormone. By definition, the hyperthyroidism is limited in severity and duration.

Subacute thyroiditis is thought to be a viral or postviral syndrome that causes inflammation and damages the thyroid. It is characterized by an acute onset severe pain in the anterior neck and is often accompanied by fatigue, fever, and malaise. The thyroid is diffusely enlarged and tender in subacute thyroiditis. Laboratory tests show a suppressed TSH, elevated fT4 and tT3, and an elevated erythrocyte sedimentation rate. Radionuclide uptake scanning shows a greatly decreased uptake, often less than 1%, as a result of thyroid destruction. Mild cases are treated with aspirin or nonsteroidal anti-inflammatory drugs as well as β-blockers to alleviate adrenergic symptoms. More severe cases are treated with glucocorticoids, which alleviate symptoms but do not alter the natural history. Antithyroid drugs are not used in the therapy of thyroiditis because the pathology is not overproduction, but release of preformed thyroid hormone.

Painless thyroiditis, as the name suggests, presents as hyperthyroidism without a painful thyroid. Patients present with the typical symptoms of hyperthyroidism but only half have any enlargement of the thyroid gland. Patients follow a similar course of thyrotoxicosis, variable hypothyroidism, with a majority returning to the euthyroid state. The treatment is again supportive. β-blockers are used to control adrenergic symptoms until the thyrotoxic state spontaneously remits. Postpartum thyroiditis is a form of painless thyroiditis that occurs in 5% to 10% of women 3 to 12 months after parturition. Upwards of 66% of women with positive thyroid antibodies develop postpartum thyroid dysfunction.

Chronic autoimmune thyroiditis (Hashimoto's) is the most common cause of hypothyroidism in adults and most common cause of goiter in women. Hashimoto's thyroiditis is caused by an autoimmune process directed against the thyroid gland. Lymphocytic infiltration and fibrosis are commonly seen on histology. The clinical manifestations are commonly those of hypothyroidism. However, transient subclinical hyperthyroidism may occur (rare). A goiter is found on physical examination, and the thyroid gland is nontender on palpation. Thyroid function tests are transiently consistent with hyperthyroidism, however, the thyroid function tests eventually develop a hypothyroid pattern.

More than 90 percent of patients with Hashimoto's thyroiditis have high serum concentrations of antithyroglobulin antibodies usually early in the disease and antithyroid peroxidase antibodies, which remain present for years. If hypothyroidism is present, patients should be treated with levothyroxine.

HYPOTHYROIDISM

Hypothyroidism is the result of a lack of circulating thyroid hormone. Hypothyroidism affects 2% of the U.S. population with a female predominance. There are more than 20 causes of hypothyroidism, and these causes can be divided into primary and secondary. Primary hypothyroidism, which accounts for 99% of all cases, is caused by failure of the thyroid to make adequate amounts of hormone; however, in secondary hypothyroidism, the pituitary does not produce enough thyroid stimulating hormone (TSH) to stimulate adequate hormone production.

Etiology

Chronic autoimmune thyroiditis is by far the most common cause of hypothyroidism and can be divided into Hashimoto's disease and the atrophic form. In both forms, there is destruction of the thyroid follicles and a high incidence of antibodies to thyroglobulin and thyroid peroxidase. In Hashimoto's disease, there is goiter formation compared to the atrophic form in which there is no goiter. The second most common cause of primary hypothyroidism is iatrogenic. Neck surgery and ^{131}I are frequent causes of iatrogenic hypothyroidism.

Clinical Manifestations

The signs and symptoms of hypothyroidism are varied and diverse (Table 66.3). They occur insidiously over months to years and are often difficult for patients to recognize until they are moderate to

TABLE 66.3 Clinical manifestations of hypothyroidism

Symptoms and signs	Frequency (%)
Weakness	99
Skin changes (dry coarse skin)	97
Lethargy	91
Slow speech	91
Eyelid edema	90
Cold sensation	89
Decreased sweating	89
Cold skin	83
Thick tongue	82
Facial edema	79
Coarse hair	76
Skin pallor	67

Adapted from Larsen PR, Davies TF, Hay ID. The thyroid gland. In: Wilson JD, Foster DW, Kronenberg HM, et al, eds. *Williams Textbook of Endocrinology*, 9th ed. Philadelphia: Saunders; 1998:461.

severe. The symptoms of hypothyroidism are similar despite the underlying cause. Fatigue is perhaps the most frequent presenting complaint. The cause of fatigue is likely multifactorial, owing at least in part to an overall slowing of the metabolic rate. Dry, cool skin occurs in two thirds of patients with hypothyroidism; however, it is also a frequent complaint in individuals without hypothyroidism. In today's age of frequent screening for hypothyroidism, many if not most patients with hypothyroidism are detected early in the disease before most or any symptoms manifest.

Physical examination findings that occur commonly include delayed relaxation phase of reflexes, generalized puffiness of the face, and skin changes.

Diagnosis

The TSH should be measured in cases of suspected hypothyroidism. If the TSH is elevated, fT4 should be obtained to confirm the diagnosis. If a goiter is present, the clinical suspicion is very high, or secondary hypothyroidism is considered, then fT4 should be measured initially along with TSH. A TSH >10 mU/L with depressed fT4 is diagnostic of primary hypothyroidism. A normal or low TSH in the face of low fT4 indicates secondary hypothyroidism caused by inadequate TSH secretion by the pituitary (Table 66.4).

Therapy

The therapy for all etiologies of hypothyroidism is replacement with synthetic L-thyroxine (L-T4). The normal replacement dose is between 75 and 125 μg/day. In otherwise healthy, young individuals, a full replacement dose can be given initially. Individuals with coronary disease should be given 12.5 to 25 μg/day initially and titrated up to full replacement dose. This recommendation is to prevent angina pectoris or myocardial infarction from increased metabolic demand and increased cardiac output.

Of note, secondary hypothyroidism caused by destruction of the pituitary gland or the hypothalamus differs clinically in that these patients are also deficient in other pituitary hormones, most notably adrenocorticotropic hormone. Because treating hypothyroidism in the setting of unrecognized adrenal insufficiency can precipitate an adrenal crisis, adrenal insufficiency should be treated before beginning therapy of hypothyroidism with T_4.

Complications

Myxedema coma, a medical emergency, is the end stage of advanced, untreated hypothyroidism. Its hallmarks are hypothermia, mental status changes, hypoventilation, and bradycardia. Ileus and hyponatremia may also occur. Precipitating events are exposure to cold weather, surgery, congestive heart failure, infection, and drugs such as anesthetics, tranquilizers, and narcotics. Diagnosis is based on classic signs and symptoms of severe hypothyroidism, hypothermia, and the features discussed earlier. In myxedema coma, a relative adrenal insufficiency may prevail due to the suppression of the pituitary-adrenal axis by advanced hypothyroidism. Therapy consists of aggressive T_4 replacement (200 to 500 mg initial intravenous bolus, followed by 50 to 100 mg daily intravenously), glucocorticoids, and supportive measures including intravenous hydration, passive rewarming, and ventilatory support

TABLE 66.4 Evaluation of hypothyroidism

	Primary hypothyroid	Secondary hypothyroid
TSH	High	Normal/low
Total T_3	Low	Low
Free T_4	Low	Low

for respiratory failure. Rapid rewarming by external electric warming blankets ushers in vasodilatation and exacerbates hypotension. Precipitating factors should be sought and treated if present.

THYROID NODULES

A common manifestation of abnormal thyroid growth is the formation of nodules. Nodules can be solitary or multiple. Approximately 5% of the population has a palpable nodule and autopsy studies of the elderly show 50% of all thyroid glands contain at least one nodule. The vast majority of these nodules are of no clinical consequence; however, 10% to 15% of palpable nodules contain thyroid cancer. The main challenge in evaluating nodules is differentiating benign and malignant growths.

Evaluation of Thyroid Nodules

The first step in evaluation of newly discovered nodules is to determine if any risk factors for thyroid cancer exist such as irradiation to the neck, male gender, extremes of age (<20 or >60 years old) and a family history of thyroid cancer or multiple endocrine neoplasia syndrome 2A or 2B. Findings on examination that suggest cancerous nodules include a firm consistence, fixation to adjacent structures, and regional lymphadenopathy. It should be noted that 20% of patients with thyroid cancer present with none of these findings and have the lesions detected on routine physical examination or imaging studies for unrelated problems (Table 66.5).

The next step in evaluation of thyroid nodules involves determining if the nodule is hyperfunctioning. This can be accomplished by measuring the TSH. A suppressed TSH indicates a nodule with autonomous function. Autonomously functioning nodules are very rarely thyroid cancer, so a suppressed TSH should lead to further investigation of hyperthyroidism.

TABLE 66.5 Features of solitary thyroid nodules associated with increased risk of malignancy

History
Age <20 or >60 years (~30% malignant)
Gender: men affected more often than women
Compression symptoms (dysphagia, hoarseness)
History of neck irradiation (~30% malignant)
Family history of medullary cancer
Physical examination
Rapid growth of nodule
Fixation
Lymphadenopathy
Course
Growth of nodule while on thyroid hormone suppression
Laboratory
Euthyroid clinical status
Imaging
Nodule cold on radionuclide scanning (10% to 15% malignant)

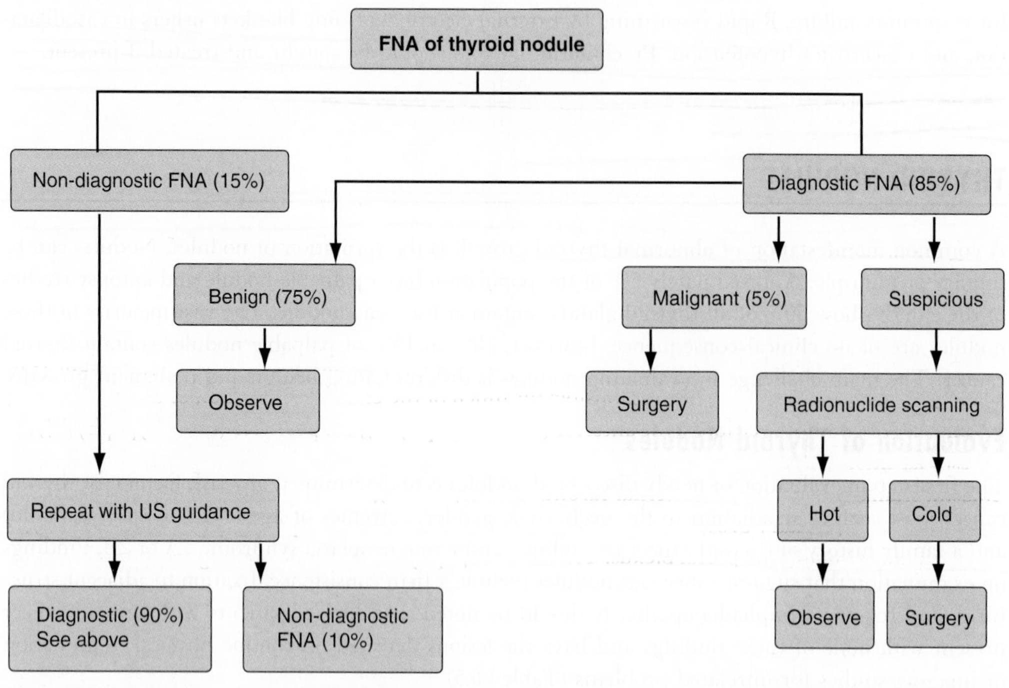

Figure 66.6 • Algorithm for evaluation and therapy of thyroid nodules. Data are percent outcomes. FNA, fine-needle aspiration.

The ultimate diagnostic test in most cases is a fine-needle aspiration (FNA) of the nodule. FNA is over 90% sensitive and specific in experienced hands. An algorithm for management of FNA results can be found in Figure 66.6.

NONTHYROIDAL ILLNESS SYNDROME

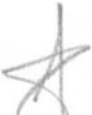

Nonthyroidal illness syndrome (NTIS), formerly known as euthyroid sick syndrome, is a term used to describe the changes in thyroid hormone levels in ill patients. In times of acute illness, particularly sepsis, there is a change in thyroid hormone levels. Despite changes in the thyroid hormone levels these patients are clinically euthyroid. The changes are likely due to impaired conversion of T_4 to T_3. As a result, T_3 levels fall and there is greater conversion of T_4 to rT_3, increasing the rT_3 levels. The TSN level in NTIS and be high, low, or normal. T_4 levels are generally low and very low levels of T_4 correlate to increased mortality. The exact physiological reason for these changes is yet to be elucidated and the usefulness of thyroid hormone therapy in this condition is unproven.

CHAPTER 67

Anterior Pituitary Diseases

Ty Carroll

The pituitary gland is located in the sella turcica at the base of the brain. Its average weight is 0.6 g. Despite its diminutive size, it is responsible for much of the endocrine function of the human body. It can be divided into three lobes: the anterior (adenohypophysis), the posterior (neurohypophysis), and a vestigial intermediate lobe. The pituitary's location in the sella turcica is surrounded by the optic chiasm, cranial nerves, and the internal carotid arteries, making these structures susceptible to damage from abnormal pituitary growth. The infundibular stalk connects the pituitary gland with the hypothalamus and contains the portal plexus. The adenohypophysial hormones are regulated by a neuroendocrine system of stimulatory and inhibitory peptides produced in the ventral hypothalamus and transported to the anterior lobe through the hypothalamic-hypophysial portal system.

The anterior pituitary produces six major hormones: prolactin (PRL), corticotropin (ACTH), growth hormone (GH), thyroid-stimulating hormone (TSH), luteinizing hormone (LH), and follicle-stimulating hormone (FSH). Their major regulatory pathways and end-organ products are shown in Figure 67.1. All of the anterior pituitary hormones, except possibly prolactin, are feedback-controlled by their end-organ secretory products, at both the hypothalamic and pituitary levels.

PROLACTIN

Prolactin is secreted in a pulsatile fashion throughout the day with the most pulses occurring during sleep. Prolactin secretion is unique as it is primarily controlled by inhibition from dopamine, which is tonically secreted. Estrogen and several other substances stimulate prolactin release. The only known function of prolactin takes place in the female breast where it initiates and maintains lactation.

CORTICOTROPIN

ACTH is a polypeptide derived from modification of a much larger precursor molecule named POMC. Its secretion from the pituitary is tightly controlled via negative feedback from cortisol. Adrenal steroidogenesis, primarily cortisol production, is the major function of ACTH.

GROWTH HORMONE

The secretion of GH is effected by several factors. Hypothalamic growth hormone releasing hormone (GHRH) stimulates secretion while somatostatin and insulin-like-growth factor (IGF)-1 inhibit its secretion. In the peripheral tissues, growth hormone's main functions are somatic growth and stimulation of metabolism. These effects are largely mediated through IGF-1.

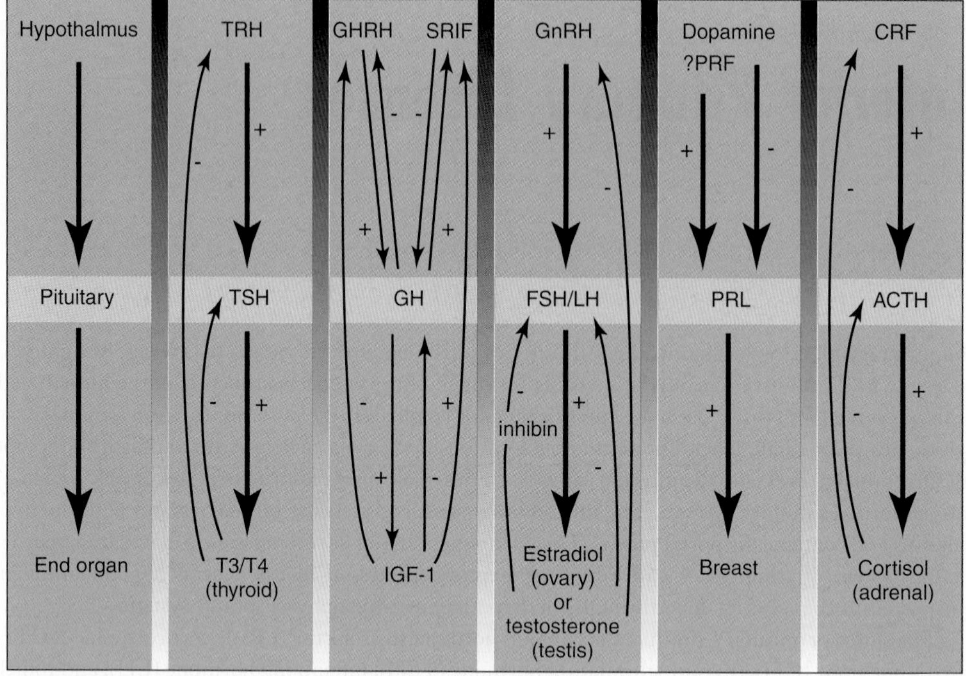

Figure 67.1 • Regulatory pathways for the six major adenohypophyseal hormones.

THYROID-STIMULATING HORMONE

The secretion of TSH is stimulated by hypothalamic thyrotropin-releasing hormone (TRH) and inhibited by the thyroid hormones T_3 and T_4. The main function of TSH is to stimulate production and secretion of thyroid hormones which ultimately effect metabolic activity.

LUTEINIZING HORMONE AND FOLLICLE-STIMULATING HORMONE

LH and FSH secretion is pulsatile and its stimulation and inhibition by gonadotropin-releasing hormone (GnRH) and sex hormones is complex. The stimulating or inhibiting nature of GnRH and sex hormones depends on the length and intensity of exposure. In general, GnRH and estrogen stimulate secretion of LH and FSH while the other sex hormones inhibit secretion of LH and FSH. The main target for LH and FSH are the gonads where they cause an increase in sex steroid production and produce germ cell maturation.

HYPOPITUITARISM

Pituitary hormonal insufficiency or hypopituitarism may involve any or all of the six major anterior pituitary hormones.

Etiology

Causes may include pituitary tumors (most common), infectious disease (tuberculosis, fungal infection), infiltrative diseases (sarcoidosis, hemochromatosis), and vascular abnormalities (Sheehan's syndrome or postpartum pituitary necrosis).

TABLE 67.1 Clinical features of pituitary insufficiency

ACTH	Adrenal insufficiency: hypotension, tachycardia, fatigue, vomiting
TSH	Hypothyroidism: cold intolerance, constipation, bradycardia Thyroid function studies: low TSH, low T3,T4
FSH/LH	Women: infertility, amenorrhea. Men: decreased libido/infertility
GH	Decreased lean body mass, and strength
Prolactin	Inability to lactate after delivery

Clinical Manifestations

The clinical features of hypopituitarism are related to the loss of pituitary hormones (Table 67.1).

The most common manifestation of pituitary hormonal deficiency depends on which hormones are deficient and to what degree. In children, growth retardation and delayed puberty are common presenting signs.

Diagnosis

Anterior pituitary hormone insufficiency is diagnosed biochemically (Table 67.2) and clinically (e.g., gonadal failure, hypothyroidism, and adrenal insufficiency).

TABLE 67.2 Evaluation for pituitary insufficiency

Pituitary hormone	Laboratory evaluation	Abnormal results
ACTH	Insulin-induced hypoglycemia/CRH stimulation test, or ACTH stimulation test	Cortisol level <18 μg/dL or a rise of <8 μg/dL from baseline
FSH, LH	Simultaneous assessment of basal FSH/LH/17 β-estradiol in females Simultaneous assessment of basal FSH/LH/testosterone in males	Low 17 β-estradiol with low or inappropriately normal FSH and LH Low total testosterone with low or inappropriately normal FSH and LH
TSH	Simultaneous assessment of TSH/free T_4	Low free T_4 with low or inappropriately normal TSH
GH	Insulin-induced hypoglycemia or GHRH-Argimine Test	GH level <7 ng/mL

CRF, corticotropin-releasing factor; FSH, follicle-stimulating hormone; GH, growth hormone; GHRH, growth hormone releasing hormone; LH, luteinizing hormone; TSH, thyroid-stimulating hormone.

TABLE 67.3 Treatment of panhypopituitarism

Pituitary hormone	Hormone replacement
ACTH	Cortisone acetate, hydrocortisone
TSH	Thyroxine: dosage adjusted to keep free T_4 in the upper normal range
FSH/LH	Men: testosterone enanthate or cypionate, testosterone patch or gel Women: estrogen therapy, oral or transdermal, adjusted to relieve symptoms
GH	Synthetic GH subcutaneous injections

Treatment

Treatment of pituitary insufficiency is shown in Table 67.3.

PITUITARY TUMORS

Pituitary tumors may be secretary or nonsecretory, are usually benign, and account for between 10% and 15% of intracranial tumors. Pituitary adenomas and their incidence are listed in Table 67.4. Prolactinomas are the most common type of secretory pituitary tumors.

These tumors are considered microadenomas if the vertical height on magnetic resonance imaging (MRI) or computed tomography (CT) is 10 mm or less, or as macroadenomas if vertical height exceeds 10 mm. Typically, a pituitary tumor presents with signs and symptoms related to mass-effect or endocrine dysfunction.

Clinical Manifestations and Diagnosis

Common clinical features of a pituitary mass include headache, visual field deficits, and cranial nerve palsies. The headache typically is retro-orbital or bitemporal. Its pathogenesis is unknown, but may be due to stretching of the dura mater. The classic visual field abnormality is bitemporal hemianopsia; it results from suprasellar tumor extension and compression of the optic chiasm. A pituitary tumor laterally invading into the cavernous sinuses may lead to dysfunction of cranial nerves III, IV, and VI, causing ophthalmoplegia, and of cranial nerves V1 and V2, causing facial pain. Pituitary tumors may also present with pituitary insufficiency.

TABLE 67.4 Incidence of pituitary adenomas

Prolactin-secreting	27%–29%
Nonsecretory or null cell	25%
GH-secreting	13%–16%
ACTH-secreting	10%–14%
Plurihormonal	8%–12%
LH/FSH/alpha subunit-secreting	2%–9%
Silent adenomas (ACTH-staining)	5%
TSH-secreting	1%

TABLE 67.5 Laboratory evaluation of pituitary tumors

Laboratory test	Value	Implication
Prolactin	>200 ng/mL	Prolactinoma
IGF-1	Elevated above normal	Acromegaly
Growth hormone level >2 ng/ml 2 hours after 75-g oral glucose load	Nonsuppressible serum GH	Acromegaly
24-hour urinary free cortisol	Elevated	Cushing syndrome
1-mg dexamethasone suppression test	8 a.m. fasting serum cortisol >5 μg/dL	Cushing syndrome
Late-night salivary cortisol	Cortisol >3 ng/dL	Cushing syndrome
TSH/T_3/T_4	Serum TSH inappropriately (normal or elevated with elevated free T_4)	TSH-secreting tumor
LH, FSH, and alpha-subunit tumor	Elevated serum LH, FSH, or alpha-subunit	FSH, LH, or alpha subunit-secreting

There are some variations, but pituitary hormones usually are lost in the following order: GH, LH/FSH, TSH, and ACTH; prolactin deficiency is rare because pituitary macroadenomas usually produce mild hyperprolactinemia (PRL of 20 to 100 ng/mL), which results from decreased dopamine inhibition due to infundibular stalk interruption.

A functional morphological classification of pituitary adenomas, which has gained wide acceptance, is useful in predicting the biologic behavior of the various tumor types and in planning appropriate treatment strategies. The initial laboratory workup of a newly diagnosed pituitary tumor is shown in Table 67.5.

Treatment

Pituitary hormone replacement is shown in Table 67.3. Although GH replacement is not routinely done in adults, some studies show positive effects on lean body mass and overall well-being.

HYPERPROLACTINEMIA

Hyperprolactinemia accounts for at least 20% of infertility in women and approximately 8% of sexual dysfunction in men, including infertility. The causes of pathologic hyperprolactinemia are diverse (Table 67.6), but a prolactin-secreting pituitary tumor is, by far, the most common cause. The pathogenesis of these tumors is unknown.

Clinical Manifestations

The clinical presentation of prolactinomas varies with the patient's age and sex. Typically, young menstruating women report irregular menses (amenorrhea, oligomenorrhea, or delayed menarche), infertility, or galactorrhea. Galactorrhea occurs in 30% to 80% of affected women. Hyperprolactinemia directly suppresses hypothalamic GnRH secretion, resulting in amenorrhea. Because they cause early disturbance in the menstrual cycle, prolactinomas typically are microadenomas at the time of diagnosis. In contrast, men and postmenopausal women usually present with macroprolactinomas that

TABLE 67.6 Causes of hyperprolactinemia

Category	Examples/disorders
Physiologic	Pregnancy, nipple stimulation/suckling, stress, exercise, sleep
Pathologic Pituitary adenoma	Prolactin-secreting pituitary tumor Plurihormonal-secreting pituitary tumor (acromegaly)
Hypothalamic-pituitary disorders causing hyperprolactinemia in the absence of a prolactinoma	Tumor (e.g., craniopharyngioma, germinoma) Histiocytosis X Sarcoidosis Pituitary stalk interruption Surgery
Adrenal insufficiency Cirrhosis Primary hypothyroidism Renal failure	
Drug-induced	Estrogens/oral contraceptives Psychotropic drugs (e.g., phenothiazines, tricyclic antidepressants) Methyldopa Metoclopramide Opiates Cimetidine Cocaine
Neurogenic	Chest wall lesions/surgery Spinal cord lesions
'Functional"/idiopathic	

produce tumor mass-related effects. Approximately 80% of affected men report decreased libido and erectile dysfunction. Galactorrhea occurs in 20% to 30% of men.

Diagnosis

A serum PRL level higher than 200 ng/mL is diagnostic of a prolactinoma. Although a slightly elevated PRL level (20 to 200 ng/mL) may be the result of a microprolactinoma, mild PRL elevations also may result from one of several secondary causes (e.g., infundibular stalk compression, renal failure, primary hypothyroidism, or drugs).

Management

The dopamine agonists, bromocriptine and cabergoline, decrease serum prolactin levels consistently and rapidly, and reduce tumor size in 80% of patients. Dopamine agonists are, therefore, the treatment of choice for all clinically significant microprolactinomas and macroprolactinomas. Many clinicians advocate initial treatment with a dopamine agonist for all patients, even those with visual abnormalities. Surgical resection is reserved for prolactinomas that do not respond to medical therapy or for patients who cannot tolerate the side effects of the dopamine agonists. External radiotherapy is reserved for the occasional patient who is refractory to or intolerant of these conventional therapies.

The ultimate goal of therapy, whether medical or surgical, is decompression of the optic chiasm, correction of cranial nerve abnormalities, and resumption of normal pituitary hormone function.

ACROMEGALY

Acromegaly, abnormal enlargement of the extremities of the skeleton caused by hypersecretion of GH after maturity, has an estimated annual incidence of three to four cases per million, without any sex predilection. It can occur at any age, but is most commonly diagnosed in the fourth or fifth decade of life. Approximately 85% of cases result from a GH-secreting pituitary macroadenoma. GH-producing pituitary tumors account for nearly 17% of all surgically resected pituitary tumors; about 30% of these tumors also secrete prolactin. Excessive GH secretion in a prepubertal child prior to the closure of the epiphyseal growth plates leads to gigantism; this condition is very rare.

Clinical Features

The manifestations of excessive GH secretion (Table 67.7 and Fig. 67.2) usually develop gradually in older patients. Because these changes are insidious, they are often missed by the patient and, instead, are first noted by someone who has not seen the patient for a long time. In younger patients, these tumors are more aggressive; thus, the characteristic features evolve more rapidly. In addition to the characteristic facial and acral soft tissue changes produced by excessive GH secretion, the sellar mass itself also may evoke symptoms from local effects. Nearly one half of patients with acromegaly harbor colonic polyps, and about 5% of all acromegalics develop colon cancer. Risk factors for neoplasia include age above 50 years, duration of acromegaly exceeding 10 years, and presence of three or more skin tags.

TABLE 67.7 Clinical manifestations of acromegaly
Coarsening facial features/soft tissue swelling
Frontal bossing
Dental malocclusion with increased spacing between teeth
Headaches
Diabetes mellitus
Excessive sweating
Soft-tissue swelling in hands/feet
Increased ring/glove size
Increased shoe size/width with thick heel pad
Skin tags
Colon polyps/cancer
Carpal tunnel syndrome
Hypertension
Hyperglycemia
Deep, resonant voice/laryngeal thickening
Obstructive sleep apnea
Galactorrhea
Osteoarthritis, especially knees and hips
Visceromegaly

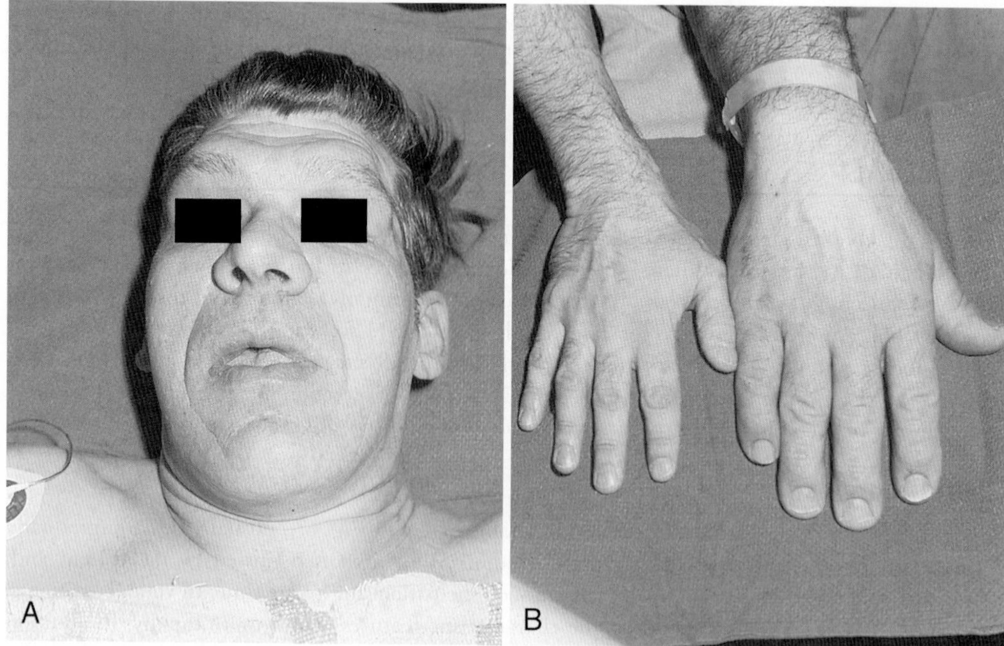

Figure 67.2 • A. A 48-year-old acromegalic man. Note the coarse facial features and prognathism. **B. Acromegaly.** The hand on the left is that of a normal man; the one on the right is that of the man with acromegaly shown in **(A)**.

Diagnosis

A serum IGF-1 level usually suffices as a screening test for acromegaly. Diagnostic biochemical criteria are elevated IGF-1 and nonsuppressible serum GH level above 2 ng/mL 2 hours after a 75-g oral glucose load (in a normal state hyperglycemia would inhibit release of GH).

Management

Acromegaly is difficult to cure. Treatment goals include lowering the serum GH level normalize the IGF-1 level, reversing associated medical problems including diabetes mellitus, hypertension, soft tissue hyperplasia, and hyperhidrosis. Management options include surgery, radiotherapy, and medications; most patients require all three. Surgical resection of the tumor remains the first line of therapy. A surgical cure can be obtained in 80% of patients with microadenomas yet in less than 30% of patients with macroadenomas. The somatostatin analogue octreotide, and the dopamine agonists bromocriptine and cabergoline, are used as medical therapy for acromegaly.

CORTICOTROPH ADENOMA OR CUSHING DISEASE

For ACTH-secreting tumors, see Chapter 69.

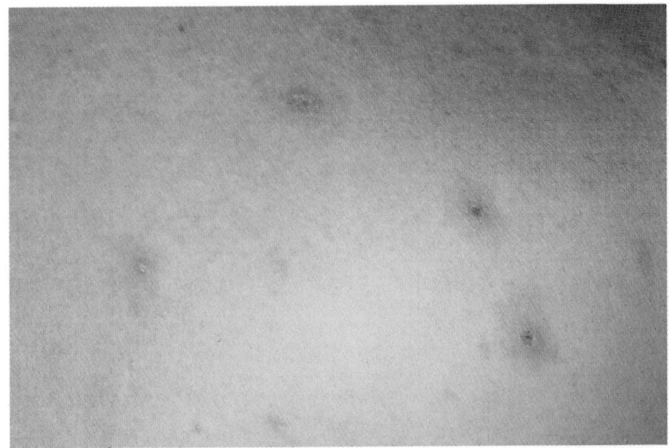

Plate 1 Varicella.
Courtesy of Janet A. Fairley, MD, University of Iowa, School of Medicine

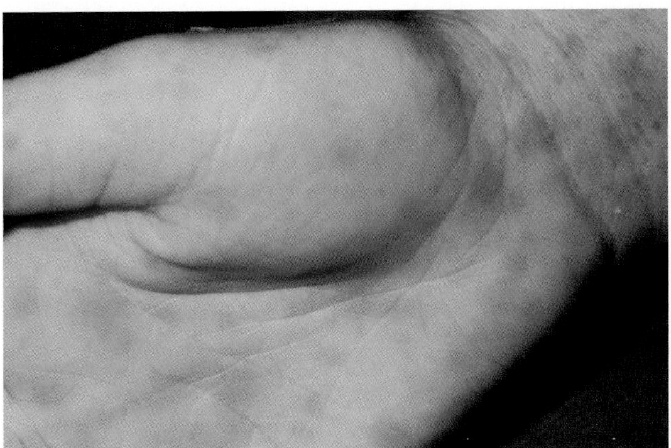

Plate 2 Meningococcemia.
Courtesy of Janet A. Fairley, MD

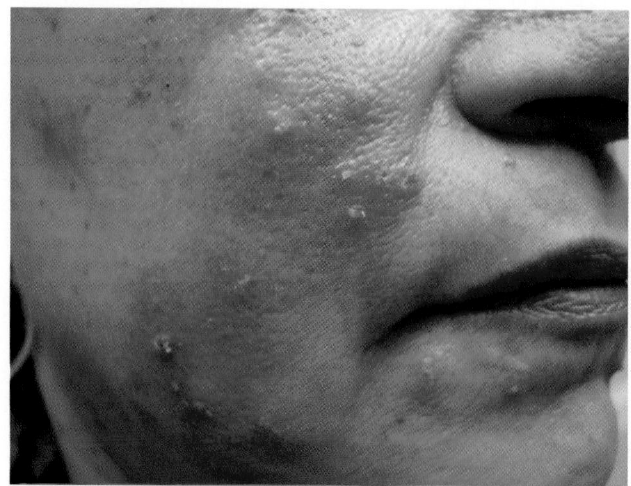

Plate 3 Herpes simplex virus infection.
Courtesy of Janet A. Fairley, MD

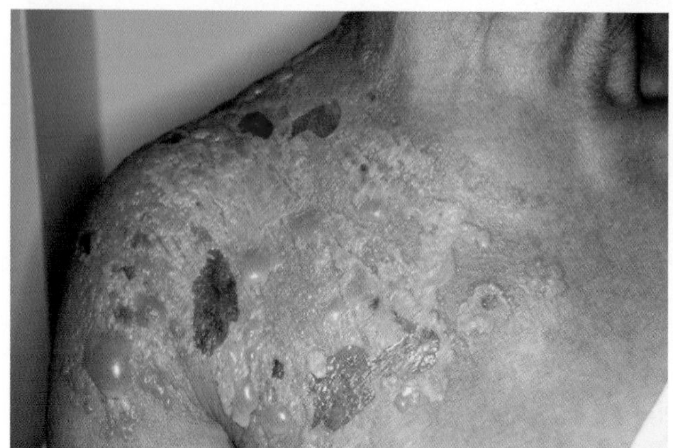

Plate 4 Herpes zoster virus infection.
Courtesy of Janet A. Fairley, MD

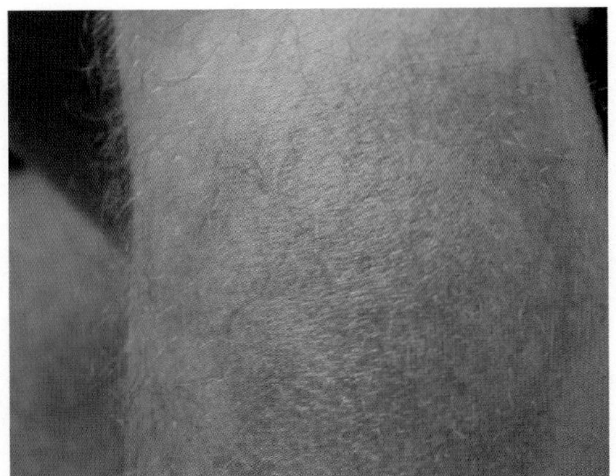

Plate 5 Erythema chronicum migrans.
Courtesy of Janet A. Fairley, MD

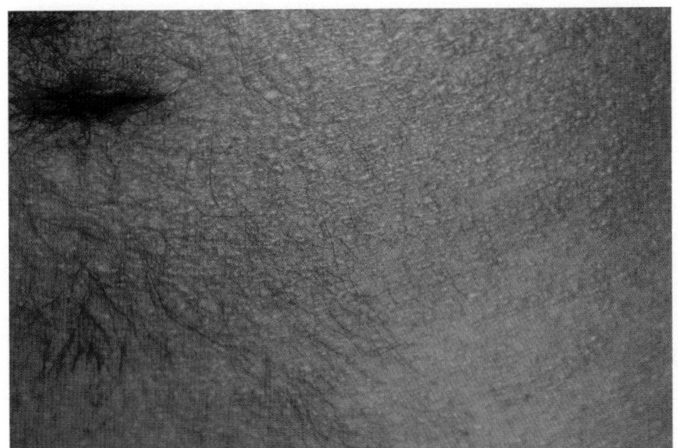

Plate 6 Drug rash.

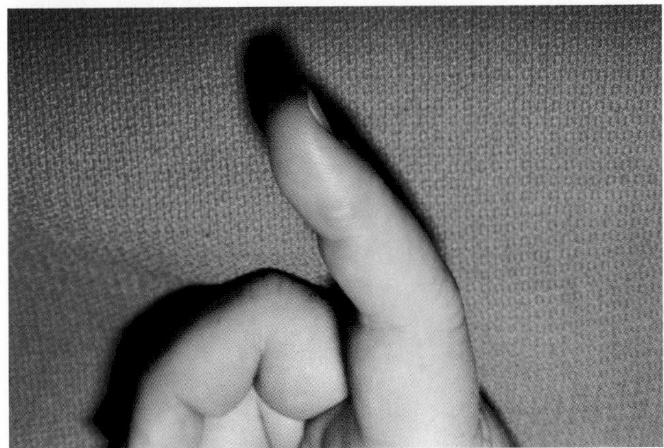

Plate 7 Coxsackie virus.
Courtesy of Janet A. Fairley, MD

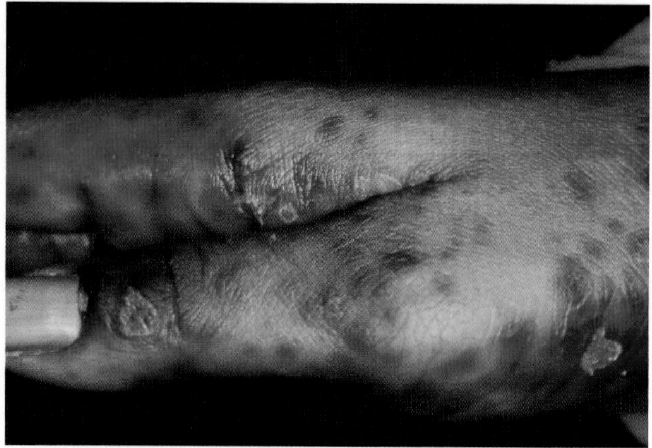

Plate 8 Secondary syphilis.
Courtesy of Janet A. Fairley, MD

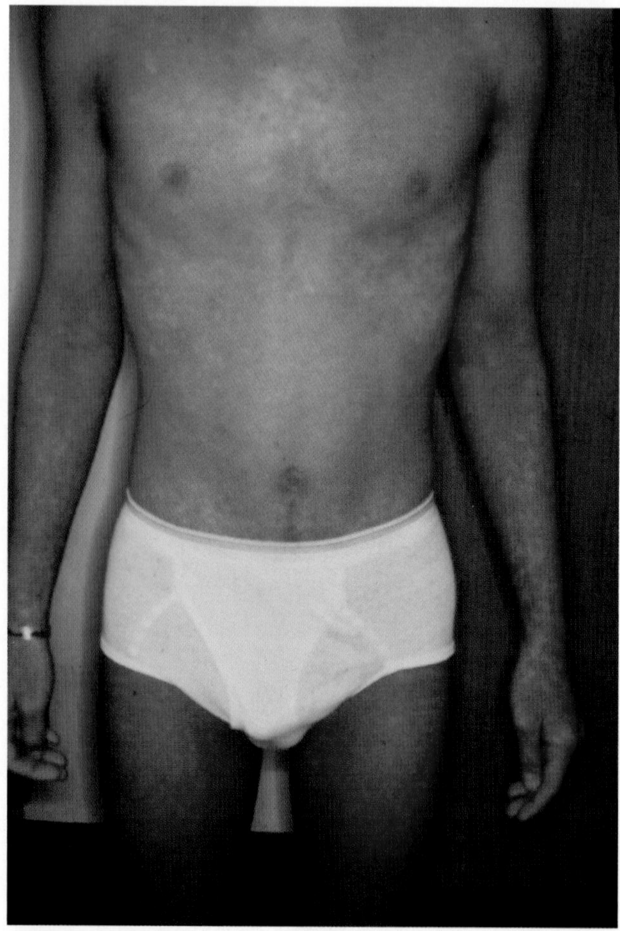

Plate 9 Mononucleosis after ampicillin.
Courtesy of Janet A. Fairley, MD

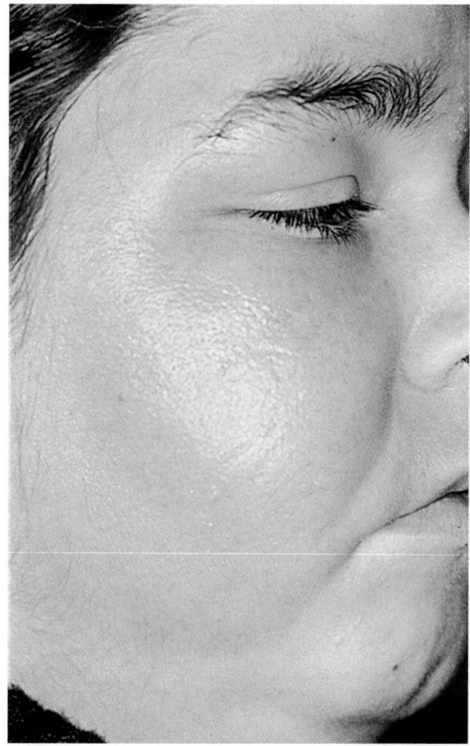

Plate 10 Erysipelas. Facial cellulites, with a well-demarcated border due to group A *b-hemolytic streptococci.*

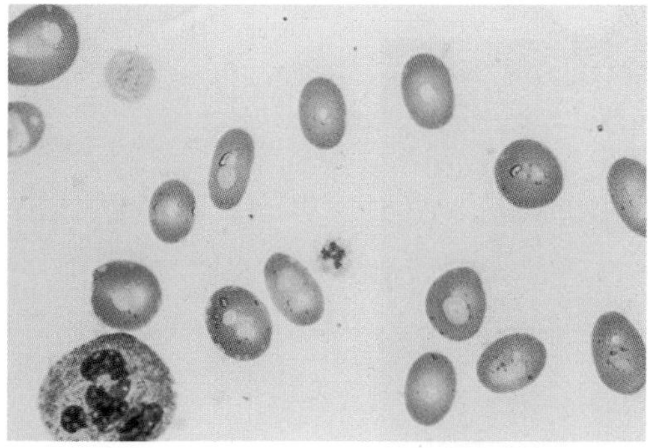

Plate 11 Pernicious anemia. The PMN has hypersegmented nuclei.

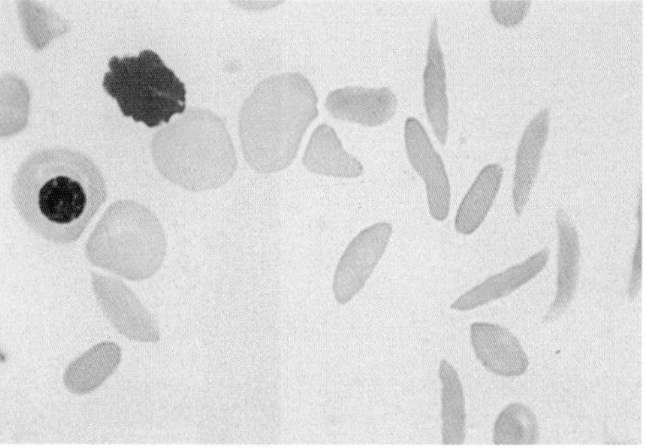

Plate 12 Sickle cell anemia showing the characteristic sickle cells.

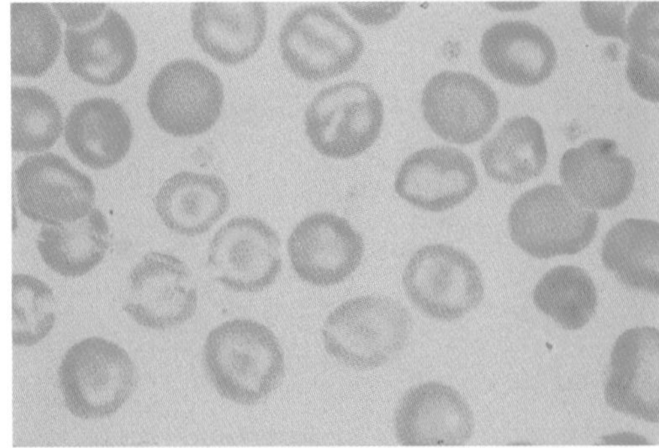

Plate 13 Hemoglobin C disease: many target cells.

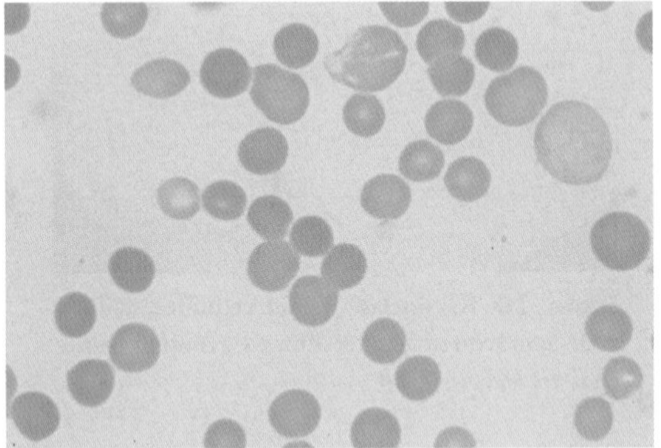

Plate 14 Peripheral smear. Spherocytes are small, globular, and without central pallor.

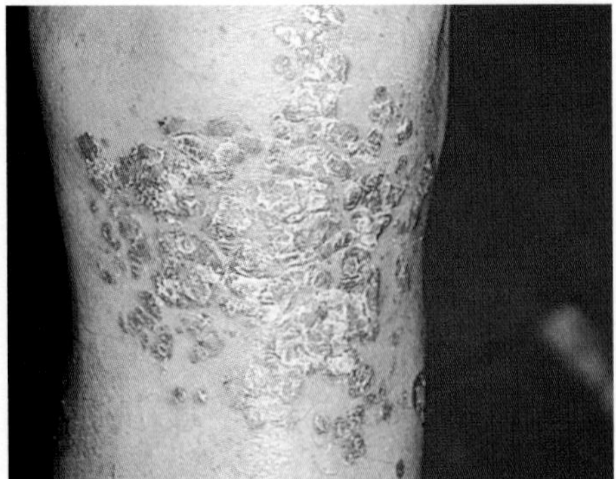

Plate 15 Psoriasis. A typical erythematous plaque over the knee. Koebner phenomenon, as the linear extension of the lesion above the knee, is seen in the site of a previous knee surgery.

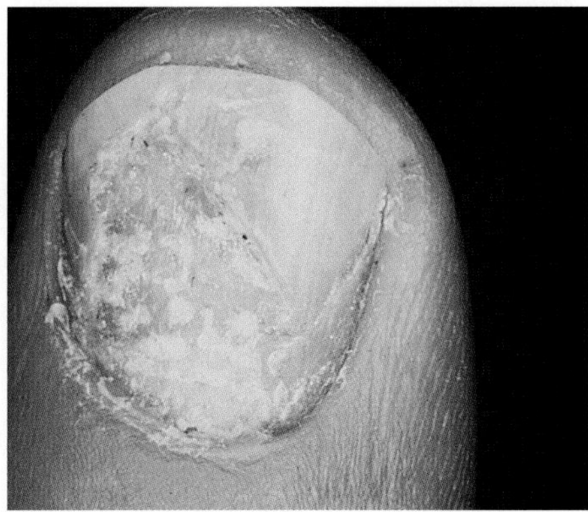

Plate 16 Psoriasis of the nails. Whitish discoloration of the nail with pits. Lifting of the nail from the plate (onycholysis) and subungual debris are also common findings in psoriatic nails.

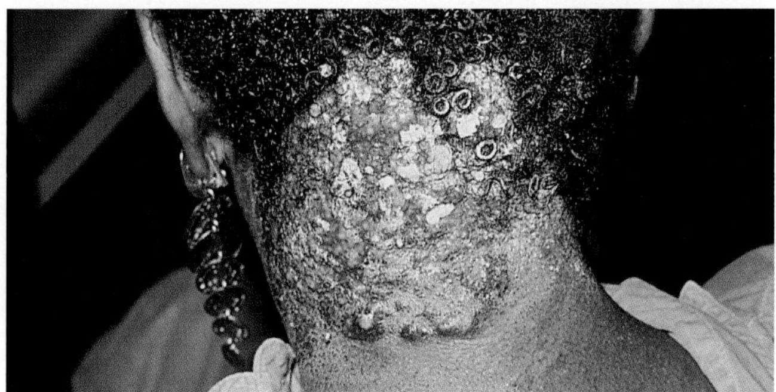

Plate 17 Tinea capitis with kerion formation owing to *Trichophyton tonsurans.*

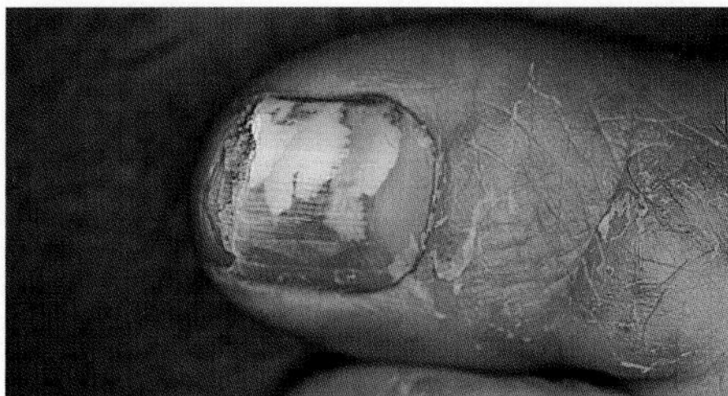

Plate 18 Onychomycosis due to *Trichophyton rubrum*. Brownish-white discoloration of the nail plate, with accumulation of subungual debris. The findings can sometimes be difficult to differentiate from those of psoriasis, and a fungal culture may be needed.

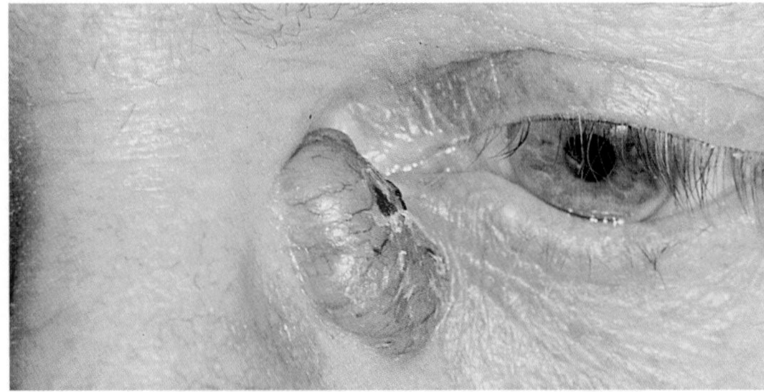

Plate 19 Basal cell carcinoma. The pearly quality of the lesion, telangiectases, and central ulceration are typical features of basal cell carcinoma of the skin.

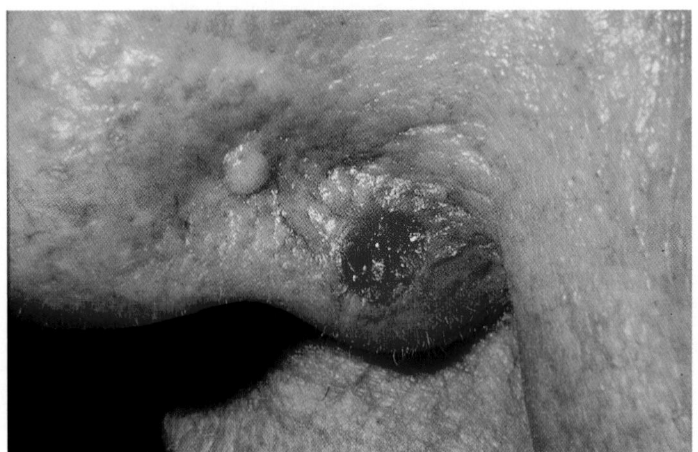

Plate 20 Squamous cell carcinoma.

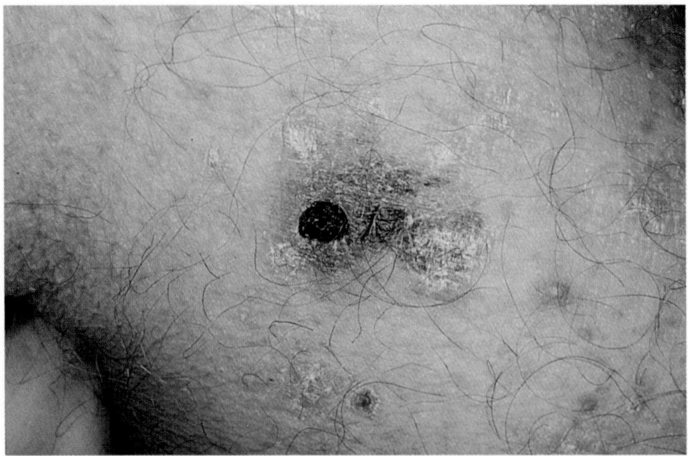

Plate 21 Malignant melanoma, superficial spreading type.

CHAPTER 68

Posterior Pituitary Diseases (Diabetes Insipidus/Syndrome of Antidiuretic Hormone)

Ty Carroll

The posterior pituitary gland is composed entirely of axons of hypothalamic neurons. It secretes two major peptide hormones, oxytocin and vasopressin (which is also known as antidiuretic hormone [ADH]). Both of these hormones are synthesized in the hypothalamus, packaged into neurosecretory granules, and transported along axons to the posterior pituitary gland where they are stored until their release into the bloodstream. Oxytocin stimulates uterine contraction, but its importance in normal parturition is unclear. Nipple stimulation by the suckling infant causes pituitary release of oxytocin, followed by milk ejection. There is little clinically significant disease caused by oxytocin excess or deficiency. Antidiuretic hormone is the major regulator of renal water excretion and, therefore, of the total body water balance. ADH causes resorption of water in the distal nephron. The most important stimulus for ADH release is increased plasma osmolality, but it is also stimulated by low blood volume and nausea. Deficiency of ADH causes diabetes insipidus (DI) with polyuria and polydipsia; excess ADH leads to the syndrome of inappropriate ADH (SIADH) with hyponatremia and oliguria. The remainder of this chapter will focus on the disorders of ADH deficiency and excess.

DIABETES INSIPIDUS

Etiology

The two major types of DI are central (hypothalamic) and nephrogenic (Table 68.1). There are two primary differences between central and nephrogenic DI: (a) the plasma ADH concentration and (b) the response to vasopressin administration. In central DI, the inappropriately low ADH concentration results in a large volume of very dilute urine. In nephrogenic DI, insensitivity of the kidney to normal or elevated ADH levels (inability to concentrate urine and reabsorb water) results in a high volume of dilute urine.

In contrast to hypothalamic DI, the key abnormality in nephrogenic DI is refractoriness to vasopressin at the level of the kidneys. Nephrogenic DI is further characterized by normal glomerular filtration rate and solute excretion, elevated plasma ADH levels, and a failure of exogenous ADH to significantly raise urine osmolality or to reduce urine volume. Lithium-induced nephrogenic DI may not be reversible, unlike nephrogenic DI due to hypokalemia, hypercalcemia, and prolonged polyuria.

Clinical Manifestations

DI is characterized by polyuria, defined as the excretion of urine in excess of 3 L per 24 hours. Large volumes of dilute urine are excreted, giving rise to severe polydipsia (abnormally large intake of fluids by mouth) and a specific craving for ice water. Biochemical and clinical hallmarks of DI are listed in Table 68.2.

TABLE 68.1 Causes of diabetes insipidus

Central/hypothalamic
Idiopathic (30%)
Postcranial syndrome (20%)
Tumors (20%)
Craniopharyngioma (most common)
Pituitary macroadenoma
Meningioma
Dysgerminoma
Metastatic carcinoma (lung, breast)
Head injury (16%)
Vascular
Sheehan's syndrome
Aneurysms
Cerebral hypoperfusion
Granulomatous disease
Sarcoidosis
Histiocytosis
Infections
Meningitis
Encephalitis
Autoimmune
Nephrogenic/renal resistant
Idiopathic
Chronic renal disease
Hypokalemia
Hypercalcemia
Drug-induced
Lithium
Demeclocycline
Methoxyflurane
Amyloidosis
Postobstructive uropathy

A third, uncommon, type of DI is primary polydipsia is an uncommon condition usually seen in psychiatric patients. It results from overdrinking in the absence of genuine thirst, with resultant polyuria and plasma dilution with appropriate ADH suppression. It requires the intake of liters of water each day. This disorder is diagnosed by demonstrating a normal osmoregulated ADH secretion and renal function during a standard water deprivation test. The treatment is fluid restriction; no therapy other than that of the underlying psychosis is required.

Diagnosis

The diagnostic approach to DI should begin with a workup for polyuria as shown in Figure 68.1. Once the diagnosis of DI is entertained, its etiology should be established and confirmed with a standard water deprivation test (see Fig. 68.1). During the first part of the test, the patient is deprived of all water intake until dehydration (defined by weight loss of at least 2% of body weight and a rise in plasma osmolality above 300 mOsm/kg) is achieved. Urine output, blood pressure, and urine

TABLE 68.2 Biochemical and clinical hallmarks of diabetes insipidus

Clinical	
Polyuria	
Mild	3 to 4 L/day
Moderate	4 to 6 L/day
Severe	>6 L/day
Polydipsia	
Especially crave very cold fluids/ice water	
Biochemical	
Urine	
Specific gravity	≤1.005
Osm_u	Inappropriately low (for high Osm_{PI})
Plasma	
Hypernatremia[a]	Serum Na^+ >145 mEq/L
Osm_{PI}[a]	>290 mOsm/L
ADH level	
Central DI	Low or inappropriately nl
Nephrogenic DI	High
Water deprivation test response to vasopressin	
Central DI	Yes
Nephrogenic DI	No

[a]Present if inadequate hypotonic fluid replacement.
OsmPL, plasma osmolality; Osm_U, urine osmolality.

osmolality are then measured every 2 hours. Normally, after water deprivation, a decrease in urine output (because ADH is stimulated by increased osmolality) and an increase in urine osmolality is expected to occur. However, in patients with central or nephrogenic DI (although ability to concentrate urine after H_2O deprivation is slightly greater in nephrogenic DI), urine output remains high and urine diluted, despite water deprivation and increased plasma osmolality. In the second portion of the test, aqueous vasopressin is given subcutaneously and urine and plasma osmolality measurements are repeated. Typical results in patients with central or nephrogenic DI and normal patients are shown in Table 68.3. Patients with nephrogenic DI lack the ability (secondary to tubular dysfunction) to concentrate urine after the administration of ADH.

Management

In acute postsurgical and traumatic hypothalamic DI, hypotonic oral or intravenous fluids are given to replace the losses and maintain hydration. Vasopressin, if needed, is given subcutaneously as a short-acting aqueous preparation. This procedure makes it possible to assess whether the DI is permanent while at the same time avoiding overtreatment, with resultant free water retention and hyponatremia. Chronic central DI is usually treated with the long-acting synthetic analogue 1-desamino-8-D-arginine-vasopressin (DDAVP, 10 to 20 μg, 1 to 2 intranasal insufflations daily or 0.1 to 0.2 mg oral daily). Other than removing the underlying cause and ensuring adequate hydration, no specific treatment exists for nephrogenic DI. Reducing the solute load by medications and restricting the patient's salt intake help reduce polyuria and minimize nocturia; thiazides are the most effective agents in this context.

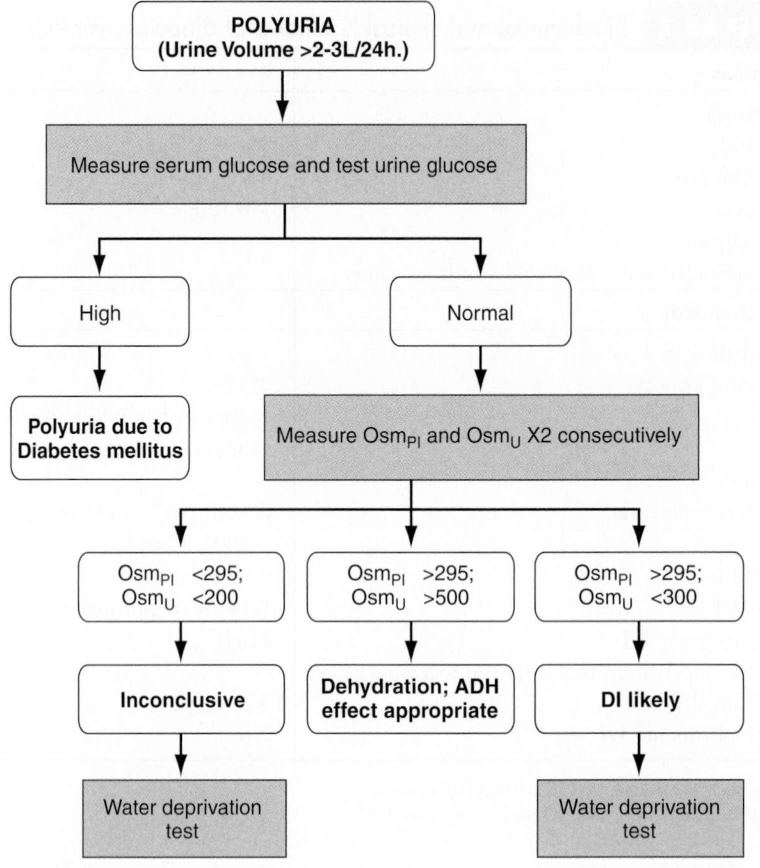

Figure 68.1 • Workup of polyuric states showing application of the water deprivation test.

TABLE 68.3 Interpretation of the standard water deprivation test

State		Urine osmolality	
	ADH level	After water deprivation, before ADH administration	After water deprivation and ADH administration
Normal	Normal	Marked increase	Normal increase
Complete central DI	Low	Minimal increase	Marked increase
Complete nephrogenic DI	High	Moderate increase	No response
Primary polydipsia	Normal (may be low)	Marked increase	Normal increase

INAPPROPRIATE ANTIDIURETIC SYNDROME

Hormone Secretion Definition

SIADH is characterized by continual ADH release in the face of subnormal plasma osmolality or in the absence of other stimuli. It accounts for more than 95% of hyponatremia in the hospitalized population.

Etiology

Many conditions affecting the lungs and brain are associated with SIADH. Small cell lung cancer is a classic and most common malignancy causing SIADH (as part of a paraneoplastic syndrome). Other underlying conditions are listed in Table 68.4.

Clinical Features

Clinical features usually are those of hyponatremia (lethargy, confusion, muscle cramps, coma, and seizures), those of the underlying cause, and, generally, diminished urine output. Volume overload edema or hypovolemia and significant thirst or excessive water intake are absent.

Diagnosis

On physical examination, the patient is eurolumic without edema. Biochemical criteria for the diagnosis of SIADH are serum Na^+ <136 mmol/L; normal renal, adrenal, and thyroid function; and normal triglycerides and glucose. Plasma, urine osmolality, and urine sodium should be ordered. Typically in SIADH, urine osmolality is higher than that of plasma. The plasma osmolality, normally

TABLE 68.4 Conditions associated with SIADH

Physiologic	Nausea, pain
Pathologic	
Tumors	Carcinoma (lung, pancreas, urinary tract) Thymoma Lymphoma, leukemia Mesothelioma
Pulmonary	Tuberculosis Pneumonia, empyema, abscess Chronic obstructive pulmonary disease
Intracranial conditions	Meningitis, encephalitis, abscess Head injury Brain tumor Cerebral hemorrhage, subdural hematoma Guillain-Barré syndrome Seizures
Drug-induced	Vasopressin preparations Carbamazepine, chlorpropamide, clofibrate, thiazides, vincristine, vinblastine, cisplatin, narcotics, phenothiazine

ranging from 275 to 290 mosmol/kg, is decreased and the urine osmolality is inappropriately elevated, >100 mosmol/kg but more commonly >300 mosmol/kg. Excessive urinary Na^+ excretion (>40 mEq/L) is usually found.

Although rarely needed, the diagnosis of SIADH may be confirmed by measuring urine osmolarity after a saline load. In SIADH, the urine osmolality remains high due to the inappropriately high levels of ADH.

Management

Mild to moderate, asymptomatic SIADH is treated by restricting fluid intake to less than the urine output, approximately 1,000 to 1,500 mL daily. If fluid restriction is unsuccessful, the antibiotic demeclocycline can be given. This agent inhibits the action of ADH at the level of the collecting duct. For details on treatment of hyponatremia, refer to Chapter 86.

CHAPTER 69

Diseases of the Adrenal Glands

Jennifer Zebrack and Albert Jochen

DISEASES OF THE ADRENAL CORTEX

The adrenal glands, located at the superior pole of each kidney, are comprised of two concentric layers: the cortex and the medulla. The adrenal cortex consists of three layers that secrete glucocorticoids, mineralocorticoids, and androgens.

GLUCOCORTICOIDS

The major regulatory system for cortisol is through hypothalamic corticotropin-releasing hormone (CRH) and pituitary adrenocorticotropic hormone (ACTH). Secretion of ACTH is pulsatile, creating a daily diurnal variation in cortisol secretion with maximal release in the morning.

MINERALOCORTICOIDS

The renin-angiotensin system is the principal regulator of aldosterone synthesis and release. Renin is produced by the juxtaglomerular cells of the kidney, which catalyzes the conversion of renin substrate to angiotensin I (A-I). Angiotensin-converting enzyme (ACE) converts A-I to angiotensin II (A-II), which stimulates aldosterone production in the adrenal cortex. Aldosterone promotes renal tubular Na^+ reabsorption and K^+ and H^+ ion excretion. The regulation of renin depends on intravascular volume. For instance, upright posture, hemorrhage, diuretics, sodium restriction, and edematous states increase renin secretion. Hyperkalemia and hyponatremia also strongly stimulate aldosterone production.

ANDROGENS AND ESTROGENS

ACTH is the major stimulator of adrenal androgen secretion. Dehydroepiandrosterone (DHEA) and androstenedione are the major androgens synthesized in the adrenals. DHEA is sulfated in the liver to yield DHEA-sulfate (DHEA-S). Androstenedione is converted to the weak estrogen estrone by peripheral aromatase.

Adrenal Insufficiency

Adrenal insufficiency can result from primary destruction of the adrenal cortices (primary adrenal insufficiency or Addison's disease), insufficient pituitary ACTH (secondary adrenal insufficiency), or decreased hypothalamic CRH (corticotropin-releasing hormone) secretion (tertiary adrenal insufficiency). Primary adrenal insufficiency results in a deficiency of cortisol and aldosterone with elevated plasma ACTH levels. Secondary and tertiary adrenal insufficiency results in a deficiency of cortisol with preserved aldosterone secretion.

ETIOLOGY

Development of the clinical manifestations of primary adrenal insufficiency (Addison's disease) requires loss or destruction of 90% or more of both adrenal cortices. In the United States, the most common cause of Addison's disease is the idiopathic type resulting from autoimmune destruction of the cortex. It is more common in women, may be familial, and is usually diagnosed in the third to fifth decades of life. This disease shows a high association with other autoimmune disorders, such as Hashimoto's hypothyroidism, Graves' hyperthyroidism, Type 1 diabetes mellitus, pernicious anemia, autoimmune hepatitis, alopecia, and vitiligo. Tuberculosis is the second most frequent cause in the United States and is a common cause in developing countries. Acute primary adrenal insufficiency occurs most commonly in a patient with underactive glands who requires increased glucocorticoid production after exposure to stress (e.g., sepsis, trauma or surgery). It also can follow acute bilateral destruction of the adrenal glands (e.g., adrenal hemorrhage or infarction) (Table 69.1).

The most common secondary cause of adrenal insufficiency is iatrogenic from prolonged use and subsequent withdrawal of prescribed exogenous glucocorticoids such as prednisone (which results in significant ACTH suppression, typically after about 30 days of administration). Other secondary and tertiary causes include any disorder of the pituitary or hypothalamus, such as trauma (infundibular stalk section), postpartum necrosis (Sheehan's syndrome), neoplasms, and inflammatory and granulomatous disorders (Table 69.1).

CLINICAL MANIFESTATIONS

The evolution of adrenal insufficiency may be gradual or catastrophically sudden. The symptoms of adrenal insufficiency are often nonspecific and include anorexia, nausea, vomiting, diarrhea, weight loss, hypotension, fatigue, weakness, fever, and confusion. In primary adrenal insufficiency, signs of dehydration due to aldosterone deficiency may be present (i.e., tachycardia, orthostatic hypotension). The characteristic hyperpigmentation of the skin (due to ACTH excess) is absent when the adrenal failure is acute, secondary, or tertiary. Hyponatremia is due primarily to an impaired ability to excrete free water; thus, it is common to any type of adrenal insufficiency. However, hyperkalemia and metabolic acidosis are absent in secondary or tertiary adrenal failure because aldosterone secretion is preserved through the renin-angiotensin system. In acute adrenal crisis, the rapid reduction in intravascular volume, vascular tone, and cardiac output can result in vascular collapse and shock.

TABLE 69.1 Etiology of adrenal insufficiency

Primary	Secondary
Idiopathic/autoimmune	Long-term glucocorticoid steroid use (abrupt withdraw)
Tuberculosis	Neoplasms
Adrenal hemorrhage	Inflammatory lesions
Bilateral infarction	Granulomatous disease
Fungal infection	Trauma (infundibular stalk section)
HIV/AIDS	Radiation
Metastatic cancer	Necrosis (Sheehan's syndrome)
Bilateral adrenalectomy	
Congenital adrenal hyperplasia	
Drugs: mitotane, ketoconazole, metyrapone	

In secondary adrenal insufficiency, patients may also have associated deficits of other pituitary hormones, such as growth hormone, follicle-stimulating hormone, luteinizing hormone, and thyroid-stimulating hormone, manifesting as growth retardation or delayed puberty in children and erectile dysfunction, amenorrhea, or hypothyroidism in adults. If a pituitary tumor is the cause, headache, visual field loss, and/or cranial nerve palsies may be present.

DIAGNOSIS

Adrenal insufficiency is best diagnosed by a rapid cosyntropin stimulation test. The test is best done between 6 a.m. and 10 a.m. Plasma samples are drawn for cortisol before and 3 to 60 minutes after administering 0.25 mg of cosyntropin intravenous (IV) or intramuscular (IM). Normally, the plasma cortisol should increase 8 μg/dL above the baseline, and it should exceed 20 μg/dL at 30 to 60 minutes. Therefore a rise of cortisol level <8 μ/g above baseline is considered abnormal. The plasma ACTH level separates primary from secondary adrenal failure; ACTH is elevated and typically exceeds 250 pg/mL in the primary type, but it is low or inappropriately normal in other types. Patients with secondary adrenal insufficiency should be tested for other pituitary hormone deficiencies as well. In the case of shock and normal adrenal function, a random plasma cortisol level should be at least 20 μg/dL; in most cases, the level exceeds 30 μg/dL. Computed tomography (CT) scan or magnetic resonance imaging (MRI) of the abdomen may suggest infection, hemorrhage, or other diffuse abnormality of the adrenal glands.

TREATMENT

If acute adrenal insufficiency is suspected, the patient should be treated immediately without waiting for confirmation of the diagnosis. Once blood specimens have been obtained for diagnosis, therapy includes prompt administration of IV fluids and IV glucocorticoid replacement, as well as treatment of the stress that precipitated the crisis. Because it does not affect plasma cortisol measurement if a cosyntropin test has been initiated, dexamethasone is often given initially. Hydrocortisone is the preferred glucocorticoid in the treatment of adrenal crisis because it exhibits the greatest mineralocorticoid activity. Mineralocorticoid replacement is unnecessary if the total daily hydrocortisone dose exceeds 100 mg. With proper treatment, patients with acute adrenal insufficiency have a very good prognosis. Left untreated, acute adrenal crisis is fatal.

Treatment of chronic adrenal insufficiency includes daily, maintenance glucocorticoid (e.g., cortisone acetate, hydrocortisone, or prednisone). Patients with primary adrenal insufficiency also require daily mineralocorticoid (i.e., fludrocortisone) replacement and unrestricted salt intake. Dosages need to be increased during illness and in the perioperative period due to the increased level of stress. Patients should be educated about the adjustment of medication during illness and wear a medical bracelet or necklace.

COMPLICATIONS/PROGNOSIS

Adrenal insufficiency is easily treatable. However, if undiagnosed or improperly treated, the consequences are often fatal, with vascular collapse and shock. In chronic adrenal insufficiency, daily replacement therapy and careful adjustment of medication during illness is necessary to avoid adrenal crisis.

Cushing's Syndrome

Cushing's syndrome is a condition caused by excess amounts of cortisol adenoma or cancer resulting from hypersecretion of the adrenal cortex which may result from a hypersecreting adrenal tumor, ectopic ACTH, or prolonged exposure to high therapeutic doses of glucocorticoids or prolonged exposure to high therapeutic doses of glucocorticoids.

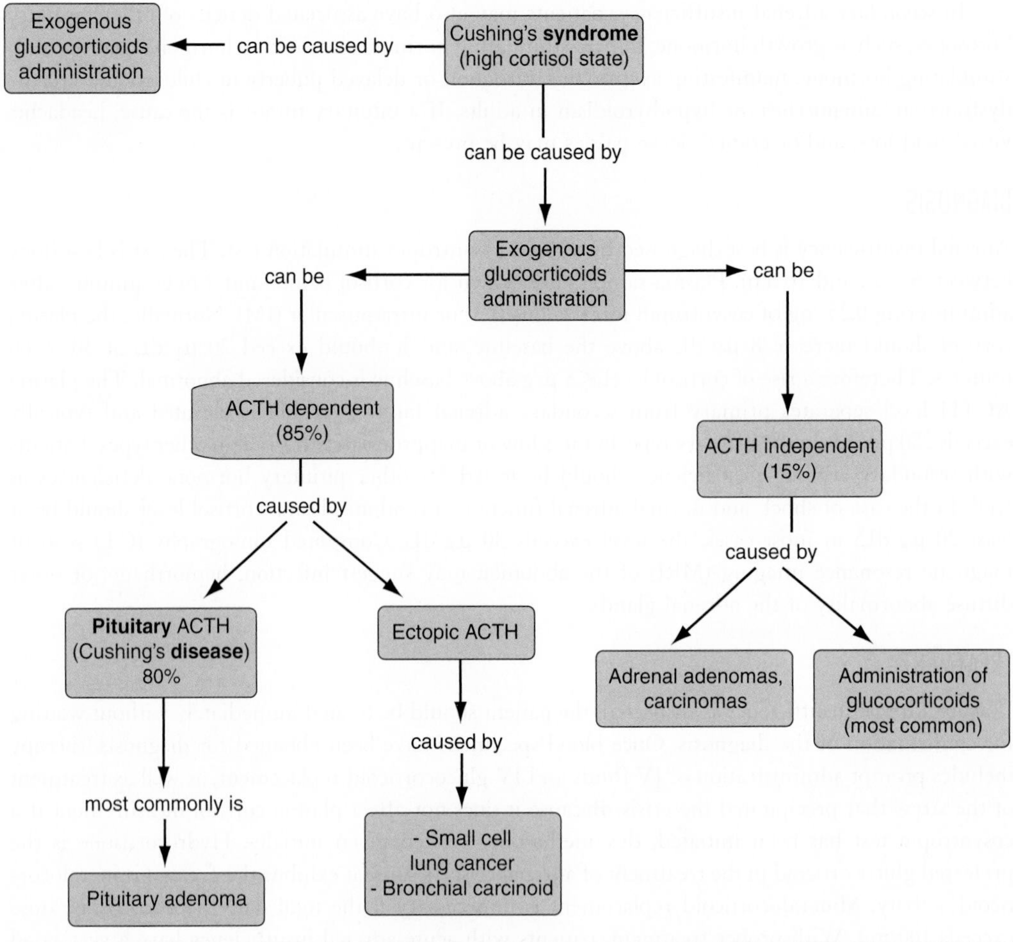

Figure 69.1 • Etiology of hypercortisolemia: Cushing's syndrome.

Cushing's disease refers to a high cortisol state caused by a pituitary ACTH hypersecreting tumor (most common cause), and less frequently pituitary hyperplasia. Cushing's disease is six times more common in women than in men; the mean age at diagnosis is in the fourth decade.

ETIOLOGY

Because of the widespread pharmacologic use of glucocorticoids, the most common cause of Cushing's syndrome is iatrogenic or exogenous glucocorticoid use. Endogenous cases (Fig. 69.1) may be either ACTH dependent (e.g., ACTH-secreting pituitary adenoma or ectopic ACTH-secreting neoplasm) or ACTH independent (e.g., adrenal adenoma, adrenal carcinoma). Benign adrenal tumors causing Cushing's syndrome predominantly produce glucocorticoids; adrenal cancers, however, often secrete high levels of adrenal androgens and glucocorticoids.

Ectopic ACTH secretion occurs in a few neoplasms (e.g., small cell carcinoma of the lung, carcinoid tumors, pancreatic islet cell tumors), usually in men in the fifth decade and beyond.

Functioning benign adrenal adenomas and adrenocortical cancers each give rise to less than 10% of cases of Cushing's syndrome. Benign adenomas are usually small and synthesize cortisol very efficiently. In contrast, functioning adrenocortical cancers are very large at diagnosis and often produce adrenal steroids inefficiently.

TABLE 69.2 Clinical manifestations of hypercortisolemia

Truncal obesity	95%
Menstrual Irregularities	80%
Hypertension	75%
Facial plethora (round face)	75%
Hirsutism/vellus type hair growth	65%
Gonadal dysfunction	50%
Violaceous striae	65%
Diabetes mellitus	65%
Hyperlipidemia	70%
Proximal muscle weakness	60%

CLINICAL MANIFESTATIONS

The clinical features of hypercortisolemia are shown in Table 69.2. They include centripetal obesity, which is caused by the accumulation of fat in trunk, face, and neck, hence the description of "buffalo hump" and "moon facies." At times, it is helpful to examine serial photographs of the patient, looking for evidence of progressive physical changes consistent with excessive cortisol exposure. The facial plethora (round face) may be subtle (Fig. 69.3) or quite obvious (Fig. 69.4).

Patients may commonly experience proximal muscle wasting and weakness, which are caused by the catabolic effect of high glucocorticoid levels on skeletal muscles. Hypertension, diabetes mellitus, osteoporosis, and depression are often present. Thin skin, easy bruisability, violaceous striae (on breasts and abdomen) and skin atrophy are some of the dermatologic manifestations of Cushing's syndrome.

Hyperpigmentation is most commonly found in sun or pressure exposed areas (elbows, knuckles, waist). It occurs most often in patients with ectopic ACTH secreting tumors and less often in patients pituitary disease (Cushing's disease). However, it is absent in high cortisol states caused by adrenal disease (Cushing's syndrome) because lack of secretion of ACTH (Table 69.3).

In benign adrenal adenomas, the signs of cortisol excess usually begin gradually. In functioning adrenocortical carcinomas, the course tends to be more acute and rapidly progressive, with prominent hyperandrogenic effects (i.e., hirsutism, virilization) and lack of typical Cushingoid features. Patients may also report abdominal, back, and flank pain and a palpable abdominal mass caused by the large tumor size.

Cushing's syndrome also can be caused as a paraneoplastic syndrome related to ectopic production of ACTH by certain cancers, classically small cell lung carcinoma. These patients more frequently present with severe proximal weakness, weight loss, and hypokalemia along with rapid development of the florid clinical manifestations of Cushing's syndrome.

DIAGNOSIS

A 24-hour urinary cortisol, or salivary cortisol and a low-dose dexamethasone suppression test, are often initially performed as the screening tests. The evaluation of a patient with suspected Cushing's syndrome is outlined in Figure 69.2.

A 24-hour urine collection for free cortisol results in very few false positive results.

Elevated salivary cortisol levels, obtained at 11 p.m., can also be used to diagnose glucocorticoid excess and to improve accuracy of low-dose dexamethasone suppression test. A low-dose 1-mg dexa-

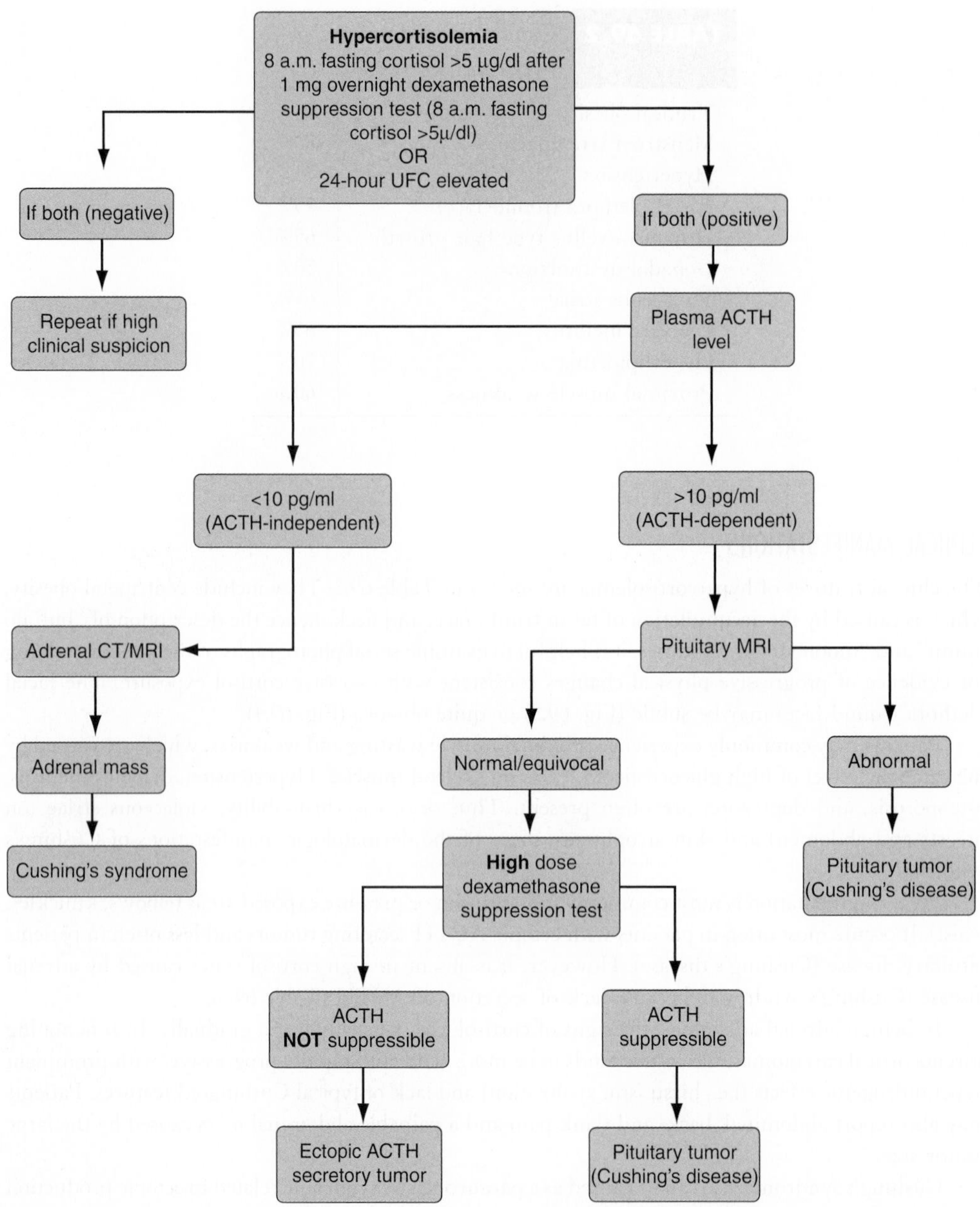

Figure 69.2 • Diagnosis, workup, and differentiation of hypercortisolemia (Cushing's disease/syndrome). UFC, urine-free cortisol.

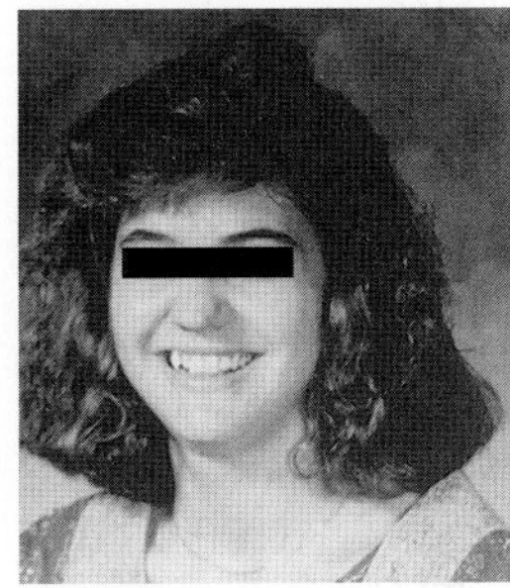
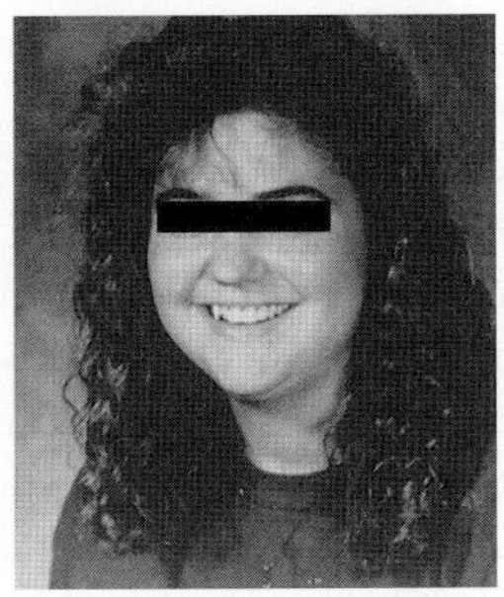

Figure 69.3 • These photographs of a young woman with Cushing's syndrome show subtle changes in the facial outlines over a 3-year period.

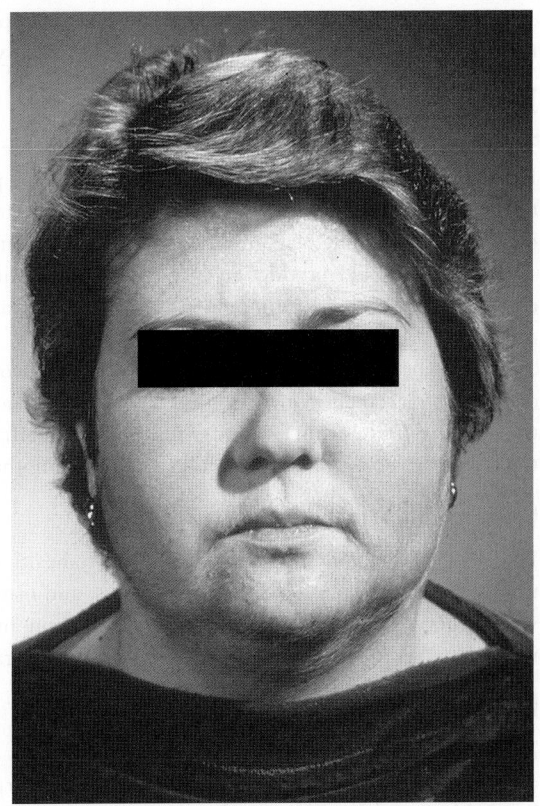

Figure 69.4 • This photograph of a middle-aged woman with Cushing's syndrome demonstrates the characteristic plethoric facies.

TABLE 69.3 Frequency of occurrence and potential causes of hypercortisolemia

Hypercortisolemia	Ectopic ACTH	Pituitary	Adrenal
Hyperpigmentation	+ +	+	−
Cause	Ectopic ACTH secreting tumor (+ACTH)	Pituitary tumor (+ACTH)	Adrenal adenoma (−ACTH)

methasone suppression test may produce false-positive results in normal subjects, in patients with obesity or depression.

Once hypercortisolemia is established, the distinction between ACTH dependence and ACTH independence should follow, based on measurement of plasma ACTH; levels exceeding 20 pg/mL indicate ACTH-dependent hypercortisolism. Patients with primary adrenal neoplasms have a suppressed or low plasma ACTH (<10 pg/mL) and adrenal mass on CT scan.

ACTH-dependent Cushing's syndrome must be further separated into a pituitary tumor or an ectopic ACTH-secreting neoplasm. A high-dose dexamethasone suppression test can be used at this time to differentiate between ectopic ACTH secreting tumor (not suppressible ACTH/cortisol secretion) versus a pituitary or adrenal ACTH secreting mass (suppressible ACTH/cortisol secretion). A normal CT or MRI of the sella cannot make exclude a pituitary-secreting tumor, because only 50% to 60% of patients with Cushing's disease (pituitary) have a sellar abnormality on head MRI or CT.

Hypercortisolemia with concomitant ACTH suppression (ACTH <10 pg/mL) and an adrenal mass seen on CT or MRI are diagnostic of a primary adrenal neoplasm.

TREATMENT

Transsphenoidal resection is the treatment of choice for the ACTH-secreting pituitary neoplasm. Remissions occur in approximately 80% to 90% of patients with Cushing's disease who undergo transsphenoidal adenoma resection. Conventional external radiotherapy is not effective as a primary treatment, but it may be combined with pituitary surgery.

Ectopic ACTH production is managed by treating the primary tumor or by using adrenolytic agents such as mitotane, aminoglutethimide, or metyrapone. These agents also are useful in inoperable cases.

Adrenalectomy is the preferred treatment in glucocorticoid-producing adrenal neoplasms. Glucocorticoid replacement is required for 1 to 2 years to avoid acute adrenal crisis due to suppression of the hypothalamus, pituitary, and atrophy of the contralateral adrenal. Malignant tumors are usually treated with debulking surgery followed by chemotherapy.

COMPLICATIONS/PROGNOSIS

Patients with Cushing's syndrome are prone to health complications related to excess cortisol production, such as hypertension, diabetes mellitus, and osteoporosis. Benign adrenal adenomas are cured with surgery. The prognosis for most adrenal carcinomas is very poor. Median survival after diagnosis in adults is 14 to 36 months; untreated, survival averages 3 months.

Primary Hyperaldosteronism

Normally, the renin-angiotensin system is the major regulator of aldosterone synthesis and release, and aldosterone promotes renal tubular Na^+ reabsorption and K^+ and H^+ ion excretion. Primary hyperaldosteronism (Conn syndrome) is an abnormal excess of mineralocorticoid production by the adrenal gland. Primary hyperaldosteronism occurs in 1% to 5% of hypertensives. It is seen most often in the third through fifth decades. In hypertensive patients with spontaneous hypokalemia (K^+ <3.5 mEq/L), 40% have some variant of primary hyperaldosteronism.

ETIOLOGY

Approximately 50% of cases of primary hyperaldosteronism are due to aldosterone-producing adenomas (APAs). Most of the remaining cases are caused by bilateral idiopathic hyperaldosteronism (IHAs). Rarely, it may be due to glucocorticoid-suppressible hyperaldosteronism or an aldosterone-secreting adrenal carcinoma. APAs are typically solitary, unilateral, small (<2 cm in diameter), and benign. In IHA, there is bilateral hyperplasia of the zona glomerulosa, possibly from hyperstimulation by an unidentified aldosterone-releasing factor.

CLINICAL MANIFESTATIONS

In primary hyperaldosteronism, the intravascular volume is typically high. Key manifestations include hypertension, spontaneous hypokalemia, metabolic alkalosis, low plasma renin activity, and an elevated plasma aldosterone level. The hypertension usually is moderate and is due to the sodium-retaining effects of the mineralocorticoid. Rarely, the hypokalemia may evoke easy fatigability, anorexia, muscle weakness, and cramps.

DIAGNOSIS

Screening for primary hyperaldosteronism should be performed in hypertensive patients with spontaneous hypokalemia below 3.5 mEq/L, or a serum K^+ below 3.0 mEq/L while taking a diuretic. The first phase of the workup includes screening tests, followed by testing to confirm the diagnosis (Table 69.4). In primary hyperaldosteronism PRA is low, PAC is elevated, and PAC/PRA ratio is >20 (elevated). Testing is optimal when the individual is salt loaded and when the hypokalemia is corrected. Before biochemical testing, the following medications should be discontinued: all antihypertensive agents except peripheral α-1 antagonists and central α-2 agonists for at least 1 week, diuretics for 4 weeks, and estrogen and spironolactone for 6 weeks.

Over 90% of cases of primary hyperaldosteronism are due to either APA or IHA, so the last phase involves differentiating between these two causes. High-resolution CT is performed initially because it localizes the APA in 70% to 80% of cases. Bilateral adrenal vein catheterization is the most definitive means to distinguish between APA and IHA.

TREATMENT

Patients with an APA who are at low surgical risk should undergo unilateral adrenalectomy. One year following a successful surgery, 80% to 90% of patients remain normotensive and normokalemic. After 5 years, however, 50% develop recurrence of the hypertension while remaining normokalemic; the reason for this is not clear. Factors predicting persistence or recurrence of hypertension after unilateral adrenalectomy include duration of hypertension and family history of hypertension.

In patients with IHA, bilateral adrenalectomy is ineffective in controlling hypertension, so medical management is the treatment of choice. Patients should follow a low-sodium diet (<80 mEq/day), exercise regularly, and maintain an ideal body weight. Potassium-sparing diuretics (e.g., spironolactone, amiloride, and triamterene) are the usual pharmaceutical agents for treating the hypokalemia of primary hyperaldosteronism. Spironolactone, the drug of choice, is often combined with nifedipine or an ACE inhibitor. If this therapy does not control the hypertension, the next step is empiric trials of other antihypertensive drugs, which usually are equally effective.

TABLE 69.4 Diagnostic tests for primary hyperaldosteronism

Screening	Level	Confirmatory	Level	Localizing
PRA (ng/mL/hour)	<2 ↓	Saline infusion test	>50	CT of the adrenals
PAC (ng/dL)	<14 ↑			MRI of adrenals
PAC/PRA (ng/dL)	>30			Adrenal vein catheterization
24-h urinary potassium (mEq)	>30			

CT, computed tomography; PAC, plasma aldosterone concentration; PRA, panel reactive antibody.

Congenital Adrenal Hyperplasia

Congenital adrenal hyperplasia (CAH) is a family of autosomal recessive disorders resulting from defects in glucocorticoid, mineralocorticoid, and androgen production. Deficient cortisol biosynthesis causes a compensatory rise in pituitary ACTH, resulting in adrenocortical hyperplasia and overproduction of the steroids that precede the enzymatic defect.

ETIOLOGY

CAH can result from any one of five enzyme deficiencies: 21-hydroxylase, 11-hydroxylase, 3β-hydroxysteroid dehydrogenase, 17-hydroxylase, or 20,22-desmolase. Classic 21-hydroxylase deficiency, the only human leukocyte antigen–linked type, accounts for more than 90% of cases of CAH. The next most common, 11-hydroxylase deficiency, accounts for almost 5% of cases.

CLINICAL MANIFESTATIONS

CAH can take two forms: a classic, congenital form with nearly total enzymatic deficiency or, more often, a late-onset form with a partial enzymatic deficiency and onset after puberty. Clinical features depend on which steroids are deficient or in excess, as well as the absolute degree of deficiency or excess. The manifestations of the most common form, 21-hydroxylase deficiency, usually include virilization in females or ambiguous genitalia, salt-wasting, nephropathy, hyponatremia, and hyperkalemia. 11-Hydroxylase deficiency typically presents with virilization in females or ambiguous genitalia, high blood pressure, and hypokalemic alkalosis.

DIAGNOSIS

In CAH, the steroid precursors to the defective enzymes are elevated; these steroids are used for diagnosis when CAH is suspected. For instance, in 21-hydroxylase and 11-hydroxylase deficiency, plasma 17-OH progesterone and 11-deoxycortisol are typically elevated, respectively. In mild or late forms, measurement of the plasma steroid precursor after exogenous cosyntropin stimulation may be necessary for diagnosis.

TREATMENT

The enzymatic defects that impair cortisol and mineralocorticoid synthesis are treated respectively with glucocorticoids and mineralocorticoids. The consequent reduction in release of pituitary ACTH results in suppression of the overproduced adrenocortical steroids.

DISEASES OF THE ADRENAL MEDULLA

Derived from embryonic neural crest cells, the adrenal medulla is composed primarily of chromaffin cells that convert the amino acid tyrosine to catecholamines (epinephrine, norepinephrine, dopamine). Released in response to stress, catecholamines are important mediators of the central and autonomic nervous systems. Because the predominant catecholamine, epinephrine, has a slightly higher affinity for β-adrenergic receptors, the main hemodynamic effect is cardiac, increasing both heart rate and contractility. Combined with an α_1-mediated vasoconstriction, these collective effects significantly raise the blood pressure. Neoplasms are the most significant of all the adrenal medullary disorders, presenting most commonly as pheochromocytomas in adults and neuroblastomas in children (one of the common solid tumors of childhood).

Pheochromocytoma

Pheochromocytomas are autonomously functioning, catecholamine-secreting, chromaffin-cell neoplasms.

ETIOLOGY

About 90% are benign solitary nodules found within the adrenal medulla itself. However, because they can arise anywhere neural crest tissue has migrated during the course of embryonic development,

TABLE 69.5 Classification of the multiple endocrine neoplasia (MEN) syndromes

MEN Syndrome	Associated disorders
MEN type I (Wermer's syndrome)	Hyperparathyroidism
	Pituitary adenomas
	Pancreatic islet cell tumor Gastrinoma VIPoma Insulinoma Glucagonoma
MEN type IIa (Sipples's syndrome)	Medullary carcinoma of thyroid
	Pheochromocytoma
	Hyperparathyroidism
MEN type IIb	Marfanoid habitus
	Pheochromocytoma
	Medullary carcinoma of thyroid
	Mucosal and intestinal neuromas

approximately 10% are located intra-abdominally in close proximity to the celiac or mesenteric sympathetic ganglia. Adrenal medullary pheochromocytomas are almost always (90%) unilateral. Bilateral lesions usually occur as familial neoplasms, as in type IIa (Sipple's syndrome) or type IIb multiple endocrine neoplasia syndrome (Table 69.5). The multiple endocrine neoplasia syndromes are transmitted as autosomal dominant diseases with incomplete penetrance and variable expression.

CLINICAL MANIFESTATIONS

The hallmark of a pheochromocytoma is hypertension. The clinical triad of episodic headaches, palpitations, and excessive diaphoresis occurring with hypertension provides the best clinical clue for this tumor (Table 69.6). If this triad and hypertension are absent, the diagnosis of a pheochromocytoma

TABLE 69.6 Clinical manifestations associated with pheochromocytomas

Symptoms	Incidence (%)	Signs	Incidence (%)
Headache	75–100	Hypertension	75–100
Palpitations	50–75	Tachycardia	50–75
Diaphoresis	50–75	Postural hypotension	50–75
Anxiety	25–50	Paroxysmal hypertension	25–50
Tremulousness	25–50	Weight loss	25–50
Chest pain	25–50	Tremor	25–50
Abdominal pain	25–50	Pallor	25–50
Nausea/emesis	25–50		
Weakness/fatigue	25–50		

can be set aside confidently. Although 80% or more of these patients are hypertensive on examination, nearly one half exhibit normotensive, symptom-free periods, interspersed with episodic and transient symptoms.

DIAGNOSIS

The most commonly used screening test is a 24-hour urine measurement of catecholamines (norepinephrine and epinephrine) or their metabolites (metanephrine and vanillylmandelic acid). Because many medications (levodopa, tricyclic antidepressants, and decongestants) influence the test results, all medications should be withheld for a minimum of 1 to 2 days, if possible, before collecting the urine sample. The sensitivity and specificity of plasma and urinary catecholamines is shown in Table 69.7. In most diagnoses of pheochromocytoma, the total urinary metanephrine and catecholamines (norepinephrine and epinephrine) exceed 1,000 μg per 24 hours and 150 μg per 24 hours, respectively.

Plasma norepinephrine, another useful screening test in pheochromocytomas, typically exceeds 2,000 pg/mL. However, because catecholamine secretion may be intermittent, single plasma catecholamine measurements may be less sensitive than urinary levels. Recently, measurement of plasma metanephrine levels has been shown to have a higher sensitivity and specificity than the level of urinary catecholamine and their metabolites for the diagnosis of both sporadic and familial pheochromocytoma.

Once a pheochromocytoma is confirmed biochemically, localization with CT or MRI should follow. Radionuclide tests with ^{131}I-meta-iodobenzylguanidine, a radioactive amine taken up and concentrated by adrenergic chromaffin cells, are useful if extra-adrenal or metastatic pheochromocytomas are suspected.

TREATMENT

Pheochromocytoma is almost always cured by surgical excision of the tumor. The recent development of laparoscopic surgical techniques has provided a safe alternative to open surgical techniques. An α-adrenergic blocking agent (e.g., phenoxybenzamine, 10 mg twice daily, then increase by 10 mg every 2 days until blood pressure is controlled) is administered for at least 14 days prior to surgery in order to avoid an intraoperative hypertensive crisis. Phentolamine (a reversible α-blocker) and nitroprusside (a direct-acting arterial vasodilator) usually are used to manage any hypertensive crises that arise during the induction of anesthesia or during surgery. When α-blockade fails to control the hypertension metyrosine, a tyrosine hydroxylase inhibitor, which reduces tumor stores of catecholamines, also may be used for preoperative management of pheochromocytoma.

Successful preoperative α-blockade lowers intraoperative fluid requirements, decreases the need for intraoperative medication to control blood pressure, and attenuates blood loss. Severe hypotension after tumor excision usually is avoided by perioperative plasma volume expansion with normal saline. Following α-blockade, β-blockers are used preoperatively to control tachycardia.

COMPLICATIONS/PROGNOSIS

Unrecognized pheochromocytomas are potentially lethal. Hypertensive crisis or shock may be precipitated by drugs, anesthetic agents, surgery for unrelated conditions, or childbirth. However, with

TABLE 69.7 Laboratory diagnosis of pheochromocytoma

	Plasma	Urinary
Sensitivity	Free metanephrine: 99%	Fractionated metanephrine: 97%
Specificity	Free metanephrine: 89%	Total metanephrine: 93% VMA: 95%

VMA, vanylmandelic acid.

early diagnosis, these patients have a very high cure rate. Inoperable or malignant pheochromocytomas are managed medically with α- and β-adrenergic blockade. If these agents fail to provide symptom relief, metyrosine may be added. In these rare patients, the 5-year survival rate is less than 50%.

Incidental Adrenal Mass

Since the advent of abdominal imaging using CT or MRI, the incidentally discovered adrenal mass (the so-called adrenal incidentaloma) has become a common radiographic finding and clinical dilemma. The incidence of detection of such adrenal masses is common and ranges from 0.5% to 10% of such imaging studies.

ETIOLOGY

Common causes of an adrenal mass can be found in Table 69.8 and include both benign adenomas and malignant tumors (primary adrenocortical carcinoma or metastatic lesions). Primary malignancies that most commonly metastasize to the adrenals include breast, lung, lymphoma, melanoma, and colon. The majority of small (<5 cm) masses are benign and nonfunctional (do not secrete hormone). Functioning adrenal tumors include pheochromocytoma and those that cause Cushing's syndrome or primary hyperaldosteronism. Between 50% to 70% of primary adrenocortical carcinomas are functional.

CLINICAL MANIFESTATIONS

Patients with small, nonfunctioning, benign adrenal nodules are typically asymptomatic, while patients with primary adrenocortical carcinoma most commonly present with abdominal pain and an easily palpable mass. Other clinical characteristics of adrenal masses depend on their functional nature; excessive cortisol is the most common secretory product for both benign and malignant functioning masses.

TABLE 69.8 Differential diagnosis of adrenal mass

Benign nonfunctional adrenal cortical adenoma
Benign functional adrenal cortical adenoma
Cushing's syndrome
Virilizing
Feminizing
Hyperaldosteronism
Primary adrenal cortical carcinoma
Nonfunctional
Functional
Tumors of the adrenal medulla
Pheochromocytoma
Ganglioneuromas/neuroblastoma
Benign adrenal cyst
Myelolipoma
Intra-adrenal hemorrhage
Metastases from other primary malignancies
Congenital adrenal hyperplasia

TABLE 69.9 Screening laboratory assessment for adrenal incidentaloma

Overnight 1-mg dexamethasone suppression test or 24-hour urinary free cortisol
Serum dehydroepiandrosterone sulfate
Serum potassium
Aldosterone: Plasma rennin activity (if serum potassium <3.5 mEq/L)
24-hour urine metanephrine, VMA, and catecholamines

VMA, vanylmandelic acid.

DIAGNOSIS

Initially, the appearance of the CT or MRI scan images taken in context with a thorough history and physical examination may provide clues to the nature of the mass. Evidence is sought for signs of Cushing's syndrome, pheochromocytoma, primary hyperaldosteronism, nonadrenal malignancies, and adrenocortical carcinoma. Initial screening tests shown in Table 69.9 should be performed. Patients who have a primary cancer elsewhere may require needle biopsy to evaluate for adrenal metastasis. A pheochromocytoma should be excluded before needle biopsy is performed.

TREATMENT

For small lesions (<5 cm) associated with normal adrenal function, evaluation typically includes serial CT scans every 3 to 6 months over a period of up to 12 to 18 months. If the lesion is stable in size, it is presumed to be a benign, nonfunctional adrenal adenoma and no further follow-up is needed. Masses 5 cm or larger are usually resected as the risk for adrenocortical carcinoma is greater.

Gastroenterology

Kia Saeian

CHAPTER 70

Peptic Ulcer Disease

Krista Wiger

Peptic ulcer disease (PUD) refers to the condition resulting in focal areas of mucosal defects extending through the muscularis mucosa attributed the affects of acid and pepsin. These ulcers most commonly occur in the duodenum and the stomach; however, they may develop in other locations such as the lower esophagus or Meckel's diverticulum.

PUD is more prevalent in men than in women with an overall lifetime prevalence estimated at 10%. Traditionally, duodenal ulcers have been 2 to 4 times as common as gastric ulcers; however, recent studies suggest that this ratio is reversing given successful treatment regimens of duodenal ulcers and decreasing prevalence of *Helicobacter pylori* infection. PUD incidence increases with age, likely secondary to an increased prevalence of nonsteroidal anti-inflammatory drugs (NSAIDs) usage and *H. pylori* infection. First-degree relatives of patients with PUD have an increased incidence in the same type of ulcer. Patients with O blood type, nonsecretors of ABO antigens, and human leukocyte antigen B5 have an increased rate of developing a duodenal ulcer. Smoking increases both ulcer types, impairs healing, and promotes recurrence. Multiple extrinsic factors such as personality type, coffee, diet, and alcohol have been implicated; however, clear evidence substantiating them as risk factors is not available. Other diseases such as cirrhosis, renal failure, chronic obstructive pulmonary disease, polycythemia vera, and hyperparathyroidism are associated with an increased incidence of duodenal ulcer.

ETIOLOGY

The mucosal defense system consists of the mucus/bicarbonate layer and epithelial cells and relies on blood flow to clear the diffused acid and supply nutrients. In addition, prostaglandins (cyclooxygenase [COX]-1) enhance these above processes and contribute to this defense system. Peptic ulcers occur when the mucosal defense system is unable to protect the mucosa from the effects of acid and pepsin. Multiple factors that affect the mucosal defense system have been implicated. These range from *H. pylori* infection to inhibition of prostaglandin production by NSAIDs. Although 30% of patients with duodenal ulcers do have an increased basal acid output, gastric ulcers may occur in normal or low acid output conditions. Nevertheless, both conditions heal with acid suppression. *H. pylori* infection and NSAIDs are the most common causes of PUD. *H. pylori* infection is associated with an increased risk of peptic ulcer disease, gastric adenocarcinoma, and gastric lymphoma. The precise mechanism of its contribution to ulcer formation continues to be defined. Increased gastrin and pepsinogen levels, immunologic factors, and genetic factors have been implicated and are under further evaluation. Risk factors for *H. pylori* infection include male sex, increasing age, Hispanic and African American race, living with children, birth in a developing country, and lower levels of education. Although approximately 10% to 15% of patients with *H. pylori* will develop peptic ulcer disease, up to 95% of patients with duodenal ulcers and 75% of patients with gastric ulcers are infected. In Western countries, the association is less robust, with approximately 80% duodenal ulcers and 60% gastric ulcers associated with *H. pylori*.

NSAIDS are the second most common cause of PUD and have been associated with a significant increase in complications such as bleeding and perforation. Prostaglandin depletion and direct cellular toxicity have been implicated as viable mechanisms. This prostaglandin depletion explains why the enteric-coated preparations still contribute to ulcer formation. The cyclooxygenase-2 selective agents such as celecoxib or rofecoxib do not involve the COX-1 pathway so are not as ulcerogenic, but they do elevate the risk of PUD. Several of these drugs have been removed from the market and are under further investigation for contributing to cardiovascular events. NSAID ulcer bleeding risk is increased with age >55 years, oral steroid use, dose and formulation, anticoagulation, and prior ulcer disease.

The third most common cause, resulting in <1% of all PUD, is the hypersecretory state of Zollinger-Ellison syndrome.

CLINICAL MANIFESTATIONS

The classic symptoms of a duodenal ulcer are epigastric abdominal burning or cramping pain that may radiate laterally or to the back. This pain occurs 2 to 4 hours after eating, is relieved by food or antacid, and may occur during sleep. Often these symptoms may be present for a few weeks, then resolve and recur weeks to months later. Patients may initially present with anorexia, nausea, or vomiting or with complications of the ulcer (i.e., bleeding, perforation, or obstruction).

Gastric ulcers are characterized by burning epigastric or occasionally back pain. Pain may be relieved or exacerbated by food, periodic, and recur in 30 to 90 minutes. However, gastric ulcers often are asymptomatic in older patients and only present with the significant complications of bleeding or perforation. On physical examination, epigastric tenderness to palpation may be detected, but this is not specific for PUD. Other than detecting complications or other disease processes, the clinical examination has been shown to have limited accuracy in making the diagnosis of PUD. The presentation of gastric adenocarcinoma, infiltrative diseases, pancreatitis, nonulcer dyspepsia, biliary disease, and anginal equivalents may mimic PUD.

Dyspepsia is an epigastric pain or discomfort with a component of fullness, bloating, distension, or nausea. This complaint is very common yet nonspecific with only 15% to 25% of these patients found to have ulcers.

DIAGNOSIS

Standard upper gastrointestinal (GI) contrast radiography detects 70% to 80% of lesions of PUD, with detection rate increasing up to 90% when the double-contrast method is employed. Currently, upper endoscopy is the diagnostic test of choice, providing 99% diagnostic accuracy and the ability to perform biopsies to rule out malignancy and evaluate for active *H. pylori* infection. The advantages of upper endoscopy must be weighed against its higher cost and invasive nature (e.g., need for sedation). Several tests are available for diagnosing *H. pylori* infection, each with its own limitations. Using endoscopy with gastric biopsy, testing may be done histologically, via culture, or tissue urease activity.

Noninvasive testing options include the ^{13}C- or ^{14}C-urea breath test, detection of *H. pylori* antigen in the stool, and serologic testing. Recent use of antibiotics, proton pump inhibitor, or bismuth may result in false-negative results. To ensure accuracy of the urea breath test, proton pump inhibitors should be held for 7 days prior to the test. In order to confirm eradication of *H. pylori*, stool antigen testing should be performed not earlier then 12 weeks after medical therapy. The serologic test using enzyme-linked immunosorbent assay technology to detect immunoglobulin (Ig) G antibody is inexpensive and unaffected by medications; however, it fails to differentiate current from prior infection and has the highest accuracy in confirming eradication only when performed 12 months after treatment.

In patients with PUD already undergoing endoscopy, a biopsy-based test is reasonable, whereas the ease and inexpensive nature of the IgG antibody make it the test of choice in screening other patients. When there is a need for confirming eradication, the urea breath tests or stool antigen are often used. Gastrin levels and acid secretory studies should only be utilized when a hypersecretory state is suspected.

Given the high prevalence of dyspepsia, the high cost of endoscopy, and limitations of clinical diagnosis, a test-and-treat strategy is advocated to optimize cost-effective evidence-based care. In this strategy, patients with warning signs such as age >55 years, weight loss, blood loss, anemia, dysphagia, hoarseness, recurrent vomiting, or family history have a higher risk of clinical disease and malignancy and therefore undergo prompt endoscopy. If endoscopy is not indicated, patients should still be tested for *H. pylori*. However, if symptoms remain refractory to treatment, an upper endoscopy is warranted (Fig. 70.1).

TREATMENT

Promoting ulcer healing, preventing recurrences, and avoiding complications are the objectives of ulcer therapy that are obtained by promoting the mucosal defense system and inhibiting acid production. NSAID usage and smoking are risk factors for poor healing, recurrence, and complications and therefore should be discontinued. Stress may delay wound healing. Although evidence of a causal relationship between alcohol and ulcer disease is not proven, abstinence is recommended.

Acid inhibition and neutralization are achieved by several different agents. Antacids buffer the acid that is already present and thereby inactivate pepsin by increasing the gastric pH. H2-receptor antagonists, such as cimetidine or famotidine, block the H2-receptor on the parietal cells. Healing rates of 90% have been documented after 8 weeks of therapy.

Proton pump inhibitors, such as omeprazole and pantoprazole, irreversibly bind to the H^+, K^+-ATPase enzyme of the gastric parietal cell and block the final pathway of gastric acid secretion and have become the first-line treatment in ulcer disease. Pantoprazole is available in intravenous formulation and are widely used in acute, intensive settings where parenteral dosing or absorption is prohibitive. Healing rates of 90% to 100% are typically achieved for duodenal ulcers at 4 weeks; however, 8 weeks is needed to achieve the rate of 90% for gastric ulcer healing. Double dosing is typically used for healing, whereas daily dosing is effective for maintenance. These medications are very well tolerated; however, some interact with the cytochrome P-450 system and can lead to drug interactions. Hypergastrinemia secondary to sustained hypochlorhydria results in enterochromaffin-cell hyperplasia that has lead to gastric carcinoid tumors in rats. Although this has not been reported in humans, development of fundic gland polyps has been associated with these medications.

Enhancement of the mucosal defense system may be achieved by either sucralfate or prostaglandins. Sucralfate is a sulfated polysaccharide-aluminum complex that forms a protective gel, which binds to the ulcer and normal mucosa and resulting in a physical barrier from acid and pepsin. Other mechanisms such as pepsin absorption, prostaglandin stimulation, and decreasing oxidant damage contribute to its efficacy. This treatment has been most effective in duodenal ulcer healing; however, frequent dosing makes it less convenient for treatment. Prostaglandin E_i, such as misoprostol, inhibits acid secretion, is cytoprotective, and has been mainly used to prevent NSAID induced ulcers. Crampy abdominal pain and diarrhea are relatively common side effects and, because of its uterotropic effect, it can induce abortion.

In patients that test positive for *H. pylori* and have documented ulcer disease, successful eradication of *H. pylori* expedites healing and essentially results in a cure. Multiple drug regimens consisting

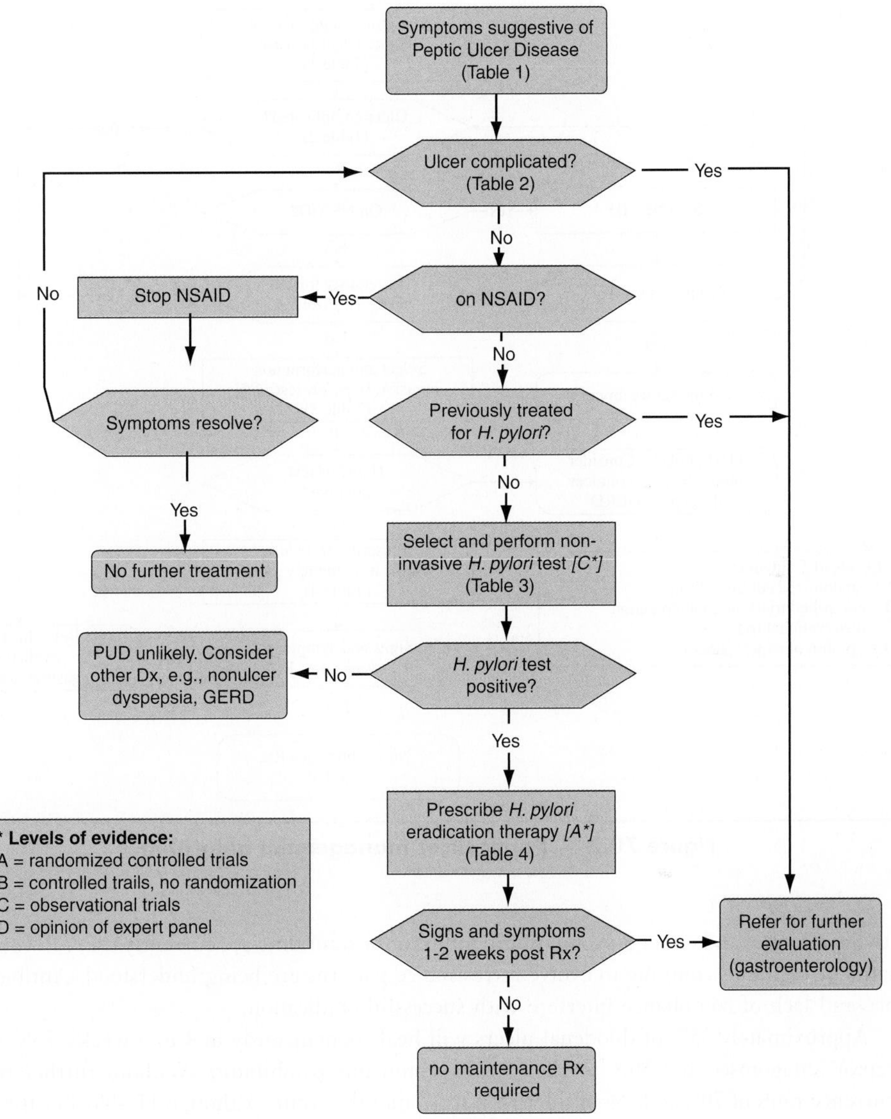

TABLE 1
Symptoms of Peptic Ulcer

- Gnawing or burning epigastric pain
- Pain relieved with food or antacids
- Pain that awakens at night or between meals when stomach is empty

(Heartburn as the predominant symptom indicates GERD, not PUD)

TABLE 2
Signs and Symptoms of Complicated Ulcer

- GI bleeding (e.g., heme positive stool, melena, hematemesis, anemia)
- Obstruction (e.g., nausea with vomiting)
- Penetration or perforation (severe abdominal pain)
- Cancer (e.g., weight loss, anorexia)
- Keep in mind, the risk of cancer increases with age

TABLE 3
***H. pylori* Tests and Charges**

Detect exposure:

- ELISA serology $15 (by clin. micro lab)
- Office serum test $24

Detect active infection:

- Stool antigen test $129
- Urea breath test $479 (special preparation required - see text)

TABLE 4
Preferred Treatment Regimen for *H. pylori* Induced PUD

- Proton pump inhibitor
- Clarithromycin
- Either amoxicillin or metronidazole

Figure 70.1 • Peptic ulcer disease in adults.

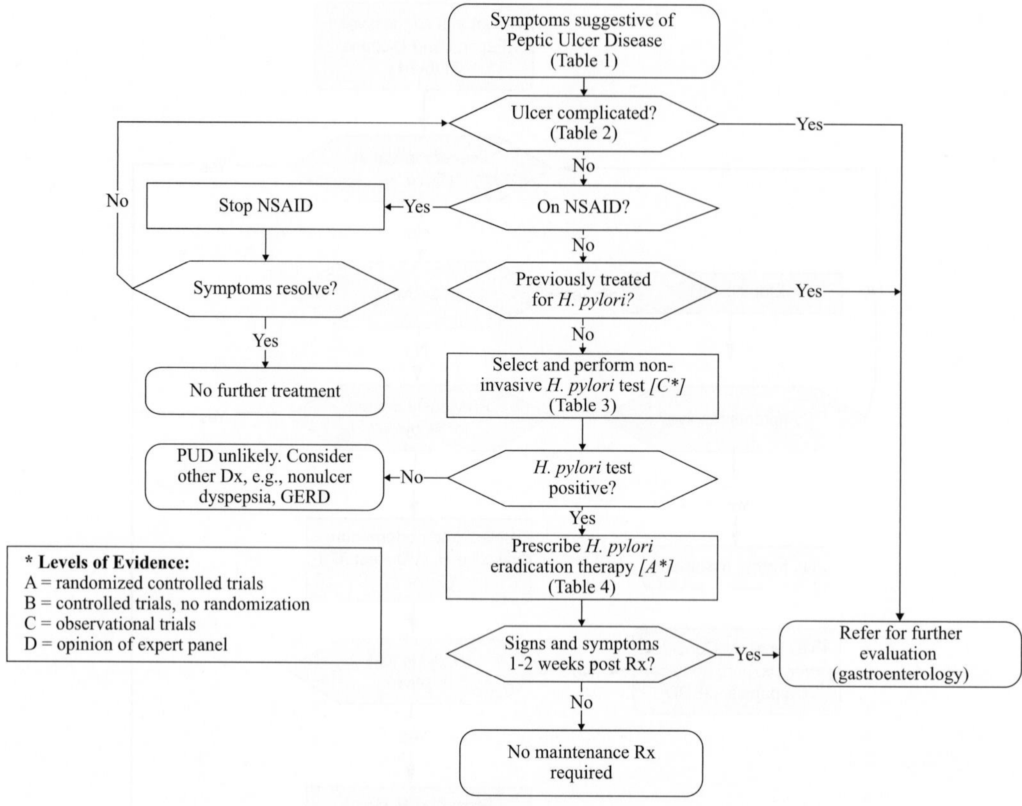

Figure 70.2 • Peptic ulcer management algorithm.

of two antibiotics and either a proton pump inhibitor or ranitidine are currently used. Recommended treatment regimens continue to evolve as resistance patterns are being understood. Antibiotic resistance and lack of compliance interfere with successful eradication.

Approximately 35% of duodenal ulcers will heal spontaneously in 4 to 6 weeks, 75% with H2-receptor antagonists, and 80% to 100% with proton pump inhibitors. Without further treatment, recurrence rates of 70% to 80% in the first 6 to 12 months occur. Although H2-blocker therapy may reduce the recurrence rate, the most efficacious way is the eradication of *H. pylori*.

H. pylori treatment failure should be considered in patients with nonhealing ulcers. Repeat testing through the urea breath test or by stool *H. pylori* antigen should be determined (see precautions above). NSAID usage and hypersecretory states should also be considered. The increase risk of malignancy in gastric ulcers necessitates that these be endoscopically followed until healing is documented. There is controversy, but some authorities regard antral ulcers at low risk for malignancy, especially if benign. Endoscopic biopsies are obtained initially; repeated endoscopy is not required for documenting healing. Multiple courses of therapy may be needed for slow-healing ulcers.

Surgery

The current success rates of medical management have significantly decreased the role of surgery in the management of peptic ulcer disease. Antiulcer operations (Billroth procedures) focus on first reducing gastric acid secretion by removing the antrum with the highest concentration of parietal cells and reconnecting the gastric body to the small intestine. Second, they reduce neural stimulation of acid secretion through a highly selective vagotomy procedure.

Complications

Complications will affect nearly one third of patients in their lifetime (Table 70.1). Intractability is defined as either the failure of ulcer healing despite 3 months of intensive therapy, recurrence of the ulcer, or complications despite maintenance therapy. NSAID usage, smoking, penetrating or obstructing ulcers, and *H. pylori* resistance have been associated. If no modifiable cause is found, surgical intervention may be warranted. Bleeding from PUD is the most common cause (~50%) of acute gastrointestinal bleeding, affects up to 15% to 20% of patients with PUD, and is the initial presentation for 20% to 30% of patients. NSAID usage, especially in the elderly, accounts for a significant increase in GI bleeding. Even though up to 80% of bleeding will stop spontaneously, the mortality rate is 6% to 10%. Diabetes, age over 60, comorbid conditions, and continued or recurrent bleeding are associated with a higher mortality. Ulceration of the posterior duodenal bulb and high lesser curvature erode large arteries and typically result in more extensive bleeding. In this setting, after adequate resuscitation, endoscopy is not only a diagnostic and potentially therapeutic intervention but also facilitates proper risk stratification of the patients. For nonsurgical candidates, angiographic embolization may be considered. In addition, medical management with aggressive oral or intravenous proton pump inhibitor therapy may facilitate platelet aggregation and has been shown to diminish rebleeding rates.

Perforation occurs in 5% to 10% of duodenal and 2% to 5% of gastric ulcer cases and may be the presenting manifestation. Risk factors for this include age, NSAID use, and ulcers in the anterior duodenal bulb or lesser curve. Typical presentation is prior vague abdominal discomfort acutely changing to severe sharp abdominal pain. Clinical examination may reveal hypotension, tachycardia, and peritoneal signs consisting of abdominal rigidity and rebound tenderness. Free air may be noted on abdominal x-ray and care must be taken to order an upright film. If the duodenal contents have spilled, hyperamylasemia can be seen. Although a small minority of patients will have spontaneous sealing, if perforation is documented or highly suspected, emergent surgical intervention is indicated. Currently, laparoscopic techniques for perforated peptic ulcers are under investigation. Given the risk of perforation extension, endoscopy is contraindicated.

Penetration is erosion from the gastric or duodenal wall into the pancreas, liver, biliary tree, or colon without perforation. Patients will present with a change in the pattern of radiation of their symptoms, depending on which area is penetrated. These penetrating ulcers may respond to medical

TABLE 70.1 Complications of peptic ulcer disease
Intractability
Bleeding
Perforation
Penetration
Gastric outlet obstruction
Complications of therapy (H2-blockers antacids of proton pump inhibitors)

Complications of surgery
  Postgastrectomy syndrome
  Dumping syndrome
  Blind-loop syndrome
  Anastomotic ulcer
  Postvagotomy diarrhea

therapy; however, complicated ulcers, such as those resulting in fistula formation, will require surgical intervention.

Gastric outlet obstruction develops in up to 2% of patients with peptic ulcer disease and is caused by either the acute inflammatory edema or spasm or the chronic process of scarring and fibrosis in the area of the pyloric channel or proximal duodenum. The resulting obstruction is a progressive process that may take weeks to develop. Emesis of retained foods, postprandial abdominal pain, bloating, early satiety, and weight loss may be the presenting symptoms. A splashing sound noted with bodily movement (succussion splash) is a suggestive sign. Laboratory tests may indicate prerenal azotemia, anemia, hyponatremia, low serum albumin, and hypokalemic alkalosis. Endoscopy is required to define the cause and exclude malignancy, although barium studies may be used to make the diagnosis. Medical management includes volume resuscitation, correction of electrolyte imbalances, and nasogastric tube drainage of the stomach. Acid suppression is more efficacious in the case of the inflammatory narrowing. Endoscopic balloon dilatation of the pylorus or surgical intervention is utilized in retention persisting beyond 5 to 7 days.

OTHER ULCER DISEASES

Zollinger-Ellison Syndrome

Zollinger-Ellison (ZE) syndrome is characterized by the hypersecretion of acid resulting from the release of gastrin by a gastrinoma. This leads to not only severe ulcerative disease in the upper GI tract, but also diarrhea and hyperchlorhydria. This entity accounts for less than 1% of peptic ulcers, is more common in men, presents between the ages of 30 to 50 years, and should be suspected in patients with multiple ulcers or ulcers beyond the duodenal bulb.

While the symptoms of ZE may mimic PUD, findings such as diarrhea, a family history suggesting multiple endocrine neoplasia (MEN)-1 association such as hyperparathyroidism, or severe progressive/ recurrent PUD may also raise suspicion. Patients who undergo PUD surgery will develop ulcerations at or beyond the anastomosis.

Approximately 90% of gastrinomas are found in the wall of the duodenum or the head of the pancreas, with slightly over one half being multiple. Almost a third of gastrinomas have a MEN-1 association, which may be associated with hyperparathyroidism and pituitary tumors. Despite their slow rate of growth, approximately 50% of gastrinomas metastasize to the regional lymph nodes and/or the liver.

A barium study or esophagogastroduodenoscopy demonstrates ulcers and may show prominent gastric and duodenal folds, thickened and widened small intestinal folds, and excessive fluid in the small bowel. Fasting serum gastrin levels and basal acid output are elevated. Computed tomography, magnetic resonance imaging, ultrasound, endoscopic ultrasound, and arteriography have 40% to 70% sensitivity in locating gastrinomas. Somatostatin receptor scintigraphy (SRS) and selective arterial secretagogue injection test (SASI test) have shown diagnostic superiority (up to 90%) and additionally may locate metastatic spread more effectively. This has now become the test of choice in this setting.

Surgical resection is the treatment; however, in patients where this is not feasible, very high dose proton pump inhibitors (4 to 8 times standard doses) or rarely a total gastrectomy can provide acid control. Chemotherapy (streptozocin, 5-FU, and Adriamycin) may decrease tumor size and gastrin production in malignant gastrinomas but does not provide a cure.

STRESS ULCERS

Severe physiologic stress can result in the compromise of the mucosal defensive system and its perfusion and therefore result in the spectrum of erosion to severe GI bleeding from ulcerations. In patients with severe burns, duodenal ulcerations (Curling's ulcers) or gastroduodenal ulcers in central nervous system trauma or serous illnesses (Cushing's ulcer) are well described. These stress ulcers have a high mortality rate and respond poorly to treatment; therefore, prevention in at-risk patients is imperative. Sucralfate, antacids, H2-antagonists, and proton pump inhibitors have been successfully utilized. If an enteral route is an option, sucralfate is preferable as it may be associated with lower rates of nosocomial pneumonia.

CHAPTER 71

Gastroesophageal Reflux Disease

Kurt Pfeifer

Gastroesophageal reflux disease (GERD) is one of the most common disorders encountered by internists, affecting up to 1 out of every 5 people in the United States. It is characterized by the clinical symptoms of gastroesophageal reflux (GER) or histopathological changes caused by reflux of gastric secretions into the esophagus. In addition to heartburn, the cardinal symptom of GERD, the disease can result in severe complications, including esophageal strictures and adenocarcinoma.

ETIOLOGY AND PATHOPHYSIOLOGY

GERD develops as a result of dysfunction of the processes responsible for preventing GER and clearing refluxed secretions from the esophagus. Normally, tonic contraction of the lower esophageal sphincter (LES), as well as diaphragmatic crural contraction, helps protect the distal esophagus from GER. When reflux does occur, esophageal peristalsis clears most of the gastric contents, preventing prolonged exposure of the esophageal mucosa to acidic secretions. Any residual gastric acids are neutralized by alkaline saliva and bicarbonate secreted from submucosal glands. Gastroesophageal reflux occurs regularly even in healthy people, but GERD develops when there is an imbalance between the damaging effects of refluxed material and the ability of the esophagus to withstand and clear it.

Gastroesophageal reflux can occur through three mechanisms. The primary mechanism of reflux in both normal individuals and those with GERD is *transient lower esophageal sphincter relaxation*.

Another cause of reflux episodes is sudden elevations in intra-abdominal pressure. In the setting of a hiatal hernia, the contribution of diaphragmatic crural contraction to distal esophageal closure is lost. A less common cause of GER is inappropriately low basal LES pressures that do not exceed intragastric pressures. Also known as hypotensive LES, this condition is caused by dysfunction of the smooth muscle within the LES. Hypotensive LES can occur in scleroderma.

A variety of clinical conditions and medications can further predispose to GER. In pregnancy, reflux is secondary to elevated intra-abdominal pressure and progesterone-induced lowering of LES pressure. Fatty meals, coffee, alcohol, and smoking can lower the LES pressure and delay gastric emptying; medications, such as calcium channel blockers and anticholinergics, also lower the LES pressure. Furthermore, reflux esophagitis has been associated with eradication of *Helicobacter pylori* in patients with peptic ulcer disease.

CLINICAL FEATURES

Most patients with GERD report frequent heartburn that can be provoked or increased by laying down, bending forward, or exercising. In addition, by the time of presentation to a physician, many patients report effectively self-treating these symptoms with over-the-counter antacids or acid-suppressing medications. However, even in those with significant reflux-induced complications, heartburn may be absent and a variety of other symptoms present. In some patients, esophageal acidification leads to hypersalivation ("water brash"), whereas others report chest pain.

Dysphagia may be a presenting symptom and is usually due to peptic esophageal stricture, although esophagitis-induced dysmotility and decreased esophageal compliance may also contribute. Finally, gastroesophageal reflux with regurgitation can lead to "sour brash" (sour taste due to regurgitation of gastric secretions into the oropharynx), chronic cough, pharyngitis, laryngitis, sinusitis, dental caries, and worsening of asthma.

DIAGNOSIS

In most cases, a thorough history is sufficient to make a diagnosis. Empiric acid suppressive therapy is not only indicated for treatment but can also confirm the diagnosis by eliminating symptoms. Diagnostic testing for GERD is typically reserved for patients with atypical symptoms or to detect complications of the disease. In these patients, barium swallow can demonstrate gross structural abnormalities (i.e., strictures) and esophageal motility disorders but is too insensitive to detect esophagitis.

Endoscopy is the most sensitive diagnostic test for detection of reflux esophagitis but is often normal in patients with GERD. It should be reserved for refractory cases, dysphagia, odynophagia, weight loss, anemia, gastrointestinal hemorrhage, and suspicion of Barrett's esophagus. For patients with normal endoscopy but persistent symptoms despite acid suppression therapy, correlation of the patient's symptoms with objective evidence of GER can help determine if GERD is truly the cause.

Ambulatory esophageal pH monitoring can be used for this purpose and utilizes a transnasal esophageal probe to monitor pH continuously for 24 hours. Several parameters are measured, but the most important are the percentage of time with a pH <4.0 and the temporal relation between GER symptoms and an acidic esophageal pH. In addition to confirming the diagnosis of GERD, this test can help determine the efficacy of acid-suppressing treatments.

MANAGEMENT

The initial treatment of GERD depends on the severity of the patient's symptoms and endoscopic evidence of esophagitis (Fig. 71.1). For patients with mild to moderate symptoms and no evidence of complications of GERD, lifestyle modifications with antacids as needed is an appropriate first step. Endoscopy is indicated to evaluate for esophagitis and exclude causes other than GERD in patients with severe symptoms or other evidence of complicated disease. If esophagitis is detected, initial therapy should include lifestyle changes and proton pump inhibitor (PPI) therapy because histamine-2 (H_2) receptor antagonists are usually inadequate for healing esophageal erosions. If no esophagitis is found on endoscopy and symptoms persist despite PPI therapy, ambulatory esophageal pH monitoring is useful for confirming a causal relationship between GER and the patient's symptoms. Patients with esophagitis may be treated with PPIs for 8 to 12 weeks and then started on an H_2 blocker for long-term therapy. However, many patients develop recurrent symptoms and require continuous treatment with PPIs. For patients with refractory GERD, antireflux surgery (fundoplication) or endoscopic antireflux procedures can be utilized.

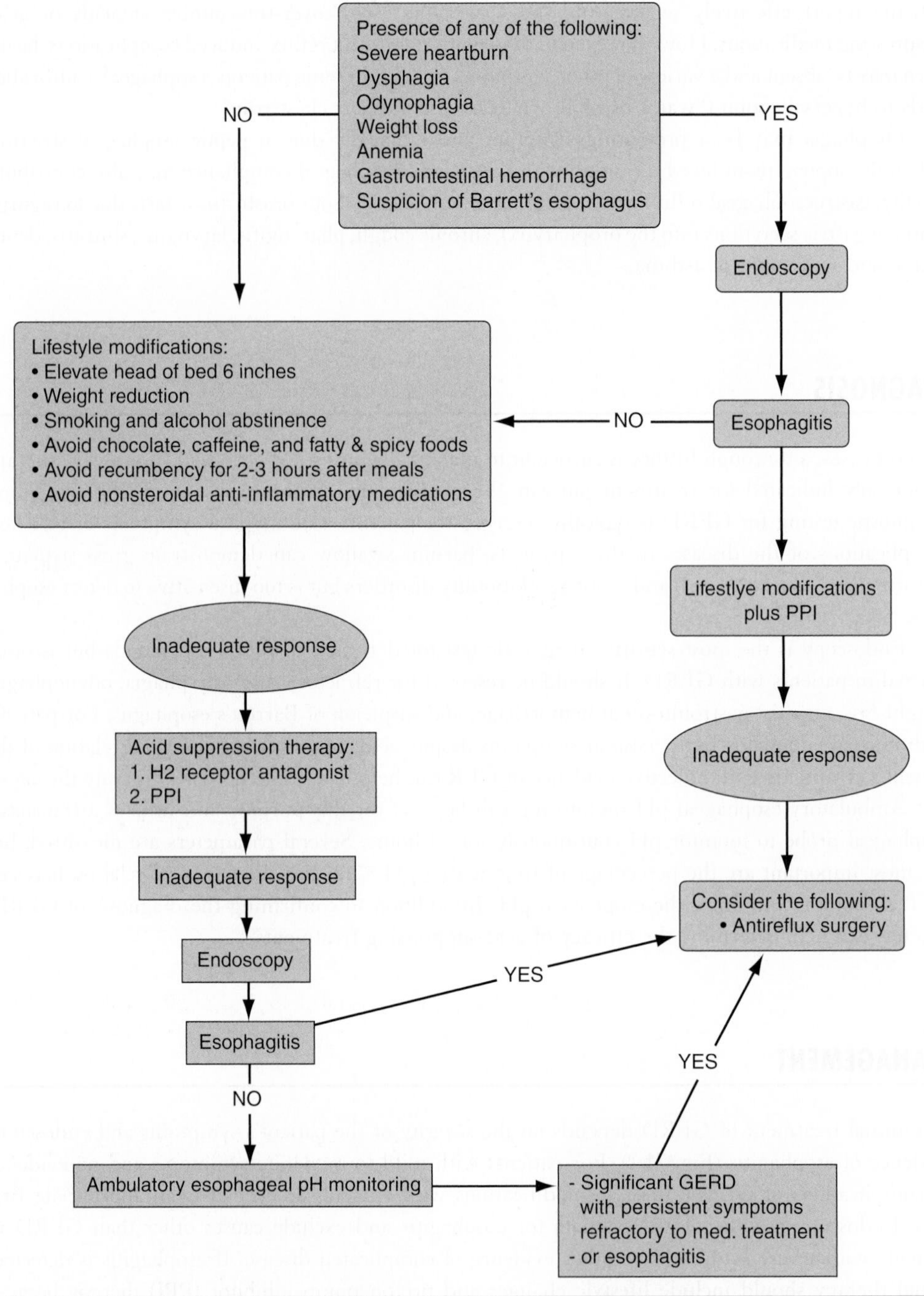

Figure 71.1 • Management of gastroesophageal reflux disease. PPI, proton pump inhibitors.

TABLE 71.1 Common complications of gastroesophageal reflux disease
Esophageal ulcers
Esophagitis
Esophageal strictures
Barrett's esophagus (precancerous lesion)

COMPLICATIONS

The reflux of gastric secretions into the esophagus can create several serious complications (Table 71.1). When reflux is particularly severe or mucosal defenses overwhelmed, patients may develop esophageal ulcers with symptoms of chest pain, odynophagia, and hematemesis. With more chronic exposure to acidic gastric contents, esophageal strictures may develop. Most patients with this complication present with slowly progressive dysphagia, although some may present acutely with food impaction. In addition to maximal antireflux therapies, these conditions must be distinguished from esophageal webs, motility disorders, and malignant strictures.

In contrast to esophageal strictures and ulcers, Barrett's esophagus develops asymptomatically and is not reversed by medical therapy for GERD. It is found more commonly in men, whites, tobacco users, and those with longstanding (>5 years) GERD. Representing one of the most serious sequelae of long-standing GERD, Barrett's esophagus is characterized by replacement of the native esophageal squamous epithelium with an abnormal columnar epithelium called *specialized intestinal metaplasia*. Although more resistant to the effects of acid reflux, the abnormal mucosa is prone to dysplasia and adenocarcinoma. The risk of esophageal malignancy is 30 to 50 times that of the general population and requires close endoscopic surveillance in an interval dictated by the degree of dysplasia. Esophagectomy is recommended for high-grade dysplasia, although photodynamic therapy (PDT) has been suggested as an option for poor operative candidates.

CHAPTER 72

Biliary Disorders

Kia Saeian

The biliary disorders described in this chapter include: cholestasis, gallstone disease (cholelithiasis, cholecystitis, choledocholithiasis, and cholangitis), primary biliary cirrhosis, and primary sclerosing cholangitis.

CHOLESTASIS

Etiology

Cholestasis is due to either impaired bile and/or flow. It is most clearly manifested clinically by jaundice, which refers to a yellow appearance of skin and eyes resulting from retention and deposition of excessive bile pigment. Liver test abnormalities are referred to as cholestatic when the alkaline phosphatase and/or bilirubin are elevated out of proportion to the aminotransferases, as opposed to a "hepatitic pattern" in which elevated amino transferases predominate. A mixed cholestatic and hepatitic pattern more likely favors a parenchymal etiology particularly in its resolution phase. The classification of cholestasis into either intra- or extrahepatic types, based on the anatomic location of impairment of bile production or flow, simplifies identification of etiology and helps in determining the diagnosis and planning management. Common causes of cholestasis are presented in Table 72.1.

Clinical Manifestations

Common symptoms of cholestasis are jaundice and pruritus. The latter may precede jaundice and even occur in the absence of hyperbilirubinemia. Hyperlipidemia, xanthomas, and xanthelasma may follow long-standing cholestasis. Other features of cholestasis include acholic stools, due to the lack of bile reaching the duodenum; steatorrhea due to the absence of bile acids in the small bowel; dark urine due to bilirubinuria; osteomalacia and osteoporosis, probably due to several factors, such as impaired vitamin D and calcium absorption from the gut; easy bruising or hemorrhage due to vitamin K malabsorption in the liver; and excoriations from scratching.

Diagnosis

Important elements to elicit in the history include presence of fever, chills, pain, and colic, suggesting mechanical obstruction and cholangitis; current and recent medication use (e.g., antibiotics, anabolic steroids, phenothiazine) suggestive of potential drug-induced liver injury; weight loss suggestive of potential malignancy; prior abdominal or biliary tract surgery; prior diseases clinically associated with cholestasis; and family history. On examination, search for evidence of jaundice, hepatosplenomegaly, an enlarged, palpable gallbladder (Courvoisier's sign), abnormal lymph nodes, and xanthomas.

Once hemolysis has been excluded in a jaundiced patient, the etiology of an elevated bilirubin, particularly when it is predominantly conjugated (or direct) hyperbilirubinemia, is likely to be hepatobiliary disease. The elevation of alkaline phosphatase and mild aminotransferase elevations are the

TABLE 72.1 Common etiologies of cholestasis

Intrahepatic	
Cholestatic	Benign recurrent intrahepatic cholestasis Drug-induced liver injury (e.g., anabolic steroids, chlorpromazine) Graft-versus-host disease Pregnancy Primary biliary cirrhosis (PBC) Sarcoidosis Sepsis
Mixed	Any hepatitis (particularly in resolution phase)
Extrahepatic	
Common bile duct obstruction	Ampullary tumors Cholangiocarcinoma Choledochal cyst Gallstone disease Pancreatic disease (e.g., malignancy, pancreatitis, pseudocyst) Sphincter of Oddi dysfunction Stricture
Other	AIDS cholangiopathy Mirizzi's syndrome Primary sclerosing cholangitis Secondary sclerosing cholangitis

rule. If there is concern as to whether the elevated alkaline phosphatase is from another source (e.g., bone, red blood cells), alkaline phosphatase isoenzymes can be checked. Even in the setting of complete bile duct obstruction, it is unusual to have elevated serum total bilirubin levels above 25 to 30 mg/dL in the absence of parenchymal liver disease and/or renal dysfunction. Interestingly, in acute biliary obstruction, the alanine transaminase is the first enzyme to rise but it then drops quickly, with the alkaline phosphatase and bilirubin rising more gradually.

When the source hyperbilirubinemia and alkaline phosphatase is established to be hepatobiliary, an abdominal ultrasound should be done to determine whether the bile ducts are dilated. The diagnostic differences between computed tomography and ultrasound are shown in Table 72.2. If there is no dilation, intrahepatic etiologies should be pursued (Table 72.1). In the setting of biliary dilation, an evaluation as outlined in Figure 72.1 should be followed. If the ultrasound shows a dilated biliary tree and identifies a distinct or suspicious etiology (e.g., choledocholithiasis), cholangiography via endoscopic retrograde cholangiopancreatography (ERCP) is the next step because it provides therapeutic and tissue biopsy options. If ERCP is not feasible or available, percutaneous transhepatic cholangiography (PTC) by an experienced radiologist should be pursued. If the ultrasound simply demonstrates a dilated biliary system without a distinct etiology, cholangiography by magnetic resonance cholangiopancreatography (MRCP) should be pursued because it has the advantage of being noninvasive although it lacks tissue diagnostic (e.g., brushings of strictures) or therapeutic (e.g., gallstone extraction) capability. Identification of a focal lesion requires further delineation by computed tomography or magnetic resonance imaging and tissue sampling if warranted. If the ultrasound

TABLE 72.2 Diagnosis of cholestasis: computed tomography versus ultrasound examination

Procedure	Advantages	Disadvantages
Ultrasound	Better at detecting gallstones in the gallbladder Accurately measures diameter of common bile duct	Only uncommonly detects gallstones in the common bile duct Less than optimal visualization of pancreatic tumor, cyst, etc.
Computed tomography	Better visualization of pancreas	Poor sensitivity for detecting gallstones within gallbladder or common bile duct

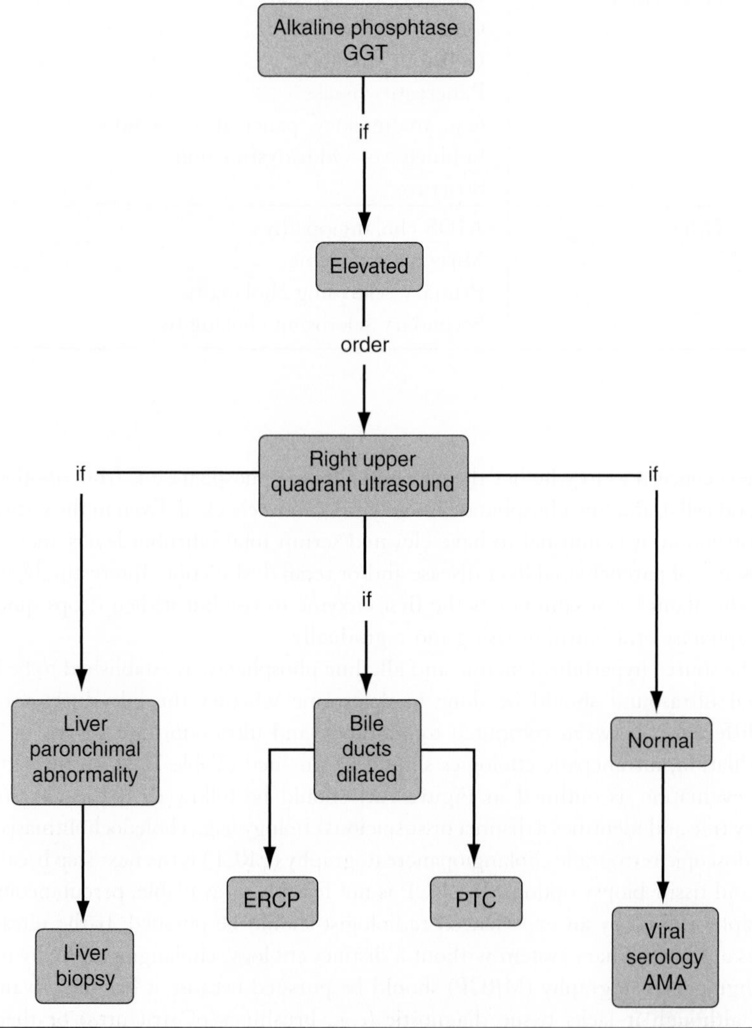

Figure 72.1 • Evaluation of elevated gamma glutamyl transferase and alkaline phosphatase. ERCP, endoscopic retrograde cholangiopancreatography; PTC, percutaneous cholangiography.

reveals a nondilated biliary system and no distinct etiology, evaluation for parenchymal liver disease (including possibly a liver biopsy) should be pursued.

Treatment

Treatment of cholestasis is aimed at the cure of the causative disorder.

GALLSTONE DISEASE

Gallstone disease afflicts 10% of Americans and is a common cause of extrahepatic cholestasis. It is more prevalent in women (about twice as common) and shows an increasing incidence with age, with up to 30% over the age of 50 years having gallstones. There appears to be a genetic predisposition, with first-degree relatives of patients with gallstone disease 4.5 times more likely to develop gallstones than controls. Certain populations including Amerindian populations of North America, Bolivia, and Chile as well as Scandinavians represent higher risk groups. Other predisposing factors are obesity, rapid weight loss, medications, and administration of total parenteral nutrition (Table 72.3).

Gallstone disease may manifest itself by cholelithiasis, acute cholecystitis, choledocholithiasis, or cholangitis.

Cholelithiasis

Although cholelithiasis is commonly encountered, only a minority of these cases result in symptomatic disease and even a smaller minority develop complications requiring intervention. In the United States and most Western countries, cholesterol gallstones predominate, whereas pigment stones account for only about 20% of gallstones.

ETIOLOGY

Cholesterol gallstones are generally large, yellow, and are characterized by cholesterol being either the only or major constituent. Cholesterol gallstone formation is caused by an excess of cholesterol in relation to phospholipids and bile acids. Cholesterol needs to be in equilibrium with phospholipids and bile acids in order to be soluble within the aqueous environment of micelles or vesicles. Therefore, an increased secretion of cholesterol or a decrease in bile acids (due to terminal ileal disease or use of cholestyramine) or reduced levels of phospholipids leads to cholesterol supersaturation and subsequent stone formation.

TABLE 72.3 Risk factors for gallstones
Advancing age
Amerindian ethnicity
White race
Female sex
Medications (estrogens, ceftriaxone, clofibrate, octreotide)
Obesity
Pregnancy
Rapid weight loss
Terminal ileal disease (e.g., Crohn's disease)
Total parenteral nutrition

Pigment stones contain less than 25% cholesterol, appear either brown or black, and are radio-opaque. Black stones have a high calcium bilirubinate concentration and are more often seen in chronic hemolytic state and cirrhosis. Brown stones consist of unconjugated bilirubin calcium salts, form due to chronic infection, and are seen in patients with chronically obstructed bile ducts, such as those with benign strictures or primary sclerosing cholangitis. Pigment stones predominate in the tropics and Southeast Asia where recurrent infectious cholangitis leads to oriental cholangiopathy.

CLINICAL MANIFESTATIONS

Poorly localized episodic right upper quadrant or epigastric pain often associated with nausea and occurring after ingestion of a meal is the typical picture of a patient with symptomatic gallstones. Symptoms from gallstones have a high rate of recurrence. The majority of patients with gallstones, however, are asymptomatic. In fact, most gallstones are detected incidentally during radiological evaluation of the abdomen.

Some gallstones do become symptomatic through a simple mechanism such as migration via the cystic duct and impaction within the common bile duct, resulting in choledocholithiasis, or through an as-yet unclear mechanism in acute or chronic cholecystitis. There is a small group of patients with biliary dyskinesia who may not have gallstones but are symptomatic due to inadequate contractility of the gallbladder.

DIAGNOSIS

In the setting of episodic postprandial, right upper quadrant pain with or without nausea, the diagnosis of cholelithiasis should be strongly considered. In the absence of cholecystitis, there may be no pain or only mild right upper quadrant tenderness to palpation. Because only 10% to 15% of gallstones, mostly pigment stones, are radio-opaque, plain abdominal radiographs are of low yield in identifying gallstones. Ultrasound is the examination of choice, has high reliability, and is particularly accurate in detecting gallstones in the gallbladder. Oral cholecystography, which requires reliable ingestion and normal absorption of the contrast medium, a healthy liver, and a patent cystic duct, is no longer used clinically. Computed tomography scans are not as reliable in identifying gallstones. Both MRCP and ERCP have excellent sensitivity for detecting gallstones but are typically reserved for identifying choledocholithiasis.

TREATMENT

The patient's age and concomitant health problems weigh heavily in the decision on appropriate therapy. In patients with asymptomatic gallstones, the cumulative probability of symptoms developing is about 10% at 5 years and no greater than 20% at 15 to 20 years. In most patients, biliary symptoms precede the onset of complications. Thus, cholecystectomy is not indicated in the asymptomatic patient. A previously practiced dictum that diabetics with asymptomatic gallstones should undergo prophylactic cholecystectomy is *not* supported by more recent data. Certain subgroups such as Native Americans, the morbidly obese, and heart and/or lung transplant recipients are at higher risk for biliary disease and its complications and should thus undergo prophylactic cholecystectomy if possible. Patients with symptomatic gallstones, even in the absence of current symptoms or one of the feared complications (e.g., cholecystitis, cholangitis, choledocholithiasis), should be considered for cholecystectomy, the most effective treatment for cholelithiasis. The introduction of laparoscopic technique for cholecystectomy has revolutionized management of cholelithiasis. Because it avoids a formal laparotomy, it minimizes hospital stay, recovery time, and provides a significant savings. Those with prior abdominal operations may not be candidates. In those with significant comorbidities and/or advanced age, it may be reasonable to avoid cholecystectomy even in the presence of significant symptoms.

Oral dissolution of cholesterol gallstones with ursodeoxycholic acid in selected patients supersaturates the bile acid pool, diminishes lithogenicity, and provides an attractive option for patients who are not operative candidates for cholecystectomy. However, such medical treatment has a high rate of recurrence and requires lifelong administration. Another option is extracorporeal shockwave lithotripsy (ESWL), which delivers high-pressure sound waves focused directly on the gallstones. The requirements are similar to those of oral dissolution therapy with the exception that ESWL may be used with stones up to 2 cm in size. Concomitant dissolution therapy with ursodeoxycholic acid is employed.

COMPLICATIONS

A complication of gallstone disease may be formation of biliary-enteric fistula due to chronic inflammation from long-standing cholelithiasis, with formation of adhesions from the duodenum or the colon at the hepatic flexure to the gallbladder. This condition has no characteristic clinical picture, but patients may present with symptoms of biliary colic or signs of cholecystitis or cholangitis. A plain abdominal radiograph may reveal air in the biliary tree (pneumobilia). Another complication is gallstone ileus, which is caused by the erosion of a gallstone into the intestinal tract with subsequent mechanical obstruction.

Acute Cholecystitis

ETIOLOGY

Cholecystitis is inflammation of the gallbladder wall. Most cases of acute cholecystitis result from impaction of a gallstone in the cystic duct obstructing outflow from the gallbladder.

CLINICAL MANIFESTATIONS

A typical attack of cholecystitis is discrete episode of abdominal pain, which may initially be located in the epigastrium or in the right upper quadrant, is sudden in onset, often occurs at night, and lasts hours to days. The patient may report a history of prior similar episodes. The pain is generally not positional, may be worsened by deep inspiration, and may be accompanied by nausea and vomiting. As cholecystitis progresses, the pain almost universally localizes in the right upper quadrant and may radiate to the shoulder and the right scapular area. Care must be taken to differentiate acute cholecystitis from the myriad other upper abdominal disorders it may mimic, including a perforated or penetrating peptic ulcer, acute pancreatitis, hepatitis, myocardial infarction, pneumonia, and right-sided pyelonephritis.

DIAGNOSIS

The diagnosis can often be made based on the above historical findings plus a suggestive examination. Tenderness to palpation in the right upper quadrant with inspiration (Murphy's sign) and an impression of a palpable mass should be sought on examination. In more advanced stages, signs of peritoneal irritation are noted. Fever and leukocytosis are common. Ultrasonography accurately detects cholelithiasis, and when gallbladder wall thickening is present in the right clinical setting, no further studies are required. False positives may be noted in patients with hypoalbuminemia who commonly exhibit thickened gallbladder walls in the absence of cholecystitis. If further confirmation is required, the hepatic dimethyl iminodiacetic acid scan is extremely sensitive and should be the next diagnostic test. In this test, the radiolabeled agent is administered intravenously, is taken up by hepatocytes, and excreted into the biliary tree. When imaged in the setting of an obstructed cystic duct, the radiolabeled agent is visualized in the biliary tree and the duodenum but fails to fill the gallbladder, signifying the presence of cholecystitis. However, total bilirubin levels over approximately 20 mg/dL do not allow for adequate excretion by the hepatocytes and preclude valid interpretation of this test.

TREATMENT

Patients with acute cholecystitis should be hospitalized, provided with analgesia and intravenous hydration, and evaluated by an appropriate surgeon. Most patients are also treated with antibiotics, particularly in the presence of fever and leukocytosis. Cholecystectomy usually is performed during the same admission and urgently if the patient is toxic. Cultures of the gallbladder and bile are positive in at least one half of patients with acute cholecystitis at surgery. The most common organisms are aerobic coliforms, streptococci, clostridia, and bacteroides. If there is concomitant choledocholithiasis, particularly in the setting of fever and leukocytosis, a preoperative ERCP with removal of the stone and probable endoscopic biliary sphincterotomy is warranted.

Choledocholithiasis and Cholangitis

ETIOLOGY

Choledocholithiasis is the presence and often obstruction of the bile duct by a stone that has typically migrated from the gallbladder via the cystic duct into the common bile duct. The stone may acutely obstruct the common bile duct with resultant jaundice, liver enzyme elevations, and/or acute pancreatitis. In Asian and African countries, where calcium bilirubinate stones predominate, many common bile duct stones arise not only in the gallbladder, but also primarily in intra- and extrahepatic portions of the biliary tract (hepatolithiasis). When there is concomitant infection due to the complete or partial obstruction, ascending cholangitis is encountered.

CLINICAL MANIFESTATIONS

Bile duct stones produce biliary colic with nausea and vomiting. However, 20% of patients with bile duct stones have no pain, and 25% to 30% of patients have no jaundice. Thus choledocholithiasis may occur in the absence of pain, jaundice, or any other symptoms. The pain from choledocholithiasis is typically epigastric rather than in the right upper quadrant. It differs from the pain of acute pancreatitis in that it typically does not radiate to the back. Charcot's triad of right upper quadrant pain, jaundice, and fever when accompanied by mental status changes and renal insufficiency is called Raynaud's pentad and indicates worsening cholangitis and more severe disease, requiring urgent decompression preferably by ERCP.

DIAGNOSIS

Elevated serum alkaline phosphatase and mild hyperbilirubinemia are the most characteristic laboratory abnormalities. Leukocytosis is common; bacteremia due to enteric organisms may occur. Plain abdominal radiographs may show an ileus and, uncommonly, gallbladder stones. Ultrasonography usually shows biliary tract dilation, but this finding may be absent in the early phase of obstruction. Small common bile duct stones may be missed on ultrasound. Both MRCP and ERCP have excellent sensitivity for detection of common bile duct stones. If the diagnosis is in question and there is no evidence of cholangitis, MRCP can be employed to document the presence of choledocholithiasis. If there is evidence of cholangitis in the proper clinical setting, even in the absence of common bile duct stones on ultrasound, ERCP should be employed as it also is the therapeutic modality of choice.

TREATMENT

Patients with symptomatic common duct stones should be treated with intravenous antibiotics, fluids, analgesics, and urgent decompression should be sought if there is any evidence of cholangitis. As soon as the patient has been stabilized, ERCP should follow to establish a diagnosis and to extract the gallstones. Following recovery, the patient should also undergo a laparoscopic cholecystectomy unless advanced age or comorbidities preclude this. If the common bile duct stones cannot be removed by ERCP, open cholecystectomy and common bile duct exploration is typically required, although skilled laparoscopic surgeons may attempt laparoscopic cholecystectomy and address the common bile duct stones laparoscopically via choledochoscopy.

COMPLICATIONS

In the setting of choledocholithiasis, the occurrence of high fevers and sepsis (Chapter 59) suggests the diagnosis of ascending cholangitis, which requires rapid diagnosis, resuscitation, and intervention.

PRIMARY BILIARY CIRRHOSIS

Primary biliary cirrhosis (PBC) is a destructive cholangiopathy that results in nonsuppurative inflammation and subsequent destruction of both small- and medium-sized bile ducts. In spite of its name, cirrhosis is not invariably present at diagnosis, and the rate of progression is quite variable. There is a strong female predominance (10:1) and the median age is approximately 50 years at the time of diagnosis. The prevalence of PBC is between 20 and 240 cases per 1 million population and appears to be highest in northern Europe, although no clear racial predominance exists.

Clinical Manifestations

Patients often are diagnosed at the presymptomatic stage based on a finding of elevated liver enzymes. Typically, alkaline phosphatase is elevated three- or fourfold, with mild elevation of the aminotransferases. The bilirubin may be normal in early disease but is an extremely useful marker of disease progression. Approximately two thirds of patients with PBC complain of fatigue, whereas only 10% of patients are jaundiced at presentation. Pruritus also is a common complaint. Osteopenia, hypercholesterolemia manifested by xanthomas (cholesterol deposits in elbows, palms, soles), xanthelasma (cholesterol deposits in periorbitol area), as well as steatorrhea, also may be encountered. Portal hypertensive bleeding may occur in the absence of cirrhosis due to presinusoidal portal hypertension. This bleeding is believed to result from obliteration of portal venules by regenerative nodules.

Diagnosis

Positive serum antimitochondrial antibody (AMA) at a titer of 1:40 or higher is highly specific for PBC and has a sensitivity of about 95%. The AMA appears to be directed against the E2 antigen of the pyruvate dehydrogenase complex on the internal mitochondrial membrane. An elevated serum quantitative immunoglobulin M level helps confirm the diagnosis. Liver histology reveals inflammatory cells infiltrating the interlobular and septal bile ducts. Granulomas, the classic florid duct lesion, and ductular proliferation may be seen.

Treatment

If PBC is untreated, cirrhosis typically follows in 15 to 20 years after initial diagnosis. An elevated serum bilirubin level, advanced age, a low albumin, elevated prothrombin time, and edema have been associated with a worse prognosis. Treatment with ursodeoxycholic acid, 13 to 15 mg/kg, has been shown to improve transplant-free survival in patients with moderate to severe PBC. The only long-term cure appears to be liver transplantation, which has excellent results.

PRIMARY SCLEROSING CHOLANGITIS

Etiology

Primary sclerosing cholangitis (PSC) is a chronic inflammatory condition of the intrahepatic and extrahepatic biliary system associated with inflammatory bowel disease. Although genetic predisposition and immunologic factors are believed to play a role, the exact etiology of PSC is unknown. Approximately 60% to 70% of all patients with PSC have inflammatory bowel disease, but only 5% to 7.5% of inflammatory bowel disease patients develop PSC. The severity of one disease does not necessarily affect the development or progression of the other.

Clinical Manifestations

Patients often present in the third decade of life and are predominantly men. Laboratory tests show cholestasis with a marked elevation of alkaline phosphatase. Hypergammaglobulinemia, positive p-ANCA, and mildly elevated aminotransferases may be seen.

DIAGNOSIS

Diagnosis is made based on cholangiography (ERCP, MRCP, or PTC) revealing strictures with intervening areas of normal-appearing bile ducts and a beaded appearance. Dominant strictures are found in a minority of patients.

Liver biopsy findings range from portal inflammation to progressive fibrosis and eventual disappearance of bile ducts and cirrhosis. The classic "onion-skin" lesion is seen in approximately 40% of biopsies. Primary sclerosing cholangitis is a progressive disease, with a mean survival ranging from 11 to 17 years after diagnosis.

PSC has a number of unique complications, including cholelithiasis and choledocholithiasis, as well as cholangiocarcinoma, which is difficult to detect and even more difficult to treat.

Treatment

Therapy for PSC involves symptomatic treatment and management of complications. Cholestyramine is the first-line agent for treatment of pruritus. Antihistamines, ursodeoxycholic acid, and rifampin are used for refractory patients. Replacement of fat-soluble vitamins and aggressive monitoring and treatment of bone disease are required. Endoscopic dilation of dominant strictures may be helpful in a minority of patients, but unnecessary biliary intervention should be avoided because of the high risk of cholangitis. Because of the diffuse nature of most strictures, biliary surgery is successful in the minority of patients with isolated extrahepatic disease. There are no satisfactory long-term medical, endoscopic, or nontransplant surgical options for most patients with PSC.

Surveillance for cholangiocarcinoma is suboptimal because biliary brushings and biopsies miss 30% to 50% of lesions, and other potential tools, such as serum CA 19-9, have not been found to be reliable. Surveillance for colonic dysplasia should not be neglected in patients with associated inflammatory bowel disease, regardless of the course of PSC. Liver transplantation provides the only means of long-term survival in patients with end-stage liver disease.

CHAPTER 73

Hepatitis

Kia Saeian

Hepatitis is inflammation of liver parenchyma resulting from numerous causes including viral infection, toxic injury (e.g., alcohol), drug-induced (e.g., acetaminophen), immunologic (e.g., autoimmune hepatitis), or metabolic (e.g., hemochromatosis or fatty liver).

Acute hepatitis typically presents with nonspecific systemic manifestations, including anorexia, nausea, vomiting, abdominal pain, and arthralgias. Jaundice is not necessarily present and patients may even be asymptomatic (Table 73.1).

Chronic hepatitis is a clinical syndrome, with chronic liver inflammation leading to necrosis and possibly progressing to fibrosis, cirrhosis, and liver failure. Prolonged enzyme elevations for at least 6 months along with compatible liver biopsy findings are essential for diagnosis and classification. Biopsy findings of chronic hepatitis include portal inflammation and interface hepatitis, with the histologic classification system including grading (the amount of inflammation) and staging (the degree of fibrosis). Chronic hepatitis develops in patients with hepatitis B and hepatitis C viruses but is not seen with the other viral hepatitides.

VIRAL HEPATITIS

Besides the six identified hepatitis viruses classified as A, B, C, D, E, and G, although hepatitis G is no longer felt to be a cause of significant disease. A number of other viruses, including the Epstein-Barr virus, herpes simplex virus, cytomegalovirus, parvovirus B19, TT virus, and adenovirus, also may cause acute hepatitis. Viral hepatitis has a wide range of presentation, from subclinical infection to fulminant hepatic failure (FHF).

Hepatitis A

Hepatitis A virus (HAV) is an RNA virus transmitted via the oral-fecal route and is the most common identified cause of infectious hepatitis. Infection is followed by an incubation period of about 30 days. The virus is detectable in stool from 2 weeks before the onset of jaundice and up to 8 days thereafter. Transmission may occur by person-to-person contact or ingestion of contaminated food. Uncooked shellfish is a particularly frequent culprit. Certain parts of the world, including Eastern Europe, Russia, Africa, the Middle East, and parts of South America, are areas of high endemicity where immunity before the age of 10 years is nearly universal.

CLINICAL MANIFESTATIONS

Patients younger than 4 years of age often are anicteric, 40% to 70% of those older than 15 years of age develop jaundice, and about 85% of patients have nonspecific symptoms. When jaundice develops, it resolves within 2 weeks in 85%. Interestingly, cigarette smokers tend to lose interest in smoking. Examination in most reveals tender hepatomegaly, splenomegaly in a small percentage, rash, and lymphadenopathy. A minority (<10%) develop a relapsing course that may lead to prolonged cholestasis. Patients with sickle cell disease are more susceptible to this particular pattern. Extrahepatic manifestations include immune-complex mediated glomerulonephritis, vasculitis, and other autoim-

TABLE 73.1 Causes of acute hepatitis

Viral hepatitis
Hepatitis A, B, C, D, E*
Epstein-Barr virus
Cytomegalovirus
Mumps
Parvovirus B19
Herpes simplex virus
Noninfectious hepatitis
Alcohol
Medications
Autoimmune
Wilson's disease
Toxins (mushroom poisoning)

*Hepatitis G is not associated with active disease.

mune phenomena. Mortality is rare among young patients, but rates as high as 1% to 2% have been reported in those over the age of 40 years. Concomitant liver disease and pregnancy appear to result in more severe disease.

DIAGNOSIS

Aminotransferases are elevated, beginning in the prodromal phase, and normalize in most patients by 2 months, although 15% of patients have persistent elevations for approximately 6 months. Diagnosis of acute infection is confirmed by detection of immunoglobulin (Ig) M anti-HAV antibody, which becomes undetectable in approximately 75% of patients at 6 months. A positive IgG anti-HAV antibody reflects resolved prior infection immunity or from vaccination. Although rarely indicated, liver biopsy findings include spotty necrosis with portal and periportal inflammation.

TREATMENT

Management consists of supportive measures with treatment of symptoms. Contrary to earlier belief, bedrest does not accelerate recovery and early ambulation should be encouraged. The great majority of patients do not require hospitalization, with the exception of those with severe or persistent anorexia, mental status changes, or coagulopathy. No specific medications are indicated for treatment of acute hepatitis A. Corticosteroid therapy may be useful in accelerating resolution of the prolonged cholestatic phase. Prevention of infection is possible via passive immunization and vaccination. Passive immunization is the method of choice for postexposure prophylaxis because immunity develops within 3 to 5 days and lasts up to 3 months. The inactivated vaccine confers immunity for at least 5 to 10 years and consists of a sequence of two injections, although some clinicians advocate a third dose to lengthen the duration of protection.

Hepatitis B

The hepatitis B virus (HBV), a double-stranded DNA virus, remains the leading cause of chronic hepatitis, with 350 million infected individuals worldwide and some 1.25 million infected individuals in the United States. In the United States, HBV is largely a disease of adulthood and is associated with parenteral and sexual exposures.

CLINICAL MANIFESTATIONS

Once an adult is infected by HBV, the outcome is variable, with the majority (about 65% to 70%) developing a subclinical, transient hepatitis followed by development of lifelong immunity, indicated by the presence of hepatitis B surface antibody (HbsAb). Another 25% develop overt hepatitis but still develop lifelong immunity and HbsAb. In contrast to neonates, approximately 90% of whom develop chronic hepatitis B infection, only about 5% of adults develop chronicity. Approximately 1% of patients develop fulminant acute hepatitis B, which has a high mortality.

DIAGNOSIS

All patients with chronic infection are at higher risk for development of hepatocellular carcinoma, although the risk is variable depending on disease activity. In the United States, HBV currently accounts for 10% to 15% of hepatocellular carcinomas and 5% to 10% of cases of end-stage liver disease. A positive hepatitis B core IgM antibody (HBcAb IgM) test indicates acute infection (Table 73.2). Among those with chronic infection, a subgroup (the so-called healthy carriers) exhibits *only* hepatitis B surface antigen (HBsAg); others with more active viral replication exhibit hepatitis B e antigen (HBeAg) and/or hepatitis B viral DNA (those with chronic active infection). "Healthy carriers" also exhibit hepatitis B e antibody (HBeAb), which indicates less viral replication. The presence of hepatitis B surface antibody (HBsAb) indicates immunity.

TREATMENT

Therapy for acute HBV infection consists of supportive measures with liver transplantation an option for fulminant hepatic failure. Treatment of chronic hepatitis B is typically reserved for those with a viral DNA load of $>10^5$ copies/ml and/or those with advanced histologic disease. Medical therapy includes interferon or nucleoside analogs such as lamivudine, adefovir, or entecavir. Treatment with interferon-based therapy has the advantage of a limited course as well as the potential of HBsAb seroconversion, but is less often employed than nucleoside analogues because of its side effects (leucopenia, thrombocytopenia) and lack of response in those patients with higher viral loads.

Acute exposure to HBV should be treated with hepatitis B immunoglobulin and vaccination unless immunity is already established.

TABLE 73.2 Hepatitis B virus markers

	Anti-HBc Total	Anti-HBc IgM	HBsAg	Anti-HBs	HBeAg	Anti-HBe	HBV DNA
Acute hepatitis B	(+)	(+)	(+)	(−)	(+)	(−)	(+)
Vaccinated for hepatitis B	(−)	(−)	(−)	(+)	(−)	(−)	(−)
Prior hepatitis B exposure: immune	(+)	(−)	(−)	(+)	(−)	(+)	(−)
Chronic hepatitis B: "healthy carrier"	(+)	(−)	(+)	(−)	(−)	(+)	(+)/(−)
Chronic hepatitis B: active replication	(+)	(+)/(−)	(+)	(−)	(+)	(−)	(+)

Hepatitis C

ETIOLOGY

Hepatitis C virus (HCV), a single-stranded RNA virus, typically is transmitted parenterally, and accounts for approximately 20% of cases of acute viral hepatitis. The two most common genotypes in the United States are 1a and 1b.

CLINICAL MANIFESTATIONS

The incubation period of HCV is 7 to 8 weeks. Acute HCV may present with nonspecific symptoms such as fatigue and malaise, and leads to jaundice in only 21% of patients. The acute hepatitis rarely is fulminant, but does lead to chronic infection in 55% to 85% of patients depending on the patient's immunologic competence. HCV is the most common cause of chronic hepatitis in the United States. Although many people with chronic HCV are asymptomatic, an estimated 25% develop cirrhosis over a span of 25 years. Factors that might promote progression to more aggressive disease include high viral load, viral genotype, 1a/1b, male gender, concomitant alcohol use, and viral coinfection. Each year, hepatocellular carcinoma develops in 1% to 3% of patients with cirrhosis due to HCV. End-stage liver disease from HCV is now the most frequent indication for liver transplantation in the United States.

DIAGNOSIS

Antibody to HCV (anti-HCV) may be detectable by the time of or up to 8 weeks after the onset of symptoms. Unfortunately, this antibody is not protective. Serologically, acute HCV can be diagnosed by the presence of HCV RNA in the serum as early as 10 days after exposure, well before the onset of alanine aminotransferase (ALT) elevation or symptoms. Once chronic HCV infection is documented, a liver biopsy is the procedure of choice in assessing the severity of the disease and determining prognosis.

TREATMENT

Routine specific treatment of acute HCV is effective, but waiting at least 3 months to determine whether chronicity develops is prudent. The best currently available therapy for chronic hepatitis C is combination therapy with alpha-interferon and the oral nucleoside analogue ribavirin (41% response rate after 48 weeks of therapy). Ribavirin is relatively well tolerated, except for most common side effect of hemolytic anemia.

No vaccine is available for HCV and immunoglobulin is *not* protective. HCV universally recurs after liver transplantation. Patients with chronic HCV, particularly those with cirrhosis, should be vaccinated against hepatitis A and B viruses.

Hepatitis D

Hepatitis D virus (HDV) is a single-stranded RNA virus that requires the presence of HBV for complete virion assembly and secretion. HDV always occurs in association with either acute or chronic HBV infection. Interestingly, in chronic HDV infection, HBV activity is suppressed. Although reported worldwide, HDV appears most frequently in the Mediterranean basin.

Diagnosis of acute HDV infection is signaled by the presence of IgM anti-HDV, although this may be transient and a positive IgG anti-HDV may be the only sign of recent infection. New polymerase chain reaction (PCR) assays for HDV RNA are available.

Management of HDV infection is similar to that of the underlying HBV infection, with alpha-interferon as the only currently approved treatment choice. Nucleoside analogues are also preventive measures, directed at prevention and eradication of HBV.

Hepatitis E

Hepatitis E virus (HEV), previously called *epidemic non-A, non-B hepatitis*, is an RNA virus most often seen in India, the Far East, the Middle East, and parts of Latin America.

CLINICAL MANIFESTATIONS

The hepatitis E virus has been associated with the largest epidemics of infectious hepatitis in the world. Transmission, symptoms, and overall clinical presentation resemble that of acute hepatitis A infection with jaundice and tender hepatomegaly. The overall fatality rate appears somewhat higher than HAV and is particularly high in pregnant women in the second and third trimester. A cholestatic picture with elevated alkaline phosphatase phase is more common than hepatitis A. Another pattern of clinical presentation characterized by ascites and other signs of FHF without encephalopathy also has been reported. Finally, chronicity is not seen with HEV.

DIAGNOSIS

A positive IgM anti-HEV confirms the diagnosis and may be positive as early as 4 days after onset of symptoms. Liver histology is indistinguishable from hepatitis A virus infection. Abnormal aminotransferases normalize over a 6-week period.

TREATMENT

As with HAV infection, management consists of supportive measures.

AUTOIMMUNE HEPATITIS

Autoimmune hepatitis (AIH) is defined as a chronic periportal hepatitis associated with hypergammaglobulinemia, positive serum autoantibodies, and absence of viral hepatitis and other causes of chronic liver disease. Autoimmune hepatitis is a rare disorder, with an incidence currently reported as 50 to 200 cases per 1 million persons in white populations. There is a female predominance with AIH, and an association with human leukocyte antigen DR3 and DR4 alleles has been noted. Approximately 70% of patients are women, with the peak incidence between 16 and 30 years of age.

Etiology

Autoimmune hepatitis is categorized into three types (I, II, III) based on the presence of specific autoantibodies.

Clinical Manifestations

About one half of patients with AIH present with acute hepatitis characterized by jaundice, nausea, vomiting, and tender hepatomegaly. Acute liver failure occasionally may be the initial manifestation. About 25% of patients present with already established cirrhosis at the time of diagnosis and suffer from its concomitant complications. Patients with AIH have an increased risk of developing hepatocellular carcinoma.

Approximately one half of patients have other coexisting autoimmune disorders. Autoimmune syndromes commonly associated with AIH include autoimmune thyroiditis, vitiligo, rheumatoid arthritis, diabetes mellitus, and ulcerative colitis. Other syndromes overlapping with autoimmune liver disease, such as primary biliary cirrhosis and primary sclerosing cholangitis, also have been reported.

Diagnosis

Marked elevation of aspartate aminotransferase (AST) and ALT is commonly present and a high level serum IgG is also found (presenting 97% of patients with type 1). However, there is no single test that documents the presence of AIH, so the diagnosis may be difficult.

Autoimmune hepatitis is categorized into three types based on the autoantibody profile. High titers of positive antinuclear antibody (ANA) or antismooth muscle antibodies (ASMA) define type 1

AIH; anti liver-kidney microsomal autoantibodies (anti-LKM) define type 2 AIH; and autoantibodies against soluble liver antigens (anti-SLA) define type 3. Biopsy findings are similar to that of hepatitis A, except for the predominance of plasma cell infiltration.

Treatment

The level of inflammation initially present, largely determines the natural history of AIH. Without treatment, the 10-year mortality of patients with a 10-fold elevation of aminotransferases and two-fold elevated IgG levels is 90%. Treatment usually is with corticosteroids alone or in combination with azathioprine. Patients need to be treated for at least 12 months.

ALCOHOLIC HEPATITIS

Alcohol remains the leading cause of cirrhosis in the Western world and causes a spectrum of disease ranging from fatty liver to alcoholic hepatitis and cirrhosis.

Etiology

For the average person, consumption of approximately 40 g of alcohol per day is required for development of alcoholic cirrhosis. One glass of wine, a half-pint of beer, or a shot glass of liquor contains approximately 7 g of alcohol. Lifelong alcoholics have a 20% to 30% risk of developing cirrhosis. Patients with underlying or concomitant liver disease are more susceptible to developing alcoholic liver disease, even with ingestion of smaller amounts of alcohol. Decreased fatty acid oxidation, increased triglyceride synthesis, and generation of acetaldehyde lead to a dose-related acute swelling of hepatocytes and development of a fatty liver. Stellate cells eventually are activated, resulting in pericellular fibrosis and development of cirrhosis.

Clinical Manifestations

Alcoholic liver disease should be suspected in patients with a history of heavy alcohol use, patients without other evident causes of liver disease, or patients with other complications of alcoholism. The clinical syndrome of acute alcoholic hepatitis has a high mortality of up to 60% in severe cases. There often is no obvious predisposing factor. Alcoholic hepatitis may present with fever, jaundice, anorexia, and hepatomegaly. In patients with alcoholic cirrhosis, stigmata of chronic liver disease such as palmar erythema, gynecomastia, and spider angiomata maybe present. Signs of portal hypertension (ascites, hepatic encephalopathy) may later develop.

Diagnosis

Acute onset of jaundice, fever, and right upper quadrant discomfort, along with markedly elevated bilirubin levels, are encountered in alcoholic hepatitis. An AST:ALT ratio greater than 2, especially one greater than 3 with ALT <300 IU, is highly suggestive. One exception is acute Wilson's disease, which may present with AST/ALT ratio of 4 or greater. The reason for the elevated ratio in alcoholic liver disease is a relative lack of ALT synthesis due to a deficiency of pyridoxal 5′-phosphate in alcoholics. The cardinal histologic features of alcoholic hepatitis include ballooning degeneration, Mallory bodies, and neutrophil infiltration of the parenchyma. Histologic confirmation rarely is required.

Treatment

Cirrhosis may already be present but is not universal in patients with alcoholic hepatitis. Continued alcohol intake has the strongest adverse impact on outcome. The presence of encephalopathy, impaired synthetic function, or variceal hemorrhage also predicts poor outcome. The severity of alcoholic hepatitis may be assessed by the discriminant function (DF), determined by: [4.6 × elongation of prothrombin time (seconds) over baseline] + bilirubin (mg/dL). Values of 32 or higher indicate very severe disease. The DF does not distinguish reversible (pure alcoholic hepatitis) from end-stage liver disease. In patients with an elevated discriminant function score over 32, pure alcoholic hepatitis, and no contraindications (e.g., active infection or gastrointestinal hemorrhage), pentoxifylline (400 mg three times per day) or corticosteroid (prednisone, 40 mg/day) therapy may enhance short-term survival. Alcohol abstinence is required, and management of other complications is similar to that for other forms of liver disease.

DRUG-INDUCED LIVER DISEASE

Etiology

The liver is a major site for biotransformation and metabolism of drugs. Drug-related hepatotoxicity arises from interaction of hepatotoxic medications and their metabolites within hepatocytes. This may be related to intrinsic hepatotoxins or may result from idiosyncratic reactions.

Clinical Manifestations and Diagnosis

The clinical syndromes and histopathology produced by drug-induced liver injury are quite varied and may mimic all known types of hepatobiliary disease. In addition, a single medication may lead to several different histologic findings; for example, methyldopa may lead to hepatitis, cholestasis, or granuloma formation. Although drug-induced liver damage is rare, it does account for 2% to 5% of hospital admissions for jaundice in the United States. Drug-induced fulminant hepatic failure may account for up to 30% of cases of FHF (Table 73.3).

Certain individuals appear to be at higher risk for development of toxicity. Reduced hepatic blood flow, decreased activity of cytochrome enzyme systems, and decreased renal clearance make elderly persons more susceptible to damage from nonsteroidal anti-inflammatory drugs and isoniazid. Obese patients are at increased risk because of prolonged exposure to fat-soluble drugs stored in adipose tissue. Depleted glutathione stores in patients with malnutrition and chronic alcohol use make them susceptible to acetaminophen toxicity (Fig. 73.1). Because of the nonspecific nature of the findings of drug-induced injury, diagnosis may be difficult. A high index of suspicion is required. The onset of illness usually occurs sometime between 4 days and 8 weeks after initial exposure.

TABLE 73.3 Drug-induced liver disease

Medication	Pattern of injury
Isonicotinyl hydrazine Valproic acid Acetaminophen	Hepatitis
Carbamazepine Amiodarone Sulfa drugs	Cholestasis
Phenytoin (Dilantin) Nitrofurantoin	Mixed (hepatitis and cholestasis)

INH, isoniazid.

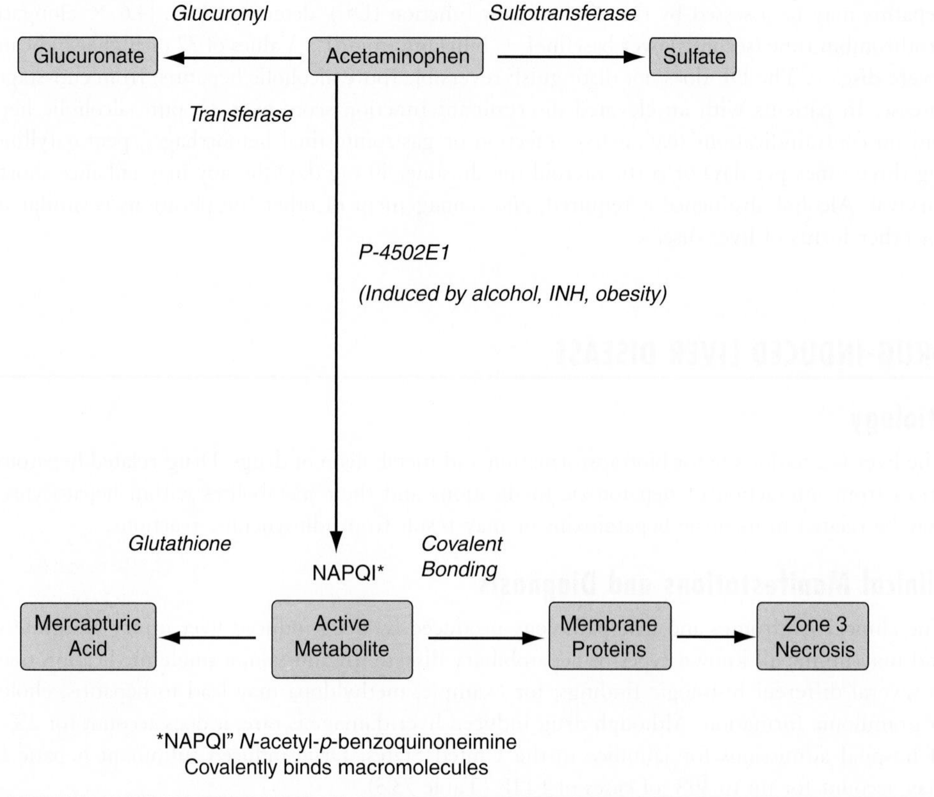

Figure 73.1 • Acetaminophen metabolism pathways.

Treatment

In most cases, improvement occurs after withdrawal of the offending medication. A drug rechallenge should be avoided. In progressive cases, however, liver transplantation may be necessary.

HEMOCHROMATOSIS

Hereditary or genetic hemochromatosis is an autosomal recessive syndrome of iron overload attributed to a defect in the *HFE* gene, which is involved in the metabolism of iron. The *HFE* gene has been identified on the short arm of chromosome 6. Most cases are attributable to a single substitution of tyrosine for cysteine at position 282 (*C282Y*) of the *HFE* gene.

Hemochromatosis should be distinguished from hemosiderosis (sometimes called secondary hemochromatosis), which refers to tissue deposition of iron and may be a consequence of iron loading from repeated transfusions.

Etiology

The defect in the *HFE* gene results in excessive intestinal iron absorption despite elevated iron stores, due to a disruption of intestinal cells. Iron deposition and, eventually, fibrosis occur not only in hepatocytes but also in cardiac tissue, pancreas, endocrine organs, and the kidney.

Clinical Manifestations

The "classic" presentation of a middle-aged man with bronzed skin, diabetes, and hepatomegaly, with or without cirrhosis, is not often seen. Abnormal liver enzymes or elevated iron studies are more common presentations that allow detection in the preclinical phase. Hypogonadotropic hypogonadism due to pituitary iron deposition, chondrocalcinosis (joint calcium pyrophosphate deposition disease [CPPD], also known as pseudogout), and metacarpophalangeal arthritis (particularly of the second and third metacarpals) also are seen. Cardiomyopathy appears to be more common in those who drink alcohol on a regular basis. Women are less affected and typically present at a later age due to the protective effects of menstrual blood loss. Patients who develop cirrhosis are at an extremely high risk for hepatocellular carcinoma

Diagnosis

A diagnostic algorithm is helpful to reach the diagnosis (Fig. 73.2). First, if hemochromatosis is suspected and no known family history of hemochromatosis is present, fasting transferrin saturation should be the first laboratory test. Second, a value greater than 45% to 50% necessitates further evaluation. Thus genetic testing for the *HFE* gene should be undertaken. A genotype result consistent with a homozygous pattern of gene *C282Y* is diagnostic of hereditary hemochromatosis; if the patient is <40 years of age with normal ALT/AST, no further testing is required. However, patients over 40 years of age with elevated AST/ALT are at significant risk for fibrosis and should still undergo biopsy for prognostic and management purposes.

Treatment

The treatment of choice is removal of excess iron stores by weekly phlebotomies. Once significant fibrosis occurs in any organ, the changes are irreversible, although iron depletion may ameliorate the severity. Screening of first-degree relatives of patients with hereditary hemochromatosis should be pursued.

WILSON'S DISEASE

Wilson's disease is a rare autosomal recessive disorder that results from a defect in copper transport. Within the liver, copper is avidly absorbed and eventually binds to the Wilson's disease protein (WDP). Copper bound to WDP is then transported and either inserted into ceruloplasmin or carried to the bile membrane for excretion. In Wilson's disease, a gene defect in chromosome 13 results in a lack of WDP, which then results in accumulation of cytotoxic copper within the liver, central nervous system, and the iris (Kayser-Fleischer rings), as well as low serum ceruloplasmin levels and enhanced urinary copper excretion.

Clinical Manifestations

Wilson's disease has a variety of clinical manifestations (Table 73.4). Approximately one half of the patients present with the liver disease (usually between the ages of 3 and 12 years), whereas the other half present with neurologic or psychiatric symptoms (usually in adolescence and early adulthood). Onset of disease is before the age of 35 years. Liver disease may present with either acute liver failure associated with hemolysis, decompensated cirrhosis, acute hepatitis, or jaundice. A high index of suspicion is required for diagnosis, and Wilson's disease should be suspected in any child or young adult with undiagnosed liver disease. Neurologic manifestations may be difficult to detect. The most common are dystonia and Parkinsonism; psychiatric abnormalities also may be seen and cognitive function initially is intact. Neurologic abnormalities actually may be exacerbated when treatment is initiated. Kayser-Fleischer rings, subtle brown-green discoloration around the periphery of the cornea,

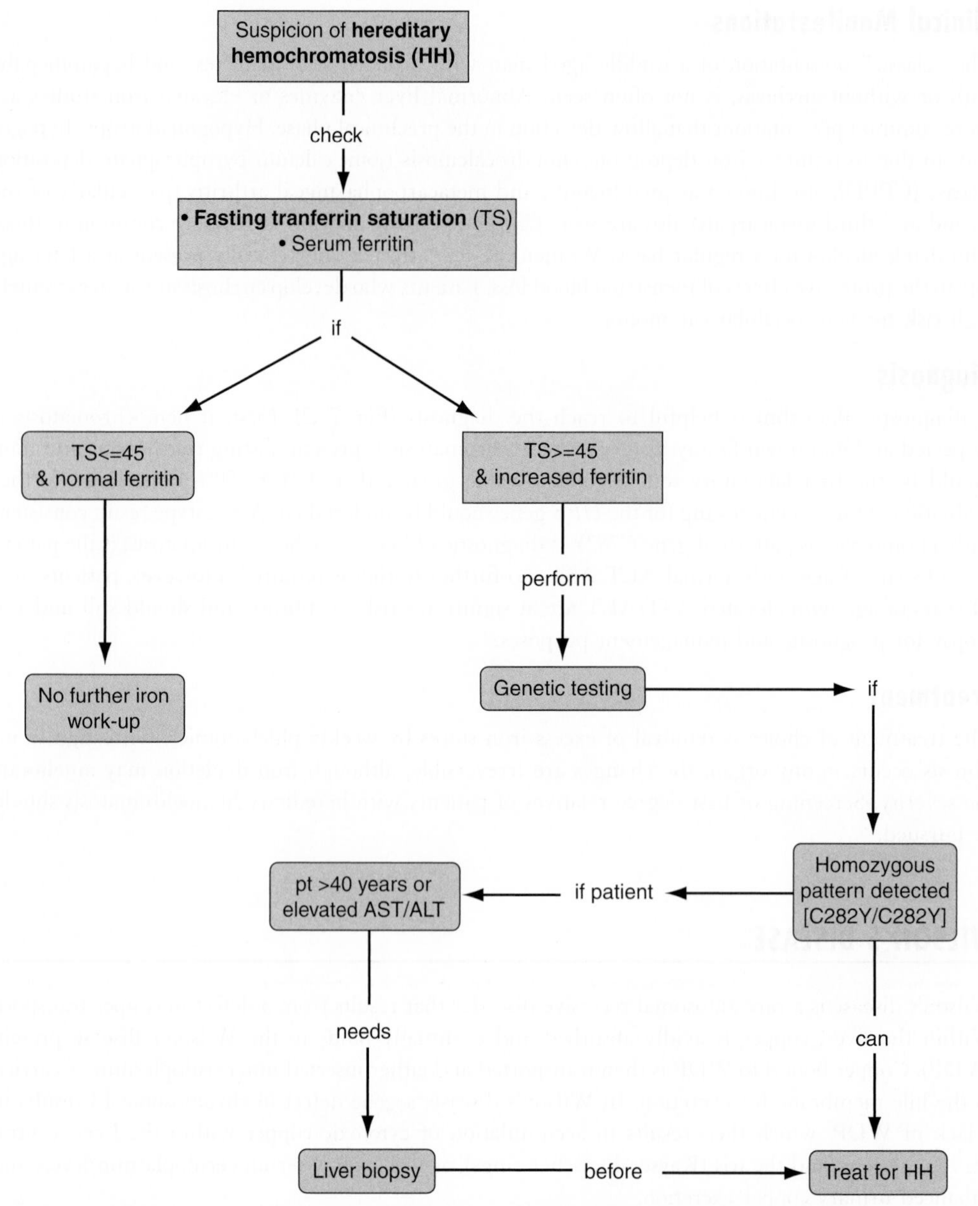

Figure 73.2 • Diagnostic algorithm for hereditary hemochromatosis.

are best seen by slit-lamp examination. They may not be detectable in patients presenting with liver disease but are present almost universally in those presenting with neurologic abnormalities. Renal manifestations include isolated proximal type 2 RTA or Fanconi syndrome. Acute hemolytic anemia, nephrocalcinosis, arthritis, and sunflower cataracts also may be seen (Table 73.4).

Diagnosis

Early diagnosis may prevent potentially lethal outcomes. Liver biopsy and slit-lamp examination should be obtained. Diagnosis requires at least two of the following features: low plasma ceruloplas-

TABLE 73.4 Clinical manifestation of Wilson's disease

Organ or system	Clinical features
Liver	Hepatitis (40%), portal hypertension, and/or cirrhosis
Central nervous system	Tremor, ataxia, rigidity, slurred speech, clumsiness
Psychiatric	Personality disorders, anxiety, irritability
Eye	Kaiser-Fleisher rings (copper deposits iris and cornea), sunflower cataracts (copper deposition in the lens)
Kidney	Isolated proximal type 2 RTA Fanconi syndrome (type 2 RTA, glycosuria, aminoacid-uria, tubular proteinuria)
Hematologic	Hemolytic anemia

min, increased urinary copper concentration, and a hepatic copper concentration greater than 250 g per gram of dry weight. Molecular techniques for genetic diagnosis are not widely available.

Treatment

The first-line treatment is oral penicillamine, which chelates copper, depletes body stores of copper, and enhances urinary copper excretion. Penicillamine may not be tolerated in cases with bone marrow suppression, an urticarial rash, drug-induced lupus, and proteinuria. Zinc also may help by decreasing copper absorption. Certain foods with a particularly high copper concentration, including chocolate, shellfish, and organ meats, should be avoided.

BUDD-CHIARI SYNDROME

Budd-Chiari syndrome is caused by obstruction of the major hepatic veins and thus hepatic venous outflow, characterized by right upper quadrant pain, hepatomegaly, and high-protein-content ascites. Occlusion may be due to myeloproliferative disorders, malignancy, hypercoagulability, oral contraceptive use, pregnancy, and an inferior vena cava "web" or malformation.

Clinical Manifestations

Rapid onset of upper abdominal pain, hepatomegaly, and ascites occurs. The course is commonly progressive, with subsequent cirrhosis or liver failure. The caudate lobe often is markedly enlarged, because its separate drainage into the inferior vena cava provides the only venous outflow for a congested liver. Patients undergoing high-dose chemotherapy and bone marrow transplantation, particularly those with pre-existing liver disease, are susceptible to a similar syndrome called *sinusoidal obstruction syndrome* (previously referred to as veno-occlusive disease).

Diagnosis

Aminotransferases are elevated and coagulopathy may denote progressive liver failure. Ultrasonography with Doppler flow imaging is diagnostic and is the first-line test. Hepatic venography documents extent of occlusion and also permits pressure measurements, which may be imperative in planning surgical intervention.

Treatment

Urgent transplantation is required for FHF or if cirrhosis develops. Treatment of the acute syndrome with thrombolytic agents occasionally is successful within the first few weeks. Decompression of the venous system with portacaval, mesocaval, mesoarial, and splenorenal shunts may be indicated in the absence of cirrhosis. The role of transjugular intrahepatic portosystemic shunting is unclear. Chronic cases with slow progression are treated with supportive measures.

CHAPTER 74

Cirrhosis

José Franco

Cirrhosis indicates progression of hepatic fibrosis to an advanced stage of nodule formation. The term *end-stage liver disease* is erroneously used for cirrhosis, but it truly should be reserved for when complications of cirrhosis such as ascites, hepatic encephalopathy, or variceal bleeding have developed ("decompensated cirrhosis"). Mortality from liver disease is the eighth leading cause of death worldwide, with approximately 800,000 deaths attributed to cirrhosis annually.

One of the earliest events that occurs in patients with cirrhosis is the development of a vasodilated state, which leads to a decrease in the effective circulating volume and an increase in splanchnic blood flow (the sum of blood passing through the liver). The increase in splanchnic blood flow coupled with increased resistance from the intrahepatic fibrosis and nodules leads to portal hypertension (portal pressure greater than 5 mm Hg). Portal hypertension directly or indirectly results in most of the complications of cirrhosis.

ETIOLOGY

The most common causes of cirrhosis in adults are chronic viral hepatitis B and C viruses, alcoholic liver disease, and nonalcoholic fatty liver disease. Less common but important causes include primary sclerosing cholangitis, primary biliary cirrhosis, autoimmune hepatitis, hemochromatosis, Wilson's disease, and alpha-1 antitrypsin deficiency.

CLINICAL MANIFESTATIONS

Physical examination findings depend on the severity of cirrhosis but may include jaundice, muscle wasting, alopecia, palmar erythema, Dupuytren's contractures, scleral icterus, spider angiomata, gynecomastia, hepatosplenomegaly, a positive fluid wave or shifting dullness from ascites, testicular atrophy, peripheral edema, altered mental status, and asterixis from hepatic encephalopathy.

The major consequences of cirrhosis include development and rupture of esophagogastric varices, ascites, spontaneous bacterial peritonitis (SBP), hyponatremia, hepatorenal syndrome (HRS), portosystemic hepatic encephalopathy (PSE), and hepatopulmonary syndrome (HPS). The Child-Turcotte-Pugh classification (Table 74.1) is the most commonly used scale to stage cirrhosis.

Esophagogastric Varices

In light of the increased resistance, collateral vessels or varices develop and bypass the liver as blood returns to the heart. When portal pressures exceed 12 mm Hg, rupture may occur. Rupture of esophageal or gastric varices may manifest with melena or massive hematemesis and represents a true emergency.

Physical examination in patients with varices may reveal findings associated with portal hypertension including a vasodilated state with a low systemic blood pressure and hyperdynamic circulation.

TABLE 74.1 Child-Turcotte-Pugh classifications score for severity of liver disease

Criterion	One point	Two points	Three points
Albumin (g/dL)	>3.5	2.8–3.5	<2.8
Bilirubin (mg/mL)	<2	2–3	>3
International normalized ratio	<1.7	1.7–2.2	>2.2
Ascites	None	Easily controlled	Poorly controlled
Encephalopathy	None	Easily controlled	Poorly controlled

Class A = 5 to 6 points; Class B = 7 to 9 points; Class C = ≥10 points.

Skin examination may reveal spider angiomata and caput medusa. Abdominal findings include hepatosplenomegaly, bulging flanks, a positive fluid wave and shifting dullness if concomitant ascites is present, and altered mental status with asterixis if hepatic encephalopathy is present.

Ascites

Ascites is the most common complication of cirrhosis and carries a 2-year survival of 50%. Ascites results from arterial underfilling with subsequent activation of vasoconstrictor and antinatriuretic factors. The end result is sodium and water retention leading to plasma volume expansion and ascites.

Physical examination in patients with ascites varies depending on the amount of fluid and can range from mild abdominal distension with bulging of the flanks and dullness on percussion to massive distension with a tense abdominal wall. As the amount of ascites increases, a positive fluid wave and shifting dullness can be detected. Umbilical hernias are common. Decreased breath sounds and hypoxemia due to pleural effusions (most commonly right-sided) may also be present.

Hepatorenal Syndrome

Hepatorenal syndrome (HRS) is characterized by decreasing urine output and rising serum blood urea nitrogen and creatinine in the absence of hypovolemia. The cause is arterial underfilling which leads to baroreceptor-mediated activation of vasoconstrictor factors ultimately leading to severe renal vasoconstriction and HRS. Type 1 HRS is rapidly progressive leading to oliguria or anuria with 80% mortality at 2 weeks. Type 2 HRS is frequently referred to as "diuretic-resistant ascites" because the renal function will vary depending on the aggressiveness of diuretic use.

Physical examination in patients with HRS is remarkable for evidence of a vasodilated state as well as volume overload manifesting as ascites, peripheral edema, pleural effusions, and vascular congestion. Mental status changes, if present, may be due to a combination of hepatic encephalopathy and uremia.

Portosystemic Encephalopathy

Portosystemic hepatic encephalopathy (PSE) can range from subtle cerebral dysfunction to deep coma and is potentially reversible. The underlying mechanism responsible for PSE is believed to be accumulation of gut-derived neurotoxins and their passage through the blood-brain barrier. These neurotoxins reach the brain through two major mechanisms: the inability of an injured liver to remove them from the circulation and by bypassing the liver altogether through varices. Implicated agents include ammonia, natural benzodiazepines, manganese, mercaptans, and aromatic amino acids. Clinically, patients with PSE present with changes in consciousness, intellectual function, personality, and neuromuscular examination (e.g., asterixis). Although there is overlap, patients with PSE can be graded into one of four categories as shown in Table 74.2.

TABLE 74.2 Grading of hepatic encephalopathy based on changes in mental status

Grade	Description
0	No alteration in consciousness, intellectual function, or behavior
1	Trivial lack of awareness, euphoria or anxiety, short attention span
2	Lethargy, disorientation, personality change, inappropriate behavior
3	Somnolence to semistupor, confusion, response to noxious stimuli
4	Coma, no response to noxious stimuli

Hepatopulmonary Syndrome

Hepatopulmonary syndrome is the result of intrapulmonary microvascular dilation, which leads to hypoxemia in the setting of cirrhosis and portal hypertension. The majority of patients with HPS have progressive dyspnea that worsens upon standing (platypnea) due to the predominance of vasodilation in the lung bases. Dyspnea on exertion is a common complaint. Examination reveals digit clubbing and, in severe cases, cyanosis and altered mental status due to hypoxemia.

DIAGNOSIS

Although classically a histological diagnosis, cirrhosis may also be diagnosed radiographically or by biochemical testing. Liver biopsy reveals the development of fibrotic nodules and loss of normal acinar structure. Abdominal imaging studies (e.g., ultrasound, computed tomography, or magnetic resonance imaging) may reveal an irregular liver surface, caudate lobe enlargement, splenomegaly, intra-abdominal or periesophageal varices, or if decompensated, the presence of ascites. The absence of these findings does not exclude early cirrhosis. The most common laboratory abnormalities include leukopenia and thrombocytopenia from splenic sequestration, anemia of chronic disease, increased prothrombin time, decreased serum albumin and total protein, and increased transaminases, alkaline phosphatase, and bilirubin. Laboratory abnormalities in conjunction with the typical examination may be sufficient to make the diagnosis of cirrhosis.

Esophagogastric Varices

Varices are diagnosed by esophagogastroduodenoscopy (EGD) and are classified as esophageal or gastric. They are present in approximately 40% of Child's A and 80% of Child's C patients. Thrombocytopenia, particularly less than 100×19^9/L, is felt by many clinicians to suggest increased probability of varices.

Ascites

Evaluation of the patient with new-onset ascites should consist of a detailed history and physical, Doppler ultrasound of the liver and hepatic vasculature to evaluate for evidence of cirrhosis and thrombosis, serologic evaluation for causes of liver disease, and a diagnostic paracentesis. The ascitic fluid should be analyzed for total protein, albumin, cell count and differential, Gram stain, aerobic cultures, and anaerobic cultures. Additional studies that may be warranted depending on clinical suspicion include amylase, glucose, lactate dehydrogenase, bilirubin, and triglycerides. The yield of ascitic fluid cytology for malignancy is low (~7%) outside of the setting of peritoneal carcinomatosis. Similarly, ascitic fluid analysis for mycobacteria is not cost effective unless the patient is immunosuppressed or has recent travel to endemic areas.

TABLE 74.3 Serum ascites albumin gradient for source of ascites

High (>1.1 g/dL)
Cirrhosis
Hepatocellular carcinoma
Budd-Chiari syndrome
Right ventricular failure
Constrictive pericarditis
Low (<1.1 g/dL)
Peritoneal carcinomatosis
Pancreatic ascites
Nephrotic syndrome
Peritoneal tuberculosis without cirrhosis

The serum albumin-ascites gradient is used to determine if ascites is the result of portal hypertension. Values greater than 1.1 g/dL are consistent with portal hypertension. Values less than 1.1 g/dL are commonly associated with nonportal hypertensive causes such as nephrotic syndrome, pancreatic ascites, tuberculosis, and carcinomatosis (Table 74.3). Ascitic protein values less than 1 g/dL indicate an increased risk of future SBP and warrant consideration of prophylactic antibiotics.

Hepatorenal Syndrome

The diagnosis of HRS is made by excluding other causes of renal dysfunction including prerenal azotemia, acute tubular necrosis, and drug-induced nephrotoxicity. Examination of urinary sediment is typically bland, the urine sodium is <10 mEq/L, proteinuria does not exceed 500 mg per day, and there is no improvement in renal function with plasma expansion.

Portosystemic Encephalopathy

The diagnosis of PSE is made by detecting neurological impairment on examination in the setting of chronic liver disease. The presence of asterixis is highly suggestive of PSE in the setting of liver disease. Laboratory studies including a chemistry panel, complete blood count, and hepatic panel should be sent. Additional tests including toxicology studies, urine analysis, blood cultures, and cerebral imaging should be obtained based on clinical suspicion. Although many clinicians obtain serum ammonia levels, there is little evidence to support a correlation between particular values and the grade of encephalopathy.

Hepatopulmonary Syndrome

The diagnosis of HPS starts with the documentation of arterial hypoxemia with pO_2 values less than 70 mm Hg and a widened alveolar-arterial oxygen gradient even when adjusted for age. Obtaining arterial blood gases in the supine and standing position may further suggest the diagnosis. Confirmation is by an agitated saline (bubble echo), which demonstrates intrapulmonary shunting, and technetium-labeled, macroaggregated albumin, which allows shunt quantitation.

TREATMENT

Esophagogastric Varices

Prophylactic treatment of esophageal varices most commonly involves the use of nonselective beta-blockers (e.g., propanolol, nadolol). Numerous studies have shown that these agents decrease the risk of first and subsequent bleeding as well as mortality by reducing portal hypertension by up to 15%. Dose titration should be performed to achieve a 20% to 25% reduction in heart rate if the patient tolerates the dose.

Ascites

Treatment of ascites involves a stepwise approach with the initial step being a 2-g (88 mmol) per day sodium restriction, which leads to complete resolution of ascites in 10% to 20% of patients. Although many clinicians introduce a fluid restriction, there is little clinical evidence to support this measure unless serum sodium values are <125 mmol/L. If ascites persists despite sodium restriction, the diuretic spironolactone should be introduced at doses of 50 to 100 mg per day in a single dose. If the ascites still persists, furosemide should be added in a 2:5 ratio with spironolactone (e.g., 40 mg furosemide per 100 mg of spironolactone). Maximum daily doses are 400 mg of spironolactone in a single dose and 160 mg furosemide in two divided doses. Higher doses of diuretics may result in electrolyte disorders, renal insufficiency, hypotension, and hepatic encephalopathy. In those intolerant of diuretics, repeated high-volume paracentesis can be performed. Transjugular intrahepatic portosystemic shunting (TIPS) is effective for refractory ascites in those intolerant of diuretics or requiring frequent paracentesis. Pre-existing hepatic encephalopathy is a contraindication to TIPS placement because encephalopathy is worsened by TIPS placement.

Hepatorenal Syndrome

Liver transplantation is the treatment of choice in patients with HRS with renal function usually improving shortly after transplant. In those who are not transplant candidates, vasoconstriction with agents such as norepinephrine, as well as the combination of midodrine, octreotide, and albumin is frequently utilized, with mixed results.

Portosystemic Encephalopathy

Patients with grade 2 PSE should be admitted to a general ward and grades 3 to 4 to the intensive care unit. Intubation to protect the airway should be considered in those with grades 3 to 4 PSE. Precipitating causes should be sought in all patients. The most common is intravascular volume depletion usually from overaggressive diuretic use. Other common precipitating causes of PSE are sleep medications, sedatives, analgesics, gastrointestinal hemorrhage, infection, constipation, hepatic necrosis, hypokalemic alkalosis, and excessive dietary protein intake. Management of encephalopathy involves treating precipitating factors by withholding diuretics, initiating gentle hydration, avoiding sedation, and investigating for an etiology. Recent data fail to show the common practice of placing patients on a protein-restricted diet to be of benefit in accelerating recovery. The mainstay of mild PSE treatment is oral lactulose titrated to 2 to 4 bowel movements per day, while those with advanced PSE should be treated with lactulose enemas due to risk of aspiration. For those patients who are refractory or intolerant to lactulose therapy, antibiotic therapy with rifaximin, a nonaminoglycoside with minimal absorption and activity against gram-positive, gram-negative, aerobic, and anaerobic pathogens, may be beneficial. Zinc supplementation may also be a useful treatment because two of the five enzymes responsible for the metabolism of ammonia to urea are zinc dependent and also because cirrhotics have high urinary zinc losses from diuretics.

Hepatopulmonary Syndrome

The only known effective treatment of HPS involves liver transplantation in appropriate candidates.

COMPLICATIONS

Variceal Bleeding

When varices bleed, patients will present with hematemesis or melena. Hemodynamic instability is common. Patients should be admitted to the intensive care unit, aggressively resuscitated, and

TABLE 74.4 Signs and symptoms in patients with spontaneous bacterial peritonitis

Abdominal pain	80%
Fever	70%
Encephalopathy	50%
Decreased peristalsis	30%
Diarrhea	20%
Septic shock	15%
Gastrointestinal bleeding	15%
Vomiting	10%
Asymptomatic	10%

pharmacological therapy (in the United States, limited to octreotide) should be initiated immediately. Once resuscitated, endoscopy should be performed. While sclerotherapy and esophageal variceal ligation or banding (EVL) are equally effective at controlling acute esophageal variceal hemorrhage, the majority of centers prefer EVL due to its ease and better complication profile. Patients should then be treated with beta-blockers and repeated EVL until variceal eradication is achieved. In the United States, effective endoscopic therapy for gastric varices is not available. Balloon tamponade with a Sangstaken-Blakemore or Minnesota tube is effective in controlling acute bleeding but is not a long-term solution.

The small number of patients who do not respond to combined pharmacological and endoscopic therapy should be considered for TIPS. TIPS creates an artificial communication between branches of the portal and hepatic veins, preferentially providing a low resistance pathway for blood through the liver rather than through varices. As with ascites management, pre-existing hepatic encephalopathy is a contraindication to TIPS placement.

Spontaneous Bacterial Peritonitis

Spontaneous bacterial peritonitis is infected ascites without an intra-abdominal source. The most common signs and symptoms of SBP are shown in Table 74.4. Common organisms responsible for SBP are *E. coli*, *K. pneumoniae*, and *Pneumococcus*, while anaerobic and fungal infections are rare. The presence of multiple organisms should raise suspicion of secondary bacterial peritonitis from a perforated viscus or abscess. The ascitic fluid cell count, differential, Gram stain, and culture results are used in diagnosing SBP (Table 74.5). The drugs of choice for SBP are the third-generation cephalosporins; a 5-day intravenous course is as effective as a 10-day course.

TABLE 74.5 Diagnosis of spontaneous bacterial peritonitis (SBP) and related conditions

Condition	Polymorphonuclear leukocytes count	Culture	Antibiotics
Culture-positive SBP	$>250/mm^3$	Positive	Yes
Culture-negative SBP	$>250/mm^3$	Negative	Yes
Bacterascites	$<250/mm^3$	Positive	Yes, may progress to SBP

Hyponatremia

Patients with ascites have impaired free water excretion resulting in increased total body water, dilution of extracellular volume and resultant hyponatremia. It is estimated that 30% of hospitalized cirrhotics with ascites will have hyponatremia. Therapy for hyponatremia is undertaken at values of 120 to 125 mmol/L and consists of fluid restriction to 1,000 to 1,500 mL per day.

Liver Transplantation

Despite continued improvements in the diagnosis and treatment of patients with cirrhosis, those with decompensation (Child's B and C) have a decreased long-term survival and should be considered for liver transplantation. Physicians caring for patients developing complications should refer them to a transplant center. Currently, the leading indications for transplant are hepatitis C virus, alcoholic liver disease, nonalcoholic fatty liver disease, biliary disease, and selected patients with hepatocellular carcinoma. Contraindications to transplant include compensated cirrhosis without complications, extrahepatic malignancy, active alcohol or illicit substance abuse, and advanced cardiopulmonary disease. Waiting times for transplant vary by region and are determined by the Model for End-Stage Liver Disease score, which is computed from the serum creatinine, total bilirubin, and international normalized ratio. The limiting factor in liver transplantation remains the significant organ shortage. Short- and long-term survival following liver transplant continues to improve as a result of better patient selection, improved immunosuppression, and advances in surgical technique, with most centers now achieving approximately 90% 1-year survival.

CHAPTER 75

Pancreatitis

Krista Wiger

ACUTE PANCREATITIS

Acute pancreatitis is the inflammation of the pancreas associated with acinar cell injury, which ranges in severity from a mild, edematous form to a severe life-threatening necrotizing pancreatitis. This process affects approximately 185,000 patients a year in the United States. Severe disease occurs in approximately 10% to 30% of patients and overall carries a mortality rate of 2% to 10%. The majority of patients, however, have a mild clinical course. Acute and chronic pancreatitis represent very distinct disorders.

In contrast to chronic pancreatitis, the function and structure of the pancreas are typically preserved in acute pancreatitis despite the fact that the latter often results in very severe disease.

Etiology

Depending on the geographic location, the incidence and etiologies of pancreatitis vary. Although the most common causes of acute pancreatitis are alcohol and gallstones, there is a growing list of etiologies (Table 75.1).

Acute pancreatitis is caused by a cascade of events resulting in autodigestion of the gland. The initial process is the activation of proteolytic enzymes in the pancreas rather than in the small intestine where it should normally occur. These activated enzymes (e.g., trypsin) digest the pancreas and result in additional activation of other enzymes such as elastase and phospholipase, leading to further digestion of membranes causing proteolysis, edema, interstitial hemorrhage, coagulation, and fat necrosis as well as vascular damage. Additional enzymes, such as bradykinins and vasoactive substances, result in further vasodilation and increased vascular permeability. The end result of all of these processes is acute necrotizing pancreatitis.

Clinical Manifestations

Patients typically present with a steady midepigastric or periumbilical pain, which radiates to the back or flanks, waxes and wanes, and is exacerbated by lying down and improved by leaning forward. Onset of the pain is rapid and may last days. Nausea, vomiting, abdominal distention, and low-grade fever are typically present. Hypotension results from increased vascular permeability, low peripheral resistance, and fluid sequestration. Abdominal examination may reveal tenderness to palpation and decreased or absent bowel sounds frequently due to the occurrence of an ileus. "Painless bruising" or ecchymotic discoloration in the periumbilical (Cullen's sign) or flank (Grey-Turner's sign) areas are uncommon (2% of cases), typically develop later in the clinical course, and have a low specificity. The latter may reflect retroperitoneal hemorrhage, yet both are associated with poor prognosis.

Diagnosis

BIOCHEMICAL FEATURES

The majority of the clinical signs and symptoms are nonspecific. Thus, the diagnosis requires a combination of high clinical suspicion and elevated pancreatic enzymes, often corroborated by compat-

TABLE 75.1 Conditions frequently associated with acute pancreatitis

Obstruction	Trauma
Choledocholithiasis	Blunt abdominal trauma
Tumors	Abdominal operations
Sphincter of Oddi stenosis	ERCP procedure
Metabolic	**Vascular**
Hypertriglyceridemia	Shock
Acute hypercalcemia	Vasculitis
Toxins	**Drugs**
Ethanol	Valproic acid
Methanol	Azathioprine (6-MP)
Scorpion venom	Metronidazole
Congenital	Sulfonamides
Pancreas divisum	Most diuretics
	Pentamidine
	Tetracycline
	Mesalamine
	ACE inhibitors
	DDI (2′ 3′ dideoxyinosine)
	Cocaine abuse

ible radiologic findings. Amylase activity rises in the first 2 to 12 hours and normalizes in 3 to 5 days. False-negatives may result from hyperlipidemia in approximately 10% of individuals who may have normal amylase levels during an episode of acute pancreatitis. Given that amylase has multiple sources (salivary glands, reproductive system) and is renally cleared, false positives may occur in bowel perforation, acute cholecystitis, renal failure, ruptured ectopic pregnancy, and many other processes, thus decreasing its overall utility (Table 75.2). Lipase peaks within the first 24 hours and has a higher specificity than amylase, particularly when elevation is one- to twofold the upper limit of normal. Higher threshold for abnormal results (three- to fivefold elevation of upper limit) increases the specificity of both amylase and lipase, but the sensitivity remains low. Nevertheless, false elevation of lipase can also be found in other diseases (Table 75.2). Finally, there is no correlation between disease severity and levels of elevation.

Leukocytosis, mild hypocalcemia, transient hyperglycemia, and aspartate transaminase elevation may also be noted. In patients with an elevated gamma glutamyl transferase, alanine transaminase, and alkaline phosphatase, gallstone pancreatitis is the most likely etiology of pancreatitis.

IMAGING

Plain abdominal x-rays may show free air, gallstones, ileus, or pancreatic calcifications. The presence of calcifications suggests chronic pancreatitis. Chest x-ray may demonstrate pleural effusions (particularly left-sided), and atelectasis related to subphrenic inflammation. Abdominal ultrasound is the initial imaging modality of choice recommended to evaluate for gallstones and/or biliary dilatation. Urgent intervention for decompression is required when ultrasound reveals evidence of new-onset (<48 hours) biliary or gallstone-induced pancreatitis. Ultrasound visualization of the pancreas itself

TABLE 75.2 Diseases associated with false elevation of amylase and lipase

Disease	Amylase	Lipase
Acute cholecystitis	+	+
Intestinal obstruction	+	+
Peptic ulcer disease	+	+
Diabetic ketoacidosis	+	+
Acute renal failure	+	+
Medications		
Furosemide	−	+
Metronidazole	+	+
Thiazide	+	+
Valproic acid	+	+
Pelvic inflammatory disease	+	−
Ruptured ectopic pregnancy	+	−
Salivary gland tumors	+	−

is limited particularly by overlying bowel gas. Computed tomography (CT) scan with oral and intravenous contrast may show pancreatic enlargement, loss of fat planes, hypodense areas, fat stranding, and presence of fluid collections. Contrast may be contraindicated in patients with allergic responses or renal impairment. CT with intravenous contrast is the modality of choice for detecting pancreatic necrosis and should be undertaken if the patient fails to improve or with any signs of clinical deterioration particularly after 48 hours have passed since onset of symptoms. Magnetic resonance imaging (MRI) is an alternative with a comparable sensitivity and specificity for severe pancreatitis; however, pancreatic necrosis may be less definitively identified.

Determining the underlying cause of acute pancreatitis enhances treatment and may potentially reduce recurrences. The underlying etiology can be ascertained in approximately 80% of individuals though a history, physical examination, focused laboratory testing, and either ultrasound or CT scans. If no cause is found, patients who have had either one severe or two mild episodes of acute pancreatitis should undergo magnetic resonance cholangiopancreatography (MRCP). Depending on the MRCP findings, an endoscopic retrograde cholangiopancreatography (ERCP) with biliary crystal analysis or in the case of patients with prior cholecystectomy, ERCP with sphincter of Oddi manometry may be warranted. Endoscopic ultrasound is considered in patients with risk factors for pancreatic cancer (age >40 years, tobacco usage, or family history of pancreatic cancer).

Disease Severity

Identifying patients with severe pancreatitis remains a challenge. Multiple classification systems based on clinical, biochemical, and/or radiographic findings are available. The Ranson and Glasgow systems require a 48-hour period for full assessment and although higher scores correlate with poorer outcomes, they have not been re-evaluated in lieu of the significant advancements in critical care medicine (Table 75.3). The Acute Physiology and Chronic Health Evaluation II (APACHE) offer evaluation at 24 hours and may be recalculated during the course of the disease or after procedures. An added assessment of obesity (APACHE-O) score further improves the positive predictive value. The Atlanta classification system is based on the clinical manifestation such as abdominal tenderness along with either score from the Ranson criteria or APACHE criteria. The cumbersome nature of the scores has limited their clinical utility.

TABLE 75.3 Acute pancreatitis scoring systems

Ranson criteria	
At admission	**48 hours after admission**
Age >55 years	Decrease in hematocrit by more than 10%
White blood cell count >16,000/uL	Fluid sequestration of >6 L
Blood glucose >200 mg/dL	Hypocalcemia (<8.0 mg/dL)
Serum lactate dehydrogenase >350 IU/L	PO_2 <60 mmHg
Serum aspartate transaminase >250 IU/L	Increase in blood urea nitrogen to >5 mg/dL after hydration
	Base deficit of >4 mmol/L
Prognostic Implications of Ranson criteria	
Score	**Mortality**
0–2	2%
3–4	15%
5–6	40%
7–8	100%
Glasgow score	
(More than three of the below factors predicts a more severe course.)	
Age >55 years old	
White blood cell count >15,000/uL	
Glucose greater than 180 mg/dL	
Lactate dehydrogenase >600 U/L	
Aspartate transaminase >100 U/L	
Blood urea nitrogen >45 U/L	
PaO_2 <60 mm Hg	
Calcium <8 mg/dL	
Albumin <3.2 g/dL	

Specific biochemical markers as tools in prognostication are being utilized and studied. C-reactive protein levels 48 hours after symptoms begin have correlated with severity. Multiple inflammatory mediators such as interleukin-6 and -8 have been evaluated however, are still in the primary stages of research. Trypsinogen activation peptide is released with the activation from trypsinogen to trypsin and correlates with disease activity. Early studies suggest that its levels may be clinically useful as a disease severity indicator.

Treatment

Medical therapy of pancreatitis is dependent on the severity of the presentation: the basic components consisting of volume repletion, pain relief and bowel rest. Studies indicate that inadequate resuscitation predisposes patients not only to renal insufficiency but also increases risk of further injury and an increased risk of developing necrosis. Nasogastric suction is utilized in patients with vomiting or a paralytic ileus. Patients need to be monitored closely for signs of complications or worsening as well as electrolyte imbalances. Stress ulcer prophylaxis may also be indicated.

Nutritional management involves the limitation of enteral feeding to avoid stimulating the exocrine function and thereby avoiding further enzymatic damage. The intake is advanced slowly as tolerated over the next few days. In patients with a prolonged, severe course, total parenteral nutrition is utilized.

Complications

Acute pancreatitis may results in a number of complications (Table 75.4). Pancreatic pseudocyst is a collection of pancreatic fluid that may form in up to one half of patients with severe pancreatitis. It takes at least 4 weeks for pseudocyst to form after an episode of pancreatitis. Most pseudocysts resolve spontaneously, but some may evolve to become persistent collections. A pancreatic abscess characterized by a collection of pus may also occur as a complication of acute pancreatitis. It may present with persistent symptoms of pancreatitis and high fevers. Percutaneous drainage is indicated for enlarging, persistent, or infected collections.

In the minority of the cases, patients may present or develop circulatory shock and require intensive care unit care. Pancreatic necrosis, gram-negative sepsis, and ascending cholangitis may also lead to sepsis syndrome.

Adult respiratory distress syndrome (ARDS) may occur due to the circulating phospholipases and free fatty acids damage to alveolar surfactant. Acute renal failure may occur due to hypoperfusion and increased renovascular resistance. Mental status changes may be related to toxic psychosis, alcohol withdrawal, or opiate effects and are challenging to clearly differentiate and medically manage.

Stone impaction in the ampulla of Vater may present with progressive jaundice followed by fevers secondary to ascending cholangitis. Prompt removal of the stone within 48 hours of onset typically endoscopically is warranted along with antibiotic coverage.

Pancreatic necrosis (PN) occurs in 80% of patients presenting with severe episodes during the second or third week of the illness. Infected PN accounts for the majority of deaths related to acute pancreatitis. CT-guided fine needle aspiration is performed and cultures are obtained, although the Gram stain has the highest sensitivity. *Escherichia coli, Klebsiella, and Enterococcus* are the most common infections, followed by *Staphylococcus* and *Pseudomonas.* Antibiotics and surgical debridement in infected PN are the standard of care.

TABLE 75.4 Complications of acute pancreatitis

Systemic	Local	Adjacent organs
Shock	Impacted common bile duct stone	Splenic vein occlusion
Acute renal failure	Pancreatic necrosis Sterile Infected	Bleeding
Adult respiratory distress syndrome	Pancreatic abscess	Pleural effusion
Sepsis	Bleeding	Pancreatic fistula
Miscellaneous	Pseudocyst	
Disseminated intravascular coagulation		
Hyperglycemia		
Hypocalcemia		

CHRONIC PANCREATITIS

Chronic pancreatitis is the consequence of progressive inflammation resulting destruction of pancreatic structure and/or function. In contrast to acute pancreatitis, this damage typically persists despite removal of the precipitating cause. The prevalence of chronic pancreatitis varies depending on geographic location, with estimates ranging from 12 to 45 cases per 100,000 individuals. There is a marked predominance for males. Approximately 10% to 20% of those with long-term heavy alcohol use are affected.

Etiology

There are multiple etiologies (Table 75.5) of chronic pancreatitis. Chronic alcoholism is the main cause, accounting for up to 70% of cases in developed countries. Amount and duration of consumption correlate with disease severity. Idiopathic pancreatitis, in which no specific cause is identified, may account for approximately 20% of etiologies.

A potential anatomic cause is pancreas divisum, which is the congenital failure of the fusion of the ducts of the ventral and dorsal pancreas in approximately 5% of the population.

Clinical Manifestations

Patients with chronic pancreatitis typically present with epigastric pain that radiates through to the back, which may be triggered by food or alcohol intake. These symptoms are typically intermittent but with time may become increasingly progressive and severe. Anorexia, weight loss, and diarrhea may be noted. Musculoskeletal complaints such as bone pain secondary to intramedullary fat necrosis or inflammation of the joints may be seen. Patients typically appear older than their stated age. Physical examination may reveal epigastric tenderness, tender subcutaneous nodules secondary to fat necrosis. If the bile duct is obstructed by edema and fibrosis of the pancreatic head, jaundice may be present. A palpable abdominal mass should raise suspicion of a pseudocyst or abscess in patients with episodes of recurrent acute pancreatitis superimposed on chronic pancreatitis.

Diagnosis

When there is a clinical suspicion of chronic pancreatitis based on symptoms and signs, specific testing should be pursued. Because of the marked destruction of pancreatic tissue, both amylase and lipase are typically normal. The sensitivity and specificity of biochemical tests is dependant on the duration and severity of the disease process. In early disease, testing for pancreatic secretion with

TABLE 75.5 Causes of chronic pancreatitis
Alcohol (70%)
Idiopathic
Metabolic hypercalcemia, hyperparathyroidism, hypertriglyceridemia
Inherited   Cystic fibrosis

Autoimmune
  Primary
  Secondary: inflammatory bowel disease, primary biliary cirrhosis, Sjögren's syndrome

Obstructive chronic pancreatitis
Pancreatic, biliary tumors, strictures, scarring, sphincter of Oddi dysfunction, pancreas divisum

serum trypsin or fecal elastase testing may be helpful although the sensitivity is poor. In severe or long-term disease, elevated serum glucose levels and 48- or 72-hour quantitative fecal fat collections demonstrating steatorrhea are supportive of the diagnosis. Over 7 grams of fat per 24-hour collection is typically considered an abnormal quantitative stool fat study with chronic pancreatitis patients with steatorrhea often exhibiting values of 20 to 40 grams fat per 24 hours. Overall, biochemical testing has a very limited role in the diagnosis chronic pancreatitis.

Because pancreatic calcifications may be found in up to 50% of patients with alcohol-induced chronic pancreatitis on a plain abdominal x-ray, this an inexpensive and reasonable first test to order. Transabdominal ultrasound is good for detection of associated biliary abnormalities such as biliary ductal dilatation, pancreatic enlargement, and possibly pseudocysts. However, visualization of the pancreas may be limited due to large body habitus or overlying bowel gas. Abdominal CT has better sensitivity for detection of pancreatic calcifications, edema, and ductal dilatations, and permits better identification of cystic and mass lesions. MRCP and ERCP better delineate ductal dilatation and may reveal a correctable obstruction.

ERCP is currently considered the gold standard for the diagnosis of chronic pancreatitis with a sensitivity and specificity of over 90%. However, ERCP is an invasive test and is indicated in patients in whom a final diagnosis cannot be established or in cases where a stone may need to be extracted to relief an obstruction that is thought to cause the pancreatitis. Potential complications of ERCP such as bleeding, perforation, and procedure-induced pancreatitis may limit its use. Endoscopic ultrasonography (EUS) is being increasingly utilized, may be more sensitive than ERCP, avoids the risk of pancreatitis, does also provide therapeutic options, and may actually represent the most sensitive modality.

Treatment

Management is typically divided into treatment and control of the underlying pain and management of the complications ranging from steatorrhea, nutritional deficiency, and diabetes to pancreatic cancer. Pain exacerbations are treated with bowel rest and analgesics with opiates required in most patients. Issues of substance abuse frequently complicate management. The efficacy of previously accepted measures is currently being studied. Decreasing pancreatic stimulation and subsequent secretion is believed to diminish pain. This may be accomplished with pancreatic enzyme supplements that are not enteric coated but is only effective in patients with mild chronic pancreatitis pain. Care must be taken to administer concomitant acid suppression to avoid deactivation of nonenteric-coated enzymes by gastric acid secretion. The use of antioxidant therapy is also under investigation.

The benefit of surgical therapy appears to be isolated to patients with dilated pancreatic ducts for whom a lateral pancreaticojejunostomy (e.g., a Puestow procedure) may relieve pain in a majority. Preliminary data suggests that patients with dilated pancreatic ducts who report pain relief after placement of temporary pancreatic stents during ERCP may benefit most from surgical decompression in this manner. Surgical partial pancreatic resection, endoscopic extraction of ductal stones, dilation of strictures, or pancreatic sphincterotomy may have short-term benefit but lack long-term data in support of their use. Celiac plexus blocks have shown variable efficacy.

Complications

Malabsorption results from a decrease in pancreatic enzyme secretion and may result in weight loss. Significant fat malabsorption is encountered, whereas little to no carbohydrate malabsorption is seen. Treatment entails supplementation with pancreatic enzyme supplements and avoiding excessive fat intake. In addition to potential fat soluble vitamin deficiencies, deficiencies of cobalamin (B_{12}) and zinc may occur.

Diabetes is a late finding and is more likely to be complicated by hypoglycemia due to a codeficiency of glucagon.

Splenic vein thrombosis may result from inflammation of the tail of the pancreas and is classically a cause of isolated gastric varices. Gastrointestinal bleeding from this and a variety of causes may occur. Biliary duct compression by a pseudocyst or fibrosis requires surgical treatment to prevent biliary cirrhosis.

Over time, chronic pancreatitis is a risk factor for the development of pancreatic carcinoma. Approximately 5% of pancreatic cancers are attributed to chronic pancreatitis. No effective screening for pancreatic cancer is currently available.

CHAPTER 76

Inflammatory Bowel Disease

Kurt Pfeifer

The term inflammatory bowel disease (IBD) primarily refers to chronic ulcerative colitis (CUC) and Crohn's disease. Both are idiopathic inflammatory disorders. Whereas in Crohn's disease inflammation may involve any part of the gastrointestinal tract, CUC disease activity is isolated to the colorectal mucosa. Despite extensive evaluation, approximately 10% of IBD colitis cannot be classified as CUC or Crohn's disease and is referred to as "indeterminate" colitis.

CHRONIC ULCERATIVE COLITIS

Chronic ulcerative colitis (CUC) is characterized by idiopathic inflammation isolated to the colorectal mucosa but with known extracolonic manifestations and associations. Although in the past CUC was most prevalent among whites, it is now seen in populations worldwide. Its incidence has been relatively stable over the past three decades with an annual incidence in North America of 6 to 14 cases per 100,000 person year. Bimodal peaks of incidence are seen with the first and largest peak in the 3rd and 4th decade and the second peak around the age of 60 years.

Etiology

The etiology of CUC is not currently known, but multiple factors are likely involved. The incidence is higher in nonsmokers and ex-smokers, and possibly in oral contraceptive users. However, appendectomy seems to be protective. A minority of patients have a family history of IBD, and the concordance rate among identical twins is low (approximately 5%). However, a geographic pattern of disease is evident in the increased incidence of CUC in more northern latitudes. No evidence favoring an infectious, allergic, immunologic, genetic, or psychosomatic cause has held up to scrutiny.

Clinical Manifestations

The symptoms of CUC vary from mild with frequent bloody rectal discharges and tenesmus (a painful, recurrent spasm of the rectum with an urge to defecate but passage of little fecal matter) to severe with debilitating systemic and abdominal symptoms. The onset of CUC is typically gradual, but the disease can present in a fulminant form with life-threatening complications (10% of cases). Fever, weight loss, anemia, and hypoproteinemia occur in more severe cases. Fecal losses of water, sodium, and potassium are not severe because bowel movements are small volume and contain only blood and mucus. Eighty percent of patients have intermittent exacerbations with total remissions, but 10% to 15% remain continuously active. Historically, 5% of patients have gone into permanent remission after the initial episode of colitis. However, many of these patients are now felt to have been suffering from hemorrhagic bacterial dysentery, most likely *Escherichia coli* O157:H7, and were misdiagnosed. A severe attack is characterized by more than six bloody stools daily with systemic signs of severe illness (fever, tachycardia, anemia, or erythrocyte sedimentation rate [ESR] >30 mm/hr).

Extracolonic manifestations occur in about 10% of patients and may occasionally precede bowel

TABLE 76.1 Frequency of occurrence and timing of extraintestinal manifestations in relation to gastrointestinal symptoms in inflammatory bowel disease

Manifestation	Chronic ulcerative colitis	Crohn's disease	Parallel disease course
Aphthous ulcers	+	+	Yes
Episcleritis	+	+	Yes
Erythema nodosum	+	+ +	Yes
Pyoderma gangrenosum	+ +	+	Yes
Asymmetric arthropathy	+	+	Yes
Primary sclerosing cholangitis	+ +	+	No
Sacroiliitis	+	+	No
Ankylosing spondylitis	+	+	No
Amyloidosis	+	+	No

+ +, occurs more commonly in one disease versus the other.

symptoms. Oral aphthous ulcers, episcleritis, uveitis, pyoderma gangrenosum (erythematous papule or pustule more common on lower extremities), erythema nodosum (raised tender, violet nodules on the anterior aspect of lower extremities) and an asymmetric, nondeforming arthropathy of large joints tend to parallel the course of the colitis. Conversely, sacroiliitis, primary sclerosing cholangitis (PSC), ankylosing spondylitis, and secondary amyloidosis may progress without active colitis and even after proctocolectomy (Table 76.1).

Diagnosis

The physical examination is often normal or demonstrates only mild, diffuse abdominal tenderness. Abdominal distention, tympany, and severe tenderness in acutely ill patients suggest fulminant colitis and possible toxic megacolon. A slightly granular texture is noted on digital rectal examination, and bloody mucus is often seen on the glove.

There are no diagnostic laboratory abnormalities, but plain abdominal radiographs can detect free intra-abdominal air and assess the colonic diameter in suspected toxic megacolon (Fig. 76.1). Barium enema can determine the extent of the disease and better define its nature. It may be nearly normal in early or mild disease. Ulcerations, usually tiny and difficult to see, often appear as fuzzy serrations or fine spiculations (Fig. 76.2), whereas large ulcerations resemble a collar button. In less active stages, the mucosal surface may be nodular and finely polypoid, reflecting inflammatory pseudopolyps. When the entire colon is involved, "backwash ileitis" is not uncommon and appears as a dilated ileal segment with smooth mucosa.

On endoscopy, the hallmark of CUC is the uniformity of inflammatory changes in the circumferential and longitudinal direction, beginning at the anal verge and ending with a clear demarcation to normal-appearing mucosa located within the colon or at the ileocecal valve. Histopathological findings also help differentiate CUC from other forms of colitis (Table 76.2).

Full colonoscopy with inspection and biopsy of the terminal ileum can supplant barium enema, but neither should be done in acute, severe colitis for risk of perforation or precipitating toxic megacolon. Instead, all patients with a dysenteric syndrome (tenesmus and frequent, bloody stools) should undergo fiberoptic sigmoidoscopy without preparation by enemas or laxatives. Beginning at the dentate line, the mucosa is uniformly friable, hyperemic, finely ulcerated, and granular. Edema obscures the usual fine tracery of blood vessels beneath the mucosa. With limited distal disease,

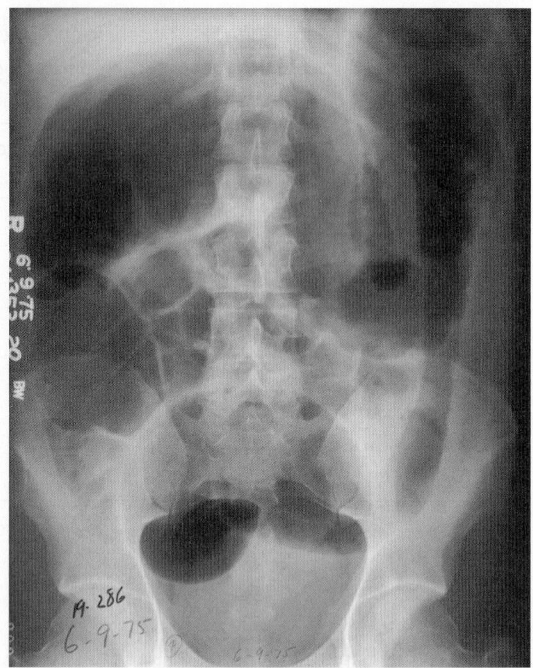

Figure 76.1 • Plain radiograph of toxic megacolon. Pronounced distension of the cecum and ascending colon are demonstrated. Note the absence of haustrations in the air-filled descending colon.

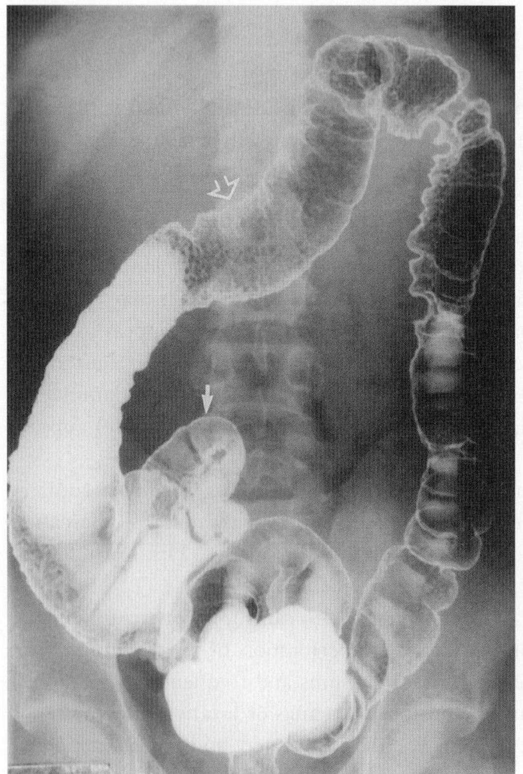

Figure 76.2 • Barium enema in acute ulcerative colitis. The colon and rectum are diffusely involved. Normal haustral pattern is lacking in the proximal and transverse colon segments. Note superficial ulcerations, causing the spiculated contours of the transverse colon (*open arrow*). The terminal ileum (*solid arrow*) is normal. (Courtesy of Edward Stewart, MD, Milwaukee, Wisconsin.)

TABLE 76.2 Differential diagnosis of ulcerative versus Crohn's colitis

	Chronic ulcerative colitis	Crohn's colitis
Distribution	Continuous	Segmental
Ileal involvement	0[a]	Diagnostic, if present
Histology		
Inflammation	Diffuse	Focal
Granulomas	0	2+ (~30%)
Transmural	0	4+
Clinical		
Perianal lesions	1+	3+
Fistulae	0–1+	2+
Strictures	1+	3+
Hemorrhage	2+	0–1+
Endoscopy		
Friability	3+	1+
Aphthoid lesions	0	4+
Granularity	3+	1+
Cobblestone	0–1+	3+
Linear, deep ulcers	1+	3+
Involvement	Uniform	Nonuniform

[a]The scale of 0–4+ indicates the frequency of a finding in each of the two diseases, with 0 being the least frequent.

these gross changes are demarcated proximally by normal mucosa within the viewing range of the sigmoidoscope.

The disease invariably begins at the anal verge with varying degrees of proximal extension. It involves only the rectosigmoid in 40% to 50% of patients, the left colon in 30% to 40%, and proximal extension beyond the splenic flexure (pancolitis) in about 20% to 40%. In 20% to 30% of patients with disease initially limited to the distal colon, there is proximal extension over time. On histopathology, inflammation is confined to the colonic mucosa and submucosa, and in acute stages, neutrophils and eosinophils invade the surface and crypt epithelium with crypt abscess formation. Changes in crypt architecture (crypt branching and atrophy) are a constant feature that separates IBD from acute infectious colitis. As the crypts are destroyed, the mucosa thins, but foci of regenerating mucosa often develop into inflammatory pseudopolyps. The chronic and recurrent inflammation often leads to shortening and stricturing of the colon ("lead-pipe" colon on barium studies). The ulceration and inflammation in fulminant cases extends into the muscle layers, with intramural plexus damage causing dilatation, impaired motor function, and ultimately, perforation—the so-called toxic megacolon.

Treatment

MEDICAL THERAPY

Medical management aims to control the acute attack, prevent recurrences, and correct nutritional, fluid, and electrolyte deficits. Although both corticosteroids and 5-aminosalicylate (5-ASA) compounds shorten acute attacks, corticosteroids act faster and are more effective; however, corticosteroids have cumulative side effects that are more serious. Patients with mild to moderate, extensive colitis may be given sulfasalazine (4 to 6 g/day) or oral prednisone (30 to 60 mg/day) if the clinical severity requires it.

Patients with acute attacks are hospitalized, closely monitored for progressive signs and symptoms, and given hydrocortisone (100 mg every 6 hours) intravenously and/or by rectal drip. Most patients tolerate only clear liquids and require parenteral nutrition. Refractory patients with CUC may respond to treatment with intravenous infusions of infliximab. Early surgical consultation is mandatory as emergency proctocolectomy is indicated in the 20% to 30% of patients who fail to improve within 1 week.

Once remission occurs, patients are maintained indefinitely on a 5-ASA drug (e.g., sulfasalazine 1 g twice daily) to reduce the risk of clinical relapse. Unfortunately, side effects are common and include nausea, vomiting, headaches, folate malabsorption, hemolytic anemia, alveolitis, hepatitis, and reversible male infertility.

Patients who are intolerant of the 5-ASA medications can be treated with immunomodulatory therapy (e.g., azathioprine, 6-mercaptopurine) in hopes of maintaining remission. Immunomodulators carry the potential risk of infection, pancreatitis, allergy, and neoplasia, and their use must be weighed against the potential benefit of a curative proctocolectomy.

SURGICAL THERAPY

Indications for surgery are toxic megacolon, acute exacerbations or chronic disease activity uncontrolled by medical therapy, and unacceptable side effects from drugs. Total proctocolectomy cures CUC. Less extensive surgical resections or temporary colon bypass procedures are not appropriate.

Complications

Chronic ulcerative colitis carries an increasing annual risk of 0.8% to 1% for developing colorectal cancer (CRC). Patients with pancolitis are at highest risk, but the risk is also increased in patients with left-sided involvement. The diagnosis of cancer in CUC is difficult because the symptoms mimic those of the underlying colitis, and radiography and endoscopy are less accurate than in the normal colon. Beginning 8 years after diagnosis, annual surveillance colonoscopy with multiple random biopsies obtained at 10-cm intervals is currently recommended for all CUC patients regardless of the extent of disease involvement. An exception is patients with concomitant primary sclerosing cholangitis, who have a particularly high risk of CRC and should undergo surveillance beginning at the time of diagnosis. Dysplastic changes of the colonic mucosa occur in many patients before CRC develops and are nearly universal when a cancer is diagnosed. If dysplasia is confirmed, evaluation for proctocolectomy is warranted. When adjusted for tumor stage at diagnosis, CRC complicating CUC has the same prognosis as CRC in general.

CROHN'S DISEASE

Crohn's disease is a chronic inflammatory disorder of unknown cause affecting the gastrointestinal tract (anywhere from mouth to anus) with secondary involvement of regional lymph nodes, liver, skin, eyes, and joints. It is often categorized as: (a) involving both the small intestine and colon, (b) isolated to small intestine (also called regional enteritis), or (c) isolated to the colon (Crohn's colitis). For uncertain reasons, the incidence of Crohn's disease has risen substantially during the past few decades. It is diagnosed before 30 years of age in 75% of patients and before 20 years of age in 30%.

Etiology

While the exact etiology of Crohn's disease has not been elucidated, it is clearly an autoimmune process. It is particularly common among Jews of Eastern European heritage and people residing in areas with a cold or temperate climate, yet more recent demographic studies suggest that all ethnic groups in "Westernized" nations are at risk. No defined pattern of inheritance is apparent, but first-degree relatives have a 5% to 15% lifetime risk of acquiring Crohn's disease. Intriguingly, studies of monozygotic twins with one affected member demonstrate that the unaffected twin has only a 50% to 60% risk of developing Crohn's disease.

Clinical Manifestations

The clinical picture is determined by the site of gastrointestinal involvement. Given the distal ileal involvement in 80% to 90% of patients, nonbloody diarrhea is the rule. Steatorrhea and vitamin B_{12} malabsorption are also common and directly proportional to the length of affected ileum. Abdominal pain (usually in the right lower quadrant) is very common. A steady ache indicates serosal extension and possible perforation, which in turn may lead to fistulae into the bowel, urinary bladder, vagina, or abdominal wall. Colicky pain that is relieved with bowel movements suggests partial ileal obstruction due to inflammatory ileal swelling or fibrotic strictures. Weight loss is also common and is caused by anorexia, fear of pain after eating, or malabsorption. Rectal bleeding most often is occult, but gross bleeding occasionally occurs, especially in young persons during their first attack with extensive Crohn's colitis.

Perineal disease may be severe, often with dusky, anal skin tags and perianal or ischiorectal abscesses, draining perineal fistulas, and anorectal stricture. Painful defecation is a harbinger of anal and perianal disease. Pneumaturia and fecal matter in the urinary sediment suggest an ileovesical or colovesical fistula, whereas dyspareunia and a brownish, malodorous vaginal discharge are clues to a rectovaginal fistula. Antroduodenal involvement may cause ulcer-like pain and pyloric or duodenal obstruction. Low-grade fever is a frequent finding, but spiking fevers should raise suspicion of an abscess.

Extraintestinal complications include erythema nodosum, arthritis, uveitis, oral aphthous ulcers, and primary sclerosing cholangitis. Malabsorption caused by ileal disease or surgical resection leads to secondary metabolic bone disease, anemia, bleeding diathesis, gallstones, and renal oxalate stones.

Diagnosis

There is no single test that confirms the diagnosis of Crohn's disease; rather, the diagnosis is made from a constellation of clinical, laboratory, histopathologic, endoscopic, and radiographic findings. Physical examination is largely nonspecific, but patients with intraabdominal abscesses may have a tender, abdominal mass. Laboratory abnormalities reflect inflammation, malnutrition (including hypoalbuminemia), blood loss, and malabsorption. Imaging of the ileum by a small bowel series or barium enema may show mucosal edema, aphthous ulceration, luminal narrowing ("string sign"), fistula formation, and inflammatory mass effect, but these findings are typical of patients with longstanding disease. In addition to these studies, abdominal and pelvic computed tomography can detect inflammatory masses, abscesses, fistulas with adjacent organs, colonic obstruction, and perforation with abscess formation.

Endoscopic evaluation with biopsies of the terminal ileum and throughout the colon may identify crypt architectural distortion, which is a hallmark feature of chronic, destructive intestinal inflammation. "Skip areas" in the colon (present in 20% of patients) and absence of rectal disease negate the diagnosis of ulcerative colitis. The rectum is affected in 60% of patients with Crohn's disease, but only 20% patients have disease limited to the colon. The small bowel, mainly the distal ileum, is solely involved in 30% of patients, and in 50% of cases ileitis contiguously extends into the colon. Duodenal and antral involvement occurs in 1% to 3% of cases.

Perianal disease with fistulas and abscesses, as well as deep anal and perineal ulcers, develop in 30% of patients at some time and are the initial presentation in 1% to 3% of patients. On histopathology, inflammation, along with edema and fibrosis, involves all layers of the gut wall, and noncaseating granulomas with giant cells are identified in one half of cases.

The distinction from CUC is important but challenging; helpful features for making the distinction are listed in Table 76.2. In 5% to 10% of patients with IBD, CUC cannot be separated from Crohn's colitis and is termed "indeterminate colitis."

Treatment

MEDICAL THERAPY

The overriding goal of treatment is to achieve and maintain clinical remission, thus preserving quality of life in patients with this chronic, recurrent disease. Pain and diarrhea respond to codeine and antidiarrheal agents (e.g., loperamide). Nutritional support corrects vitamin and mineral deficiencies and ensures adequate caloric intake. Liquid formula diets are useful in some cases of severe and extensive disease, and patients with narrow strictures should avoid high-residue foods (e.g., corn, cabbage, pulp of citrus fruit, enteric-coated tablets). Parenteral alimentation may be needed in preparation for surgery or as part of short-term therapy to induce a remission.

A few medications can help induce clinical remission but do not help in managing complications, such as abscesses and bowel strictures. In patients with mild disease, 5-ASA can reduce the risk of exacerbations, and the choice of 5-ASA formulation depends on the location of the patient's disease activity. Enteric-coated 5-ASA (mesalamine) products begin to release the active agent in the small bowel, while the release of 5-ASA from sulfasalazine and olsalazine occurs entirely within the colon.

In patients with moderate to severe disease, prednisone (20 to 40 mg per day) is useful but does not prevent recurrences, and its use should be limited to less than 4 months. Chronic steroid use is associated with multiple adverse reactions, including adrenal insufficiency, bone demineralization, and avascular necrosis of major joints.

Patients who require steroids for the induction of remission should be considered for immunomodulator therapy, such as azathioprine, 6-mercaptopurine, and methotrexate. Their use must be weighed against their serious potential side effects (bone marrow suppression, pancreatitis, and predisposition to infections, allergies, and neoplasia).

Maintenance therapy with therapeutic doses of mesalamine or immunomodulators (e.g., azathioprine, 6-MP) may lower the 1-year relapse rate from about 60% to 25%.

In patients with moderate to severe disease unresponsive to immunomodulators, newer biologic agents such as infliximab, a monoclonal antibody to TNF-α, have emerged as alternatives for rapidly inducing remission and preventing relapses.

High-dose metronidazole, given for many months, can promote temporary fistula closure, but the drug may induce peripheral neuropathy, particularly in doses over 1 g per day.

SURGICAL THERAPY

Surgery by an experienced surgeon is reserved for treating intractable disease and local complications (e.g., abscesses, bowel obstruction, enterocutaneous fistulas, incapacitating pain unresponsive to medical measures, and severe perirectal and anal disease). The lifetime risk of requiring surgery is about 70%, and 30% to 50% of patients require multiple surgeries. The implications of proctocolectomy for Crohn's colitis differ from those for CUC. The disease may not be eradicated, and 20% to 50% of patients later develop Crohn's disease in the remaining terminal ileum.

Complications

The risk of colorectal carcinoma in extensive Crohn's colitis approaches that in CUC. As in CUC, surveillance colonoscopy with multiple biopsies is widely practiced. In addition, several cases of adenocarcinoma of the ileum have been reported in patients with ileal Crohn's disease, but no guidelines exist for regular surveillance of the small bowel for premalignant changes or early cancer.

CHAPTER 77

Diverticular Disease of the Colon

Kurt Pfeifer

Colonic diverticular disease is a clinical condition in which patients develop symptoms or complications caused by multiple diverticula of the colon (*diverticulosis*). The manifestations of diverticular disease range from uncomplicated diverticulosis, which is often asymptomatic, to diverticulitis and diverticular bleeding. Up to two thirds of the population develops diverticulosis by age 85 years, and approximately 15% of these patients will eventually develop symptomatic diverticular disease.

ETIOLOGY

Diverticula develop as a result of herniation of the mucosa and submucosa through areas of weakness in the muscular layer of the colon. Because the herniations do not include all layers of the bowel wall, they are not true diverticula. The exact pathophysiology is not certain, but three factors are likely major contributors to diverticulosis: colonic wall compliance, elevated intraluminal pressures, and low-fiber diet. With aging and in medical conditions such as Marfan's disease, the strength and integrity of the colonic wall weakens as a result of loss of normal collagen and other extracellular protein content. Loss of colonic wall compliance is asymmetric and most pronounced in the left colon, consistent with the clinical predominance of left-sided diverticulosis. In addition to colonic wall weakening, patients with diverticulosis may have elevated intraluminal pressures generated by abnormally intense and closely spaced contractions called *segmentation*. Segmentation may create intraluminal pressures sufficient to cause herniation of colonic mucosa through vulnerable points in the muscular wall. Dietary fiber can reduce the intensity of segmentation, and it is the loss of this protective effect in low-fiber diets that has been implicated as the cause of the high incidence of diverticulosis in Western countries.

CLINICAL MANIFESTATIONS

Most patients with uncomplicated diverticulosis are asymptomatic, but a minority report episodic abdominal bloating and pain, typically in the left lower quadrant, lasting several days and often temporarily relieved by bowel movements. On palpation, the area of reported pain may be tender, but the remainder of the physical examination is usually unremarkable and laboratory evaluation unrevealing. Diverticulitis occurs in as many as 10% of patients with diverticulosis and results from perforation of one or more diverticula causing extracolonic inflammation. These microperforations may be further complicated by formation of abscesses, sinus tracts and fistulae, and (rarely) by free perforation and peritonitis.

Hemorrhage from penetrating blood vessels within the herniated colonic mucosal tissue may result in diverticular bleeding. As a result of herniation, changes occur within these blood vessels that leaves them more vulnerable to injury and bleeding. Up to 70% of all rectal bleeding in elderly patients is due to proximal colonic diverticular disease. Patients with diverticular bleeding present with self-limited, painless, bright to dark red blood mixed with stool. The right colon is the most common site of diverticular bleeding, which has a 50% reoccurrence rate in patients who had a previous bleeding episode.

The clinical features of diverticulitis are severe, abrupt onset of left lower quadrant abdominal pain, low-grade fever, and change in bowel habits (most often constipation). On physical examination, left lower quadrant tenderness may be elicited. Rebound tenderness and abdominal rigidity should raise the suspicion of peritonitis caused by perforation. Diffuse abdominal pain accompanied by abdominal distention and high fevers may be the result of a diverticular abscess causing bowel obstruction.

DIAGNOSIS

Uncomplicated diverticulosis is often diagnosed incidentally on either colonoscopy or barium enema examination (Fig. 77.1). Mild to moderate leukocytosis may be present in patients with diverticulitis.

An upright plain radiograph of abdomen and chest may detect the presence of bowel obstruction or perforation (free air under the diaphragm) occurring as a result of complicated diverticulitis.

Computed tomography scan of the abdomen has become the test of choice for the diagnosis of diverticulitis. Findings of bowel wall thickening and soft tissue inflammation seen on computed tomography scan are highly suggestive of diverticulitis. The presence of a soft tissue mass may

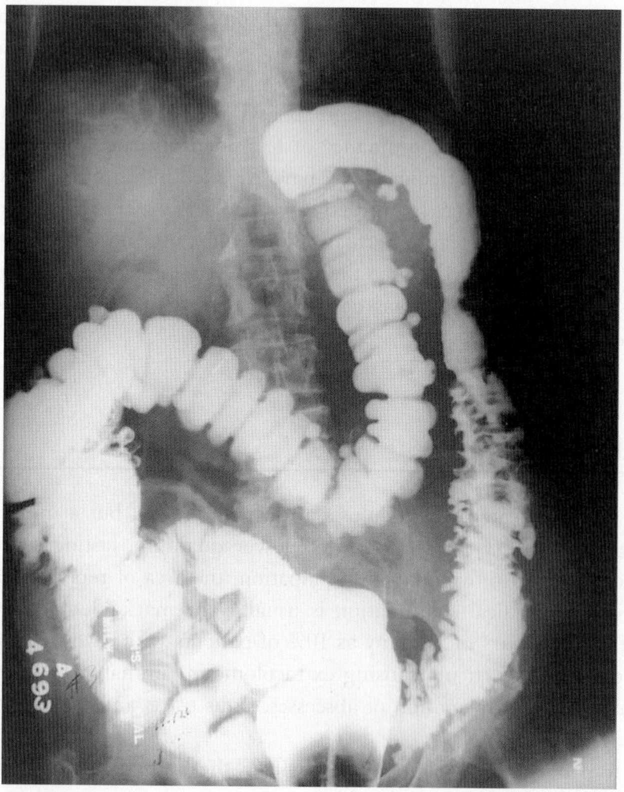

Figure 77.1 • Barium enema showing diverticulosis of the colon.

represent a diverticular abscess. Barium enema should be avoided in the acute phase because of the risk of peritonitis that may result from barium leaking into the peritoneum through microperforations. A colonoscopy is usually not performed during an episode of acute diverticulitis due to possible risk of perforation.

In a patient with diverticular bleeding and stable hemodynamics, urgent colonoscopy (<18 hours after onset) should be the initial diagnostic (and possibly therapeutic) modality and may allow localization of the site of bleeding. If colonoscopy is unrevealing and bleeding persists, a nuclear scan or angiography may be warranted.

TREATMENT

Increased dietary intake of fiber, such as unprocessed wheat bran, may help relieve symptoms, but the amount necessary (up to 20 g daily) may cause intolerable abdominal bloating and flatulence. Methylcellulose or psyllium are also useful and are better tolerated, albeit more expensive.

Recurrent hemorrhage is common in diverticulosis, and other than increasing fiber intake and avoiding anticoagulants, little can be done to prevent recurrence. Repetitive, severe bleeding is an indication for partial colectomy after correct preoperative localization of the bleeding site.

Most episodes of diverticulitis are mild and can be managed medically as an outpatient. Oral intake is restricted to clear liquids, and empiric antibiotic therapy is given for 10 days to target anaerobic and gram-negative organisms (i.e., metronidazole plus ciprofloxacin). Patients with intolerance of oral intake, fever, pain requiring narcotic analgesia, or evidence of abscess or other complications require hospitalization for intravenous fluids and broad-spectrum antibiotics (i.e., ertapenem).

Peritonitis is an indication for urgent surgical intervention, while abscesses can be drained surgically or under ultrasound or computed tomography guidance, followed by nonurgent bowel resection when the inflammation has subsided. Recurrent attacks or onset before age 35 years also warrant elective resection of the involved segment, usually the sigmoid colon.

COMPLICATIONS

Several complications may develop in the setting of diverticulitis. They include diffuse peritonitis, perforation, partial or compete obstruction, and diverticular abscesses. Sigmoid diverticulitis may result in fistula formation.

CHAPTER 78

Bowel Obstruction

Kurt Pfeifer

Mechanical bowel obstruction and adynamic ileus represent two of the most common gastrointestinal problems encountered by physicians in the hospital. Small bowel obstruction accounts for up to 20% of surgical admissions in the United States, and treatment of ileus costs over half a billion dollars annually.

ETIOLOGY

Mechanical bowel obstruction and adynamic (or paralytic) ileus have similar presentations but fundamentally different causes. Mechanical obstruction results from anatomical abnormalities impeding the flow of bowel contents despite normal intestinal smooth muscle contractility. In adynamic ileus, no physical obstruction to flow is present. Instead, generalized hypomotility of intestinal smooth muscle results in stasis of bowel contents.

Mechanical Bowel Obstruction

Mechanical bowel obstruction can result from either intraluminal blockade (i.e., tumors, foreign bodies, gallstones) or extrinsic compression (i.e., adhesions, extraluminal tumors, volvulus). The leading cause of small bowel obstruction is postsurgical adhesions, particularly after colorectal, gynecologic, and upper gastrointestinal procedures. Other less common etiologies include malignancy (both gastrointestinal and metastatic), hernias, volvulus, and Crohn's disease. Mechanical obstruction of the large bowel is less common and more likely to be due to malignancy.

Blockade of intestinal flow results in the accumulation of gastrointestinal secretions and partially digested food or fecal matter proximal to the obstruction. Dilatation of the proximal bowel stimulates further mucosal secretion and peristalsis, causing worsening abdominal distention and cramping abdominal pain. As this vicious cycle continues, the risk of bowel rupture with resultant peritonitis and septic shock increases. Other potential complications are sepsis from bacterial translocation and strangulated bowel due to hyperactive peristalsis, causing the distended bowel to twist and occlude its mesenteric blood supply.

Adynamic Ileus

The most common cause of adynamic ileus is intraperitoneal surgery, especially colon resections. Postoperative bowel hypomotility is physiologic, but when the duration exceeds 2 to 3 days, it is considered paralytic ileus. Aside from a surgical complication, ileus can be a consequence of sepsis, electrolyte derangements, intra-abdominal inflammation, and medications (opioids). Additionally, acute colonic pseudo-obstruction (Ogilvie syndrome) is adynamic ileus affecting only the colon that classically arises in elderly patients suffering any severe illness.

TABLE 78.1 Features of mechanical obstruction and paralytic ileus

	Mechanical obstruction	Paralytic ileus
Abdominal pain	Colicky, occurs in bouts that reach a peak	Usually absent; discomfort and dyspnea depend on extent of distention
Other symptoms	Nausea, vomiting, abdominal distention, and obstipation	Nausea, vomiting, abdominal distention, and obstipation
Abdominal examination	Soft and tympanitic, visible outlines of dilated intestinal loops, borborygmi (early); bowel sounds are absent in late disease complicated by peritonitis	Abdomen distended and characteristically silent
Radiographs	Single or multiple loops of distended small bowel with air-fluid levels; may have a "cut-off" sign where air is not seen distal to a segment of bowel	Multiple, distended, gas-filled small and large intestinal loops (colon distention only in Ogilvie syndrome), with gas present in the rectum
Course and treatment	Progressive unless obstruction relieved with conservative or surgical intervention	Often self-limited; responds to correction of the underlying illness through intestinal decompression and management of fluid/electrolyte problems

CLINICAL FEATURES

The features of mechanical bowel obstruction and adynamic ileus are compared in Table 78.1. Key distinguishing characteristics are based on the history and physical examination. Abdominal pain, a major complaint in the patient with bowel obstruction, is usually absent in patients with ileus. Furthermore, bowel sounds will be markedly decreased or absent in ileus but hyperactive in the setting of a mechanical obstruction.

DIAGNOSIS

Although the history and physical examination frequently identify the cause of a patient's abdominal distention, plain supine, upright, and lateral abdominal radiographs should be obtained for confirmation and to document the severity of the problem. Besides an abnormal number of air-fluid levels (Fig. 78.1), bowel gas patterns might suggest inguinal or other internal hernias, volvulus, or air in the portal vein (bowel infarction). Laboratory analysis is useful for detecting potential contributors to ileus or complications of obstruction, including electrolyte abnormalities and acid-base disturbances. In select cases, a cautiously performed barium enema can show the level and nature of mechanical colon obstruction, and in sigmoid volvulus, is often the treatment of choice.

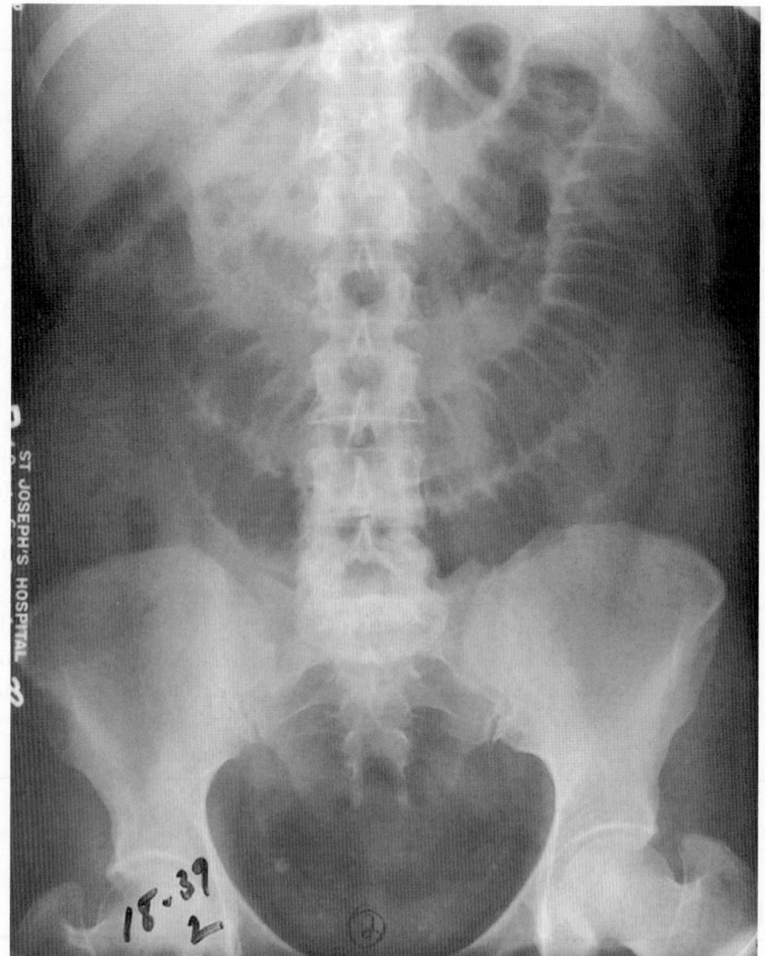

Figure 78.1 • Plain x-ray of abdomen showing small bowel obstruction.

MANAGEMENT

For both adynamic ileus and mechanical obstruction, initial treatment consists of correcting fluid and electrolyte imbalances, relieving nausea and emesis, and limiting medications that slow gut motility. Decompression of the bowel with intermittent nasogastric suction is also an important early intervention in patients with severe bowel dilatation or emesis. Patients suffering from acute colonic pseudo-obstruction refractory to the above measures in addition to repeated enemas and increased mobilization often require colonoscopy for decompression tube placement. Recent studies in patients without advanced cardiopulmonary disease have also shown that intravenous neostigmine is equally efficacious. In suspected mechanical obstruction, early surgical consultation should be considered before strangulation (creating a nonviable bowel segment) or perforation occurs.

When the patient's symptoms significantly improve, a slow return to their previous diet can be initiated. Most cases of ileus and bowel obstruction resolve with nonsurgical therapies, but the patient remains at risk for recurrence in the future.

Nephrology

Virginia Savin

CHAPTER 79

Acute Renal Failure

Robert Riniker

Acute renal failure (ARF) is a sudden decline in renal function. Glomerular filtration rate (GFR) has been viewed as the primary measure of renal function, with blood urea nitrogen (BUN), creatinine, and urine output (UO) as surrogate markers. ARF has been defined by either azotemia (retention of nitrogenous wastes such as BUN and creatinine) and/or oliguria (urine output <400 to 500 mL per day) regardless of the need for renal dialysis. Typical definitions have specified an increase in creatinine of 0.3 to 0.5 mg/dL or 50% above previous baseline. The Acute Dialysis Quality Initiative (ADQI) (an international consensus group) established definition of risk, injury, failure, loss, and end-stage kidney disease (RIFLE) shown in Table 79.1. Criteria include three levels of acute deterioration based on serum creatinine, GFR, or urine output, and two levels of outcome based on the duration of need for dialysis. These criteria are intended for classification of patients in the acute care situation and not to those with intrinsic renal disease such as acute glomerulonephritis. The RIFLE criteria appear to be useful in predicting mortality and duration of hospitalization and may permit quantifying severity of renal injury in studies of therapy and outcome.

ETIOLOGY

Normal renal function depends on renal blood flow and intraglomerular pressure, intact glomeruli and tubules, and patent ureters and urethra. Dysfunction at any of these points will result in renal insufficiency. Disease processes may compromise one or several of these functions. ARF is usually divided into categories of prerenal (diminished renal perfusion), renal (structural injury), and postrenal (obstruction). Prerenal processes are common in hospitalized patients.

Prerenal

Prerenal ARF is a failure to perfuse the kidney at adequate pressure (Table 79.2). It may occur in patients with severe intravascular volume depletion due to gastrointestinal (GI) losses, bleeding, or urinary losses associated with diuretics or uncontrolled diabetes mellitus. Prerenal ARF also occurs in shock or during obstruction of renal vasculature. Shock is usually easily recognized by hypotension and dysfunction of organs including kidneys, lungs, liver, or GI tract. Relative hypotension occurs when a decline in blood pressure (BP) to low normal values (such as a systolic BP of 100 to 110 mm Hg) can no longer drive blood across a fixed obstruction of the renal artery or distally, within the renal parenchyma. Effective renal perfusion is also diminished in heart failure and liver disease. During intravascular volume depletion or hypotension, inhibition of ANG II by angiotensin converting enzyme inhibitors, or angiotensin receptor blockers and nonsteroidal antiinflammatory agents (NSAIDS) decrease glomerular filtration pressure and GFR.

Renal

Renal ARF is due to intrinsic abnormalities in the kidneys. Intrinsic ARF is due to acute glomerulonephritis (AGN), acute interstitial nephritis (AIN), or acute tubular necrosis (ATN).

TABLE 79.1 RIFLE definitions of acute renal failure

Levels of impairment		
	GFR criteria	**Urine output criteria**
Risk	50% increase in serum creatinine or 25% decrease in GFR	<0.5 mL/kg/hour for 6 hours (<35 mL/hour for 70-kg adult)
Injury	100% increase in serum creatinine or 50% decrease in GFR	<0.5 mL/kg/hour for 12 hours (<35 ml/hour for 70-kg adult)
Failure	200% increase in serum creatinine or 75% decrease in GFR or serum creatinine >4.0 mg/dL	<0.3 mL/kg/hour for 24 hours (<20 mL/hour for 70-kg adult) or anuria for 12 hours
Levels of outcome		
Loss	Persistent acute renal failure: dialysis >4 weeks	
End-stage renal disease	End-stage kidney disease: dialysis >3 months	

GFR, glomerular filtration rate.

GLOMERULONEPHRITIS

AGN presents as ARF and is usually accompanied by hypertension, hematuria with red blood cell (RBC) casts, and proteinuria (nephritic sediment). Rapidly progressive glomerulonephritis (RPGN) indicates nephritis with progression of renal failure over weeks or months. Both AGN and RPGN are immune mediated. Prompt diagnosis and therapy of underlying infection or autoimmune disorders may improve renal function and prevent progression to chronic renal failure. Classification and etiology of AGN and RPGN are discussed in the chapter on glomerulonephritis (Chapter 81).

ACUTE INTERSTITIAL NEPHRITIS

AIN is an inflammatory process in the interstitium. This is typically due to an allergic reactions to drugs (Table 79.2), although it can also be seen with various infections (viruses, bacteria, rickettsia, leptospira, toxoplasmosis, mycobacterium tuberculosis [MTB]) and sarcoid.

ACUTE TUBULAR NECROSIS

ATN is by far the most common intrinsic renal cause of ARF (>90%). ATN may be due to ischemia or nephrotoxins (Table 79.2). The renal tubules have a high oxygen demand that makes certain segments susceptible to hypoxic injury. Ischemic ATN is, in fact, the result of prerenal ARF, with the so-called intermediate syndrome occurring when prerenal failure progresses through ischemia to cause ATN, with features of both prerenal ARF and ATN present. Nephrotoxic ATN is usually due to drugs or pigments (hemoglobin, myoglobin). ATN may also result from myeloma casts in paraproteinemias such as multiple myeloma.

Postrenal

Postrenal ARF is due to obstruction to urine flow. This can occur at the renal pelvis, ureter, or urethra. The renal pelvis can be obstructed by stones, clots, tumors, or sloughed renal papilla. The ureters may be obstructed by these processes or by external compression from retroperitoneal fibrosis, radiation fibrosis, or tumor. Females may have ureteral obstruction due to cervical cancer. The most common cause of urinary obstruction is urethral obstruction due to benign prostatic hypertrophy or prostate cancer.

TABLE 79.2 Causes of acute renal failure

Prerenal failure
Volume depletion: poor fluid intake, diuretics, gastrointestinal loss, hemorrhage
Decreased renal perfusion:
Decreased cardiac output: acute myocardial infarction, congestive heart failure, pericardial tamponade
Peripheral vasodilation: sepsis, liver failure, neurogenic shock
Altered renal hemodynamics: anaesthesia, surgery, NSAID, ACE-I, ARB, cyclosporine, hepatorenal syndrome
Renal vasculature occlusion: fixed obstruction: renal artery stenosis, thromboembolic disease, intrarenal atherosclerosis, vasculitis, atheroemboli
Intrinsic renal failure
Renal vascular disorders: malignant hypertension, atheroemboli, vasculitis, thrombotic TTP, HUS, scleroderma renal crisis, toxemia of pregnancy
Glomerular diseases: acute postinfectious GN, rapidly progressive GN, SLE, Goodpasture's syndrome
Acute tubular necrosis:
Ischemia (severe hypotension)
Nephrotoxins (aminoglycosides, amphotericin B, cisplatin, radiocontrast, certain cephalosporins), pigments (hemoglobin, myoglobin), cast nephropathy (multiple myeloma, light chain disease)
Acute interstitial nephritis:
Drugs (NSAID, diuretics, penicillins, cephalosporins, rifampin, acyclovir, phenytoin, captopril, interferon)
Bacterial and viral infections of the kidney (legionella, staphylococcus, streptococcus, gram-negative bacteria, brucellosis, TB, CMV, HIV, EBV, toxoplasmosis, fungi) infiltrative diseases (sarcoid, lymphoma, leukemia).
Postrenal failure
Ureteral obstruction (bilateral or involving single functioning kidney): retroperitoneal fibrosis or tumor, ureteral calculi, postoperative strictures, radiation fibrosis/strictures
Bladder obstruction: bladder cancer, bladder stones, neurogenic bladder
Urethral obstruction: BPH, prostate cancer, cervical cancer, urethral stricture

BPH, benign prostatic hypertrophy; CMV, cytomegalovirus; EBV, Epstein-Barr virus; GN, glomerulonephritis; HIV, human immunodeficiency virus; HUS hemolytic uremic syndrome; NSAID, nonsteroidal anti-inflammatory drug; SLE, systemic lupus erythematosus; TB, tuberculosis; TTP, thrombotic thrombocytopenic purpura.

Special Etiologies

Several other etiologies are discussed elsewhere, but warrant brief mention as causes of ARF. Hemolytic-uremic syndrome (HUS) and thrombotic thrombocytopenic purpura (TTP) (Chapter 97) both present with microangiopathic hemolytic anemia, uremia, and thrombocytopenia; TTP is often associated with fever and neurologic symptoms. Atheroembolic disease can cause ARF following endovascular instrumentation (for example, cardiac catheterization), often days to weeks afterward; it may also occur spontaneously. Renal vein thrombosis can occur with severe dehydration, hypercoagulable states (especially with nephrotic range proteinuria), or renal cell carcinoma. Renal vein thrombosis may be associated with flank pain, hematuria, or pulmonary embolism. Hepatorenal syndrome occurs as either an acute or subacute deterioration in renal function in patients with advanced liver disease.

CLINICAL MANIFESTATIONS

Initial symptoms of ARF are limited to decreased urine output. The diagnosis of ARF is usually made based on laboratory tests including elevated BUN and/or serum creatinine. Additional laboratory findings include development of metabolic acidosis, progressive hyperkalemia, hypocalcemia, and hyperphosphatemia. Hyponatremia usually occurs only with administration of hypotonic intravenous solutions. Physical findings are absent initially but later may include evidence of volume expansion, hypertension, and edema. Symptoms and signs of uremia develop only after a number of days and include altered mental status, pericarditis, and GI bleeding.

History should be reviewed for potential causes of ARF (hypotension, medications, congenital kidney diseases, procedures requiring radiocontrast or risking emboli), previous baseline chronic renal insufficiency (CRI), urinary signs (abnormal color, dysuria), and sequelae (volume overload, bleeding diathesis). Examination should concentrate on volume status to rule out prerenal causes, evidence of postrenal obstruction (pelvic examination in females, rectal examination in males, bladder scan or possible Foley catheter), urine output (anuric, oliguric, or nonoliguric), sequelae (volume overload, uremic pericarditis), and evidence of related diseases (rash with vasculitis or embolic process, murmur with endocarditis).

DIAGNOSIS

The diagnosis of ARF is approached in a stepwise fashion (Fig. 79.1). Prerenal ARF due to shock should be addressed first. The BUN and creatinine should be rechecked and nonrenal causes of elevated BUN and creatinine assessed (Table 79.3). Oliguria should be confirmed and bladder outlet obstruction ruled out by bladder scan or Foley catheter. Significant residual urine volume is >100mL to 300 mL. Of note, serum creatinine will rise by about 1 mg/dL a day if GFR is nearly zero.

Chronic kidney disease (CKD) should be assessed using prior records and previous BUN and serum creatinine. Additional indicators of CKD include anemia, hypocalcemia, and hyperphosphatemia. Ultrasound showing small kidneys (<9 cm), cortical thinning, or multiple cysts is suggestive of CKD. Nephritic sediment suggests an acute process needing urgent evaluation. If there is any doubt about chronicity, it is prudent to assume the process is acute until proven otherwise.

The urinalysis is a pivotal initial test. Findings in the urinalysis and use of urine chemistries are summarized in Table 79.4. In prerenal ARF, urinalysis shows increased specific gravity (SG) and hyaline casts. Urine typically has high osmolality and urea with decreased urine sodium. In glomerulonephritis or vasculitis urinalysis includes proteinuria, hematuria (with dysmorphic RBC), and RBC casts. In acute interstitial nephritis, urine may or may not be concentrated; white blood cells (WBCs), including eosinophils, and WBC casts may be present. In ATN, many granular casts, tubular cells and cellular casts may be present, urine SG is low (1.010), and urine sodium concentration is high. Tubular cells, cellular casts, and granular casts that appear dark (so-called muddy brown casts) may be seen; true pigmented casts are seen in hemolysis and rhabdomyolysis.

There are a number of renal indices used to assess tubular function (Table 79.4). The fractional excretion of sodium (FENa) is probably the most widely used and is calculated as:

$$\text{FENa} = (\text{U sodium / P sodium})/(\text{U creatinine/ P creatinine}) \times 100$$

FENa <1% suggests good tubular function; FENa >3% suggests acute tubular necrosis; Interpretation of FENa between 1% and 3% is indeterminate. Prerenal ARF (including hepatorenal

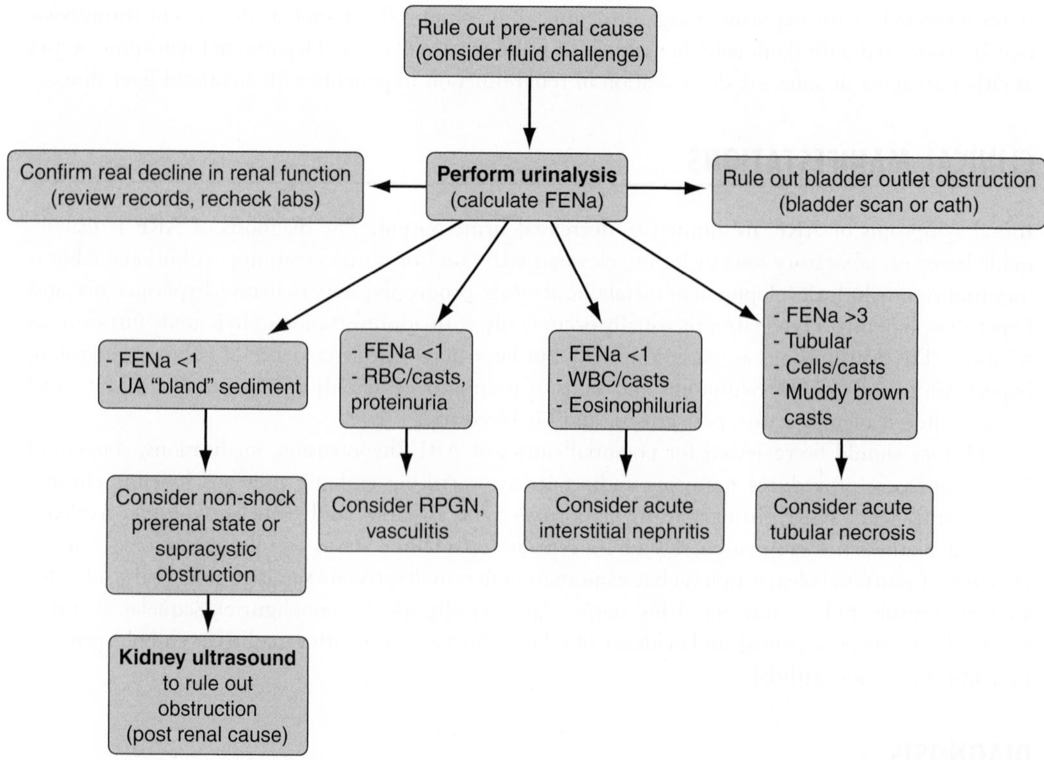

Figure 79.1 • Approach to the diagnosis of acute renal failure (ARF). FENa, fractional excretion of sodium.

syndrome), glomerulonephritis, vasculitis, acute interstitial nephritis, radiocontrast, and pigment-induced ATN have low FENa (<1%). Prerenal ARF with progression to ischemic ATN will initially show low FENa (usually for the first 48 hours). About 10% of nonoliguric ATN also have a low FENa. The FENa may be >1% in advanced CKD, diuretic use, diuresis induced by glucose, mannitol, bicarbonaturia, and in acute volume expansion. Fractional excretion of urea can be used as an alternative measure, with FEUrea <35% suggesting a prerenal process and >55% and 65% suggesting ATN.

A multisystem process should be evaluated. Common examples are hepatorenal syndrome, HUS/TTP, embolic process, and hypertensive crisis. Prerenal and postrenal processes should be identified and treated. Postrenal obstruction above the level of the urethra can usually be safely and definitively identified with a abdominal ultrasound. Differentiating nonshock prerenal ARF from intrinsic renal ARF can be difficult and requires analysis of the entire clinical picture.

TREATMENT

Treatment varies according to the type and etiology of ARF. One of the mainstays of treatment in patients who have developed ESRD is hemodialysis. Prevention of ARF is also important.

It is possible to prevent certain forms of ATN. Radiocontrast-induced ATN can, to some extent, be avoided by excluding high-risk patients, using lower doses of iso-osmotic agents, and pretreating with intravenous infusion of saline or bicarbonate solutions. N-acetylcysteine may decrease the risk

TABLE 79.3 Nonrenal causes of abnormal blood urea nitrogen and creatinine

Compounds interfering with creatinine secretion
Cimetidine
Trimethoprim
Quinine
Compounds falsely increasing creatinine in certain assays
Acetoacetic acid in ketoacidosis
Cefoxitin
Flucytosine
Ascorbic acid
Uric acid
L dopa
Myeloma proteins
Creatine ingestion
Nonrenal causes of elevated blood urea nitrogen
Increased urea generation
High protein intake
Gastrointestinal bleeding
Catabolic states with increased tissue breakdown
Myocardial infarction
Glucocorticoids
Slow urine flow rate
Causes of low blood urea nitrogen
Decreased urea generation
Severe liver disease
Malnutrition—low protein intake
Increased glomerular filtration rate
Anabolic hormones
Pregnancy
Acromegaly
Syndrome of inappropriate antidiuretic hormone
Decreased tubular reabsorption of urea
Diuresis (high urine flow rate without volume depletion)

of ATN (600 mg twice daily, orally beginning the day before the radiocontrast). Toxic injury due to therapeutic agents can be minimized by adjusting doses appropriately and, in the case of amphotericin B, by using lipophilic preparations.

Prerenal

Prevention of progression of prerenal ARF to ATN requires increased renal perfusion. Fluid depletion should be corrected and, if hypotension is present, it should be treated with fluids and vasopressors. Initial fluid replacement should be with isotonic rather than hypotonic solutions. Norepinephrine is currently the preferred vasopressor. Drugs that decrease renal blood flow and those that are nephrotoxic should be stopped. Clinical studies do not support the use of "renal dose" dopamine for

TABLE 79.4 Laboratory characteristics of acute renal failure

Parameter	Pre-renal	Tubular necrosis	Acute interstitial nephritis
FENa (%)	<1	>3	
Urine sodium (mEq/L)	<10–20	>20–40	
Sediment	Normal or hyaline casts	Tubular cells/casts "Muddy brown" casts	WBC/casts eosinophils
BUN/CT	>20	<20	
Urine osmolality	>500	<350–400	
Urine SG	>1.015	<1.015	
FEUrate (%)	<12	>20	
FEUrea (%)	<35	>50–65	

prerenal ARF. Diuretics can be used to increase urine flow rate after fluid depletion and hypotension have been corrected.

Renal

Treatment of ATN includes restoring renal perfusion and stopping any toxic agents. Treatment with loop diuretics or mannitol may increase urine output but do not alter the course of renal failure. ATN may be oliguric (<400 mL per day) or nonoliguric. Nonoliguric ATN is easier to manage than oliguric ATN and has a better outcome. Loop diuretics may be indicated in the first 24 hours of oliguric ATN to convert to the condition to nonoliguric ATN and perhaps limit damage. After this, the only role for diuretics is in an attempt to control volume.

GN and, in particular, RPGN require urgent consultation with a nephrologist and evaluations to establish a specific diagnosis. Kidney biopsy may be required. Treatment is dictated both by the severity and the etiology of the condition. AGN after infection requires treatment of the infection. AGN or RPGN of autoimmune origin are treated with immunosuppression.

AIN is treated by stopping the offending agent. If systemic symptoms of allergy are severe, corticosteroids may be indicated. Renal function returns gradually over several days or weeks and steroid therapy is not proven to hasten recovery.

Postrenal

Postrenal ARF requires elimination of the obstruction by catheters, stents, or surgical interventions. Renal failure occurs only if both kidneys are affected. Obstruction may affect one kidney and renal failure may occur when the second kidney is obstructed. Percutaneous nephrostomy tubes may be placed by interventional radiologists while ureteral stents require urology consultation. If the obstruction is of short duration, renal function is recovered rapidly; with more chronic obstruction, recovery is delayed and may be incomplete.

Indications for hemodialysis are outlined in Table 79.5.

Indications for Dialysis

Dialysis is indicated for metabolic acidosis, hypervolemia that is refractory to diuretics, hyperkalemia, hyponatremia, uremic symptoms (anorexia, nausea/vomiting, encephalopathy, seizures), and uremic

TABLE 79.5 Potential Indications for hemodialysis

Volume overload (refractory to therapy)
Severe hyperkalemia (potassium >6.5)
Uremic pericarditis with tamponade
Metabolic acidosis and increased anion gap
Refractory hypertension
Anuria/oliguria (not responding to fluids)
Uremic encephalopathy (altered mental status, seizures)
Sever hypo/hypernatremia (Na <120 or Na >155)
Elevated blood urea nitrogen (>80)

pericarditis. Dialysis is usually delayed until these indications develop. Prophylactic early dialysis may actually worsen outcome. Frequent dialysis is often required to permit nutrition without volume overload and continuous therapies are often used if the patient is hemodynamically unstable. The specific prescription for dialysis is dictated by availability of the required equipment and expertise.

COMPLICATIONS

Complications of ARF include infection, which is the most common cause of death. Electrolyte problems include metabolic acidosis, an increased anion gap, hyperkalemia, hypocalcemia, hyperphosphatemia, hypermagnesemia, and, if hypotonic fluids are given, hyponatremia. Volume overload occurs if the patient is oliguric and sodium and fluids are given. Platelet dysfunction develops, resulting in bleeding disorders. Uremic pericarditis with tamponade can occur. Uremic symptoms develop after 5 days or more and include anorexia, nausea, vomiting, seizures, and uremic encephalopathy. Iatrogenic problems can develop if the doses of renally cleared medications are not properly reduced.

CHAPTER 80

Chronic Renal Failure

Shibin Jacob and Virginia Savin

Chronic renal failure, or chronic kidney disease (CKD), is the persistent and usually progressive reduction in glomerular filtration rate (GFR; less than 60 mL/min/1.73 m^2). There are multiple causes of CKD and progression to end-stage renal disease (ESRD) may occur. CKD results in limited ability to maintain homeostasis of salts and water and of water-soluble waste products including urea and nonvolatile acids. As renal function declines, endocrine functions of the kidney, including synthesis of erythropoietin and vitamin D and catabolism of insulin, are impaired.

ESRD is a characterized by irreversible loss of renal function that results in life-threatening uremia. In the United States, renal replacement therapy using dialysis or transplantation is offered to most patients with ESRD.

The prevalence of CKD has doubled in the United States from 697 per million in 1990 to 1,424 per million in 2001. This increase may be related to increased recognition of CKD and to increasing survival of people with chronic diseases and the elderly. Diabetes and hypertension are the two most common causes of CKD and ESRD in the United States. CKD is associated with excess cardiovascular risk with an increase of cardiovascular events of more than 10-fold in patients with GFR $<$30 mL per minute versus those with GFR $>$60 mL per minute.

ETIOLOGY

Chronic renal failure or CKD may result from renal ischemia or injury to renal vasculature, from intrinsic renal disease due to inflammatory or other disorders, or from partial or total urinary obstruction. These conditions correspond to the categories often used in analysis of transient causes of renal failure, namely prerenal azotemia, renal injury, and postrenal or obstructive dysfunction.

Two most common causes of CKD are diabetes and hypertension. The risk factors of CKD include increased body mass index, hypertension, smoking, diabetes, low high-density lipoprotein cholesterol, and lead exposure. The most common hereditary etiologies of renal disease are autosomal dominant polycystic renal disease and Alport's syndrome. Rarer diseases include medullary cystic renal disease and Fabry's disease.

CKD is divided into various internationally accepted stages based on decline in GFR (Table 80.1). This staging helps in diagnostic and management approaches, including evaluation of risk factors in patients with CKD. The normal rate of decline in GFR in adults is about 1 mL/year, with a GFR of about 70 mL per minute in males by the age 70 years. Albuminuria is a key adjunctive tool used to monitor CKD and response to treatment.

CKD may lead to uremic syndrome. Uremic syndrome is a constellation of derangements that affects many organ systems (Table 80.2). Uremia can be caused either by accumulation of

TABLE 80.1 Chronic kidney disease: a clinical action plan

Stage	Description	Glomerular filtration rate (mL/min/1.73 m^2)	Symptoms	Action
	At increased risk due to diabetes mellitus, family history of CKD	≥90 (with CKD risk factors)	None	Screening for CKD. Risk reduction by stopping smoking, weight loss, exercise. Control of blood sugar, blood pressure, lipids
1.	Kidney damage with normal or ↑ GFR	≥90	None	Diagnosis and treatment of comorbid conditions, slowing progression, cardiovascular disease risk reduction
2.	Kidney damage with mild ↓ GFR	60–89	None	Estimate progression Tight glycemic control if diabetes mellitus Control blood pressure to 130/80 mm Hg or less
3.	Moderate ↓ GFR	30–59	None Possible nocturia	Refer to nephrologist Evaluate and treat anemia, bone disease, malnutrition
4.	Severe ↓ GFR	15–29	Fatigue Decreased appetite for meat Insomnia, loss of concentration Edema of face or feet Dry skin, itching	Preparation for dialysis or transplantation Education, place dialysis access

(continued)

TABLE 80.1 Chronic kidney disease: a clinical action plan (*Continued*)

Stage	Description	Glomerular filtration rate (mL/min/1.73 m²)	Symptoms	Action
5.	Kidney failure	<15 (or dialysis)	Same as 4 with more severe fluid retention, loss of appetite, decline in mental function, peripheral neuropathy	Replacement using dialysis or transplantation

For staging purposes, the GFR is estimated using Cockroft and Gault or Modification of Diet in Renal Disease 2 equations.
Recommended equations for estimation of glomerular filtration rate from plasma creatinine concentration (P_{Cr}):
1. Equation from the Modification of Diet in Renal Disease study[a]
Estimated GFR (mL/min per 1.73 m²) $= 1.86 \times (P_{Cr})^{-1.154} \times (\text{age})^{-0.203}$
Multiply by 0.742 for women, Multiply by 1.21 for blacks
2. Cockcroft-Gault equation

$$\text{Estimated creatinine clearance (mL/min)} = \frac{(140 - \text{age}) \times \text{body weight } (kg)}{72 \times P_{Cr}\ (mg/dL)}$$

Multiply by 0.85 for women
CKD, chronic kidney disease; GFR, glomerular filtration rate.

TABLE 80.2 Uremic manifestation by organ system

Systems	Manifestations
Fluid and electrolytes	Extracellular fluid volume expansion Hypocalcemia, hyperkalemia
Acid-base	↑ Anion gap Metabolic acidosis
Hematologic	Anemia Bleeding disorder
Musculoskeletal & endocrine	Bone disease (osteitis fibrosa and osteomalacia) Amenorrhea Hyperlipidemia Secondary hyperparathyroidism (hypocalcemia, ↑ parathyroid hormone)
Cardiovascular disease	Coronary artery disease, peripheral vascular disease Pericarditis Cerebrovascular accident
Gastrointestinal	Peptic ulcer disease Gastritis
Neurological	Encephalopathy Seizures Peripheral neuropathy
Dermatological	Pruritus Yellow skin

products of protein metabolism or loss of other renal functions, such as fluid and electrolyte homeostasis, and hormonal abnormalities.

CLINICAL MANIFESTATIONS

Clinical features and therapies of uremic syndrome are summarized in Table 80.2.

Fluids, Electrolytes, and Acid-Base Abnormalities

Metabolic acidosis is common in patients with advanced CKD. With advancing renal disease, net excretion of nonvolatile acids is limited to 30 to 40 mmol per day, which causes a modest drop in the pH and plasma bicarbonate. This can usually be partially corrected by modest doses of $NaHCO_3$ or sodium citrate. Hypocalcemia, hyperphosphatemia, and hyperkalemia are commonly present.

Patients with stable CKD have modest increases in total body sodium and water that may not be clinically apparent. This extracellular fluid expansion contributes to intraglomerular hypertension and accelerates further renal damage. The weight gain from the increased extracellular fluid volume is often masked by the loss of lean body mass. Hyponatremia is unusual and water restriction is required only if hyponatremia is documented.

Assessment of protein and energy malnutrition should commence in stage 3 CKD to prevent nutritional complications that lead to muscle wasting. Uremic fetor seen in patients with uremia is due to breakdown of urea in saliva to ammonia.

Hematologic Abnormalities

Normocytic normochromic anemia is usually seen in stage 3 CKD (GFR 30 to 59 mL/min) and is almost always present in stage 4. The primary cause of anemia is erythropoietin deficiency. Chronic inflammatory states with impaired response to erythropoietin are common and uremia itself contributes to erythropoietin resistance. Additional contributing factors to anemia include nutritional deficiencies of iron or folate, hyperparathyroidism, aluminum toxicity, and shortened red cell survival due to inflammation or blood loss. The treatment of anemia depends on supplementation of recombinant erythropoietin. It is necessary to maintain adequate iron stores and folate levels during erythropoietin therapy.

Bleeding disorders may occur in stage 4 or 5 CKD. Hemostatic abnormalities are prolonged bleeding time due to abnormal platelet function and impaired prothrombin consumption. These can be treated with cryoprecipitate, desmopressin, or conjugated estrogens if required.

Musculoskeletal and Endocrine Abnormalities

Bone disease associated with CKD (renal osteodystrophy) includes osteitis fibrosa, which results from secondary hyperparathyroidism (Chapter 65), osteomalacia, or adynamic bone disease. The pathophysiology of secondary hyperparathyroidism (increased parathyroid hormone [PTH]), is related to abnormal calcium, phosphate, and vitamin D metabolism. Decreased GFR causes a decrease in inorganic phosphate excretion leading to a high phosphate level that stimulates PTH, suppressing calcium levels via decreased calcitriol production. Decreased calcitriol levels decrease gastrointestinal absorption of calcium, resulting in hypocalcemia, which will further increase PTH secretion. These bone diseases can lead to pain and increased risk of fractures. With progression of renal disease, the parathyroid mass increases and can lead to a pattern of diffuse hyperplasia, monoclonal nodular growth, or diffuse monoclonal hyperplasia. Abnormal Ca/PO_4 metabolism can also lead to extraosseous calcifications in soft tissues and blood vessels, which may be contribute to increased cardiovascular mortality in CKD. Calciphylaxis is the severe form of soft tissue and vascular calcification, which can lead to skin and soft-tissue necrosis.

Secondary hyperparathyroidism and osteitis fibrosa are best prevented or treated by decreasing the phosphate levels to normal by dietary restriction, phosphate binders (e.g., calcium carbonate, calcium acetate, and sevelamer), and adding vitamin D as calcitriol or other preparations. Aluminium-based phosphate binders were used in the past but are generally avoided because of the risk of bone accumulation and resulting osteomalacia.

Cardiovascular Disease

Cardiovascular disease is the leading cause of morbidity and mortality in patients with CKD and ESRD. The risk is often 10- to 200-fold depending on the stage of disease and other risk factors. Left ventricular hypertrophy (LVH) and dilated cardiomyopathy are the strongest predictors of cardiovascular mortality. About one third of patients reaching ESRD already have advanced cardiovascular complications (occlusive coronary disease, cerebrovascular, and peripheral vascular disease). The major cardiovascular complications include ischemic heart disease, congestive cardiac failure, left ventricular hypertrophy, and pericarditis. In patients with ESRD, pulmonary edema may be precipitated in the absence of volume overload due to an increase in alveolar capillary membrane permeability.

Hypertension in patients could be pre-existing hypertension, which has been worsened by renal disease or new hypertension due to CKD. Intraglomerular hypertension further hastens the progression of renal disease. Correction of anemia with administration of erythropoietin or transfusion increases blood pressure and may exacerbate hypertension in CKD. Hypertension needs to be treated to a goal of 125/75 mm Hg in patients with proteinuria and 130/85 mm Hg in patients without proteinuria. Angiotensin-converting enzyme (ACE) inhibitors and angiotensin receptor blockers (ARBs) have a higher benefit in patients with proteinuria. Contraindications to ACE inhibitors or ARBs (intractable cough, anaphylaxis, hyperkalemia that cannot be controlled by diet) may warrant use of calcium channel blockers. Diltiazem and verapamil are superior in antiproteinuric and renal protective effects to nifedipine. The goal of treatment in this setting is to decrease the progression of renal disease and to decrease the cardiovascular complications (Chapter 133). Control of dyslipidemia to the National Cholesterol Education Program guidelines is also extremely important in this population to decrease the cardiovascular morbidity and mortality. Statins are also associated with an increased risk of rhabdomyolysis in patients with CKD and ESRD.

Neurologic Effects

Neurological abnormalities, including central, peripheral, and autonomic neuropathy, are common in patients with Stage 4 CKD and ESRD. The early manifestations of central nervous system dysfunction include impaired memory, loss of concentration, and insomnia and daytime somnolence. Autonomic neuropathy may contribute to gastric motility disorders, including delayed gastric emptying. Central nervous system symptoms usually resolve with dialysis, whereas peripheral neuropathy (if severe) may improve, persist, or even progress. Renal transplantation may further improve neuropathies.

Gastrointestinal Disease

Gastritis, peptic ulcer disease, and mucosal ulceration are common. Patients with polycystic kidney disease have a higher incidence of diverticulosis.

Dermatological Disease

Pruritus is common in patients with CKD. A yellow discoloration of the skin is also typical of uremia. Nail discoloration and splinter hemorrhages may also occur. Such symptoms respond to renal replacement therapy.

DIAGNOSIS

The history and physical examination is important to detect possible etiologies or initial symptoms and signs of uremia. Drugs of particular significance are analgesic use (often ignored or underestimated by the patient), nonsteroidal anti-inflammatory drugs, antimicrobials, lithium, and ACE inhibitors. Physical examination should include blood pressure, fundoscopy, abdominal bruits, edema, neuropathy, asterixis, muscle weakness, prostatic masses in men, and pelvic masses in women.

The diagnosis of chronic renal failure is primarily based on laboratory data as symptoms associated with chronic kidney disease (CKD) are conspicuous by their absence until the late stages of the disease. Laboratory data should be divided into two groups: those to evaluate the likely etiology of renal disease and those to monitor the progression of renal disease itself. This includes serial measurements of serum creatinine, urinary protein excretion, estimations of GFR, urea, calcium, phosphate, bicarbonate, alkaline phosphatase, monitoring for anemia, and lipids.

The most useful imaging study in the initial evaluation of patients with CKD is renal ultrasound. It can verify the presence of two kidneys, renal size including presence or absence of disparities between sides, renal masses, and obstruction. Symmetric small kidneys imply renal scarring and chronic irreversible renal disease, although normal-sized kidneys may be present in patients with polycystic kidney disease, amyloidosis, diabetes, and human immunodeficiency virus–associated renal disease. Asymmetric renal size implies a unilateral process, either developmental or chronic. Renal vascular imaging may be done through renal Doppler or magnetic resonance angiography to evaluate the feasibility of revascularization. Spiral computed tomography without contrast may be useful in evaluating renal stones.

Renal biopsy is done in patients when a clearcut diagnosis cannot be made on clinical grounds and the possibility of reversible renal disease is still not ruled out. Extent of tubulointerstitial scarring is the most reliable predictor of progression towards ESRD. In advanced CKD progressing to ESRD, the renal biopsy may not be warranted due to the lack of potential therapeutic significance. Patients are often surprised about the diagnosis as symptoms pertaining to the kidneys are conspicuous only by their absence. It is important to find the etiology of the renal disease.

TREATMENT AND PREVENTION

The treatment of CKD falls into three broad categories: (a) treatments aimed toward resolution of the primary cause of the renal disease (e.g., removal of obstructing renal calculi, optimal treatment of diabetes and hypertension including lifestyle modifications, avoidance of analgesics, immunomodulation in patients with lupus or vasculitis); (b) treatments aimed toward stabilizing or slowing the progression of renal disease (treatment of proteinuria with ACE inhibitors, ARB, revascularization for renal artery stenosis, protein restriction, optimal control of comorbidities including diabetes and hypertension), and minimizing the effects on other organ systems; and (c) renal replacement therapy.

Doses of commonly used medications may need dose adjustments in patients with CKD. Reduc-

TABLE 80.3 Prevention and early treatment to slow progression of chronic kidney disease

For patients with diabetes or hypertension and chronic disease:

- Prescribe angiotensin converting enzyme inhibitor or angiotensin receptor blocker to protect kidney function
- A diuretic should usually be part of the hypertension regimen
- Keep blood pressure below 130/80 mm Hg

It is also important to:

- Provide referral for dietary counseling (Medicare will pay for nutrition counseling for chronic kidney disease)
- Monitor and treat traditional cardiovascular risk factors, particularly smoking and hypercholesterolemia
- Refer patients to a nephrologist for an early opinion
- Team with a nephrologist once the glomerular filtration rate is 30 mL/min/1.73 m^2 or less

Most people may not have any severe symptoms until their kidney disease is advanced. However, you may notice that you:

- feel more tired and have less energy
- have trouble concentrating
- have a poor appetite
- have trouble sleeping
- have muscle cramping at night
- have swollen feet and ankles
- have puffiness around your eyes, especially in the morning
- have dry, itchy skin
- need to urinate more often, especially at night

Adapted from the National Institutes of Health website, http://nkdep.nih.gov/professionals/index.html.

TABLE 80.4 Treatments to slow the progression of chronic kidney disease in adults

	Diabetic kidney disease	Nondiabetic kidney disease	Kidney disease in the transplant patient
Strict glycemic control	Yes[a]	NA	Not tested
Angiotensin-converting enzyme inhibitors or angiotensin-receptor blockers	Yes	Yes (greater effect in patients with proteinuria)	Not tested
Strict blood pressure control	Yes <125/75 mm Hg	Yes <130/85 mm Hg (in patients without proteinuria) <125/75 mm Hg (in patients with proteinuria)	Not tested
Dietary protein restriction	Inconclusive	Inconclusive	Not tested

[a]Prevents or delays the onset of diabetic kidney disease.

tions in GFR mandate dose adjustments or omissions of commonly used hypoglycemic agents. Two medications that need to be avoided entirely are meperidine and metformin.

Renal replacement therapy, which includes dialysis and/or renal transplantation, has been the treatment of ESRD for the last few decades and has prolonged lives. Dialysis should be started sufficiently early to prevent serious complications of uremic state. There is no clearcut GFR or creatinine level at which patients develop uremic symptoms. Dialysis is generally started when the serum creatinine is >8 mg/dL or the creatinine clearance is <10 ml/μm. Some clear indications for dialysis include uremic pericarditis, uremic neuropathy or encephalopathy, refractory muscle irritability, anorexia, nausea despite protein restriction, acid-base disturbances, volume overload unresponsive to diuretic therapy, and hyperkalemia unresponsive to dietary restriction. Prevention may play an important part in slowing the progression of CKD (Tables 80.3 and 80.4).

Renal transplantation offers a near complete resolution of the adverse processes associated with ESRD. All possible attempts should be made to correct any reversible causes of the renal disease in order to stabilize CKD, or decrease the rate of progression. Monitoring progression of CKD and treating associated disorders may decrease morbidity and mortality and delay the need to implement renal replacement therapies.

CHAPTER 81

Glomerulonephritis

Virginia Savin

Glomerulonephritis (GN), literally meaning inflammation of glomeruli, is a leading cause of renal failure worldwide. Inflammation is characterized by infiltration by leukocytes, edema, and vascular fragility.

Glomerular disease may manifest by three major syndromes: nephritic syndrome, nephrotic syndrome, and rapidly progressive glomerulonephritis (RPGN). Nephritic syndrome consists of sudden onset of hematuria and nonnephrotic range proteinuria (<1.5 g/day), active sediment with red blood cell (RBC) casts or dysmorphic RBCs, acute renal failure, and hypertension. Nephrotic syndrome is characterized by heavy proteinuria (>3.5 g/day), edema, hypoalbuminemia, and hyperlipidemia (Chapter 82). RPGN is characterized by active sediment (RBC casts and dysmorphic RBCs), and rapid development of acute renal failure usually over a period of weeks to months (Fig. 81.1).

GN is mediated by immune processes that include deposition of antibodies and complement within the glomerulus, with resulting injury to intrinsic glomerular cells and infiltration by leukocytes and damage to the capillary walls.

GN accounts for the majority of progressive renal disease in many parts of the world.

ETIOLOGY

GN has diverse etiologies related to disorders of the immune system, including abnormal immunoglobulin regulation and abnormal complement regulation. Intraglomerular deposits of immunoglobulins and complement components are seen in some—but not all—forms of GN. Progression of glomerular scarring can occur after severe injury; this may be slowed by nonimmunological interventions aimed at control of glomerular hemodynamics (reduction in systemic blood pressure and inhibition of the renin/angiotensin/aldosterone system). The pathological features of GN are listed in Table 81.1

CLINICAL MANIFESTATIONS OF GN

Signs and symptoms of GN include disorders in the major glomerular functions, filtering water and small solutes, and providing a barrier impermeable to plasma proteins and blood cells (Table 81.2). Hematuria is a key manifestation of glomerulonephritis. Glomerular inflammation leads to glomerular hemorrhage where blood enters the Bowman's space and erythrocytes are incorporated into RBC casts. Thus RBC casts are the hallmark of glomerular injury and are nearly always present in acute glomerulonephritis. RBC casts may persist for an indefinite period after an acute injury but will generally decrease in number as inflammation resolves. A careful review of urinary sediment by an experienced observer may be required to document their presence.

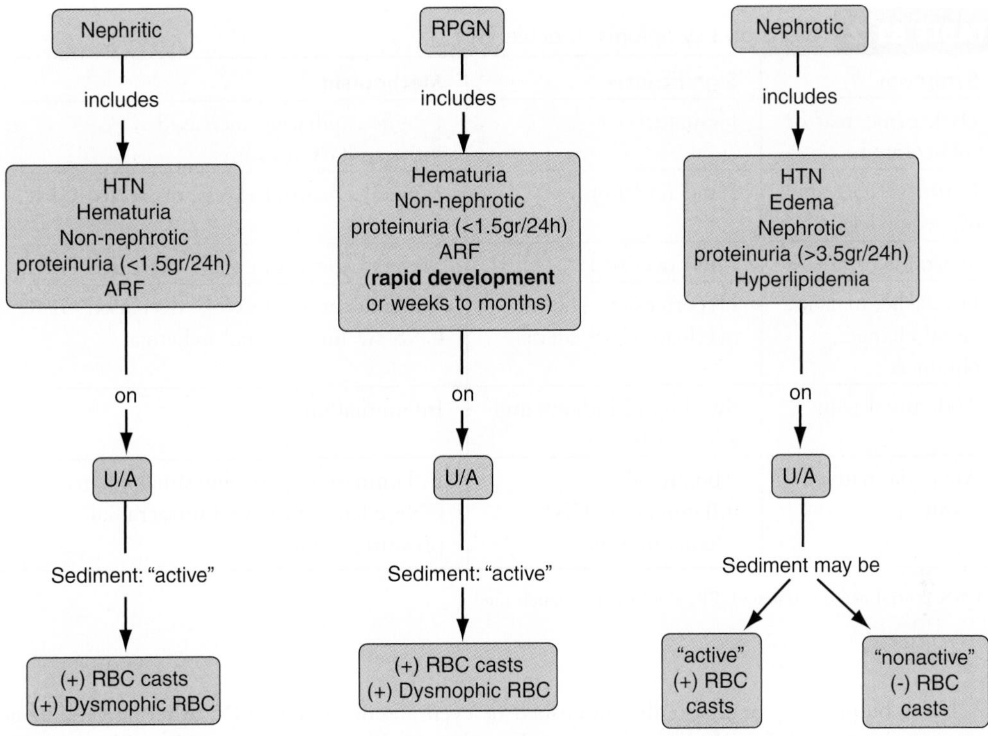

Figure 81.1 • Clinical features and urinalysis findings of the three major classes of glomerular disease. U/A, urinalysis.

Hypertension is a frequent sign of GN. Hypertension arises from two mechanisms: release of renin due to inflammation and impaired renal perfusion, intravascular volume expansion caused by mineral corticoid-induced fluid retention and/or renal insufficiency. Malignant hypertension (Chapter 87) with central nervous system manifestations of headache, confusion, blurred vision, or blindness may occur.

Flank pain or nonspecific abdominal pain may occur because of stretching of the renal capsule or inflammation of perinephric tissues. This may be so severe as to suggest renal stones or an acute abdomen or may be absent. Loss of appetite or vomiting may indicate edema of gastrointestinal tissues or may be signs of increased intracerebral pressure or of uremia.

TABLE 81.1 Pathologic features of glomerular disease

Focal	<50% of glomeruli contain the lesion
Diffuse (global)	Most glomeruli (>50%) contain the lesion
Segmental	Only a part of the glomerulus is affected by the lesion (most focal lesions are also segmental, such as focal segmental glomerulosclerosis)
Proliferation	An increase in cell number of one or more of the resident glomerular cells, with or without an inflammatory cell infiltration
Membranous changes	Capillary wall and matrix thickening
Crescent formation	Epithelial cell proliferation and mononuclear cell infiltration in Bowman's space

TABLE 81.2 Signs and symptoms in acute GN

Symptom	Significance	Mechanism
Dark urine, tea- or cola-colored	Hematuria	Fragile capillaries, increased intracapillary pressure
Puffiness, edema of face or legs	Fluid retention	Mineralocorticoid excess, decreased GFR
Shortness of breath	Fluid overload	Mineralocorticoid excess, decreased GFR
Headache, malaise, visual changes, blindness	Hypertension, volume overload, CNS edema	Mineralocorticoid excess, decreased GFR, CNS swelling, retinal ischemia
Abdominal pain	Swelling of kidneys and adjacent tissues	Inflammation
Anorexia, nausea, vomiting	Abdominal inflammation, CNS edema, uremia	Inflammation, gastrointestinal edema, CNS edema, increased intracranial pressure, uremia

CNS, central nervous system; GFR, glomerular filtration rate.

Urine output may be markedly diminished or even absent in acute GN. Alternatively, urine output can be normal. In either case, intravascular volume is likely to be increased, and hemoglobin and hematocrit reduced, because of increased plasma volume. Because of fluid retention, pulmonary vascular congestion may be present and frank pulmonary edema may occur suddenly.

Nephritic Syndrome

POSTSTREPTOCOCCAL OR POSTINFECTIOUS GN

The classical presentation of poststreptococcal glomerulonephritis includes the sudden onset of gross hematuria, RBC casts in the urine, and nonnephrotic proteinuria. Signs and symptoms generally occur 1 to 2 weeks after a pharyngitis or 3 to 6 weeks after a skin infection with Group A β-hemolytic streptococci. Weight gain with edema formation, hypertension that can be malignant, flank or abdominal pain, decreased urine output, and renal failure are common and fluid retention may result in pulmonary edema. Nephrotic syndrome occurs only in 5% of newly diagnosed patients. Throat and skin culture may yield β-hemolytic streptococci if no antibiotic therapy has been given. Recent streptococcal infection may be confirmed by elevated anti-streptolysin O (ASO) titers and anti-DNase antibodies. Serum complement levels are depressed for 8 weeks or longer.

In most cases of poststreptococcal glomerulonephritis, frank renal failure does not occur and the serum creatinine does not exceed 4 mg/dL. However, marked oliguria and renal failure requiring dialysis can occur. Severe symptoms may be associated with crescentic GN and with incomplete recovery and later progression to renal failure. Most patients recover renal function within 2 months but hematuria may persist for many months and may be more evident during viral or febrile illnesses or after vigorous exercise.

Similar forms of GN occur with other bacterial and viral infections. Common organisms include *Pneumococcus*, *Staphylococcus aureus*, Coxsackie virus, and hepatitis B virus in the early period or in the setting of both acute and chronic endocarditis.

Rapidly Progressive GN

RPGN is a clinical syndrome rather than a pathological diagnosis. It defined as loss of renal function of more than 50% over a period of 3 months in patients with hematuria and proteinuria indicating

TABLE 81.3 Causes of rapidly progressive glomerulonephritis

Anti-GBM disease
With lung hemorrhage (Goodpasture's syndrome)
Without hemorrhage (anti-GBM nephritis)
Complicating membranous nephropathy
Immune complex–mediated glomerulonephritis
Postinfectious glomerulonephritis
Poststreptococcal
Endocarditis
Visceral abscess
Collagen-vascular disease
Systemic lupus erythematosus
Cryoglobulinemia
Henoch-Schönlein purpura
Primary renal disease
Membranoproliferative glomerulonephritis
Immunoglobulin A nephropathy
ANCA-associated glomerulonephritis
Polyarteritis nodosa (p-ANCA)
Wegener's granulomatosis (c-ANCA)
Idiopathic crescentic glomerulonephritis

ANCA, antineutrophilic cytoplasmic antibody.

glomerular injury. The rapid progression connotes a severe form of primary or secondary glomerular disease, examples of which are listed in Table 81.3.

GOODPASTURE SYNDROME

One form of RPGN is Goodpasture's syndrome (the most common form of anti-GBM disease). Goodpasture's syndrome is characterized by pulmonary hemorrhage and acute or subacute renal failure, often occurs in children and young adults, and is eight times more common in men than women. In Goodpasture's syndrome, antibodies are directed against glomerular and alveolar basement membrane, causing nephritis and pulmonary hemorrhage. This pulmonary-renal syndrome can present as an isolated pulmonary or renal disorder, with the other organ affected subclinically or later in the disease course. Pulmonary symptoms, which are present in approximately two thirds of cases, include hemoptysis, dyspnea on exertion, cough, and pulmonary infiltrates on chest x-ray. Renal manifestations involve hematuria, RBC casts, volume overload, hypertension, and uremia. Fever, arthritis, and abdominal pain may occur. Prognosis for recovery of renal function is poor when the disease is already in the advanced stage at the initial presentation.

ANTINEUTROPHILIC CYTOPLASMIC ANTIBODY GN

A second form of RPGN is antineutrophilic cytoplasmic antibody (ANCA) associated glomerulonephritis, which is not immune mediated. Wegener's granulomatosis (Chapter 52) and polyarteritis nodosa (Chapter 52) can present with glomerulonephritis and may be associated with positive blood test for ANCA. The antigens for these antibodies have been identified as myeloperoxidase (MPO;

c-ANCA) and proteinase 3 (PR3; p-ANCA). The presence of c-ANCA has a high specificity for the pulmonary renal syndrome of Wegener's granulomatosis, while p-ANCA is more likely to present as a preglomerular lesion with polyarteritis nodosa (Chapter 52).

OTHER

A third form of RPGN, in contrast with ANCA-associated GN, has an immune complex–mediated mode of glomerular injury, which can be found in systemic lupus erythematosus (SLE; Chapter 48) and Henoch Schönlein purpura (HSP). HSP is characterized by hematuria, RBC casts, fever, abdominal pain, and a typical petechial rash over buttock and lower extremities.

Nephrotic Syndrome

MEMBRANOUS GLOMERULAR DISEASE

Membranous glomerular disease is the most common cause of nephrotic syndrome in adults, accounting for up to 50% of cases. Affected people usually are between the ages of 30 and 50 years, with men affected more commonly than women. The GFR usually is normal or slightly decreased. If the history and physical examination are abnormal, malignancy should be sought, especially adenocarcinoma of the lung, colon, and breast.

Other secondary causes of membranous nephropathy include hepatitis B, SLE, and drugs such as gold, penicillamine, captopril, and nonsteroidal anti-inflammatory drugs. No definitive therapy exists, but immunosuppression may induce remission and prolong survival in selected patients.

MINIMAL CHANGE DISEASE

Minimal change disease accounts for 20% of all cases of nephrotic syndrome in adults and 75% to 80% of all cases in children. The peak age of onset is 2 to 6 years of age; however, it also may be seen as late as 15 to 18 years of age. A second peak occurs in adults around the age of 50 years. This disease is characterized by the absence of hypertension. It can occur, rarely, with malignancy (mainly lymphomas) as well as with medications such as nonsteroidal anti-inflammatory drugs. It is treated with oral corticosteroid therapy.

Other GN

MEMBRANOPROLIFERATIVE GLOMERULONEPHRITIS

Membranoproliferative glomerulonephritis (MPGN) accounts for about 12% of all cases of nephrotic syndrome in adults in the United States. It is defined by histological features of mesangial matrix accumulation and immune deposits into the capillary wall. It occurs with equal frequency in males and females in their teens and 20s.

MPGN may be idiopathic or may occur in association with other diseases including chronic hepatitis B virus, hepatitis C virus, autoimmune diseases including SLE, rheumatoid arthritis (RA), scleroderma, celiac disease, cirrhosis, TTP, scleroderma, or malignancies. Three types are identified: Type I is associated with hepatitis C and with cryoglobulinemia; Type II, or dense deposit disease, is associated with genetic or acquired deficiencies in Factor H and with partial lipodystrophy; and Type III associated with antibodies to complement (C3 nephritic) factors. MPGN may present with nephrotic syndrome in 50% of cases, or a nephritic picture with hematuria, RBC casts, hypertension, and decreased GFR associated with a low C3 level. Fifty percent of patients with MPGN and nephrotic syndrome progress to end-stage renal disease within 10 years, while only 15% of those without nephrotic syndrome reach ESRD at 10 years.

IMMUNOGLOBULIN A NEPHROPATHY

Worldwide, immunoglobulin (Ig) A nephropathy is the most common glomerular disease, accounting for about 40% of biopsied patients in Asia, 20% in Europe, and 10% in North America. The disease

TABLE 81.4 Systemic diseases with renal involvement
Diabetes mellitus (most common)
Systemic lupus erythematosus
Multiple myeloma
Polyarteritis nodosa
Wegener's granulomatosis
Scleroderma
Hemolytic-uremic syndrome
Thrombotic thrombocytopenic purpura (TTP)
Amyloidosis
Cryoglobulinemia
Postpartum renal failure
Disseminated intravascular coagulation
Human immunodeficiency virus
Sickle cell anemia

is characterized by recurrent attacks of gross hematuria, often following a nonspecific viral illness, commonly an upper respiratory infection. The course varies widely, ranging from asymptomatic hematuria without progression to rapidly progressive GN. Hypertension and nephrotic syndrome are uncommon and, if present, portend a poor prognosis. IgA nephropathy has a sixfold greater incidence in men and most patients are younger than 35 years at the time of diagnosis. Serum IgA concentration may be elevated and serum complement is normal. Skin biopsies may show mesangial deposits of IgA.

DIABETIC NEPHROPATHY

Diabetic nephropathy is the most common cause of end-stage renal disease in the United States. Microalbuminuria, defined as albumin excretion of 30 to 300 mg per 24 hours is the first indication of diabetic nephropathy. Urine should be monitored for microalbuminuria every 6 to 12 months in all diabetic patients, and those exhibiting it should be treated with an angiotensin-converting enzyme (ACE) inhibitor, regardless of blood pressure, to forestall renal failure. ACE inhibitors and calcium channel blockers, along with a diuretic, are the treatment of choice for controlling hypertension in the diabetic angiotensin receptor blockers (ARB) also reduce proteinuria. When proteinuria appears and impaired renal function develops (serum creatinine ≥2 mg/dL), referral to a nephrologist is recommended to assist in preserving renal function and preparing the patient for end-stage renal disease care. Early and aggressive control of blood sugar and arterial pressure preserves renal function. The hallmark morphologic change seen in diabetic nephropathy is mesangial matrix expansion; when nodular, it is called nodular sclerosis or Kimmelstiel-Wilson lesion. However, this is only seen in 20% of patients. Other systemic diseases that can present with glomerular involvement are listed in Table 81.4.

DIAGNOSIS

History and physical examination play an important part in the diagnosis of glomerulonephritis, particularly to establish onset, duration, and temporal pattern of symptoms (for example, in relation to an infection or administration of a drug) and or the presence of systemic disease such as SLE, diabetes, hepatitis C virus, multiple myeloma, or amyloidosis.

TABLE 81.5 Serum complement levels in glomerular diseases

Low	Normal
Postinfectious glomerular nephritis	Immunoglobulin A nephropathy
Membranous proliferative glomerular nephritis	Rapidly progressive glomerular nephritis
	Goodpasture's syndrome
	Wegener's granulomatosis

Urinalysis and careful microscopic examination of urinary sediment is a key diagnostic test to detect glomerular injury. Hematuria, cardinal feature of glomerular injury, defined as the presence of more than 3 RBC per high-power field on microscopic examination of the urine sediment, has a broad differential diagnosis (Chapter 17).

Gross hematuria is an insensitive indicator of the degree of blood loss, because as little as 1 mL of blood is enough to change the color of 1 L of urine to red or brown. Hemoglobinuria caused by hemolysis and myoglobinuria caused by rhabdomyolysis also can cause a red or brown urine and yield a positive hemoglobin dipstick. However, in myoglobinuria, the spun specimen has a red color (supernatant) but no red blood cells in the urine sediment. Thus, true hematuria can be diagnosed only by microscopic examination.

Microscopic examination of the spun urine showing the presence of red blood cell casts is diagnostic of glomerulonephritis (Fig. 81.1). However, the absence of red blood cell casts does not rule out glomerular disease. Dysmorphic red cells also correlate highly with glomerulonephritis. Dysmorphic red blood cells and acanthocytes result from cell membranes traumatized either by passage through the glomerular capillary or by osmotic trauma as they pass through the nephron. Finally, dipstick results indicating 4+ proteinuria are highly suggestive of glomerular disease. Serum complement levels can also be helpful in differentiating glomerular nephritis (Table 81.5). Definitive diagnosis and histological typing of GN can be made only through the use of renal biopsy.

TREATMENT

General Treatment

Primary goals include control of hypertension and volume overload, and treatment of the underlying disease, if any. Treatment of ongoing infections is mandatory and is often sufficient to result in resolution of GN. Treatment of underlying autoimmune disorders in SLE, RA, Wegener's granulomatosis, Goodpasture's syndrome, and systemic vasculitis may result in arrest and reversal of glomerular injury. A variable degree of renal scarring may remain. Proteinuria, hypertension, and renal insufficiency may return and progress after months or years.

Specific Treatment

Treatment of GN is determined by the clinical manifestations and the etiology of the condition (Table 81.6).

Antibiotics are advised for treatment of poststreptococcal GN to eliminate residual streptococci. The glomerular injury is not altered by antibiotics.

Treatment of anti-GBM nephritis and Goodpasture's syndrome is most effective when started early in the course of disease, specifically when creatinine is less than 6 mg/dL. Treatment should include corticosteroids, immunosuppression, and plasmapheresis. Renal transplantation can be carried out successfully after the anti-GBM antibodies have gone away.

TABLE 81.6 Treatment of selected types of glomerulonephritis

	Antibiotics	Glucocorticoids	Immuno-suppression	Plasmapheresis
Postinfectious	If infection is current	Not usually	No	No
Systemic lupus erythematosus	No	Yes	Yes	No
Vasculitis antineutrophilic cytoplasmic antibody	No	Yes	Yes	In severe acute injury
Anti-GBM	No	Yes	Yes	Yes

Treatment of ANCA and vasculitis includes intravenous or oral cyclophosphamide, usually in combination with intravenous steroids. Therapy should be continued for a minimum of 1 year and at least 6 months after all clinical evidence of disease has disappeared.

Treatment of IgA nephropathy is generally supportive, and most patients have recurrent episodes of hematuria. Only about 25% of all patients progress to end-stage renal disease. Poor prognostic indicators include male gender, older age, hypertension, proteinuria exceeding 2 g per day, and impaired renal function at the time of presentation. Treatment with ACE inhibitors and ARBs lowers blood pressure, decreases proteinuria, and may prolong survival; fish oil (omega-3 fatty acids, 12 g/day); or with vitamin E may also improve outcome. Patients with proliferative GN or crescents and those with nephrotic syndrome should be treated with prednisone for about 6 months. Renal transplantation is effective in IgA nephropathy, although patients have a 20% to 60% risk of recurrence on a histological basis and about a 10% risk of slowly progressive renal failure and loss of graft function.

COMPLICATIONS

Complications include acute hypertension, volume expansion, or renal failure. Late complications include progressive renal insufficiency. Additional manifestations may include involvement of other organs if the GN is due to systemic disease such as SLE, granulomatosis, Goodpasture's syndrome, and systemic vasculitis.

CHAPTER 82

Nephrotic Syndrome

Robert Riniker

Nephrotic syndrome (NS) is defined by the presence of proteinuria greater than 3.5 g per day (about 3 g protein per 1 g creatinine in a random urine collection), hypoalbuminemia, and edema. Idiopathic nephrotic syndrome (INS) is more common in children and young adults, whereas diabetes mellitus (DM) is the most common cause of secondary NS in older adults.

ETIOLOGY

The causes of nephrotic-range proteinuria are listed in Table 82.1. Historically, the most common primary renal causes of NS are minimal change disease in children and membranous glomerulopathy in adults. Focal segmental glomerulosclerosis (FSGS) is increasingly common in children and has become the most common cause of INS in adults less than 40 years old. DM is the most common systemic cause of nephrotic syndrome; proteinuria in DM begins as microalbuminuria (a small amount of albumin excreted in the urine) and increases in amount as kidney injury progresses.

NS may be idiopathic (INS), that is, not associated with systemic disease or with glomerulonephritis, or may occur in patients with underlying systemic diseases such as type I or type II diabetes mellitus (DM), immunological disorders including systemic lupus erythematosus and rheumatoid arthritis, human immunodeficiency virus or acquired immune deficiency syndrome, malignancies including solid tumors and hematological malignancies, and other chronic inflammatory diseases or infections.

CLINICAL MANIFESTATIONS

Nephrotic proteinuria (>3.5 g per 24 hours) occurs because of failure of the glomerular capillary to prevent filtration of plasma proteins. Albumin and other proteins are lost in the urine. The characteristics of the filtration barrier depend on contributions by the glomerular basement membrane and the endothelial and epithelial cells (podocytes). Changes in podocyte function are responsible for the marked increase in filtration in NS. Hypertension and renal insufficiency may be present and hyperlipidemia is common, as is venous thrombosis. Renal damage in patients with NS may lead to renal failure requiring dialysis or transplantation.

Patients with NS most often present with edema due to hypoalbuminemia and fluid retention. Adult patients, especially males, may note foamy urine. Edema is most prominent in soft tissues; facial or periorbital edema is evident in the morning, whereas lower extremity edema is greater in the evening after being upright. Severe edema may involve the entire lower extremities, genitalia, and abdominal wall and may affect the gut, liver, and the kidneys themselves. Ascites may be a prominent feature. Edema is less prominent in patients with lesser degrees of hypoalbuminemia, and in young men who have good nutrition, tight fascia, and little subcutaneous tissue.

TABLE 82.1 Causes of nephrotic syndrome

Primary glomerular diseases
Minimal change disease
Membranous nephropathy
Focal segmental glomerulosclerosis
Membranoproliferative glomerulonephritis
Secondary glomerular diseases
Postinfectious: poststreptococcal, endocarditis, syphilis, hepatitis B virus, cytomegalovirus, protozoa, parasitic
Metabolic: diabetes mellitus, myxedema
Connective tissue diseases and vasculitis: systemic lupus erythematosus, Sjögren's syndrome, polyarteritis nodosa, Goodpasture's syndrome, Henoch-Schönlein purpura, scleroderma, dermatomyositis
Neoplastic: solid tumors, lymphoma, leukemia
Drugs: gold, penicillamine, mercury, probenecid, nonsteroidal anti-inflammatory drugs, captopril
Allergens: poison ivy, insect bites
Systemic diseases: amyloidosis, malignant hypertension, sarcoidosis, severe congestive heart failure, constrictive pericarditis
Inherited diseases: sickle cell disease, Fabry disease
Miscellaneous: thrombotic thrombocytopenic purpura, hemolytic-uremic syndrome, pre-eclampsia

Hypertension may occur, especially when renal failure is present or there is a component of glomerular inflammation or scarring. Alternatively, patients who are severely volume depleted may be hypotensive.

Hypercholesterolemia and hypertriglyceridemia, the other components of nephrotic syndrome, occur because of increased hepatic cholesterol synthesis and decreased peripheral metabolism.

DIAGNOSIS

Urinalysis is essential to the diagnosis of NS. Proteinuria is confirmed by urine dipstick and formal measurement of urinary protein concentration. Microscopic hematuria may also be present. Urine concentration is often high during edematous states; pH varies within the normal range. Leukocytes are generally absent and leukocyte esterase negative. Quantitative protein is traditionally measured in a 24-hour urine collection, but calculation of protein/creatinine ratio is useful in screening and in monitoring the efficacy of treatment or occurrence of relapse.

Microscopic examination of the urine shows oval fat bodies and smaller fat bodies, representing the residual lipid that was filtered bound to albumin and that has not been completely metabolized by tubular cells. Cholesterol polarizes light and is evident as bright particles with a "Maltese cross" configuration in a dark field when crossed polarizing filters are used. Fat may also be present in casts.

A small amount of hematuria is common, especially when glomerular scarring is present, but red blood cell casts are usually rare or absent.

Urine protein electrophoresis is useful in determining the composition of proteins. Only albumin is present in the "selective proteinuria" of early INS. The finding of a monoclonal peak is diagnostic for plasma cell dyscrasia.

Renal biopsy is required to determine the etiology, plan therapy, and provide prognosis in most adults with NS. However, children and younger adults who do not have renal insufficiency, hematuria, or serological evidence for systemic disease may be treated with a short course of oral corticosteroids and biopsy deferred in those who have prompt complete remission of proteinuria.

TREATMENT

Treatment of the nephrotic syndrome has two aims: first, to treat and reverse the cause of proteinuria; and second, to ameliorate the clinical symptoms and potential complications of hypoproteinemia, edema, hypercoagulable state, and hypercholesterolemia. Treatment of the underlying disease requires defining the process and etiology, most often by renal biopsy. Treatment of MCNS, FSGS, membranous nephropathy, and most autoimmune disorders usually begin with corticosteroids. Immunosuppressive therapy may be needed.

Proteinuria may also be decreased by angiotensin-converting enzyme inhibitors or angiotensin receptor blockers, regardless of the etiology or histological diagnosis. Dietary protein restriction may also decrease proteinuria, whereas higher protein intake may exacerbate proteinuria.

Edema can be treated with diuretics, sodium restriction, and local therapies including elevation of legs.

Hypercholesterolemia should be treated with lipid-lowering agents such as HMGco-A inhibitors.

COMPLICATIONS

Nephrotic syndrome may be the cause of several complications. First, hypercoagulable state may occur because of urinary losses of factors that maintain clotting homeostasis, such as antithrombin III. This may lead to thrombosis of peripheral veins or renal veins. Acute flank pain with a significant rise in proteinuria should alert one to the possibility of renal vein thrombosis, an entity that may complicate nephrotic syndrome. Second, patients with nephrotic syndrome have an increased susceptibility to infections. Third, acute renal failure may occur in nephrotic syndrome caused by minimal change disease. Finally, protein malnutrition, manifested by decreased lean body mass, can develop as a result of massive proteinuria.

Long-term complications include accelerated rates of atherosclerotic disease and progressive renal insufficiency.

Renal failure requiring dialysis or transplantation 20 years after diagnosis occurs in less than 15% of patients with minimal change nephrotic syndrome but occurs in nearly 50% of patients with FSGS. Patients with NS due to diabetes mellitus have advanced glomerular lesions and, although progression may be slowed, have a poor long-term prognosis for renal survival.

CHAPTER 83

Acute Interstitial Nephritis

Virginia Savin

Tubulointerstitial nephritis affects primarily the tubules and interstitium, rather than glomeruli or renal vasculature. It may be responsible for 10% to 15% of kidney disease and may lead to chronic renal failure.

ETIOLOGY

The causes of acute interstitial nephritis (AIN) include reactions to drugs including penicillins and sulfonamides, diuretics, nonsteroidal anti-inflammatory drugs, and other agents (Table 83.1). Systemic infections with viruses, bacteria, fungus, or other agents, as well as acute bacterial pyelonephritis, also cause acute tubulointerstitial nephritis. The renal dysfunction in these cases may not be recognized because of the other severe clinical manifestations. Acute transplant rejection is also characterized by AIN. The renal involvement in the syndrome of cholesterol embolization also involves interstitial nephritis. AIN is a part of the involvement in many systemic and autoimmune disorders.

CLINICAL MANIFESTATIONS

The major clinical finding in acute tubulointerstitial nephritis is the development of acute renal insufficiency. One third of patients develop the triad of fever, skin rash, and peripheral eosinophilia with arthralgias, whereas as many as 50% have peripheral eosinophilia alone. The absence of these features does not exclude the possibility of acute tubulointerstitial nephritis. Hypertension and edema are important features of acute glomerulonephritis but usually are not seen in acute tubulointerstitial nephritis. AIN causes a rapid decline in renal function over several days or weeks and is commonly due to hypersensitivity or immunologic responses.

DIAGNOSIS

The history of previous drug use and the occurrence of urine abnormalities renal insufficiency within 3 to 10 days of starting an offending agent should raise the suspicion of AIN. Urinalysis should be performed first. It may show hematuria, more commonly in cases with a drug-induced etiology. Urine leukocytes and white blood cell casts may also be found. The presence of eosinophiluria as noted by Hansel stain or Wright stain may be helpful, but this usually is present only within the first 5 to 7 days of the disease. Eosinophiluria is not pathognomonic for tubulointerstitial nephritis because it is also seen in atheroembolic disease and rapidly progressive glomerulonephritis (RPGN).

TABLE 83.1 Causes of acute interstitial nephritis

Drug-related	Systemic infections	Primary renal infections	Immune disorders
Antimicrobial drugs	Streptococcal infections	Acute bacterial pyelonephritis	Acute glomerulonephritis
Penicillins (especially methicillin)	Cytomegalovirus		Systemic lupus erythematosus
Rifampin	Infectious mononucleosis		Transplant rejection
Sulfonamides	Legionnaire's disease		
Nonsteroidal anti-inflammatory drugs	Leptospirosis		
Allopurinol			
Loop diuretics			

The presence of red blood cell casts indicates glomerulonephritis rather than tubulointerstitial nephritis. If the diagnosis is still uncertain, a renal biopsy may be needed to confirm AIN.

TREATMENT

A short course of corticosteroids may be effective in shortening the course of tubulointerstitial nephritis. Cessation of the offending drug is the mainstay of treatment. In patients with drug-induced interstitial nephritis, renal function begins to normalize 1 to 2 weeks after stopping the offending agent.

CHAPTER 84

Polycystic Kidney Disease

Ellen McCarthy

Autosomal dominant polycystic kidney disease (ADPKD) is the most common dominantly inherited disease in the United States, affecting approximately half a million people, and more than 10 million people worldwide. ADPKD occurs with equal frequency in all racial and ethnic groups.

Autosomal recessive polycystic kidney disease (ARPKD) is much rarer than ADPKD, and occurs in 1 in 20,000 live births. Affected children typically are diagnosed in utero, with large echogenic kidneys and evidence of poor urinary output.

Another form of hereditary cystic disease includes medullary cystic disease. Acquired cystic disease of the kidney can occur in the setting of chronic kidney disease; and, following toxic insult, it carries an increased risk of renal carcinoma.

ETIOLOGY

Polycystin-1 and polycystin-2 are the proteins mutated in *PKD1* or the less common and less severe *PKD2*, respectively. The gene for polycystin-1 is found on chromosome 16.

CLINICAL MANIFESTATIONS

Clinical presentation of ADPKD usually occurs in adulthood. Common clinical manifestations of ADPKD include abdominal or flank pain, hematuria, and hypertension. Hypertension is often present prior to increase in plasma creatinine levels. Extrarenal manifestations may include cerebral "berry" aneurysms (10%), hepatic cysts, valvular heart disease, and colonic diverticula. Anemia and an increased risk of renal cancer may be present. The disease progresses to end-stage renal disease in about 25% of individuals by age 50 years and 50% by age 70 years.

Medullary cystic kidney disease is an autosomal dominant condition characterized by development of end-stage renal disease (ESRD) and gout. Medullary sponge kidney is a benign condition of unclear etiology associated with the development of renal stones, especially calcium oxalate stones.

DIAGNOSIS

ADPKD is often diagnosed on screening ultrasound or computed tomography scan in patients with a known family history of the disorder, as part of a radiological workup of hematuria, or on radiological studies ordered for an unrelated reason. Radiological evaluation by ultrasound or computed tomography scanning reveals bilaterally enlarged kidneys with multiple cysts and, in up to one third of patients, the presence of hepatic cysts. A urinalysis may show hematuria or proteinuria.

It is now possible to screen patients for ADPKD through genetic linkage analysis. Although this can predict the likelihood with a 99% certainty, it is quite expensive and requires cooperation from family members. Moreover, because there is no definitive therapy for ADPKD, testing should be reserved for individuals who can afford it and have the desire to know.

TREATMENT

There is no definitive treatment for ADPKD or ARPKD at this time. Aggressive treatment of hypertension is important. ESRD in these disorders is best treated with renal transplantation in suitable candidates.

CHAPTER 85

Nephrolithiasis

Jeffrey Wesson

Nephrolithiasis, also known as kidney stones or renal calculi, is a common disorder characterized by the formation of aggregates of microscopic crystals into solid objects (stones) ranging from millimeters to centimeters in linear dimension. Between 5% and 15% of people in the United States suffer at least one episode of nephrolithiasis during their lifetime, with substantial variations in rates between regions. The disease typically appears during middle age, with men more commonly affected than women by 2 to 1. The risk of recurrent stones approaches 50% in 3 to 5 years.

ETIOLOGY

The pathophysiology of nephrolithiasis remains poorly defined, beyond the recognition that crystals form and aggregate to make stones. Crystals can form when the concentration of the constituents of the crystals exceed their solubility in urine, but most people do not form crystals or stones in the urinary tract despite relatively high concentrations of these constituents, due in part to the limited time urine spends in the body after formation (a few hours) and in part to the presence of natural inhibitors of crystal formation (citrate and various proteins). Several different types of crystals can be found within a single kidney stone, and preventative treatments need to target the type of crystals being formed. Crystals that form naturally in people include various forms of calcium oxalate salts, calcium phosphate salts, uric acid salts, struvite (magnesium ammonium phosphate), and cystine crystals, but stones also can be formed from crystals of pharmaceutical agents (acyclovir, indinavir, and many others). Conditions that favor low urine volumes increase the risk for all forms of stones, whereas high concentrations of the constituents forming the crystals are addressed in ways specific to the stone type.

Calcium Stones

Calcium stones, including all forms of calcium oxalate and calcium phosphate crystals, are radiopaque and account for more than 80% of all kidney stones. Calcium stones are associated with diets rich in oxalate-containing foods, salt, protein (particularly meat), and surprisingly, they are also associated with dietary calcium restriction. Normal dietary calcium intake has been shown to be protective against calcium stone formation. Excessive calcium intake (milk-alkali syndrome) is rarely seen anymore, with effective drugs for blocking stomach acid production. Vitamin C abuse can lead to hyperoxaluria and calcium stone formation.

Associated medical conditions include polycystic kidney disease, medullary sponge kidney, distal renal tubular acidosis, hyperparathyroidism, and conditions leading to chronic diarrhea (surgical "short gut", Crohn's disease, or other malabsorption syndromes). A positive family history of stones is common, but a genetic link has not been established yet. Serum studies are generally normal, but if hypercalcemia is present, hyperparathyroidism (1% to 3% of calcium stone cases) should be considered, along with sarcoidosis, hyperthyroidism, multiple myeloma, or other malignancy. Hypercalciuria is the most commonly found urine abnormality (roughly 50% of patients), but it does not predict stone disease. Uric acid crystals may serve as the nidus for calcium stone formation in some mixed composition stones.

Uric Acid Stones

Uric acid stones are the only radiolucent stones and account for about 10% of the cases. Uric acid stones are formed in hyperuricosuric states, volume depletion, and acidic urine, which reduces the solubility of uric acid. Alkalinizing the urine may dissolve uric acid stones. Uric acid stones are associated with protein rich diets (particularly meat), which increase both uric acid production and urine acidity. Fifty percent of patients with uric acid stones also have gout.

Struvite Stones

Struvite stones are composed of radiopaque, magnesium ammonium phosphate crystals and account for about 10% of cases. These stones are unique in that they are associated with chronic urinary tract infection with urea-splitting organisms, such as *Proteus* spp, which raise the urine pH. Consequently, they are routinely found in people with abnormal urinary drainage, such as those with ureteral reflux, neurogenic bladder, other forms of bladder dysfunction, or ureteral diversions. Surgical stone removal may be required to treat the predisposing infection adequately.

Cystine Stones

Cystine stones also are radiopaque and are created by an inherited defect in the renal tubular absorption of cystine that results in cystinuria. These crystals are found in 1% to 3% of stone samples, and they recur frequently in most affected individuals. The diagnosis is suggested by a positive urine nitroprusside test and confirmed by stone analysis. Urine sediment may show the characteristic hexagonal cystine crystals and crystal formation is favored in acidic urine.

CLINICAL MANIFESTATIONS

Severe colicky flank and/or abdominal pain and hematuria (microscopic or gross) are the two most common presenting symptoms of kidney stones, and these occur when the stone causes partial or full obstruction while passing through the ureter. However, an increasing number of asymptomatic patients are identified as stone formers by the incidental discovery of stones in an abdominal computed tomography or ultrasound examination for other purposes. Stones in the renal pelvis usually are painless unless infection or obstruction is present; they may cause stuttering episodes of pain due to intermittent blockage. Ureteral stones, on the other hand, cause nausea, vomiting, and severe abdominal and/or flank pain radiating into the groin, urethra, or genitalia in nearly all patients. Stones at the ureterovesical junction may result in dysuria, frequency, and urgency, even in the absence of infection. Once in the bladder, stones are normally passed out of the body without difficulty, but they can be retained and grow to very large sizes in patients with bladder dysfunction. Fever and pyuria suggest associated urinary tract infection, but need to be confirmed by culture. If complete obstruction is present, pyuria may not occur. Chronic and complete obstruction can result in hydronephrosis and eventually loss of function in the affected kidney.

DIAGNOSIS

The gold standard for diagnosis of nephrolithiasis is the noncontrast helical computed tomography scan of the abdomen and pelvis, typically using 5-mm segments through the kidneys and lower urinary tract, which routinely defines the size and location of any stones in the urinary tract. Under special circumstances, an abdominal ultrasound or intravenous pyelogram (IVP) may be used, but they generally have inferior sensitivity and specificity to the computed tomography scan. A simple x-ray of the abdomen has limited diagnostic utility, but may be useful to track progression of previously diagnosed radiopaque stones. In the setting of the acute pain syndrome, a basic chemistry profile should be obtained to check for acute renal failure due to obstruction and related electrolyte disorders. Urine should be obtained for routine urinalysis to confirm the presence of blood and check for evidence of infection. Crystals seen in the urine sediment of stone formers are predictive of the stone type, so the urinary sediment should be examined under the microscope. Any passed stones should be saved for analysis. Metabolic evaluation of kidney stones should always be performed before starting on a therapeutic regimen.

The clinical evaluation of stone formers should include a personal and family history of stone disease and a review of medical conditions related to stone formation. Because calcium stones account for the vast majority of stone formers, a review of dietary habits contributing to increased risk for stone formation should be obtained, including intake of food high in calcium (principally dairy products) or oxalate (spinach, beets, rhubarb, nuts, some beans, rutabagas, and chocolate), as well as salt and meat intake.

Laboratory tests should include serum studies for renal function, electrolytes, calcium, magnesium, phosphate, and uric acid, and urine should be obtained for urinalysis and microscopic examination for crystals. If hypercalcemia is present, a parathyroid hormone level should be obtained. Urine culture should be obtained when clinically indicated. Stone analysis should be performed whenever possible because preventative therapies vary with the type of crystal formed. Because many dietary risk factors and therapies are well established for calcium stones, there is some debate about the utility of further evaluation in first time calcium stone formers; however, all recurrent and noncalcium stone formers should have two 24-hour urine collections to focus risk modification strategies. The analysis should include evaluation of urine volume, creatinine, crystal forming components (calcium, oxalate, phosphate, uric acid, and cystine when appropriate), crystallization modifiers (pH, citrate, and magnesium), and markers of dietary intakes (sodium and potassium).

TREATMENT

Acute Management

In an acute episode of nephrolithiasis, an effective analgesic must be given; opiates may be needed. Water intake should be increased to maintain a daily urine output of 2 L or more. If this is not possible, intravenous fluids should be given to increase urinary output. Stone removal strategies are based on the size of the stone. Most small stones (<5 mm in maximum dimension) will pass spontaneously. Surgical removal would only be attempted if the stone passage becomes complicated. Complicating features include failure to pass in 3 to 7 days, acute renal failure, gross hematuria with clots, or infection. Larger stones (>5 mm) generally require urologic intervention. Initially, a ureteral stent may be placed to guarantee urine flow from the obstructed kidney. Extracorporeal shock wave lithotripsy to fragment the stone into pieces <5 mm remains the most common treatment modality, but ureteroscopic and percutaneous approaches have become increasingly common. Open surgical procedures are performed very rarely.

Chronic Management

Chronic management of renal calculi to prevent new stone formation is also important.

All forms of stones respond to increasing urine volumes (dilution), which reduces supersaturation. Fluid intake should be increased until daily urine output exceeds 2 to 3 L. Calcium-containing stones should be addressed first by diet modifications to reduce risks (as cited above) and this may be the only therapy required in first time or infrequently recurrent stone formers (>5 years between episodes). Thiazide diuretics, such as 12.5 to 25 mg of hydrochlorothiazide, reduce urinary calcium excretion and are most effective in hypercalciuric calcium stone formers. Potassium citrate (60 mEq per day) in divided doses is routinely used in hypocitraturia, but also may help prevent recurrence in patients with normal urinary citrate levels. Patients with hyperuricosuria (>1,000 mg of uric acid per 24 hours) and normal serum calcium can be benefited by 100 to 200 mg per day of allopurinol to reduce uric acid synthesis. Patients with acquired hyperoxaluria secondary to disease, restriction, or bypass of the small intestine may benefit from oral calcium supplements with meals to precipitate dietary oxalate within the intestine or from cholestyramine (4 g three times a day), which binds oxalate in the gut. Patients with primary hyperoxaluria may be helped by pyridoxine, which reduces endogenous oxalate synthesis.

Treatment of patients with uric acid stones includes increased water intake as above, and alkalinization of the urine to a pH of 7 or above to increase uric acid solubility and potentially dissolve uric acid crystals. Therapies include supplementation with potassium citrate, potassium bicarbonate, or sodium bicarbonate in divided doses, or acetazolamide may be used to alkalinize the nocturnal urine. Allopurinol should be given for hyperuricemia in doses of 200 to 300 mg per day to reduce the formation of uric acid. Purine-rich foods such as beef and liver should be avoided.

Prevention of recurrent cystine stones is aimed at decreasing urinary concentration of cystine below the solubility limit of 200 to 300 mg/L. Besides the methods already described, alkalinization of the urine to a pH above 7.5 is critical. This usually can be achieved with Shohl's solution, which contains sodium citrate.

CHAPTER 86

Fluid and Electrolyte Disorders

Virginia Savin

DISORDERS OF WATER BALANCE

Serum sodium is the predominant cation in plasma. Its concentration is generally expressed as mEq/L and is often used to make an estimate of plasma osmolality. Clinically, changes in serum sodium concentration almost always reflect changes in water balance rather than changes in sodium balance. In healthy persons, the plasma osmolality is maintained between 285 and 300 mOsm/kg. Regulation of osmolality depends on central nervous system functions of thirst, which result in behaviors leading to water ingestion or avoidance, and stimulation or suppression of release of antidiuretic hormone (ADH), which results in regulation of renal urinary concentration and dilution. Changes in intravascular volume comprise additional physiological stimuli for thirst and ADH release. Intravascular volume depletion leads to thirst and ADH release, whereas intravascular volume expansion leads to suppression of both thirst and ADH release.

ADH is the nonapeptide arginine vasopressin. It is synthesized in the hypothalamus, stored in the posterior pituitary, and released in response to increased osmolality or to decrease in intravascular volume. ADH rises with increased osmolality (most often water loss, leading to an increase in serum sodium concentration) and falls with decreased osmolality (most often water intake, leading to a decrease in serum sodium concentration). An increase in plasma osmolality of less than 5% causes increased ADH secretion, which results in an increase in urine concentration and in conservation of water. The regulation is very sensitive and renal responses are rapid so that little change in osmolality is evident. Similarly, a small decrease in plasma osmolality (and serum sodium concentration) decreases ADH and leads to decreased urine concentration and loss of water.

Thirst, like ADH release, is stimulated by hyperosmolality and suppressed by hypo-osmolality. Thirst is a very strong drive and people will attempt to drink to correct hyperosmolality even if potable water is not available; aversion to water is also strong and people will refuse to drink when they are hypo-osmolar. The intact thirst mechanism accounts for the fact that people with renal failure will generally maintain normal serum sodium even when they have no urine output.

Hyponatremia

Hyponatremia and hypernatremia are most often disorders of water balance. Plasma osmolality, expressed in mOsm per kilogram of H_2O, can be measured directly using instruments that measure the freezing point depression or vaporization point elevation, physical properties that are varied by the number of particles in a solution. Osmolality is often estimated using the following formula:

$$P_{osm} = 2\,[Na^+] + BUN/2.8 + glucose/18$$

In this formula, Na^+ is expressed in mEq/L and blood urea nitrogen (BUN) and glucose in mg/dL. Na^+ and its accompanying anion, Cl^-, are the most important determinants of plasma osmolality.

Hyponatremia is defined as plasma $[Na^+]$ less than 135 mEq/L. It usually indicates a hypo-osmolal state and results in a shift of water into cells (cell swelling). Mild stable hyponatremia (128 to

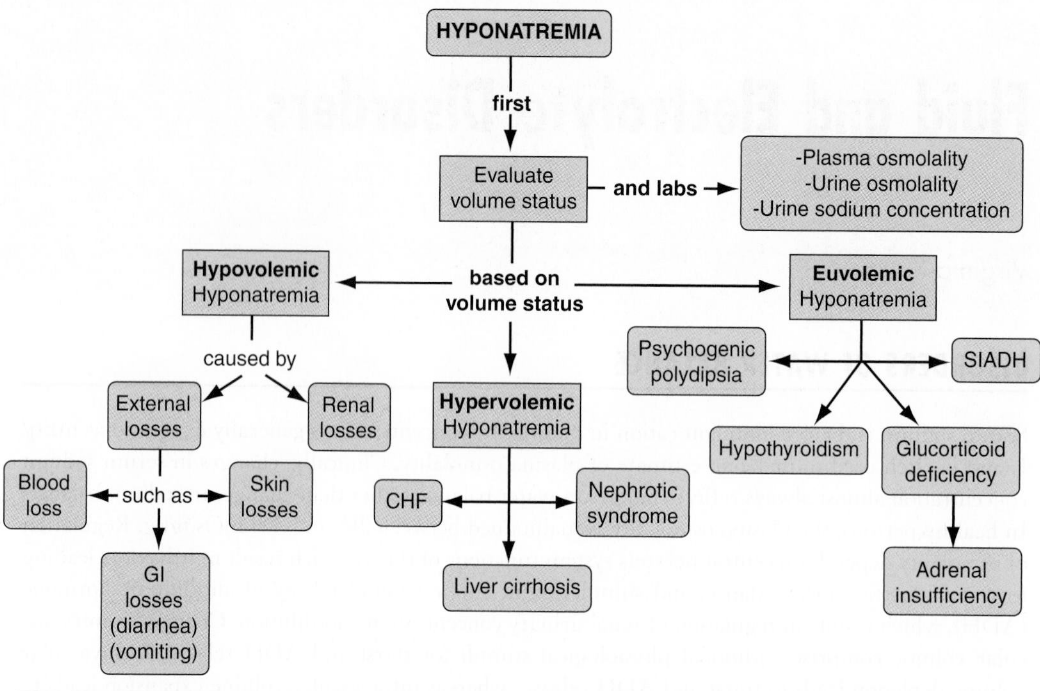

Figure 86.1 • Causes and initial evaluation of hypotonic hyponatremias.

135 mEq/L) is common in hospitalized patients, is not in itself dangerous, and is often not investigated. Progressive hyponatremia or serum sodium less than ~125 mEq/L warrants analysis and correction of the underlying cause. Hyponatremia commonly occurs in systemic illnesses including congestive heart failure, liver failure, and edematous states. As noted above, it is unusual in either acute or chronic renal failure unless injudicious intravenous fluids have been given (Fig. 86.1).

ETIOLOGY OF ALTERED SERUM SODIUM

Determination of plasma osmolality is an important step in evaluating disorders of serum sodium (Table 86.1). Hyperglycemia is the most common cause of hyponatremia with normal or elevated osmolality; other causes include ingestion of alcohols or infusion of mannitol or glycine. These osmotically active solutes cause hyponatremia by pulling water out of cells. Extreme elevations of

TABLE 86.1 Types of hyponatremia based on plasma osmolality

Elevated osmolality (hypertonic hyponatremia)
Hyperglycemia
Glycine infusion
Mannitol infusion
Normal osmolality (pseudohyponatremia)
Severe hyperlipidemia
Severe hyperproteinemia
Low osmolality (true or hypotonic hyponatremia)

lipids (usually triglycerides increased by more than 500 mg/dL) or proteins (e.g., multiple myeloma or Waldenstrom macroglobulinemia, with increase in protein level of >4 g/dL) may lead to artifactual hyponatremia (pseudohyponatremia). These artifacts are largely prevented by use of modern techniques for measuring serum sodium concentration that measure Na^+ concentration in the aqueous phase of plasma.

CLINICAL MANIFESTATIONS

Symptoms of hyponatremia are primarily neurologic and can include lethargy, confusion, seizures, and coma. The severity of symptoms is related to the degree of hyponatremia and to the rate of development of hyponatremia. Acute hyponatremia is more likely to cause symptoms due to brain swelling. In contrast, symptoms may be mild or absent with chronic hyponatremia because adaptive processes (involving the cellular extrusion of electrolytes and "osmoles") minimize the degree of brain swelling.

DIAGNOSIS

Hypotonic hyponatremia is a common type of sodium disorder. When hypotonic hyponatremia is present, volume status needs to be assessed to determine its cause and to choose the appropriate therapy. Hypotonic hyponatremia may occur in association with hypovolemia (for example, after gastrointestinal losses), with euvolemia (for example, syndrome of inappropriate antidiuretic hormone [SIADH]) or with hypervolemia (for example, congestive heart failure) (Table 86.2).

Hypovolemic hyponatremia occurs when total body Na^+ is depleted in relation to total body water (TBW). This can occur with either renal or nonrenal Na^+ loss. Nonrenal Na^+ loss is common among ill and hospitalized patients and can occur with diarrhea, vomiting, or bleeding. Renal losses occur in response to diuretics, in uncontrolled diabetes mellitus, and in the rather uncommon syndromes of renal salt wasting. In each of these settings, hypovolemia induces the release of ADH, which promotes the reabsorption of water from urine. Hyponatremia then occurs as a result of the loss of Na^+ and the retention of water. Urinary electrolytes may be useful in distinguishing between renal and nonrenal losses. With renal losses, urinary Na^+ usually exceeds 20 mEq/L. In contrast, with nonrenal Na^+ loss, urinary Na^+ usually is less than 20 mEq/L.

In euvolemic hyponatremia, volume status is normal and hyponatremia is due to an excess of water. The most common cause of euvolemic hyponatremia is SIADH (Chapter 68). Common causes of SIADH include cancers, pulmonary disease, intracranial disease, and medications. Urinary Na^+ typically exceeds 20 mEq/L and the urine is inappropriately concentrated (U_{osm} >100 mOsm/kg)

TABLE 86.2 Causes of hyponatremia

Decreased ECV	Normal ECV	Increased ECV
Renal losses	SIADH	Nephrotic
Diuretics		Congestive heart failure
Salt-losing nephropathy	Hypothyroidism	Cirrhosis
Hypoaldosteronism		
Gastrointestinal losses Diarrhea Vomiting		
Skin losses Fever, burns		

ECV, extracellular volume; SIADH, syndrome of inappropriate antidiuretic hormone.

for the degree of plasma hypo-osmolality. Another two causes of euvolemic hyponatremia are severe hypothyroidism and adrenal insufficiency (more common in primary than in secondary adrenal insufficiency).

Hyponatremia also may occur with expanded extracellular fluid in congestive heart failure, cirrhosis, and nephrotic syndrome. These conditions are characterized by decreased effective circulatory volume despite a higher than normal TBW. The decrease in effective circulatory volume results in secretion of ADH, which, in turn, leads to water retention and dilutional hyponatremia. In these settings, hyponatremia usually serves as a marker of the severity of the underlying disease and occurs only when severe disease is present. For example, the plasma sodium might fall to about 130 mEq/L when the cardiac index is 1.5 L/min/m^2 or less. In such conditions, urine Na^+ concentrations are less than 20 mEq/L because of avid Na^+ reabsorption.

MANAGEMENT

In treatment of hyponatremia, the rate and magnitude of correction must be controlled because central nervous system (CNS) injury, including central pontine myelinolysis, can be caused by too-rapid correction. A consensus has emerged that acute hyponatremia should be corrected more rapidly than chronic hyponatremia. Acute hyponatremia is characterized by CNS symptoms and fairly rapid correction to a level at which symptoms have abated is indicated. The goal of therapy is to raise the plasma Na^+ 1 to 2 mEq/L/hour until the patient becomes asymptomatic, which generally corresponds to a plasma Na^+ of 120 to 125 mEq/L (Table 86.3).

TREATMENT

In chronic hyponatremia, adaptive processes have normalized brain water. Because of this, slower correction is indicated. Fluid restriction (1,000 to 1,500 ml/day) may be all that is needed to treat chronic hyponatremia. The rate of increase in plasma Na^+ should not exceed 0.5 to 1.0 mEq/L/hour or more than 12 mEq/L over 24 hours. Overcorrection of plasma Na^+ (>135 to 140 mEq/L) should be avoided. Correction should occur over 48 to 72 hours. In all cases of hyponatremia, underlying diseases should be treated and offending medications stopped.

TABLE 86.3 Treatment of hyponatremia

I. Determine the rate of correction
Acute hyponatremia
Rapid correction at a rate of 1 to 2 mEq/L/hr until plasma Na^+ 120 mEq/L
Chronic hyponatremia
Slow correction at a rate of 0.5 mEq/L/hr until plasma Na^+ 120 mEq/L
II. Determine the mode of correction
Hypovolemic hyponatremia
Saline
Euvolemic hyponatremia
Fluid restriction; furosemide alone or with saline to replace urine N+ losses
Demeclocycline in SIADH if above is insufficient
Hypervolemic hyponatremia
Treat underlying disease
Fluid restriction
Furosemide alone or with saline to replace urine Na+ losses if above is unsuccessful

SIADH, syndrome of inappropriate antidiuretic hormone.

The specific mode of therapy to raise the plasma Na^+ is best determined by the type of hyponatremia. To correct hypovolemic hyponatremia, the Na^+ deficit may be calculated as follows:

$$Na^+ \text{ deficit} = (\text{desired plasma } Na^+/\text{actual plasma } Na^+) \times \text{TBW}$$

Intravenous saline may be given to restore circulating volume, thereby turning off the volume-mediated stimulus to ADH secretion.

To correct euvolemic hyponatremia, it is useful to know the free water excess, which can be derived as follows:

$$\text{Desired TBW} = (\text{actual plasma } Na^+/\text{desired plasma } Na^+) \times \text{actual TBW}$$

$$\text{Free water excess (in liters)} = \text{actual TBW} - \text{desired TBW}$$

Restriction of water intake corrects the hyponatremia by a percentage per day, equal to the net water balance divided by the total body water. A net negative water balance of 500 mL in a 60-kg woman, for example, raises the plasma sodium by 0.5/30, or 1.6%. If that subject's starting plasma sodium is 120 mEq/L and no other change in water metabolism occurs, the next day's plasma sodium will be 122 mEq/L.

Hypervolemic hyponatremia should be managed by treating the underlying condition. However, free water restriction is the treatment of choice for edematous states such congestive heart failure and cirrhosis.

Hypernatremia

Hypernatremia is a plasma Na^+ level greater than 150 mEq/L. It is relatively uncommon because the thirst mechanism protects against its development. As a result, most cases occur in individuals who lack access to water; hypernatremia is most likely to occur in very young, elderly, and comatose patients. Occasionally, hypernatremia can occur in patients with a defective thirst mechanism secondary to a central nervous system disease.

Hypernatremia virtually always indicates hyperosmolal state. It reflects water loss that has not been replaced except in unusual circumstances of intravenous administration of sodium solutions that are isotonic or hypertonic to plasma. It is most commonly seen in persons who have ongoing losses of hypotonic fluids and who are unable to replace the water loss.

Hypotonic fluid losses—including evaporation from respiratory tract and skin, upper and lower gastrointestinal losses, and sweat—stimulate thirst and lead to ingestion of liquids. Thus, hypernatremia is common only in persons who are unable to drink because of debility, paralysis, gastrointestinal obstruction, or lack of access to water. CNS processes may impair thirst and are common in nursing home patients; many of these patients also are unable to express thirst or to obtain water because of debility.

ETIOLOGY

Hypernatremia, like hyponatremia, can be categorized according to the associated volume status. Common causes are listed in Table 86.4.

CLINICAL MANIFESTATIONS

As with hyponatremia, symptoms are mostly neurologic and are more severe when the disorder is acute than when it is chronic. Initially, the increase in plasma osmolality pulls water from the intracellular space and leads to cellular dehydration. Symptoms can include twitching, seizures, and coma. In infants, subdural hemorrhage may occur as a result of ruptured bridging veins. After 12 to 24 hours of hypernatremia, cellular loss of water is counteracted by an increase in intracellular solute, including both electrolytes and organic molecules. Severe hypernatremia carries a grave prognosis; the in-hospital mortality rate is greater than 50% for adults with plasma Na^+ greater than 160 mEq/L.

TABLE 86.4 Causes of hypernatremia

Hypervolemic
Administration of sodium loads
Euvolemic
Diabetes insipidus
Nephrogenic
Central
Hypovolemic
Gastrointestinal losses (diarrhea)
Renal losses
Osmotic diuresis (glucose, mannitol)
Loop diuretics
Insensible losses (burns, fever)

DIAGNOSIS

Hypernatremia most often occurs because of hypotonic losses of Na^+ and water. This condition is termed *hypovolemic hypernatremia*. Losses may be gastrointestinal, renal, or insensible losses. With nonrenal losses, because aldosterone promotes tubular reabsorption of Na in response to hypovolemia, urine Na^+ is low (<20 mEq/L) and urine osmolality is high (>400 mOsm/kg) as a result of ADH responses to hyperosmolality and hypovolemia.

Euvolemic hypernatremia is seen with diabetes insipidus (DI) and is the result of pure water loss. It is important to stress that in DI, hypernatremia is a complication seen only in patients with limited access to water or a thirst defect. That is, both the ADH feedback loop and the thirst feedback loop must fail for hypernatremia to develop in DI.

Diabetes insipidus may be central or nephrogenic (Chapter 68). In central DI, ADH secretion by the posterior pituitary is absent or incomplete. Central DI may occur as a result of surgery, trauma, cancer, encephalitis, or granulomatous disease (such as sarcoidosis), or it may be idiopathic. In nephrogenic DI, there is an impairment of the tubular response to ADH. Commonly, it is an acquired disorder and may be due to tubulointerstitial diseases (e.g., sickle cell disease), metabolic disorders (hypokalemia, hypercalcemia), or drugs (lithium, demeclocycline). With both central and nephrogenic DI, urine osmolality is inappropriately low for the degree of hypernatremia. Water deprivation testing and the responsiveness to exogenously administered ADH are useful in distinguishing nephrogenic from central DI. If diagnostic uncertainty persists, the serum ADH level should be measured.

Hypervolemic hypernatremia is an uncommon type of hypernatremia. It may be caused by intravenous administration of hypertonic saline, sodium bicarbonate, or by hypertonic feedings. Patients with this condition have an increase in total body Na^+. If they have access to water, they will minimize the effect of sodium administration by drinking fluids and by excreting sodium in their urine.

MANAGEMENT

It is prudent to correct hypernatremia at a rate no greater than 0.5 mEq/L/hour because rapid correction may lead to cerebral edema. In planning therapy, it is useful to estimate the free water deficit, which can be derived as follows:

TABLE 86.5 Treatment of hypernatremia

Hypervolemic	Discontinue administration of hypertonic load; use loop diuretics if needed, replace water loss
Euvolemic	Free water replacement Central DI: antidiuretic hormone analogue (DDAVP) Nephrogenic DI: salt restriction, thiazide, ± NSAIDs
Hypovolemic	Saline until euvolemic, then free water

DDAVP, ADH analogue desmopressin acetate; DI, diabetes insipidus; NSAID, nonsteroidal anti-inflammatory drugs.

$$\text{Actual TBW} = \text{body weight (kg)} \times 0.6 \text{ (0.5 for women)}$$

$$(\text{Actual plasma Na}^+ / \text{Desired plasma Na}^+) \times \text{actual TBW} = \text{desired TBW}$$

$$\text{Free water deficit (in liters)} = \text{desired TBW} - \text{actual TBW}$$

Specific therapy for hypernatremia is dictated by the associated volume status and the underlying etiology. With hypervolemic hypernatremia, administration of Na^+ should stop. If necessary, loop diuretics such as furosemide can be given and urinary water loss replaced with free water so that there is a net loss of Na^+. If renal failure is present, dialysis may be necessary to correct the hypernatremia.

Patients with central DI are best managed using the ADH analogue desmopressin acetate (DDAVP), which is administered by nasal insufflation (0.1 to 0.4 ml) once or twice daily. Nephrogenic DI is resistant to the use of ADH. If the cause of nephrogenic DI cannot be eliminated and if polyuria is symptomatic, treatment may be needed. The goal of therapy is to induce a state of mild volume depletion, which limits the volume of filtrate delivered to the diluting segment (the thick ascending limb of Henle) and thus reduce the degree of polyuria. This can be accomplished using a low Na^+ diet, thiazide diuretics, and occasionally, nonsteroidal anti-inflammatory agents.

When hypovolemia is present, normal saline should be administered until euvolemia is restored and then fluids can be given to replace the free water deficit (Table 86.5).

DISORDERS OF POTASSIUM BALANCE

Potassium (K^+) is the most important intracellular cation, with an intracellular concentration of approximately 150 mEq/L. Extracellular K^+ accounts for only about 2% of total K^+ stores, and the plasma K^+ level does not always provide an accurate estimate of total K^+ stores.

Potassium homeostasis is influenced by intake, excretion, and cross-membrane shifts. Daily intake of K^+ usually is 50 to 100 mEq/day. Excretion of potassium occurs through sweat, the gastrointestinal tract, and skin. In the face of hypokalemia, the daily excretion can decrease to about 10 mEq/day. Approximately 90% of dietary K^+ is excreted in the urine as a result of the distal tubular secretion of K^+. The delivery of an adequate amount of Na^+ to the distal nephron and the actions of aldosterone are important in renal K^+ excretion.

Acid-base disturbances cause changes in plasma potassium levels due to transcellular shifts in potassium. Acidosis increases plasma potassium by 0.7 mEq/L for every 0.1 unit decrease in pH, and alkalosis decreases plasma potassium by 0.7 mEq/L for every 0.1 increase in pH.

Hypokalemia

Hypokalemia is plasma K^+ below 3.5 mEq/L, with a decrease in total body potassium.

ETIOLOGY

Hypokalemia (Table 86.6) can be due to decreased K^+ intake, increased K^+ loss, and intracellular K^+ shifts. Gastrointestinal and renal K^+ losses are minimized when the intake of K^+ is low. Eventually, however, hypokalemia does develop if potassium intake is very low (<20 to 30 mEq per day) for a prolonged period. This can occur in malnourished alcoholics and in elderly patients consuming a "tea-and-toast" diet. Hypokalemia due to decreased intake is uncommon, because K^+ is present in many foods.

A common cause of hypokalemia is long-term use of diuretics, either thiazides or loop. These enhance distal nephron's sodium delivery, which in turn enhances sodium-potassium exchange at that site and causes kaliuresis. Causes of hypokalemia (in relation to blood pressure) are shown in Figure 86.2.

CLINICAL MANIFESTATIONS

Symptoms of hypokalemia are related to changes in membrane polarization. Cardiac, neuromuscular, and renal manifestations dominate. Electrocardiographic changes of hypokalemia can include T-wave flattening, U-waves, ST segment depression, and PR prolongation. Hypokalemia can predispose patients to arrhythmias, which can include atrioventricular block, paroxysmal atrial tachycardia, and rarely, ventricular tachycardia. Hypokalemia also can predispose patients to digoxin toxicity.

Patients with hypokalemia may have muscle cramps and weakness. Leg weakness may occur first and then involve ascending muscle groups. In severe cases, weakness can progress to paralysis. Severe hypokalemia may even result in rhabdomyolysis. Effects on smooth muscle can lead to ileus. Hypokalemia also may evoke a resistance to the kidney tubular action of ADH and result in nephrogenic diabetes insipidus and associated polyuria and polydipsia.

MANAGEMENT

Therapy must be directed at the underlying cause of hypokalemia and at replacing the K^+ deficit. A decrease in plasma K^+ from 4.0 to 3.0 mEq/L suggests a total body deficit of 550 to 600 mEq in

TABLE 86.6 Principal causes of potassium depletion

Deficient dietary intake
Excessive Losses
Gastrointestinal
• Protracted vomiting
• Diarrhea
• Fistual
• Laxative abuse
Renal
• Metabolic alkalosis
• Diuretics
• Hyperaldosteronism
• Tubular dysfunction (renal tubular acidosis)

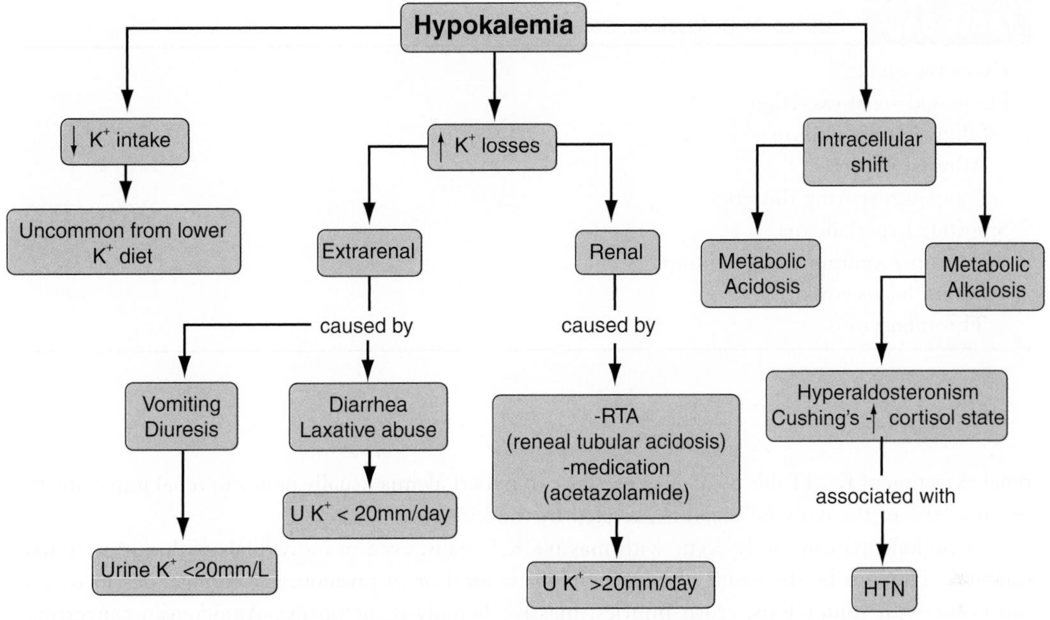

Figure 86.2 • Causes and pathophysiology of hypokalemia associated with hypertension.

a healthy 100-kg male, or a deficit of 110 to 120 mEq in an emaciated 45-kg man or woman. Potassium levels less than 2.0 mEq/L may represent a deficit exceeding 1,000 mEq. When acidosis is present and the plasma K^+ is low, it is important to provide K^+ replacement before correcting the acidosis, because the K^+ level will fall further as the pH rises. This effect is compounded by the effect of bicarbonate in enhancing urinary potassium excretion.

For most nonurgent situations, it is preferable to use oral potassium replacement because it is the safest route of therapy. Oral doses can vary from 20 to 120 mEq per day. Potassium usually is administered as potassium chloride. Other available forms include potassium bicarbonate, citrate, and gluconate. When life-threatening hypokalemia is present or if the patient cannot tolerate oral replacement, intravenous K^+ replacement may be necessary. Administration through a peripheral line should not exceed a rate of 10 mEq per hour, with a concentration no greater than 40 mEq/L of potassium in the infused fluid. If necessary, rates of up to 20 to 40 mEq per hour can be given via a central line with continuous cardiac monitoring.

Hyperkalemia

Hyperkalemia is a plasma K^+ level greater than 5.0 mEq/L. In the clinical approach to hyperkalemia, spurious or pseudohyperkalemia must first be excluded. Pseudohyperkalemia is defined as hyperkalemia that develops in the blood sample after the blood is drawn. It usually is due to hemolysis resulting from improper venipuncture technique (prolonged tourniquet application or excessive fist clenching), marked leukocytosis (>70,000/mL), and thrombocytosis (>1 million/mL). This can be distinguished from true hyperkalemia by measuring plasma potassium levels. This occurs because the clot that is formed with serum may release intracellular K^+ into the serum, whereas plasma is collected in an anticoagulated tube and clotting will not occur.

CLASSIFICATION AND ETIOLOGY

Once pseudohyperkalemia is excluded, the etiology of hyperkalemia must be determined. Hyperkalemia can be due to increased K^+ intake, shifts of K^+ from the intercellular space, or decreased

TABLE 86.7 Causes of potassium excess

Excessive intake
Decreased renal excretion
Oliguric renal failure
Adrenal failure
Potassium-sparing diuretics
Spurious hyperkalemia
Improper venipuncture technique
Severe leucocytosis
Thrombocytosis

renal excretion of K^+ (Table 86.7). The presence of hyperkalemia usually points to renal impairment, because 90% of the daily K^+ load is excreted by the kidneys.

Hyperkalemia can rarely occur with massive K^+ loads, even in individuals with normal renal function. This can be the result of exogenous loads (oral or intravenous) or endogenous loads (as can occur with tumor lysis, crush injuries, massive hemolysis, or burns). Angiotensin-converting enzyme inhibitors or angiotensin II receptor blockers may cause hyperkalemia by blunting the synthesis of aldosterone, an effect that is compounded by the effect of these medicines to lower the glomerular filtration rate. Nonsteroidal arthritis medicines such as ibuprofen or naproxen inhibit prostaglandin synthesis, thus also reducing glomerular filtration rate as well as aldosterone synthesis. These effects are especially apt to occur in subjects with already reduced kidney function.

CLINICAL MANIFESTATIONS

Symptoms of hyperkalemia usually develop when the plasma K^+ rises above 6.5 mEq/L. They are related to changes in membrane polarization. Cardiac manifestations are the most serious. On the electrocardiogram, peaked, symmetrical T-waves are seen earliest. Later findings can include PR prolongation, QRS widening, ventricular fibrillation, complete heart block, and asystole. Weakness, paralysis, and respiratory failure also may occur because of hyperkalemia.

MANAGEMENT

Therapy for mild hyperkalemia should include dietary K^+ restriction and cessation of any drugs that interfere with K+ excretion. In addition, diuretics (loop diuretics or thiazides) may be used to increase renal K^+ excretion. In the treatment of hypoaldosteronism, mineralocorticoid replacement is useful.

Life-threatening hyperkalemia requires immediate attention. When electrocardiogram changes are present, calcium should be given to antagonize the effect of hyperkalemia on the cell membrane. It can be given intravenously as 10% calcium gluconate (10 mL over 15 minutes) and the dose can be repeated in 5 to 10 minutes. Calcium has a rapid onset and the duration of action is about 30 minutes.

At the same time, K^+ must be shifted into the intracellular space. This can be accomplished with insulin. Typically, 25% to 50% dextrose and insulin (5 to 10 units) may be given together intravenously and repeated in 15 minutes as required. Use of albuterol or other beta-mimetic inhaled drug may lower the plasma potassium by 0.5 mEq/L.

As a third component of therapy, K^+ removal can be facilitated with the use of the cation exchange resin sodium polystyrene sulfonate (Kayexalate). Orally, 30 to 50 g can be given in sorbitol (to prevent constipation) and repeated every 3 to 4 hours as needed. When the oral route is not feasible, it may be given as a retention enema. Sodium retention is a potential complication because each gram of the resin releases 1 to 2 mEq of Na^+ for each 1 mEq of K^+ that is bound. Finally, hemodialysis may be needed when volume overload, severe acidosis, or uremia is present. Maximal K^+ removal rate with hemodialysis is about 1 mEq per minute. Peritoneal dialysis is a far less efficient method of treating hyperkalemia.

CHAPTER 87

Hypertensive Emergencies

Shibin Jacob and Virginia Savin

Hypertensive crisis is the acute and severe elevation of blood pressure including hypertensive emergencies and hypertensive urgencies. Hypertensive emergency (also called malignant hypertension) is defined by severe hypertension (usually in the range of systolic blood pressure [SBP] >220 mm Hg and diastolic blood pressure [DBP] >125 mm Hg) with acute organ damage including central nervous system (CNS) dysfunction or intracerebral hemorrhage, visual changes with hemorrhages, exudates and papilledema of the optic fundus, myocardia infarction, pulmonary edema, or renal insufficiency. The term hypertensive urgency applies to patients with SBP >220 mm Hg and DBP >125 mm Hg who have no evidence of end-organ (target organ) damage.

Many episodes of hypertensive emergencies develop in patients who have been treated for hypertension but have decreased or stopped treatment.

ETIOLOGY

Hypertensive urgency and emergency occur most frequently in patients with essential hypertension that has been treated ineffectually. For secondary causes of hypertension, see Chapter 133.

Arterial and arteriolar vasoconstriction occur with mild to moderate increases in the blood pressure. This autoregulatory mechanism protects organs from hyperperfusion and consequent capillary leak. Autoregulation is especially important in the brain, kidney, and heart. The autoregulatory mechanisms work well in a narrow range of 50 to 150 mean arterial pressure (MAP). With increasing hypertension, systemic hypertension is transmitted to the end organs through the smaller distal vessels and leads to increased perfusion that varies directly with MAP. This increased perfusion leads to edema and hemorrhage from small vessels in the brain and kidney. In addition, the increased pressures and flow in small arterioles and capillaries can lead to endothelial injury causing marked vasoconstriction. Plasma constituents enter the vascular wall and result in fibrinoid necrosis of small arterioles, a marker of long standing failure of the autoregulatory process and of hyperperfusion.

In patients with chronically elevated blood pressures, the range of autoregulation is shifted to a higher level. Although these patients are relatively protected from higher pressures, they are prone to tissue hypoperfusion even in the "low normal range" of MAP. Patients with longstanding hypertension develop hypertensive emergency around diastolic blood pressure of 130 mm Hg, whereas previously normotensive patients who develop acute hypertension can develop symptoms at diastolic blood pressure of 100 mm Hg or less.

If hypertension is not treated effectively, hypertensive emergency may ensue. Hypertensive urgency is characterized by rapid increase in blood pressure; the acuity of the increase is more important than the absolute pressure in determining the severity of the condition and the urgency of treatment. Co-existing conditions such as renal insufficiency, congestive heart failure (CHF), coronary artery disease, or retinal changes increase the risk of progression to hypertensive emergency.

TABLE 87.1 Clinical features: manifestations of target organ damage associated with hypertensive emergency

Target organs	Clinical manifestations
Central nervous system	Altered mental status Seizures Cerebrovascular accident Encephalopathy Headache Intracranial hemorrhage
Ophthalmologic	Blurred vision Diplopia Retinal hemorrhages Papilledema
Renal	Acute renal failure Hematuria
Cardiovascular	Angina (chest pain) Congestive heart failure Pulmonary edema Aortic dissection
Hematologic	Microangiopathic hemolytic anemia

CLINICAL MANIFESTATIONS

In the setting of hypertensive emergency, many organ systems are affected (Table 87.1). CNS manifestations of hypertensive emergency include headaches, altered mentation, retinal hemorrhages, optic disc edema, encephalopathy, hemorrhagic stroke, and coma. The cardiovascular manifestations are angina, myocardial infarction, pulmonary edema, and aortic dissection. In the kidneys, acute renal insufficiency (or acute worsening of chronic renal insufficiency) and hematuria can be present. Eclampsia may occur in pregnant women, when the rise in blood pressure may be associated with edema, proteinuria, disseminated intravascular coagulation, and seizures. The patient may also report headache, blurred vision, visual field cuts, or blindness.

Patients with hypertensive crisis most often have an increased intravascular volume as well as increased peripheral resistance due to vasoconstriction. Hematological manifestations, including intravascular platelet aggregation and microangiopathic hemolytic anemia are also seen as a result of endothelial injury.

DIAGNOSIS

History provides some of the key information needed for the evaluation of patients with hypertensive urgency/emergency. Prior diagnosis of hypertension and poor control of blood pressure are common. The use of nonsteroidal anti-inflammatory agents, cocaine or amphetamines, or of tyramine-containing foods in patients on monamine oxidase inhibitors should be sought. Family history of hypertension, renal insufficiency, CHF, CAD, diabetes, and dyslipidemia increase risk of hypertensive emergency.

Gathering information about CNS symptoms (headache, diplopia, blurred vision, confusion, weakness, seizures), cardiovascular symptoms (dyspnea, chest pain, palpitations), and renal symptoms (anuria, hematuria) that often precede or accompany hypertensive crisis is important.

A focused physical examination should be performed. Physical findings include elevated blood pressure assessed using an appropriately sized cuff or intra-arterial monitoring. Neurological examination may show focal weakness or loss of motor skills, confusion, or somnolence. Visual examination should include funduscopic examination for evaluation of retinal changes. Grade III (retinal exudates, hemorrhage) or grade IV (optic disc edema) retinopathy suggest hypertensive emergency, whereas Grade II retinopathy is seen in uncontrolled hypertension. Hyperreflexia and edema in a pregnant woman may signify pre-eclampsia. Cardiovascular examination should include evaluation of bruits (carotid, renal), murmurs, and heart sounds. The presence of a third heart sound may signify ventricular failure, and S4 may imply noncompliant left ventricle. Evaluation for aortic dissection and coarctation of aorta should also be done.

Diagnostic studies include basic metabolic panel (BMP) to evaluate renal function and electrolytes and an electrocardiogram to detect presence of ischemic changes. Urinalysis with microscopy may allow detection of hematuria, red blood cell casts, or other abnormalities indicative of renal disease. A complete blood count with peripheral smear may be useful to assess for microangiopathic hemolytic anemia and the finding of a widened mediastinum on chest x-ray may raise the suspicion of aortic dissection. Additional diagnostic evaluation is done based on the available clinical data, which could include computed tomography of the head, serum and urine drug screen, renal doppler, and renal biopsy.

TREATMENT

Hypertensive Emergencies

The goal of treatment is to achieve a graded 20% to 25% reduction of MAP in 30 to 60 minutes to decrease the target organ damage, guided by the patient's clinical condition. Effective treatment of blood pressure may lead to improvement in glomerular filtration rate and improved long-term survival. This is supported by improved survival since introduction of more potent antihypertensive agents in the 1980s. A variety of agents are available for use in hypertensive emergency (Table 87.2).

Sodium nitroprusside is a rapidly acting arterial and venodilator, decreasing the preload, afterload, and myocardial oxygen demand. Rate of onset is extremely rapid, with a plasma half-life of 3 to 4 minutes. Nitroprusside is metabolized into thiocyanate by the liver, and excreted through kidneys. In patients with renal disease, this can lead to thiocyanate toxicity if used for >24 to 48 hours. Cyanide toxicity is rare, but can occur in patients with renal failure. Nitroprusside is the drug of choice for most patients with hypertensive emergency, with a few exceptions. Because nitroprusside crosses the placenta, it is contraindicated in patients with eclampsia or pre-eclampsia.

Labetalol is a selective alpha-1 blocker and a nonselective beta-blocker that decreases the peripheral vascular resistance. Onset of action is in 1 to 5 minutes when given intravenously, and the half-life is about 12 minutes. It is metabolized via the liver. The oral bioavailability is about 25%, and the elimination half-life is about 8 hours. Labetalol does not cause reflex tachycardia or a decrease in cerebral perfusion. It is ideal for use in patients with excessive catecholamine stimulation, and can be safely used in patients with cardiovascular and cerebrovascular disease. This can be used as the primary drug and then switched to oral dose. The contraindications include second- or third-degree heart block and bronchospasm. Abrupt discontinuation of labetalol may precipitate anginal symptoms or myocardial infarction in patients with ischemic heart disease.

Esmolol is an ultrashort-acting (elimination half-life of 9 minutes) beta-blocker that lacks alpha-blocking properties. It is used as an infusion, and the effects are rapidly reversed on discontinuation

TABLE 87.2 Selected intravenous drugs for hypertensive emergencies

Drugs	Dose	Important side effects
Diazoxide (Hyperstat)	50–100 mg bolus or 15–30 mg/min infusion	Hypotension, tachycardia, angina, vomiting, hyperglycemia
Enalaprilat (Vasotec)	1.25–5 mg every 6 hours	Hypotension, renal failure if bilateral renal artery stenosis is present
Fenoldopam (Corlopam)	0.1–1.0 μg/kg/min	Myocardial infarction, congestive heart failure, hypokalemia, arrhythmias, leukocytosis
Furosemide (Lasix)	40–160 mg every 4–6 hours	Hypotension, hypokalemia, hyperglycemia on prolonged use
Labetalol (Normodyne, Trandate)	20–80 mg by bolus every 10–15 min or 0.5–2 mg/min infusion	Hypotension, bronchoconstriction, heart block, bradycardia
Sodium nitroprusside (Nipride)	0.25–10 μg/kg/min (maximum dose for 10 min only)	Vomiting, twitching, thiocyanate intoxication, methemoglobinemia, cyanide poisoning
Nitroglycerin (Nitro-Bid IV)	5–100 μg/min	Headache, vomiting, methemoglobinemia, tolerance

of the infusion. Esmolol does not cause reflex tachycardia; it can be used as a single agent or as a supplemental agent in patients with myocardial ischemia who cannot tolerate reflex tachycardia. It should be avoided in patients with cocaine-induced hypertension because of its relative sparing of alpha receptors leading to paradoxical hypertension, and in patients at risk of bronchospasm. In patients with cocaine-induced hypertensive emergency, it may be used as an adjuvant once alpha blockade with another agent is achieved. It is currently rarely used in the setting of hypertensive urgency.

Intravenous nitroglycerin is an arterial and venodilator, with greater action as a venodilator. Onset of action is rapid and elimination half-life is 4 minutes. The main indication is in the setting of myocardial ischemia or pulmonary edema. Main adverse effects include headache and reflex tachycardia. Nitroglycerin is usually used in combination with a beta-blocker to decrease reflex tachycardia.

Nicardipine is a dihydropyridine calcium channel blocker that reduces afterload by reducing the peripheral vascular resistance. It has greater vasodilating properties on coronary vessels and reduces cerebral vasospasm. It is preferred over other agents in patients with stable angina and subarachnoid bleed.

Other agents commonly used include hydralazine (a direct vasodilator, preferred in eclampsia or pre-eclampsia), enalapril (an intravenous angiotensin-converting enzyme inhibitor with rapid onset of action and short half-life), and fenoldopam (a selective dopaminergic receptor agonist).

Hypertensive Urgencies

The goal in treating hypertensive urgencies is reduction in blood pressure by oral agents in about 24 hours. If there is a history of noncompliance with treatment, it is important to restart therapy and to choose medications that do not cause rebound hypertension. During acute treatment, blood pressure response should be monitored closely and required doses may be lower than those previously prescribed.

Common agents used to treat hypertensive urgencies include clonidine (a central alpha-2 agonist with onset of action in 30 to 60 minutes, preferred in cocaine withdrawal, can interact with other drugs causing postural hypotension and severe rebound hypertension on withdrawal) sublingual nitroglycerin (rapid onset of action, agent of choice in myocardial ischemia, can cause headache and reflex tachycardia). Captopril (an angiotensin-converting enzyme inhibitor with onset of action in 30 to 60 minutes; lasts 4 to 6 hours without change in cardiac output, cerebral blood flow, or heart rate; preferred in renovascular hypertension), and losartan (angiotensin II blocker, half-life of 2 hours, has active metabolite with half life of 6 to 9 hours). Angiotensin-converting enzyme inhibitors and angiotensin II blockers should be avoided in pregnancy.

The key to decreasing the incidence of recurrent hypertensive urgency or emergency is patient education. The importance of sodium restriction, medication compliance, and regular follow-ups cannot be overemphasized. Early follow-up after acute treatment is required because regression of endothelial injury may lead to increased sensitivity to therapy while increased activity and increased dietary sodium will lead to resistance. Patients who have access to follow-up by a primary care clinician and to appropriate medications are more likely to have a good long-term outcome than those who do not get follow-up. Five-year survival of untreated malignant hypertension is nearly zero and is improved to 80% to 90% with use of currently available antihypertensive agents.

COMPLICATIONS

Complications of severe hypertension include hypertensive encephalopathy, cerebral infarction, intracerebral or subarachnoid hemorrhage, acute pulmonary edema, acute congestive heart failure, acute myocardial infarction or unstable angina, aortic dissection, and acute renal failure. Early diagnosis and treatment are directed toward prevention of these complications and prolonging survival.

Hematology

John Adamson

CHAPTER 88

Acute Leukemias

John Charlson

Acute leukemia is a malignancy of immature hematopoietic cells in which a malignant clone of leukocytes proliferates, but fails to mature. The immature cells accumulate in the bone marrow and suppress normal hematopoiesis. Left untreated, acute leukemia is rapidly fatal, with most patients dying of infection or bleeding within several months of diagnosis.

ACUTE MYELOGENOUS LEUKEMIA

Acute myelogenous leukemia (AML) is a disease of advancing age, with a slightly higher incidence in men. More than 50% of all cases occur in patients over 60 years of age. The etiology of AML is unknown, but heredity, radiation exposure, and exposure to certain chemicals and drugs are implicated. Patients with Down's syndrome are 20 times more prone to acute leukemia (AML and acute lymphoblastic leukemia) than normal. Increased risk prevails in other diseases as well (e.g., Fanconi's anemia, Bloom's syndrome).

Acute leukemias usually are classified by the morphologic, histochemical (for example, peroxidase-positive granules in the cytoplasm indicate myeloid lineage), immunophenotypic (based on variable expression of cell-surface antigens), and cytogenetic (chromosomal abnormalities, point mutations) characteristics of the malignant cells.

The French-American-British (FAB) classification relies on morphology and the results of cytochemical stains to differentiate the various leukemias, including differentiation of myeloid versus lymphoid origin (Table 88.1). In the older FAB classification system, AML has seven subtypes, with some of relevant clinical features discussed below. The more recent World Health Organization (WHO) classification incorporates information regarding cytogenetics (Table 88.2). This type of classification is increasingly important, because cytogenetic findings may have even more impact on prognosis and treatment than FAB subtype (Table 88.3).

Acute promyelocytic leukemia, classified as AML M3 subtype in the FAB system, is classified as AML with recurrent cytogenetic abnormalities by the WHO. The 15:17 translocation is invariably present. The coagulation system is virtually always activated, with disseminated intravascular coagulation either at diagnosis or with the initiation of treatment; patients require aggressive blood and platelet support in addition to consumed factor replacement. Overall, patients are younger and survival is greater than 70% with current therapy. Recognition of this subtype is important before the initiation of induction therapy, so that the coagulopathy is treated early and serious bleeding prevented.

Clinical Features

The clinical features of acute leukemia are related to the depression of normal blood counts or infiltration of organs by leukemic blasts. Most symptoms are related to the disruption of hematopoiesis by rapid expansion of the leukemic blast population. Fatigue and weakness are common manifestations and can be due in part to anemia. Mucosal bleeding, bruising, and petechiae result from decreased

TABLE 88.1 French-American-British classification: subtypes of acute lymphoblastic leukemia

Subtype	Morphology	Cytochemistry	Immunophenotype	Complete remission (%)	3-Year Remission (%)
L1 (Childhood)	Small uniform blasts Small nucleoli	Myeloperoxidase Periodic acid-Schiff (+ +)	CD 10+ (CALLA+)	85	40
L2 (Adult)	Larger blasts, irregular nucleoli	Myeloperoxidase Periodic acid-Schiff (+)	Same as L1	35	
L3 (Burkitt-like)	Large blasts, basophilic cytoplasm, vacuolated large nucleoli	Myeloperoxidase Periodic acid-Schiff (−)	CD 10− CD 19, 20+	10	

TABLE 88.2 World Health Organization classification of acute myeloid leukemia

	Description	Monoclonals	Cytogenetics
M0	Undifferentiated	CD13+ CD14+ CD33+ CD34+	
M1	AML with minimal differentiation	CD13+ CD14+ CD33+ CD34+	Various, includes +8, del7
M2	AML with differentiation (granules, Auer rods)		T(8;21)
M3	Acute promyelocytic leukemia: disseminated intravascular coagulation		T(15;17)
M4	Acute myelomonocytic M4EO: with eosinophils		11q Inv(16) T(16;16)
M5	Acute monocytic leukemia		T(9;11)
M6	Erythroleukemia		Del(7a) Del(5a)
M7	Megakaryocytic leukemia	Antiplatelet GP11b/111a	

AML, acute myeloid leukemia.

platelet production. Severe or recurrent infection result from lack of mature functional neutrophils. These symptoms often arise and progress over a matter of a few weeks. Acute monocytic leukemia has a tendency to infiltrate tissues, such as the gums, central nervous system (CNS), or skin (Fig. 88.1). Megakaryocytic leukemia is associated with Down's syndrome. AML with differentiation typically has Auer rods.

Presentations that require urgent treatment may occur. Hyperleukocytosis (blood blast counts

TABLE 88.3 Cytogenetic abnormalities and prognosis in acute myeloid leukemia

Favorable	Inv(16), t(15;17), t(8;21)	Complete remission 84% 5-year overall survival 57%
Unfavorable	−5/del(5q), −7/del(7q), abnormal(3q, 9q, 11q, 20q, 21q, 17p), t(6;9), t(9;22), complex cytogenetics (3+ abnormalities)	Complete remission 55% 5-year overall survival 23%

Inv, inversion; t, translocation; del, deletion. From Slovak ML, Kopecky KJ, Cassileth PA, et al. Karyotypic analysis predicts outcome of preremission and postremission therapy in adult acute myeloid leukemia: a Southwest Oncology Group/Eastern Cooperative Oncology Group Study. *Blood* 2000;96:4075, with permission.

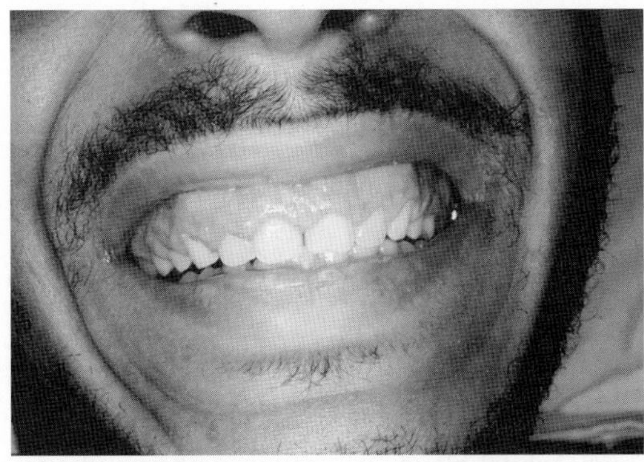

Figure 88.1 • Gum hypertrophy.

of 100,000/mm^3 or more) predisposes to *leukostasis syndrome*, in which aggregates of blast cells occlude small arteries in multiple organs. The features of this rapidly fatal syndrome include coma, obtundation, confusion, intracranial hemorrhage, massive hemoptysis, respiratory failure, and myocardial infarction. Patients with acute promyelocytic leukemia (MB leukemia) present with features of DIC (low platelets, prolonged PT, PIT fibrinogen and severe hemorrhage).

Diagnosis

Anemia and thrombocytopenia are common laboratory findings. The white blood cell count may be either low or high, but the presence of early precursor cells (or "blasts") in the circulating blood is a strong indicator of leukemia. Diagnosis and classification of AML rests on examination of bone marrow samples. The bone marrow is usually hypercellular; if more than 20% of the cells are blasts, a diagnosis of acute leukemia can be made. Cytogenetic studies are routinely performed on bone marrow samples, including examination of the karyotype and sometimes fluorescence in situ hybridization assays for specific mutations. Presence of certain cytogenetic abnormalities can have impact on prognosis.

Management

Initial treatment includes stabilization of the patient with transfusion of blood products, correction of coagulopathy, antibiotics for infection. Therapy of AML, with the exception of M3, initially involves induction therapy and some postinduction "consolidation." The goal of induction therapy is to attain a complete remission. Typically, a combination of chemotherapy agents, cytarabine and an anthracycline, are given to produce profound bone marrow hypoplasia. Complete remission occurs when the marrow regenerates normally (<5% blasts and normal morphology) and the peripheral counts have recovered. The incidence of mortality during induction, usually as a result of infection or uncontrolled bleeding, is nearly 10%, although it may be 60% to 80% in older (>65 years) persons.

Consolidation chemotherapy follows achievement of complete remission. Without it, the leukemia invariably recurs within 4 to 18 months. Consolidation therapy improves both the duration of remission and overall survival. The median survival is 18 to 24 months. Approximately 15% to 20% of all AML patients appear to achieve long-term remission and, possibly, cure. Bone marrow transplant may be indicated for some patients who have achieved remission.

ACUTE LYMPHOBLASTIC LEUKEMIA

Acute lymphoblastic leukemia (ALL) is most common in children, with a peak incidence between 2 and 6 years. The term *adult ALL* usually refers to patients older than 15 to 18 years, and it is biologically different from childhood ALL. Acute lymphoblastic leukemia has a second peak incidence in adults over the age of 60 years.

Clinical Features

In general, the clinical features of acute lymphoblastic leukemia are similar to AML, with the signs and symptoms of bone marrow failure, including fatigue, bleeding, or fever, depending on the degree of cytopenias at the time of the diagnosis. As a result of tissue infiltration by malignant lymphoblasts, ALL manifests testicular enlargement, skin nodules, lymphadenopathy, splenomegaly, and cranial nerve palsies.

Diagnosis

The peripheral blood may show dramatically high white blood cell count with circulating lymphoblasts, or it may show neutropenia and few abnormal cells. Diagnosis again depends on bone marrow biopsy and analysis. The bone marrow usually is hypercellular because of the lymphoblastic infiltration, and normal marrow elements may appear to be completely absent. The diagnosis of ALL is also based on the morphology of the malignant blasts, plus their immunophenotypic, histochemical, and cytogenetic characteristics.

Management

Conventional treatment of ALL in general involves a sequence of induction; consolidation and intensification (given several times in sequence); and maintenance chemotherapy (for 1 to 2 years). All therapy regimens in ALL include some type of prophylactic treatment of the CNS. Leukemia recurs in the CNS in 30% of untreated cases, and 5% of adults present initially with CNS disease.

Twenty-five percent of adults with ALL are cured with conventional chemotherapy. Allogeneic bone marrow transplantation currently is reserved for patients following their first relapse, or for certain high-risk patients after achieving first remission.

CHAPTER 89

Myeloproliferative Disorders

John Charlson

Hematologic malignancies are divided into lymphoid and myeloid processes, and each of these is further classified as acute or chronic. Conceptually, each of these classifications reflects abnormalities at different steps in the differentiation and maturation of pluripotent hematopoietic stem cells (Table 89.1).

Myeloproliferative disorders include chronic myeloid disorders characterized by the expansion of terminal myeloid cell lines in the peripheral blood. The major categories of chronic myeloproliferative disorders include chronic myelogenous leukemia, polycythemia vera, essential thrombocythemia, and agnogenic myelofibrosis with myeloid metaplasia (also known as chronic idiopathic myelofibrosis). These disorders are considered preleukemic and have varying probabilities of evolving into acute leukemia. Chronic neutrophilic leukemia and chronic eosinophilic are also chronic myeloproliferative disorders but are very rare and will not be discussed further.

CHRONIC MYELOGENOUS LEUKEMIA

Chronic myelogenous leukemia (CML) is a chronic myeloproliferative disorder that results from a reciprocal translocation of chromosomes 9 and 22 creating the Philadelphia chromosome (Ph). This results in production of the *BCR/ABL* oncogene, which codes for a protein with unregulated tyrosine kinase activity, leading to altered cellular proliferation and survival. The median age at diagnosis is 67 years. CML accounts for 15% to 20% of all leukemias and an estimated 4,600 cases were diagnosed in the United States in 2005. The vast majority of cases transform to acute myelogenous leukemia. Prior to the introduction of imatinib, patients who did not undergo bone marrow transplant had median survival of 5 to 7 years.

Etiology

Ionizing radiation is a risk factor for CML. As noted above, the *BCR/ABL* oncogene promotes malignant proliferation of mature myeloid cells.

Clinical Manifestations

The onset of CML is asymptomatic. Routine laboratory testing may reveal leukocytosis. Slowly developing mild anemia leads to fatigue and decreased exercise intolerance. Early satiety, a feeling of abdominal fullness, and left upper quadrant discomfort can be related to splenomegaly. As the disease progresses, patients may experience bruising or mucosal bleeding due to thrombocytopenia. Splenomegaly, often massive, is the outstanding physical sign. Hepatomegaly and bony pain and tenderness (from increased intramedullary pressure causing pressure on nerve-rich endosteum) may be noted. Pallor, fever, weight loss, and lymphadenopathy are late manifestations.

Early CML is described as being in *chronic phase*, and over time it evolves to *accelerated-phase* CML and then *blast-phase* CML, which is similar to acute leukemia. There are several different criteria for determining disease stage, but in general, chronic phase is characterized by neutrophilic

TABLE 89.1 Organization of hematologic malignancies

Lymphoproliferative disorders	Myeloid disorders
	Acute myeloid leukemia
Multiple myeloma	Chronic myeloid disorders
Acute lymphocytic leukemia	A. Myelodysplastic syndromes
Hodgkin's lymphoma	B. Chronic myeloproliferative disorders
Non-Hodgkin's lymphoma	Polycythemia vera
Plasma cell dyscrasias	Essential thrombocythemia
Chronic lymphoid leukemias	Chronic myelogenous leukemia
Hairy cell leukemia	Myelofibrosis w/myeloid metaplasia (also know as chronic idiopathic myelofibrosis)
	Chronic neutrophilic leukemia
	Chronic eosinophilic leukemia

leukocytosis, thrombocytosis, basophilia, and a blood and bone marrow blast count of <10%. Accelerated phase CML is defined by a blood or bone marrow myeloblast count of 10% to 19%, blood basophilia (>20%), and thrombocytopenia or thrombocytosis (>1 million/μL). Blast phase (or blast crisis) occurs when the blood or bone marrow blast count is more than 20%. Extramedullary involvement, in sites such as lymph nodes, skin, central and nervous system, can occur in up to 10% of patients in blast phase. Infections may become more common as mature neutrophils are replaced by more immature cells.

Diagnosis

Laboratory findings include mild anemia and an elevated white blood cell (WBC) count, sometimes more than 100,000/μL (normal range up to 12,000/μL). The WBC differential includes granulocytes at all stages of development, with the blast count typically less than 5%. The platelet count is elevated in 15% to 35% of chronic phase patients. Thrombocytopenia can signal progression of disease. The leukocyte alkaline phosphatase (LAP) score is low, which distinguishes CML from other myeloproliferative disorders. Serum uric acid may be increased due to cell turnover. A bone marrow biopsy, although rarely needed for diagnosis, may differentiate CML from myelofibrosis, or help detect the Ph chromosome, especially if there are few proliferating cells present in the peripheral blood. The bone marrow is hypercellular, with increased granulopoiesis. Routine karyotyping detects the Philadelphia chromosome in more than 90% of cases

Management

First-line therapy for CML is imatinib, which inhibits the tyrosine kinase *BCR/ABL*. Treatment effect is monitored in terms of hematologic response, cytogenetic response, and molecular response (Table 89.2).

Bone marrow transplantation, which has been considered the only curative treatment for acute myelogenous leukemia (AML), may be an option for patients who fail imatinib therapy and have a suitable donor. Standard antileukemic chemotherapy is not very effective against blast-phase CML. Cytotoxic chemotherapy such as hydroxyurea may be used to reduce markedly elevated cell counts, but it does not prolong survival or alter disease course.

TABLE 89.2 Response criteria to treatment for chronic myelogenous leukemia

Hematologic response	WBC $<$10,000/μL with persistent immature forms (blasts, promyelocytes, myelocytes)
Partial hematologic response	Persistent thrombocytosis or splenomegaly, but $\geq$50% reduction. WBC $<$10,000/μL with no immature forms
Complete hematologic response	Normal platelet count No sign of disease
Cytogenetic response Minor cytogenetic response	35% to 65% of metaphases with Ph chromosome positivity
Major cytogenetic response	1% to 35% of metaphases with Ph chromosome positivity
Complete cytogenetic response	No metaphases with Ph chromosome positivity
Molecular response	$>$3 log-fold reduction in quantitative polymerase chain reaction copies of BCR-ABL Associated with higher rate of progression free survival

POLYCYTHEMIA VERA

Like the other chronic myeloproliferative disorders, polycythemia vera (PV) represents a clonal stem cell disease resulting in expansion of all myeloid cell lines, but predominantly the erythroid lineage. Production of red blood cells (RBCs) is normally regulated by erythropoietin, but the red blood cells in PV proliferate independent of the actions of erythropoietin. The median age at diagnosis is 60 to 65 years.

Etiology

Radiation exposure is associated with an increased risk of the disease. Recent research has demonstrated a specific mutation in the *JAK2* gene (JAK2V617F mutation) in the majority of PV patients, as well as some of the other myeloproliferative disorders.

Clinical Manifestations

At presentation, 80% of patients with PV are symptomatic. Common complaints include headache, dizziness, dyspnea, and painful paresthesias (erythromelalgia) and are caused by the increased red blood cell (RBC) mass and hyperviscosity. Pruritus, especially after a hot shower, is caused by histamine release from neutrophils. The peptic ulcers that develop in 10% of patients are also attributed to increased histamine. Risk of arterial or venous thrombosis is increased, and up to one fifth of patients present with thrombotic complications such as stroke, myocardial infarction, or deep venous thrombosis. Physical findings include splenomegaly in the majority of patients, facial or conjunctival plethora, and less commonly hypertension and hepatomegaly.

Diagnosis

The first step in making a diagnosis of PV is to document an increase in red cell mass (RCM). Red cell volume can be assessed by labeling a sample of the patient's RBCs with ^{51}Cr radiotracer, and this can help in determining if the RCM is truly increased or if it is only relatively increased due to decreased plasma volume. Formal RCM determination is not required if hemoglobin is more than

TABLE 89.3 Causes of secondary erythrocytosis

Congenital	Mutant high-oxygen-affinity hemoglobin Autonomous high erythropoietin production (including Chuvash polycythemia) Autosomal dominant polycythemia (e.g., erythropoietin receptor mutation)
Acquired hypoxemia	High altitude Chronic lung disease Cyanotic congenital heart disease Sleep apnea Smoking Carbon monoxide poisoning, chronic Hepatoma
Hepatic lesions	Cirrhosis Hepatitis Renal tumors
Renal lesions	Cysts Renal artery stenosis Postrenal transplantation Wilms tumor
Other tumors	Cerebellar hemangioblastoma Uterine fibroids Bronchial carcinoma Adrenal tumors Pheochromocytoma Androgens, anabolic steroids
Drugs/chemicals	Nickel Cobalt

18.5 g/dL in men or 16.5 g/dL in women, because these values are almost never achieved by plasma volume depletion alone.

The second step is to differentiate PV from secondary erythrocytosis (Table 89.3). Serum erythropoietin level is an important test, because in many of the secondary types of erythrocytosis, erythropoietin levels are elevated or high-normal, whereas in PV, erythropoietin production is suppressed. Tissue hypoxia is one cause of secondary erythrocytosis, and so evaluation should include assessment of smoking history and for other types of cardiac or pulmonary disease. Testing can include arterial blood gas analysis (oxygen saturation below 92% suggests a secondary cause) and carboxyhemoglobin determination. An oxygen dissociation curve (P_{50}) may be determined to identify high-affinity mutant hemoglobin; this is useful if the patient has a family history of erythrocytosis, raising the possibility of congenital erythrocytosis. Hepatic and renal cysts or tumors can be associated with increased erythropoietin levels; therefore, the workup might include abdominal ultrasound (which can also be used to document splenomegaly). Bone marrow biopsy is not necessary to make the diagnosis of PV, but it may be useful for cytogenetic analysis and for demonstrating characteristic features of PV such as increased erythroid and megakaryocytic proliferation. Diagnostic criteria for PV are listed in Table 89.4.

TABLE 89.4 Diagnostic criteria for polycythemia vera

A1	Red cell mass >25% above mean normal predicted value or hemoglobulin >18.5 g/dL in men, 16.5 g/dL in women
A2	Absence of causes of secondary polycythemia
A3	Palpable splenomegaly
A4	Clonality marker (abnormal karyotype or X-linked polymorphism)
B1	Thrombocytosis (platelet count >400,000/μL)
B2	Neutrophil leukocytosis (neutrophil count >10,000/μL, or >12,500/μL in smokers)
B3	Splenomegaly documented by ultrasound or isotope scanning
B4	Low serum erythropoietin level, or endogenous erythroid colony growth

A1 + A2 + A3, or A1 + A2 + A4 establishes the diagnosis; A1 + A2 + two of B criteria establishes the diagnosis.
Adapted from American Society of Hematology Self-Assessment Program, 2nd ed, 2005.

Management

Therapy for PV includes phlebotomy to lower the hemoglobin, aspirin for thromboprophylaxis, and cytoreductive agents to treat thrombocytosis and painful splenomegaly. Phlebotomy is done at least weekly initially to achieve a hematocrit <45% for men and <42% for women. Aggressive phlebotomy is associated with an initially increased risk of thrombosis, particularly in patients who are elderly or have history of thrombosis, and so cytoreductive therapy is indicated along with phlebotomy. Choices of cytoreductive therapy include hydroxyurea, anagrelide, and interferon-alpha. Hydroxyurea is often avoided in patients less than 60 years old because of some concern about the drug being associated with development of leukemia, although this is controversial. Low-dose aspirin (81 to 100 mg per day) is effective in reducing the risk of thrombosis and death from cardiovascular causes, and it also improves vasomotor symptoms such as erythromelalgia. Allogeneic stem cell transplant is the only curative therapy; however, this treatment is rarely used.

Complications

With treatment, the median survival of newly diagnosed patients less than 40 years old ranges from 10 to 18 years, and the survival of patients older than 65 years is not significantly shortened. Thrombosis and bleeding (such as gastrointestinal bleeding) are the major causes of death. After a number of years, PV evolves from a proliferative disease to a condition with progressive marrow fibrosis, pancytopenia, and extramedullary hematopoiesis in organs such as the spleen, known as postpolycythemic myeloid metaplasia (PPMM). A small percentage of patients (varying depending on which cytoreductive therapy was used) may experience transformation to AML.

ESSENTIAL THROMBOCYTHEMIA

The platelet count may rise in a variety of clinical situations (e.g., infectious or inflammatory disorders, occult cancer, postsplenectomy state, or severe iron deficiency). If all of these causes of secondary thrombocytosis are excluded, what remains is essential thrombocythemia (ET). Essential thrombocythemia is comparable to polycythemia vera because it represents the clonal expansion of a transformed myeloid stem cell. The laboratory findings are dominated by the elevated platelet count that often exceeds 1 million/μL. It occurs predominantly in people over age 50 years.

Clinical Manifestations

ET usually is asymptomatic. When symptoms do develop, they usually are of a thromboembolic nature. However, ET also causes hemorrhage because the platelets, although abundant, are abnormal and dysfunctional. The thrombosis may occur at various sites, including the central nervous system, myocardium, mesentery, and peripheral veins or arteries. Splenomegaly is the only outstanding physical sign. Patients with exceptionally large spleens may develop painful splenic infarctions. Eventual transformation to acute leukemia is rare.

Laboratory results show platelet counts that are very high (they must exceed 800,000/mm^3 with upper limit of normal 400,000/mm^3). Hematocrit and RBC counts usually are normal in ET, but if hematocrit is >48% or RBC count is $>6.0 \times 10^{12}$/L, the possibility of PV should be considered. Peripheral blood smear reveals an increased number of large platelets, sometimes clumped. The bone marrow is hypercellular in ET, with clumps of megakaryocytes that may be enlarged and dysplastic appearing. Marrow iron stores are normal; absent stainable iron suggests iron deficiency as the cause of thrombocytosis. Marrow fibrosis is minimal or absent. Cytogenetic analysis is done to assess for the Ph chromosome (because CML may also present with thrombocytosis) and abnormalities associated with myelodysplastic syndrome.

Diagnosis

Diagnosis of ET is based on complete blood count and bone marrow findings, along with a thorough clinical evaluation that excludes causes of secondary thrombocytosis as shown in Table 89.5. Presence

TABLE 89.5 World Health Organization diagnostic criteria for essential thrombocythemia

	Positive Criteria
1.	Sustained platelet count ≥600,000/μL
2.	Bone marrow specimen showing predominantly proliferation of the megakaryocytic lineage, with increased number of enlarged, mature megakaryocytes
	Exclusion criteria
3.	No evidence of polycythemia vera Normal RCM; Hgb <18.5 g/dL in men and <16.5 g/dL in women Stainable iron in marrow; normal serum ferritin; normal MCV If above condition unmet, failure of iron trial to increase RCM or Hgb to polycythemia vera range
4.	No evidence of chronic myelogenous leukemia No Ph chromosome and no BCR-ABL fusion gene
5.	No evidence of chronic idiopathic myelofibrosis Collagen fibrosis absent Reticulin fibrosis minimal or absent.
6.	No evidence of myelodysplastic syndrome No del(5q), t(3;3)(q21;q26), inv(3)(q21;q26)
7.	No evidence that thrombocytosis is reactive, due to: Underlying infection or inflammation Underlying neoplasm Prior splenectomy

Hgb, hemoglobulin; MCV, mean corpuscular volume; RCM, red cell mast.

of JAK2 V617F mutation in patients with ET is associated with higher hemoglobin and WBC levels, and possibly increased likelihood of transforming to AML or developing thrombosis.

Management

Treatment of ET is based on symptoms or the assessed risk of thrombosis and bleeding, and therapy is given with the goal of lowering the platelet count to 400,000 to 600,000/μL range. Platelet-lowering treatment is given to patients with thrombotic risk factors (>60 years old, cardiovascular risk factors), platelet counts over 1.5 million/mm^3, or past or current thrombotic events. Platelet-lowering therapy usually consists of hydroxyurea or anagrelide; both agents have been shown to significantly decrease thrombotic events. Anagrelide is sometimes chosen as therapy in younger patients due to the concern that long-term hydroxyurea use may lead to secondary leukemia. Patients with active digital ischemia or ischemic stroke should be considered for immediate platelet reduction with plateletpheresis. Low-dose aspirin may be used to help prevent thrombosis, if there are no contraindications. However, aspirin is avoided in patients with platelet counts over 1.5 million/mm^3 because these patients are at increased risk for bleeding.

MYELOFIBROSIS WITH MYELOID METAPLASIA

Idiopathic myelofibrosis (IMF) with myeloid metaplasia (also known as chronic idiopathic myelofibrosis) is the least common of the chronic myeloproliferative disorders, and it carries the worst prognosis. Annual incidence of the disease is 0.2 to 1.5 cases per 100,000 population, with a median survival of 3.5 to 5.5 years. Seventy percent of cases are diagnosed in patients older than 70 years. IMF is characterized by marrow fibrosis and extramedullary hematopoiesis, typically in the spleen resulting in splenomegaly. Benzene exposure and radiation have been associated as risk factors. JAK2 gene mutation is noted in 43% to 57% of patients with AMM; the neoplastic hematopoietic stem cell proliferates within the marrow, and cytokines are produced that cause a reactive proliferation of fibroblasts.

Clinical Manifestations

Symptoms are often related to anemia, splenomegaly, and the hypercatabolic state (Table 89.6). A number of other symptoms occur less commonly. On physical examination, an enlarged spleen is noted in 85% to 100% of patients, and up to one third of patients eventually develop massive splenomegaly.

TABLE 89.6 Clinical features of idiopathic myelofibrosis with myeloid metaplasia

Mechanism	Sign/symptom
Anemia	Dyspnea, light-headedness
Splenomegaly	Pain, early satiety
Hypercatabolic state	Fatigue, weight loss, night sweats, pruritus
Portal hypertension/ascites	Abdominal distension/pressure, peripheral edema
Splenic infarct	Acute left upper quadrant pain, fever, nausea
Esophageal varices	Gastrointestinal bleeding
Thrombocytopenia	Bleeding (particularly mucosal), bruising
Hyperuricemia	Monoarticular arthritis, nephrolithiasis

Anemia may be moderate or severe, with variable WBC and platelet counts. On examination of the peripheral smear, one finds teardrop-shaped RBCs (poikilocytes) and fragmented cells. Immature WBC and normoblasts may be seen. Bone marrow usually cannot be aspirated (so-called dry tap on bone marrow biopsy). Diagnosis requires bone marrow biopsy using a specialized needle, which shows bundles of fibrous tissue and many residual megakaryocytes. The Ph chromosome is absent unless the myelofibrosis has evolved from CML.

Management

For many patients, treatment is largely supportive. Anemia is the major hematologic complication and it may be multifactorial. Patients who have not progressed to transfusion-dependence may respond to exogenous erythropoietin, androgen supplementation, or low-dose thalidomide. Symptomatic massive splenomegaly may be treated with splenectomy or splenic irradiation. Thalidomide is sometimes given to control spleen size, but it must be titrated based on WBC and platelet count. Younger patients (<55 years) with high-risk features (hemoglobulin <10 g/dL, abnormally low or high WBC count, >1% circulating blasts) should be considered for myeloablative stem cell transplant. In recent studies of allogeneic transplant, 40% to 58% of patients survived more than 2 years.

Complications

Complications include bone marrow failure, hypersplenism, thrombosis, and evolution to AML. The risk for transformation to AML is increased in patients with severe anemia and high numbers of immature myeloid cells in the circulation.

CHAPTER 90

Iron Deficiency Anemia

John Charlson and Jenny Petkova

Iron is a critical element of the porphyrin compounds (myoglobin and hemoglobin) as well as of the respiratory enzymes in the mitochondria. About one tenth of dietary iron is absorbed into the body via the duodenum. Bound to transferrin, iron is transported to the liver and the bone marrow for storage or use in erythropoiesis. In the mitochondria of the normoblasts, the ferrous iron is joined with protoporphyrin to form heme, which is then transported to the ribosomes where four heme moieties combine with two alpha and two beta globin chains to create the complete hemoglobin molecule. Hemoglobin synthesis decreases as erythroblasts mature and stops with the extrusion of the nucleus and the cessation of RNA-directed protein synthesis. Without a nucleus, the lifespan of the red blood cell (RBC) is limited and, after approximately 120 days, red cells are phagocytosed by the cells of the reticuloendothelial system. Most of the iron is recycled back to the bone marrow for new hemoglobin synthesis. The rest is stored in the liver, the spleen, and the bone marrow in the form of ferritin and hemosiderin. Ferritin is present in all cells and tissue fluids. Its concentration in blood correlates roughly with total-body iron stores and can be used as a marker of iron deficiency or overload. Hemosiderin is found predominantly in macrophages.

Total body iron is 3 to 4 g in the form of hemoglobin (2 g), proteins and enzymes (400 mg), transferrin (3 to 7 mg), and ferritin/hemosiderin (1 g). Adult men lose about 1 mg of iron daily, which is easily replaced because a normal diet provides more than 10 mg of iron daily. In women, the daily loss is higher (1.5 mg). This is further exacerbated during pregnancy; each pregnancy incurs about 700 mg iron loss to the mother. The minimal daily iron requirements are summarized in Table 90.1.

ETIOLOGY

Iron deficiency is caused by two broad categories of conditions: (a) inadequate intake due to diet poor in iron or malabsorption and (b) chronic blood loss.

In adults, the most common sites of chronic gastrointestinal bleeding are peptic ulcers, gastritis, hiatal hernia, hemorrhoids, angiodysplasia, and stomach or colon cancers. Menstrual blood loss is a common cause of iron deficiency. Fibroids or endometrial cancer can cause bleeding and are associated with iron deficiency. Urinary losses can cause iron deficiency in patients with renal stones or malignancy of kidney, ureters, or bladder. Uncommon causes of iron deficiency are intravascular hemolysis and urinary hemosiderin loss in patients with paroxysmal nocturnal hemoglobinuria (presenting with hemolytic anemia and thrombosis) or malfunctioning mechanical heart valves.

Dietary iron deficiency is a common cause of iron deficiency in infants. Milk products are poor in iron and infants on prolonged breastfeeding or milk formula diets can develop iron deficiency without iron supplementation. Typical American diets are poor in iron and place young women and children at risk for developing iron deficiency anemia.

Iron malabsorption is relative rare. It is seen in patients with celiac sprue, chronic atrophic gastritis, achlorhydria, and after gastrointestinal surgery.

TABLE 90.1 Minimal daily iron requirements

Population groups	Minimal amount of oral iron (mg)
Infants	10
Children	5
Women of childbearing age	20
Pregnant women	30
Men and postmenopausal women	10

Modified from Lichman MA, Beutler E, Kausnansky K, et al. *Williams Hematology*, 7th ed. New York: McGraw-Hill, 2005.

CLINICAL PRESENTATION

The clinical picture of iron deficiency is influenced by the degree of anemia and the rapidity with which it develops. Symptoms may be completely absent or the patient may present with exercise intolerance, light-headedness, palpitations, dyspnea, or muscle weakness. Signs of iron deficiency are pallor and brittle nails. Pica (an appetite for nonfoods items such as chalk or paper, or an abnormal appetite for items that are related to foods such as flour and raw potato) and pagophagia (eating ice) can be present regardless of the degree of anemia. Cheilosis (fissures at the corners of the mouth) and koilonychia (spooning of the nails) are signs of advanced tissue iron deficiency.

DIAGNOSIS

Serum ferritin is an easily available and commonly used marker for assessing iron stores. Levels less than 15 μg/L are diagnostic of iron deficiency. Total iron binding capacity (TIBC), an indirect measure of the circulating transferrin, is increased in iron deficiency anemia. Serum iron is decreased. Transferrin saturation, calculated by dividing the serum iron by the TIBC and multiplying it by 100, is decreased below 15% in iron deficiency.

Another marker for iron deficient hematopoiesis is erythrocyte zinc protoporphyrin, an intermediate of heme synthesis. Although it is a very sensitive test, it is not very specific and can be elevated in other conditions such as chronic lead poisoning, sideroblastic anemia, and anemia of chronic inflammation. Although rarely needed, the criterion standard in diagnosing iron deficiency remains the absence of stainable iron stores on bone marrow biopsy.

Stages of Iron Deficiency

The first stage is *negative iron balance*. During this stage, the iron deficit is compensated for by mobilizing storage iron. At this point serum iron, TIBC and RBC protoporphyrin levels are normal. The serum ferritin level is decreased as well as stainable iron on bone marrow aspirate. If iron losses continue, the iron stores are being depleted and *iron-deficient erythropoiesis* begins. During this stage, TIBC may begin to increase. As long as the serum iron is normal, hemoglobin production is unimpaired. When the transferrin saturation falls below 15% to 20%, hemoglobin synthesis is impaired. Hemoglobin and hematocrit begin to fall and *iron deficiency anemia* develops. In moderate anemia (hemoglobin [Hb] 10 to 13 g/dL), the bone marrow (Table 90.2) is hypoproliferative. With worsening of the anemia (Hb 7 to 8 g/dL) erythroid hyperplasia develops. On peripheral smear, the RBCs are small and hypochromic. Reactive thrombocytosis can be present.

Differences in irons studies for iron deficiency anemia, thalassemias, and chronic anemia are shown in Table 90.3.

TABLE 90.2 Stages of iron deficiency and their laboratory findings

	Early iron deficiency without anemia	Mild anemia	Advanced anemia
Hemoglobin (g/dL)	12–14	9–12	<6
MCV(fL)	>80	<80	<80
MCH (pg)	>32	28–32	<27
RDW	14–18	14–18	>18
Serum iron (μg/dL)	>60	60–40	<40
Total iron binding capacity (μg/dL)	250–350	350–400	>410
Ferritin (μg/mL)	15–20	10–20	<10
Transferrin saturation (%)	>30	30–15	<10
Erythrocyte protoporphyrin (ng/mL red blood cells)	30–70	>100	100–200
Bone marrow iron	Absent	Absent	Absent
Red cell morphology	Normal	Normocytic, hypochromic	Microcytic hypochromic

Modified from Kutty K, Kochar MS. *Kochar's Textbook of Internal Medicine*, 4th ed. Baltimore: Lippincott, Williams, and Wilkins, 2003.

TREATMENT

Before treating iron deficiency anemia, its cause must be identified because it can be the presentation of gastrointestinal cancer or other life-threatening illness. Iron deficiency anemia in a male or post-menopausal female mandates an evaluation for gastrointestinal sources of blood loss, especially cancer. Iron is replaced with oral preparations, which most patients are able to tolerate. The recommended daily dose is 100 to 200 mg of elemental iron, which can be achieved with one tab 3 to 4 times a

Table 90.3 Comparison of iron studies in iron deficiency, beta thalassemia, and anemia of chronic inflammation

	Iron deficiency anemia	Beta thalassemia	Anemia of chronic inflammation
Serum ferritin	↓	Normal	Normal or ↑
Serum iron	↓	Normal or ↑	Normal or ↓
Transferrin sat (%)	↓	Normal or ↑	↓
Total iron binding capacity	↑	Normal	Normal or ↓
Mean corpuscular volume	Low	Low	Normal or low

day. Patients who are unable to tolerate oral iron may start from a lower dose and gradually increase it to the recommended level, switch to a liquid preparation, or take the iron with food (although this will decrease the absorption). This therapy will predictably cause reticulocytosis in 5 to 7 days and a rise in the hemoglobin by approximately 1 g/dL within the first 2 weeks of treatment. The patient should be treated for 3 to 6 months after correction of anemia to replenish iron stores. Failure to respond appropriately or inadequate rise of the hemoglobin may be due to noncompliance, poor absorption, excessive blood loss, or incorrect diagnosis.

Patients unable to tolerate oral iron or with malabsorption should be treated with parenteral iron. Available parenteral forms of iron therapy include iron sucrose, iron dextran, and sodium ferric gluconate. Common side effects include hypotension, cramps, dizziness, nausea, vomiting, and allergic reactions. Life-threatening hypersensitivity reactions are rare, but can occur with the iron dextrans.

Packed RBC transfusion is rarely indicated in iron deficiency. It is reserved for patients with symptomatic anemia, cardiovascular instability, or in preparation for surgery. Transfusions correct the anemia acutely as well as provide iron for future use.

CHAPTER 91

B_{12} Deficiency and Other Megaloblastic Anemias

John Charlson

Macrocytosis is a condition in which red blood cells (RBCs) appear large, with a corresponding increase in mean corpuscular volume (MCV). In addition to vitamin B_{12} or folate deficiency, macrocytosis can occur in a variety of disorders, including liver disease and alcohol ingestion (extra cholesterol adsorbed into RBC membrane), reticulocytosis (immature RBCs are larger and may increase MCV), and myelodysplastic syndromes.

ETIOLOGY

The etiology of megaloblastic anemias is diverse, but a common basis is impaired DNA synthesis. Megaloblastic anemias occur because vitamin B_{12} or folic acid is not available for DNA synthesis because of deficiency or inability to appropriately incorporate folic acid (often due to antimetabolite medications). Diminished DNA synthesis interferes with mitosis and effective proliferation, producing a population of RBCs that is smaller in number and larger in size than normal.

The most common causes of megaloblastic anemia are cobalamin (vitamin B_{-12}) and folate deficiencies. Cobalamin is an important cofactor in converting homocysteine to methionine to produce methyl groups. Folic acid transports these methyl groups to the site of cellular proliferation in order to convert uridylate (RNA base) to thymidylic acid (DNA base). With deficiency of either vitamin B_{12} or folic acid, DNA synthesis becomes defective and cytoplasmic RNA accumulates.

Cobalamin deficiency develops slowly because adult daily requirements are only 1 to 2 μg, and normally there are large stores in the liver. Strict vegetarians may manifest cobalamin deficiency after many years of that dietary lifestyle. In the gastrointestinal tract, cobalamin is bound in the stomach by intrinsic factor (IF) secreted by parietal cells. Cobalamin is then released by IF in the terminal ileum, where the cobalamin is absorbed. Partial gastrectomy and ileal disease or resection interfere with this process and, over time, can lead to cobalamin deficiency. Less commonly, bacterial overgrowth in intestinal blind loops or the fish tapeworm *Diphyllobothrium latum* may consume the available cobalamin. Pernicious anemia is a condition in which autoantibodies to gastric parietal cells cause gastritis and decreased production of IF, as well as interference with the vitamin B_{12}-binding sites on IF (see Color Plate 11).

Folic acid deficiency is more often related to dietary insufficiency because of the higher daily requirement for folic acid relative to folate stores. Deficiency develops most quickly in patients with high demand for folic acid (e.g., pregnant women) or poor intake (e.g., alcoholics).

CLINICAL MANIFESTATIONS

The hematologic pictures of vitamin B_{12} and folic acid deficiency are indistinguishable from each other. However, vitamin B_{12} deficiency can also cause serious neurologic disturbances because of vitamin B_{12}'s unique role in providing fatty acids to protect the spinal cord. It is important to distinguish between the two deficiencies because presumptively supplementing folic acid may correct the macrocytic anemia of a vitamin B_{12} deficiency, while allowing progressive and possibly irreversible neurologic damage to occur.

The anemia of vitamin B_{12} deficiency develops slowly, allowing for cardiovascular compensation. As the anemia becomes severe, patients may develop pallor, dyspnea, high-output heart failure, dizziness, or syncope. The neurologic consequences of vitamin B_{12} deficiency include peripheral neuropathy, subacute combined degeneration of the spinal cord (hyporeflexia, impaired vibration, and position sense), and mental status changes. Pernicious anemia typically occurs in the elderly and can be associated with other autoimmune diseases such as subacute thyroiditis. Gastric cancer develops in 8% of patients with pernicious anemia, which is a rate greater than in the general population. In both folic acid and B_{12} deficiencies, there may be glossitis and mild icterus, the latter due to the increased rate of red cell destruction within the bone marrow and the moderate shortening of the red cell survival in the circulation.

Findings on a complete blood count include anemia, often accompanied by leukopenia and thrombocytopenia, macrocytosis, and an increased red cell distribution width. Morphologically, the RBCs vary in size (anisocytosis) and shape (poikilocytosis), with the presence of macro-ovalocytes (large, oval-shaped RBCs). Neutrophils are also large, with hypersegmented nuclei. The bone marrow is hypercellular and also displays megaloblasts, indicating a high degree of ineffective erythropoiesis.

DIAGNOSIS

The serum vitamin B_{12} or RBC folate levels are usually low if there is deficiency. Serum homocysteine levels are increased in both deficiency states, whereas serum and urine methylmalonic acid (MMA) levels are elevated primarily in the setting of vitamin B_{12} deficiency and not in folic acid deficiency. Homocysteine and MMA elevations can be seen before overt anemia develops and while vitamin B_{12} levels are still in the low-normal range, indicating subclinical vitamin B_{12} deficiency. If both of these tests are normal, deficiency of these vitamins is essentially ruled out.

The diagnosis of pernicious anemia should be attempted first by checking for anti-intrinsic factor (IF) antibodies. The presence of anti-IF antibodies has specificity close to 100%, and so a positive test confirms the diagnosis.

Traditionally, the Schilling test was done to diagnose pernicious anemia. With this test, radiolabeled vitamin B_{12} is given to a patient; if less than the normal amount is later excreted in the urine, it indicates a problem with B_{12} absorption. In the second step of the test, oral intrinsic factor is given along with the radiolabeled vitamin B_{12}. If urinary excretion of the vitamin B_{12} now normalizes, it indicates that the initial poor absorption was due to lack of intrinsic factor (i.e., pernicious anemia). If added intrinsic factor does not correct the problem, it suggests the presence of a more general malabsorption problem (e.g., sprue or pancreatic insufficiency). The Schilling test is not commonly performed because it is a fairly cumbersome test.

MANAGEMENT

Folic acid deficiency is treated with oral replacement, 1 mg daily for several months or until blood counts normalize. Again, it is important to rule out concomitant vitamin B_{12} deficiency because folic acid may correct the hematologic abnormalities associated with B_{12} deficiency, but leave the neurologic manifestations untreated. Pernicious anemia is typically treated with intramuscular vitamin B_{12}. It may also be treated with high-dose oral vitamin B_{12}; this requires good patient compliance and close monitoring of serum levels of vitamin B_{12} and MMA.

CHAPTER 92

Anemia of Chronic Disease

John Charlson

ETIOLOGY

Mild to moderate anemia is a characteristic feature of many acute or chronic infectious and inflammatory disorders, as well as some malignancies. It is the second most prevalent type of anemia after iron deficiency anemia. The conditions most commonly associated with anemia are summarized in Table 92.1.

The anemia of chronic disease (also termed anemia of inflammation [AI]) results from the decreased ability of the body to compensate for the mildly decreased lifespan of the erythrocytes. Red blood cell (RBC) lifespan is reduced by release of cytokines, which affects iron availability for erythropoiesis and impairs production of endogenous erythropoietin, as well as the erythroid cells' response to it.

The proliferation and differentiation of erythroid progenitor cells is also impaired in AI. Normally, the physiologic response to decreased hemoglobin and decreased tissue oxygenation is an increase in erythropoietin production. It appears that inflammation also causes a state of resistance to erythropoietin, which results in AI.

CLINICAL PRESENTATION

The clinical picture of AI is dominated by the signs and symptoms of the underlying condition, which is characterized by acute or chronic immune activation. Moderate anemia with hemoglobin

TABLE 92.1 Common causes for anemia of inflammation

Infectious	Inflammatory	Malignancy
1. Viral infections including human immunodeficiency virus 2. Bacterial (acute and chronic): tuberculosis, osteomyelitis, abscess 3. Parasitic: malaria 4. Fungal	1. Autoimmune diseases: rheumatoid arthritis, systemic lupus erythematosus, vasculitis, sarcoidosis, inflammatory bowel disease 2. Chronic rejections of solid organ transplants 3. Systemic inflammatory response syndrome	Solid tumors Multiple myeloma Lymphomas

Modified from Lichman MA, Beutler E, Kausnansky K, et al. *Williams Hematology*, 7th ed. New York: McGraw-Hill, 2005.

TABLE 92.2 Common laboratory findings in anemia of inflammation

	Anemia of inflammation	Iron deficiency anemia	Both
Iron	Low	Low	Low
Mean corpuscular volume	Normal	Low	Low
Transferrin	Low to normal	High	Low
Transferrin saturation	Low	Low	Low
Ferritin	Normal to high	Low	Low to normal

Modified from Lichman MA, Beutler E, Kausnansky, et al. *Williams Hematology*, 7th ed. New York: McGraw-Hill, 2005 and NEJM 352;10 Anemia of Chronic disease.

less than 10 g/dL may exacerbate preexisting heart or respiratory disease increasing fatigue and exercise intolerance.

DIAGNOSIS

AI usually is normocytic and normochromic, but can become microcytic and hypochromic in its advanced stages. Because in AI there is no iron deficiency but abnormal handling of iron, patients present with low serum iron, normal or low total iron binding capacity and transferrin saturation of 15% to 20%. The serum ferritin level is the most distinguishing feature between iron deficiency anemia and AI (Table 92.2).

Ferritin is low in iron deficiency anemia, reflecting the depleted iron stores and normal or high in AI. The bone marrow aspirate shows presence of stainable iron; however, most of it is in the macrophages. The morphology of the RBCs on peripheral smear is nonspecific. The reticulocyte count is inappropriately low for the degree of anemia. Leukocytosis and thrombocytosis can be present.

TREATMENT

AI rarely is severe enough to necessitate periodic packed RBC transfusions, except to prepare for surgery. Long-term use of blood transfusions is associated with complications such as iron overload. The management of AI is directed toward the underlying inflammatory disorder if possible. The use of recombinant erythropoietin is recommended for some patients and, if a component of iron deficiency exists, supplemental iron therapy should be considered (patients with a low serum ferritin; for example, in the setting of AI). The goal for the hemoglobin should be around 11 to 12 g/dL; higher levels have been associated with increased thrombotic and vascular adverse events.

CHAPTER 93

Sickle Cell Disease

Jenny Petkova

Sickle cell disease (SCD) is a homozygous inherited hemoglobinopathy caused by a genetic mutation in a single autosomal gene, resulting in substitution of valine for glutamine at the position of the sixth amino acid of the beta-globin chain.

ETIOLOGY AND PATHOGENESIS

In SCD, the product—hemoglobin (Hb) S—is poorly soluble when deoxygenated. Deoxygenated HbS polymerizes into a ropelike fiber, which then aligns with other polymer fibers causing distortion of the biconcave red blood cells (RBCs) into a crescent shape together with a marked decrease in erythrocyte deformability. Subsequent changes in the cellular volume, membrane structure and function, and increased adherence to the vascular endothelium contribute to the occlusion of small blood vessels that characterizes SCD. In addition, sickle cells are rapidly hemolyzed and have a short life of about 10 to 20 days (normal is 120 days).

CLINICAL MANIFESTATIONS

The clinical presentation of sickle cell disease varies markedly among the different genotypes. Individuals with sickle cell trait (SCT; heterozygous for the HbS gene) usually are asymptomatic and do not develop symptoms under physiological conditions and have a normal lifespan. Patients who are homozygous for HbS develop vaso-occlusive, infectious, and hematological crises that characterize SCD. Anemia is present in all patients with SCD. It is due to the chronic hemolysis that can be complicated by folate deficiency. Extramedullary erythropoiesis can cause bone malformations. Chronic hemolysis can lead to premature formation of pigmented bile stones that can cause biliary colic or cholecystitis.

Most individuals with SCD have their first presentation before the age of 10 years; dactylitis (acute pain of the hands and the feet) is the most common initial symptom. Patients also present with strokes, leg ulcers, splenomegaly, and painless hematuria caused by papillary infarcts. However, sickle cell crises are a typical feature of this disease and include vaso-occlusive, hematological, and infectious crises.

Vaso-occlusive crises are the hallmark of clinical presentation of patients with SCD. Over time, they occur in every organ system, compromising blood supply, causing hypoxia, and leading to tissue death and localized pain. Fever is often present. The most commonly affected tissues are bone, chest, and abdomen, causing typical painful episodes. The incidence of painful episodes peaks between 20 and 40 years of age. The painful episodes can be precipitated by infection, dehydration, stress, menses, alcohol use, and hypoxemia; however, the majority of painful episodes are without identifiable cause. They can affect any area in the body—back, chest, abdomen, or extremities—and cause mild to excruciating pain. On occasion, avascular necrosis of the bone can develop.

A particularly painful and life-threatening complication is the acute chest syndrome. It usually is caused by vaso-occlusion but can be secondary to lung infarction, pulmonary fat embolism due to bone marrow infarction, or bacterial pneumonia. The patient presents with fever, chest pain, and a new pulmonary infiltrate. Chronic pulmonary arterial hypertension and right-sided heart failure are due to chronic pulmonary artery vaso-occlusion.

Splenic infarcts are so common early in the course of the disease that by adulthood most patients have very small scarred spleens (autosplenectomy), which places them at risk for infectious crises.

Vaso-occlusive crisis can also occur in the vessels of the brain, causing stroke. Leg ulcers are a common complication frequently leading to physical disability. Priapism is an unwanted painful erection that occurs in up to 35% of the males with SCD, usually before the age of 25 years. If lasting over 3 hours, it is considered an emergency and requires urological intervention.

The kidney is the organ most susceptible to the effects of the sickling. Up to 50% of patients have radiographic abnormalities of the kidneys; however, renal failure is usually a late complication of SCD. Recurrent renal infarctions of the kidney medula can cause isosthenuria, the inability of the kidney to concentrate urine.

Liver disease can be acute (benign cholestasis of SCD and acute hepatic crisis) or chronic, secondary to viral hepatitis infection or iron overload from repeated blood transfusions.

Hematological crisis is related to splenic sequestration crises due to acute massive pooling of erythrocytes in the spleen. It occurs more commonly in children but can occur in adults as well. It can be complicated by hypovolemic shock. A related hematological crisis—an aplastic crisis—is characterized by a sudden decrease in hemoglobin and reticulocyte count. It most frequently is caused by Parvovirus B19 infection of the bone marrow or folate deficiency.

Infectious crises are due to underlying functional asplenia in most adults with sickle cell anemia, leading to defective immunity against encapsulated organisms (e.g., *Haemophilus influenzae, Streptococcus pneumoniae*). Individuals with infectious crisis also have lower serum immunoglobulin M levels and impaired opsonization and complement pathway activation. Accordingly, persons with sickle cell anemia also exhibit increased susceptibility to other common infectious agents, including *Mycoplasma pneumoniae*, *Salmonella typhimurium*, *Staphylococcus aureus,* and *Escherichia coli*.

DIAGNOSIS

The chronic intravascular hemolysis in SCD is associated with mild anemia (Hb 8 to 10 g/dL), reticulocytosis (3% to 15%), high mean corpuscular volume (because of the high reticulocyte count), high unconjugated (indirect) bilirubin, elevated lactate dehydrogenase, and low haptoglobin. The peripheral smear reveals sickle cells (see Color Plate 12), reticulocytosis, and frequently Howell-Jolly bodies indicative of hyposplenism. The RBCs are normochromic unless there is a concomitant iron deficiency. If the mean corpuscular volume is within normal limits, the possibility of another hemoglobinopathy or iron deficiency must be excluded.

Newborn screening for SCD is currently available in 44 states. It is a DNA-based test performed within 72 hours of life, with a second screening at 1 to 2 weeks. Testing is by isoelelectric hemoglobin electrophoresis and abnormal results are confirmed by DNA analysis.

MANAGEMENT

Patients with SCD should be seen regularly by a physician as a part of a comprehensive health care program by a multidisciplinary team. The program should include infection prophylaxis and treatment, transfusion therapy, and pain management of the acute painful episodes and for chronic pain, which might require long-term narcotic therapy. Genetic counseling for patients with SCD or SCT is essential. Immunization with the pneumococcal and influenza vaccines is recommended in addition to the usual childhood immunizations. Daily prophylaxis with penicillin V 125 mg twice daily is recommended until the age of 3 years, followed by penicillin V 250 mg twice daily until the age of 5 years to prevent pneumococcal sepsis.

RBC transfusions lower the percent of HbS by three mechanisms: dilution, suppression of erythropoietin production and thus suppression of HbS production, and by the increased lifespan of the normal RBC.

Transfusions are recommended to increase the oxygen-carrying capacity of the blood and restore volume in splenic sequestration, acute chest syndrome, and sepsis or to improve the rheologic properties of the blood in patients with cerebral thrombosis. Simple transfusion is required to replace the oxygen-carrying capacity. Partial exchange transfusions should be performed in case of acute chest syndrome and for chronic transfusions to improve viscosity and reduce the risk of iron overload. The hemoglobin should not be raised above 10 g/dL with any technique to avoid increased viscosity and risk of vaso-occlusive episodes.

Treatment of acute chest syndrome is supportive: oxygen, antibiotics, pain control, and volume repletion. Exchange transfusion in adults is recommended if PaO_2 cannot be maintained above 70 mm Hg with supportive measures only. The goal is to lower the HbS to below 50%.

Acute pain episodes usually require hospitalization, aggressive rehydration, pain control usually with narcotics, and judicious use of blood transfusions. There is a high addiction potential in these patients and nonnarcotic agents should be used when possible. Some patients with SCD develop chronic pain syndrome. They should be treated like cancer pain patients with long-acting oral morphine preparations and fentanyl patches.

Early recognition and improvement in the management of SCD has lead to significant improvement in the mean survival of patients with SCD, with a median survival of >50 years.

COMPLICATIONS

SCD has many complications, some of which can be life threatening. Severe drug (narcotic) addiction is a common sequelae of sickle cell disease. Iron overload secondary to repeated transfusions can also occur due to the longer median survival of these patients compared to the past.

Most common causes of death are infection (48%), stroke (10%), complications from transfusion reactions (7%), splenic sequestration (7%), thromboembolism (5%), renal failure (4%), and pulmonary hypertension (3%).

CHAPTER 94

Thalassemias

Jenny Petkova

Thalassemia is a heterogeneous group of disorders classified according to the hemoglobin chain involved, beta or alpha. They are the cause of an inherited form of anemia, in which there is a defect in the synthesis of hemoglobin. Hemolytic anemia results from the abnormal hemoglobin.

BETA THALASSEMIA

The synthesis of beta chains of globin is encoded by two genes located on chromosome 11. Beta thalassemia is an inherited disorder caused by a group of mutations causing abnormal transcription of the beta chain gene. The production of the beta chains is decreased, thus creating an excess of alpha chains. The excess alpha chains are unable to form soluble polymers on their own, precipitate in the red blood cell (RBC), and disrupt the RBC cytoskeleton, producing a wide array of clinical manifestations.

Depending on the degree of decrease of beta-chain production, beta thalassemia is divided into three groups: beta thalassemia major, beta thalassemia intermedia, and beta thalassemia minor (Fig. 94.1).

In patients with beta thalassemia major, the beta chains are completely absent. Newborns with this condition have no manifestations because beta chains are not essential in utero. However, during the first year of life, the production of hemoglobin (Hb) A ($\alpha 2\beta 2$) becomes more important while the levels of fetal hemoglobin (HbF – $\alpha 2\gamma 2$) decrease. In the absence of beta chains, the child develops severe anemia, signs of extramedullary erythropoiesis, and chronic hemolysis caused by the excess of insoluble alpha chains.

Patients with thalassemia intermedia are a heterogeneous group who usually are compound heterozygotes of two thalassemia variants and have a milder syndrome and longer life expectancy compared to the patients with thalassemia major. However, they are symptomatic with different degrees of severity.

Patients with one normally functioning gene present with thalassemia minor or thalassemia trait. These patients are entirely asymptomatic, but can have abnormal blood parameters easily confused with iron deficiency anemia—hypochromia and microcytosis.

Clinical Manifestations

The clinical picture of thalassemia major is dominated by severe anemia, chronic hemolysis, extramedullary hematopoiesis, and, eventually, iron overload from increased iron absorption from the gastrointestinal tract and chronic transfusions.

Children present in their first year of life with growth retardation, irritability, and pallor. Skeletal abnormalities result from the expansion and extension of hematopoiesis into bones skull, long bones, and jaw. This causes delayed bone maturation, thinning of bone cortex, and osteoporosis. The children exhibit the typical "chipmunk facies," shortening of the limbs, particularly the upper limbs, and pathologic fractures. Hepatosplenomegaly is prominent primarily because of extramedullary hematopoiesis.

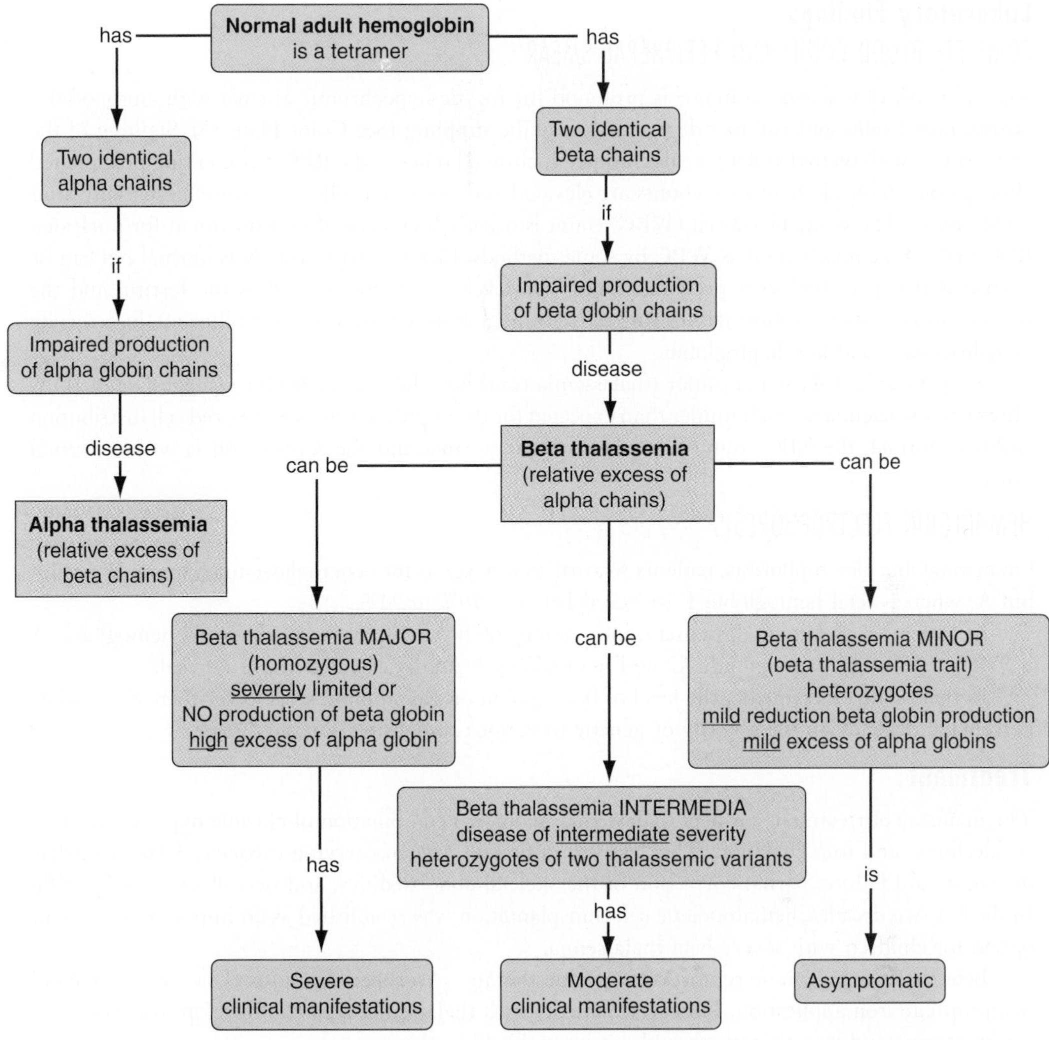

Figure 94.1 • Pathophysiology and clarification of thalassemias.

Kidneys may be enlarged because of extramedullary hematopoiesis. Chronic hemolysis causes jaundice, formation of pigment bile stones early in life, and biliary tract inflammation. Iron overload causes a clinical picture indistinguishable from idiopathic hemochromatosis. It is due to the accelerated iron turnover and increased iron absorption through the gut and chronic transfusions. High output heart failure and arrhythmias are frequent causes of death.

Patients with thalassemia intermedia usually do not require chronic transfusion therapy; they have chronic anemia, hepatosplenomegaly, and signs and symptoms of iron overload (such as skin hyperpigmentation, liver disease, diabetes mellitus, or dilated cardiomyopathy) because of increased absorption of dietary iron. Chronic hypoxia is commonly present in these patients, which leads to increased pulmonary vascular resistance, pulmonary hypertension, and heart failure.

Patients with thalassemia minor are asymptomatic, but commonly show a microcytic hypochromic anemia.

Laboratory Findings

COMPLETE BLOOD COUNT AND PERIPHERAL SMEAR

The hallmark of thalassemia major is profound microcytic hypochromic anemia with anisopoikilocytosis, target cells, and variable degree of basophilic stippling (See Color Plate 13). Staining of the blood smear with methyl violet reveals clumped inclusion bodies in the RBC representing precipitated alpha globin chains. Reticulocyte counts are elevated and nucleated cells are common especially after splenectomy. The white blood cell (WBC) count is usually high even after adjustment for nucleated RBC that can be miscounted as WBC by some methods. Platelet count usually is normal but can be decreased if hypersplenism is present. Serum iron level is elevated as well as the ferritin and the transferrin saturation. Abnormalities suggestive of hemolysis are high indirect bilirubin, high lactate dehydrogenase, and low haptoglobin.

Patients with thalassemia minor (thalassemia trait) have laboratory findings suggestive of IDA. However, the anemia is much milder than expected for the degree of microcytosis, red cell distribution width is normal, the RBC count is normal or near normal and the serum iron is within normal range.

HEMOGLOBIN ELECTROPHORESIS

On hemoglobin electrophoresis, patients who are homozygous for beta thalassemia have no hemoglobin A, whereas fetal hemoglobin F ($\alpha 2\gamma 2$) is between 10% to 90%.

In patients with beta thalassemia minor, hemoglobin A may reach 90% (normal hemoglobin A is 95% to 98%) with hemoglobin A2 and hemoglobin F mildly elevated above normal.

In thalassemia intermedia, the level of hemoglobin on electrophoresis is lower then 90% and its percentage depends on the severity of genetic mutations responsible for the disease.

Treatment

The mainstay of treatment for beta thalassemia major is a combination of chronic hypertransfusion, splenectomy, and iron chelation. This leads to improved oxygen-carrying capacity, delay of cardiac dilatation and failure, partial correction of the skeletal abnormalities, and overall improved health. In the last two decades, hematopoietic cell transplantation was established as an important treatment option for children with severe beta thalassemia.

Beta thalassemia minor requires no specific therapy. A proper diagnosis is necessary to avoid inappropriate iron application. However, patients with thalassemia trait can develop true iron deficiency anemia and iron therapy should not be withheld in them.

Beta thalassemia intermedia patients must be monitored closely for worsening anemia or development of complications from chronic hemolysis or extramedullary hematopoiesis. Chronic transfusion therapy is eventually needed in these patients, but can be delayed by splenectomy until the third or even fourth decade of life. However, due to the risk of iron overload unrelated to transfusions, they should be monitored with regular ferritin checks and iron chelation therapy should be initiated if ferritin exceeds 1,000 ng/mL.

Genetic counseling is very important for parents with beta thalassemia trait. Because only one copy of the beta chain gene is inherited from each parent, the fetus has a 25% chance of having beta thalassemia major, a 25% chance of having a normal genotype, and a 50% chance of being a carrier. The introduction of DNA-based antenatal diagnosis has led to almost complete eradication of new cases of severe beta thalassemia in Italy, Greece, and Cyprus.

ALPHA THALASSEMIA

The four alleles controlling alpha-chain synthesis are located on chromosome 16. Depending on the number of deleted alleles, there are four types of alpha thalassemia syndromes: (a) alpha thalassemia-

2 trait, caused by the loss of one allele, alpha; (b) thalassemia-1 trait, caused by the loss of two alleles; (c) hemoglobin H disease with only one functional allele; (d) hydrops fetalis with Bart's hemoglobin and no functional gene. Some mutations produce unstable alpha globins like hemoglobin Constant Spring, which is an alpha thalassemia variant common in Asia.

Clinical Manifestations

Alpha thalassemia-2 trait, also called alpha thalassemia minima, is a carrier state that is completely asymptomatic. The complete blood count, hemoglobin electrophoresis, and peripheral smear can be normal.

Alpha thalassemia-1 trait is also called alpha thalassemia trait. It presents with a clinical picture similar to beta thalassemia trait. The mean corpuscular volume is low and hypochromia, microcytosis, and target cells are present on peripheral smear but hemoglobin electrophoresis is normal.

Patients with hemoglobin H disease in whom three of the four alpha globin chains is impaired have an excess of beta globin chains. Unlike alpha chains that are extremely insoluble, beta chains are able to form a homotetramer–hemoglobin H ($\beta 4$). Hemoglobin H has a left-shifted oxygen dissociation curve and does not contribute to oxygen transport. It also is unstable and causes chronic hemolytic anemia that starts in utero. Patients present at birth with prolonged neonatal jaundice and anemia. Later in life, children exhibit signs of a chronic hemolytic state, including hepatosplenomegaly, early onset biliary pigment stones, biliary inflammatory disease, and leg ulcers. The skeletal deformities typical of beta thalassemia are rare. Most patients do not require chronic transfusions during the first decade of life. Because hemoglobin H is readily oxidized, the patients' hemolytic process worsens with oxidative stress such as an infection or with exposure to certain medications (e.g., sulfa drugs, antimalarials). Because of the high RBC turnover, iron absorption is increased and the patients are at risk for developing iron overload.

Hydrops foetalis with formation of Bart's hemoglobin ($\gamma 4$) is fatal in utero. Lack of fetal hemoglobin ($\alpha 2\gamma 2$) and the extremely left-shifted oxygen dissociation curve of Bart's hemoglobin cause profound tissue ischemia of the developing fetus. Edema is a result of the high-output heart failure that ensues. Fetal death occurs usually in the second to midthird trimester. Mothers are at risk for polyhydramnios and other obstetrical complications.

Diagnosis

LABORATORY FINDINGS AND HEMOGLOBIN ELECTROPHORESIS

Patients with alpha thalassemia minima (two traits) have only mild hypochromia and microcytosis. Hemoglobin Bart's is not present at birth.

The peripheral smear of patients with alpha thalassemia trait (one trait) shows hypochromia and microcytosis; however, the hemoglobin electrophoresis is normal and Hemoglobin A2 is not elevated. Hemoglobin Bart's can be present at birth, but disappears during maturation. Hemoglobin H is not present.

In patients with hemoglobin H disease, the peripheral smear reveals hypochromia and anisopoikilocytosis. Reticulocytes are elevated up to 5% because of chronic hemolysis. Hemoglobin H is between 5% an 40% of the total hemoglobin. Hemoglobin Bart's can be present as well. Hemoglobin A2 is usually slightly low.

In patients with hydrops foetalis, the peripheral smear shows severe hemolysis and many nucleated RBC. Hemoglobin consists mainly of hemoglobin Bart's. Usually hemoglobins A and F are not found.

Treatment

Alpha thalassemia-1 and -2 traits (alpha thalassemia minima and alpha thalassemia trait) require no treatment. Proper diagnosis is important to avoid misdiagnosis of IDA and unnecessary iron supplementation therapy. Parents with these conditions require genetic counseling.

Management

Management of hemoglobin H disease is similar to that of beta thalassemia intermedia—transfusions as needed and monitoring for signs of iron overload. Hydrops fetalis with hemoglobin Bart's is almost always lethal in utero. Because maternal morbidity is high in this condition, prenatal diagnosis and early termination of pregnancy should be considered.

CHAPTER 95

Hereditary Spherocytosis

Jenny Petkova

Hereditary spherocytosis (HS) is a form of hemolytic anemia caused by a red blood cell (RBC) membrane defect. Its incidence is about 200 to 300 per million in northern Europeans; however, this may be an underestimate because mild cases are often asymptomatic. Males and females are affected equally. The disease is autosomal dominant in about 75% of the cases.

ETIOLOGY AND PATHOPHYSIOLOGY

The hallmark of HS erythrocytes is loss of membrane surface area relative to increased intracellular volume, causing the characteristic spheroidal shape. The loss of surface area results from increased membrane cytoskeletal fragility caused by defects in proteins of the erythrocyte membrane—spectrin and other proteins (Fig. 95.1).

Spectrin deficiency in HS is due to decreased synthesis (mutations in the spectrin genes) or decreased incorporation into the membrane (mutations in the ankyrin gene). The severity of the HS correlates well with the degree of spectrin deficiency.

Hemolysis is due to RBC membrane instability and a process called "conditioning" that occurs in the spleen. The increased fragility and a decrease in RBC surface area results in spherocytic shape and hence destruction of cells, caused by a repeated passage through the spleen (splenic conditioning). The pivotal role of the spleen in the pathophysiology of HS is clearly demonstrated by splenectomy, which virtually eliminates the hemolysis, anemia, and the need for transfusions in moderate to severe cases of HS.

CLINICAL PRESENTATION

The most common clinical features of hereditary spherocytosis are hemolytic anemia, jaundice, and splenomegaly. There are three forms characterized by the severity of the clinical presentation.

Mild HS occurs in 20% to 30% of patients. The patients have reticulocytosis, mild jaundice, and splenomegaly but no anemia. This form may often go unrecognized until adulthood when patients can present with complications such as cholelithiasis and cholecystitis.

Moderate HS is seen in 60% to 75% of patients. These patients usually are diagnosed in childhood and present with anemia, elevated reticulocyte counts, elevated bilirubin, and splenomegaly. Diseases that cause further splenomegaly (infectious mononucleosis, for instance) may worsen the hemolysis. Patients with moderate HS may require transfusions when the bone marrow is unable to compensate for the hemolysis (e.g., during pregnancy or parvovirus infection).

Severe HS occurs in the remaining 5% of the cases. The patients present with marked hemolysis, anemia, hyperbilirubinemia, and splenomegaly. Without treatment, they are transfusion dependent and may develop complications of severe uncompensated anemia including growth retardation, de-

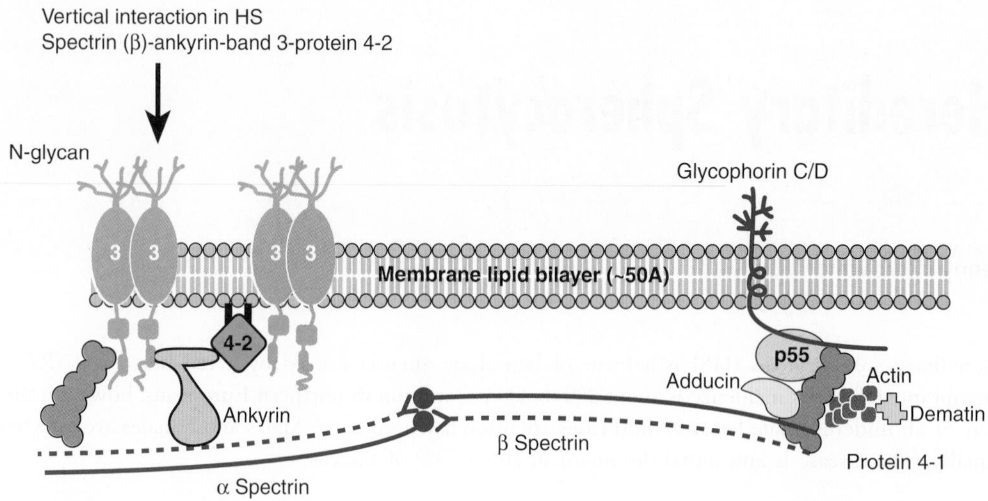

Figure 95.1 • Red cell cytoskeleton. (From Bolton-Maggs PHB, Stevens RF, Dodd NJ. Guidelines for the diagnosis and management of hereditary spherocytosis. *Br J Haematol* 2004;126:455–474, with permission.)

layed sexual maturity, and features of thalassemic facies. The inheritance in these cases is almost always recessive and the parents are asymptomatic.

DIAGNOSIS

Laboratory values reveal anemia with appropriate reticulocytosis (5% to 20% depending on the severity of the anemia). The mean corpuscular volume is normal or low, especially for the degree of the reticulocytosis. The red cell distribution width is high, accounting for the two very different erythrocyte populations—spherocytes (small, globular, and without central pallor; see Color Plate 14) and reticulocytes (larger, bluish, polychromatophilic cells).

Pseudohyperkalemia can be present because of the high rate of potassium leak out of the RBC as the blood cools after the blood draw. Rapid separation of the RBC from the plasma reveals that the actual potassium level is normal.

The increased osmotic fragility typical for HS can be demonstrated by placing the patient's RBCs in a series of hypotonic solutions. HS cells begin hemolyzing at a saline concentration of 0.64% and are completely hemolyzed at 0.5% saline—a concentration at which normal RBC are just beginning to lyse (osmotic fragility test). Coombs test is negative. The bone marrow shows normoblastic hyperplasia unless aplastic crisis or concomitant folate deficiency is present.

COMPLICATIONS

Acute worsening of the chronic anemia can be caused by aplastic crisis (which may be due to parvovirus B19 or other viral infection), increased hemolysis accompanying acute viral illness (probably because of increased splenic activity), and ineffective red cell production secondary to folic acid insufficiency.

Bilirubin gall stone formation is a common complication of HS. Its incidence increases with the age of the patients and the severity of the hemolysis. Much rarer complications are leg ulcers, extramedullary hematopoiesis, and hypertrophic cardiomyopathy.

TREATMENT

Like other chronic hemolytic anemias, treatment of HS is supportive. Folic acid is given to prevent deficiency of that vitamin. Blood transfusions may be necessary for extreme drop of the hemoglobin. Splenectomy should be considered in patients with moderate or severe HS. Postsplenectomy spherocytosis and increased osmotic fragility persist, but by removing the primary site of red cell destruction, splenectomy nearly normalizes the lifespan of erythrocytes and significantly decreases the number of reticulocytes. It decreases or even eliminates the need for chronic RBC transfusions and significantly decreases the incidence of cholelithiasis. The risk of sepsis is significant in the very young patients for whom partial splenectomy is recommended initially, followed by complete splenectomy later in life. Immunization against *Streptococcus pneumoniae*, *Haemophilus influenzae,* and *Meningococcus* should be performed 4 to 6 weeks prior to splenectomy.

CHAPTER 96

Autoimmune Hemolytic Anemia

Jenny Petkova

Autoimmune hemolytic anemia (AHA) is characterized by decreased erythrocyte lifespan and the presence of autoantibodies directed toward autologous red blood cells (RBC). These autoantibodies result in the immunologic destruction of RBCs. The clinical manifestations of this group of diseases, called autoimmune hemolytic anemia (AIHA), depend greatly upon the type of antibody that is produced by the abnormal immune reaction.

The annual incidence of warm-antibody AHA is 1 per 75,000 to 80,000 population. It is difficult to estimate the incidence of primary AHA because it can be the initial presentation of an underlying condition like systemic lupus erythematosus or malignant lymphoma. Approximately 50% of the cases are idiopathic.

Warm-antibody AHA has been diagnosed in all age groups; however, the majority of the patients are older than 40 years and the highest incidence is in the seventh decade.

Cold-antibody AHA is less common than warm-antibody AHA with prevalence of 14 per 1,000,000. Women are affected more frequently than men. Drug-induced hemolytic anemia had been estimated to account for 18% to 20% of all immune hemolytic anemias. Approximately 88% of the cases results from second- and third-generation cephalosporins.

ETIOLOGY, CLASSIFICATION, AND PATHOGENESIS

AHA can be classified according to the temperature at which the autoantibodies display optimal reactivity with the human RBC. The majority of cases of AHA in adults (80% to 90%) is caused by warm-acting antibodies (warm agglutinins) that react optimally at 37°C (98.6°F) (Table 96.1). The remainder of the cases are due to cold-acting antibodies (cold agglutinins) that react optimally at lower temperatures. This distinction is important because the pathophysiology and the therapeutic approach are different. An even smaller group of AHA is caused by both warm and cold reactive autoantibodies

Classification of AHA is also based on the presence or absence of an underlying disorder. When there is no recognizable underlying disorder, the AHA is termed *primary*. When AHA is a manifestation or complication of another disease process, it is considered *secondary* (often a malignancy or collagen vascular disease).

In warm antibody AHA, the antibodies that mediate RBC destruction are predominantly polyclonal immunoglobulin (Ig) G, which have high affinity for human erythrocytes at 37°C. In primary warm-antibody AHA (the most common type), the antibodies are often specific for a single erythrocyte membrane protein. In secondary AHA (i.e., systemic lupus erythematosus, rheumatoid arthritis, scleroderma, dermatomyositis, ulcerative colitis, and other autoimmune diseases), there is a fundamental disturbance in immune regulation, which allows for the production of antibodies against multiple self-antigens. When RBCs are coated with IgG autoantibodies, they assume a spherical shape, become more rigid and further fragmented, and eventually are destroyed during subsequent passages through the spleen.

In cold-antibody AHA, the autoantibodies are produced either by a malignant clone of B cells in lymphomas and Waldenström macroglobulinemia or by polyclonal B-cell activation in response

TABLE 96.1 Classification of autoimmune hemolytic anemia

I. Warm-antibody type (warm agglutinins)	A. Primary (idiopathic) warm AHA B. Secondary warm AHA 1. Associated with lymphoproliferative disorders (Hodgkin's and non-Hodgkin's lymphoma) 2. Associated with rheumatic disorders (systemic lupus erythematosus) 3. Associated with nonlymphoid neoplasms (ovarian cancer) 4. Associated with chronic inflammatory diseases (ulcerative colitis) 5. Associated with drugs (α-methyldopa)
II. Cold-antibody type (cold agglutinins)	A. Primary (idiopathic) cold AHA B. Secondary cold AHA 1. Postinfectious: *Mycoplasma pneumoniae*, infectious mononucleosis 2. Associated with malignant B-cell lymphoproliferative disorders 3. Mediated by cold hemolysins a. Primary (idiopathic) paroxysmal cold hemoglobinuria b. Secondary i. Associated with acute viral syndrome in children ii. Associated with congenital or tertiary syphilis
III. Mixed autoantibodies	A. Primary (idiopathic) mixed AHA B. Secondary mixed AHA 1. Associated with rheumatic disorder (systemic lupus erythematosus)
IV. Drug-induced immune hemolytic anemia	A. Hapten or drug adsorption mechanism B. Immune complex mechanism (ternary complex mechanism) C. True antibody mechanism

AHA, autoimmune hemolytic anemia.
Modified from Lichman MA, Beutler E, Kausnansky K, et al. *Williams Hematology*, 7th ed. New York: McGraw-Hill, 2005.

to infections such as *Mycoplasma pneumoniae* or infectious mononucleosis. The pathogenicity of cold agglutinins depends on their ability to bind to RBCs and activate complement. Complement fixation by cold agglutinins can cause erythrocyte injury by direct lysis or destruction by splenic macrophages.

Certain medications can cause injury to the RBC through an immune mechanism (drug-related immune hemolysis) that can be hapten, immune complex, or an autoantibody-mediated mechanism as shown in Table 96.2.

CLINICAL PRESENTATION

Presenting features of warm-antibody AHA usually are related to anemia (e.g., fatigue, decreased exercise tolerance). Most patients have an insidious onset over several months. Occasionally, patients present with acute onset of fever, pallor, jaundice, hepatosplenomegaly, tachypnea, tachycardia, or

TABLE 96.2 Mechanisms of drug-mediated autoimmune hemolytic anemia

Mechanism	Role of the drug	Drug affinity to cell membrane	Antibody to the drug	Antibody class	Mechanism of red cell destruction	Examples of drugs acting through this mechanism
Hapten or drug adsorption mechanism	Binds to the red cell membrane	Strong	Present	IgG	Splenic sequestration of IgG coated RBC	Penicillins Cephalosporins 6-mercaptopurin Carbromal Tolbutamide
Immune complex mechanism (Ternary complex mechanism)	Forms ternary complex with antibody and a component of the red cell membrane	Weak	Present	IgM IgG	Direct lysis by complement and splenic clearance by complement bound RBC	Cephalosporins Rifampicin Amphoteracin B Diclofenac Quinidine Chlorpropamide Probenecid
Autoantibody mechanism	Induces formation of antibody against native red cell antigen	None	Absent	IgG	Splenic sequestration	Cephalosporins L-dopa α-methyldopa Procainamide Diclofenac Fludarabine

Ig, immunoglobulin; RBC, red blood cell.
Modified from Lichman MA, Beutler E, Kausnansky K, et al. *Williams Hematology*, 7th ed. New York: McGraw-Hill, 2005.

heart failure. In secondary AHA, the symptoms of the underlying disorder can be the presenting symptoms. Occasionally, patients with warm-antibody AHA present with immune thrombocytopenia. These patients have Evans' syndrome, which is characterized by the combination of autoimmune hemolytic anemia and thrombocytopenia caused by antibodies against RBCs and the platelets.

Most patients with cold-antibody AHA have chronic anemia with or without jaundice. In other patients, the main feature is episodic, acute hemolysis and hemoglobinuria after cold exposure. The presentation depends on the temperature at which the cold antibody binds to RBCs and to complement. Cold-mediated vasoocclusive phenomena like acrocyanosis are caused by sludging of RBCs in the small vessels of the skin. Skin necrosis and infections, however, are rare. Patients with paroxysmal cold hemoglobinuria have a distinctive presentation. A few minutes to hours after cold exposure, the patients develop pain in their back or legs, abdominal cramps, and occasionally headache. This is followed by fever and chills. The urine passed after the episode contains hemoglobin. The constitutional symptoms and the hemoglobinuria last a few hours and may be followed by jaundice.

The clinical picture of drug-induced immune hemolytic anemia is variable with severity of symptoms depending on the rate of hemolysis. In general, patients with immune hemolysis caused by the hapten or drug-adsorption mechanism and autoimmune mechanism have a more insidious onset after repeated exposure to the drugs over a period of days to weeks. In contrast, patients with hemolysis caused by the ternary complex mechanism have an acute presentation after even one dose of the drug if they have had previous exposure to the drug. These patients present with acute severe hemolysis and hemoglobinuria and can develop acute renal failure.

DIAGNOSIS

Patients with AHA should be assessed for a underlying illnesses such as a malignancy or collagen vascular disease depending on the clinical circumstances.

Complete Blood Count with Peripheral Smear and Other Laboratory Values

Patients with AHA present with different degrees of anemia, from life-threatening to mild. All have an increased reticulocyte count. Leukopenia and neutropenia can be present in patients with drug-mediated immune hemolytic anemia.

A review of peripheral smears of patients reveals spherocytosis and polychromasia due to reticulocytosis. In the absence of hereditary spherocytosis, this finding suggests an immune hemolytic process. Reticulocytosis may be absent in patients with secondary AHA when bone marrow function is compromised by an underlying process, such as with lymphoproliferative disease or malignancy invading the bone marrow.

Hyperbilirubinemia, mostly due to elevated nonconjugated (indirect) bilirubin, is suggestive of hemolysis; however, its absence does not exclude the diagnosis. Serum haptoglobin levels are low and lactate dehydrogenase levels are increased. Urinary urobilinogen is increased. Urinary hemoglobin is rare in patients with warm-antibody AHA, more common in patients with cold-antibody disease, and characteristic in patients with paroxysmal cold hemoglobinuria.

Coombs' Test (Direct Antiglobulin Test)

Diagnosis of AHA or drug-mediated immune hemolytic anemia requires demonstration of immunoglobulin and/or complement bound to the patient's RBCs; this is done through the direct antiglobulin test (DAT), also called the Coombs' test. Initially, a screening test is performed with a reagent containing antibodies against both immunoglobulins and complement components. If it is positive, a second series of tests is performed with reagents against IgG or C3. Specific reagents against IgM or IgA are also available. The most common DAT patterns are presented in Table 96.3.

TABLE 96.3 Common direct antiglobulin test patterns

Reaction pattern	Type of immune injury
IgG alone	Warm-antibody AHA Hapten drug adsorption or autoantibody-type drug-mediated immune hemolytic anemia
Complement alone	Cold agglutinin disease Paroxysmal cold hemoglobinuria Ternary complex–type drug-mediated immune hemolytic anemia
IgG and complement	Warm antibody AHA Autoantibody-type drug-mediated immune hemolytic anemia
IgM and complement	Secondary cold agglutinin hemolytic anemia due to *M. pneumoniae* and infectious mononucleosis

Ig, immunoglobulin; AHA, autoimmune hemolytic anemia.
Modified from Lichman MA, Beutler E, Kausnansky K, et al. *Williams Hematology*, 7th ed. New York: McGraw-Hill, 2005 and Kutty K, Kochar MS. *Kochar's Textbook of Internal Medicine*, 4th ed. Baltimore: Lippincott, Williams, and Wilkins, 2003.

TREATMENT

Patients who develop rapidly progressive anemia with circulatory collapse, and patients in whom anemia can worsen an underlying condition such as coronary artery disease, benefit from packed RBC transfusion.

Treatment of warm-antibody AHA includes corticosteroids, splenectomy, and immunosuppressive medications such as steroids. The 10-year survival of these patients is estimated at 73%. Corticosteroids such as prednisone are the mainstay of treatment. They cause marked decrease in the hemolysis in two thirds of the patients and induce a complete remission in 20%. After hemoglobin begins to increase, the prednisone dose should be tapered slowly over the next few months. Therapy should be continued until the DAT becomes nonreactive. The patients should be followed for several years after the discontinuation of the prednisone because relapse may occur.

Splenectomy removes the primary site of erythrocyte sequestration and destruction; approximately two thirds of splenectomized patients will have a complete or partial remission. The relapse rate, however, is high and many patients continue to require steroids, although usually in smaller doses. Vaccines against *Neisseria meningitis*, *Streptococcal pneumoniae*, and *Haemophilus influenzae* should be given prior to splenectomy.

Patients with cold-agglutinin AHA and mild chronic hemolysis benefit from avoiding cold exposure. Patients with idiopathic cold agglutinin disease usually have a benign course. In symptomatic patients, rituximab has been used with good response. Plasma exchange can provide temporary improvement of the hemolysis in critically ill patients.

Treatment of drug-mediated AHA consists of discontinuation of the causative agent. Immune hemolysis caused by drugs usually is benign and self limiting after the drug is discontinued.

COMPLICATIONS

Common complications of AIHA, which can eventually result in death, are pulmonary emboli and infections. Episodes such as deep venous thrombosis or splenic thromboses are common during the acute episodes.

CHAPTER 97

ITP/TTP/HUS

Jenny Petkova

IDIOPATHIC THROMBOCYTOPENIC PURPURA

Idiopathic thrombocytopenic purpura (ITP) is an acquired disorder presenting with isolated thrombocytopenia without apparent cause. It is a common disorder, with an incidence of 32 per million per year for symptomatic patients (55 per million per year if asymptomatic patients with platelet counts less than 50,000 are included). Older data suggested that there is female predominance; however, newer studies do not support such a sex predisposition.

Etiology and Pathophysiology

Thrombocytopenia in ITP is caused by accelerated immune-mediated platelet destruction in the spleen. The majority of the antiplatelet antibodies are class immunoglobulin G. Antibody-coated platelets are destroyed by macrophages located primarily in the spleen and, occasionally, in the liver and the bone marrow. Bone marrow responds to thrombocytopenia with increased platelet production; however antiplatelet antibodies can also interfere with megakaryocyte maturation.

Clinical Presentation

In children, ITP usually has an acute onset 3 to 4 weeks after a viral infection, although in adults its onset can be acute or insidious. Patients can present with severe bleeding or be completely asymptomatic and the thrombocytopenia is an incidental finding. The bleeding manifestations of ITP are mucocutaneous, unlike the slow visceral bleeds associated with coagulation disorders. Patients with ITP can present with petechiae, nonpalpable purpura, or easy bruisability. Epistaxis, gingival bleeding, and menorrhagia are common. Overt gastrointestinal blood loss or gross hematuria is rare. Intracranial hemorrhage is extremely rare.

Diagnosis

Two criteria are required for making the diagnosis of ITP. First, severe thrombocytopenia, with otherwise normal complete blood count and white blood cell differential, including a normal peripheral smear, is present. Second, there are no clinically apparent conditions or medications that could cause the thrombocytopenia. There is no gold standard for diagnosing ITP and the diagnosis is partly one of exclusion of other causes of thrombocytopenia (Chapter 25).

A presumptive diagnosis of ITP is made when the history, physical examination, complete blood count, and the peripheral smear are unrevealing for other etiologies (Table 97.1).

The only recommended further workup for these patients is testing for human immunodeficiency virus and hepatitis C virus in patients with risk factors for these conditions and bone marrow biopsy in patients over 60 years of age to rule out myelodysplasia.

TABLE 97.1 Clinical and laboratory features of disorders that may resemble idiopathic thrombocytopenic purpura

Thrombotic thrombocytopenic purpura/hemolytic uremic syndrome • Symptoms of fever, mental status changes, and renal failure • The peripheral smear reveals schistocytes
Disseminated intravascular coagulation • Associated with sepsis, trauma, or malignancy • Signs and symptoms of consumptive coagulopathy (prolonged clotting times) • Signs of macroangiopathy (schistocytes) on the peripheral smear
Thrombocytopenia in liver disease • Accompanied by other signs and symptoms of portal hypertension • Splenomegaly
Gestational thrombocytopenia • During late gestation in up to 5% of all pregnancies and resolves after delivery • Platelet number is typically above 70,000/μL • Not associated with fetal thrombocytopenia (15% of the infants with low platelets may have idiopathic thrombocytopenic purpura)

Bone marrow examination also is recommended for patients with poor or no response to therapy. In typical ITP, the overall bone marrow cellularity is normal. The number of megakaryocytes can be normal or increased, with a shift toward younger precursors.

Treatment

The natural history of ITP is very different in children and adults, with 70% to 80% of children recovering within 6 months without any specific treatment. Treatment with corticosteroids, intravenous immunoglobulin (IVIG), or anti-D(WinRho) may speed platelet recovery, but spontaneous remissions occur in less than 10% of adults with ITP.

The goal of treatment for ITP is to provide a platelet count sufficient to prevent major bleeding, which is rare with platelet counts above 10,000/μL.

In asymptomatic patients, the morbidity from the side effects exceeds the possible benefits of the therapy. There is no accepted platelet count that is an indication for initial treatment. Patients with platelet counts greater than 30,000 to 50,000/μL rarely develop more severe thrombocytopenia. These patients require careful monitoring, but no specific initial therapy. Asymptomatic patients with even lower platelet counts (greater than 10,000/μL) can be managed in a similar manner.

Treatment should be initiated in patients with moderate or severe thrombocytopenia who are actively bleeding or at a high risk for bleeding. Initially, prednisone 1 to 2 mg/kg/day is given until the platelets counts are back to normal. This is followed by slow tapering and eventually prednisone is stopped. Patients who do not respond to initial therapy, who require large daily doses, or who become steroid-dependent should undergo splenectomy. With splenectomy, up to two thirds of the patients will have a remission. Patients with good initial response to steroids are more likely to have a remission after splenectomy.

If splenectomy fails, further treatment with IVIG or Anti-D (WinRho) should be attempted.

THROMBOTIC THROMBOCYTOPENIC PURPURA AND HEMOLYTIC UREMIC SYNDROME

Thrombotic thrombocytopenic purpura (TTP) and hemolytic uremic syndrome (HUS) are thrombotic microangiopathies that present with small-vessel thrombosis, consequent microangiopathic hemolytic anemia, and consumptive thrombocytopenia.

The incidence of TTP is estimated to be 11 cases per million per year. Idiopathic TTP accounts for 37% of the cases. Peak incidence of idiopathic TTP is between 30 to 50 years of age. It is rare before the age of 20 years. Females are affected twice as often as males. Drug-associated TTP occurs in 13% of all patients with TTP. Another 13% are associated with autoimmune diseases, 7% are sepsis related, infections account for 7%, and 4% occur after hematopoietic cell transplantation.

Diarrhea-associated HUS can occur in any age, but is most common in children less than 10 years of age. It can be sporadic or epidemic. About 80% of the cases are associated with *Escherichia coli* O157:H7, but it can be caused by other Shiga toxin–producing *E. coli* serotypes and by *Shigella dysenteriae* type I. Diarrhea-negative HUS is much less common.

Etiology and Pathogenesis

In TTP, the microangiopathy and tissue injury usually present with fever and neurological signs. Although renal involvement is common, oliguric renal failure is rare.

In HUS, the main site of damage is the kidney and the patients typically present with acute oliguric renal failure. Diarrhea-associated HUS is caused by enteric infection with Shiga toxin–producing gram-negative bacilli, whereas diarrhea-negative or atypical HUS occurs in patients without predisposing conditions. Secondary thrombotic microangiopathy can be seen in association with advanced cancer, infections, organ and bone marrow transplantation, and exposure to drugs (Table 97.2).

The hallmark of TTP-HUS pathology is hyaline microthrombi comprised primarily of platelets. Platelet activation can be triggered by variety of stimuli using different pathways. Endothelial injury, auto-induced antibodies, or drug-induced antibodies can trigger secondary TTP. Idiopathic TTP is associated with congenital or acquired ADAMTS13 deficiency—a metalloprotease responsible for cleaving vWF multimer. ADAMTS13 deficiency inhibits this mechanism and causes microvascular platelet aggregation and thrombosis.

Most patients with HUS have normal levels of ADAMTS13. Shiga toxin produced by *E. coli* or other bacteria causes the release of ultralarge vWF multimers in the circulation and delays their cleavage by the enzyme ADAMTS13. Nondiarrhea-associated HUS is caused by inherited deficiency of protein regulating the alternative complement pathway. Deficiency of factor H, factor I, or membrane cofactor protein leads to increased endothelial deposition of C3b causing activation of the complement pathway and microvascular thrombosis.

Clinical Presentation

The five classic clinical features of TTP are microangiopathic hemolytic anemia, consumptive thrombocytopenia, acute renal failure, neurologic abnormalities, and fever. HUS typically presents with acute onset anemia, thrombocytopenia, and renal impairment. The clinical features of TTP and HUS can overlap and diagnosis cannot be made by the clinical presentation alone.

The onset of TTP can be acute or chronic, developing over days or even weeks. Diarrhea-associated HUS develops 1 to 2 weeks after hemorrhagic diarrheal illness.

Approximately one third of the patients with TTP present with symptoms of hemolytic anemia caused by mechanical destruction of the red blood cells in the small thrombosed blood vessels.

Thrombocytopenia usually causes petechiae or purpura. Gastrointestinal or genitourinary bleeding is uncommon.

TABLE 97.2 Thrombotic microangiopathies

I. Idiopathic	A. Congenital: due to inherited ADAMTS13 deficiency B. Acquired: with or without ADAMTS13 deficiency
II. Secondary	A. Associated with infections 1. Bacterial: *Streptococcus pneumoniae*, Group A streptococci, *Staphylococcus aureus, Campylobacter jejuni, Enterobacter, Escherichia coli, Salmonella typhi, Shigella dysenteriae* 2. Viral: Coxsackie B, cytomegalovirus, Epstein-Barr virus, herpes simplex, human immunodeficiency virus, human T-cell lymphotrophic virus 1, influenza, parvovirus B19 3. Fungal: *Aspergillus fumigatus, Blastomyces, Candida* species B. Associated with tissue transplant: rejection, graft vs. host disease C. Associated with malignancy: Trousseau's syndrome D. Pregnancy associated: HELLP syndrome, eclampsia, pre-eclampsia E. Autoimmune: systemic lupus erythematosus, other vasculitides, antiphospholipid syndrome F. Drug-associated: ticlopidine, clopidogrel, quinine, cyclosporine, tacrolimus, gemcitabine G. Postoperative: after cardiovascular surgery H. Malignant hypertension
III. Hemolytic uremic syndrome	A. Diarrhea-positive: Shiga toxin–associated B. Diarrhea-negative: due to inherited complement regulating protein deficiency

Modified from Lichman MA, Beutler E, Kausnansky K, et al. *Williams Hematology*, 7th ed. New York: McGraw-Hill, 2005.

Microangiopathy can affect any organ. Neurologic signs can be transient or persistent and range from mild confusion and headache to focal deficits, seizures, and coma. Cardiac microangiopathy presents with myocardial infarction, arrhythmias, or heart failure. The kidney is a common site of injury. Patients with TTP usually present with abnormal urinalysis and preserved renal function, whereas acute anuric renal failure requiring dialysis is more typical for HUS. About 25% of theses patients may have persistent renal insufficiency with creatinine clearance less than 40 mL/min.

Fever is less frequently present and may be suggestive of sepsis and its complications rather than idiopathic TTP-HUS.

Diagnosis

In the diagnosis of TTP and HUS, it is important to consider the clinical and diagnostic features of other disorders (Table 97.3).

Almost all patients present with signs of hemolytic anemia: low hemoglobin, elevated indirect bilirubin and lactase dehydrogenase, decreased haptoglobin, schistocytosis, and reticulocytosis. The direct antiglobulin test (Coombs test) is always negative. Thrombocytopenia is common (mean platelet count around 25,000/μL) and can be severe. Most patients have normal prothrombin time, partial thromboplastin time, and fibrinogen reflecting an intact coagulation system.

Urinalysis reveals proteinuria, a few red cells, and red cell casts. Creatinine can be elevated to the point of requiring dialysis.

Severe ADAMTS13 deficiency (<5%) usually is present in patients with idiopathic TTP. Assays for it and its inhibitor are available; however, low ADAMTS13 level is not specific for TTP and

TABLE 97.3 Comparison of clinical and diagnostic features of ITP, TTP, HUS, DIC, and HIT

	Idiopathic thrombocytopenic purpura (ITP)	Thrombotic thrombocytopenic purpura (TTP)	Hemolytic uremic syndrome (HUS)	Disseminated intravascular coagulation (DIC)	Heparin-induced thrombocytopenia (HIT)
Preceding conditions	None	Idiopathic or due to drugs, posttransplant, associated with autoimmune diseases or sepsis	Diarrhea caused by Shiga toxin–producing bacteria	Sepsis, major trauma, burns, malignancies	Exposure to heparin
Pathophysiology	Immune-mediated platelet destruction in the spleen	Platelet activation by vWF	Platelet activation by vWF Factor H deficiency	Activation of coagulation	Platelet activation by heparin-induced antibodies
Clinical presentation	Mucocutaneous bleeding	Microangiopathic hemolytic anemia, consumptive thrombocytopenia, acute renal failure, neurologic abnormalities, fever	Acute onset anemia, thrombocytopenia, renal impairment	Bleeding with or without thrombosis in acute DIC, thrombosis in chronic DIC	Thrombosis
Thrombocytopenia	Present	Present	Present	Present	Present
Anemia	Not present	Present	Present	Not present	Not present
Signs of microangiopathy (schistocytes)	Not present	Present	Present	Can be present	Not present
PT/PTT	Normal	Normal	Normal	Elevated	Normal
d-dimer	Normal	Normal	Normal	Elevated	Normal
Lactase dehydrogenase	Normal	High	High	Can be elevated	Normal

DIC, disseminated intravascular coagulation; PT, prothrombin time; PTT, partial thromboplastin time.

can be decreased in other conditions such as disseminated intravascular coagulation, idiopathic thrombocytopenic purpura, sepsis, and systemic lupus erythematosus. At this time, measuring the ADAMTS13 level is not essential for making the diagnosis and treatment should not be delayed pending the results.

Treatment

The mainstay of therapy for idiopathic and some secondary TTP is plasma exchange. It removes the antibodies against ADAMTS13 and replenishes its level. Plasma exchange should be instituted immediately after the diagnosis has been made clinically pending any confirmatory testing. It should be continued until complete remission is achieved: platelets >150,000 /μL, no signs of hemolysis (normal lactase dehydrogenase), and resolution of the nonstroke-associated neurological symptoms. At this time, the optimal tapering management is not clear.

Plasma exchange usually is not beneficial in diarrhea-associated HUS. Most patients recover with supportive treatment only. The role of antibiotic therapy for hemorrhagic *E. coli* is controversial because some reports suggest increased incidence of HUS after antibiotic treatment.

Corticosteroids can be used as an adjunct in patients with idiopathic TTP.

Platelet transfusions are relatively contraindicated because they can cause further expansion of the thrombotic process and thus worsen TTP-HUS. They should be reserved for patients with life-threatening bleeding or prior to surgery.

Refractory idiopathic TTP-HUS can respond to immunosuppression therapy. Rituximab (monoclonal antibody against CD20) has been successfully used with or without cyclophosphamide.

Splenectomy can result in remission or decrease the number of relapses in patients who do not improve with any other therapy. Splenectomy can be done laparoscopically in most patients.

TTP is a progressive disease with mortality rates as high as 90% if no treatment is initiated. Plasma exchange treatment decreases the mortality dramatically to 10% to 20%. Most deaths occur within the first week after presentation and almost all occur during the first month. Most patients improve within 1 to 3 weeks after initiation of plasma exchange. Renal insufficiency can become chronic in about 25% of the cases. Relapses occur in 30% of the patients during the first year after presentation and usually respond well to plasma exchange. Diarrhea-associated HUS has a more benign course with 9% mortality and 3% of patients developing end-stage renal disease requiring hemodialysis.

CHAPTER 98

Disseminated Intravascular Coagulation

Jenny Petkova

Disseminated intravascular coagulation (DIC) is a systemic process characterized by thrombosis and hemorrhage. It is initiated by a number of disorders (mostly commonly sepsis and trauma). DIC is not a disease but a coagulation abnormality that complicates these primary disorders.

ETIOLOGY

Numerous disorders can trigger DIC, with sepsis and trauma accounting for the majority of cases (Table 98.1). DIC is caused by activation of the coagulation, the fibrinolytic system, and platelet system. DIC results from massive activation of the coagulation cascade due to exposure of blood to procoagulants.

In normal hemostasis, this process is localized at the site of endothelial wall injury and thrombin formation is tightly regulated by multiple antithrombotic pathways existing in the plasma and the endothelium (antithrombin and tissue factor pathway inhibitor). In DIC, thrombin production exceeds the ability of the antithrombotic pathways; thrombin circulates in the entire body causing disseminated intravascular coagulation. The pathophysiology of the development of DIC is shown in Figure 98.1.

CLINICAL MANIFESTATIONS

The clinical picture of DIC can be very different depending on the nature of the underlying disorder. There are two clinical forms of DIC: acute and chronic.

Acute DIC is associated with sepsis, major trauma, and burns. The most common symptom is bleeding—oozing from venipuncture sites, gastrointestinal blood loss, and intracranial or pulmonary hemorrhage. DIC can be considered an example of organ dysfunction from sepsis, similar to other forms of sepsis-related organ dysfunction (e.g., acute respiratory distress syndrome, ileus).

Severe organ damage results from microvascular thrombosis in both arterial and venous vessels. Thrombosis of major vessels is rare. Skin involvement presents with hemorrhagic bullae, limb gangrene, and necrosis. Renal dysfunction is caused by thrombosis of the afferent glomerular arterioles or acute tubular necrosis due to hypotension or sepsis. A total of 25% to 65% of all patients develop oliguria, anuria, and azotemia. Hepatocellular dysfunction with jaundice is present in 22% to 57% of patients with DIC and is caused by microangiopathy, underlying infection, and hypotension. Central nervous system involvement presents with coma, delirium, transient focal deficits, and meningeal signs. Acute promyelocytic leukemia is associated with acute DIC.

Chronic DIC is much less common that acute DIC and usually is associated with a solid tumor, frequently adenocarcinoma. Bleeding is rare in chronic DIC and the clinical picture is dominated by thrombosis. The most common presentation is deep venous thrombosis with or without pulmonary embolism and superficial migratory thrombophlebitis (Trousseau's syndrome). Arterial thrombotic events such as renal infarcts, strokes, or digital ischemia are rare.

TABLE 98.1 Causes of disseminated intravascular coagulation

Infection
Gram-negative and gram-positive bacteremia, viruses (herpes, Lassa, dengue), Rocky Mountain spotted fever, fungi (*Candida* spp., *Aspergillus* spp.), and others (clostridia, toxic shock syndrome, malaria)
Trauma
Crush injuries, brain injuries, thermal injuries
Vascular injuries
Giant hemangioma, aortic aneurysm, vasculitis, aortic balloon pump, acute myocardial infarction, pulmonary embolism, malignant hypertension
Obstetric complications
Abruptio placentae, eclampsia, amniotic fluid embolism, hydatidiform mole, uterine rupture, retained dead fetus/missed abortion
Malignancies
Adenocarcinomas, tumor lysis syndrome, acute leukemia
Other
Adult respiratory distress syndrome, amyloidosis, inflammatory bowel disease, cirrhosis, fulminant hepatic necrosis, pancreatitis, snake bites, Reye's syndrome, hypovolemic/hemorrhagic shock

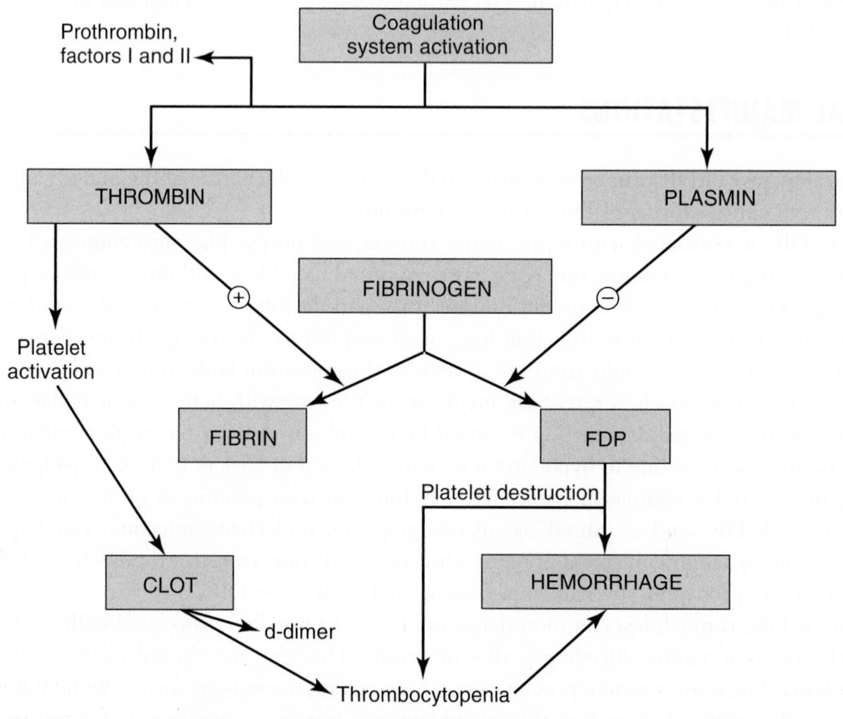

Figure 98.1 • The evaluation of disseminated intravascular coagulation.

DIAGNOSIS

The diagnosis is suggested by the history of the underlying disorder, the clinical presentation, moderate thrombocytopenia, and often times, microangiopathy (schistocytes) found on the peripheral blood smear. The diagnosis is confirmed by laboratory tests suggestive of increased thrombin generation and fibrinolysis. Elevated fibrin degradation products and D-dimer are markers for fibrinolysis. Fibrinogen is usually decreased and prothrombin time (PT) and partial thromboplastin time (PTT) are prolonged, reflecting the consumption of clotting factors. In chronic DIC, the typical laboratory markers can be variable. Because of the slower rate of consumption, enhanced synthesis can compensate for the lost clotting factors and platelets. In such patients, platelets counts can be only mildly decreased; PT, PTT, and fibrinogen can be normal; and the diagnosis is based on an elevated D-dimer and evidence of microangiopathy on the peripheral smear.

TREATMENT

Treatment is supportive with platelet and clotting factor replacement therapy if needed. The key to management of DIC and a favorable prognosis is effective treatment of the underlying disease that has initiated the DIC.

Acute DIC is associated with high mortality rate determined in part by the primary process causing DIC. The mortality rate ranges from 40% to 80% depending on the severity of the underlying condition. The focus is treatment of the underlying cause of the DIC. Patients require supportive measures (treatment of sepsis in the case of infection). Most improve with resolution of the primary disorder without specific therapy for the DIC.

Patients with DIC complicated by severe thrombocytopenia (<20,000/μL), moderate thrombocytopenia, and serious bleeding or who need surgery or other invasive procedures require platelets and coagulation factor replacement. Platelet transfusion should be given. Fibrinogen should be replaced using cryoprecipitate and maintained above 100 mg/dL. Fresh frozen plasma should be given to replace the remaining coagulation factors.

CHAPTER 99

Hemophilia/von Willebrand Disease

Jenny Petkova

HEMOPHILIA A

Hemophilia A is an X chromosome–linked recessive disorder. It is caused by decreased synthesis of factor VIII or synthesis of nonfunctional factor VIII. Its estimated incidence is one in every 5,000 to 7,000 live male births. It occurs in all ethnic groups and has no geographic predilections. Approximately 30% of the mutations occur de novo. Multiple alterations of the factor VIII gene have been reported that lead to hemophilia A.

Etiology and Pathogenesis

Factor VIII is a cofactor for factor IX activation. When activated by thrombin, factor VIIIa forms a trimer in complex with calcium. Factor VIIIa and the activated factor IX (IXa) associate on the surface of platelets to form a functional factor X–activating complex called ten-ase (X-ase). In the absence of factor VIII, the rate of activation of factor X is dramatically decreased. In patients with hemophilia, clot formation is delayed because of markedly reduced thrombin generation (due to factor X activation rate). The clot that is formed is friable and easily lyses (Fig. 99.1).

Clinical Manifestations

Soft-tissue hematomas and crippling hemarthroses are characteristic of hemophilia A. Based on the level of factor activity, hemophilia A is classified as severe (<1% of normal activity), moderate (1% to 5%), and mild (5% to 20%) as shown in Table 99.1

SEVERE DISEASE

Most patients with severe hemophilia present with bleeding during the first year of life. Approximately 5% of the infants develop intracranial hemorrhage during delivery. Around 50% of nondiagnosed hemophiliacs have significant bleeding during circumcision.

Easy and excessive bruising, hematomas, and hemarthrosis occur as children start ambulating. Hemarthrosis involves (in decreasing order of frequency) knees, elbows, shoulders, wrists, and hips. After a minor trauma and sometimes spontaneously, the joint becomes progressively painful, swollen, and warm. Mild fever can be present; however, high sustained fever should trigger an investigation for superimposed joint infection. Symptoms resolve within a few days after the bleeding stops. Without treatment, recurrent hemarthroses lead to chronic hemophilic arthropathy by young adulthood, often complicated by muscle atrophy and soft-tissue contractures.

Soft-tissue hematomas are characteristic of coagulation factor deficiencies. In patients with severe hemophilia, hematomas can occur with minimal trauma or spontaneously. They can stabilize and slowly resorb or enlarge progressively. Retroperitoneal hematomas can cause renal insufficiency by obstructing the ureters. Pharyngeal and retropharyngeal hematomas can complicate common colds and cause airway compromise. Hemorrhages into the muscle can occur in calves, thighs, buttocks, and forearms and can lead to muscle contractures and atrophy, as well as nerve paralysis.

Almost all patients with severe hemophilia experience hematuria. Renal colic can occur if a clot

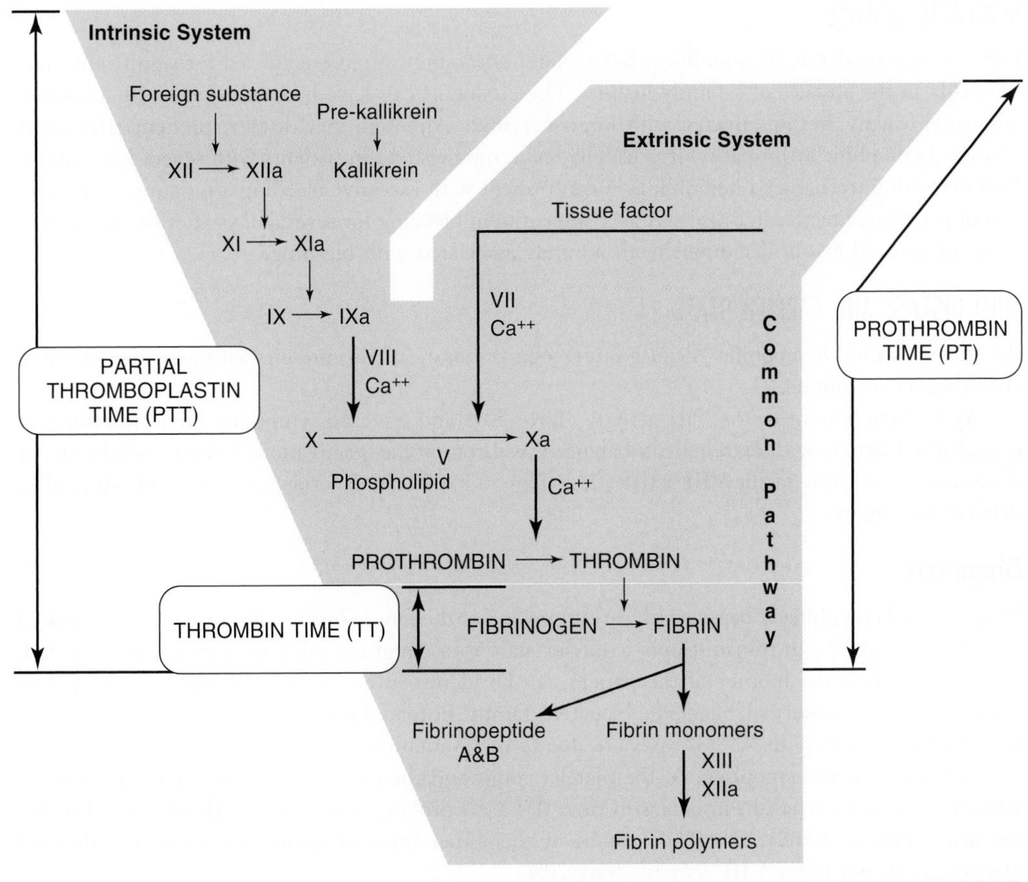

Figure 99.1 • Coagulation cascade.

obstructs the ureters. Intracranial hemorrhage usually follows trauma, but can be spontaneous. It should be suspected in any hemophilic patient presenting with a headache. Bleeding from mucous membranes is common in patients with severe hemophilia. Epistaxis and hemoptysis are common. Peptic ulcer disease is five times more common in patients with hemophilia than in the general population. Patients with severe hemophilia can present with later onset and less severe bleeding episodes if a coinherited factor V Leiden mutation is present.

TABLE 99.1 Clinical bleeding in relation to coagulant factor levels in hemophilia

Severity	Coagulant factor activity (%)	Type of bleeding
Severe	<1	Spontaneous bleeding
Moderate	1–5	Severe bleeding after minor injury, occasional spontaneous bleeding
Mild	5–20	Severe bleeding after major hemostatic stress, no spontaneous bleeding

MODERATE DISEASE

Patients with moderate hemophilia A have a later onset and can go undetected for significant time, especially in the absence of a family history. These patients can have hemarthroses and hematomas associated usually, but not always, with known trauma. Although they do develop hemarthropathy (chronic hemophilic arthropathy) it is usually less crippling than in patients with severe hemophilia. Patients with unrecognized hemophilia A can present with excessive bleeding after surgery. Extraction of permanent teeth can cause excessive intermittent bleeding for several days after the procedure; however, natural loss of deciduous teeth is rarely associated with bleeding.

MILD DISEASE AND CARRIER STATE

Patients with mild hemophilia A can go unrecognized and can also present with excessive bleeding after surgery or trauma.

Most carriers have factor VIII activity above 50% and have no symptoms even after surgical procedures. Carriers with extremely imbalanced X-chromosome inactivation, Turner's syndrome, or X mosaicism can have factor VIII activity less than 50% and can experience excessive bleeding after delivery or surgery.

Diagnosis

Diagnosis of hemophilia A begins with careful review of the family history. Because it is an X-linked disorder, the father can transmit only a carrier state to a daughter, whereas sons are not affected. In most instances, the mother of the patient can be identified as a carrier because of personal or family history of abnormal bleeding. Negative family history does not rule out the diagnosis of hemophilia because up to 30% of cases are due to new mutations.

In patients with hemophilia A, the platelet count and the prothrombin time (PT) are normal, whereas activated partial thromboplastin time (PTT) is prolonged as factor VIII is involved in the intrinsic pathway. Rarely, the PTT can be at the upper limit of normal in patients with mild hemophilia A and factor VIII activity above 20%.

A definitive diagnosis of hemophilia A is based on decreased factor VIII activity measured by one-stage clotting assay or chromogenic assays.

It is important to distinguish hemophilia A from other bleeding disorders that may present with similar symptoms. Hemophilia A can be distinguished from von Willebrand based on the features presented in Table 99.2.

The presence of acquired factor VIII deficiency (for example, secondary to SLE or malignancy) can be differentiated from hemophilia A with decreased factor VIII activity, by mixing plasma from the affected patient with normal plasma. If PTT normalizes, the patient has hemophilia A with factor VIII deficiency. If PTT does not normalize, factor VIII inhibitor is present.

TABLE 99.2 Comparative laboratory abnormalities between hemophilia A and von Willebrand disease

Tests	Hemophilia A	von Willebrand disease
Factor VIII levels	Decreased	Decreased
Partial thromboplastin time	Prolonged	Prolonged
Prothrombin time	Normal	Normal
Bleeding time	Normal	Prolonged
Ristocetin cofactor activity	Normal	Decreased

Factor IX deficiency (hemophilia B) has family history and clinical presentation very similar to hemophilia A. Measuring the activity of factors VIII and IX allows one to distinguish between the two conditions.

TREATMENT

With the use of factor VIII replacement, the morbidity and mortality of patients with hemophilia A have decreased significantly and their lifespan now approaches that of healthy individuals.

Patients with hemophilia A should be advised against the use of medications that can interfere with platelet aggregation such as aspirin and nonsteroidal anti-inflammatory agents. Pain should be controlled with acetaminophen and judicious use of narcotic agents. Hemorrhagic episodes are managed by replacing factor VIII. Both fresh frozen plasma and cryoprecipitate contain factor VIII; however, infusion with these products requires large volumes and allows only an approximation of the amount of factor VIII provided.

Patients with severe hemophilia A should receive prompt infusion of factor VIII to decrease the occurrence of extensive joint degeneration, deformity, and muscle wasting. Life-threatening bleeds, such as retropharyngeal, retroperitoneal, and intracranial hemorrhages, should be treated aggressively by raising factor VIII level to normal to near normal levels; its level should be maintained until the bleeding stops and the hematoma begins to resolve. Asymptomatic patients with head trauma should receive a prophylactic dose of factor VIII before further diagnostic procedures such as computed tomography scan of the head are performed.

In patients with mild to moderate hemophilia, the synthetic vasopressin analog desmopressin acetate (DDAVP) can be used. It increases factor VIII level two- to threefold above the baseline by stimulating the endothelium to stimulate factor VIII activity. Patients with severe hemophilia A do not respond to it. A potential side effect is hyponatremia due to desmopressin acetate's antidiuretic activity, especially in patients whose free water intake exceeds 1 L per day. Cardiovascular adverse effects associated with desmopressin acetate include increased heart rate, hypertension, and myocardial infarction.

For major surgical procedures, factor VIII should be raised to normal and maintained for 7 to 10 days until healing is underway. Prophylactic therapy is available for severely affected patients. It improves the clinical condition and the quality of life of the patients. Liver transplantation successfully cures hemophilia A and at this time can be an option for patients with chronic hepatitis and liver failure.

COMPLICATIONS

Prior to 1985, transmission of hepatitis B and C and human immunodeficiency virus (HIV) was a major complication, and liver failure and acquired immunodeficiency syndrome became a leading cause of death in older patients with hemophilia. Screening of donor populations, instituting heat- or solvent-detergent sterilization techniques, and development of recombinant factor VIII concentrates have significantly reduced the risk of viral or prion transmission.

HEMOPHILIA B

Hemophilia B also is an X-linked recessive disorder caused by decreased clotting activity of factor IX (also called Christmas factor or plasma thromboplastin component) clinically indistinguishable from hemophilia A. It occurs in 1 of every 25,000 to 30,000 male births. Like hemophilia A, it affects all ethnic groups and has no geographic predilection.

Clinical Manifestations

Depending on factor IX activity, hemophilia can be classified as severe (<1% of normal factor IX level), moderate (1% to 5%), and mild (5% to 40%). Bleeding episodes in patients with hemophilia B are very similar to those of patients with hemophilia A. Untreated recurrent hemarthroses may lead to crippling arthropathy and muscle wasting. Soft tissue hematomas and mucous membrane bleeding are common.

Diagnosis

In most cases of hemophilia B, the PT is normal and PTT is prolonged. Bleeding time usually is within the normal range. Specific assay of factor IX clotting activity is necessary for definitive diagnosis.

Other inherited or acquired disorders associated with deficiency of vitamin K–dependent factors, such as liver disease or the pharmacological effects of warfarin, must be distinguished from hemophilia B. In these conditions, not only factor IX, but all vitamin K–dependent coagulation factors (thrombin, VII and X) will be decreased.

Treatment

Like hemophilia A, the basic treatment of hemophilia B is factor replacement.

Several different products are available. They include prothrombin complex concentrates (factor IX, factors VII and X, and proteins C and S), which in their activated form can cause thromboembolic events and disseminated intravascular coagulation (DIC). Highly purified factor IX concentrates prepared from human plasma (after viral inactivation) or through recombinant DNA technology can also be used.

Complications

Unless treated properly, patients with hemophilia B have the same complications as patients with hemophilia A. In addition to joint deformities, hepatitis B and C and HIV are common in patients treated before 1985. Patients treated after 1985 are unlikely to be infected with these viruses and can expect to have a relatively normal lifespan.

VON WILLEBRAND DISEASE

von Willebrand factor (vWF) is an important component of hemostasis. It serves as a carrier for factor VIII and a link between platelets and the disrupted vessel wall. Abnormalities in vWF level or activity result in von Willebrand disease (vWD), the most common inherited bleeding disorder in humans. vWD is an extremely heterogeneous and complex disorder, with over 20 different subtypes. The vWD gene is located on chromosome 12. Both autosomal dominant and autosomal recessive inheritance have been described. Some of the characteristic features of the five major subtypes are summarized in Table 99.3.

Etiology and Pathogenesis

vWF, a multimeric protein, is synthesized in megakaryocytes and vascular endothelial cells. The most severe form of vWD, type 3, is due to complete deficiency of vWF. Type 1 vWD is caused by a quantitative decrease in vWF multimers. Type 2 vWD is due to a qualitative defect in vWF multimers. Type 2B is due to increased affinity of vWF for platelet-binding sites, causing accelerated clearance of these platelets from the plasma, resulting in thrombocytopenia. von Willebrand disease can be classified as inherited or acquired (associated with other diseases).

TABLE 99.3 Classification, laboratory features, and frequency of von Willebrand disease by type

	Type 1	Type 2A	Type 2B	Type 3	Pseudo (platelet type)
Prothrombin time	Normal	Normal	Normal	Normal	Normal
Bleeding time	↑	↑	↑	↑↑	↑
Partial thromboplastin time	↑	↑	↑	↑	↑
Platelet count	N	N	N or ↓	N or ↓	N or ↓
Inheritance	AD with incomplete penetrance	AD	AD	AR or codominant	AD
Frequency	Most common (>70 %)	Clinically significant (10% to 15%)	Uncommon (<5%)	Rare	Rare
Molecular defect	Partial quantitative vWF deficiency	Qualitative vWF defect, decreased large vWF multimers	Qualitative vWF defect, increased vWF-platelet interaction	Severe quantitative vWF deficiency	Platelet defect, decreased vWF-platelet interaction
vWB factor	↓	↓	↓	↓↓↓ or absent	↓ or N
Ristocetin cofactor activity	↓	↓	↓ or N normal	↓↓↓ or absent	↓
RIPA	↓ or normal	↓	↑ to low concentrations of ristocetin	Absent	↑ to low concentration to ristocetin
vWF multimers	Normal	Large multimers reduced to absent	Large multimers absent	Absent	Large multimers absent
Platelet count	N	N	N or ↓	N or ↓	N or ↓

AD, autosomal dominant; AR, autosomal recessive; N, normal; RIPA, ristocetin-induced platelet aggregation; vWF, von Willebrand factor.
Modified from Lichman MA, Beutler E, Kausnansky K, et al. *Williams Hematology*, 7th ed. New York: McGraw-Hill, 2005 and Kutty K, Kochar MS. *Kochar's Textbook of Internal Medicine*, 4th ed. Baltimore: Lippincott, Williams, and Wilkins, 2003.

Clinical Presentation

Mucocutaneous bleeding is the most common symptom in patients with vWD. Sixty percent of the patients with type 1 vWD present with epistaxis, 40% have easy bruising and hematomas, 35% have menorrhagia, and 35% have gingival bleeding. Gastrointestinal bleeding occurs in approximately 10% of the patients. Mucocutaneous bleeding after trauma (such as teeth extraction, delivery, or surgery) is common. Hemarthroses in patients with moderate disease are rare and occur only after major trauma.

Patients with type 3 vWD present with severe mucocutaneous bleeding episodes and can experience hemarthroses, joint deformities, and muscle hematomas similar to those of patients with hemophilia A.

Thrombocytopenia is a typical feature of type 2B vWD. Thrombocytopenia can be worsened by conditions increasing vWF production or secretion—such as physical exercise, pregnancy, infection—perioperatively or in the neonatal period.

Patients with certain disorders, such as myeloproliferative disorders, benign or malignant B cell disorders, hypothyroidism, autoimmune disorders, solid tumors (Wilms' tumor in particular), cardiac or vascular defects (aortic stenosis), and exposure to drugs including ciprofloxacin and valproic acid can develop a rare, acquired form of vWD. Such patients present with late-onset bleeding without prior bleeding history and negative family history.

DIAGNOSIS

Up to 20% of normal individuals have a positive bleeding history; hence, a detailed family history should always be performed.

Laboratory Values

The following tests are routinely performed in patients with suspected vWD: factor VIII activity assay, vWF antigen, and ristocetin cofactor activity. Bleeding time, although usually prolonged, varies significantly with the experience of the operator and should not be used as a screening test in patients with possible vWD or other platelet abnormalities. PT is normal in all forms of vWD because none of the factors in the extrinsic pathway are affected.

A decrease in factor VIII levels correlates well with the decrease in vWF. Patients with type 1 and type 2 have only mildly to moderately decreased levels of factor VIII, whereas patients with type 3 vWD have much lower levels of factor VIII. As factor VIII levels are affected in all forms of vWD, PTT is always prolonged.

Ristocetin cofactor activity quantifies the ability of plasma vWF to agglutinate platelets in the presence of ristocetin. Ristocetin cofactor activity usually is reduced and correlates well with the decrease in the vWF level. It is the most sensitive and specific single test for detection of vWD.

Ristocetin-induced platelet aggregation (RIPA) measures the affinity with which vWF binds to its platelet receptor. This activity is generally reduced in all patients with vWD.

Platelet-type (pseudo) vWD is caused by a platelet defect and phenotypically mimics vWD. Typical laboratory findings are decreased large multimer levels, hyperresponsiveness to RIPA, and thrombocytopenia (Table 99.3).

Acquired vWD (secondary to malignancies, autoimmune disorders, or medications) can be difficult to differentiate from inherited vWD because testing for the associated antibodies is not readily available. The diagnosis is based on the late onset of the disease, negative family history, and the identification of an underlying condition.

Treatment

The main treatment modalities are desmopressin (DDAVP), which induces secretion of both vWF and factor VIII, and replacement therapy. The choice of treatment depends on the type of vWD and the hemostasis needs.

Type 1 patients are most often treated with desmopressin alone; type 3 patients require vWF concentrates; and types 2A and 2B patients are treated with a combination of DDAVP and vWF-containing factor VIII products. Prophylaxis usually is not needed except in preparation for surgical and dental procedures and in patients with severe type 3 vWD who present with hemarthroses and hematomas.

Patients with thrombocytopenia associated with vWD may require platelet transfusions in addition to factor VIII and vWF-containing products. Fibrinolytic inhibitors, such as ϵ-aminocaproic acid, can be used in conjunction with DDAVP or vWF replacement concentrates in patients with significant bleeding or who are undergoing dental extraction.

Estrogen and oral contraceptives have been used empirically for treatment of menorrhagia. In addition to their effect on the ovaries and uterus, they increase plasma vWF levels most likely by increasing production of vWF in the endothelium.

Acquired vWD usually improves with treatment of the underlying disorder. Refractory cases can be treated with corticosteroids, plasma exchange, intravenous gammaglobulin, DDAVP, and vWF-containing factor VIII concentrates.

Oncology

Christopher Chitambar

CHAPTER 100

Multiple Myeloma

John Charlson

MULTIPLE MYELOMA

Multiple myeloma is a malignancy of mature plasma cells. These B-cells proliferate in the bone marrow and produce monoclonal immunoglobulins, called serum monoclonal (M) protein.

Multiple myeloma accounts for roughly 10% of hematologic malignancies. The estimated incidence in the United States in 2005 was approximately 16,000 cases. The incidence is twice as high in African Americans as in whites. The median age at onset is 66 years; only 2% of patients are less than 40 years old at diagnosis.

Etiology

Ionizing radiation is the most strongly associated environmental risk factor; other potential risk factors include exposure to nickel, agricultural chemicals, petroleum products, and benzene. Genetic mutations associated with multiple myeloma and monoclonal gammopathy of undetermined significance (MGUS) include partial deletions of chromosome 13 and translocations involving chromosome 14. Chromosome 13 abnormalities have been thought to lead to a poorer prognosis.

Clinical Manifestations

Common presenting symptoms of multiple myeloma include bone pain, fatigue, and recurrent bacterial infections. Typical laboratory abnormalities include anemia, renal insufficiency, and hypercalcemia.

BONE LESIONS/PAIN

This is the most common presenting symptom. Pain due to an incidental pathologic fracture can be sudden and severe. Vertebral compression fractures can result in back pain, neurologic symptoms from spinal cord compression, and even loss of height. Radiographs reveal osteolytic or "punched-out" lesions that can be widespread and distributed throughout the skeleton. Less commonly, diffuse osteoporosis is seen rather than lytic lesions. Lytic lesions increase in size and number as the disease progresses. Skeletal radiographs are preferred to radionuclide bone scans because the lytic bone lesions in myeloma are not associated with an osteoblastic response and are not usually visualized on bone scan. Hypercalcemia in multiple myeloma is related to lytic bone lesions.

BACTERIAL INFECTIONS

Most patients with myeloma secrete antibodies; however, these antibody products are aberrant. Synthesis of functioning, polyclonal antibodies is decreased. This results in an increased susceptibility to bacterial infections, particularly pneumococcal infections.

RENAL INSUFFICIENCY

Impaired renal function is noted in up to 80% of cases of myeloma and may be the presenting feature. Renal insufficiency in multiple myeloma is most commonly related to tubular damage caused by reabsorption of large amounts of monoclonal light chains known as Bence-Jones proteins. Amyloid deposition secondary to myeloma can also contribute to renal insufficiency.

ANEMIA

Anemia is present in 70% of patients with myeloma and is multifactorial. Anemia of chronic disease secondary to malignancy and renal insufficiency, along with replacement of normal bone marrow function by malignant cells are possible causes.

NEUROLOGIC SYMPTOMS

All levels of the nervous system can be affected in some way by multiple myeloma. Peripheral neuropathy can result from amyloid infiltration. Vertebral compression fractures can cause nerve root symptoms or spinal cord compression, which is a medical emergency. Confusion may be a result of hypercalcemia, uremia, or hyperviscosity.

Diagnosis

As noted above, laboratory findings can include anemia, hypercalcemia, and renal insufficiency. Erythrocyte sedimentation rate may be markedly elevated. Rouleaux formation may be noted on peripheral blood smear.

A number of clinical scenarios may prompt workup for multiple myeloma: unexplained anemia or renal failure, lytic bone lesions or pathologic fracture, recurrent infection, nephrotic syndrome, or peripheral neuropathy.

INITIAL WORKUP

Initial workup should include serum protein electrophoresis (SPEP), urine protein electrophoresis (UPEP), immunofixation, radiographic skeletal survey, and assessment for end-organ damage (renal failure, anemia, and hypercalcemia). UPEP should ideally be based on 24-hour urine collection. Measurement of free light chains in the serum provides additional useful information. Bone marrow biopsy should be considered if a monoclonal protein is found in blood or urine. Beta-2 microglobulin, albumin, C-reactive protein, and lactate dehydrogenase have prognostic value for multiple myeloma.

Monoclonal immunoglobulins can be identified in a few conditions other than multiple myeloma: chronic lymphocytic leukemia (<5% of cases), non-Hodgkin's lymphomas (rare), and incidentally in other chronic illnesses. Nonsecretory multiple myeloma comprises 3% of myeloma cases; these patients do not have detectable monoclonal protein in serum or urine. Measurement of free light chains in the serum can be useful in this setting for diagnosis and monitoring treatment response.

DIAGNOSTIC AND STAGING CRITERIA

Diagnostic criteria for multiple myeloma and MGUS are outlined in Table 100.1. These are based on International Myeloma Working Group recommendations. The International Staging System divides patients into three stages and prognostic groups based on albumin and beta-2 microglobulin levels (Table 100.2).

Treatment

There is no evidence that treating smoldering multiple myeloma or MGUS prevents or slows the development of multiple myeloma. Observation alone is recommended. Active treatment of multiple myeloma can include chemotherapy and autologous stem cell transplant. Allogeneic stem cell transplant is used less often and mainly in the setting of clinical trials. Chemotherapeutic agents used for multiple myeloma include corticosteroids (dexamethasone and prednisone), thalidomide (and

TABLE 100.1 Diagnostic criteria for multiple myeloma and monoclonal gammopathy of undetermined significance

Multiple myeloma
(Diagnosis requires 1 major and 1 minor, or 3 minor, criteria.)
Major criteria
Monoclonal (M) protein: IgG >3.5 g/dL; IgA 2.0 g/dL
Marrow plasmacytosis >30%
Plasmacytoma
Minor criteria
Lytic bone lesions
Marrow plasmacytosis 10% to 30%
Monoclonal (M) protein quantity less than above levels
Decrease in other immunoglobulin levels
Monoclonal gammopathy of undetermined significance
Monoclonal (M) protein: <3 g/dL
Urine light chains <1.0 g per 24 hours
Marrow plasmacytosis <10%
No lytic bone lesions

lenalidomide, which is an analogue of thalidomide with less toxicity), melphalan, and bortezomib (a proteasome inhibitor, approved for patients with refractory and relapsed myeloma). Initial therapy often includes steroids and thalidomide. Melphalan is avoided in stem cell transplant candidates because its alkylating function may interfere with stem cell mobilization.

Autologous stem cell transplant (ASCT) is a procedure in which patients have their hematopoietic stem cells harvested and preserved and then receive high-dose chemotherapy. The patient's bone marrow is essentially shut down after high-dose chemotherapy, and so the stored stem cells are given back to restore hematopoietic function. ASCT prolongs overall survival by approximately 12 months, with a mortality rate of 1% to 2%. Characteristics that may exclude patients as candidates for ASCT include advanced age, poor performance status, and medical comorbidities.

TABLE 100.2 International Staging System for multiple myeloma

Stage	Frequency (%)	Median survival (months)
Stage I (Serum albumin $\geq$3.5 g/dL and β_2-microglobulin <3.5 μg/mL)	29	62
Stage II (Not stage I or III)	38	44
Stage III (serum β_2-microglobulin $\geq$5.5 μg/mL)	34	29

Adapted from Rajkumar SV, Kyle RA. Multiple myeloma: diagnosis and treatment. *Mayo Clin Proc* 2005;80: 1373–1382.

Complications

Hypercalcemia, skeletal lesions, renal insufficiency, anemia, and hyperviscosity are clinical manifestations of multiple myeloma that can be apparent at presentation or develop with disease progression.

Symptoms of *hypercalcemia* include somnolence, confusion, nausea/vomiting, and volume depletion. Initial treatment is hydration. Intravenous bisphosphonates such as pamidronate and zoledronic acid are effective at normalizing calcium levels within several days.

Focal pain due to *skeletal lesions* uncontrolled by analgesics may be treated with radiation therapy. Pathologic fractures or impending pathologic fractures in long bones may require surgical fixation. Spinal vertebral lesions can lead to painful compression fractures, which may be treated with vertebroplasty or kyphoplasty (substances or devices inserted into collapsed vertebrae to restore height and relieve pain). Spinal cord compression can develop secondary to compression fractures or plasmacytoma in the spinal canal. Symptoms could include lower extremity weakness or numbness, back pain, and bowel or bladder dysfunction. This is considered an emergency that should be evaluated by magnetic resonance imaging or computed tomography myelogram and urgently treated with corticosteroids and radiation. Bisphosphonates (pamidronate, zoledronic acid) are recommended for myeloma patients with at least one lytic bone lesion for the prevention of progression of bone lesions.

Renal insufficiency can develop due to light chain cast nephropathy. It is important to keep in mind that a number of factors may contribute to renal failure in patients with this predisposition: nonsteroidal anti-inflammatory agents, volume depletion, and radiographic contrast media. *Anemia* may improve with treatment of the underlying disease or improvement of renal failure. Concurrent causes of anemia, such as deficiency of iron, folate, or vitamin B12, need to be ruled out. Patients with symptomatic anemia may benefit from administration of erythropoietin or darbepoetin.

Hyperviscosity may present with symptoms such as confusion or visual disturbances. Plasmapheresis should be done to remove the paraproteins causing the increased viscosity.

WALDENSTRÖM'S MACROGLOBULINEMIA

Waldenström's macroglobulinemia is a low-grade malignant lymphoma of plasmacytoid lymphocytes that secrete excessive amounts of a monoclonal immunoglobulin (Ig) M paraprotein. Bone marrow, lymph node, spleen, and liver infiltration are typical.

Clinical Manifestations

Most patients present with symptoms due to anemia or the presence of the macroglobulin, such as cryoglobulinemia (e.g., Raynaud's phenomenon), hyperviscosity, and protein-protein interaction (e.g., platelet dysfunction with petechiae and ecchymosis). Unlike multiple myeloma, renal failure and bone lesions are uncommon.

Diagnosis

Diagnosis depends on demonstration of a monoclonal IgM paraprotein on SPEP and characteristic infiltration of plasmacytoid lymphocytes in the bone marrow or lymph nodes.

Treatment

Waldenström's macroglobulinemia may be treated with plasmapheresis and or chemotherapy.

OTHER

The malignant proliferation of plasma cells results in a variety of clinical syndromes: MGUS is considered an asymptomatic, premalignant process that culminates in multiple myeloma in about

10% to 15% of patients. It is characterized by the presence of a serum monoclonal (M) protein <3 g/dL and an absence of end-organ damage or bone marrow abnormalities.

Smoldering multiple myeloma (like MGUS) is considered a premalignant disorder. There is a serum monoclonal (M) protein ≥3 g/dL and bone marrow plasmacytosis, but no end-organ damage (e.g., anemia, bone lesion). The risk of progression to multiple myeloma is much higher from smoldering multiple myeloma than with MGUS.

Solitary plasmacytoma is myeloma isolated to a single bone or soft-tissue site.

CHAPTER 101

Lymphomas

John Charlson

HODGKIN'S LYMPHOMA

Hodgkin's lymphoma (previously termed Hodgkin's disease) is a malignancy of the lymphoid system. Most of the tumor mass is composed of nonmalignant lymphocytes, histiocytes, granulocytes, plasma cells, eosinophils, and fibrosis, each apparently reactive (unlike non-Hodgkin's lymphomas). The disease is characterized by Reed-Sternberg cells and their variants, although they form only a minority of the cellular component of the lymph node.

Hodgkin's lymphoma is relatively uncommon: 7,300 cases occurred in the United States in 2005. There is a striking bimodal age distribution, with the first peak occurring in young adulthood and a second peak after age 50 years.

Etiology

The disease is more common in upper socioeconomic groups and in persons with a prior history of infectious mononucleosis. Epstein-Barr viral DNA has been detected in the genome of Reed-Sternberg cells, suggesting an etiologic relationship to this agent. The Reed-Sternberg cell is now known to be of B-cell origin.

There are four main histologic types of Hodgkin's lymphoma. These include, in order of decreasingly favorable prognosis: lymphocyte predominant, nodular sclerosis, mixed cellularity, and lymphocyte depletion subtypes. The first three subtypes tend to present with more limited disease, whereas lymphocyte-depleted Hodgkin's lymphoma often is widespread by the time of diagnosis. Nodular-sclerosing Hodgkin's lymphoma has a predilection for the mediastinum, especially in young women. Hodgkin's lymphoma of unfavorable cell types (e.g., mixed cellularity and advanced stage) is commonly observed in HIV-infected patients.

Clinical Features

Most patients with Hodgkin's lymphoma present with the complaint of a painless mass, usually in the neck but occasionally in the axilla or groin. On examination, rubbery, usually painless lymphadenopathy is noted. Occasionally, an abdominal mass, representing enlarged retroperitoneal nodes, or splenomegaly is the initial finding. Some patients are totally asymptomatic and the physician may discover lymphadenopathy during the course of a routine physical examination or detect mediastinal adenopathy on a chest radiograph obtained for other indications (Fig. 101.1).

Occasionally, extensive lymphadenopathy causes symptoms by compression of adjacent organs, (e.g., venous obstruction in an extremity, hydronephrosis [and renal failure if both ureters are compressed], superior vena cava syndrome, tracheal compression, dysphagia due to esophageal compression, and spinal cord compression).

A minority of patients (about 25%) present with characteristic paraneoplastic systemic "B" symptoms, such as unexplained fever, weight loss, and night sweats. The presence of B symptoms implies a less favorable prognosis in any given stage. Another occasionally noted symptom is pruritus, which typically is intense and refractory to symptomatic treatment.

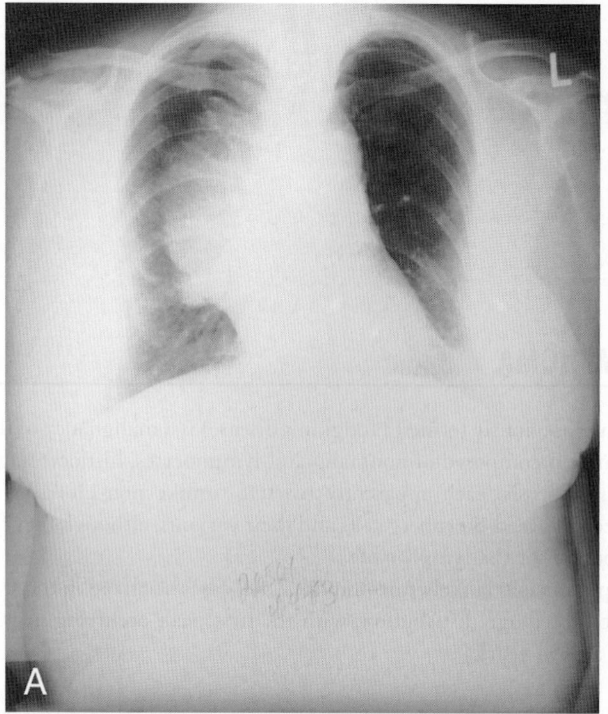

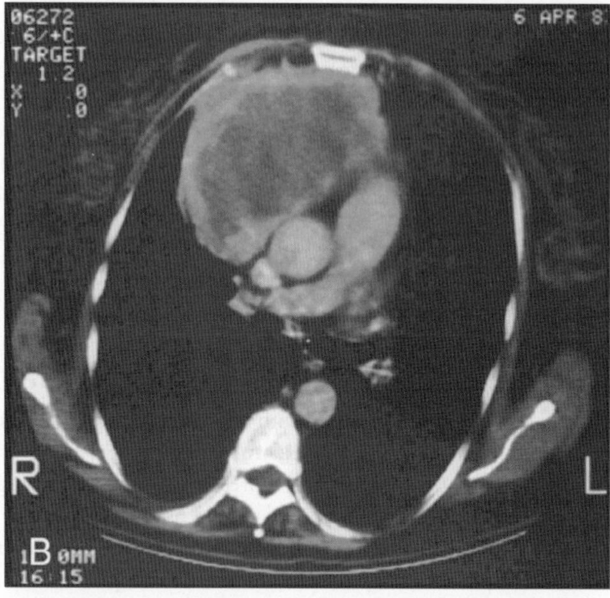

Figure 101.1 • Hodgkin's disease presenting as a mediastinal mass. **A.** Posteroanterior chest radiograph shows a large mass to the right of the ascending aorta. **B.** Computed tomography scan showed it was an anterior mediastinal mass.

Diagnosis

The diagnosis of Hodgkin's lymphoma is based on careful pathologic analysis of an adequate tissue sample. Reed-Sternberg cells are the hallmark of Hodgkin's lymphoma, but their presence alone is insufficient for diagnosis, because similar cells may be seen in other conditions (e.g., lymphomas, carcinomas, infectious mononucleosis, and toxoplasmosis). The use of immunologic markers (immunophenotype) aids in the diagnosis.

Staging of Hodgkin's lymphoma is facilitated by the knowledge that it spreads most commonly by contiguous extension to adjacent nodal groups and structures. Initial assessment includes a careful history and physical examination and selected laboratory studies (complete blood count with differential, platelet count, erythrocyte sedimentation rate, and liver and renal function tests). In addition to determining the risk of extranodal disease in bone marrow or liver, laboratory studies help assess whether anemia of chronic disease, nephrotic syndrome, or other rare manifestations of Hodgkin's lymphoma (or concomitant independent disease) are present.

Imaging studies, including computed tomography (CT) scans of the neck, chest (Fig. 101.1), abdomen, and pelvis and positron emission tomography (PET) scans, are used in combination for staging of disease and for assessing response to treatment.

Bone marrow involvement is evaluated by iliac crest biopsy; such involvement is important to identify, but is rare without extensive, widespread adenopathy, B symptoms, a positive bone scan, or an elevated alkaline phosphatase.

The modified Ann Arbor staging system is shown in Table 101.1.

Treatment

Treatment options for Hodgkin's lymphoma include radiation alone, radiation plus chemotherapy, and chemotherapy alone. Treatment decisions are based on stage more than histology. A simplified outline of treatment decisions by stage is shown in Table 101.2.

In contrast to the poor survivals seen in the 1960s, the overall survival rate today for patients with early-stage Hodgkin's lymphoma is 75% to 90%, and for those with disseminated disease, it is 50% or greater.

Complications

The complications of Hodgkin's lymphoma are myriad. Infectious complications are more prevalent in Hodgkin's lymphoma because of inherent immunodeficiency, which is temporarily worsened by extensive radiotherapy and chemotherapy.

TABLE 101.1 Modified Ann Arbor Staging of Hodgkin's lymphoma and non-Hodgkin's lymphomas

Stage	Definition
I	Involvement of a single node group
IE	Stage I, accompanied by a single extranodal site
II	Two or more involved nodal groups on the same side of the diaphragm
IIE	Stage II accompanied by a single extranodal site
III	Involved nodes on both sides of the diaphragm
III_1	Upper abdominal nodes or spleen (S) involved
III_2	Periaortic, iliac, or mesenteric nodes involved
IV	Extranodal disease beyond that indicated by E

The suffix A or B may be used with any stage. *A* indicates no systemic symptoms; *B* indicates documented fever, night sweats, or weight loss of >10% of body weight.

TABLE 101.2 Treatment regimens for Hodgkin's lymphoma

Stage	Treatment alternatives	5-year disease-free survival (%)
IA, IIA (includes E)	Extended-field radiotherapy	80 to 90
IB, IIB	Chemotherapy alone, or extended field radiotherapy if pathologically staged	60 to 85
IIA with bulky mediastinal disease	Combination chemotherapy plus mantle radiotherapy	80
$IIIA_1$	Extended-field radiotherapy	60 to 85
$IIIA_2$	Combination chemotherapy and total lymphoid radiotherapy	70 to 85
IIIB	Combination chemotherapy	60 to 80
IVA, IVB	Combination chemotherapy	50 to 70

Radiotherapy causes early local complications such as sore throat, dysphagia, nausea, and diarrhea as well as later complications such as radiation pneumonitis or fibrosis, pericardial effusion, pericardial constriction, coronary artery disease, radiation spinal cord damage, hypothyroidism, and late-onset solid tumors of the skin, lung, esophagus, and breast.

NON-HODGKIN'S LYMPHOMAS

The non-Hodgkin's lymphomas (NHL) are a heterogeneous group of malignant neoplasms of the immune system that, despite diverse origins, share a common link in the characteristic monoclonal proliferation of malignant B or T lymphocytes. In contrast to the predominantly reactive polymorphic cells of Hodgkin's lymphoma, those of the NHLs are monomorphic and monoclonal. Unlike Hodgkin's lymphoma, which tends to spread by contiguity, NHL often spreads hematogenously to involve diverse sites important in immune regulation and lymphocyte proliferation. NHLs can arise in diverse extranodal sites and the bone marrow often is involved. Thus, the site of presentation and spread of NHL are more unpredictable and widespread than in Hodgkin's lymphoma. Most patients present with stage III or IV disease, thus rendering NHL somewhat less curable.

Malignant lymphomas account for 6% to 7% of malignancies. It is estimated that 56,390 new cases will be diagnosed in 2005. The incidence increases with age, although NHLs occur in all age groups. High-grade lymphomas are common in younger patients, with the frequency of indolent (low-grade) lymphomas increasing with age. States of immunosuppression (e.g., acquired immunodeficiency syndrome [AIDS], rheumatoid arthritis, Sjögren's syndrome, and a history of Hodgkin's lymphoma, prior transplantation and immunosuppressive therapy) are all associated with an increased incidence of NHL.

Etiology

The precise etiology of most cases of NHL is elusive. African Burkitt's lymphoma, the posttransplant lymphomas, and lymphomas associated with AIDS are strongly associated with Epstein-Barr virus (EBV) infections. The human T-cell leukemia virus 1 (HTLV-1) is implicated in adult T-cell leukemia and the lymphomas endemic in southwestern Japan and the Caribbean basin. Other infectious pathogens have been implicated in the pathogenesis of NHL as well, including *Helicobacter pylori*, hepatitis C virus, *Chlamydia psittaci*, and *Campylobacter jejuni*. Agricultural chemicals and ionizing radiation have been associated with increased incidence of NHL. Prior treatment for Hodgkin's lymphoma increases risk for NHL by 20-fold.

Clinical Manifestations

The manifestations of NHL can best be described as protean. This group of diseases should always be included in the differential diagnosis of a patient with an unidentified organ disease process. NHL commonly presents with lymphadenopathy similar to Hodgkin's disease, although hepatosplenomegaly and widespread palpable adenopathy are more common. Conversely, clinically or radiographically significant mediastinal lymphadenopathy is less frequent. The adenopathy may be bulky and large abdominal masses may be felt. Massively enlarged nodes may cause organ compression or obstruction. The nodes are usually described as discrete or rubbery, unlike the hard nodes of metastatic carcinoma. The bone marrow is commonly involved (20% to 40% of cases), more frequently when hepatosplenomegaly or hematologic abnormalities are present and especially when the histology is low grade.

Classification of NHLs is according to the WHO (World Health Organization) classification system (Table 101.3). This classification system divides NHL into B-cell and T/NK-cell groups, with each of these groups subdivided into mature and precursor cell types. Some authors further characterize lymphomas as indolent, aggressive, or highly aggressive. Precursor T- and B-cell lymphomas are highly aggressive. Indolent lymphomas almost invariably arise from B cells, whereas a sizable portion of the intermediate and high-grade lymphomas are of T-cell origin.

Lymphomas with a large-cell component and a diffuse histologic growth pattern are known collectively as aggressive or high grade. They are more likely to show invasive characteristics. Indolent lymphomas are typically comprised of more mature appearing lymphocytes and behave less aggressively.

High-grade NHLs may involve the central nervous system, manifesting as a parenchymal mass or infiltration of the meninges and cranial or spinal nerve roots, with resultant nerve dysfunction. Diplopia and facial weakness, myelopathy, or radiculopathy at any level may occur.

The presentations of extranodal lymphomas are widely variable, mimicking tumors of the brain, thyroid, gastrointestinal tract, lung, or genital tract of either gender.

The B symptoms characteristic of Hodgkin's lymphoma occur in NHL as well.

Diagnosis

The diagnosis of NHL is established by biopsy of an involved lymph node or other tissue, including bone marrow and the many extranodal sites where lymphomas may arise. The hallmark of malignancy, a clonal lymphocyte population, is established by immunohistochemical study, flow cytometry, or DNA analysis. Light microscopy can define the cell size and architecture.

The evaluation of patients with NHL is similar to that of Hodgkin's lymphoma. History, physical examination, and laboratory tests are performed initially. PET scan and CT scans of neck, chest, abdomen, and pelvis are used to help define disease stage, as well as to monitor during and after treatment.

Bone marrow biopsy is required. The marrow is involved in most disseminated low-grade lymphomas but is not as prognostically important. In intermediate and high-grade lymphomas, marrow involvement is less frequent, but, when present, it is more ominous. Additional investigation may be necessary, such as examination of the cerebrospinal fluid or gastrointestinal tract.

The Ann Arbor staging system, is also applied to non-Hodgkin's lymphoma. The E category is used often in extranodal lymphomas. Indolent, low-grade lymphomas rarely present with localized disease (stages I or II), but intermediate and high-grade lymphomas are localized in up to 40% of cases.

TABLE 101.3 World Health Organization classification of lymphoid malignancies

Classification	Percentage of total cases	Classification	Percentage of total cases
Precursor B-cell neoplasms		**Precursor T-cell neoplasms**	
Precursor B-cell lymphoblastic leukemia/ lymphoma		Precursor T-cell lymphoblastic leukemia/ lymphoma	1.7
Mature B-cell neoplasms		**Mature T-cell and NK-cell neoplasms**	
CLL/SLL	6.7	T-cell prolymphocytic leukemia	
B-cell prolymphocytic leukemia		T-cell large granular lymphocytic leukemia	
Lymphoplasmacytic lymphoma	1.2	Aggressive NK-cell leukemia	
Splenic marginal zone lymphoma	<1	Adult T-cell leukemia/ lymphoma	<1
MALT lymphoma	7.6	Extranodal T/NK-cell lymphoma, nasal type	
Nodal marginal zone lymphoma	1.8	Enteropathy-type T-cell lymphoma	
Follicular lymphoma	22.1	Hepatosplenic T-cell lymphoma	<1
Mantle cell lymphoma	6.0	Subcutaneous T-cell lymphoma	
Diffuse large B-cell lymphoma	30.6	Mycosis fungoides	<1
Mediastinal large B-cell lymphoma	2.4	Primary cutaneous anaplastic large cell lymphoma	
Intravascular large B-cell lymphoma		Peripheral T-cell lymphoma, unspecified	
Primary effusion lymphoma		Angioimmunoblastic T-cell lymphoma	
Burkitt's lymphoma/ leukemia	<1	Anaplastic large cell lymphoma	2.4
B-cell proliferation of uncertain malignant potential		**T-cell proliferation of uncertain malignant potential**	
Posttransplant lymphoproliferative disorder		Lymphomatoid papulosis	
Lymphomatoid granulomatosis			

Adapted from Ansell SM, Armitage J. Non-Hodgkin lymphoma: diagnosis and treatment. *Mayo Clin Proc* 2005;80: 1087–1097.

TABLE 101.4 International Prognostic Index for diffuse large B-cell lymphoma

Factor		Adverse prognosis	
Age		>60 years	
Ann Arbor stage		III or IV	
Serum LDH level		Above normal	
Number of extranodal sites		≥2	
ECOG performance status		≥2	
Number or risk factors	**Complete response rate (%)**	**5-year disease-free survival (%)**	**5-year survival (%)**
0 or 1	87	73	70
2	67	51	50
3	55	49	43
4 or 5	44	40	26

ECOG, Eastern Cooperative Oncology Group.

The International Prognostic Index (IPI) for aggressive non-Hodgkin's lymphoma was designed to use easily obtainable clinical data to define various risk groups (Table 101.4).

Treatment

Treatment of lymphomas is complex, because the biology of disease varies with the subtype. Unlike Hodgkin's lymphoma, in which treatment decisions depend primarily on the stage of disease, in NHL, histologic features often are more important than stage in treatment strategies. Several clinically important types are discussed below.

Follicular lymphoma, which is the second most common type of NHL, is an example of indolent lymphoma (histologic grades I and II). Indolent lymphomas are almost always stage III or IV disease at presentation. Initially, even patients with stage IV disease often can be observed without treatment. Palliative radiotherapy can be used for stage I or II disease, and chemotherapy can be used for more advanced disease that is symptomatic or progressing. Rituximab, a monoclonal antibody to the CD20 protein on B-cells used alone or with chemotherapy, is an effective treatment option. Median survival averages 8 to 12 years. The "watch-and-wait" approach is commonly employed.

Diffuse large B-cell lymphoma, considered an aggressive lymphoma, is the most commonly diagnosed type of NHL. Localized disease is managed with excisional biopsy, followed by combination chemotherapy and consolidative radiation, an approach particularly suitable for extranodal presentations (stages IE and IIE).

In stage III or IV disease, chemotherapy is the treatment of choice. CHOP (cyclophosphamide, doxorubicin, vincristine, and prednisone) with Rituxan is the standard treatment in the United States, and it offers approximately 50% chance of cure.

Precursor T- and B-cell lymphomas are lymph and tissue mass manifestations of the same immature cells seen in acute lymphoblastic leukemia. The diagnosis of lymphoma (versus leukemia) is made in patients with predominantly lymph node or soft-tissue disease and less than 25% bone marrow involvement. These are highly aggressive diseases that require intensive chemotherapy.

CHAPTER 102

Breast Cancer

John Charlson

Breast cancer is the most common cancer in women and the second leading cause (following lung cancer) of cancer-related death in women. Its incidence has been slowly increasing over the past 30 years, with a marked increase in the number of diagnoses since 1990 due to wider screening.

In 2005, there were an estimated 211,240 new cases of breast cancer diagnosed and 40,870 deaths from breast cancer occurred in the United States. Males accounted for 1,870 of the new cases. Western countries have the highest incidence rates, and this is likely related to dietary factors and other socioeconomic variables.

Various factors contribute to an individual's risk for developing breast cancer (Table 102.1). The current estimate of an overall lifetime incidence for women is around 12%, with the greatest risk concentrated in the sixth decade and beyond.

ETIOLOGY

Numerous risk factors for breast cancer have been defined. Hereditary susceptibility accounts for 5% to 20% of cases and can be associated with specific germline mutations, including the breast cancer genes 1 (BRCA-1) and 2 (BRCA-2). These mutations are transmitted in autosomal dominant fashion and indicate a markedly elevated risk of breast and ovarian cancer.

Hormonal factors appear to play an important role in disease development and progression. The effect of early menarche, delayed pregnancy, and late menopause is to prolong cyclic stimulation. Diet and obesity may lead to a relative state of excess estrogens and alcohol may alter estrogen metabolism. In these instances, prolonged estrogen stimulation probably acts as a promoter to more fundamental molecular perturbations. Prolonged estrogen therapy (e.g., hormonal replacement therapy), with or without progestins, is a minor risk factor.

Almost all breast cancers are adenocarcinomas. Invasive breast cancer comprises 75% to 85% of breast neoplasms. Infiltrating ductal carcinoma, which arises from ductal tissue, accounts for 85% of invasive breast cancer cases. Carcinoma arising from the secretory lobules is termed infiltrating lobular carcinoma and accounts for about 5% to 10% of cases. The remaining types of invasive breast cancer include mucinous, medullary, and tubular carcinoma, based on their cellular origins. Carcinoma in situ, comprising approximately 15% to 25% of breast neoplasms, is a tumor that has remains confined within the ducts or lobules. Whereas lobular carcinoma in situ (LCIS) is considered premalignant, with a 25% chance of progression into malignancy, ductal carcinoma in situ (DCIS) is considered a malignancy. DCIS is six times more common than LCIS.

CLINICAL FEATURES

The usual clinical presentation is a painless lump or localized thickening (fibrosis) in the breast. Most breast masses, however, are not cancer. Breast masses in premenopausal women usually are due to

TABLE 102.1 Risk factors for breast cancer

Risk factor	Estimated risk magnitude (relative risk)
Female	Overwhelming
Age	>10 for elderly
Obesity	2.0 for postmenopause
Regular alcohol intake	1.0 to 1.5 with daily use
History of previous breast cancer	Risk is 1% annually in opposite breast
Previous premalignant breast disease	
Hyperplasia	1.6
Atypical hyperplasia	>4.0
Lobular carcinoma in situ	20% to 25% cancer risk in either breast over two decades
Heredity	
One affected first-degree relative	1.5
Two affected first-degree relatives	3.0
Premenopausal bilateral cancer in first-degree relatives	8.0
Hormonal factors	
Age at menarche <12	1.5 to 1.7
Age at menopause >54	2.0
First pregnancy after age 30 to 35 years	1.5 to 2.0
Nulliparity	1.5
Early pregnancy, age <21	Increases risk by 60%
Early castration without hormone replacement	Marked reduction in risk
Prolonged hormone replacement	1.3
Prolonged oral contraceptives	Debatable effects

fibrocystic disease or fibroadenoma. Nonmalignant causes of masses in the postmenopausal age group are sclerosing adenosis, fibrocystic disease, fibroadenomas, or fat necrosis due to unappreciated trauma. Because age is the most important risk factor, suspicion should be adjusted accordingly.

Pain or discomfort, while more common in nonmalignant breast conditions, may be a presenting symptom in breast cancer. Rarely, the patient will report an axillary mass with or without an evident breast abnormality. Nipple discharge most often is due to benign intraductal papillomas, but cancer must always be excluded.

Typically, the physical examination reveals a localized, firm mass or thickening of the breast tissue. In more advanced cancer, there may be dimpling or puckering of the overlying skin, distortion of the breast or nipple, or palpable axillary or supraclavicular nodes. More locally advanced cancer is characterized by skin fixation, ulceration, and adjacent skin nodules. Rare forms of breast cancer include Paget's disease of the nipple, which presents as eczematoid dermatitis caused by infiltration of the nipple with an underlying carcinoma, and inflammatory breast carcinoma, a distinct clinical entity presenting as erythema and edema of the overlying skin due to extensive involvement of the dermal lymphatics from an underlying aggressive ductal carcinoma.

With screening, early breast cancer may present as a mammographic abnormality before it is detectable on breast examination.

Metastases cause symptoms related to the organ of involvement (e.g., bone pain, jaundice, cough, central nervous system symptoms).

DIAGNOSIS

When a breast mass is discovered, either clinically or on mammography, the diagnosis must be established pathologically. In premenopausal women, a painful, cystic mass may be observed for resolution through one menstrual cycle to exclude the possibility of fibrocystic disease, but any persistent or suspicious mass must be biopsied promptly.

Mammography is always done before biopsy to evaluate the appearance of the mass and both breasts (Fig. 102.1). Ultrasonography is useful for distinguishing solid from cystic masses and showing small lesions in women with dense breast tissue. Breast magnetic resonance imaging (MRI) is highly sensitive and is used mainly for screening of high-risk patients (e.g., BRCA positive), and for resolving questions left by conventional imaging. Positron emission tomography (PET) scan is used to evaluate for distant metastatic disease.

Tissue examination to confirm a diagnosis of breast cancer is required before treatment. Tissue is often obtained by fine-needle aspiration or core-needle biopsy. Also important in treatment planning is knowledge of whether cancer has spread to regional, draining lymph nodes. Sentinel node biopsy,

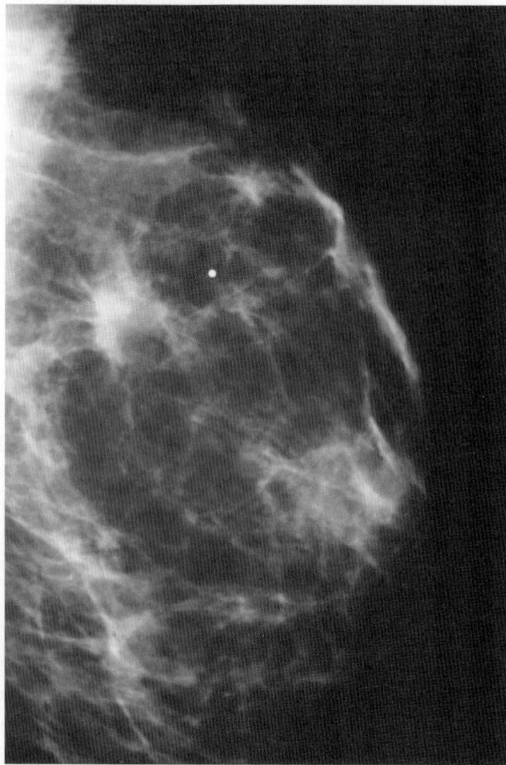

Figure 102.1 • Mammographic findings in breast cancer. The characteristic findings associated with cancer are a spiculated irregular mass or clustered microcalcification. Only a biopsy procedure can establish whether a mammographically detectable lesion is benign or malignant.

TABLE 102.2 Tumor-node-metastasis (TNM) staging of breast cancer

Tumor	
Tis	Carcinoma in situ
T1	Tumor <2 cm in diameter
T2	Tumor >2 cm but <5 cm
T3	Tumor >5 cm
T4	Extension to chest wall; skin edema, ulceration, satellite nodules on breast; inflammatory carcinoma
Node	
N0	No clinically palpable nodes
N1	Movable ipsilateral axillary nodes
N2	Nodes (ipsilateral) fixed to one another or to axillary structure
N3	Internal mammary nodes
Metastasis	
M0	No metastases
M1	Metastases, including ipsilateral supraclavicular node

From the American Joint Committee on Cancer. *Manual for Staging of Cancer*. 4th ed. Philadelphia: JB Lippincott; 1992, with permission.

performed at the time of resection of the breast mass, is a procedure in which a radionuclide and visible blue dye are injected into the tumor bed, allowing the surgeon to identify the lymph node or nodes draining the tumor site. With very careful histologic and immunohistochemical study of these nodes, it is possible, with about 95% accuracy, to rule out lymph node involvement. If the sentinel nodes are involved, more extensive lymph node dissection is required to document the extent of lymph node involvement. When sentinel node biopsy is negative, the morbidity of extensive lymph node dissection can frequently be avoided. With the above information, tumor-node-metastasis staging can be completed (Table 102.2), which is important for predicting the risk of recurrence and directing postsurgical, adjuvant treatment. Additional staging tests may include radionuclide bone scan or brain MRI.

The size of the tumor and the presence of involved axillary nodes remain the principal prognostic factors (Table 102.3). The presence of estrogen receptor (ER) and progesterone receptor (PR) also are important prognostic factors, and are key in deciding whether to use adjuvant hormone therapy. Overexpression of Her-2/neu, a cell surface tyrosine kinase-like molecule, has prognostic and therapeutic importance as well, due to the availability of a monoclonal antibody trastuzumab. Overexpression of Her-2/neu, which occurs in 15% to 20% of breast cancers, is associated with worse prognosis. Molecular assays for expression of specific genes involved in breast cancer (gene-expression profiling) are another promising prognostic tool (Table 102.4).

Screening is done to diagnose breast cancer at earlier stages when cure is more likely. Major expert groups in the United States recommend annual screening with mammography and clinical breast exam on an annual basis starting at age 50 years. There is some disagreement about the 40- to 49-year-old patient group, but most experts recommend screening mammogram every 1 to 2 years for this group. Breast self-examination has not been proven effective as a screening tool.

TABLE 102.3 Survival by stage of breast cancer

Stage	Tumor-node-metastasis category	10-year disease-free survival (% without systemic therapy)
0	Tis, N0, M0	98
I	T1, N0, M0	80 (all stage I patients)
	T<1cm	90
	T 1-2 cm	80–90
IIA	T0, N1, M0; T2, N0, M0	60–80
IIA	T1, N1, M0	50–60
IIB	T2, N1, M0	5–10 worse than IIA above
IIB	T3, N0, M0	30–50
IIIA	T0-T2, N2, M0 or T3, N1, M0	10–40
IIIB	T4, N0-N2, M0	5–30
IIIC	Any T, N3, M0	15–20
IV	Any T, Any N, M1	<5

TREATMENT

Management of Noninvasive (In Situ) Carcinoma

Lobular carcinoma in situ rarely presents as a palpable mass or discrete mammographic findings but usually is discovered as an incidental histologic finding in biopsy specimens taken for other reasons. It signifies increased later cancer risk in either breast (20% to 30% incidence over 15 to 20 years). Careful annual screening for cancer is recommended. Prophylactic bilateral mastectomy is the only alternative for women unwilling to accept the risk of subsequent cancer, but this is considered a drastic step. Use of tamoxifen prophylaxis is of benefit.

Ductal carcinoma in situ may present as a lump or mammographic abnormality. Tumor excision (lumpectomy) followed by radiotherapy reduces the risk of local relapse; however, there is no proven survival benefit the addition of radiotherapy. A mastectomy usually is curative, but for most patients it is cosmetically less desirable than a "breast-sparing" lumpectomy and radiotherapy.

TABLE 102.4 Prognostic factors in operable breast cancer

Factor/criterion	Favorable	Unfavorable
Nodal status	Histologically negative nodes	Increasing number of positive nodes
Tumor size	<1 cm	Increasing tumor size
Tumor grade	Well-differentiated	Poorly differentiated
Hormone receptors	ER%/PR%, ER!/PR%	ER%/PR!, especiallyER!/PR!
Oncogene amplification	HER2/NEU –	HER2/NEU +

ER, estrogen receptor; PR, progesterone receptor.

Local Therapy for Invasive Cancer

Surgery, radiotherapy, and systemic adjuvant therapy are all used in the treatment of localized breast cancer. Survival with "breast-conserving" therapy (lumpectomy with axillary sampling plus radiation) is comparable to that with a total mastectomy and axillary lymph node dissection for the treatment of most stage I and II cancers.

Systemic Adjuvant Therapy for Resected Breast Cancer

Relapse after primary locoregional therapy usually occurs in distant sites and is primarily the result of prior occult micrometastases. Recurrent breast cancer is, with rare exception, incurable. Adjuvant chemotherapy (prophylactic, after primary resection) can reduce the risk of relapse. Most patients with tumors larger than 1 cm or with evidence of metastasis in the lymph nodes (node-positive) are potential candidates for adjuvant therapy, and the selection of treatments is based on whether or not the tumor is endocrine-responsive and whether Her-2/neu is expressed at high levels (Table 102.5).

Patients with endocrine-unresponsive tumors may receive combination chemotherapy following surgery. In patients with ER- and PR-positive tumors, hormonal treatment options may include the estrogen agonist tamoxifen, chemical or surgical ovarian ablation, or one of the aromatase inhibitors in postmenopausal women. A patient with high risk of recurrence may receive chemotherapy before initiating hormonal therapy. Trastuzumab is a monoclonal antibody the Her-2 receptor, and has been shown to decrease recurrence and improve survival when combined with adjuvant chemotherapy in patients that overexpress Her-2/neu.

In contrast to the excellent prognosis in patients with minimal disease (i.e., a small primary lesion and no nodal involvement), the prognosis worsens in patients with positive axillary nodes; more than 85% of patients with 10 or more positive nodes would eventually relapse if not treated with systemic adjuvant therapy. Fortunately, such treatment can reduce the risk of relapse by about 30% to 45%.

Management of Locally Advanced Breast Cancer

Locally advanced disease is defined as tumors or axillary lymph nodes with fixation to the chest wall, extensive ulceration or satellite cutaneous nodules, or inflammatory cancer with diffuse dermal involvement. In all these presentations, mastectomy alone rarely effects local control. However, com-

TABLE 102.5 Adjuvant therapy for operable breast cancer

Therapy	Application
Adjuvant therapy in general	Tumor >1 cm High-risk features
Hormone therapy	ER/PR positive Follows chemotherapy with or without trastuzumab Sole adjuvant therapy in older, node-negative patients
Tamoxifen	Pre- or postmenopausal
Aromatase inhibitor	Postmenopausal
Chemotherapy	Consider in all patients with tumor >1 cm Exceptions: elderly, node-negative, medically unfit
Trastuzumab	Her2/neu overexpression Lymph-node positive

bining initial or neoadjuvant chemotherapy with subsequent radiotherapy or surgery leads to control of disease in 30% to 40% of patients.

Follow-Up after Primary Treatment

Long-term follow-up after primary treatment is essential. New cancers occur in the contralateral breast at the rate of 1% annually, a risk that can be reduced by the administration of tamoxifen. In patients who undergo a breast-sparing procedure, a relapse of the first cancer or a new cancer ultimately will develop in 5% to 20% of patients. Thus, previously treated patients must be followed carefully and screened with annual breast examinations and mammography.

Being relapse-free for 5 years does not guarantee cure in breast cancer. Adjuvant therapy reduces the relative risk of recurrence by about 50%, so the absolute risk ranges from <5% to 50%, depending on initial risk factors, but the risk of metastasis is lifelong. The most common sites of metastatic spread are bone (40% to 50%), soft tissue, regional lymph nodes (10% to 30%), and lung or pleura (25%).

Management of Metastases

In general, aggressive diagnostic evaluation is appropriate when relapse is suspected. If possible, biopsy documentation should be established. The diagnosis of metastatic disease has serious implications, because it is rarely curable. The median survival of patients with relapsed breast cancer is 2 to 3 years. Therapeutic options include chemotherapy, hormonal therapy, and trastuzumab, depending on whether hormone receptors are present and Her-2 overexpressed.

COMPLICATIONS

Surgery with axillary dissection may result in postoperative lymphedema swelling of the arm due to blockage of lymphatic vessels, which may develop months or even years later. Radiotherapy causes minor, transient, acute erythema and edema of the breast in most patients; later, scarring, shrinkage, and distortion of the breast, delayed lymphedema, radionecrosis of ribs or clavicle, and brachial plexus neuropathy may follow. Chemotherapy produces transient nausea or vomiting and anorexia; alopecia, fatigability, and myelosuppression are common in most patients. Leukemia is a rare late complication of chemotherapy. Tamoxifen therapy produces or worsens a hypoestrogenic state with menopausal-like symptoms, increases risk of deep venous thrombosis, and may, in rare cases, induce the development of endometrial cancer (although the reduction in risk of breast cancer relapse far outweighs the possible risk of inducing endometrial cancer).

PREVENTION OF BREAST CANCER

Primary prevention by early pregnancy or dietary modification is neither feasible nor of proven value. Selective estrogen receptor modulators (SERMs), tamoxifen and raloxifene, have antiestrogenic effects on breast tissue and have been shown to decrease the incidence of invasive breast cancer in high-risk patients. Tamoxifen is approved by the U.S. Food and Drug Administration for this purpose; concerns about adverse effects, including increased incidence of endometrial cancer and venous thromboembolic disease, may explain why it is not used more widely for primary prevention. Carriers of BRCA1 and BRCA2 mutations comprise a different high-risk group, and preliminary data suggest that tamoxifen significantly decreases risk of invasive breast cancer, particularly in BRCA2 carriers.

CHAPTER 103

Colon Cancer

Jenny Petkova

EPIDEMIOLOGY

Colorectal cancer (CRC) is the third most common cancer in both sexes and the third cause of cancer-related death in the United States in both sexes. It is rare before the age of 40 years and its incidence increases with age, reaching 3.7 in 1,000 by the age of 80 years. Most patients diagnosed with colorectal cancer are older than 50 years.

ETIOLOGY

Most colorectal cancers arise from polyps (any visible protrusion from the mucosa of the gastrointestinal tract). Histologically, these polyps can be divided into nonneoplastic (i.e., hyperplastic polyps) and neoplastic (adenomatous polyps or adenomas). Adenomatous polyps are premalignant and a minority (<1%) become malignant, although most colon cancers are believed to arise from adenomatous polyps. The probability of an adenoma becoming malignant depends on the histology, the size, and the gross appearance of the lesion. Villous adenomas become malignant three times more often than tubular adenomas. Sessile adenomas undergo malignant transformation more often than pedunculated (stalked) ones. The likelihood of adenomas containing invasive cancer is 10% for adenomas >2.5 cm and less than 2% for adenomas <1.5 cm in size.

RISK FACTORS

A number of conditions are associated with an increased incidence of CRC, including inflammatory bowel disease with pancolitis or active disease for over 10 years, personal history of adenomas or CRC, one or more first-degree family members or two or more second-degree relatives with CRC, and genetic syndromes predisposing to CRC. Some dietary and environmental factors possibly modifying the risk of developing colon cancer are listed in Table 103.1.

CLINICAL PRESENTATION

The clinical presentation of CRC depends largely on the anatomical site of the tumor. In the ascending colon, stool is liquid and lesions in that area can be asymptomatic. Because CRC tends to bleed intermittently, stool testing for occult blood may be negative and patients may present with asymptomatic hypochromic microcytic anemia or with signs and symptoms of anemia such as palpitations, exercise intolerance, dyspnea on exertion, or muscle weakness. Unexplained hypochromic microcytic

TABLE 103.1 Risk factors for colon cancer

Risk factors	Possible preventive factors
Sedentary lifestyle	Aspirin and possibly other nonsteroidal anti-inflammatory drugs
Obesity	Hormone replacement therapy, statins
Diet rich in red meats	Vitamin B6, folic acid
Cigarette smoking	Diet rich in vegetables, fruits, and fiber
Alcohol use	Calcium, magnesium

anemia in an adult (with the possible exception of premenopausal women) warrants endoscopic or thorough radiographic visualization of the entire large bowel.

In the descending colon, the stool becomes more concentrated, so tumors in that area may present with signs of abdominal obstruction (abdominal pain, cramping, abdominal distention, constipation or diarrhea, nausea, vomiting) or bowel perforation and peritonitis.

Cancer of the rectosigmoid area often presents with hematochezia, tenesmus, and a narrowing of the stool caliber.

Rare presentations include fever of unknown origin, *Streptococcus bovis* or *Clostridium septicum* bacteremia, and formation of a malignant fistula into adjacent organs (bladder or small bowel). CRC is ultimately proven to be the originating site of 6% of all adenocarcinomas of unknown primary.

Screening

Benign adenomas progress to invasive cancer over a prolonged period of time, usually around 10 years. This long premalignant interval provides the rationale for colon cancer screening. For individuals at average risk, initial screening is recommended after the age of 50 years. The choice of screening method should be discussed with the patient, taking into consideration side effects, safety, convenience, and cost. The following options are recommended: annual fecal occult blood testing, flexible sigmoidoscopy every 5 years, double-contrast barium enema every 5 years, or colonoscopy every 10 years. Other methods like virtual colonoscopy are currently under investigation. For patients with increased risk of CRC, screening should be done by colonoscopy every 5 years starting at the age of 40 years (or 10 years earlier than the age of presentation of a relative with CRC). The risk stratification for colorectal cancer is shown in Table 103.2.

TABLE 103.2 Relative risk factors for colon cancer

High risk	Moderate risk	Average risk
Familial polyposis	First-degree relative with colorectal cancer	All individuals above the age of 50 years
Hereditary nonpolypous colorectal cancer	History of breast, uterine, or ovarian cancer	
Inflammatory bowel disease		

DIAGNOSIS

CRC can be suspected in a patient presenting with any of the above symptoms or may be discovered during a routine screening. Colonoscopy is the single best diagnostic test in a symptomatic patient. It allows for detection and biopsy of suspicion lesions. If a colonoscopy is not possible due to technical difficulties, a double-contrast barium enema can reveal characteristic "apple core" constricting lesions. Further preoperative evaluation may include computed tomography (CT) scan of the abdomen and pelvis to determine the extent of regional tumor growth, lymphatic involvement, and metastatic spread. Evaluation by magnetic resonance imaging may be useful in patients with rectal cancer because of its ability to better characterize the mesorectal lymph nodes. A positron emission tomography scan may aid in the evaluation of suspected recurrence after a conventional workup has been nonrevealing and in the assessment of potentially resectable isolated liver metastasis. Chest CT is indicated for evaluation of rectal cancer because, unlike colon cancer that predictably metastasizes to the liver first, rectal cancer may metastasize to the lung directly. The serum level of carcinoembryonic antigen (CEA) is elevated in about one third of the patients with early-stage tumors and in 90% of the patients with metastatic disease. It is not a useful screening test but can be used to detect recurrence following resection of CRC.

STAGING AND TREATMENT

Surgery is both diagnostic and curative for patients with early stages of colon cancer. The type and extend of surgery depends on the location of the tumor and the involvement of lymph nodes and adjacent organs found during the surgery. The tumor-node-metastasis system and Duke's stages are defined after the surgical resection and pathology evaluation of both the primary tumor and the regional lymph nodes. The staging system is shown in Table 103.3. In general, a curative surgical operation includes removal of the involved bowel segment with disease-free margins at both ends, and en-block removal of the applicable vessels and lymphatics. If needed, temporary colostomy may be placed. However, patients with extensive bowel involvement, tumors adhering to adjacent organs or located <5 cm from the anal verge require a permanent colostomy. A subtotal or total colectomy is performed if more than one tumor is present or if multiple polyps exist. Patients with advanced metastatic disease can require limited bowel resection to prevent obstruction, perforation, or continuous bleeding. If resection is impossible, a diverting colostomy is placed.

TABLE 103.3 Staging system for colon cancer

Stages			Pathology
Duke's	TNM	Numerical	
—	TisN0M0	0	Carcinoma in situ
A	T1N0M0	I	Cancer limited to the mucosa and submucosa
B1	T2N0M0	I	Cancer extending into muscularis mucosae
B2	T3N0M0	II	Cancer extends into the serosa
C	TxN1M0	III	Involvement of the regional lymph nodes
D	TxNxM1	IV	Distant (hematogenous) metastasis: liver, lung

TMN, tumor-node-metastasis.

TABLE 103.4 Survival in colon cancer based on stage

Stage	Percent survival
I	93
II	72 to 85
III	44 to 64
IV	8

Adjuvant chemotherapy is warranted in all patients with Duke's C stage and possibly in a subset of Duke's B patients. It decreases the risk of local recurrence and improves survival. The therapeutic regimen includes 5-fluoruracil, combined with leucovorin with or without irinotecan or oxaliplatin.

In patients with metastatic disease at the time of diagnosis, chemotherapy improves overall survival and the progression-free survival compared to the best supportive care only. Radiation therapy is indicated in all patients with rectal cancer and colon tumors arising <25 cm from the anal verge. It improves local control and possibly improves survival. It can be combined with chemotherapy (5-FU acts as a radiosensitizer) to further decrease the risk of relapse and improve survival.

Selected patients with isolated hematogenous metastases to the lung or the liver at the time of presentation, recurrence at the surgical anastomotic site, or new primary tumors can benefit from surgical resection. Up to 15% to 25% of patients with less than five liver metastases can be cured by such "metastectomies."

After the initial curative surgery, the patient should be followed with history and physical examination every 3 to 6 months for the first 3 years, every 6 months for the next 2 years, and annually thereafter. CEA levels and CT of the chest and abdomen should be done in patients with stage II and III CRC. If not done preoperatively, surveillance of the remaining colon is carried out by a colonoscopy within 1 year after the surgery and, if negative, every 3 to 5 years subsequently.

PROGNOSIS

Unlike other cancers, the prognosis of colorectal cancer is not influenced by the size of the primary tumor. Poor prognostic factors include lymphatic involvement at the time of surgical resection, higher number of lymph nodes involved, penetration through the intestinal wall, perforation, tumor adherence to an adjacent organ, venous invasion, poorly differentiated histology, aneuploidy, specific chromosomal changes, and high CEA levels prior to surgery. Five-year survival rates are summarized in Table 103.4 stratified by risk.

Most recurrences after a curative resection occur within 4 years, thus 5-year survival is a good predictor for cure. Prognosis is best for patients with stage I tumors; more than 90% of them are cured. For patients with stage III (Duke's stage C) CRC, adjuvant chemotherapy decreases recurrence by 40% and improves survival by 20%. Less benefit from adjuvant chemotherapy occurs in patients with Duke's B stage. Patients with advanced disease that respond to chemotherapy have longer survival than nontreated patients and about 5% of them survive more than 5 years.

CHAPTER 104

Lung Cancer

John Charlson

Lung cancer was rare until cigarette smoking became endemic. The age-adjusted lung cancer mortality in men has risen from 11 per 100,000 in 1940 to 77.9 per 100,000 in 2001. In women, whose endemic smoking patterns began a generation later, the rate rose from 5 per 100,000 in 1960 to 40.8 per 100,000 in 2001. With 172,570 new cases and 163,510 deaths yearly, lung cancer is by far the most common cancer in the United States. The incidence and mortality of these cancers finally began to decrease in the 1980s in men. The incidence in women has leveled off in recent years after increasing for decades.

ETIOLOGY

Cigarette smoking continues to be the major cause of lung cancer. The relative risk of lung cancer in a long-term smoker is 10 to 30 times that of a nonsmoker. Cigar and pipe smoking increase the risk of lung cancer to a lesser degree. Certain occupational hazards predispose to lung cancer; these include asbestos exposure, uranium mining, and exposure to arsenic and nickel. Known or suspected cofactors include exposure to radon, beryllium, and various hydrocarbons. Lower-level environmental exposure to radon has also been associated with increased cancer risk. Passive smoke inhalation by the spouses of heavy smokers may account for as many as 8,000 cases annually.

Patients should be strongly encouraged and taught to stop smoking. Smoking cessation lowers the risk after 15 years by 80% to 90%, but an increased relative risk, about 1.5 to 2.0 compared to nonsmokers, remains indefinitely.

PATHOLOGY

The four basic types of lung cancer are adenocarcinoma, small cell, squamous cell, and large cell (Fig. 104.1). A simple, widely used classification divides lung cancers into small cell and nonsmall cell types, reflecting the generally systemic nature of small cell lung cancer, which entails a minor role for surgery. With the exception of adenocarcinomas, which often occur in peripheral lung zones, most lung cancers arise in proximal bronchi.

CLINICAL FEATURES

The usual signs and symptoms of lung cancer are outlined in Table 104.1. Asymptomatic solitary nodules, discovered incidentally or on screening x-ray, are important because of their potential for cure.

Lung cancer symptoms may come from the primary lesion, intrathoracic extension, distant

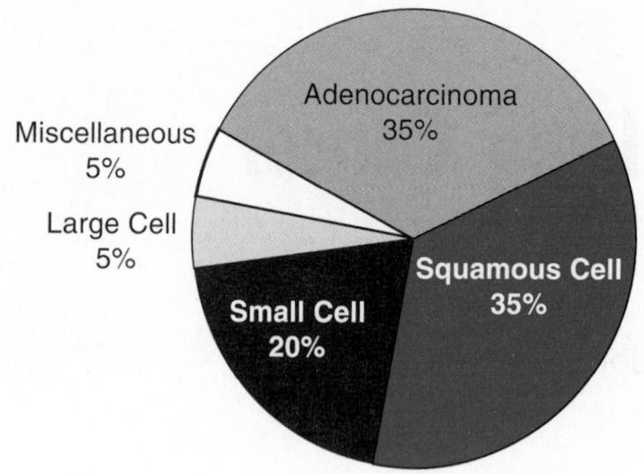

Figure 104.1 • Lung cancer cell types.

metastases, or paraneoplastic syndromes. Primary symptoms with all cell types include cough, dyspnea, sputum production, and hemoptysis. These symptoms are nonspecific and can be associated with other conditions such as chronic obstructive pulmonary disease; changes from baseline can indicate a superimposed process. Persistent pneumonia or a lung abscess may be the initial clue to underlying bronchial obstruction by tumor.

Intrathoracic extension of tumor with chest wall invasion causes pain. Mediastinal invasion can cause dyspnea or entrapment of the recurrent laryngeal nerve(s), producing a voice change due to vocal cord paralysis. If right-sided, it can cause the superior vena cava syndrome, featuring pain and swelling in the face and upper extremities. Cancers arising from the apex of the lung (Pancoast tumor) may invade the brachial plexus, leading to shoulder and arm pain or weakness. Pleural effusion, causing dyspnea or pain, can be caused by pleural involvement of mediastinal lymphatic obstruction.

Metastatic disease is seen at presentation in most patients, justifying an extensive preoperative workup. Lung cancer most often metastasizes to the bones, brain, liver, and adrenal glands. Related paraneoplastic syndromes are listed in Table 104.1.

TABLE 104.1 Clinical features and common paraneoplastic syndromes of lung cancer

Presentation	Features
Solitary pulmonary nodule	Asymptomatic
Primary symptoms	Cough, hemoptysis, dyspnea, wheezing
Regional effects	Hoarseness, esophageal compression Superior vena cava syndrome Superior sulcus invasion Horner syndrome Pleural and pericardial effusions Phrenic nerve paralysis
Metastasis	Brain, bone, liver, adrenal gland
Systemic (paraneoplastic)	Syndrome of inappropriate antidiuretic hormone, Cushing's syndrome (small cell) Eaton-lambert syndrome (small cell) Hypertrophic pulmonary osteoarthropathy (adenocarcinoma) Gynecomastia, weight loss Hypercalcemia (squamous cell)

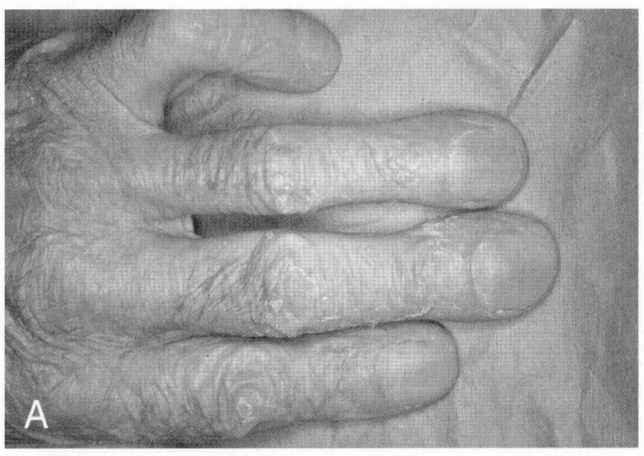

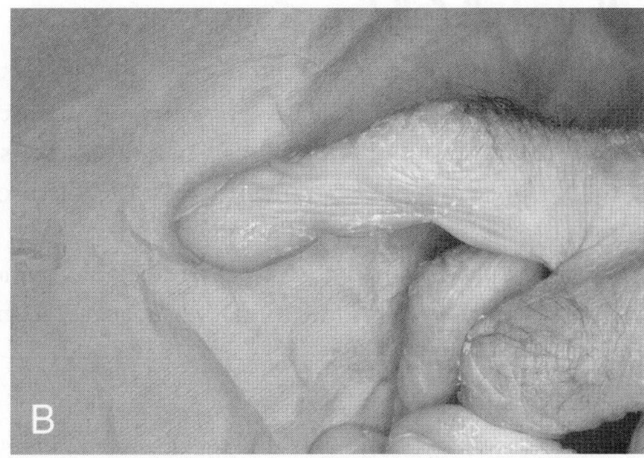

Figure 104.2 • Finger clubbing in bronchogenic carcinoma. **A.** Frontal view. **B.** Profile.

DIAGNOSIS

When lung cancer is suspected, diagnostic workup is done to confirm a histopathologic diagnosis and to define the extent of disease (staging). Physical examination may detect supraclavicular adenopathy, pleural effusion or atelectasis, the localized wheeze of bronchial obstruction, weight loss, clubbing of the fingers (Fig. 104.2), or signs of gross metastatic disease. Laboratory testing is performed to uncover anemia, hepatic dysfunction, hypercalcemia, and hyponatremia.

Cytologic examination of sputum may provide a definitive, noninvasive clue, especially in central lesions arising from the bronchi. Cytologic and histologic specimens are obtained from peripheral lesions through transthoracic fine-needle aspiration or core biopsy, under computed tomography (CT) or ultrasound guidance. Centrally located tumors are usually accessed via bronchoscopy.

Imaging studies used during preinvasive diagnostic workup or as staging studies after diagnosis include chest radiographs; CT scans of the chest, abdomen, and pelvis; radionuclide bone scans; and a CT or magnetic resonance scan of the brain. Positron emission tomography scan also is useful for evaluating solitary pulmonary nodules and for staging.

Small cell lung cancer is staged as limited (confined to the ipsilateral thorax and supraclavicular nodes) or extensive, based on the same tests used for all lung cancer patients. Regardless of the clinical stage, this disease nearly always is biologically disseminated. Thus, all patients undergoing treatment receive systemic chemotherapy. In contrast, nonsmall cell lung cancer disseminates later in its course; thus, meticulous thoracic and mediastinal staging is required because of the potential for surgical cure.

TREATMENT

Small Cell Lung Cancer

One cannot overemphasize the systemic nature of small cell cancer and the necessity of systemic chemotherapy, even in patients with limited stage disease. Untreated patients with this cancer have a median survival of only a few months. Patients with disease limited to the one side of the thorax respond to chemotherapy in almost 90% of cases. Instead of a median survival of only 2 to 4 months in untreated cases, average survival in treated patients exceeds 1 year; most importantly, a small subset of patients (15% to 30%) are alive and free of disease at 2 years and are potentially cured.

Patients with extensive stage disease also respond to therapy; about 80% of patients have a meaningful regression of disease with improvement in their cancer symptoms. Their survival also is prolonged from 1 to 3 months to 8 to 12 months.

Non-small Cell Lung Cancer

Nonsmall cell cancer is treated surgically, if possible. Unfortunately, the prognosis is still dismal for most patients. Most patients present with disease that is unresectable because it is too far advanced. Furthermore, only about 50% of patients successfully undergoing such surgery are truly cured, due to the presence of subclinical metastatic disease. Chemotherapy and radiation therapy add small benefit in terms of overall survival.

Patients believed to have unresectable tumors, due to extensive locoregional disease, or who have medical contraindications to surgery can be treated with radiation therapy, with or without chemotherapy.

CHAPTER 105

Cervical, Endometrial, and Ovarian Cancers

Jenny Petkova

CERVICAL CANCER

In 2005 in the United States, there were approximately 10,000 new cases of invasive cervical cancer and 3,700 deaths from this disease (1.3% of all cancer related deaths). There has been a decrease of 75% in the incidence and mortality from cervical cancer during the past 50 years due to the institution of screening and cancer prevention programs. In developing countries without such programs, 370,000 new cases are diagnosed each year with mortality rate as high as 50%.

The occurrence of cervical cancer is age related; it is extremely rare before the age of 20 and peaks in women 45 to 50 years of age. Women over 75 years of age account for 10% of the cases.

Etiology

The major risk factors for invasive cervical cancer as well as cervical intraepithelial neoplasia (the premalignant precursor of cervical cancer) include early onset of sexual activity and multiple sexual partners. Other risk factors are history of sexually transmitted diseases, multiple pregnancies, low socioeconomic status, and immunosuppression. Cervical cancer is nearly always associated with human papilloma virus (HPV) infection, which is transmitted during sexual activity. HPV-16 and HPV-18 are most associated with cervical cancer. Cigarette smoking or exposure to environmental smoke is also associated with increased risk among HPV-infected women, suggesting that components of tobacco are promoters of abnormal growth of HPV-infected cells.

Cervical intraepithelial neoplasia is a preinvasive lesion that can slowly progress into cancer. The majority (95%) of cervical carcinomas are squamous cell, typically arising from the squamocolumnar junction of the cervical epithelium. Adenocarcinoma, neuroendocrine, and small cell carcinomas are rare.

Cervical cancer progressively invades the surface, then the base, of the cervix, followed by extension to the parametrium and pelvic sidewalls. Involvement of the regional lymphatics, including the obturator and iliac nodes, follows. Locally advanced disease invades the bladder and rectum.

Clinical Manifestations

Cervical intraepithelial neoplasia and carcinoma in situ usually are asymptomatic and are diagnosed incidentally during routine Papanicolaou (Pap) smear screening or during the evaluation of inflammatory or infectious diseases of the genital tract. The most common symptoms are abnormal vaginal bleeding, postcoital bleeding, and vaginal discharge that is watery, mucoidal, or purulent. Vaginal discharge can be mistaken for severe cervicitis, especially because inflammation on cervical cytology sear is commonly present in overt malignancy. Locally advanced disease causes pelvic or lower back pain and urinary symptoms such as hematuria or ureteral obstruction. Edema of one or both lower extremities may occur. Vaginal passage of stool or urine is uncommon.

Diagnosis

SCREENING

Because the premalignant phases of this disease normally span years, there is ample time for detection of premalignant changes, allowing successful treatment of dysplasia and carcinoma in situ before invasive disease develops. Annual pelvic examinations with a Pap smear from the cervix should begin at the onset of sexual activity or at age 18 years. After two to three negative annual examinations, and if dysplasia and HPV infection are not present, the frequency of screening can be reduced to every 2 to 3 years. If premalignant changes have not developed on routine screening by age 65 years, invasive cancer is unlikely during remaining life. Conversely, patients with HPV infection should be screened more often and indefinitely.

In symptomatic women or after a positive screening smear, a pelvic examination should be performed. On cervical examination, most women have a visible cervical lesion ranging from superficial ulceration to exophytic tumors. A punch biopsy taken from the edge of the tumor usually confirms the diagnosis. If the cervix appears normal, colposcopy and direct biopsy should be performed. Conization is performed after a nondiagnostic colposcopy. Benign tumors that can be mistaken for cervical carcinoma include Nabothian cysts, glandular hyperplasia, mesonephric remnants, inflammatory glandular changes, and endometriosis.

STAGING

The tumor-node-metastasis (TNM) classification, staging, and survival for cervical cancer are summarized in Tables 105.1 and 105.2, respectively.

TABLE 105.1 Tumor-node-metastasis classification for cervical cancer

Stage	Description
Tumor	
T0	No evidence of primary tumor
T1	Cervical carcinoma confined to the uterus
T1a	Microscopic invasive carcinoma
T1b	Macroscopic tumor
T2	Cervical carcinoma extending beyond the uterus, but not to the pelvic wall or the lower third of the vagina
T2a	Involving the upper one third of the vagina
T2b	Involving the parametrium
T3	Tumor involving the pelvic wall or the lower one third of the vagina
T3a	Involving the lower third of the vagina
T3b	Involving the pelvic walls and/or causing hydronephrosis
T4	Spread to an adjacent organ (bladder/rectum)
Node	
N0	No lymph-node involvement
N1	Regional lymph nodes involved
Metastasis	
M0	No distant metastases
M1	Distant metastatic spread

TABLE 105.2 Staging and survival in cervical cancer

Stage	Tumor-node-metastasis stage	5-year survival rate (%)
IA	T1a N0 M0	90
IB	T1b N0 M0	70–90
IIA	T2a N0 M0	75–85
IIB	T2b N0 M0	60–65
IIIA	T3 N0 M0	30–50
IIIB	anyT N1 M0	20–30
IVA	T4 anyN M0	<20
IVB	anyT anyN M1	<5

Management

Cervical intraepithelial neoplasia, carcinoma in situ, and very early microscopic cervical cancer can be treated with conization only. Women with stages I and IIA can be cured with radical hysterectomy with lymphadenectomy or definitive radiation therapy (combined external beam and intracavitary brachytherapy). Radical trachelectomy (removal of the cervix and parametria with preservation of the uterus and ovaries) can be an alternative to radical hysterectomy in women who wish to preserve fertility. Adjuvant chemotherapy is recommended for women with stage I and IIA with bulky tumors or positive resection margins. Chemoradiation therapy is the preferred approach for patients with locally advanced disease: stages IIB, III, and IVA. Patients with disseminated disease (stage IVB) should be offered palliative radiation and/or chemotherapy to alleviate the pain or uterine bleeding.

Prevention

In 2006, the U.S. Food and Drug Administration approved a vaccine against HPV types 6, 11, 16, and 18, which are responsible for about 70% of cervical cancers and 90% of genital warts. The vaccine has been found to be almost 100% effective in preventing diseases caused by the four HPV types covered by the vaccine, including precancers of the cervix, vulva and vagina, and genital warts. Regular Pap tests and follow-up can prevent most, but not all, cases of cervical cancer. The only sure way to prevent HPV is to abstain from all sexual activity. Condoms may help reduce the risk of cervical cancer.

ENDOMETRIAL CANCER

Endometrial carcinoma is the most common gynecological malignancy in the United States and accounts for 6% of all cancers in women. The incidence between 1992 and 2000 was close to 30 cases per 10,000 women; however, when corrected for prevalence of hysterectomy, the incidence is almost 50 cases per 10,000 women per year.

Etiology

Endogenous risk factors include obesity, diabetes mellitus, hypertension, polycystic ovaries, and prior granulosa cell tumors. Exogenous risk factors include hormone replacement therapy with unopposed estrogen, which increases the risk 4- to 10-fold. The concomitant administration of progestins markedly reduces this risk. Prolonged treatment with the weak estrogen agonist tamoxifen in breast cancer appears to increase the risk of endometrial cancer by 2- to 4-fold.

A familial predisposition has been suggested for first-degree relatives. Other familial conditions associated with endometrial cancer are Lynch syndrome and familial breast cancer.

The most common type of endometrial cancer is adenocarcinoma (75% to 80%). Clear cells and papillary serous tumors are highly aggressive cancers that account for 1% to 5% and 5% to 10%, respectively. Mucinous and squamous cell carcinomas account for less than 2% of all endometrial cancers.

Clinical Presentation

Abnormal vaginal bleeding is the primary symptom, so that all women with postmenopausal bleeding require investigation. Premenopausal women should be investigated if they have other risk factors for endometrial cancer (obesity, hypertension). Advanced disease leads to pelvic and abdominal pain. Metastases may appear as supraclavicular adenopathy, hepatic metastases, or pulmonary nodules. Physical examination may reveal an enlarged uterus or pelvic masses.

Diagnosis

Cytologic assessments of the vaginal and cervical surfaces may be positive but are unreliable for screening. Although endometrial sampling is better, a thorough dilatation and curettage is the most accurate test, and must be done if symptoms of endometrial cancer are present.

Clinical staging should include a chest radiograph to evaluate lung involvement and a computed tomography scan of the abdomen and pelvis if there is a suspicion of extrapelvic disease. Contrast-enhanced magnetic resonance imaging is the best imaging modality to assess myometrial invasion and cervical involvement; however, it can be falsely negative in 1% to 10% of patients with deep myometrial invasion and should not be used as a substitute for the surgical staging.

Surgical staging requires inspection of the entire abdomen, biopsies of all suspicious sites, collection of peritoneal fluid for cytology, and evaluation of the pelvic and paraaortic lymph nodes. The TNM classification, staging, and survival for endometrial cancer are summarized in Tables 105.3 and 105.4.

Management

Surgical treatment involves total abdominal hysterectomy and bilateral salpingo-oophorectomy with peritoneal washings and pelvic and periaortic node sampling. External beam and intracavitary radiation is an alternative to surgery in patients with poor surgical risks and as an adjunct to surgery in patients with high-risk stages I and II disease. Patients with advanced stages III or IVA should receive radiotherapy. Medroxyprogesterone or megestrol (progestational agents) are used for palliation in patients with metastatic disease if their tumor expresses progesterone receptors. Staging and survival are shown in Table 105.4.

OVARIAN CANCER

Ovarian cancer is the second most common gynecological malignancy, but the most common cause of death among women with gynecological malignancies and the fifth most common cause of cancer-related death in women in the United States. Its incidence rises sharply after age 40 years, peaking at about 70 years. Hereditary ovarian cancer accounts for 5% of cases and may be associated with hereditary breast, ovarian, endometrial, or colon cancers.

Etiology

The different types of ovarian neoplasms are shown in Table 105.5. Eighty percent of malignant ovarian tumors arise from the surface epithelium (epithelial tumors). Half of these are papillary serous

TABLE 105.3 Tumor-node-metastasis classification for uterine cancer

Stage	Description
T0	No primary tumor
Tis	Carcinoma in situ
T1	Tumor not extending outside of corpus uteri
T1a	Cancer limited to the endometrium
T1b	Less than one half of the myometrium involved
T1c	More than one half of the myometrium involved
T2	Tumor not extending outside of the uterus
T2a	Endocervical glandular involvement
T2b	Cervical stromal involvement
T3	Extrauterine invasion without local organ invasion
T3a	Involvement of uterine serosa and/or adnexa
T3b	Vaginal involvement
T4	Tumor invading bladder or bowel mucosa
N0	No local lymph node involvement
N1	Metastasis to pelvic in para-aortic lymph nodes
M1	Distant metastatic spread including involvement of lymph nodes other than the pelvic and para-aortic

TABLE 105.4 Staging and survival in uterine cancer

Stage	Tumor-node-metastasis	5-year survival (%)
Stage I		
Stage IA	T1a N0 M0	>90
Stage IB	T1b N0 M0	85–90
Stage IC	T1c N0 M0	80
Stage II		
Stage IIA	T2a N0 M0	75
Stage IIB	T2b N0 M0	70
Stage III		
Stage IIIA	T3a N0 M0	60
Stage IIIB	T3b N0 M0	30
Stage IIIC	anyT N1 M0	50
Stage IV		
Stage IVA	T4 anyN M0	15
Stage IVB	anyT anyN M1	10

TABLE 105.5 Ovarian neoplasms

Origin	Histopathology
Epithelium	Serous Cystadenoma Cystadenocarcinoma Mucinous: benign or malignant Endometrioid Adenosarcoma Mesodermal mixed tumor Clear cell tumors: benign or malignant Transitional cell tumors Brenner tumor benign or malignant Transitional cell carcinoma
Sex cord	Granulosa stromal cell tumors Granulose cell tumors Thecoma-fibroma tumors Sertoli-Leydig cell tumors Gynandroblastoma Lipid cell tumors
Germ cells	Teratoma: solid or cystic Dysgerminoma Yolk sac tumors Choriocarcinoma Mixed germ cell tumors

cystadenocarcinomas. Mucinous papillary cystadenocarcinomas and endometrioid or undifferentiated tumors each account for 10% to 15% of cases. Stromal and germ cell tumors are uncommon and include granulosa cell tumors and arrhenoblastomas. Germ cell tumors are responsible for only 1% to 2% and include dysgerminomas, malignant teratomas, embryonal carcinomas, and the rare choriocarcinoma. Borderline tumors are very low-grade primary epithelial ovarian tumors that may have a prolonged clinical course of years or even decades, regardless of whether they are localized or metastatic.

Women in the United States have 1.4% to 1.8% lifetime risk of developing ovarian cancer. Nulliparity has been identified as a major risk factor. Infertility (but not infertility treatment), endometriosis, early menarche, and late menopause are also associated with higher rates of developing ovarian cancer. Multiple births, prolonged lactation, tubal ligation (and hysterectomy to lesser degree), and oral contraceptive use are protective. Mutations in the genes involved in the DNA repair (BRCA1 and 2, MDH-2, PMS1 and 2) appear to cause increased risk of cancer, with BRCA mutations accounting for 90% of the hereditary ovarian cancers.

Clinical Presentation

Early ovarian cancer evokes few symptoms; as a result, most patients present with more advanced stage II or III disease. Early symptoms like lower abdominal pain, cramping, bloating, constipation, indigestion, nausea, fatigue, urinary complaints, dyspareunia, and irregular vaginal bleeding are nonspecific and may be confused with nonmalignant conditions. Acute symptoms due to ovarian torsion or rupture are rare. Advancing disease causes single or multiple mass effects. With spread to peritoneal and diaphragmatic serosal surfaces, ascites and pleural effusion develop. Ascites may be the presenting complaint and may be erroneously thought to be due to liver disease. Three fourths of patients have disease disseminated throughout the peritoneum at diagnosis (stage III or IV). Death usually results from bowel obstruction, often at multiple sites. Additional complications include cachexia, refractory ascites, or renal failure from ureteral obstruction.

Diagnosis

A pelvic (ovarian) mass in a postmenopausal woman requires open or laparoscopic biopsy. In premenopausal women, masses smaller than 8 cm are usually functional cysts and should be observed for regression over 2 to 3 menstrual cycles. Masses exceeding 8 cm should be diagnosed promptly, especially if there are features suggestive of malignancy—solid fixed, irregular mass. Ultrasound is the most useful initial test for further evaluation of ovarian mass. CA-125 levels are elevated in patients with advanced disease, but are of limited value in young premenopausal women and in nonepithelial ovarian cancers. Computed tomography or magnetic resonance imaging of pelvis and abdomen can be used to evaluate metastatic spread and help plan the surgical intervention. Gene expression profiling by microarrays, a promising technology to identify cancer gene upregulation, is currently under investigation. The International Federation for Gynecology and Obstetrics staging for ovarian cancer is summarized on Table 105.6.

Treatment

Surgery is necessary for diagnosis, staging, and treatment of ovarian cancer. Optimal surgical debulking of tumors is the key to successful treatment and includes total abdominal hysterectomy, bilateral salpingo-oophorectomy, omentectomy, lymph node sampling, and removal of all visible disease. The few patients with borderline malignancy or stage I disease without penetration of the ovarian capsule usually are cured by surgery. In more advanced disease, even when complete resection is not possible, tumor reduction (debulking), with excision of all apparent abdominal disease, results in a more favorable prognosis with subsequent chemotherapy. With adjuvant chemotherapy, a group of stage

TABLE 105.6 Staging system for ovarian cancer

Stage	Description
Stage I	Tumor not extending beyond the ovaries
IA	Single ovary involved
IB	Both ovaries involved
IC	Surface spread on one or both ovaries, rupture during surgery, positive cytology of peritoneal fluid/washings
Stage II	Tumor extending into the pelvis
IIA	Extension into the uterus or the fallopian tubes
IIB	Extension to other pelvic structures
Stage III	Extrapelvic spread
IIIA	Micrometastases to peritoneum (only microscopically diagnosed)
IIIB	Gross spread to serous surfaces outside the pelvis smaller than 2 cm
IIIC	Gross spread >2 cm or positive retroperitoneal lymph nodes
Stage IV	Distant metastatic spread including cytologically positive pleural effusion, parenchymal liver metastasis

II patients also can be cured. Chemotherapy is the current principal treatment for advanced stages of ovarian carcinoma. The overall 5-year survival is 60% to 85% for patients with stage I ovarian cancer and 5% to 15% for stage IV. At 10 years, only about 10% of stage III patients are alive and disease free. There is no evidence that careful screening of asymptomatic women effectively detects early-stage disease. All tests, including pelvic examination, pelvic ultrasound, and CA-125 measurements, are limited by their lack of specificity or sensitivity for early ovarian cancer.

CHAPTER 106

Prostate Cancer

Jenny Petkova

Prostate cancer is the most frequently diagnosed cancer among American men (except for nonmelanoma skin cancer). With the introduction of prostate-specific antigen (PSA) screening in the early 1990s, a large number of asymptomatic patients with occult disease are being identified. Because the clinical behavior of prostate cancer ranges from an indolent tumor with little clinical importance to invasive metastatic cancer, its early detection poses a complex management dilemma.

About 30% of men above the age of 50 years are estimated to have prostate cancer. Autopsy series of males who have died of causes unrelated to cancer have revealed that almost all men above the age of 90 years have one or more foci of cancer in the prostate gland. Prostate cancer before the age of 40 years is rare and accounts for less than 1% of all cases. Most clinically symptomatic cancers occur after the age of 60 years and death from prostate cancer is most common among 75-year-old men. The estimated lifetime risk of developing prostate cancer is 20%, whereas the risk of dying from it is 4%. The incidence of prostate cancer in African American men is 1.5 times higher than that in white men and the mortality is twice as high in the former population. In contrast, the incidence of prostate cancer in Asian men is one half that of white males.

ETIOLOGY

Prostate cancer does not occur in castrated men indicating that androgens play a permissive role in its development. Racial variations of the tissue level of 5-α-reductase, an enzyme that converts testosterone into its more potent derivative dihydrotestosterone, may explain racial differences in the incidence of prostate cancer. The highest values are found in African American men, whereas Asian men have lower values. A family history of prostate cancer is associated with a twofold increase in the risk of this disease.

Histologically almost all prostate cancers are acinar adenocarcinomas. Small cell (neuroendocrine) tumors, squamous cell carcinomas, transitional cell carcinomas, and lymphomas are rare. The Gleason grading system classifies the prostate carcinomas into well-differentiated (score 2 to 4), moderately differentiated (score 5 to 7), and poorly differentiated (8 to 10).

Unlike benign prostatic hypertrophy (BPH), which arises in the central periurethral zone, prostate cancer usually originates from the periphery of the gland (the posterior lobe is the most common initial site). As the disease advances, the tumor extends locally and eventually invades the prostate capsule; if not treated, it invades the local structures, the pelvic walls and the seminal vesicles. The regional pelvic nodes are involved first followed by the periaortic nodes.

CLINICAL PRESENTATION

Low-grade, low-stage prostate cancer may remain asymptomatic throughout a patient's life. Initial evidence of disease may be an elevated PSA found on screening or a prostate nodule detected on digital rectal examination. Because prostate cancer arises from the periphery of the gland, it rarely causes obstructive urinary symptoms until it is locally advanced. Hematuria and hematospermia are caused by bladder or seminal vesicles invasion. Bone pain can occur from metastatic disease. Leukoerythroblastic anemia is typical for bone marrow invasion. Ureteral obstruction may result in postrenal kidney failure.

DIAGNOSIS

The diagnosis of prostate cancer is most commonly suspected after an elevated PSA is discovered on a screening examination. Less frequently, the diagnostic evaluation is triggered by an abnormal digital rectal exam. PSA is a proteolytic enzyme secreted by the prostate acinar cells that serves to liquefy the seminal plasma coagulum. Cancer cells secrete up to three times greater amounts of PSA than normal prostate cells. In healthy men, the PSA level is <4 ng/mL. It increases moderately in benign prostatic hypertrophy (4 to 10 ng/mL); values greater than 10 ng/mL should raise a high level of suspicion for prostate cancer. The level of PSA is related to the volume of cancer present and it can also roughly predict the stage of the tumor. Patients with a PSA level of 4 to 10 ng/mL have a 20% to 25% chance of having prostate cancer. Almost invariably, this is early treatable cancer. A PSA level >10 ng/mL indicates 60% chance of having cancer, while a level >20 ng/mL portends a 95% chance of having prostate cancer. Almost all of these patients have advanced nonresectable or metastatic disease.

Once prostate cancer is suspected because of a positive digital examination or an elevated PSA, a transrectal ultrasound (TRUS) should be performed. This can differentiate cancerous nodules from BPH, infection, or calcifications. TRUS can also guide the urologist in taking biopsies for prostate staging and grading analysis. Typically multiple biopsies are obtained from both prostate lobes. Even when TRUS is suggestive of prostate cancer, only 15% to 30% of the patients have a positive biopsy.

The tumor-node-metastasis classification and the clinical staging are summarized in Tables 106.1 and 106.2.

TREATMENT

Patients with very early nonaggressive cancers (stage I) can be managed by "watchful waiting." Over the subsequent 10 years, only 15% of them will have progressive disease and will require therapy. Elderly patients with asymptomatic disease and multiple comorbidities, high operative risk, or who refuse therapy should be managed in the same way.

Patients with localized prostate cancer (stage II) can be treated with curative beam radiation or radical prostatectomy. Both entities offer similar survival rates in 10 years; however, local recurrence may be higher after radiation. Treatment selection is based also on the patient's preference and the complication rate. Radical prostatectomy entails 1% mortality, 1% to 5% incontinence, and 100% impotence. Recent "nerve-sparing" prostatectomy techniques for early-stage patients appear to reduce the postoperative impotence rate to less than 50%. The late complications of curative beam radiotherapy are significant chronic radiation cystitis or proctitis in 2% to 5% of patients as well as impotence in about 50%. Brachytherapy is a relatively new radiotherapy modality that renders results similar to the classic treatment options for patients with well-differentiated tumors, but seems to be inferior in patients with high Gleason scores. All patients should be counseled extensively about the risks and benefits of both treatment options and older patients (>75 years) should have the option of watchful waiting.

Patients with capsule invasion but without hematogenous metastases (stage III) should be treated

TABLE 106.1 Tumor-node-metastasis classification for prostate cancer

Stage	Description
Local extend	
T1	Incidental histological finding of nonpalpable, nonvisualized by imaging tumor
T1a	Tumor found in <5% of the resected tissue
T1b	Tumor found in >5% of the resected tissue
T1c	Tumor found on needle biopsy
T2	Tumor confound to the prostate
T2a	Tumor involving less than half of one lobe
T2b	Tumor involving the whole lobe
T2c	Tumor involving both lobes
T3	Tumor extending through the prostate capsule
T3a	Tumor extending through the capsule
T3b	Tumor invading the seminal vesicles
T4	Tumor invading adjacent structures other than the seminal vesicles (bladder, rectum) or extending to the pelvic walls
Lymph node involvement	
Nx	Lymph nodes not assessed
N0	No regional lymph nodes metastasis
N1	Metastatic spread to regional lymph nodes
Distant metastasis	
M0	No distant metastasis
M1	Distant metastasis present
M1a	Nonregional lymph nodes
M1b	Bone metastasis
M1c	Other organs

TABLE 106.2 Staging system for prostate cancer

Stage	Tumor-node-metastasis	Gleason score
Stage I	T1a N0 MO	<2
Stage II	T1-2 N0 M0	Any
Stage III	T3 N0 M0	Any
Stage IV	T4 N0 M0 Any T N1 Any T, any N, or M1	Any

with radiation. Patients with stage IV based on positive distant lymph node involvement without bone or other organ metastases can be treated in a similar fashion. Patients with bone metastases should receive hormonal therapy. Orchiectomy is the simplest, cheapest method and has the fasted onset of affect; however it remains the least popular. Monthly or quarterly injections of (luteinizing hormone releasing hormone) (LHRH) agonists have comparable effects and side effects. In addition, their effect is reversible and avoids the patient's image of castration. Because a flare of the disease may occur from a transient rise of androgens soon after therapy starts, a short course of an antiandrogen should accompany LHRH therapy. When used alone, the nonsteroidal antiandrogens (Flutamide and Casodex) are of limited value. Exogenous estrogen therapy, although cost-effective and avoiding the hypoandrogenic syndrome ("male menopause"), is rarely used because of its risks of gynecomastia and thromboembolic disease. It is contraindicated in patients with known hypertensive or atherosclerotic cardiac disease. Patients whose metastatic prostate cancer is no longer responsive to antiandrogen therapy may benefit from treatment with the chemotherapeutic drug docetaxel.

PROGNOSIS

The prognosis depends on the stage and grade of tumor in localized disease. The 5-year survival is 88% to 95% for localized prostate cancer, 70% to 85% for locally advanced disease, and 20% to 30% for metastatic disease. Radical prostatectomy and radiation series achieve survival in the range of 70% to 75% at 10 years for stage I and II disease, but only 25% to 30% of patients with stage III disease survive 10 years (although a subset of patients with low-grade disease have prolonged survivals without active intervention). Fifty percent of patients with metastatic prostate cancer live 2 to 3 years, 20% survive 5 years, and only a few survive 10 years.

SCREENING

The asymptomatic period of prostate cancer can be longer than 10 years; the group of men most involved is of advanced age and will die of other causes rather than prostate cancer. Based on these facts, in Europe early-stage patients are not treated and there are no recommendations for screening. In the United States, there is a consensus that because early-stage cancers are potentially curable, men with a life expectancy of more than 10 years should be identified and treated. Screening with an annual digital rectal examination in addition to PSA testing is recommended for all African American men older than 45 years, all white men older than 50 years, and for all men older than 40 years with an affected first-degree relative.

Neurology

Martin Muntz, Safwan Jaradeh, and Diane Book

CHAPTER 107

Ischemic Stroke

Diane Book and Martin Muntz

Stroke is the third-leading cause of death and the leading cause of adult disability in the United States. It is increasingly considered a serious neurologic emergency warranting expedient evaluation, acute treatment, and carefully considered preventive measures. Just as effective medical and surgical interventions for coronary artery disease have evolved over the past several decades, so has management of cerebrovascular disease evolved away from a nihilistic "watch-and-wait" attitude toward an increasingly interventional and analytical approach, bolstered by the results of multiple recent successful clinical trials and advances in neuroimaging, allowing better patient selection for acute therapies.

Stroke is a sudden neurologic deficit or symptom attributable to vascular disease of the central nervous system, encompassing many diverse entities, including transient brain ischemia, brain infarction, brain hemorrhage, subarachnoid hemorrhage, and vascular disease of the spinal cord. The most common of these by far is ischemic brain infarction. Brain infarction follows cerebral blood vessel occlusion resulting from thrombosis and/or embolism. The term *transient ischemic attack* (TIA) has traditionally been defined as clinical syndromes of focal brain ischemia lasting less than 24 hours. However, most TIAs lasting more than 1 hour are associated with some degree of brain infarction, so the definition of TIA is now changed to transient clinical symptoms of stroke without evidence of infarction on brain imaging.

ETIOLOGY

Ischemic stroke results from occlusion of cerebral blood vessels, depriving the local brain tissue of oxygen and nutrients required for normal metabolic function. Vascular occlusion usually induces a territory of ischemia with the most severe deficits in blood flow at the core of this territory. Surrounding this core is tissue with varying degrees of ischemia, depending on the availability of collateral perfusion. This region, called the ischemic penumbra, may be salvageable if adequate perfusion is restored before cell death occurs. The ultimate infarction or "stroke" reflects those areas in which cell death ensued, with TIA representing the mildest end of the spectrum in which no cell death results. This exquisitely time sensitive potential to rescue ischemic penumbra from infarction drives all acute stroke therapies.

Many factors may ultimately lead to the occlusion of a cerebral blood vessel. Cerebral occlusion may result from local atherosclerosis, thrombosis, or embolism of a remote thrombus to the brain. Therefore, stroke can be viewed as the final product of diverse factors that ultimately lead to vascular occlusion. These stroke risk factors are common with cardiovascular risk factors, including hypertension, diabetes, cigarette smoking, hypercholesterolemia, alcohol abuse, and obesity. Additionally, stroke can reflect a complication of heart disease, as in atrial fibrillation or acute myocardial infarction causing cerebral embolism. Other stroke risks emerging from recent research include hypercoagulable states, specific inflammatory markers, endothelial factors, and genetic predisposition.

Clinical stroke syndromes represent the specific patterns and territory of vascular occlusion resulting from thrombosis or embolism to either small penetrating end vessels or to large vessels

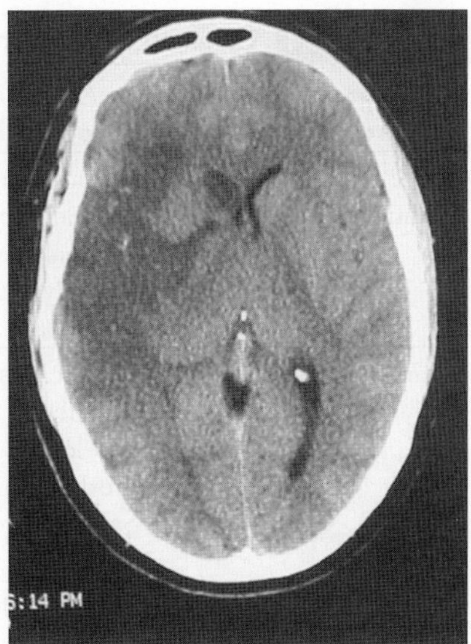

Figure 107.1 • Large vessel stroke. Computed tomography scan of brain showing a large area of ischemic infarction involving the right frontal and parietal lobes, in the territory of the middle cerebral artery (ischemic cerebrovascular accident).

(internal carotid, vertebral, middle/anterior/posterior cerebral or basilar arteries). All ischemic strokes can be categorized into one of five underlying mechanisms of stroke: embolism, large vessel disease, small vessel occlusion, cryptogenic, and other defined but unusual causes. Cryptogenic stroke is applied to unknown causes after an appropriate evaluation is unrevealing, whereas other unusual causes of stroke might include dissection, arteritis, venous infarction, or infection (Fig. 107.1).

Embolism causes ischemic stroke in one third or more of cases. Potential sources of emboli include the heart (atrial fibrillation, sick sinus syndrome, myocardial infarction with mural thrombus, dysfunctional or artificial valves, dilated cardiomyopathy, and infective endocarditis), the proximal internal carotid and vertebral arteries, the aortic arch, and the deep venous system. Patent foramen ovale is increasingly recognized as a conduit for paradoxical embolism. Emboli from the aortic arch and cervical vessels may arise from the irregular surface of atherosclerotic lesions. Hypercoagulable states, including pregnancy, oral contraceptive therapy, and antiphospholipid syndrome may increase the likelihood of embolization by promoting thrombus formation at any of these sites. Emboli most typically cause large (>1 cm) infarcts involving the cortical surface, basal ganglia, or cerebellum.

The small vessel or lacunar stroke, seen in roughly 20% of ischemic strokes, reflects disease of the small penetrating end-arterioles which have no collateral sources of flow. Occlusion arises gradually following hypertension-induced necrosis, atherosclerosis, and lipid deposition. Because the area supplied by the affected vessel is small, occlusion causes a small (<1 cm) infarct, located typically in the basal ganglia, internal capsule, thalamus, or pons (Table 107.1).

Large vessel disease represents atherosclerosis and stenosis of large feeding arteries, both extracranial (internal carotids and vertebrals) and intracranial (Circle of Willis vessels). Ischemia may result from atherosclerotic occlusion or tight stenosis of a large artery that limits cerebral perfusion distally. In that case, infarction may be visible in the cortex or deep white matter "watershed" areas (boundaries between main vascular territories). Alternatively, large vessel disease may result in local thrombosis from slow flow and endothelial factors that promote thrombosis or plaque rupture, occluding the artery and/or allowing distal embolization of the thrombus or plaque. These infarcts tend to be cortical and wedge shaped, reflecting the entire territory of the occluded artery. Other large vessel sources of ischemic stroke typically seen in younger patients include arterial dissection, vasospasm due to migraine, and cerebral vasculitis.

TABLE 107.1 Common lacunar stroke syndromes

Lacunar stroke syndrome	Clinical manifestations	Neuroanatomical location of ischemia
Pure motor hemiparesis	• Unilateral motor deficit of face, arm, and leg • Normal sensation • Mild dysarthria may be present • No aphasia, apraxia, or agnosia	Posterior limb of the internal capsule, basal pons, medial medulla, or corona radiata
Pure sensory stroke	• Unilateral sensory loss and/or paresthesia in face, arm, trunk, and leg • Normal muscle strength • Symptoms often out of proportion to examination	Thalamus (especially the ventroposterolateral nucleus) or pontine tegmentum
Ataxic hemiparesis	• Unilateral leg > arm weakness • Ipsilateral ataxia of arm and leg • Speech and facial muscles generally unaffected	Posterior limb of internal capsule, basal pons, or thalamus
Dysarthria-clumsy hand syndrome	• Unilateral supranuclear facial weakness • Tongue deviation • Dysarthria • Dysphagia • Impaired fine motor testing of the hand • Normal sensation	Basal pons or genu of internal capsule

Although more than 20 distinct syndromes have been described, these are the most prevalent.

CLINICAL MANIFESTATIONS

Neurologic symptoms of ischemic stroke begin suddenly, most often without warning or pain. Patients often minimize the urgency of their symptoms because there is no pain. The neurologic deficit may be maximal at onset in the case of acute embolism, or progress over several minutes in evolving thrombosis. Regardless, the symptoms generally peak within minutes, distinguishing ischemic infarction clinically from the evolving symptoms of migraine or focal seizure. After the initial symptoms plateau acutely, stroke signs may further evolve depending on the size of the infarct and volume of edema. Generally, in larger infarcts, symptoms progress over the first 48 to 72 hours due to focal mass effect from edema before the final deficits stabilize. In small infarcts, the neurologic deficits usually plateau within the first hours and remain stable thereafter. In most strokes, any eventual clinical recovery occurs after the insult over months and years.

The specific focal neurological deficits associated with a stroke vary by the vascular territory involved, and the extent of collaterals to the involved region (Table 107.2). For example, unilateral weakness (hemiparesis or hemiplegia) is the most frequent sign of stroke, usually from involvement of the corticospinal tract anywhere along its course descending from motor cortex through the white matter and internal capsule to the brainstem. Other common symptoms of brain ischemia include

TABLE 107.2 Stroke signs and symptoms by vascular territory

Cerebral artery	Brain area	Signs/symptoms
Anterior cerebral	Medial frontal lobes, motor cortex leg	Paralysis contralateral leg/foot Impaired gait
	Premotor cortex and anterior frontal lobes	Lack of spontaneity, poor decision-making and insight, difficulty with voluntary motor tasks, slowness of thought, cognition, urinary incontinence, grasp and suck reflexes
	Medial parietal lobes, sensory cortex leg	Sensory loss contralateral leg/foot
Middle cerebral	Lateral frontal lobe, motor cortex arm/face or basal ganglia	Paralysis contralateral arm/face Conjugate eye deviation
	Lateral parietal lobe, sensory cortex arm/face	Sensory loss contralateral arm/face
	Lateral inferior frontal, Broca's area	Nonfluent aphasia (Broca's aphasia)
	Superior temporal gyrus	Fluent aphasia (Wernicke's aphasia)
	Temporal lobe white matter, optic radiations	Homonymous hemianopia
	Parietal cortex, dominant	Acalculia, left-right disorientation, finger agnosia, agraphia
	Parietal cortex, nondominant	Hemi-inattention, anosognosia (denial of deficit)
Posterior cerebral	Occipital and medial Temporal lobes	Contralateral hemianopia, color anomia, memory deficits
	Corpus callosum (posterior)	Alexia without agraphia
	Thalamus	Contralateral sensory loss, dysesthesia, pain, memory deficits, aphasia, contralateral paralysis
	Midbrain, cerebral peduncles	Contralateral hemiplegia, oculomotor palsy
Vertebral and basilar	Cerebellum	Truncal or limb ataxia, nystagmus, vertigo, nausea, emesis
	Brainstem	Cranial nerve palsies (diplopia, facial motor/sensory, dysphagia, dysphonia, dysarthria, gaze palsy), hemiparesis, hemisensory loss

unilateral visual field deficit in both eyes (hemianopia) reflecting temporal or occipital ischemia, impaired speech production or comprehension (aphasia) from dominant hemisphere cortical injury, and unilateral sensory deficit with either parietal or thalamic ischemia. Some patients particularly with right hemispheric lesions may be unaware or only gradually aware of their own deficits (anosognosia). Brainstem ischemia (vertebrobasilar system) may cause nausea and vomiting, vertigo, gait imbalance, diplopia, dysphagia, dysarthria, or ptosis. Ischemic stroke may impair alertness or cause sudden disorientation, inability to remember new information, deviation of the eyes or head to one side, or inability to read. These features may be isolated or combined with other impairments. While not a stroke by definition, retinal ischemia (brief monocular blindness or amaurosis fugax) may be associated. Lightheadedness is not a symptom of stroke and is possibly due to anemia, hypovolemia, autonomic dysfunction, vasovagal phenomena, or cardiac arrhythmia.

DIAGNOSIS

Stroke diagnosis includes the initial decision that acute focal neurologic deficits stem from a cerebrovascular cause, then the subsequent evaluation to determine the specific mechanism of the stroke. Acute stroke is still largely a clinical diagnosis, with imaging serving to exclude other stroke mimics and to contribute to the mechanism evaluation. A stroke diagnosis rests primarily on an appropriate history and neurologic exam. The initial history must focus on the exact time of symptom onset, a description of deficits, and the exclusion of facts that indicate a stroke mimic. An accurate history of time of symptom onset often requires interview of witnesses and first responders in addition to the patient. Stroke mimics include migraine aura, focal seizure, brain tumor (unusually), hypoglycemia, and nonorganic deficits such as conversion or factitious disorder. Migraine and seizure are indicated by a history of deficits evolving over minutes to hours, often gradually progressing, reaching a plateau, and gradually remitting in reverse order. Stroke, by contrast, presents with acute and immediate deficits without a graduated time course. Brain tumor most often presents with subacute onset over days or weeks, but can sometimes present with acute deficits, requiring imaging to distinguish from stroke. Nonorganic or psychiatric strokelike presentation can be diagnosed by a careful examination to disclose nonphysiologic and effort-dependent patterns of neurological deficit.

The neurologic examination should efficiently identify the new deficits. The examiner must consider the likely vascular territories involved and tailor their examination to unmask related deficits not evident by history. For example, patients with right hemisphere stroke and anosognosia (lack of awareness of deficit) may not report any specific deficits, yet a careful examination discloses a left visual field cut and hemi-inattention to the left. A patient with fluent aphasia cannot provide an intelligible history and may just appear delirious, yet focused examination will disclose an isolated language disturbance without altered attention and arousal and intact motor function consistent with isolated temporal lobe dysfunction. Therefore, the initial history will significantly direct the initial neurologic examination.

Once the clinical history and examination suggest stroke and exclude any likelihood of stroke mimics, urgent brain imaging is required mainly to distinguish hemorrhagic from ischemic stroke and to more definitively exclude mass lesions. The current standard of care is emergency noncontrast head computed tomography (CT) scan. This test is highly sensitive to brain hemorrhage, but very insensitive to acute brain ischemia. Thus, the diagnosis of ischemic stroke remains clinical based on history and exam, as the initial brain CT merely excludes hemorrhage or mass. However, magnetic resonance imaging (MRI) is gradually replacing CT as the initial imaging test in suspected stroke because of increasing availability and certain advantages over CT. MRI can now sensitively screen for acute blood using gradient–echo sequences, and has the advantage of exquisite delineation of acute ischemia. Diffusion-weighted MRI can reveal ischemic brain tissue within minutes of onset.

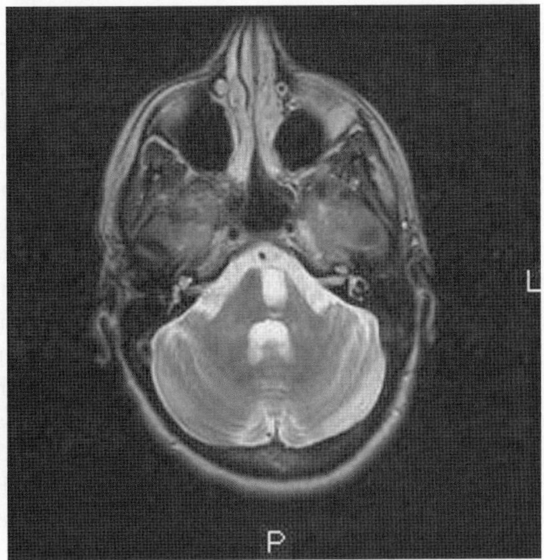

Figure 107.2 • Small vessel stroke. Magnetic resonance imaging scan of brain (T2 weighted) at the level of the lower pons. This slice demonstrates a bright wedge-shaped lesion in the ventral left pons (*arrow*), consistent with an infarction resulting from occlusion of one of the small penetrating arteries that are end arteries fed by the basilar artery, supplying the pons.

Furthermore, newer MRI and CT techniques being studied can help distinguish reversibly ischemic brain (penumbra) from infarcted brain, allowing for more careful selection of candidates for hyperacute therapies. Nevertheless, MRI takes longer to perform, requires a still patient, and is contraindicated or not tolerated in a variety of conditions, so CT will remain a necessary first imaging study for some.

After the clinical history, examination, and initial brain imaging indicate stroke (or TIA) as the diagnosis, an expedient evaluation should follow to clarify the specific stroke mechanism and modifiable risk factors. Imaging of the brain with MRI most reliably distinguishes embolic, lacunar, and watershed infarctions (Fig. 107.2). A growing variety of vascular imaging modalities are used to identify severe atherosclerotic lesions. Extracranial vessels can be imaged with duplex Doppler studies, magnetic resonance angiography (MRA), or CT angiography (CTA). Intracranial large vessels are imaged with MRA, CTA, or transcranial Doppler. Catheter angiography is now reserved for cases requiring interventional therapy (stents or intraarterial thrombolytics) or for diagnostic dilemmas such as vasculitis or hemodynamic insufficiency. Cardiac imaging with transthoracic ECHO in most cases is performed to assess the left ventricle as a potential embolic source.

Transesophageal ECHO is superior for detecting patent foramen ovale and for visualizing the left atrium, atrial appendage, and aortic arch. It should be performed in patients with suspected embolism in whom the transthoracic ECHO is not revealing. All patients should undergo 12-lead electrocardiogram and cardiac telemetry monitoring to detect myocardial ischemia and rhythm disturbances, particularly atrial fibrillation. All patients should be evaluated for hypertension, diabetes, hypercholesterolemia, smoking, and heart disease. Other commonly ordered laboratory evaluations include complete blood count, serum creatinine, and C-reactive protein. In young patients (<50 years) and older patients with no clear cause for stroke, a workup for occult hematologic abnormalities is recommended; this includes prothrombin time, partial thromboplastin time, antinuclear antibodies, serum protein electrophoresis, serological tests for syphilis, erythrocyte sedimentation rate, lupus anticoagulant, anticardiolipin antibody, factor V Leiden, homocysteine, prothrombin gene mutation, and activity of protein C, protein S, and antithrombin III. Ultimately, the risk-factor profile, vascular pathology and specific pattern of brain infarction (usually clarified with MRI) will determine which type of stroke has occurred: large vessel, small vessel, embolic, other, or cryptogenic.

MANAGEMENT

Management of ischemic stroke involves three concurrent goals. Acute treatments aim to restore cerebral perfusion and/or salvage reversibly ischemic brain tissue to limit the infarct. Stroke prevention includes the evaluation of stroke mechanism, identification of risk factors, and management of each. Promotion of stroke recovery encompasses the supportive care required to limit complications and the specific rehabilitative strategies to facilitate long-term recovery. All strokes, regardless of subtype, warrant that each of these three components be addressed in the most expedient setting possible. This usually requires acute hospitalization, where careful consideration of swallow evaluation, deep venous thrombosis prophylaxis, fall risks, and early mobilization and rehabilitation can be performed. TIA patients should similarly be urgently evaluated to institute stroke prevention therapies immediately, given the great opportunity to prevent permanent deficits.

Acute management of ischemic stroke includes airway protection as needed, electrocardiogram, and telemetry to evaluate for arrhythmia and myocardial ischemia, urgent CT to exclude hemorrhage, and neurology consultation. Correction of anemia, dehydration, hypoxemia, and glucose abnormalities is vital. Most patients with acute stroke are hypertensive at presentation, which may in part be a normal physiological pressor response to ischemia. Antihypertensive medications generally should be avoided or used with great caution acutely, and only if the systolic pressure persists above 220 mm Hg or if another medical condition warrants lowering blood pressure (for example, acute heart failure). Some form of deep venous thrombosis prophylaxis is also necessary.

Acute thrombolytic therapies to restore cerebral perfusion have become standard, with a growing menu of drug and route options. The only U.S. Food and Drug Administration–approved thrombolytic therapy is intravenous tissue plasminogen activator (tPA) administered within 3 hours of ischemic stroke. Careful evaluation is necessary before this drug is administered, given the significant risk of cerebral hemorrhage. Although still experimental, intra-arterial delivery of tPA requiring emergency catheter angiography is increasingly applied in acute stroke up to 6 hours, often in combination with early intravenous tPA. Other thrombolytic and neuroprotective agents are currently being evaluated for their ability to minimize brain injury.

Antithrombotic and anticoagulant agents are administered to prevent a second stroke, which is most likely within the first week of a stroke. Intravenous heparin is recommended for patients with cardiogenic embolism (except bacterial endocarditis), due to the significant risk of recurrent embolism during the first 2 weeks after cardiogenic stroke. The risk of fatal hemorrhage is high in patients with a very large infarct (half of a hemisphere or larger), and this outweighs the benefit of heparin in such patients. Heparin is usually given as a constant infusion, beginning with 800 to 1,000 units per hour, without a loading bolus. Heparin may also be used in patients with cranial arterial dissection, as the usual mechanism of stroke in such patients is embolism from the dissection site. Cardioembolic stroke patients are then converted to oral warfarin anticoagulation for long-term stroke prevention. Dissection usually is treated with a several-month course of warfarin while the vessel intima presumably heals. Most other stroke patients, however, have no definite indication for anticoagulation, so instead receive antiplatelet agents from the start. These agents have been shown to reduce subsequent stroke risk by 20% to 30%. The first-line options include aspirin (50 to 325 mg daily), combination aspirin (50 mg) and sustained-release dipyridamole (400 mg), and clopidogrel (75 mg daily).

Risk-factor modification represents the most potent strategy for stroke secondary prevention. Aggressive treatment of hypertension to targets less than 135/85 mm Hg, low-density lipoprotein cholesterol to less than 100 mg/dL, and diabetes, as well as tobacco cessation, are the primary interventions. Patient and family education about stroke risk factors, pharmacologic modifications, and behavioral modifications represent pivotal tasks but also major challenges. Beyond risk factors, specific vascular lesions can be modified with a growing menu of revascularization techniques. Patients with large vessel stenosis benefit from revascularization. With high-grade (>70%) carotid stenosis, carotid endarterectomy surgery is superior to aspirin in preventing stroke recurrence. Carotid angioplasty with stenting is favored in patients with high surgical risk factors. This catheter-based technology is being increasingly used in vascular beds other than the extracranial carotid artery, including intracranial vessels that are not accessible surgically. Studies to determine safety and efficacy of these procedures are ongoing.

COMPLICATIONS

Common complications of stroke include the sequelae of the focal neurologic deficits, aspiration pneumonia, deep vein thrombosis, falls, and depression. Focal neurologic deficits are entirely dependent on the location and volume of the infarct. Recovery patterns range from minimal recovery to full recovery, with the most dramatic improvements in the first several months, and more subtle recovery over years. Indeed, the absence of significant improvement in the first months predicts poor prognosis for recovery. The most common deficit, contralateral motor weakness, usually presents with initial flaccidity complicated after days or weeks by chronic spasticity, abnormal response to plantar stimulation, hemiparetic posturing with gait, and dependent edema. Deep vein thrombosis usually occurs in patients rendered bedridden or immobile by motor or sensory deficits, and dysarthria and dysphagia predict aspiration. Sensory loss can be complicated by painful neurogenic dysesthesias and temperature distortions, which can become progressively worse over time as affective neuronal circuits reorganize. Visual deficits can be diverse affecting all stimuli within a hemifield, or isolated to moving targets, colors, or certain patterns. Language deficits can range from mild word finding trouble to global aphasia. While the fluent aphasic patient with comprehension deficits (Wernicke's type) is most impaired functionally, it is the nonfluent aphasic (Broca's type) with full understanding of their limitations that most often become depressed. The possible cognitive deficits from stroke are diverse and often under recognized. Attention deficits including frank hemineglect often improve with behavioral therapies, while amnestic disorders, personality change, and behavioral syndromes are less responsive. Motor, sensory, and behavioral deficits each predispose patients to falls and subsequent traumatic injuries.

CHAPTER 108

Intracerebral and Subarachnoid Hemorrhage

Diane Book and Martin Muntz

Hemorrhagic stroke represents only 15% to 20% of all strokes. Hemorrhagic stroke includes two main subtypes: intracerebral hemorrhage (ICH) and subarachnoid hemorrhage (SAH). Risk of death and major disability from hemorrhagic stroke is much greater than from ischemic stroke.

INTRACEREBRAL HEMORRHAGE

Intracerebral hemorrhage (ICH) refers to extravasation of blood, most commonly from an arterial source, into brain parenchyma forming a hematoma.

Etiology

The most common type of intracerebral hemorrhage is the hypertensive bleed, which occurs when a small, deep vessel weakened by chronic hypertension (Bouchard's aneurysm) ruptures. These are the same vessels that may also occlude in ischemic small vessel stroke. Typical locations for hypertensive hemorrhage are deep gray matter regions supplied by the penetrating end arteries, namely the basal ganglia (especially putamen), thalamus, cerebellum, and pons. A bleed in the hemispheric white matter is not usually due to hypertension. These hemorrhages result from amyloid angiopathy in the elderly, vascular malformation, brain tumor, mycotic aneurysm, cerebral venous thrombosis, coagulopathy, anticoagulant and thrombolytic agents, hemorrhage into a cerebral infarct (so-called hemorrhagic infarction), vasculitis, and sympathomimetic drugs (including cocaine). In the elderly, amyloid angiopathy is the usual cause of recurrent hemispheric cerebral hemorrhage.

Clinical Manifestations

The classic presentation of ICH is sudden focal neurological deficit, headache, nausea, vomiting, hypertension, and early neurological deterioration. Compared to ischemic stroke, patients with intracerebral hemorrhage tend to be younger, more hypertensive, and more stuporous. Headache is more frequent than with ischemic stroke, and the neurologic deficits are more likely to progress. Nevertheless, hemorrhage should be differentiated from infarction by computed tomography (CT) scan rather than by the clinical presentation. A large bleed may raise intracranial pressure sufficiently to impair consciousness, or cause brain herniation and death. Patients who survive the acute bleed, even a fairly large one, often recover remarkably well, because permanent damage usually is limited to the ischemic zone immediately surrounding the bleed.

The focal clinical signs of ICH are the same as those listed for ischemic stroke; however, several clinical syndromes occur often, correlating with the typical locations of cerebral hemorrhage. Putaminal hemorrhage presents with contralateral hemiparesis, gaze deviation, hemisensory loss, hemianopia, and either aphasia or neglect (dominant or nondominant hemisphere). Thalamic hemorrhage produces contralateral hemisensory loss, hemianopia, some hemiparesis, and gaze palsies. Cerebellar hemorrhage induces severe nausea, vomiting, vertigo, ataxia, headache, and can cause brainstem compression and death. Signs of pontine hemorrhage include coma with extensor posturing, eye movement deficits, pinpoint pupils, and paralysis.

Diagnosis

Diagnosis of cerebral hemorrhage is based on imaging. In any acute stroke syndrome, urgent CT scan is indicated to identify hemorrhage, which appears as hyperdense (Fig. 108.1). For those with unexplained bleed and without hypertension, a search for the cause of bleeding is performed. Magnetic resonance imaging (MRI) with gadolinium contrast will detect most vascular malformations and brain tumors. Catheter angiography is often necessary to detect or exclude aneurysm, vasculitis, venous thrombosis, and very small vascular malformations. Mass effect from the hematoma during the acute period may obscure small aneurysms, tumors, and malformations. Definitive exclusion of

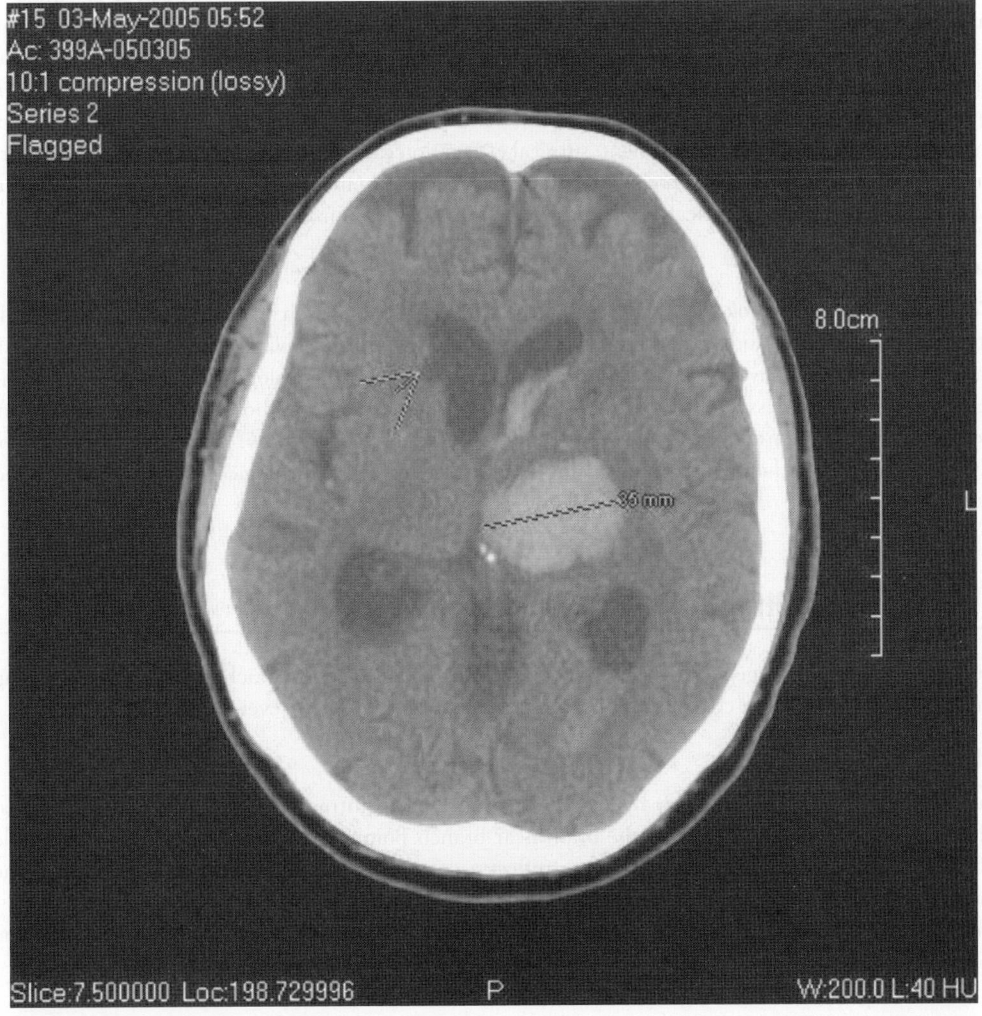

Figure 108.1 • Intracerebral hemorrhage. Computed tomography scan of brain showing intracerebral hemorrhage into the left thalamus from hypertension with extension of blood into the frontal and temporal horns of the lateral ventricle. Note the blood in the temporal horn layering with gravity in the supine patient (*white arrow*). The black lines reflect a measuring tool of the dimensions of the hematoma in the left thalamus, and mark an incidental chronic small vessel stroke on the right.

these causes requires follow-up magnetic resonance imaging and angiogram after resorption of the hematoma.

Treatment

Emergency evaluation includes CT scan, electrocardiogram, coagulation tests (including prothrombin time, partial thromboplastin time, and complete blood count with platelet count), and consideration of airway management with endotracheal intubation. Toxicology screen is useful, especially in young patients. Blood pressure, if elevated, is treated gently to maintain a mean arterial pressure below 130 mm Hg, and lower postoperatively. Urgent neurology or neurosurgery consultation should be obtained. Coagulation defects should be corrected with plasma and vitamin K. Some patients are candidates for a new drug containing Factor VII which promotes coagulation, limiting expansion of the hematoma. Alert patients with small hemorrhages may be observed on a general inpatient ward with frequent monitoring of vital signs and mental status. Patients with impaired alertness or large hemorrhages should be admitted to an intensive care unit experienced in ICH management. These patients are at high risk for deterioration, brain herniation, and death from increased intracranial pressure (ICP). Aggressive ICP management includes ICP monitoring, osmotherapy, hyperventilation, and barbiturate sedation. In patients with hemispheric intracerebral hemorrhage who deteriorate despite intensive medical treatment, surgical evacuation can relieve elevated intracranial pressure but remains controversial. In cerebellar hemorrhage, if the hematoma exceeds 3 cm in diameter, surgical evacuation is more clearly recommended to prevent brainstem compression.

Complications

Cerebral hemorrhagic stroke causes death in nearly 50% of patients, with only 20% reaching independence by 6 months. A major contributor to the mortality of ICH is elevated ICP. Elevations of ICP cause cerebral edema, hydrocephalus, herniation, and concurrent neurological deterioration. All the sequelae of critical illness may further complicate these cases, such as pulmonary embolism, infection, decubitus skin ulcers, and prolonged intubation requiring tracheostomy. Other complications of ICH are similar to ischemic infarction including permanent focal neurological deficits, seizures, and disability.

SUBARACHNOID HEMORRHAGE

Subarachnoid hemorrhage refers to leakage of blood initially into the subarachnoid space surrounding the brain, but can also be complicated by cerebral hemorrhage when severe.

Etiology

Subarachnoid hemorrhage (SAH) results from rupture of an intracranial saccular aneurysm, most of which are located at the base of the brain near branch points of the major arteries of the Circle of Willis. These aneurysms are thought to reflect a congenital defect in the muscular wall of the artery. Cerebral aneurysms are more prevalent in people with a family history of saccular aneurysms, fibromuscular dysplasia, polycystic kidney disease, coarctation of the aorta, and connective tissue diseases including Marfan syndrome.

CLINICAL MANIFESTATIONS

Subarachnoid hemorrhage is a medical emergency requiring rapid identification. The cardinal symptom of SAH is sudden, extremely severe pain in the head or neck, and it is often associated with brief loss of consciousness, nausea, vomiting, stiff neck, and focal neurological signs. Bleeding into the subarachnoid space causes the headache and meningeal signs through elevation of intracranial pressure and meningeal irritation. The focal neurologic signs—most commonly hemiparesis, aphasia, and paralysis of third and/or sixth cranial nerves—occur from local pressure or ischemic effects on nearby brain tissue and exiting nerves. The diagnosis of SAH is missed in roughly 25% of cases. Misdiagnosis is particularly common when symptoms are less severe. The combination of neck stiffness and nausea may resemble a viral syndrome, while that of headache, nausea, and photophobia may simulate migraine. One should consider SAH when there is abrupt neck pain or headache, particularly if the patient perceives the pain symptoms to be new or in any way different from past experiences.

DIAGNOSIS

Urgent CT must be done immediately when SAH is suspected. It is positive in the first 24 hours in nearly 90% of cases, with subarachnoid blood appearing as a bright area lining the brain or settling within the ventricular system on noncontrast images. Because CT may miss a small bleed, diagnostic lumbar puncture should be performed in suspicious cases to screen for xanthochromia, indicating breakdown of red blood cells in the cerebrospinal fluid. Xanthochromia in the cerebrospinal fluid may take 3 to 4 hours to appear after symptom onset, and may persist for more than a week.

Selective catheter angiography is then performed to identify the aneurysmal source of SAH. However, the initial angiogram is negative in at least 20% of cases, so repeat angiography at 1 week may be performed with a small yield. Rapid advancements in magnetic resonance angiography and CT angiography may allow these noninvasive tests to replace catheter angiography in diagnosis of some ruptured aneurysms in the future.

TREATMENT

Once SAH is diagnosed, patients should be transferred urgently to a hospital with an intensive care unit with specialized neurovascular expertise. Bed rest, stool softeners (to prevent straining with bowel movements, as Valsalva can increase ICP), analgesia, and treatment of high blood pressure are undertaken to minimize the risk of recurrence of bleeding. Nimodipine, a lipophilic calcium channel blocker, is effective in reducing brain injury from vasospasm after SAH, in a dose of 60 mg every 4 hours, given for 14 to 21 days after onset.

Definitive treatment for SAH consists of surgical clipping of the aneurysm. Additionally, catheter-delivered intravascular detachable coils are increasingly used in cases inaccessible surgically. Catheter angiography is required to locate the aneurysm and for planning a treatment approach. The trend is for surgery to be performed at the earliest possible opportunity. Many experienced centers now recommend urgent angiography and surgery on the first day after bleeding. After the aneurysm is secured, intravascular volume expansion with hypervolemia/hemodilution/hypertension therapy can lower the risk of vasospasm. When vasospasm does occur, transluminal angioplasty may effectively improve patient outcomes.

COMPLICATIONS

The most serious complications of aneurysmal SAH are rebleeding and vasospasm. Recurrent hemorrhage manifests as rapidly declining neurologic status and carries a 70% mortality rate. The risk of recurrent hemorrhage is highest in the first 24 hours and remains high for 4 weeks. Vasospasm, by contrast, is delayed to between 3 and 14 days after initial hemorrhage, and is demonstrated by repeat angiography or by transcranial Doppler ultrasound. Symptomatic vasospasm causes delayed focal ischemic symptoms leading to frank infarction in 50% of cases. Early aneurysm clipping (or coiling) and then institution of hypervolemia/hemodilution/hypertension therapy represent key measures to avoid these complications. Other common complications of aneurysmal SAH include obstructive hydrocephalus from intraventricular blood, hyponatremia, and seizures.

CHAPTER 109

Seizures

Martin Muntz and Diane Book

Seizures are defined as sudden excessive electrical discharge in the brain leading to abnormal movement, sensation, or behavior, or an alteration in consciousness. Seizures are relatively common, with the lifetime prevalence of an initial seizure approaching 10%. A seizure is not a diagnosis; rather, it is often a symptom of a structural brain abnormality or toxic or metabolic insult. Epilepsy or seizure disorder refers to a predisposition to having repetitive seizures; this may be inherited or due to underlying brain pathology.

ETIOLOGY

Structural brain abnormalities can lead to seizure. Previous stroke—either ischemic or hemorrhagic—can cause seizure, as can subdural or epidural hemorrhage. Intracranial arteriovenous malformations and aneurysms are other potential etiologies of seizures. Meningitis, encephalitis, and brain abscesses are potential infectious causes. Brain tumors, either primary or secondary, can lead to seizure—generally in the setting of progressive neurologic dysfunction over a period of days to months. A previous history of head trauma or anoxic injury can also predispose to seizure.

Toxic insults and metabolic abnormalities are also frequent causes of seizure. Intoxication with drugs such as cocaine and theophylline can cause seizure, whereas other medicines like imipenem, lithium, quinolone antibiotics, and tricyclic antidepressants (especially bupropion) can lower the seizure threshold. Seizures are also common in withdrawal from alcohol and other central nervous system depressants like benzodiazepines. Electrolyte abnormalities such as hypoglycemia, hypercalcemia, and hyponatremia are another potential cause of seizure.

CLINICAL MANIFESTATIONS

Generalized tonic-clonic seizures are caused by abnormal electrical discharges in both brain hemispheres. These seizures typically begin with sudden tonic posturing and loss of consciousness that often leads to a fall, and tonic contraction of the diaphragm leads to apnea. Alternating flexion and extension of the limbs follows. Dilated pupils, tongue biting, and urinary incontinence are also seen. Eventually, the tonic-clonic movements cease and respirations resume. The postictal period is typically marked by confusion and impaired responsiveness, which can often help in differentiating seizure from syncope. Amnesia for the time during and just prior to the seizure is also common.

The neuroanatomic location of the abnormal electrical discharge determines the manifestations of a focal seizure. In focal motor seizures, electrical disturbances in the motor cortex lead to repetitive contralateral movements. Ictal phenomena may be sensory if the abnormal discharge originates in the sensory cortex, and olfactory hallucinations can be related to seizure activity in the medial temporal lobe. Auras experienced by patients are manifestations of focal seizure as well. Alterations in consciousness can occur if the electrical disturbance involves the temporal lobe (partial complex seizure), but—in contrast to generalized seizures—falls are not usually seen. Stereotypical movements such as picking at objects or staring often accompany the state of impaired consciousness. The electrical discharges often spread quickly to contiguous areas of the brain, associated with spreading of the motor and sensory manifestations. Focal seizures can also secondarily generalize, leading to bilateral tonic-clonic motions and loss of consciousness.

Postictal paralysis, or Todd's paralysis, is a transient neurologic deficit that follows some seizures. Usually, these episodes of focal neurologic dysfunction last for minutes to hours after a seizure, but may rarely be persistent for over a day. The deficit often corresponds to the region of the brain in which a focal seizure originates, but the clinical presentation may be variable.

DIAGNOSIS

The differential diagnosis of seizure (Chapter 22) includes syncope, complex migraine, cardiac arrhythmia, transient ischemic attack, encephalopathy, and pseudoseizure. While there is no *sine que non* for seizure, the diagnosis usually is a clinical one; investigations like continuous electroencephalogram (EEG) monitoring are usually reserved for diagnostic dilemmas.

EEG and magnetic resonance imaging (MRI) are typically recommended for evaluation of a first seizure. These are not done to make the diagnosis of seizure, but rather to identify a structural or electrical abnormality that could be the causative agent. MRI is more sensitive than computed tomography scan for identifying lesions such as cerebrovascular accident, brain tumor, and vascular abnormalities that can lead to seizure. Routine laboratory testing to evaluate for electrolyte abnormality and hypoglycemia is usually done, and drug testing of the blood and urine is performed if clinically indicated. Lumbar puncture for cerebrospinal fluid analysis can be done if the clinical scenario suggests central nervous system infection.

TREATMENT

Treatment of acute seizures begins with basic life support measures—maintaining airway, breathing, and circulation. Blood glucose should be checked to rule out hypoglycemia-induced seizure, which is treated with intravenous dextrose. Intravenous benzodiazepines and fosphenytoin are often prescribed acutely to terminate a seizure. Propofol and barbiturates can also be used in patients with refractory status epilepticus.

The choice of antiepileptic medications for suppression of seizures is based on the type of seizure experienced, and the decision to start long-term medical treatment can be a controversial one based on the risk of seizure recurrence and the potential toxicity of therapy. Clinical characteristics that increase the risk of recurrent seizure include a history of traumatic brain injury, abnormal neuroimaging, focal neurologic deficit, abnormal EEG, and presentation with partial seizure. If the decision is made to begin chronic antiepileptic therapy, a single agent is started initially; dosage increases are made and/or additional medications are added incrementally in an attempt to minimize both seizure recurrence and medication toxicity. Phenytoin, carbamazepine, valproic acid, and topiramate are often chosen as first-line agents for patients with recurrent generalized tonic-clonic seizures and partial seizures, with gabapentin and lamotrigine commonly chosen as initial treatment of partial seizures as well. Drug therapy for seizure disorder is evolving rapidly, and consultation with a neurologist is usually recommended.

Multiple surgical therapies for seizure disorder refractory to antiepileptic medications are available. Cerebral foci of epileptiform activity can be resected or isolated from normally functioning brain tissue. Vagus nerve stimulators have also been implanted under the skin of the chest wall, leading to a reduction in seizures by up to 50% in half of patients who undergo the procedure.

COMPLICATIONS

Acute complications of seizure include falls and accidents during the acute event, leading to traumatic injuries. The repetitive muscle contractions themselves can cause dislocations of joints and rhabdomyolysis. The injuries obviously have the potential to be more severe if the patient is driving or operating other machinery; injuries to bystanders can also occur. Laws restricting drivers' licenses in patients with seizures vary widely by state.

Status epilepticus is defined as one single seizure lasting longer than 5 to 30 minutes or multiple frequent seizures without return to clinical baseline between ictal periods. Complications of status epilepticus include aspiration, neurogenic pulmonary edema, and long-term disability from neurologic deficits due to neuronal death. Mortality in patients presenting with a first episode of status epilepticus approaches 20%.

CHAPTER 110

Headaches

Martin Muntz and Diane Book

The symptom of pain in the face or head is one of the most common reasons for a person to be evaluated by a physician. Although patients with infrequent, minor headaches often treat themselves without seeking medical attention, a subset of the population has chronic headaches or symptoms caused by a serious underlying condition. People with chronic headache disorders not only have morbidity related to symptoms, but there is also a significant economic impact on society as a whole in lost productivity at work and school.

ETIOLOGY

The most common primary headaches are migraine headache, tension-type headache, and cluster headache. Migraine headaches often begin in young adulthood and have familial predisposition. Women are more commonly affected than men. Many stimuli have been implicated as triggers for migraine, such as menstruation, hunger, foods, caffeine, weather changes, and stress. The etiology of other primary headache disorders like cluster headache and tension-type headache are less well understood. Cluster headache occurs more commonly in men than women.

Many disorders lead to secondary headache. Irritation of pain-sensitive areas of the head and neck—such as the scalp, muscles, dura, arteries, cervical nerves, and cranial nerves III, V, VI, and VII—can lead to headache pain. Headache can also be a sign of serious disease, such as brain tumor, temporal arteritis, or hemorrhage (subarachnoid, subdural, epidural, cerebellar, or intracerebral).

CLINICAL MANIFESTATIONS

The most common primary headache disorder is tension-type headache. These headaches are typically bilateral and not exacerbated by daily activities. Photophobia and phonophobia are rare, and vomiting is atypical. Patients often describe the pain as tightness in a bandlike distribution around the head. Headache secondary to musculoskeletal disorders like cervical osteoarthritis, radiculopathy, and temporal-mandibular joint syndrome must be considered as well in a patient with these symptoms.

Migraine headaches are recurrent headaches that typically are unilateral and pulsating. They may last 4 to 72 hours; patients will often avoid the activities that exacerbate these headaches, such as physical activity, loud noises, and bright lights. Sleep may end the pain. Nausea and vomiting may occur during the attack, and an aura may precede the headache by up to an hour. Auras may consist of localized paresthesias or numbness, dysarthria, or vision problems like scintillations (bright shapes that expand through the visual field). Auras develop gradually over about 5 minutes and may last between 5 minutes to an hour.

Cluster headaches present with excruciating unilateral pain and associated autonomic dysfunction, commonly in the form of tearing, conjunctival injection, rhinorrhea, and even a transient

Horner's syndrome. These headaches often are short-lived, reaching peak intensity within 15 minutes, with the pain classically described as sharp and stabbing rather than pulsating. These headaches occur recurrently in "clusters" that last weeks to months.

Patients with headache secondary to other conditions may have symptoms that follow certain patterns as well. Subarachnoid hemorrhage (SAH) typically presents as an acute headache that is described as the worst in a patient's life. This "thunderclap headache" may be preceded by a less severe headache that denotes a sentinel bleeding event. SAH may be accompanied by photophobia, neck stiffness, meningeal signs, focal neurologic deficits, and even coma. New headaches of progressively worsening severity suggest brain tumor, subdural hemorrhage, or pseudotumor cerebri. New-onset headache in an elderly patient suggests the possibility of temporal arteritis, especially in the presence of jaw claudication, myalgias, and fever. Retro-orbital pain may be associated with glaucoma, and sinusitis can cause fever and facial tenderness, especially in the maxillary teeth. Papilledema is a sign of elevated intracranial pressure and may be seen in patients with brain tumor or hydrocephalus. Focal neurologic deficits in patients with headache suggest serious disorders like brain tumor, intracranial bleeding, or abscess.

DIAGNOSIS

A thorough and accurate history and physical examination is imperative for a clinician in the diagnostic evaluation of a patient with headache (Chapter 15). Laboratory and imaging tests are done based on the clinical presentation. The presence of focal neurologic deficits on examination or sudden and atypical features by history should prompt evaluation for secondary headache causes. Acute onset of severe headache suggests the possibility of SAH. Diagnostic evaluation often begins with computed tomography (CT) scan without contrast, but small bleeds may be missed; thus, lumbar puncture to evaluate for red blood cells is often recommended in these patients with negative CT scans. Cerebrospinal fluid analysis is also useful in patients with fever, headache, and negative neuroimaging. Contrast CT or magnetic resonance imaging can be done to evaluate for tumor or other pathology in patients with negative noncontrast CT scans with focal neurologic deficits or papilledema. Patients with papilledema and negative neuroimaging may have pseudotumor cerebri, diagnosed with elevated opening pressures on lumbar puncture. Elevated erythrocyte sedimentation rate is seen in patients with temporal arteritis, and temporal artery biopsy is done to confirm the diagnosis.

TREATMENT

Pain medication is given for symptom control in patients with headache, and the underlying cause should be discovered and treated when possible. Therapy for migraine headache has two components: acute management and prophylaxis. Some patients with migraine can be treated acutely with nonsteroidal anti-inflammatory drugs and rest, although this is usually ineffective in severe migraine. In patients inadequately treated with this regimen, 5-hydroxytryptamine-1b/d receptor agonists, such as sumatriptan, have generally replaced ergot derivatives as first-line specific therapy for migraine; oral, sublingual, intranasal, and subcutaneous preparations are available. Preparations containing opiates and barbiturates may be used in patients with symptoms resistant to these therapies, but with the added risk of rebound headache if overused. Prophylaxis of migraines is done in patients with frequent symptoms that are severe enough to limit the ability to work and do other daily activities, with agents that are able to decrease the frequency of migraines by at least 50% in most patients. These prophylactic medications include antidepressants (selective serotonin reuptake inhibitors and tricyclic antidepressants), antiepileptic medications (valproic acid and topiramate), and antihypertensives (calcium-channel blockers and beta-blockers). Pain medications often are used for treatment of patients with tension-type headache, and low-dose daily tricyclic antidepressants are also often prescribed. High-flow oxygen by face mask is recommended for acute management of cluster headache.

COMPLICATIONS

Complications of primary headache disorders typically are related to decreased productivity related to absences from work and school. Obviously, the complications of secondary headache disorder are diverse and potentially devastating depending on the underlying disorder.

CHAPTER 111

Normal Pressure Hydrocephalus

Martin Muntz and Diane Book

Normal-pressure hydrocephalus (NPH) is a rare cause of dementia, but the potential for treatment makes this an important diagnosis to consider. NPH most commonly affects patients during their sixth and seventh decade, but it has rarely been described in children and young adults.

ETIOLOGY

NPH is idiopathic, but secondary hydrocephalus can be due to disorders such as head trauma, brain tumor, intracerebral hemorrhage, and meningitis. Progressive impairment of the periventricular blood flow, especially in vessels affected by atherosclerotic disease, is hypothesized to cause the clinical deterioration in NPH.

CLINICAL MANIFESTATIONS

NPH typically manifest with the clinical triad of gait disturbance, cognitive deterioration, and urinary incontinence together with enlargement of the ventricular system on neuroimaging. The signs and symptoms of NPH, however, are insidious and progressive. The gait disturbance of NPH usually is the first to manifest, and it has been described as bradykinetic, shuffling, and "short-stepped." Patients may initially complain of difficulty with rising from a seated position, as well as ascending or descending stairs (called apraxic gait). A "giving-way" phenomenon of the lower extremities is often described. As the disease progresses, turning during ambulation often becomes difficult and may require multiple small steps—known as turning en bloc. Abnormal step cadence and height may be seen on examination, but weakness usually is not evident on manual muscle testing.

The cognitive impairment in patients with NPH can range from mild to severe and profound. Deficits in memory, recall, and concentration may occur; however, these are often overshadowed by apathy and bradyphrenia (slowed thought processes). Aphasia, apraxias, and agnosias typically are absent. As with early Alzheimer dementia, the cognitive impairment can be difficult to differentiate from depression in some cases (Table 111.1).

Urinary incontinence typically occurs late in the course of NPH, if at all. Increased urinary frequency, however, is almost always present. The stretching of the periventricular nerve fibers in NPH is hypothesized to cause partial loss of the normal inhibition of bladder contractions.

DIAGNOSIS

In patients with NPH, neuroimaging with computed tomography scan or magnetic resonance imaging typically reveals ventricular enlargement that is out of proportion to the degree of cerebral

TABLE 111.1 Comparison of clinical features of normal pressure hydrocephalus, Parkinson's disease, and Alzheimer's dementia

	Normal pressure hydrocephalus	Parkinson's disease	Alzheimer's disease
Gait abnormalities	+	+	–
Aphasia, apraxia	–	–	+
Incontinence	+	–	–
Dementia	+	–	+

atrophy. Opening pressure is normal to slightly increased during lumbar puncture; this is in contrast to the increased opening pressure seen in acute and secondary cases of hydrocephalus. Removal of 40 to 50 mL of cerebrospinal fluid (CSF) during lumbar puncture may lead to a temporary or sustained clinical improvement in the gait disorder; this is not only supportive diagnostic data, but also may predict whether a patient will respond favorably to a surgical CSF shunt. In patients who have continuous CSF pressure monitoring performed, B waves—transient increases in intracranial pressure—may be seen. Neuropsychological testing is often used as an adjunctive test to differentiate the cognitive delay of NPH from that seen in other causes of dementia, such as Alzheimer's dementia.

TREATMENT

The treatment for NPH is a surgical shunting procedure. Patients with good response to CSF removal at lumbar puncture and those with more mild symptoms are more likely to have significant improvement with a shunt. Gait abnormalities are more likely than cognitive impairment to respond favorably to CSF removal. A shunt procedure is not recommended for all patients, however. Intracerebral hemorrhage is the most feared immediate complication of the procedure, and delayed morbidity is observed due to subdural hematoma, infection, shunt obstruction, headache, and seizure. Due to these complications, patients with an unfavorable risk-to-benefit ratio—such as those with profound dementia and those with severe cerebral atrophy or white matter disease on magnetic resonance imaging—are often not offered the procedure.

COMPLICATIONS

Disability related to progressive dementia and gait abnormalities is the usual complication of NPH. Surgical shunts can also become obstructed, leading to recurrent hydrocephalus; CNS infections related to surgical shunts can be life threatening and are difficult to treat.

CHAPTER 112

Parkinson's Disease

Martin Muntz and Safwan Jaradeh

Idiopathic Parkinson's disease (PD) is the most common extrapyramidal disorder and is characterized by resting tremor, bradykinesia, rigidity, and postural instability.

PD is a neurodegenerative disorder that preferentially affects the elderly with a prevalence approaching 1% in people over the age of 65 years and 2% in people 85 years of age and older. While symptomatic treatments have improved, PD is still a significant cause of disability and increased mortality.

ETIOLOGY

Degeneration of dopaminergic neurons in the basal ganglia—especially in the substantia nigra—leads to the features of parkinsonism in PD. Cytoplasmic inclusions called Lewy bodies are present in the remaining dopaminergic neurons on pathologic examination. Although several genes have been linked to PD, about 85% of patients do not have an affected first- or second-degree relative. There is no definite environmental cause of PD, and the incidence of PD seems to be decreased in both cigarette smokers and people who drink caffeine. Despite active research, the mechanism of neuron degeneration is still unknown.

Drug-induced parkinsonism typically manifests symmetric findings, which can help differentiate this entity from idiopathic PD. Neuroleptic antipsychotics like haloperidol and antiemetics such as metoclopramide can lead to parkinsonism. This is an acute self-limited disorder, although clinical resolution can be delayed for weeks to months after discontinuation of the etiologic agent. Rarely, other conditions may present with parkinsonism, such as hydrocephalus, head trauma, and cerebrovascular disease.

CLINICAL MANIFESTATIONS

Tremor is a common presenting complaint in PD, but the other classic features (bradykinesia, rigidity, and postural instability) are often more difficult to elicit when taking a history. Patients with PD may describe asymmetric limb weakness, clumsiness, stiffness, and aching as manifestations of both rigidity and bradykinesia. Turning in bed and opening jars may also be difficult. Gait is often slow to initiate, and patients may describe difficulty in rising from a seated position. Impairment of fine repetitive tasks—such as brushing teeth, fastening buttons, and tying shoes—is a common presenting complaint.

The tremor of PD is a rest tremor, and it should be observed with patient's hands resting on the table or the patient's knees. It is a slow tremor (typically 4 to 6 oscillations per second) and it is often asymmetric, especially at its onset. Repetitive flexion and extension of the second finger against the thumb produces the classic pill-rolling tremor of parkinsonism. The tremor abates when the patient is asleep, and it is worsened during times of emotional distress. Patients often exhibit small and irregular handwriting (micrographia), which can help differentiate the tremor of PD from that of essential tremor where large and tremulous handwriting is common.

Rigidity refers to involuntary limitation of skeletal muscle movement. Stiffness and pain with passive range of motion is commonly seen on physical examination with the patient relaxed. Often, there is cog-wheel rigidity or involuntary resistance to range of motion that is intermittent and jerky, similar to the movement of gears and cogs.

Bradykinesia, like tremor, often begins asymmetrically in patients with PD. Although patients may describe weakness, manual muscle strength testing and reflexes are normal in the absence of a second diagnosis. Physical examination shows difficulty with fine repetitive motion, such as tapping the fingers and toes, twiddling the thumbs, and making circles with the hands. These movements are slow and have irregular cadence and low amplitude in patients with parkinsonism.

Gait is also often abnormal in PD; this is a manifestation of postural instability. The "get up and go test" is done by having a patient stand up from a seated position without the use of the arms, which are kept at the patient's side. It is frequently difficult for patients with PD to perform this task, despite normal muscle strength. Patients become stooped and the normal swinging motion of the arms during walking is lost—the arms frequently are kept at the patient's side. Later in the disease process, steps are short and shuffling, and freezing and falls are not uncommon. Patients may also walk at an increasing speed in attempt to prevent falling due to the abnormal center of gravity from stooped posture; this is the so-called festinating gait. Initiating and stopping gait is often difficult. The distance between the feet is usually normal or narrow, and a wide-based gait suggests an alternate diagnosis.

The Myerson's sign (abnormal glabellar reflex testing) can be another clue to the diagnosis of PD. The glabellar reflex test is performed by repeatedly tapping the skin of the forehead between the eyes. In normal subjects, there is reflex orbicularis oculi muscle contraction causing the eyes to blink; however, the reflexive blinking normally stops after 5 to 6 taps on the forehead. In patients with PD, however, blinking is persistent; this is referred to as Myerson's sign.

DIAGNOSIS

The diagnosis of PD is clinical and based on careful history and physical examination. Although ancillary tests are occasionally done to rule out other diagnoses, there are no specific imaging or laboratory tests needed to make the diagnosis in most cases. Response to a therapeutic trial with levodopa has been used as a diagnostic test occasionally, but the symptoms of patients with mild disease often do not justify treatment. The diagnosis is more evident in patients with more severe disease; thus, therapeutic trial with levodopa is often unnecessary for diagnosis in these patients.

The differential diagnosis of PD and parkinsonism is important (Table 112.1). Parkinsonism is a syndrome where Parkinson-like signs have different etiologies such as vascular or degenerative diseases. Up to a quarter of patients receiving an initial diagnosis of PD are misdiagnosed. Signs and symptoms that should suggest alternate diagnoses include marked autonomic dysfunction, abnormal eye movements, Babinski's sign, urinary retention, and falls or dementia early in the disease course. Development of disability within 5 years of the appearance of symptoms also should prompt further evaluation for other diseases. The so-called Parkinson-plus syndromes where Parkinsonism is associated to other neurobiological diseases, such as multisystem atrophy and progressive supranuclear palsy are commonly initially misdiagnosed as PD, but respond poorly to therapy and progress more rapidly than PD. Evaluation by a neurologist is necessary if one of these disorders is suspected.

TABLE 112.1 Comparison of primary and secondary clinical features for Parkinson's disease

	Primary idiopathic Parkinson's disease	Secondary Parkinson's disease or Parkinsonism (due to small vessel disease, or other degenerative disorders)
Bradykinesia	+	+
Tremors	+	+/−
Gait impairment	+	+
Systemic increase of muscle tone	+	−
Autonomic dysfunction	−	+
Response to levodopa treatment	+	−

TREATMENT

Many nonpharmacologic therapies are available for patients diagnosed with PD. Education about the variable course of disease and rate of progression can be helpful, and many support groups are available both for patients and family members of patients with PD. Exercise and physical therapy, especially gait and balance training, may improve patients' ability to perform activities of daily living in the short term.

Several different medications are available to treat symptoms of PD, but the optimal timing for beginning drug therapy is uncertain. Short-term clinical trials suggest that the medications do not cause neuron toxicity, but some neuroimaging studies have shown a reduction in dopamine transporters after treatment. Thus, drug therapy generally is reserved until the point when symptoms become significantly bothersome or begin to cause disability. Dopamine agonists and levodopa, a dopamine precursor, are usually utilized as first-line agents for motor symptoms of PD. Levodopa is often combined with carbidopa (a peripheral decarboxylase inhibitor) to decrease the conversion of levodopa to dopamine before the drug reaches the brain. Failure to respond to an adequate dose of levodopa after a 3-month period occurs in less than 10% of patients. Motor fluctuations and other side effects, such as dyskinesias and painful dystonias, seen with levodopa therapy can limit the utility of this medication. The "on-off phenomenon" is a severe form of motor fluctuations with sudden shifts between mobility and immobility toward the end of the levodopa dosing interval.

Dopamine agonists, such as pramipexole, ropinirole, and pergolide, seem to be slightly less efficacious than levodopa, and they are often avoided in patients with dementia due to somnolence and hallucinations that are seen with these agents. However, a significantly lower rate of motor fluctuations is reported with dopamine agonists. Anticholinergic agents, monoamine oxidase B (MAO-B) inhibitors, and amantadine are less effective than dopamine agonists but are used as second-line agents or added when tremor becomes increasingly severe. Side effects such as confusion and hallucinations often limit their utility, especially in the elderly. Some clinical trials have suggested that MAO-B inhibitors, dopamine agonists, and coenzyme Q10 are neuroprotective agents that can slow the progression of PD, but further studies are needed to clarify this effect.

Potential surgical treatments for PD include thalamotomy or implantation of a deep-thalamic brain stimulator for tremor that is severe and unresponsive to medical therapy. Pallidotomy and subthalamic deep-brain stimulators can improve all aspects of PD, but are generally reserved for ambulatory patients with advanced disease due to cost and potential complications such as hemorrhage and infection.

COMPLICATIONS

Motor disability is the major complication of PD. Gait and balance dysfunction worsen as the disease progresses, leading to falls and limited ability to ambulate. Tremor can impact even the simplest of daily activities. Motor fluctuations caused by drug therapy often worsen and become debilitating with ongoing administration after 4 to 6 years. Sleep disturbances and hallucinations are other medication side effects that can be particularly disabling. Dementia also is frequently diagnosed in patients with advanced PD.

CHAPTER 113

Peripheral Neuropathy

Martin Muntz and Safwan Jaradeh

Peripheral neuropathy is a common neurologic disorder that is defined generally as any disease of the peripheral nervous system. Its prevalence rises from 2.4% in the general population to about 8.0% in people over the age of 55 years. Because peripheral neuropathy has many different causes and variable manifestations, a careful clinical examination and logical selection of diagnostic tests is crucial in the evaluation of patients suspected of having this problem. Classification into the distinct subtypes of mononeuropathy, mononeuritis multiplex, and polyneuropathy is a necessary step in the diagnosis and management of this heterogeneous disease.

ETIOLOGY

The list of etiologic agents for peripheral neuropathy is long, and this section should not be interpreted as a comprehensive list; rather, some of the more common causes will be discussed here. Diabetes mellitus is the leading cause of peripheral neuropathy in the United States and other developed countries, while leprosy is another common cause of neuropathy in some underdeveloped countries. Vitamin B_{12} deficiency and renal insufficiency are examples of metabolic derangements that can cause peripheral neuropathy. Infectious diseases such as human immunodeficiency virus, West Nile virus, and Lyme disease can also lead to neuropathy. Medication lists of patients should be examined closely, as common medications such as amiodarone, hydralazine, metronidazole, and phenytoin are just a few examples of the long list of drugs that can cause peripheral neuropathy. Several antiretroviral medications (nucleoside reverse transcriptase inhibitors) and chemotherapeutic antineoplastic agents (paclitaxel, cisplatin, and vincristine) have also been identified as etiologic agents. Toxins such as ethanol, organophosphates, and heavy metals (lead, arsenic, and mercury) can produce peripheral neuropathy as well.

Peripheral neuropathy can be a paraneoplastic syndrome, especially in patients with small cell lung cancer and breast cancer, and it can be a manifestation of hematologic diseases like multiple myeloma, lymphoma, and cryoglobulinemia. Vasculitis typically causes mononeuritis multiplex, as can systemic diseases like sarcoidosis and amyloidosis. Genetic disorders like subtypes of Charcot-Marie-Tooth disease cause neuropathy as well. Table 113.1 describes etiologies of acquired polyneuropathy.

CLINICAL MANIFESTATIONS

Patients with peripheral neuropathy have diverse symptoms and findings, and the constellation of manifestations in a particular patient is important in distinguishing among the subtypes and in tailoring the evaluation. There is usually some combination of pain, weakness, paresthesia, anesthesia, muscle atrophy, and autonomic dysfunction. Neuropathic pain is often described as burning and

TABLE 113.1 Etiological diagnosis of acquired polyneuropathy

I	Immune: acute inflammatory demyelinating polyneuropathy or Guillain-Barré syndrome, chronic inflammatory demyelinating polyneuropathy, sarcoidosis, connective tissue disorders
N	Nutritional deficiencies and malabsorption: vitamins B_1, B_6, B_{12}, folate, and vitamin E
D	Diabetes mellitus
I	Infections: leprosy, Lyme disease, HIV, herpes zoster, diphtheria
C	Cancer ad dysproteinemia
A	Alcoholism
T	Toxic-metabolic: pharmaceutical or environmental, renal or hepatic failure
E	Endocrine causes: hypothyroidism, acromegaly

shooting, and patients often complain of "electric shock" sensations. Allodynia—pain due to a stimulus that would generally not be painful—and exaggerated pain sensations to a noxious stimulus (hyperalgesia) can be present and may be disabling.

A focal neuropathy that affects a single peripheral nerve is known as mononeuropathy, and this can occur at essentially any peripheral nerve. Compression, trauma, and entrapment are the most common causes of mononeuropathy. Pain, weakness, and/or paresthesias localized in a peripheral nerve distribution suggest this diagnosis. Entrapment of the median nerve in the carpal tunnel causes the most common mononeuropathy—carpal tunnel syndrome.

Mononeuritis multiplex is characterized by the involvement of several distinct peripheral nerves simultaneously or serially. This subtype of neuropathy is often rapidly progressive and associated with systemic illnesses such as vasculitis, cancer, sarcoidosis, and infection—making expedient identification and evaluation important. Diabetic amyotrophy is characterized by acute pain and asymmetric weakness of the lower extremities; it mimics mononeuritis multiplex and is likely caused by vasculitis of lumbosacral plexus nerves.

Polyneuropathy, the third subtype of peripheral neuropathy, is a diverse collection of peripheral neuropathies. Distal symmetric polyneuropathy, the most common variety of this disorder, affects peripheral nerves in a length-dependent manner. Because nerves to the hands and feet are among the longest in the body, there is often a "stocking and glove" distribution of symptoms at the onset of the disease. The signs and symptoms then often progress proximally. Metabolic derangements and toxins are the most common causes of polyneuropathy, with diabetic polyneuropathy being the prototype.

DIAGNOSIS

In patients with typical history and physical findings of a common peripheral neuropathy like carpal tunnel syndrome or diabetic polyneuropathy, no further diagnostic testing is required. Laboratory testing is based on the clinical scenario. Electrodiagnostic testing can be done if the diagnosis is in doubt, and also to objectively clarify the anatomic sites of involvement in certain cases. Investigation of the underlying etiology is also important, especially in patients with mononeuritis multiplex; peripheral nerve biopsy is often done in these patients to evaluate for vasculitis. Autonomic testing can also be performed in specialized centers to evaluate patients with symptoms of autonomic instability.

TREATMENT

If an underlying medical disorder or anatomic lesion is discovered, therapy should be directed against the specific etiology. In the case of vasculitis-induced mononeuritis multiplex, immunosuppressive agents like steroids are often used. Control of symptoms such as neuropathic pain is also important, and several classes of medications have been used with varying degrees of success. Antiepileptics, such as gabapentin and carbamazepine, and antidepressant medications are often utilized, but opioid pain medications are often given if first-line agents fail.

COMPLICATIONS

Like the clinical manifestations, complications of peripheral neuropathy vary based on subtype and etiology. Foot ulcers often complicate diabetic neuropathy, and falls can complicate neuropathy associated with decreased proprioception or autonomic dysfunction.

CHAPTER 114

Multiple Sclerosis

Martin Muntz and Safwan Jaradeh

Multiple sclerosis (MS) is a central nervous system (CNS) autoimmune disorder characterized by at least two demyelinating lesions separated in space (location in the CNS) and time. The typical onset is in the third or fourth decade of life, and women are twice as likely as men to acquire the disease. The clinical manifestations, as well as the prognosis, are variable. The relapsing-remitting type of MS accounts for about 80% of patients; it is characterized by acute signs and symptoms that evolve and then improve spontaneously or with treatment. Conversely, the other 20% of patients typically present with CNS dysfunction that slowly evolves over months at the onset; this is called primary progressive MS. Secondary progressive MS occurs when patients with relapsing-remitting MS experience ongoing worsening of neurologic dysfunction without recovery between episodes.

ETIOLOGY

Pathologically, the hallmark of disease is the demyelinated plaque due to a loss of myelin with preservation of axons. These plaques, on magnetic resonance imaging (MRI), are usually round or oval-shaped with finger-shaped projections called Dawson's fingers, which typically run perpendicular to the periventricular white matter. The impulses conducted along the demyelinated axons are delayed compared to the rapid saltatory conduction of unaffected axons, and leading to the manifestations of MS.

Genetic predisposition certainly plays a role in the pathogenesis of MS. The concordance rate for monozygotic twins approaches 31%, as compared to 5% in dizygotic twins. There is a 5% risk of developing MS for people who have a first-degree relative with the disease, significantly higher than that of the general population.

In addition to the genetic predisposition, environmental factors are believed to contribute to the development of MS. These factors are not well understood, but many epidemiologic studies have demonstrated regional variation in the incidence of the disease. MS is most common in northern Europe, Australia, and the central portion of North America, where the prevalence is more than 30 per 100,000; also, the risk of developing MS seems to be modified by emigrating from a low-risk region to a high-risk region, or vice versa. Infectious etiologies, such as *Chlamydia pneumoniae* and human herpesvirus 6, have been suggested but are yet unproven.

CLINICAL MANIFESTATIONS

The initial signs and symptoms of MS, like the clinical course, are variable and unpredictable. One of the common presenting clinical scenarios is optic neuritis, which is characterized by painful monocular vision loss. Other patients present with weakness, paresthesias, ataxia, and impaired gait. An-

TABLE 114.1 Common clinical presentation patterns of MS and related pathophysiologic mechanisms

Clinical presentation	Pathophysiologic mechanism
Optic neuritis with monocular blindness (may be associated with transverse myelitis) Diplopia due to internuclear ophthalmoplegia	Cranial nerve dysfunction
Unilateral weakness (hemiplegia) Paresthesias (sensory changes) Generalized weakness or fatigue	Involvement of pyramidal and sensory pathways
Ataxia, vertigo, clumsiness	Cerebellar dysfunction

other classic symptom heralding the diagnosis of MS is diplopia, suggesting internuclear ophthalmoplegia. The onset of this neurologic dysfunction may be gradual or sudden (Table 114.1).

Besides the presenting complaints discussed above, patients with MS may describe other symptoms. Lhermitte's sign is an "electrical" sensation that travels down the spine and into the limbs with flexion of the neck. Symptoms of neurogenic bladder and bowel are common, as are clumsiness, vertigo, and fatigue. Increase in the severity of complaints with transient increase in body temperature—after a hot bath, for example—or with fever is called Uhthoff's symptom and is suggestive of MS. Paroxysmal episodes of pain, paresthesias, clumsiness, dysarthria, or tonic limb posturing also suggest the diagnosis. These recurrent stereotypical phenomena typically last a couple of minutes and occur after specific movements or sensory input.

The physical examination of a patient with MS is also variable and dependent on the distribution of clinical CNS involvement. Focal weakness and ataxia are common with relapses. An afferent pupillary defect suggests current or prior optic neuritis, and this is elicited with a swinging flashlight test. The examiner shines a light in alternating eyes, and the pupil of the affected eye constricts when the light is shone in the opposite eye (consensual response) and appears to dilate when the light source is quickly shone in the affected eye due to decreased direct response. Internuclear ophthalmoplegia can be detected by testing horizontal gaze. Adduction is decreased in one eye, and concurrent nystagmus is observed in the abducting eye, leading to the diplopia described by the patient. This may be unilateral or bilateral. Spasticity often dominates the physical examination of patients with progressive disease, but all types of upper motor neuron focal neurologic deficits may be present. Tremor is common in patients with cerebellar disease.

DIAGNOSIS

The initial signs and symptoms of MS often resolve spontaneously; thus, an increased index of suspicion is required to make an early diagnosis in many cases. The diagnosis is based on CNS lesions or "attacks" that are disseminated in space and time in patients with relapsing-remitting disease. The first attack must be clinical, but the second lesion required for diagnosis may be clinical or based on diagnostic testing (MRI, cerebrospinal fluid analysis, and evoked potentials). Demyelinating plaques appear in the white matter as hypointense lesions on T1-weighted images and hyperintense on T2-weighted images (Fig. 114.1). Enhancement with gadolinium is associated with acute demyelination and can help suggest age differences among lesions on MRI. Plaques on MRI are about 15 times more frequent than new clinical events, and these plaques often do not correspond to any specific clinical complaint.

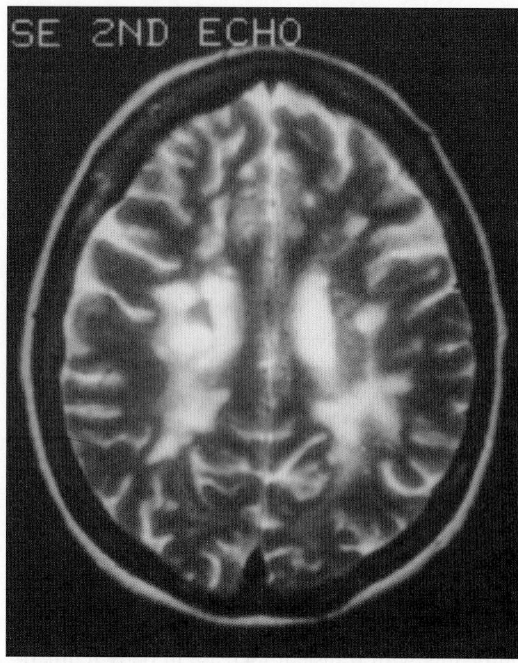

Figure 114.1 • T2-weighted image of head MRI from a patient with multiple sclerosis, showing the presence of foci of hyperintense signal in the periventricular white matter bilaterally ("Dawson's fingers").

Cerebrospinal fluid (CSF) analysis is another helpful adjunctive test that can be useful in the diagnosis of MS. Oligoclonal immunoglobulin G bands are seen on CSF electrophoresis in about 90% of patients with MS. These bands are absent on serum electrophoresis in these patients, representing inflammation specifically in the CNS. CSF analysis is especially helpful to exclude infectious and neoplastic etiologies of neurologic dysfunction. Lymphocytic pleocytosis with fewer than 50 white blood cells is frequently seen in the CSF of patients with MS as well.

Somatosensory and visual evoked potentials can provide physiologic evidence of subclinical demyelination, thus aiding in the diagnosis by documenting a second lesion that is distinct from the initial clinical event. Visual evoked potentials may be the most helpful, as it may provide evidence of a previous episode of optic neuritis that is not evident on MRI.

TREATMENT

There are several goals of MS therapy, including attenuation of the severity and duration of relapses, reduction of relapse frequency, prevention of disability related to progressive disease, and symptomatic management of complications and disability. Corticosteroids are the mainstay of treatment of acute MS relapses; there is good evidence that steroids hasten recovery. Infection must first be ruled out as the underlying etiology of a patient's exacerbation of neurologic dysfunction, as resultant immunosuppression from steroid therapy may worsen the inciting infectious process. There is no evidence to suggest the optimal dose, form, or duration of steroid therapy, but intravenous methylprednisolone is often given for 5 days followed by a short tapering course of oral prednisone. There is also evidence to suggest benefit of plasmapheresis treatment in severe steroid-unresponsive MS exacerbation. Patients with bulbar muscle weakness should be monitored closely to ensure proper airway protection and oropharyngeal secretion clearance.

Several therapies have been shown to have some efficacy in decreasing the frequency of exacerbations in relapsing-remitting MS. Interferon beta-1a (Avonex), interferon beta-1b (Betaseron), and glatiramer acetate (Copaxone) have all been shown to reduce the rate of clinical relapse and the development of new lesions on MRI.

Several symptomatic treatments are available for patients with MS. Mild spasticity can be managed with stretching and physical therapy. Muscle relaxants like baclofen and tizanidine can be used to treat patients with spasticity unresponsive to physical therapy, and intrathecal administration of baclofen with an indwelling pump can be helpful in patients whose muscle spasm is resistant to other therapies. Education to avoid high temperatures and prevent viral illnesses can reduce Uhthoff's symptom, which may resemble an exacerbation of the disease. Paroxysmal symptoms—paresthesias and tonic posturing, for example—can be treated with antiepileptic therapy such as phenytoin or carbamazepine. Amantadine and modafinil have been used for fatigue associated with MS, with some success.

Treatment of neurogenic bladder with oxybutynin or tolterodine can reduce symptoms of urgency and incontinence, but indwelling or intermittent catheterization may be needed eventually. Sexual dysfunction, as a result of MS or therapies for depression, is often treated with medications such as sildenafil or similar agents.

COMPLICATIONS

Depression and disability from fixed neurologic deficits are the commonly observed complications of MS, and a multidisciplinary approach to these problems is recommended. After the initial diagnosis is made, education should be provided on the disease manifestations, clinical course, variability, and potential for disability characteristic of MS. Physical, occupational, and speech therapists, along with psychologists and social workers, all play a significant role in optimal management of these patients, and they should be consulted early in the course of the disease.

CHAPTER 115

Amyotrophic Lateral Sclerosis

Martin Muntz and Safwan Jaradeh

Amyotrophic lateral sclerosis (ALS), or Lou Gehrig's disease, is a progressive neurodegenerative disorder characterized by the presence of both upper and lower motor neuron signs. The average life expectancy of this fatal disease is 3 to 5 years after the onset of symptoms, and there is no known cure. The prevalence is between 5 and 7 per 100,000 and it afflicts individuals over the age of 20 years, most often in the sixth decade of life.

ETIOLOGY

Pathologically, astrocytic gliosis replaces the degenerating motor neurons in ALS. The underlying inciting factor is unknown in sporadic cases, which make up the great majority of patients. About 5% to 10% of cases are familial, with defects in the superoxide dismutase 1 gene and other chromosomal abnormalities identified. Historically, weakness due to motor neuron degeneration was observed after lead and mercury intoxication; however, monitoring of occupational lead and mercury exposure has prevented this occupational health risk.

CLINICAL MANIFESTATIONS

The initial clinical manifestations of ALS depend on the regional site of involved motor neurons: cervical, thoracic, lumbosacral, or bulbar. Often only one site—frequently one limb—is affected at the onset of disease, and patients have progressive regional complaints prior to involvement of other regional sites. Patients with cervical or thoracic disease may describe difficulty with fine motor activities such as buttoning clothes and writing. Clumsiness while walking or climbing stairs is a typical complaint of those presenting with lumbosacral disease. Bulbar disease often leads to hoarseness, dysarthria, or dysphagia. Other patients initially complain of fatigue, dyspnea, muscle cramping, or weight loss.

Classically, both upper and lower motor neuron signs are evident on the physical examination. Lower motor neuron (LMN) findings such as weakness on manual muscle testing, muscle atrophy, and fasciculations are typical. Upper motor neuron (UMN) signs include hyperreflexia, spasticity, clonus, and Babinski's sign or other pathologic reflexes. Sensory abnormalities, dementia, and autonomic nervous system dysfunction are very rare in ALS, and alternative diagnoses should be considered if these are present.

Weakness of the respiratory muscles leads to hypoventilation, initially at night. Poor sleep, nightmares, morning headaches, and daytime somnolence can occur in patients with hypercarbia at night, similar to patients with obstructive sleep apnea. Frank dyspnea during the day may occur as respiratory muscle weakness progresses. Periodic pulmonary function testing is recommended to identify patients who may need treatment of hypoventilation.

DIAGNOSIS

There is no specific serologic or radiologic test for ALS—the diagnosis is mainly clinical. Both LMN and UMN findings must be present, and there must be evidence of progressive spread within one region (cervical, thoracic, lumbosacral, and bulbar) or to other regions. Evidence of other disease processes on imaging or electrodiagnostic tests that could explain the findings of a particular patient must also be absent.

Electrodiagnostic testing with nerve conductions and electromyelogram documents the presence and extent of lower motor neuron loss. It also aids in differentiating ALS from other conditions such as multifocal motor neuropathy, although the latter does not cause UMN findings on exam. UMN lesions can sometimes be seen with magnetic resonance imaging.

TREATMENT

There is only one medication approved by the U.S. Food and Drug Administration for ALS. The glutamate antagonist riluzole has been shown to prolong survival by an average of 3 to 6 months in two trials. There was no benefit, however, in any functional or symptomatic measurements in either trial. Treatment of depression, which is believed to be very common in patients with ALS, is frequently recommended. Several types of noninvasive ventilation, such as bilevel positive airway pressure, can be used at home to improve quality of life for patients with respiratory complaints. Nutritional support can be provided with tube feeding in the setting of progressive dysphagia.

COMPLICATIONS

Progressive muscle weakness and respiratory failure are the major complications of ALS. Worsening dysphagia from bulbar muscle weakness leads to weight loss and aspiration. After the diagnosis of ALS is made, the physician must counsel the patient on the progressive and fatal nature of this disease. There should be ongoing discussions regarding many issues, including advanced directives and goals of care. The potential risks and benefits of prolonged mechanical ventilation and tube feeding must be included in these ongoing discussions.

CHAPTER 116

Guillain-Barré Syndrome

Martin Muntz and Safwan Jaradeh

Guillain-Barré syndrome (GBS) is a polyneuropathy of acute onset with an annual incidence of between 1 and 4 cases per 100,000 population worldwide. Several distinct subtypes of the syndrome have been described, including acute inflammatory demyelinating polyradiculoneuropathy (AIDP), which will be discussed in this chapter. AIDP is the most common subtype of GBS, comprising about 95% of cases in North America and Europe. It is caused by an immune attack directed mainly at peripheral nervous system myelin sheaths, leading to the extensive demyelination that accounts for the ascending paralysis and other clinical manifestations of the disease.

ETIOLOGY

About one third of cases are idiopathic, as no obvious trigger is identified. In most cases, infections such as upper respiratory tract infections or especially *Campylobacter jejuni* precede the condition. *Mycoplasma pneumoniae* and viruses—including cytomegalovirus and Epstein-Barr virus—have also been implicated as triggers of GBS. Immunizations—including tetanus toxoid, influenza vaccine, and rabies vaccine—have been suspected of causing GBS as well. Clusters of GBS cases have occurred in association with other illnesses and events (such as surgery, childbirth, or immunization), leading to the proposal of causative relationships. Signs and symptoms of GBS typically occur within 6 weeks of the manifestations of the infection, which often include gastroenteritis and flulike symptoms. It is hypothesized that antibodies synthesized in response to certain infections crossreact with myelin sheath or Schwann cell components, resulting in peripheral nerve demyelination.

CLINICAL MANIFESTATIONS

GBS should be suspected in patients who complain of acute muscle weakness and other neurologic symptoms, especially after a recent febrile illness. Most cases begin with numbness, paresthesia, and weakness in the distal extremities; rapid proximal progression of ascending paralysis is typical. On physical examination, deep tendon reflexes are absent or hypoactive, and muscle weakness is usually symmetric. Muscle wasting is often delayed, but can be detected in severe cases. Also frequently affected are cranial and autonomic nerves, and dysfunction of the latter can lead to hypertension, cardiac arrhythmia, postural hypotension, urinary retention, and ileus. Inability to protect the airway and facial muscle weakness are frequent manifestations of cranial nerve involvement in patients with GBS.

Severity of disease peaks between 2 and 4 weeks in most patients; respiratory muscle weakness leads to hypoventilation and the need for mechanical ventilation in up to 25% of cases. After a plateau phase of variable length, improvement in proximal muscle strength begins. Over weeks to months, neurological recovery progresses in the opposite direction of the onset of the disease, from proximal to distal.

DIAGNOSIS

The differential diagnosis for a patient with acute flaccid paralysis is extensive. However, data from neurophysiologic electrodiagnostic studies and cerebrospinal fluid (CSF) analysis in the setting of a patient with typical clinical manifestations can help confirm the diagnosis of GBS. Neurophysiologic studies are important not only in diagnosing GBS, but also in differentiating among its subtypes and in the prognosis. In AIDP, the findings on nerve conduction studies demonstrate the demyelination that produces the clinical manifestations. These electrodiagnostic studies can be normal early in the disease, but testing becomes diagnostic in all but the most mild of cases as the disease progresses; thus, they should be repeated serially and expanded to include more nerves if the initial testing is normal.

Lumbar puncture with CSF analysis can also assist with making the diagnosis. There is an elevated CSF protein concentration without associated pleocytosis; this phenomenon is known as albuminocytologic dissociation and is characteristic of GBS. An elevated CSF white blood cell count associated with acute muscle weakness is suggestive of an alternative diagnosis, especially infectious or neoplastic. The timing of the lumbar puncture is important, as the CSF protein level can be normal for the first 48 hours after symptoms begin. Also, the sample should preferably be obtained before treatment is begun, since intravenous immunoglobulin therapy may cause aseptic meningitis with elevated CSF white blood cell count.

Differentiation between GBS and chronic inflammatory demyelinating polyradiculoneuropathy (CIDP) is based on the timing of the nadir of disease. When the progression of disease extends beyond 4 weeks, patients are likely to have CIDP, as opposed to those who develop a disease severity nadir before 4 weeks consistent with GBS. Patients with CIDP are likely to have a relapsing-remitting or a more chronic course of disease than that of patients with GBS.

TREATMENT

Both supportive and specific therapies are important in the treatment of GBS. Multidisciplinary supportive measures are essential in detecting and managing the potentially fatal consequences of this disease. Serial vital capacity and negative inspiratory force should be monitored closely with transfer to an intensive care unit for early endotracheal intubation and mechanical ventilation if these parameters worsen, as respiratory failure may occur in about one-quarter of GBS cases. Abnormalities in cardiac rhythm and vital signs are often the first signs of autonomic complications of the disease; thus, it is important to closely monitor this aspect of patient care. Prophylaxis for peptic ulcer and deep venous thrombosis is warranted, as is early detection and management of urinary retention, ileus, and pain. Consultation with physical, occupational, and speech therapy are integral in the management of patients with GBS.

Specific therapies for patients with GBS are directed toward the autoimmune pathogenesis of the disease. Although corticosteroids have been found to be largely ineffective in patients with GBS, plasma exchange and intravenous immunoglobulin (IVIg) have been shown to decrease the percentage of patients who require mechanical ventilation and increase the number of patients who have recovered full strength after 1 year. The ease of administration of IVIg has made this the treatment of choice instead of plasma exchange in many hospitals, given the similar efficacy of the two treatments. Debate on the indication for specific therapies is ongoing, even though IVIg or plasmapheresis is generally recommended in adult patients when ambulation becomes limited. Influenza vaccine is often avoided in patients with a previous history of postvaccination GBS.

COMPLICATIONS

As previously mentioned, respiratory and autonomic failure are the most feared acute complications of GBS, leading to a reported mortality of between 4% and 15%. Persistent weakness is more common, leading to disability in up to 20% of patients after 1 year despite receiving standard treatment. Elderly patients, those who require mechanical ventilation for respiratory failure, and patients who are bedbound from their weakness are more likely to suffer from ongoing disability. Chronic fatigue, even in those patients who have recovered muscle strength clinically, can be a long-term complication of GBS; this is possibly related to persistent subclinical abnormalities that are present on electrodiagnostic testing.

CHAPTER 117

Myasthenia Gravis

Martin Muntz and Safwan Jaradeh

Myasthenia gravis (MG) is an autoimmune disorder that causes dysfunction at the neuromuscular junction, usually due to antibodies directed against the postsynaptic nicotinic acetylcholine receptor (AChR). Classically, this leads to "fatigable" muscle weakness that becomes progressively worse with repetitive stimulation or exertion. With improved diagnostic testing, the annual incidence of myasthenia gravis now approaches 2 per 100,000, and diagnosis of patients over the age of 60 years has significantly increased.

ETIOLOGY

There is no specific cause identified in most cases of myasthenia gravis; however, large family studies suggest a genetic predisposition to autoimmune diseases. About 10% to 15% of MG patients have a thymoma, whereas thymic lymphoid hyperplasia occurs in 60% to 70% of cases. Thyroid disease occurs in about 10%, often in association with antithyroid antibodies. Penicillamine treatment for diseases such as Wilson's disease and rheumatoid arthritis can lead to the development of AChR antibodies and clinical manifestations of MG, which typically resolve with discontinuation of the drug. The Lambert-Eaton syndrome is another rare neuromuscular junction disorder clinically similar to myasthenia gravis, but is due to presynaptic neuromuscular blockade. In 50% to 60% of cases, it is a paraneoplastic syndrome most often associated with small cell lung cancer.

CLINICAL MANIFESTATIONS

The classic painless fatigable muscle weakness may be mild and thus difficult to elicit when taking a patient's history; however, weakness may be described as becoming more pronounced after repetitive tasks or at the end of the day. There is variation among patients in the muscle groups affected. Cranial nerve involvement is common and may present with ptosis, diplopia, or difficulty with facial expression. The history of a patient's voice becoming difficult to understand during prolonged speaking is also suggestive of myasthenia gravis. Weakness of proximal muscles and intrinsic muscles of the hands are typical of limb involvement; this may lead to difficulty with ambulation, brushing or washing hair, and fine motor activities with the hands. Dyspnea may signify hypoventilation due to respiratory muscle weakness.

The physical examination can be very helpful in making the diagnosis of myasthenia gravis. Ptosis that improves with even very short rest—such as blinking—is characteristic; this can be elicited by asking a patient to stare at an object on the wall without blinking. Ptosis should occur while staring at the object and resolve with blinking, and it is often asymmetric. A positive peek sign, consisting of separation of the eyelids with resultant exposure of the sclera despite the patient's

TABLE 117.1 Clinical presentations and diagnostic tests in amyotrophic lateral sclerosis, Guillain-Barré syndrome, and myasthenia gravis

Features	Amyotrophic lateral sclerosis	Guillain-Barré syndrome	Myasthenia gravis
Preceding event	Absent	Upper respiratory infection	Absent
Clinical manifestations	Hyperreflexia Asymmetric limb weakness Spasticity Fasciculations Respiratory muscle weakness	Areflexia Ascending paresis (symmetric) Paresthesias Respiratory muscle weakness	Ptosis Weakness worsening with repetitive stimulation Dysarthria/Dysphagia Respiratory muscle weakness Associated with thymoma
Diagnostic tests	EMG	EMG + cerebrospinal fluid (↑ protein) analysis	EMG/RNS Anti-acetylcholine receptor antibody

EMG, electromyelogram; RNS, repetitive nerve stimulation

attempt to keep the eyes closed, signifies orbicularis oculi weakness that is suggestive of myasthenia gravis. Weakness of the neck and shoulders can be tested by asking the patient to hold an antigravity position, such as holding the head off of a pillow while lying supine or holding the arms above the head while sitting. Again, weakness is often asymmetric. Repetitive manual muscle testing with progressive weakness can be helpful but difficult to detect reliably. The deep tendon reflexes and sensory exam will be normal unless there is another coexisting disease process.

Often, patients with MG experience a relapsing-remitting course of their symptoms. Exacerbations may be triggered by acute medical illness like infection, surgery, as well as by medications. Sedative medications and general anesthetic agents are most often linked to exacerbations, but common agents such as beta-blockers, verapamil, and aminoglycoside antibiotics have also been linked to worsening muscle weakness in patients with MG.

Clinical features of MG and other neuromuscular diseases such as amyotrophic lateral sclerosis and Guillain-Barré syndrome are compared and listed in Table 117.1. Manifestations and diagnostic testing of the above diseases and multiple sclerosis are also described in Figure 117.1.

DIAGNOSIS

Serologic testing for MG with AchR antibodies is positive in about 85% of patients with generalized disease, and the sensitivity approaches 100% in patients with a thymoma. It is less sensitive for patients with localized ocular disease. For the subset of patients with MG who are AchR antibody-negative—also known as seronegative myasthenia gravis—antibodies against other components of neuromuscular transmission, such as muscarinic tyrosine kinase, can frequently be detected to aid in diagnosis.

Anticholinesterase testing (Tensilon test) can be a useful diagnostic test at the bedside. Acetylcholinesterase inhibitors, such as edrophonium, act to increase the concentration of acetylcholine at the

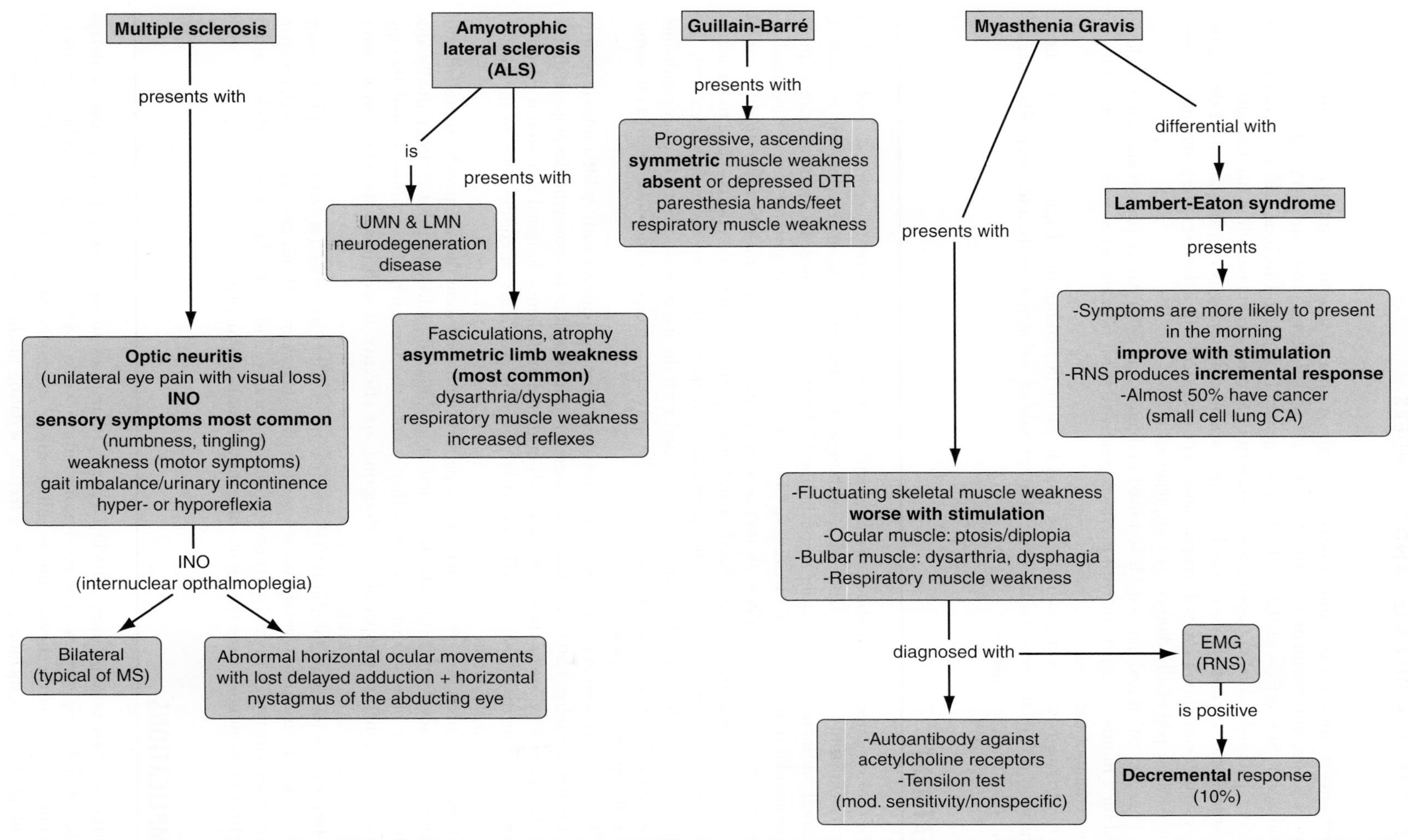

Figure 117.1 • Clinical characteristics of common neurological syndromes.

neuromuscular junction and, thus, muscle strength. Within 30 seconds of intravenous edrophonium administration, improvement in manual muscle strength testing, ptosis, or extraocular movements should occur. Side effects of the medication are generally mild and include salivation, lacrimation, sweating, and abdominal cramping; however, serious adverse events including bradycardia, asystole, and bronchoconstriction do occur rarely. Thus, cardiac monitoring is clearly warranted during this test. A syringe containing 2 mg of atropine should be prepared before the test to be given intravenously if any of these potentially dangerous complications occur.

The "ice test" is another bedside test used in diagnosis of MG. An ice pack is applied to a closed eyelid for 2 minutes in a patient with ptosis. A positive test for myasthenia is resolution or significant improvement of the ptosis.

Electrodiagnostic testing can also be used to assist in making the diagnosis. Repetitive nerve stimulation reveals incremental decrease in amplitude of action potentials, and single-fiber electromyography is more sensitive.

TREATMENT

Initial oral cholinesterase inhibitor therapy, with medications like pyridostigmine, is preferred for patients with mild symptoms from MG. Although the number of viable acetylcholine receptors is decreased, an increase in available acetylcholine (Ach) at the neuromuscular junction can improve neuromuscular transmission and weakness. Cholinergic crisis can occur with overuse of these medications and presents paradoxically with increased weakness; thus, care must be taken to differentiate this from worsening myasthenia. Diarrhea and other gastrointestinal side effects—due to the action of Ach at muscarinic receptors in the gastrointestinal tract—are more commonly seen with this medication class. However, they can be counteracted with the use of medications like propantheline, which is an anticholinergic agent that is specific for muscarinic receptors and does not affect transmission at the nicotinic receptors.

Thymectomy is often recommended for treatment of young patients with AchR antibody positive MG and for generalized MG. Available data suggests little benefit in patients who develop the disease after the age of 65 years or those with antibody-negative myasthenia. Surgical resection is generally recommended for thymomas as well, especially given the possibility of compression or invasion of vital structures in the chest.

Immunosuppression is recommended for patients with symptoms that are poorly controlled with the above therapies. Corticosteroids are started at low doses initially and titrated up gradually, due to the possibility of exacerbation of myasthenia with the initiation of high-dose steroid therapy. Steroid-sparing therapies, especially azathioprine, are effective as well in an attempt to avoid long-term consequences of corticosteroid use.

Intravenous immunoglobulin (IVIg) and plasma exchange are effective but have only transient benefit. They are useful in several clinical situations that include myasthenic crisis (see below), preoperatively in anticipation of thymectomy or other major surgery, and as "bridge" therapy while awaiting the effect of immunosuppressive agents like steroids and azathioprine.

COMPLICATIONS

Myasthenic crisis is respiratory muscle weakness that leads to endotracheal intubation or delays extubation following surgery. The respiratory muscle weakness is often complicated by inability to maintain and protect the airway due to bulbar muscle weakness. Myasthenic crisis can be triggered by multiple stressors, including surgery, infection, sedating medications, or weaning of immunosuppressive agents, or there may be no obvious precipitating event.

Patients with respiratory symptoms suggestive of myasthenic crisis should generally be treated in an intensive care unit, and serial measurements of forced vital capacity and negative inspiratory force should be monitored, along with assessment of airway maintenance. Endotracheal intubation for mechanical ventilation and airway protection should be done early if symptomatic or objective parameters of respiratory function worsen.

Aggressive management of respiratory failure should be combined with specific treatments for myasthenia gravis, such as acetylcholinesterase inhibitors, plasma exchange, IVIg, and immunosuppression. With improvements in intensive care management and specific therapies for myasthenic crisis, the mortality has decreased from about 75% to <5% since the 1960s, but there is still significant morbidity related in part to prolonged mechanical ventilation and difficulties with ambulation.

Psychiatry

Jon Lehrmann

CHAPTER 118

Depression

Kimberly Stoner and Jon Lehrmann

A large epidemiologic survey in 2005 found that major depressive disorder had a prevalence of 5.3% and a lifetime incidence of 13.2%. Nearly one third of patients seen in primary care clinics have significant depressive symptoms. Female patients are twice as likely to be affected. Depression reduces quality of life, costs employers over $30 billion per year due to decreased productivity of affected workers, increases the risk of suicide, and also may increase mortality in some medical conditions such as coronary artery disease.

The majority of patients with depression are treated by primary care physicians rather than mental health providers. Depressed patients often present with somatic complaints, such as headaches or pain, in concert with their emotional symptoms, which they may not divulge spontaneously. Depression is a common comorbid condition among patients with chronic pain, human immunodeficiency virus, cancer, and fibromyalgia. Restrictions imposed by health insurance policies, the shortage of psychiatrists in some geographic areas, and the social stigma associated with mental health problems reinforce the trend of depressed patients first presenting to the primary care practitioner. The U.S. Preventive Services Task Force recommends screening adults for depression, but despite this recommendation up to half of patients remain undiagnosed. Primary care physicians must be familiar with the diagnosis and management of depressive disorders as they are so often the first professional to evaluate the patient's complaints.

ETIOLOGY

The etiology of depression is multifactorial. Genetic studies have shown high concordance rates among twins and first-degree relatives for both major depressive disorder and bipolar affective disorder. Alterations in serotonin, norepinephrine, and dopamine have been described with low levels of 5-hydroxyindoleacetic acid, a serotonin metabolite, being found in the cerebrospinal fluid of patients who have attempted suicide by a violent method. Major psychosocial stressors such as the death of a spouse, divorce, or loss of a job may precipitate depressive episodes in vulnerable individuals. Hormonal influences may explain some of the higher prevalence of depression among women. Major depressive disorder with postpartum onset is well defined and more recently premenstrual dysphoric disorder has been recognized as a distinct clinical syndrome in the literature. Medical conditions such as cerebrovascular accidents and lupus seem to precipitate depression in some individuals. Patients with hypothyroidism also appear to be at higher risk for depression.

CLINICAL MANIFESTATIONS

In light of the prevalence of depression, physicians ought to maintain a high index of suspicion for mood disorders during clinical encounters. Patients with somatic complaints including fatigue, insomnia, gastrointestinal upset, vague aches and pains, a heightened degree of impairment relative to their symptoms, or symptoms that prove refractory to standard treatments should be evaluated for depression. Patients with chronic medical illness, especially painful conditions or those causing progressive disability, should be monitored for the development of depression. While the physical examination is often normal, it should be performed to rule out associated illnesses such as thyroid dysfunction (Chapter 66), pancreatic cancer, or Cushing's disease (Chapter 67 and 69). It is not necessary, however, to perform an exhaustive battery of tests to exclude medical illness before making the diagnosis of depression, particularly in patients with a low pretest probability of concomitant disease.

DIAGNOSIS

Although the diagnosis of depression can be made on history alone, the majority of depressed patients will not present to clinicians with depression as their chief complaint. Screening patients with the mood module of the Primary Care Evaluation of Mental Disorders increases the rate of detection. It is a quick and sensitive tool that utilizes items based on Diagnostic and Statistical Manual of Mental Disorders (DSM) criteria (Table 118.1). Alternatively, many clinicians use the mnemonic **SIG E CAPS** to recall the DSM criteria while performing the patient history: **S**leep, **I**nterest, **G**uilt, **E**nergy, **C**oncentration, **A**ppetite, **P**sychomotor Agitation/Retardation, and **S**uicide.

In addition to major depressive disorder, there are several other mood disorders that may present with depressive symptoms. In addition to excluding medical conditions, clinicians should also review medications and inquire about substance abuse to evaluate for the possibility of a substance-induced mood disorder. Alcohol abuse may induce depression. Stimulants, such as cocaine, have also been implicated in depression because chronic use is thought to deplete catecholamines, and because of

TABLE 118.1 Diagnostic criteria for selected mood disorders

Major depressive episode	Manic episode	Dysthymic disorder
Five or more symptoms, lasting at least 2 weeks, (must include A or B): A. Depressed mood B. Loss of interest or pleasure C. Appetite/weight change D. Sleep disturbance E. Psychomotor agitation or retardation F. Fatigue/loss of energy G. Feeling worthless or inappropriately guilty H. Impaired concentration or indecisiveness I. Thoughts of death	A. At least 7-day period of elevated or irritable mood B. Three of the following symptoms, 4 if mood is irritable: 1. Inflated self-esteem 2. Decreased need for sleep 3. Increased talking 4. Racing thoughts 5. Distractibility 6. Increase in goal-directed activity or psychomotor agitation 7. Indulgence in pleasurable activities without regard for consequences	A. Depressed mood for majority of day, most days for 2 years B. Two or more of the following symptoms: 1. Change in appetite 2. Sleep disturbance 3. Low energy/fatigue 4. Low self-esteem 5. Impaired concentration or indecisiveness 6. Hopelessness C. Symptoms cause clinically significant distress or impairment in functioning

Adapted from *Diagnostic and Statistical Manual of Mental Disorders,* 4th Revision. Washington, DC: American Psychiatric Association; 1994.

the intense dysphoric feelings that occur during the withdrawal phase. Abstinence from substances is an essential part of the treatment plan for these patients. Medications can also induce depression. Reserpine is one of the more notorious agents that may precipitate depression, but mood disturbances have been reported with use of other medications as well.

Clinicians should inquire about prior episodes of mood disturbance in depressed patients. Patients with a chronic (greater than 2 years), low-grade depression could be suffering from dysthymia. They may have difficulty pinpointing when their depression started and report that they have felt depressed for as long as they can remember. Dysthymic patients frequently have a coexisting personality disorder, but they also respond to pharmacological treatment and selective serotonin reuptake inhibitors (SSRIs) may be useful. Any patient who has ever met the criteria for a manic episode should be diagnosed with bipolar affective disorder rather than major depression. This is a clinically significant distinction because these patients require treatment with a mood stabilizer and monotherapy with an antidepressant may cause the patient to cycle into a manic episode. In patients presenting with major depressive symptoms, it is prudent to inquire about prior manic episodes to rule out a bipolar disorder before you initiate pharmacotherapy.

During the evaluation of depression, clinicians should consider the timing and psychosocial context of the patient's symptoms. Patients who report onset of depression in the fall or early winter with remission in the spring may be suffering from seasonal affective disorder and benefit from light therapy. Women who experience depressive symptoms during the luteal phase of their menstrual cycles may have premenstrual dysphoric disorder (PMDD). Several of the SSRIs have shown efficacy in clinical trials for the treatment of PMDD. Patients with minor depressive symptoms following the death of a loved one may have bereavement (which may not require any treatment, but only monitoring). If an identifiable stressor precipitated a patient's distress and functional impairment, then the diagnosis of an adjustment disorder with depressed mood should be made if the criteria for a major depressive episode are not fulfilled.

TREATMENT

Many new antidepressant medications have come to the market in recent years. These new medications often have fewer drug interactions, cleaner side-effect profiles and significantly less toxicity in overdose than the older monoamine oxidase inhibitors and tricyclics. Primary care physicians frequently prescribe these newer agents and should be familiar with their pharmacologic properties (Table 118.2).

Several principles should be kept in mind when utilizing antidepressants. No single agent has been proven more efficacious than the others and on average there is about a 66% chance of a particular patient responding to a particular medication. Studies do suggest that if a patient has a family member with depression who has responded well to an agent, then the patient will likely respond well to the same medication. With efficacy being considered equal and most medications having a convenient once-daily dosing option, selection of which drug to use is based primarily on side-effect profile, cost, or potential for drug interactions. Antidepressants should be started at a low dose, especially in elderly patients or those with hepatic impairment, and titrated up gradually to a therapeutic dose over a period of weeks. Patients should be informed that it will take several weeks after a therapeutic dose is reached to realize the full benefit of the medication. Once depressive symptoms have remitted, the medication should be continued at its full therapeutic dose for at least 6 months, preferably 1 year, in order to prevent relapse. Although antidepressants are not "addictive," it is recommended to taper the dose gradually over several weeks prior to discontinuation to monitor for the re-emergence of depressive symptoms. Patients with a history of three or more major depres-

TABLE 118.2 Antidepressant medications

Name of drug	Dosing	Targeted neurotransmitter	Advantages	Disadvantages
Citalopram (Celexa)	10–60 mg once daily	Serotonin	Very low risk of drug interactions	Nausea
Escitalopram (Lexapro)	5–20 mg once daily	Serotonin	Ease of titration of dose	No generic available
Fluoxetine (Prozac, Sarafem, Prozac Weekly)	10–80 mg once daily or 90 mg weekly	Serotonin	Very long half-life minimizes withdrawal, allows less than daily dosing	P450 drug interactions
Paroxetine (Paxil, Paxil CR)	10–60 mg once daily or CR 12.5 mg to 75 mg once daily	Serotonin	Might be less activating than other SSRIs, making it well suited for anxious patients	P450 drug interactions, most anticholinergic, weight gain, severe withdrawal, birth defects reported
Sertraline (Zoloft)	25–200 mg once daily	Serotonin	Safety in pregnancy	Diarrhea
Venlafaxine (Effexor XR)	37.5–225 mg once daily	Serotonin, norepinephrine	Affects additional neurotransmitters as dose increases	Nausea, hypertension, sexual side effects, withdrawal syndrome, adjust dose in hepatic and renal impairment
Duloxetine (Cymbalta)	20–60 mg daily total, once or twice per day dosing	Serotonin, norepinephrine	Approved for diabetic neuropathy	Twice daily dosing is preferable, no generic available
Mirtazapine (Remeron)	7.5–45 mg at bedtime	Norepinephrine serotonin	Improves insomnia, low risk of sexual dysfunction	Weight gain, constipation, dry mouth, dyslipidemia, rarely neutropenia
Bupropion (Wellbutrin SR, Wellbutrin XL)	SR 100–400 mg divided twice daily, 150–450 mg every morning for XL	Dopamine, norepinephrine	Approved for smoking cessation, does not cause sexual dysfunction	Seizures, headache, insomnia if taken later in day, dry mouth

sive episodes should stay on medication indefinitely since the relapse rate for patients with recurrent episodes is very high upon discontinuation.

SSRIs are the most commonly prescribed class of antidepressant medication. All SSRIs have been reported to cause gastrointestinal side effects, headache, drowsiness, tremor, and increased sweating. Sexual dysfunction is a very common, dose-related side effect. Some patients report feeling sedated, while an equal number report feeling "activated" after taking an SSRI. In anxious patients, it is important to start at the lowest dose and titrate slowly to avoid worsening anxiety. Although an uncommon side effect, SSRIs have been associated with syndrome of inappropriate antidiuretic hormone. SSRIs have a flulike withdrawal syndrome and must be tapered gradually prior to discontinuation.

Americans are increasingly using herbal medications. There are two agents that may be of some benefit in the treatment of depression, although clinical trial outcomes are mixed and there is not a general consensus as to their use. St. John's Wort is taken 300 to 1,000 mg daily in divided doses. Side effects are rare with St. John's Wort, but it is a potent CYP3A4 inhibitor so patients taking other medications can suffer adverse effects from drug interactions. S-adenosyl-methionine, marketed as SamE, is taken in a dose of 150 to 2,400 mg daily. A meta-analysis found that SamE is as effective as tricyclics for the treatment of depression, with few if any side effects. These agents may be an

TABLE 118.3 Mood-stabilizing agents

Name of drug	Dosing	Minor side effects	Medically serious side effects
Lithium	300–2,400 mg daily	Tremor, nausea, vomiting diarrhea, weight gain, acne	Toxicity from use of angiotensin-converting enzyme inhibitors, angiotensin-receptor blockers, nonsteroidal anti-inflammatory drugs, renal dysfunction, hypothyroidism, Ebstein's anomaly in offspring
Valproic acid (Depakote, Divalproex)	250–3,000 mg total in divided doses daily	Nausea, weight gain, hair loss	Hepatotoxicity, hyperammonemia, polycystic ovary syndrome, pancreatitis, thrombocytopenia neural tube defects
Carbamazepine Tegretol	200–1,600 mg daily divided in 2 to 4 doses	Ataxia	Aplastic anemia, hypersensitivity syndrome, leukopenia, hepatotoxicity, hyponatremia, neural tube defects, Stevens-Johnson syndrome, drug interactions
Lamotrigine Lamictal	25–400 mg divided twice daily (start at 25 mg and titrate slowly)	Rash	Stevens-Johnson syndrome
Olanzapine Zyprexa	2.5–40 mg daily	Sedation, dry mouth	Type 2 diabetes, weight gain, dyslipidemia

TABLE 118.4 Risk factors for suicide

Demographic factors	Patient history or symptoms	Comorbid conditions	Psychosocial precipitants
1. White race 2. Gender, females attempt more but males more often complete 3. Living alone 4. Marital status: widowed→ divorced→single→ married 5. Older age	1. Prior attempts 2. A detailed and feasible plan 3. Hopelessness 4. Family history of suicide 5. Suicidal talk or threats 6. Most recent psychiatric hospitalization involuntary 7. Firearm in the home	1. Chronic medical illness 2. Substance abuse or dependence 3. Any Axis I or II psychiatric diagnosis	1. Acute alcohol intoxication 2. Legal problems 3. Marital discord 4. Loss of job 5. Financial problems 6. Estrangement from family 7. Bereavement 8. Lack of social support system

option for patients who will not consider taking traditional medications or psychotherapy. However, due to the lack of regulation governing herbal supplements, it is difficult to generalize the findings of the clinical trials due to varying levels of the active compounds in different batches of the product. Physicians should warn patients of the lack of regulation in the preparation of herbal supplements.

Psychotherapy can be used in conjunction with medication or as an alternative to medication in the treatment of depression. Cognitive-behavioral therapy is the most extensively tested form of therapy and can be as efficacious as medication for the treatment of depression. For patients experiencing difficulty in a relationship, interpersonal therapy is another reasonable form of therapy. If the patient's depression was precipitated by a specific stressor, participation in a support group with others facing a similar problem may be beneficial. The combination of psychotherapy and antidepressant often is more effective than either by itself.

In patients with bipolar affective disorder, pharmacotherapy for a major depressive episode should include a mood-stabilizing agent rather than using an antidepressant drug as monotherapy. Many bipolar patients are under the care of a psychiatrist who will serve as the prescriber of medications. Mood stabilizers have a number of medically serious potential side effects. Primary care physicians may assist psychiatrists in the monitoring of mutual patients or in their treatment in cases when medically serious side effects occur. Table 118.3 provides a brief summary of side effects.

COMPLICATIONS

The most troubling outcome of depression is suicide. Despite extensive research, there is no reliable algorithm that can accurately predict which patients will commit suicide. Table 118.4 provides a listing of risk factors associated with suicide. Studies have demonstrated that discussing suicide during a clinical encounter will not foster suicidal thinking or intent, and therefore the topic should not be avoided. Utilization of a suicide contract, in which a patient agrees to call before making a suicide attempt, does not seem to lower the rate of completed suicides. It is still reasonable to discuss with the patient what to do should suicidal thoughts arise and document the plan in the medical record.

CHAPTER 119

Anxiety Disorders

Kimberly Stoner and Gunnar Larson

Anxiety disorders are collectively the most prevalent psychiatric disorders in the United States. The lifetime prevalence rate of anxiety disorders is 14.6% with associated treatment costs of billions of dollars. Due to a relatively young age of onset (most commonly childhood or early adulthood), untreated anxiety disorders cause a significant number of productive years of life to be lost or impaired, which carries a high cost for society. Anxiety disorder sufferers experience an array of somatic symptoms, oftentimes prompting them to seek care from medical rather than mental health care physicians. For this reason, it is important for all primary care physicians to be familiar with the diagnosis and management of anxiety disorders.

ETIOLOGY

W.B. Cannon's theory asserts that humans evolved with the tendency for emergency situations to provoke an increase in sympathetic nervous system activity, commonly known as the fight-or-flight response. Consequently, the experience of anxiety is ubiquitous among all people exposed to fear provoking situations. Distinguishing normal anxiety from an anxiety disorder therefore requires determining if the anxiety is excessive, irrational, or leads to functional impairment rather than serving as an adaptive response.

Many anxiety disorders seem to involve alterations in the physiology of the hypothalamic-pituitary-adrenal axis. However, it is likely that the different anxiety disorders have related but not identical etiologies. Specific phobias tend to occur in first-degree relatives, although it is unclear if this represents a nature or nurture effect. The concordance rate for panic disorder among monozygotic twins is 31%, suggesting a heritable genetic predisposition that manifests in anxiety disorder given certain environmental prompts. Obsessive-compulsive disorder (OCD) appears to have a genetic basis that results in dysfunction in specific neuroanatomic areas.

Because of its localization, OCD is one of very few conditions for which psychosurgery (cingulotomy) may still be considered a treatment option in refractory cases. Posttraumatic stress disorder (PTSD) requires exposure to a significant traumatic event in order to develop and be diagnosed. Efforts to predict who will develop PTSD and attempts to intervene following traumas to prevent its development have generally yielded disappointing results. Like PTSD, generalized anxiety disorder (GAD) is also thought to be more attributable to environmental exposures (particularly in early childhood) rather than a fully genetic attribution.

CLINICAL MANIFESTATIONS

While a patient's history may vary based on the type of anxiety disorder he or she suffers from, there are several key components of the history that need to be addressed when assessing any patient for a possible anxiety disorder. It is unusual for patients who present for medical care to state that their chief complaint is anxiety. While obtaining a history of present illness or review of systems, an array of somatic symptoms may be reported by the patient. Anxiety may manifest as insomnia, chest pain, palpitations, dyspnea, gastrointestinal distress, tremors, myalgias, headaches, lightheadedness, or sweats. Panic attacks may also occur in patients who are diagnosed with a variety of other anxiety disorders including panic disorder, specific phobias (such as when a patient with a fear of flying boards an aircraft), or social anxiety disorder (such as when the patient is faced with giving a speech) and when they do occur they typically present with more physiologic than psychological symptoms (Table 119.1).

During the history of present illness, it may be difficult to establish a definitive duration of symptoms unless the patient is able to identify a specific event as a trigger. Patients with anxiety disorders may report longstanding worry or shyness that dates back as long as they can remember and only seek care after their condition has become disabling. The patient's past medical history should be reviewed for conditions such as pulmonary embolism or hyperthyroidism that may cause anxiety. Medication history should include inquiry about prescribed drugs such as methylphenidate and theophylline, or herbal remedies such as ephedra that have stimulant properties. Social history should include legal stimulant use, such as caffeine or nicotine, as well as the use of cocaine and methamphetamine. Twenty percent of patients diagnosed with anxiety disorders abuse substances, some of which may represent an attempt to "self-medicate" their condition. During the social history, clinicians should also inquire about significant psychosocial stressors that may have precipitated the onset of symptoms. Patients will also frequently have a family history of anxiety disorders.

The physical examination of patients with anxiety disorders is most often normal, but it is necessary in order to help rule out other medical etiologies. If a patient experiences anxiety or a panic attack in the presence of the physician, then signs of increased sympathetic nervous system activity may be noted. Vital signs may reveal tachycardia, hyperventilation, or an increase in blood pressure. The patient may appear ashen or become diaphoretic. The pupils may appear more dilated. It is important to remember that these findings are not specific for anxiety disorders,

TABLE 119.1 *Diagnostic and Statistical Manual of Mental Disorders, Fourth Revision* criteria for panic attack

A discrete period that includes four or more of the following, with symptoms peaking at ≤10 minutes

1. Palpitations, heart pounding, or accelerated heart rate
2. Sweating
3. Trembling or shaking
4. Shortness of breath or smothering sensation
5. Choking sensation
6. Chest pain or discomfort
7. Nausea or abdominal distress
8. Feeling dizzy, unsteady, lightheaded, or faint
9. Derealization or depersonalization
10. Fear of losing control or going crazy
11. Fear of dying
12. Paresthesias
13. Chills or hot flashes

but rather simply indicate an adrenergic surge. Because patients experiencing a myocardial infarction may present with similar findings, an appropriate medical investigation should be performed prior to narrowing the differential diagnosis to an anxiety disorder.

DIAGNOSIS

An important first step in making the diagnosis of an anxiety disorder is to ensure that a medical condition such as hypoxemia or hypoglycemia is not responsible for the patient's anxiety. Physicians should also consider whether or not the anxiety may be related to use of, or withdrawal from, a prescribed drug or illicit substance. Clinicians should look for a temporal relationship between time of ingestion and the onset of anxiety symptoms. Urine drug screens may also be helpful when substance use is suspected, but keep in mind they are often comorbid conditions and the presence of abuse does not indicate a causal relationship to their complaints of anxiety. Once medical and pharmacologic causes have been ruled out, a history that elicits the *Diagnostic and Statistical Manual of Mental Disorders, Fourth Revision* criteria for anxiety disorders may be used to make the diagnosis (Table 119.2).

TREATMENT

After performing a thorough history and conducting an appropriate medical evaluation, the first step of treatment is to discuss the diagnosis of an anxiety disorder with the patient and provide education about the condition. The majority of patients will usually already have some insight into the fact that their symptoms are related to stress or that their worrying is excessive. In panic disorder, in contrast, many patients after exhaustive cardiac and neurologic evaluations continue to believe that they are suffering from a life-threatening, undiagnosed medical illness. This may be due to the acutely distressing nature of panic attacks and the intensity of their somatic symptoms. Therefore, clinicians ought to avoid presenting the diagnosis of panic disorder with a dismissive or overly reassuring attitude, despite having conducted an unrevealing medical workup.

For most anxiety disorders, a combination of medication and psychotherapy is often the most effective approach. For some disorders, particularly OCD and panic disorder, medications will likely alleviate but not completely eliminate symptoms. Selective serotonin reuptake inhibitors (SSRIs) are generally used first line for OCD, GAD, and panic disorder and often must be titrated to higher doses than what is typically effective for depression. Psychotherapy has also been proven beneficial in clinical trials for symptom reduction and to help patients cope with fear provoking situations. Cognitive behavioral therapy has been studied the most rigorously.

Benzodiazepines, although prescribed less frequently because of their abuse potential, also have an important role in the management of anxiety disorders (Table 119.3). For patients with specific phobias with infrequent exposures (such as having to fly on a plane or have blood drawn a few times a year), it is more appropriate to prescribe a benzodiazepine for use prior to exposure in conjunction with behavior therapy for desensitization rather than prescribing a daily SSRI. Benzodiazepines may also be used during the initiation of treatment with an SSRI and gradually tapered while the SSRI is being titrated up to an effective dose. This combined medication strategy may provide patients with more immediate symptom relief, since most SSRIs will not reach their full therapeutic benefit for several weeks to months after initiation.

Counseling patients about the initial increase in anxiety they may experience when starting an SSRI can be couched in terms that it is a sign that the medication is starting to work. When

TABLE 119.2 Diagnostic criteria for anxiety disorders

Specific phobia	Panic disorder	Social phobia (social anxiety disorder)
Unreasonable fear of a specific object or situation Exposure to object or situation provokes anxiety Patient recognizes that their fear is excessive Avoids the object or situation Leads to impairment of functioning or altered routine	Recurrent panic attacks Attack has been followed by 1 month of one or more of the following: 1. Concern about additional attacks 2. Worry about implications or consequences of attack 3. Change in behavior related to attack	Fear of scrutiny and social situations due to risk of embarrassment Exposure to social situations provokes anxiety Patient recognizes that their fear is excessive Avoidance of social situations Leads to impairment of functioning
Obsessive-compulsive disorder	**Posttraumatic stress disorder**	**Generalized anxiety disorder**
Either obsessions (recurrent, intrusive, distressing thoughts that are not worries about real-life problems, which the patient attempts to ignore or neutralize) or compulsions (repetitive behaviors the patient is driven to perform and that reduce distress) Patient realizes obsessions and compulsions are excessive/unreasonable Obsessions and compulsions are time consuming and impair functioning or routine	Patient was exposed to trauma that threatened injury and provoked fear or helplessness Trauma is re-experienced as recollections, dreams, or flashbacks triggered by environmental cues with physiologic reactivity Avoidance of stimuli associated with trauma and numbness (i.e., impaired recall of event, loss of interest in activities, sense of foreshortened future) Persistent increased arousal (i.e., insomnia, anger, hypervigilance) One-month duration Impaired functioning	Excessive worry about multiple things most days for 6 months Patient cannot control the worry Anxiety associated with three or more of the following: 1. Feeling restless or on edge 2. Fatigue 3. Impaired concentration or mind going blank 4. Irritability 5. Muscle tension 6. Disturbed sleep Worry causes significant distress or impairment of functioning

Adapted from the *Diagnostic and Statistical Manual of Mental Disorders, Fourth Revision*. Washington, DC: American Psychiatric Association; 2000.

a clinician is concerned that a patient's risk of addiction or misuse of benzodiazepines is too high, buspirone may be prescribed in conjunction with an SSRI if symptom relief with the SSRI alone is not adequate in generalized or social anxiety disorders. Buspirone does not have a quick onset of action and patients should be counseled that improvement in their symptoms will come with time (2 to 6 weeks).

TABLE 119.3 Commonly prescribed benzodiazepines

Name	Starting dose	Dosing schedule	Half-life
Alprazolam (Xanax)	0.25–0.5 mg	2–4 times daily	Short
Chlordiazepoxide (Librium)	5–10 mg	3–4 times daily	Long
Clonazepam (Klonopin)	0.25–0.5 mg	2–3 times daily	Long
Diazepam (Valium)	2–5 mg	2–4 times daily	Long
Lorazepam (Ativan)	0.5–1 mg	3–4 times daily	Midduration
Oxazepam (Serax)	10–15 mg	3–4 times daily	Short

COMPLICATIONS

Complications of anxiety disorders generally arise from failure to make the diagnosis or from inadequate treatment. Anxiety disorders are associated with increased utilization of healthcare services and can be immensely disabling. Patients with OCD are sometimes unable to leave their homes without performing several hours of checking rituals and patients with panic disorder who have become agoraphobic may be unable to leave their homes at all. Functional impairment may also result from chronic sleep disturbance that commonly occurs in PTSD and GAD. Social anxiety disorder leads to impairment in occupational and interpersonal settings resulting in isolation. An anxiety disorder may have a significant negative impact on a patient's quality of life. Clinicians should be aware that anxiety disorder patients are at risk for the development of depression, substance abuse, and suicidality.

CHAPTER 120

Schizophrenia

Kimberly Stoner and Gunnar Larson

The prevalence of schizophrenia is 1%; however, even prominent psychotic symptoms (hallucinations and/or delusions that often manifest with a lack of insight) should not be considered pathognomonic for the illness. Schizophrenia has three subgroups of symptoms: positive (i.e., hallucinations, delusions, disorganized speech), negative (i.e., decreased emotional display, impaired social functioning, apathy), and cognitive (i.e., impaired concentration, difficulty completing tasks, memory problems). Individual patients will present with different ratios of symptoms from each subgroup. Patients with mood disorders, delirium, substance intoxication or withdrawal, or a wide variety of neurological conditions may exhibit psychotic features that require treatment and differentiation from schizophrenia in a general medical setting. All physicians will likely encounter patients with acute psychotic symptoms and familiarity with the appropriate management is particularly important in the hospital setting to ensure a good outcome.

Clinicians should also be familiar with the medical care of schizophrenics. Unlike psychosis from medical or substance-related etiologies, schizophrenia is a chronic illness with a relatively early age of onset in the late teenage years or early 20s for males, and later 20s for most females. For children less than 10 years of age and adults over 40 years of age, new onset of schizophrenia is less common. Schizophrenics who have negative symptoms present with social and occupational impairment that make it difficult to access the healthcare system and impairs their efforts at treatment compliance. Schizophrenics have a much higher rate of smoking than the general population (2 to 3 times higher). Some studies have shown that smoking may positively impact some of the attentional and visuospatial working memory deficits they have. Although smoking may be of some mild benefit for their cognitive impairment, the attendant rise in cardiovascular and pulmonary health problems can be catastrophic. Schizophrenics have a reduced life expectancy of up to 20% compared to the general population, with the chief cause of these early deaths being coronary heart disease. Clinicians must also be prepared to deal with medically serious side effects associated with the newer atypical antipsychotic medications including weight gain, type 2 diabetes mellitus, and cardiac dysrhythmias.

ETIOLOGY

Twin and adoption studies suggest that genetics account for ~50% of the risk of developing schizophrenia. There does not appear to be a single locus, but rather multiple sites on different chromosomes that may contribute to its development. Environmental factors also play a role in the pathogenesis. Perinatal insults and traumatic brain injuries of varying severity during childhood often precede the development of schizophrenia in genetically predisposed individuals, as have maternal viral infections suffered during pregnancy. Stressful psychosocial events and substance abuse have also been reported as possible inciting events for exacerbation or initiation of the illness. Schizophrenia generally is a lifelong illness and studies have found many schizophrenics have subtle impairment in social functioning predating the full onset of illness and diagnosis. The dopamine theory was one of the first neurochemical theories of the cause of schizophrenia and is supported by the efficacy of first-generation antipsychotic medications, which strongly block dopamine receptors. Subsequent studies have revealed that other neurotransmitters are also involved, and neuroimaging techniques have demonstrated differences between the brains of schizophrenics and controls in a number of anatomical areas.

The potential etiologies of psychotic symptoms not associated with a diagnosis of schizophrenia are innumerable. Medical illness in the elderly, postoperative states, use of hallucinogenic drugs, Parkinson's disease (Chapter 112), encephalitis, metabolic derangement, seizure disorders (Chapter 22), and dementias may all predispose patients to experience hallucinations or paranoid ideation. Identification of the correct etiology of patient's psychotic symptoms is an important first step in management.

CLINICAL MANIFESTATIONS

Many clinicians can feel intimidated when faced with performing a history and physical examination on a patient exhibiting psychotic symptoms. While psychotic patients have the potential for violence, the media tends to overemphasize violent acts committed by mental health patients. Schizophrenics are no more likely to commit homicide than the general population, but they are more likely to be victims of violent crime. The rate of completed suicide is 10%, which is markedly higher than the general population's rate of 0.01%. More than half of schizophrenics will make a suicide attempt at some point during the course of their illness.

The majority of psychotic patients are willing to cooperate and able to provide some valuable information during clinical encounters. The history should focus on the most relevant components first, in case the patient becomes too symptomatic during the course of the interview to continue. In an acute setting, reviewing medical problems, prescribed medications and their compliance and substance use should be the first priority. As in most medical interviews, patients should be given a brief opportunity initially to describe their primary concerns even when the history they provide is very disorganized or not based in reality. A current social history can be essential for formulating a feasible treatment plan and a family history may help narrow the differential diagnoses. Often this information is available from chart review or family members and may be deferred to avoid overburdening an acutely psychotic patient with questions. Detailed questioning about hallucinations and delusions, especially in patients displaying a high level of distress and a low level of insight, is often best left to mental health professionals.

A thorough assessment of the patient's general appearance is a valuable portion of the physical examination in psychotic patients. Is the patient appropriately groomed and dressed? Is there evidence of poor nutrition, exposure to the elements, or trauma? Is the patient inattentive during the interview or avoiding eye contact? Does the patient reach out as if to grab invisible objects, engage in conversation with an unseen person, or respond to an unheard voice? Much can be learned from a brief period of unobtrusive observation. Ask the patient permission to perform the physical examination before approaching him or her with a stethoscope or other examination equipment, particularly in paranoid individuals. A neurological examination may reveal saccadic movements of the eyes because impaired smooth ocular pursuit is a common finding in schizophrenics. Clinicians should evaluate patients for abnormal movements secondary to antipsychotic medications including rigidity, akathisia (an inner sense of restlessness accompanied by an inability to stay still), bradykinesia, or involuntary movements (tardive dyskinesia), which often first appear periorally.

DIAGNOSIS

Making the diagnosis of schizophrenia involves interviewing the patient to elicit compatible symptoms. Acutely psychotic patients can be unable to provide a reliable history and in those cases collateral

TABLE 120.1 Diagnostic criteria for schizophrenia

A. Two or more of the following symptoms persistently present for 1 month: delusions, hallucinations, disorganized speech, disorganized or catatonic behavior, negative symptoms
B. Social or occupational dysfunction relative to baseline performance
C. Six-month duration of disturbance

Delusions can often be classified religious, grandiose, erotomanic, jealous, persecutory, paranoid, or somatic. Negative symptoms include flat affect, poverty of speech, apathy, and asociality.

Adapted from the *Diagnostic and Statistical Manual of Mental Disorders, Fourth Revision.* Washington, DC: American Psychiatric Association; 2000.

information must be obtained from family members or friends. The *Diagnostic and Statistical Manual of Mental Disorders* provides guidelines, which help clinicians to distinguish schizophrenia from other psychotic disorders (Table 120.1).

After ruling out medical causes and other mental health disorders, if a patient's psychotic symptoms have been present for less than 1 month, then the correct diagnosis may be brief psychotic disorder. If the psychotic symptoms have persisted for 1 to 6 months, then schizophreniform disorder is diagnosed. Most patients with schizophreniform disorder will eventually fulfill the criteria for schizophrenia when observed over time. Clinicians need to ensure that patients with psychotic symptoms are not abusing substances or suffering from a medical condition that may cause psychotic symptoms before making the diagnosis of schizophrenia. If a psychotic patient has prominent mood symptoms, then major depressive disorder with psychotic features, bipolar affective disorder, and schizoaffective disorder should be included in the differential diagnosis. It is important to evaluate patients for these disorders prior to starting treatment for schizophrenia because the appropriate medication strategy will often include an antidepressant or mood stabilizer in addition to antipsychotic medication.

TREATMENT

Antipsychotic medications are the first-line treatment for schizophrenia (Table 120.2). Psychotherapy, vocational rehabilitation, and social skills training programs may also help to improve functioning. Haloperidol, despite being an older medication, is still quite commonly used, especially for the treatment of hospitalized patients who become acutely psychotic. It is a potent dopamine antagonist, which can be administered orally, intramuscularly, or intravenously and titrated relatively easily. There is also a long-lasting decanoate form that can be given as a monthly injection, making it well suited for the treatment of schizophrenic patients who are noncompliant. Extrapyramidal symptoms (acute dystonia, parkinsonism, akathisia), sedation, weight gain, and prolactin elevation are common side effects. Seizures and QT prolongation occur uncommonly. Rare side effects include neuroleptic malignant syndrome in the short term and tardive dyskinesia in the long term. While infrequent, clinicians should monitor for these conditions as the former is potentially lethal and the latter largely irreversible.

The development of atypical antipsychotics (which are serotonin and dopamine antagonists, except for aripiprazole, which has partial agonist activity) was an exciting breakthrough in pharmacotherapy. In addition to reducing hallucinations and delusions, these medications may be more efficacious at reducing the negative symptoms of schizophrenia for some patients.

TABLE 120.2 Atypical antipsychotic medications

Medication	Dosing (starting/maximum)	Side effects
Clozaril (clozapine)	12.5 mg bid/900 mg daily	Weight gain, diabetes, orthostasis, agranulocytosis, dry mouth
Zyprexa (olanzapine)	2.5–5 mg daily/40 mg daily	Weight gain, diabetes, dyslipidemia, sedation, dry mouth
Seroquel (quetiapine)	25 mg bid/800 mg daily	Sedation, hypotension, cataracts reported in animal studies
Risperdal (risperidone)	0.5–1 mg bid/8 mg daily	Extrapyramidal side effects, elevated prolactin, increased stroke risk
Geodon (ziprasidone)	20 mg bid/80 mg bid	QT prolongation
Abilify (aripiprazole)	10–15 mg daily/30 mg daily	Headache, nausea, vomiting

Atypical antipsychotics are frequently better tolerated, although their higher cost may limit their availability in some care settings. Atypical antipsychotics have also been associated with the development of type 2 diabetes mellitus and marked weight gain, particularly olanzapine and clozapine.

COMPLICATIONS

Despite advances in therapy, schizophrenia still has a relatively poor prognosis, with the majority of patients experiencing a chronic course with multiple relapses. Only about one quarter of patients improve enough with treatment to achieve relatively normal social and occupational functioning.

CHAPTER 121

Eating Disorders

Kimberly Stoner and Jon Lehrmann

Over 5 million Americans suffer from eating disorders. While historically eating disorders have been considered a disease of young white women, there is growing recognition that eating disorders may also affect males and patients of all races and ages. The overall prevalence of anorexia nervosa and bulimia nervosa has been estimated to be around 1% each. *Diagnostic and Statistical Manual of Mental Disorders, Fourth Revision* (DSM-IV) also lists criteria for the diagnosis of eating disorder not otherwise specified, which has a prevalence of up to 5%. The epidemic of obesity in the United States has prompted interest in recognizing binge eating disorder as a distinct clinical diagnosis. Eating disorders are associated with significant morbidity from the development of medical complications. A meta-analysis of anorexia found an annual mortality rate of 0.56%, which represents a 10-fold increase in the risk of death among anorexics compared to young women without the disease. Patients suffering from eating disorders are often quite secretive about their behavior. It is important for physicians to recognize the signs and symptoms of eating disorders before significant medical complications have occurred.

ETIOLOGY

There does not appear to be a single, specific cause of eating disorders. Studies suggest rather that eating disorders develop from a complex combination of genetic, cultural, biological, psychological, familial, and environmental factors. Twin studies have found a higher concordance rate for eating disorders among monozygotic than dizygotic twins. Young women with a first-degree relative who suffers from an eating disorder are at an eightfold increased risk. Whether this is related to genetics or learned behavior from watching an affected mother or sister's eating behaviors is unclear. Eating disorders are more prevalent in industrialized countries. The idealization of thinness in American media, including unrealistic portrayals of body size and shape and heavy marketing of diet and weight loss aids, may contribute to the problem. Participation in certain activities such as gymnastics, figure skating, and running increase the risk of developing an eating disorder. Eating disorders are also more prevalent among models, ballet dancers, wrestlers, and horse jockeys. Certain personality characteristics have been implicated in the etiology; anorexia is more common among achievement-oriented individuals who exhibit perfectionistic tendencies. There have been a number of studies examining neurochemical differences in patients suffering from eating disorders. However, determining if the neurochemical alterations predisposed the individual to develop the disorder or merely represent a consequence of starvation can be challenging.

CLINICAL MANIFESTATIONS

In patients who are willing to discuss their eating behaviors openly, the diagnosis of an eating disorder can be made on history alone. Anorexic patients are often preoccupied with food and have strict, self-imposed guidelines for which foods can be eaten based on fat, carbohydrate, or caloric content. They have a rigid schedule of eating and/or exercising, have unrealistic perceptions of their own body, and express a fear of being fat. Anorexics often have poor insight and do not realize that their dieting is excessive and may quickly become defensive or irritable when others express concern. In contrast, bulimic patients usually recognize that their binging and purging behavior is markedly abnormal. They often feel guilty, ashamed, or embarrassed about their behavior and may be extremely secretive. It is not unusual for bulimic patients to have stolen food or laxatives. A nonjudgmental and empathic approach during the history may help to elicit more sensitive subject matter.

There are several components of an eating disorder history. It may help to start by obtaining objective information, such as a family history of eating disorders; the patient's menstrual history; the patient's current, highest, and goal weights; and a pertinent review of systems (common complaints include cold intolerance, constipation, lightheadedness, and palpitations). The history can then gradually be steered toward more personal subject matter such as how the patient feels about his/her body or if a specific stressor precipitated the dieting. A weight comment made in jest by a coach, parent, or significant other frequently becomes an eating disorder patient's driving motivation. It is important to try to obtain a detailed dietary history including types of food eaten and specific quantities. Patients with anorexia nervosa, binge-eating/purging subtype, may consider two slices of bread with peanut butter a "binge" in contrast to patients with bulimia, for whom a binge may be a large pizza and a half gallon of ice cream. Anorexic patients often keep a detailed daily journal of their intake. Finally, inquire about compensatory behaviors such as fasting, overexercise, inducing vomiting or using laxatives, diuretics, or enemas. This component of the history is sometimes the most shameful for the patient to discuss but is vitally important since specific behaviors are associated with different medical complications.

A thorough physical examination should be performed on all eating disorder patients. Vital signs may reveal hypothermia, bradycardia, hypotension, and orthostasis. Weight should be recorded and percentage of ideal body weight calculated. Skin findings in anorexia may include lanugo, brittle hair and nails, dryness, yellowish discoloration secondary to hypercarotenemia, or acrocyanosis. Russell's sign (abrasions, callouses, or scarring on the dorsum of the hand) may be seen in patients who self-induce vomiting. These patients may also have parotid enlargement and erosion of dental enamel on head, ears, eyes, nose, and throat (HEENT) examination. The cardiac examination may reveal a midsystolic click consistent with mitral valve prolapse, which has a higher reported frequency in eating disorder patients. Bowel sounds may be decreased in starvation, or hyperactive if the patient has recently ingested laxatives. Patients with a thin habitus and constipation often have palpable stool in the left lower quadrant. Anorexic patients will frequently have breast atrophy and atrophic vaginitis from a chronic, low estrogen state. It is important to examine the lower extremities for evidence of edema. The process of refeeding may precipitate congestive heart failure or a refeeding syndrome in some patients undergoing rapid increases in daily caloric intake.

DIAGNOSIS

Obtaining a history which elicits the DSM-IV criteria is an efficient approach for diagnosis (Table 121.1).

In patients who meet most but not all of the criteria for anorexia or bulimia, the appropriate diagnosis is eating disorder, not otherwise specified. This diagnosis also applies to patients with other abnormal eating behaviors such as chewing and spitting out food without swallowing or using compensatory behaviors to prevent weight gain after consuming normal quantities of food.

Laboratory tests are used most often to monitor for medical complications of eating disorders.

TABLE 121.1 Eating disorders diagnostic criteria

Anorexia nervosa	Bulimia nervosa	Binge eating disorder[a]
1. Weight less than 85% of ideal body weight (either due to loss or failure to gain during growth period) 2. Fear of gaining weight or becoming fat despite being underweight 3. Distorted perception of one's own body 4. Absence of at least three consecutive menstrual cycles Subtypes: Restricting (patients that do not binge or purge) or binge-eating/purging type	1. Recurrent binge eating (consuming an excessive amount of food in a short time while having the sense of a lack of control) 2. Compensatory behavior to prevent weight gain 3. Behavior occurs at least twice weekly for 3 months 4. Self evaluation influenced excessively by weight and body shape 5. Disturbance does not occur exclusively during episode of anorexia nervosa	1. Recurrent binge eating 2. Binges associated with three or more features: a. Rapid eating b. Eating until uncomfortably full c. Eating when not hungry d. Eating alone because of embarrassment e. Feeling disgusted, depressed, or guilty after 3. Distress over binging 4. Occurs twice weekly over 6 months 5. No compensatory behavior

[a]Diagnosis based on research criteria.
Adapted from the *Diagnostic and Statistical Manual of Mental Disorders, Fourth Revision.* Washington, DC: American Psychiatric Association; 2000.

However, laboratory tests may be of diagnostic value in patients presenting with a seemingly unreliable history because of inconsistencies or contradictions with reports from family members. For example, hypochloremic metabolic alkalosis with hypokalemia would be indicative of vomiting in a patient who had denied recent purging behaviors. An electrocardiogram should be obtained in every patient with either anorexia or bulimia nervosa. Sinus bradycardia, T-wave inversion, ST depression, and QT prolongation may be noted.

TREATMENT

Comprehensive care of eating disorder patients often involves a multidisciplinary team including a medical physician, a mental health professional, and a registered dietician. When anorexia patients are 20% or more below the expected weight for their height, hospitalization is required to help restore the patient's nutritional state and hydration. Referral to a mental health professional for cognitive behavioral psychotherapy is the mainstay of treatment for all eating disorders. Additionally family therapy appears to be beneficial for adolescent anorexic patients and trials of supportive, interpersonal, and group psychotherapy have demonstrated efficacy in the treatment of bulimia. Drug trials in the treatment of anorexia nervosa have had disappointing results. Selective serotonin reuptake inhibitors (SSRIs) may be used to treat comorbid depression or obsessive-compulsive disorder in anorexic patients. In contrast, numerous medications have been found to be beneficial in the treatment of bulimia. Fluoxetine titrated to a dose of 60 mg daily is often used first-line because of its favorable side-effect profile. Randomized controlled trials of several SSRIs in the treatment of binge eating disorder have also reported promising results. While the majority of eating disorder

TABLE 121.2 Medical complications of eating disorders

Body system	Complication	Presenting context
Metabolic	Hypophosphatemia	Refeeding syndrome
	Hyperphosphatemia	Vomiting
	Hypokalemia	Vomiting
	Hyponatremia	Water intoxication or due to diabetes insipidus
	Hypomagnesemia	Starvation
	Hypercarotenemia	Starvation
	Hypochloremic metabolic alkalosis	Vomiting
	Metabolic acidosis	Laxative abuse
	Hypocalcemia	Purging
Gastrointestinal	Mallory-Weiss tears/esophageal rupture	Vomiting
	Gastric rupture	Binge eating
	Rectal prolapse	Laxative abuse
	Impaired motility	Starvation
	Melanosis coli	Use of anthracin laxatives
	Gallstones	Rapid weight loss
	Elevated transaminases	Starvation
	Superior mesenteric artery syndrome	Anorexia or bulimia
Cardiac	Cardiomyopathy	Chronic ipecac ingestion
	Cardiac muscle wasting	Starvation
	Dysrhythmias/sudden death	Related to electrolyte disturbance, prolonged QT
	Congestive heart failure	Refeeding syndrome
Pulmonary (rare)	Aspiration pneumonia	Vomiting
	Pneumomediastinum	Vomiting
Reproductive	Low birth weight	Starvation while pregnant
	Hypothalamic amenorrhea	Starvation
Renal	Nephrolithiasis	Dehydration
	Azotemia	Dehydration
Endocrine	Osteoporosis/osteopenia	Starvation
	Dental Caries/parotid enlargement/ hyperamylasemia	Vomiting
	Euthyroid sick syndrome	Starvation
	Hypercortisolemia	Starvation
	Hypoglycemia	Starvation
Hematologic	Anemia	Bone marrow depression secondary to starvation, B12, iron or folate deficiency
	Leukopenia	
	Thrombocytopenia	
Neurologic	Cognitive impairment	Starvation
	Seizures	Electrolyte disturbance
	Peripheral neuropathy	Starvation
Immunologic	Impaired cell-mediated immunity	Starvation

patients will recover with treatment, the disorder can have a chronic course in 20% to 30% of patients. Close collaboration between the primary care provider and the mental health care provider is most beneficial for patients with eating disorders.

COMPLICATIONS

Numerous medical complications of eating disorders have been described in Table 121.2.

Dermatology

Priya Young, Robert Krippendorf, and Janet Fairley

CHAPTER 122

Psoriasis

Robert Krippendorf, Priya Young, and Janet Fairley

The overall prevalence of psoriasis is 2%, but it ranges from 0% in Samoan populations to 12% in the Arctic Kasach'ye. In the United States, the prevalence is 1.4% to 4.7%, but lower in African Americans. There is a hereditary predisposition, with 50% of the siblings of persons with psoriasis being affected when both parents had the disease. There are seven susceptibility loci that have been discovered on genetic testing.

ETIOLOGY

The disease appears to be mediated by effector T cells of the immune system, but what triggers this is not known. Effector T cells release multiple cytokines and chemokines, which have complex, cascading interactions and effects that lead to increased vascularity, increased leukocyte recruitment, and decreased cell adhesion.

CLINICAL MANIFESTATIONS

The hallmarks of psoriasis are the red, sharply demarcated papules and plaques covered by thick, silvery-white scales. Individual lesions can number anywhere from one to hundreds, and they vary in size and shape from small guttate papules to large circinate plaques (see Color Plate 15). Symmetrically distributed, the lesions show a predilection for the scalp, genitals, nails, and extensor aspects of the arms and legs. Secondary excoriations or lichenification may develop with pruritic eruptions.

The nails may develop pitting (see Color Plate 16), onycholysis (lifting of the nail plate from the nail bed), brown "oil spots," subungual hyperkeratosis, grooving, and crumbling. The Koebner phenomenon, in which typical lesions form at the site of minor trauma, is characteristic.

Psoriasis has numerous clinical variants, including eruptive or guttate, inverse, pustular, and erythrodermic types. Guttate psoriasis is characterized by 0.5- to 1.5-cm red papules and plaques that may be provoked by infections, particularly streptococcal ones. Inverse psoriasis is localized to the axilla, groin, and skin folds rather than the classic sites.

Pustular psoriasis can be localized or generalized. The generalized form has an acute onset with crops of pustules and associated fever and leukocytosis.

Erythroderma of any cause, including psoriasis, disrupts thermoregulation and fluid balance and thus signals a potential emergency. Erythrodermic psoriasis has many of the constitutional features of generalized pustular psoriasis. The inflammatory arthritis associated with psoriasis is discussed in Chapter 51.

DIAGNOSIS

The diagnosis is most often made by history and physical examination, but in some instances skin biopsy is performed to confirm the diagnosis. Psoriasis may be confused with nummular eczema, cutaneous T-cell lymphoma, secondary syphilis, pityriasis rosea, or tinea infections.

THERAPY

Most patients with localized disease respond to topical treatment with steroids, calcipotriene (a vitamin D analogue), coal tar, or retinoids. More severe disease, such as patients with 20% to 30% affected body surface area, warrant more aggressive therapy with light, oral retinoids, methotrexate, cyclosporine, or one of the newer biologic agents.

COMPLICATIONS

Individual patients may develop psoriatic arthritis, which especially affects the hands or feet. Erythrodermic psoriasis can be life threatening and may lead to dehydration and electrolyte imbalance from fluid loss through the compromised skin, as well as temperature dysregulation. It may require inpatient treatment.

CHAPTER 123

Seborrheic Dermatitis

Robert Krippendorf, Priya Young, and Janet Fairley

Seborrheic dermatitis is a common inflammatory skin disorder characterized by red macules and irregular patches surmounted by yellow-white, fine, greasy scales. This dermatitis affects all ages from infant to adult without predilection for either sex.

ETIOLOGY

Although no causative agent has been clearly demonstrated, *Pityrosporum ovale*—a lipophilic, pleomorphic fungus from scalp lesions—has been often isolated. Patients with human immunodeficiency virus may present with severe disease, suggesting a role for immune dysfunction in the disease.

CLINICAL MANIFESTATIONS

The classic presentation is erythematous macules or patches with overlying powdery scales on the scalp. Other areas that are commonly involved include the nasolabial folds, eyebrows, eyelids and eyelashes ears, central chest, axilla, inframammary creases, and groin. Scaly red patches on the edges of the eyelids (marginal blepharitis) may be accompanied by conjunctivitis. In severe cases, an acute eczematous eruption develops on the trunk, and may evolve into erythroderma. The course is chronic with exacerbations and remissions. The lesions often improve after exposure to sunlight during the summer, and the disease is aggravated by cold winter weather and stress.

DIAGNOSIS

A potassium hydroxide examination will distinguish seborrheic dermatitis from an atypical dermatophyte infection. The appearance is classic, but it may be difficult to distinguish from psoriasis and tinea (dermatophytosis).

TREATMENT

Scalp disease usually responds to shampoos containing selenium sulfide, salicylic acid, zinc pyrithione, tar, or ketoconazole. Topical steroid solutions may be applied once or twice daily in resistant cases. On the face and in intertriginous areas, the inflammation may be treated with mild topical steroids, antifungals, or immunomodulators such as pimecrolimus or tacrolimus.

CHAPTER 124

Impetigo

Robert Krippendorf, Priya Young, and Janet Fairley

Impetigo, also called impetigo contagiosa, is a common superficial cutaneous infection with two basic subtypes: bullous and nonbullous. Both subtypes, which are exacerbated by hot and humid weather, are more frequent in children aged 2 to 5 years than in adults.

ETIOLOGY

Bullous impetigo, in which the blistered and denuded areas are a cutaneous response to the bacterial toxin, termed exfoliatin, is caused by *Staphylococcus aureus* of phage group II and commonly seen with type 71. Exfoliatin cleaves a cell adhesion molecule in the skin, desmoglein 1, leading to blister formation. Nonbullous impetigo is due to group A β-hemolytic streptococci *(Streptococcus pyogenes),* often along with *S. aureus.*

CLINICAL MANIFESTATIONS

Nonbullous impetigo is the most frequent skin infection in children, with lesions developing at sites of injury—for example, insect bites, abrasions, or other trauma. Poor hygiene, overcrowding, humidity, and warm environments favor its development. The highest incidence is during the summer, when a higher likelihood of injuries and factors that favor the development of lesions exists. Preferred sites of involvement are the face, extremities, and neck. The primary lesion, a red macule, evolves into a papule or vesicle and rapidly becomes crusted. Typical findings are multiple, thick, honey-colored crusts, ulcers, and erosions. Bullous impetigo is less common. Lesions develop on normal skin, most commonly in the axillae, groin, and hands. They consist of superficial, fragile, subcorneal bullae containing yellow-white opaque fluid. The bullae rupture rapidly, exposing erosions that are covered by thin, yellow-brown crusts.

DIAGNOSIS

Although the thick, honey-colored crusts of nonbullous impetigo are pathognomonic, the lesions of bullous impetigo, with their thinner amber crusts, are less distinctive. The Nikolsky's sign (spreading of a blister when pressure is applied to the surrounding skin) is negative, which distinguishes bullous impetigo from primary blistering diseases (like pemphigus) with secondary infection. A culture of the blister fluid or the ulcer base confirms the diagnosis.

TREATMENT

Impetigo is effectively treated by suitable antibiotics and topical skin care. A beta-lactamase resistant antibiotic (dicloxacillin or cephalosporin) is recommended, given the need to treat staphylococci and streptococci. For superficial impetigo, topical mupirocin 2% ointment is as effective as oral antibiotics. Extensive or deep lesions mandate oral agents. Gentle cleansing and warm compresses can remove crusts. To minimize autoinoculation and contagion, patients should practice good hygiene. Patients with recurrent infections may require evaluation for potential carriage of nasal or perioral *S. aureus*.

COMPLICATIONS

In nonbullous impetigo, glomerulonephritis (caused by nephritogenic strains of streptococci) may occur. Scarlet fever is rarely seen as a sequela.

CHAPTER 125

Dermatophytosis

Robert Krippendorf, Priya Young, and Janet Fairley

Dermatophytosis (tinea or ringworm) is a superficial fungal infection of the skin, hair, or nails. The primary types of dermatophytoses are tinea capitis, tinea faciei, tinea barbae, tinea pedis, tinea manus, tinea corporis, tinea cruris, and onychomycosis. Some infections are inflammatory with fluctuant plaques and pustules, and others cause minimal scaling and erythema.

ETIOLOGY

Dermatophytes live in the superficial, cornified epidermal cells. They are ubiquitous in the environment and the source of an individual infection may be difficult to determine if there has not been family or animal contact. The host response to the infection in humans is influenced by the origin of the organism; species acquired from the soil or from animals induce a vigorous response, but those acquired from humans induce little inflammation. Three genera of dermatophytes exist: Microsporum, Trichophyton, and Epidermophyton. The organisms causing a given type of infection vary with time and geographic location. The etiologic agents responsible for each type of dermatophytosis are shown in Table 125.1. In addition, it is important to remember that nearly 5% of people in the United States have had an episode of tinea versicolor.

CLINICAL MANIFESTATIONS

Tinea pedis is the most prevalent dermatophytosis in adult and has several distinct clinical presentations: the interdigital form; a sharply circumscribed "moccasin" distribution; and an acute inflammatory, vesiculobullous eruption on the soles of the feet.

Tinea versicolor is one of the most common dermatophytes causing superficial infections, particularly in adolescents and young adults (15 to 30 years of age). The agent causing tinea versicolor is *Malassezia furfur* (*Pityrosporon orbiculare*). Nearly 5% of people in the United States have had an episode of tinea versicolor.

Tinea versicolor presents as multiple, oval, hypopigmented or hyperpigmented patches with fine scale distributed on the trunk, proximal arms, and face. Although mild pruritus may occur, tinea versicolor is asymptomatic in most cases. Many patients present during the summer months when they note the contrast between tanned and lesional skin. The race and complexion of the individual influence the color of the lesions. The inhibition of melanin production and transfer by azelaic acid produced by the fungus causes hypopigmentation, and the stimulation of melanogenesis by the inflammatory response causes hyperpigmentation.

Tinea manum often coexists with bilateral tinea pedis or fingernail involvement and resembles the dry, scaly noninflammatory form of tinea pedis. Tinea capitis is characterized by scaling patches of alopecia (see Color Plate 17). Tinea unguium or onychomycosis presents with yellow-brown

TABLE 125.1 Characteristic clinical features of dermatophytoses

Subtype	Characteristics	Comments	Causative organism
Tinea pedis	The most prevalent dermatophyte infection in adults	May be complicated by lymphangitis and cellulitis	Trichophyton rubrum
Interdigital form	Maceration, scaling, and fissuring between the fourth and fifth toes; painful infection	Most common subtype; often extends to involve additional web spaces	Trichophyton rubrum
	Sharply circumscribed, red, scaly plaques with a hyperkeratotic surface on the soles and lateral aspects of the feet in a "moccasin" distribution		Trichophyton mentagrophytes
Vesiculobullous type	Vesicles/bullae and eczematous changes in the soles of the feet	Acute inflammatory eruption; likely to be symptomatic with pruritus, burning, and tenderness	Trichophyton mentagrophytes
Tinea manum	Lesions most frequent on the palms and thumb web space in a unilateral distribution	Resembles the dry, scaly noninflammatory form of tinea pedis; often seen in conjunction with bilateral tinea pedis or fingernail involvement	Trichophyton mentagrophytes
Tinea cruris (jock itch)	Arcuate, red, generally symmetric, scaly patches with sharp margins, involving the inner thighs, inguinal folds, and rarely the perineum, buttocks, and scrotum; the enlarging rings are macerated, crusted, vesicular, or scaly	Heat and humidity perpetuate the infection; men affected more frequently than women; risk factors are obesity, tightly fitted clothing, and frequent, strenuous activity	Epidermophyton floccosum
Tinea capitis (Color Plate 17)	Initial lesions are erythematous, scaling patches of alopecia; variable inflammation; small patches of alopecia; hairs broken at the level of the skin, creating "black dots" (black-dot tinea); sharply circumscribed, boggy, highly inflammatory, tender mass (kerion); onset acute; papules and pustules often cover the surface	Superficial fungal infection of the scalp; occurs primarily in children, less common in infants, adolescents, or adults; incidence greater in boys and African American children; lymphadenopathy often present even with subtle cutaneous findings (important diagnostic clue for tinea capitis)	Most cases due to *Trichophyton tonsurans*, *Microsporum canis*, and *Trichophyton violaceum*

Tinea corporis	Single or multiple annular, erythematous plaques with fine white scale; vesicles or pustules may be present on the surface of some acute inflammatory plaques; sharply demarcated, raised borders; they enlarge progressively	Lesions are localized to glabrous (non–Bhair-bearing) skin (palms, soles, groin, and beard area excluded)	Most cases due to Trichophyton rubrum, Microsporum canis, and Trichophyton tonsurans
Tinea faciei	Erythematous lesions often have poorly defined borders; the scaling may be minimal	Unusual fungal infection to the cheeks and forehead	Trichophyton rubrum
Tinea barbae	Papules, pustules, nodules, and erythematous plaques in the beard area; with established infection, loosened and broken hairs form irregular patches of alopecia and crusting; fluctuant-draining abscesses occur in some cases	Uncommon disorder, seen almost exclusively among male farm workers; spread by contaminated razors	Trichophyton mentagrophytes, Trichophyton verrucosum
Tinea unguium (onychomycosis) (Color Plate 18)	Gradual onset with a small patch of yellow, white, or brown discoloration forming at the edge of the nail; onycholysis develops as the nail plate lifts from the nail bed with the creation of crumbly subungual debris; with further infection, the nail becomes thickened and broken	Chronic dermatophyte infection of the fingernails or the toenails	Trichophyton rubrum, Trichophyton mentagrophytes

discoloration of the nail resulting in nail thickening as the infection progresses (see Color Plate 18).The clinical features associated with the different types of fungal infections are shown in Table 125.1.

DIAGNOSIS

Dermatophyte infections are diagnosed with a potassium hydroxide preparation using scales from the surface of the lesion. When tinea capitis is suspected, hairs from the periphery of the patches are inspected for spores. However, the potassium hydroxide (KOH) examination is rarely helpful without alopecia (hair loss) or with intense inflammation. A fungal culture will confirm the diagnosis. When *Malassezia audouinii* and *Malassezia canis* commonly caused tinea in the past, the Wood's lamp examination rapidly diagnosed tinea by observing a blue fluorescence. Because these are less common etiologic agents in tinea currently, the Wood's lamp is now rarely used to diagnose tinea.

TABLE 125.2 Dermatophytosis and other dermatologic disorders to be considered in the differential diagnosis

Dermatophytosis	Differential diagnosis
Tinea corporis	Folliculitis Impetigo Trichotillomania Seborrheic, contact dermatitis Psoriasis Systemic lupus erythematosus Secondary syphilis Pityriasis rosea
Tinea barbae	Bacterial and herpetic infections Contact dermatitis
Tinea cruris	Candidal intertrigo Seborrheic dermatitis Psoriasis Irritant dermatitis
Tinea pedis and tinea manum	Psoriasis Contact dermatitis Irritant dermatitis Dyshidrotic eczema Candidiasis
Tinea unguium	Trauma Lichen planus Psoriasis Damage from nail polish Other primary nail dystrophies
Tinea faciei	Contact dermatitis Seborrheic dermatitis Systemic lupus erythematosus

The diagnosis of tinea versicolor is usually evident by the characteristic cutaneous eruption. When the findings are subtle, the skin may be viewed in a darkened room with a Wood's lamp, which will enhance the differences in the lesional and uninvolved skin. The best confirmatory test is the KOH examination. Dermatologic disorders that should be considered in the differential diagnosis are listed in Table 125.2.

TREATMENT

Tinea capitis, unguium, and barbae, and severe or recalcitrant infections of the palms, soles, groin, or glabrous skin, require systemic antifungal therapy. Topical therapy usually suffices for tinea pedis, tinea manum, tinea corporis, and tinea cruris. The most common systemic agents are terbinafine, itraconazole, and griseofulvin. A large number of topical agents are available to treat localized tinea infections. Some examples are ciclopirox, miconazole, and clotrimazole. It should be noted that where nystatin is ineffective in *Candida* (yeast) infections, it will not treat dermatophytes.

CHAPTER 126

Acne

Robert Krippendorf, Priya Young, and Janet Fairley

ACNE VULGARIS

Acne vulgaris, a very common skin disorder, is a self-limited inflammatory disorder of the pilosebaceous unit. Usually, it begins at puberty and affects mostly adolescents (85% of persons between 12 and 25 years of age). However, the median age for consultation is 24 years and 10% of patients are aged 35 to 44 years. In girls, it may precede menarche. The peak prevalence is age 14 to 17 years in girls and 16 to 19 years in boys, with a higher frequency and severity in boys. Most patients note significant improvement by age 20 to 23 years, but in 8% to 10%, some activity continues into the fifth decade. The inheritance pattern of acne vulgaris has not been established, but most experts invoke an autosomal dominant trait with variable penetrance or a polygenic trait involving many genes. Genetics may play a role because whites are affected more often than Japanese or African Americans.

Etiology

Acne develops from the interaction of multiple factors. Lipid is released into the follicular canal as part of a complex mixture called sebum that lubricates the skin. In acne, sebum is produced in excess, perhaps due to changes in androgen levels. The sebum composition is altered compared to those without acne, with a significantly lower level of linoleic acid. This abnormality may encourage the cohesion of cornified cells; their accumulation in sebaceous follicles results in comedones. These noninflammatory lesions are transformed into inflammatory lesions by *Propionibacterium acnes* in the follicular canal. *P. acnes* incites inflammation by generating free fatty acids and by recruiting lymphocytes and neutrophils, which release inflammatory mediators. The inflammatory products and sebum exert pressure on the epithelial wall, causing the follicle to rupture; inflammatory papules, pustules, and nodules follow.

Clinical Manifestations

Acne vulgaris predominantly appears in areas where the pilosebaceous follicles are the most dense, namely the face, neck, and upper trunk. Acne vulgaris has a number of clinical variants, with combinations of comedones, papules, pustules, nodules, and cysts. An open comedone is black due to the oxidation of accumulated material and the presence of melanin. A closed comedone is a flesh-colored papule with a minute ostium that inhibits the discharge of keratin debris. This is the primary lesion in the formation of inflammatory papules and pustules. In severe cases, nodules, cysts, and granulomatous lesions develop progressively. This intense inflammation finally leads to fibrosis, scars, and occasionally keloids. Individual papules and pustules resolve with transient erythema and postinflammatory hyperpigmentation, which can be particularly prominent in African Americans and takes months to improve.

Diagnosis

A complete history should be obtained to establish the cause, duration, localization, and severity. In susceptible individuals, the onset or exacerbation of acne is influenced by a family history of acne;

TABLE 126.1	Severity of acne according to number and type of lesions
Severity	**Lesions**
Mild	Less than 10 pustules
Moderate	10 to 40 pustules
Moderately severe	40 to 100 with inflammation
Severe	Nodulocystic acne

menses; occupational exposure to oils, tars, greases, chlorinated hydrocarbons, and waxes; medications such as oral contraceptives, corticosteroids, iodides, isoniazid, lithium, phenytoin, and trimethadione; cosmetics or hair preparations; and androgen excess denoted by hirsutism or menstrual irregularities. While typically distributed eruptions are diagnostic, acneiform lesions may occur in rosacea, perioral dermatitis, miliaria rubra, impetigo contagiosa, and folliculitis. The severity of acne is judged by the number of lesions and severity of inflammation (Table 126.1).

Treatment

The treatment regimen is determined by the severity of the disease and the predominant type of lesion. Topical and systemic agents can reduce bacterial load, inhibit inflammation, decrease sebaceous gland activity, and impede corneocyte adhesion. Dietary restrictions have no role. Inflammatory papules, pustules, and nodules are controlled with systemic antibiotics. They eliminate *Proprionobacter acne* from the skin, thus decreasing the free fatty acids in the sebaceous glands. Tetracycline, 1.0 g daily, tapered as clinical improvement occurs, is a safe, effective, and inexpensive initial choice. Significant response may take 4 to 6 weeks. Alternative agents are erythromycin, doxycycline, minocycline, and sulfonamides. Persons receiving tetracycline should avoid sun exposure. The only medication likely to produce a remission in patients with recalcitrant severe acne is isotretinoin (Accutane), a vitamin-A derivative. All forms of acne respond to it but the side-effect profile restricts its use to only the most severe cases. Isotretinoin is given in a dose of 0.5 to 2 mg/kg/day; doses less than 1 mg/kg/day enhance the likelihood of recurrence. Its teratogenicity precludes its use in pregnancy. Other common complications are dry skin and mucous membranes, hyperlipidemia, mucositis, and cheilitis. An increased risk of pseudotumor cerebri exists, especially when tetracyclines are given simultaneously.

Comedonal acne is best treated by the topical retinoids, which normalizes keratinization in the follicles and suppresses bacterial proliferation. The formation of new follicular plugs is inhibited and existing plugs are eliminated. Tretinoin is applied in a thin layer every night to dry skin. Early complications include burning, erythema, and peeling. The concentration of the preparation is increased according to response and tolerance. It is indicated for all types of acne because comedones are a common component.

The use of benzoyl peroxide as a topical bactericidal agent either alone or combined with tretinoin or antibiotics significantly reduce the density of *P. acne* on the skin. Many different preparations contain benzoyl peroxide, with concentrations varying between 2.5% and 10%. Irritation is the most important side effect, related to the concentration of benzoyl peroxide and the vehicle. Another treatment option in mild to moderate acne vulgaris is topical antibiotics to decrease the population of *P. acne*, the most effective ones being 1% clindamycin and 2% erythromycin. Bacterial resistance may follow topical and systemic antibiotic use. Selected patients may use oral corticosteroids, oral contraceptives, and dapsone.

Acne surgery is the physical removal of the contents of comedones, pustules, and cysts to promote rapid improvement while the patient awaits the gradual effects of topical or systemic therapy. The intralesional injection of triamcinolone acetonide into large inflammatory cysts, pustules, and nodules leads to resolution of lesions with less scarring.

ACNE ROSACEA

Rosacea, a chronic vascular and inflammatory disorder, occurs primarily on the central region of the face and has two major components: (a) the vascular component consisting of erythema and telangiectases; and (b) the acneiform component consisting of papules, pustules, and sebaceous gland hyperplasia. The inflammatory lesions exacerbate and remit and, when deep, may heal with scarring. Although associated with menopause and observed most commonly in women aged 30 to 50 years; rosacea is more severe in men. It is rare in African American patients.

Etiology

The cause of rosacea is unknown. Vascular instability, with a consistent tendency to blush and flush easily, is an important element. Celtic origin and a fair complexion are also risk factors. Vasodilators (e.g., hot liquids, alcohol, spicy foods, and sun exposure) exacerbate it. Although patients with increased numbers of *Demodex folliculorum* might improve as the organism is eliminated by treatment, the association with *Demodex* is inconsistent. Sebaceous gland activity is stimulated, but not as the primary event. Unlike acne vulgaris, abnormal keratinization is absent.

Clinical Manifestations

The cheeks, chin, nose, forehead, eyes, and, less often, the seborrheic areas of the chest, scalp, and posterior ears are involved. The disease evolves from intermittent episodes of flushing and blushing to persistent erythema and telangiectasia on the nose and cheeks. This may occur as early as the second decade. Crops of papules and pustules develop and the orifices of sebaceous glands become prominent. In severe cases, the nose becomes thickened and disfigured with the formation of rhinophyma. Rarely, inflammatory nodules are seen, which may be granulomatous or connected by sinus tracts, furuncles, and abscesses. The eyes are commonly involved, and blepharitis, conjunctivitis, iritis, keratitis, iridocyclitis, and hypopyon are common.

Diagnosis

Acne vulgaris, seborrheic dermatitis, lupus erythematosus, and carcinoid syndrome simulate acne rosacea. Lack of comedones and distribution in the medial face help distinguish it from acne vulgaris. The lesions of seborrheic dermatitis are red or pink macules covered with greasy yellow scales and localized to the eyebrows, nasolabial folds, scalp, chest, and ears. Lupus erythematosus and carcinoid syndrome can be established by estimating antinuclear antibodies and 5-hydroxyindoleacetic acid, respectively, especially in atypical cases.

Treatment

Rosacea has a spectrum of severity and its course is punctuated by exacerbations and remissions. However, even aggressive therapy rarely resolves all lesions completely. The use of a broad-spectrum sunscreen should always be encouraged. Mild disease needs no treatment except avoiding sun exposure and other vasodilatory agents. Moderate disease often responds well to oral tetracycline with or without topical metronidazole. Usually, tetracycline (1.0 g per day) for 4 to 6 weeks will suffice until the flare remits; it is then tapered to the smallest maintenance dose.

Alternative agents are erythromycin, minocycline, or oral metronidazole. Traditional acne therapy with benzoyl peroxide and topical erythromycin or clindamycin solutions may benefit some, but the benzoyl peroxide and the alcohol vehicle of these solutions may irritate sensitive, fair skin. Although topical steroids will initially help in cases of erythema, they should be used cautiously because their long-term use may worsen the telangiectases.

Rhinophyma and granulomatous lesions respond to isotretinoin, but relapses are frequent when the drug is discontinued. Additional options are pulsed dye laser or electrosurgery for telangiectases, laser or surgical therapy for rhinophyma, and antiparasitic drugs for exacerbations of rosacea due to *Demodex* infestation. Ketoconazole cream sometimes elicits good results owing to its anti-inflammatory and antibiotic properties.

CHAPTER 127

Basal Cell Carcinoma, Actinic Keratoses, Squamous Cell Carcinoma, and Malignant Melanoma

Robert Krippendorf, Priya Young, Janet Fairley

Skin cancer is the most common cancer in the United States, with over 1 million cases diagnosed annually. Nonmelanoma skin cancers are the most common, with basal cell carcinoma comprising about 80% and squamous cell approximately 20%. Melanoma is less prevalent, but its frequency has been increasing. Multiple genetic and environmental factors likely interact and contribute to the development of these diseases. Other precancerous skin disorders such as actinic keratosis will also be described in this chapter.

BASAL CELL CARCINOMA

Etiology

Risk factors for basal cell carcinoma include light skin color, blond or red hair, and blue or green eyes. Exposure to ultraviolet light, especially intense unprotected exposure in childhood or adolescence, as well as arsenic ingestion or coal tar exposure is associated with the disease. The contribution by smoking is controversial. Immunosuppression (such as with renal or cardiac transplant patients) also increases the risk. Research has shown possible role of decreased tumor suppressor gene function, as well as mutations in activating genes.

Clinical Manifestations

These cancers are usually located on the sun-exposed areas of the head and neck and to a lesser extent on the trunk and extremities. There are four general forms: nodular, superficial, morpheaform-type and pigmented basal cell carcinoma. The nodular type presents classically as a lesion with heaped borders, a pearly appearance with telangiectasias on the surface and a central ulcer or crusting. Superficial basal cell may look like a scaly, erythematous patch or plaque. Morpheaform type (also called fibrosing, infiltrative or sclerosing type) may appear as a hypopigmented, indurated patch or like a scar with unclear margins (see Color Plate 19).

Diagnosis

Skin biopsy is required for diagnosis. Other considerations to consider for the nodular subtype include: squamous cell carcinoma, keratoacanthoma, and sebaceous hyperplasia. For the superficial subtype, psoriasis, eczema, and tinea infection should be considered. For morphea-like subtype, consider localized scleroderma and for the pigmented subtype, consider nevus or melanoma.

Treatment

Many options for treatment exist and depend on the clinical setting. Curettage and electrodesiccation, excisional biopsy, Mohs' micrographic surgery (especially for larger lesions), topical therapy with 5-fluorouracil, imiquimod, photodynamic therapy, or radiotherapy may be used depending on the size and location of the cancer as well as the relative health or illness of the patient. The Mohs' micrographic technique of surgical excision is preferred therapy of choice when the face is involved.

ACTINIC KERATOSIS

Actinic keratoses are common premalignant lesions that develop on chronically sun-exposed areas. Related to cumulative sun exposure, they are the first clinical stage in the evolution of a squamous cell carcinoma. Risk factors for their development include fair skin type, failure to protect the skin with sunscreen, and exposure to high-intensity solar irradiation. Older adults with blue eyes, freckling, and a fair complexion who live in sunny, warm regions are at greatest risk for developing actinic keratoses and skin cancer. In high-risk persons, these keratoses may occur even at the age of 20 or 30 years.

Clinical Manifestations

Unless irritated or traumatized, the lesions usually cause no symptoms. The face, ears, dorsal hands, and forearms are the most commonly involved sites. The 1- to 10-mm flesh-colored, pink, or red macules or scaly papules are more easily felt by palpation than identified visually. The surface is verrucous or hyperkeratotic with variable amounts of fine white scale. Hypertrophic actinic keratoses may form cutaneous horns; squamous cell cancer may develop later in the base. Other signs of excessive sun exposure may also be seen, such as telangiectases, lentigines, and excessive wrinkling.

The rate of neoplastic transformation of actinic keratoses ranges from 5% to 15%. These squamous cell cancers are generally not aggressive, and their metastatic potential is limited. However, lesions in specific sites (e.g., the hands, ears, and lips) may be more aggressive, thus having a higher metastatic potential.

Diagnosis

Seborrheic keratosis (a benign cutaneous tumor) and squamous cell cancer may cause diagnostic confusion. Seborrheic keratosis has distinctive plugs on its surface and a "stuck on" appearance. Squamous cell cancers are more indurated. Erosion, ulceration, and progressive enlargement are more typical of squamous cell cancer.

Treatment

Daily use of broad-spectrum sunscreens should be recommended to all patients with actinic keratoses. Lesions in limited numbers are often treatable with cryoablation with liquid nitrogen. Surgical excision, although rarely indicated as primary therapy, may sometimes be needed to establish the diagnosis. Topical 5-fluorouracil (T5-FU), 1% or 5% cream, applied twice daily is the most effective therapy for multiple lesions or large areas of involvement. T5-FU elicits an inflammatory reaction at the site of precancerous and cancerous lesions. Generally, the T5-FU creams are used for 2 to 3 weeks, or for 3 days after the most intense inflammation; topical steroids may be applied in conjunction with the T5-FU to reduce the severity of the reaction.

SQUAMOUS CELL CARCINOMA

Squamous cell carcinoma, an epithelial neoplasm, evolves from a clone of atypical keratinocytes. Squamous cell carcinomas represent nearly 20% of all nonmelanoma skin cancers. They most commonly afflict older persons, persons with a fair complexion, and men.

Etiology

Many factors, particularly ultraviolet radiation, influence the incidence of squamous cell carcinoma. Patients receiving long-term immunosuppression, such as organ transplant patients, are also at high risk. Long-standing ulcers are another setting in which squamous cell carcinoma of the skin may arise.

Clinical Features

Squamous cell carcinomas frequently arise on sun-exposed sites as well-demarcated red plaques or nodules with a scaly, verrucous, or papillated surface. Compared with basal cell carcinomas, a predilection exists for the dorsal hands, scalp, and pinna. As the cancer cells invade the dermis and subcutis, the plaques become firm, indurated, and fixed to underlying structures. Ulceration and bleeding are common (see Color Plate 20). These lesions often run an indolent course with many years of radial growth. Solar lentigines, actinic keratoses, and other signs of sun damage are usually seen on the surrounding skin.

The other common settings that harbor these cancers are scarred or chronically inflamed tissues. Lesions originating within burn scars, radiation ports, chronic ulcers, or sinuses behave aggressively, although they frequently are present for many months or years prior to diagnosis. The rate of metastasis is much greater in these patients. Invasive squamous cell carcinoma occurs in 5% to 15% of solar keratoses.

Many of the same factors that are predictive of recurrence and metastasis for basal cell carcinomas apply also to squamous cell carcinomas. Large, deep, and poorly differentiated lesions are more likely to be aggressive. The ear, lip, and inner canthus of the eye are sites with particularly high rates of recurrence and increased metastatic potential. Other poor prognostic factors are perineural spread, previous recurrence with adequate treatment, and formation within a scar. Widespread disease begins with lymph node involvement.

Diagnosis

The diagnosis frequently requires a biopsy. Clinical suspicion is aroused by the appropriate setting and presentation; however, the differential diagnosis may be challenging and include basal cell carcinomas, verrucous lesions (warts and seborrheic keratoses), metastatic neoplasms, plaques of psoriasis or eczema, and verrucous melanomas.

Management

The treatment of squamous cell carcinoma is similar to that of basal cell carcinoma. Superficial lesions may be removed by excision, electrodesiccation and curettage, or cryosurgery using probes to assess the depth of tissue necrosis with freezing. Tumors that are large, deep, or localized to sites with a high risk of invasion are treated with Mohs' micrographic surgery, which is also preferred for lesions with neurotropism or basosquamous histology.

MALIGNANT MELANOMA

Although melanoma comprises a small fraction of all skin cancer, it is the most feared type of cancer and its prevalence has been on the rise.

Etiology

Risk factors are similar to those for basal cell and squamous cell, but history of early age, intense (blistering) sun damage to skin is particularly important. Median age at diagnosis is 57 years and the incidence is higher in men than in women. Likely genetic (decreased tumor suppressor gene activity or sporadic point mutation with increased tumor promoter activity, or both) and environmental factors interact.

Clinical Manifestations

Features of a melanocytic lesion suggesting malignant melanoma are termed the "ABCDs:" A = asymmetry; B = borders, irregular or notched; C = color, multiple shades of tan, brown, and black; and D = diameter, exceeding 6 mm. Among the four primary clinical subtypes with divergent histologic findings and clinical courses (Table 127.1), the outcome best correlates with the depth of

TABLE 127.1 Clinical subtypes of malignant melanoma and their characteristics

Subtype	Characteristics	Appearance of lesions	Frequency	Comments
Superficial spreading melanoma (Color Plate 19)	Radial growth phase 1 to 5 years; predilection for the trunk in men and the lower extremities in women; median age at diagnosis is the fifth decade.	Flat papule or plaque, <3 cm in diameter, irregular borders, and patches of pink, brown, black, or white and areas of regression.	70% of all cases	Dysplastic or congenital nevi are precursor lesions. Regression may also reflect depth inaccurately and underestimate the tumor growth.
Nodular melanoma	Brief or absent radial growth and rapid vertical extension; most develop in 6 to 18 months. Men more affected than women; the trunk, head, and neck are the favored sites; the mean age of onset is in the sixth decade.	Symmetric blue, gray, or black dome-shaped nodules or pedunculated papules, with average size of 1 to 2 cm. Pedunculated ones are particularly aggressive. A small fraction are amelanotic.	15% to 30%	Aggressive lesions
Lentigo maligna melanoma	Slowly evolving. Present for 3 to 15 years at diagnosis. Most common in older women on the sun-exposed skin of the head and neck. Patients usually in the seventh decade of life.	Initially a tan macule, gradually enlarges to >3 cm. Exhibits asymmetry and varied color, and flecks of pigment may be noted within the brown or tan areas. After years of progression, the surface becomes irregularly elevated.	5% of all cases	Low risk of metastasis. Some clinicians designate the flat lesion as lentigo maligna and the elevated lesion as lentigo maligna melanoma.

(*continued*)

TABLE 127.1 Clinical subtypes of malignant melanoma and their characteristics (*continued*)

Subtype	Characteristics	Appearance of lesions	Frequency	Comments
Acral lentiginous variant	Involves the palms, soles, mucosa, nail bed, and periungual regions. The sole is the most frequently described location. Affects older individuals of both genders.	Nail bed melanomas produce a visible, pigmented band. Pigmentation of the proximal nail fold (Hutchinson's sign) is useful diagnostically. Diameter is often >3 cm. May initially resemble lentigo maligna type. Ulceration and hyperkeratosis observed in the nodular sections of the neoplasm.	1% to 10% among whites. Most common type in Asians, Hispanics, and American Indians.	Aggressive lesions. Often develop in 6 months.

tumor invasion (using the Breslow scale or Clark correlation measurement; see Differential Diagnosis and Management section) at diagnosis. Superficial spreading melanoma (see Color Plate 21) may show signs of regression; because both favorable and adverse outcomes are related to regression, its relevance is controversial. Nodular melanoma often has a worse prognosis, probably because of the melanoma's greater depth at diagnosis. The acral lentiginous variant also has a poor outcome because its recognition is often delayed. Metastases in melanoma follow local extension and occur by lymphatic or hematogenous invasion.

Diagnosis

Excisional biopsy is essential for a definitive diagnosis and important for tumor staging. Other conditions that may look like melanoma are pigmented basal cell, dysplastic nevus, and seborrheic keratosis to name a few. There are four types of melanoma based on histopathology. These are superficial spreading (the most common), nodular melanoma, lentigo maligna, and the acral lentiginous variant. Depth of melanoma is important. The Breslow depth relies on tumor thickness; less than 0.76 mm is favorable. Clark levels are based on skin anatomy. Clark level I is confined to the dermis, level II to the papillary dermis, level III extends to the junction of the reticular dermis, level IV extends into the reticular dermis, and level V extends into the subcutaneous tissue.

Treatment

Treatment depends on stage. There are guidelines for how wide a margin to resect and when to have sentinel node biopsy done, but this is beyond the scope of this text.

Complications

Metastases to lymph nodes, lung, gastrointestinal tract, brain, or other sites may occur. Survival rates at 5 years for regional spread (stage III) were 60% and in distant metastases (Stage IV) less than 15%.

CHAPTER 128

Urticaria

Robert Krippendorf, Priya Young, and Janet Fairley

Urticaria is commonly known as "hives" and may occur at any age. There are various types classified by what triggers them and how long they last; most often, the cause is not known.

ETIOLOGY

Acute urticaria has a duration of less than 6 weeks; the swelling and erythematous wheals may last from 30 minutes to 2 hours per episode. When a cause is found, it is often allergen mediated. This may be due to food, a drug, or contact with a chemical. Chronic urticaria is defined as lasting 6 weeks or more. Sixty percent of cases are idiopathic, but the remaining have immunoglobulin (Ig) G autoantibodies directed against the alpha subunit of the IgE receptor. The autoantibodies cause crosslinking of the IgE receptor, which triggers mast cell degranulation. Other chemokines and chemoattractants are released and skin biopsies have shown perivascular lymphocytes (predominately CD4+), increased monocytes, and variable levels of neutrophils and eosinophils. No definite evidence for infection has been demonstrated for chronic urticaria.

CLINICAL MANIFESTATIONS

Urticarial lesions are pruritic, erythematous papules or nodules that generally arise on the trunk and extremities. Some may coalesce and have a serpiginous appearance. Each individual lesion persists for less than 24 hours, although the overall eruption may be very persistent. Physical urticaria is brought about by cold, heat, pressure, or vibration. Angioedema (swelling of lips, tongue, and/or face) may be present in up to 40% of patients with chronic urticaria. It is usually asymmetric and a finding neither the patient nor the examiner can ignore.

DIAGNOSIS

Most often, the clinical diagnosis is easily made by good history and characteristic physical examination findings. For acute onset urticaria, the history should include questioning about any drug use (prescribed, over the counter, or otherwise obtained), any relation to certain foods, and topical exposure to chemicals. Sources of infection should also be sought including viral (acute hepatitis B virus) or bacterial infections. For chronic urticaria, dermatographism and collagen vascular diseases (urticarial vasculitis; for example, secondary to systemic lupus erythematosus) may be included in the differential diagnosis. Depending on the history and other physical examination findings, serologic tests for or a skin biopsy may be done.

TREATMENT

Histamine blockade with H1 blockers (e.g., diphenhydramine, hydroxyzine, fexofenadine) and H2 blockers (e.g., cimetidine, ranitidine or famotidine) can be used. If these are inadequate, then leukotriene esterase inhibitors (zafirlukast or montelukast) may be added. In some cases, oral steroids (e.g., prednisone) may be used if refractory to drugs from the other therapeutic classes. Systemic side effects from steroids such as hyperglycemia and fluid retention may be a problem, as well as psychiatric side effects (dysphoria, psychosis); these should be monitored.

COMPLICATIONS

Chronic urticaria may be associated with autoimmune thyroid disease in close to a third of cases. Hashimoto's disease is most strongly associated and Graves' disease less so. Testing for thyroid function is reasonable.

III

Ambulatory Medicine

Jerome Van Ruiswyk

CHAPTER 129

Disease Prevention and Screening

Jerome Van Ruiswyk

Three quarters of all deaths in the United States are related to eight primary causes of death (Table 129.1), with heart disease and cancer accounting for the majority of deaths. Prevention consists of intervention, lifestyle modification, or evaluation to prevent or delay the onset of pathologic processes or illnesses, or to modify the course of established disease in an individual.

When measures prevent the development of a specific disorder (for example, vaccination against poliomyelitis) the process is called primary prevention. When patients are evaluated for diseases at an early asymptomatic stage (for example, mammograms to detect breast cancer and fecal occult blood testing to detect colon carcinoma), this screening process is called secondary prevention because it prevents morbidity and mortality but not the disease itself. When measures are undertaken to slow the progress of disease in patients with known disease (for example, the patient who needs to modify lifestyle and risk factors after recent coronary artery bypass surgery), the process is called tertiary prevention.

In situations in which an equally efficacious intervention could be applied in any of the three modes of prevention, primary prevention has a greater public health impact than either secondary or tertiary preventive measures. For example, providing immunizations to prevent infectious diseases and motivating individuals to avoid exposures or reduce risk factors by changing their lifestyle or health habits can prevent morbidity and mortality in far more individuals than efforts to detect undiagnosed disease in asymptomatic individuals or efforts to prevent progression of established disease. Therefore, the effective preventive health clinician must be skilled at assessing individuals' health risks, motivating them to change their health-related behaviors, and giving them the necessary knowledge and skills to make the required changes.

TABLE 129.1 Major causes of death in the United States

Cause of death	Number of deaths
Diseases of heart	654,092
Malignant neoplasms	550,270
Cerebrovascular diseases	150,147
Chronic lower respiratory diseases	123,884
Accidents	108,694
Diabetes mellitus	72,815
Alzheimer's disease	65,829
Influenza and pneumonia	61,472

2004 estimates from the National Center for Health Statistics (www.cdc.gov/nchs/data/hestat/preliminarydeaths04_tables.pdf#2).

ETIOLOGY

Common preventable diseases are caused by a variety of genetic and environmental factors. Effective prevention requires individualized assessment for these factors, focusing on modifiable factors that are most likely to cause morbidity and mortality, employing interventions that have proven net benefits in similar patients, and which are accepted by the patient after they are informed of the intervention's risks, benefits, and alternatives.

A prerequisite to primary prevention is knowledge of the pathophysiology of the disease and the risk factors for development of the disease. An understanding of the pathophysiology of a disease enables the physician to intervene and block the effects of specific disease-causing agents before they lead to disease development; likewise, an understanding of the risk factors for a disease is necessary to facilitate interventions that reduce the risk of disease by reducing or mitigating the effects of the risk factors. Therefore, primary prevention strategies must be targeted to the subset of identified genetic and environmental factors that are modifiable through patient or provider action.

However, screening (or secondary prevention) can be applied to patients who have an increased risk for disease morbidity or mortality due to either modifiable or nonmodifiable (e.g., genetic) factors. But to be effective against any targeted disease, screening should satisfy all the following conditions:

1. The disorder is relatively prevalent.
2. The screening test is reasonably safe, inexpensive, and acceptable to the patient.
3. The test identifies most patients with the disorder (high sensitivity), while mislabeling few normal patients as having the disorder (high specificity).
4. Follow-up confirmation tests are safe and, ideally, noninvasive and affordable.
5. Treatment of the disorder in its asymptomatic stage will improve the patient's prognosis compared with those patients who have a similar disorder and are treated only when the disease becomes symptomatic.
6. The ultimate outcome of the disorder has grave consequences for the patient's well-being, in terms of either morbidity or mortality.

Of these conditions, the two that are most difficult to evaluate and quantify are the sensitivity/specificity of the screening test, and the enhanced efficacy of treating disease diagnosed in its asymptomatic stage. Ideally, screening tests should have perfect sensitivity so that no opportunities for early intervention are missed; in reality, all screening tests have less than perfect sensitivity. Imperfect sensitivity of a screening test can lead to inappropriate security when false-negative results are obtained in individuals with the underlying disease. Conversely, imperfect specificity can lead to the negative consequences of labeling and unnecessary follow-up tests in normal patients with false-positive results. Overall accuracy and efficiency of screening tests can be improved by targeting their use toward higher-risk individuals.

There are two main errors that can complicate estimates of the true efficacy of screening strategies involving treatment of early-stage disease. Both of these may be illustrated by potential pitfalls of prostate cancer screening in elderly men. Whereas proponents argue that earlier detection of cancer will lead to its cure, opponents argue that cancers have their own finite prognosis that is unaffected by the time of detection, and that the improvement in survival time after diagnosis is merely a reflection of the cancer being detected earlier in its natural history (lead-time bias). The second potential error when estimating the effectiveness of screening is related to the fact that cancers have their own intrinsic growth rate. Given that premise, periodic screening is more likely to detect asymptomatic cancers that are inherently slower growing, because faster-growing tumors cause symptoms that lead to their detection before the next screening episode. In other words, the probability that screening will detect prostate cancer before it causes symptoms (i.e., in the preclinical phase) is inversely related to its rate of progression. Therefore, comparisons of screened to unscreened populations that are not adjusted for rate of cancer growth are biased in favor of screening (length bias). Randomized trials of screening followed by early treatment and adjustment for rates of disease progression are the best ways to avoid these biases.

In clinical practice, especially in elderly patients, the benefits and risks of screening and early treatment of disease must be individually assessed in each patient, taking into account their risk of disease-related morbidity and mortality, any comorbidities that may impact their benefit or potential for harm from early treatment, and their competing mortality risks. In general, targeting screening to high-risk populations can increase the positive predictive value (the proportion of individuals with positive tests who have underlying disease) of diagnostic testing, while increasing the likelihood that the benefit from treatment of asymptomatic disease will surpass the risks of treatment side effects.

CLINICAL MANIFESTATIONS

Preventive health guidelines have been issued by several groups, including government agencies, task forces, health-related organizations, and subspecialty societies. The recommendations of the Centers for Disease Control and Prevention (CDC) Advisory Committee on Immunization Practices (www.cdc.gov/nip/publications/ACIP-list.htm) are a useful resource on recommended immunizations. A commonly quoted set of screening and other preventive recommendations is compiled by the United States Preventive Services Task Force (USPSTF; www.ahrq.gov/clinic/prevenix.htm). Other guidelines on specific prevention practices or prevention within specific patient populations with various underlying diseases (e.g., individuals with human immunodeficiency virus infection) can be found by searching the National Guidelines Clearinghouse (www.guideline.gov). All of these guidelines must be periodically updated to reflect evolving information about the effectiveness of preventive measures.

The set of preventive procedures that physicians recommend to their patients should be based on an individualized assessment of the most likely causes of premature morbidity and mortality within their patient population. The practicing physician can implement prevention during specific prevention-focused visits or during any patient encounter. The periodic health examination is a comprehensive prevention-focused history and physical examination, accompanied in the same visit by counseling if unhealthy behaviors are detected, immunizations if required, and indicated screening procedures (e.g., cervical Papanicolaou smear, breast examination, and flexible sigmoidoscopy). Alternatively, clinicians can perform preventive interventions during any encounter for either acute illnesses or routine follow-up of chronic conditions. This strategy helps reduce the number of missed prevention opportunities in patients whose only physician visits are for injuries or acute illnesses.

DIAGNOSIS

Physicians practicing in primary care specialties have the unique opportunity to implement systems that facilitate primary, secondary, and tertiary preventive interventions targeted to the patient population they serve. Primary care practitioners can improve the efficiency of prevention and screening efforts within their practice by involving all team members in improvement efforts to achieve prevention benchmarks such as the Healthy People 2010 goals (www.healthypeople.gov). Tracking rates of completion of indicated preventive care is becoming an accepted indicator of the quality of primary care.

The CDC's Community Guide to Preventive Services (www.thecommunityguide.org) provides tips on effective implementation of prevention interventions. Surveys and other case-finding tools can be used to reach out to and identify populations that could benefit from preventive care. To reap their full benefits, positive screens should receive prompt and thorough follow-up. Patient recall systems or computerized reminder systems can be used to prompt patients to seek, and clinicians to complete, indicated preventive measures.

TREATMENT

As the patient's primary care doctor, the physician must know the benefits, risks, and limitations of each measure recommended for the prevention, early detection, or mitigation of disease. Some mea-

TABLE 129.2 Advisory Committee on Immunization Practices current recommendations for adult immunizations

Vaccine	Indications and comments
Human papilloma virus	All woman ≤26 years. Not recommended during pregnancy.
Tetanus, diphtheria (Td)	All adults once every 10 years.
Measles, mumps, rubella	One dose, for individuals born after 1956 who lack evidence of immunity. Pregnancy is absolute contraindication.
Varicella	Two doses for healthy adults with no history of varicella infection, susceptible health care workers, day care workers, family contacts of immunocompromised individuals. Pregnancy is contraindication.
Influenza	Annually for all individuals age >50 and patients at high risk for significant morbidity and mortality (e.g., those with diabetes mellitus, heart disease, pulmonary disease, renal disease, and those who are immunocompromised), health care personnel, residents of chronic care facilities. Contraindicated in persons with a history of allergy to egg yolk.
Pneumococcal	One dose, for groups similar to those for influenza vaccine. Other indications are asplenia (anatomic or functional), alcoholism, sickle cell disease, Hodgkin's disease, and nephrotic syndrome.
Hepatitis A virus	Two doses in persons living in or traveling to areas where the disease is endemic, homosexually active men, intravenous drug abusers, military recruits.
Hepatitis B virus	Three doses in individuals with high risk of exposure (e.g., health care workers, individuals at biomedical research laboratories, homosexually active men, intravenous drug abusers, hemodialysis patients).
Meningococcal	One dose in patients with asplenia, terminal complement deficiencies, military recruits, and first-year college students living in dormitories.

TABLE 129.3 Counseling recommendations related to Healthy People 2010 objectives

Objective area	Leading health indicators	Patient recommendations
Physical activity	Increase proportion of adults who engage regularly, preferably daily, in moderate physical activity for at least 30 minutes per day.	Moderate physical activity at least 30 minutes daily
Overweight and obese	Reduce the proportion of adults who are obese.	Follow Dietary Guidelines for Americans; see Chapter 132
Tobacco use	Reduce cigarette smoking by adults.	See Chapter 130
Substance abuse	Reduce the proportion of adults using any illicit drug during the past 30 days. Reduce the proportion of adults engaging in binge drinking of alcoholic beverages during the past month.	Reduce binge drinking and stop illicit drug use; see Chapter 131
Responsible sexual behavior	Increase the proportion of sexually active persons who use condoms.	Increase abstinence, or use of condoms if sexually active; see Chapter 139. Use contraceptives to prevent unintended pregnancy; see Chapter 142.
Mental health	Increase the proportion of adults with recognized depression who receive treatment.	See Chapter 118.
Injury and violence	Reduce deaths caused by motor vehicle crashes. Reduce homicides.	Use seatbelts, do not drive under the influence, gun safety.
Environmental quality	Reduce the proportion of persons exposed to air that does not meet the U.S. EPA health-based standards for ozone. Reduce the proportion of nonsmokers exposed to environmental tobacco smoke.	Support community and political efforts addressing these problems.
Immunization	Increase the proportion of noninstitutionalized adults who are vaccinated annually against influenza and ever vaccinated against pneumococcal disease.	See Table 129.2.
Access to health care	Increase the proportion of person with health insurance Increase the proportion of persons who have a specific source of ongoing care. Increase the proportion of pregnant women who begin prenatal care in the first trimester of pregnancy.	Support community and political efforts addressing these problems.

TABLE 129.4 United States Preventive Services Task Force recommendations for cancer prevention

Type of cancer	General recommendations
Breast cancer	Mammography every 1 to 2 years, with or without clinical breast examination, for women aged 40 years or older Chemoprevention with tamoxifen or raloxifene in women with high risk of breast cancer and low risk of adverse effects of chemoprevention
Cervical cancer	Papanicolaou smear every 1 to 3 years, from commencement of sexual activity in all women with a cervix
Colorectal cancer	Annual fecal occult blood testing and flexible sigmoidoscopy every 3 to 5 years starting at age 50 years

sures have been found definitely effective in well-designed studies, whereas other measures have not been shown conclusively to reduce morbidity or mortality when applied to either individuals or populations. Some preventive measures, while proven effective in populations, are not without risks in individual patients. Under these circumstances, physicians should educate patients about these key factors and allow them to make an informed decision about whether to accept recommended measures.

Vaccinations and immunizations best exemplify the primary prevention of infectious diseases. When administered to an individual, a vaccine, which is a derivative from protein components of a microbe, stimulates the individual's immune system to form antibodies against that microbe, providing protection from disease caused by infection with that microbe. The process is effective in preventing specific infectious diseases (e.g., influenza, pneumococcal pneumonia from certain strains, mumps, measles, rubella, hepatitis B virus, tetanus, and rabies).

Table 129.2 describes the recommendations for routine booster and primary immunizations in general populations of adults. Many of the primary immunizations are given early in life, when the person is younger than 6 years of age. However, adults who have not received primary immunizations need them, and adults who have been immunized previously sometimes require booster immunization (e.g., to prevent tetanus and hepatitis). Several different vaccines may be given at the same visit. The currently recommended immunizations fulfill the basic tenets of preventive medicine: efficacy, safety, and cost-effectiveness.

Modification of risk factors is another exciting example of primary prevention. By working with the patient to modify a lifestyle habit or effectively treat a risk factor, the physician can positively intervene to prevent or delay the development of disease. The effectiveness of patient counseling can be improved by framing benefits of the change from the patient's perspective; engaging the patient in setting jointly agreed upon, specific, attainable goals; teaching them the specific skills or behaviors they will need to succeed in the changes; involving other health care staff in counseling for change or compliance along with physician reinforcement of the message, because physician recommendations carry the greatest weight and often are the primary reasons patients give for accepting preventive measures; monitoring progress through follow-up contacts; or any combination of these strategies. While counseling interventions are often not extensively studied, they are low-risk interventions. Table 129.3 lists adult counseling recommendations related to the Healthy People 2010 goals.

Many screening interventions in adults involve the early detection of cancer, cardiovascular disease, infections, or other prevalent conditions that cause significant morbidity and mortality. Because illnesses detected at early stages have a better prognosis and often can be treated using less

TABLE 129.5 United States Preventive Services Task Force recommendations for noncancer prevention

Intervention	Recommendation
Screen for AAA	Men aged 65 to 75 years who have ever smoked
ASA prophylaxis to prevent coronary heart disease	Discuss aspirin use in patients with 5-year risk ≥3%
Screen for hypertension	All adults
Screen for/treat hyperlipidemia	Screen adults aged 20 or older; treat abnormal lipids in men 35 or older and women 45 or older who have an increased risk of coronary heart disease
Screen for type 2 diabetes	Adults with hypertension and hyperlipidemis
Screen for bacteruria	Pregnant women at 12 to 16 weeks gestation
Screen for chlamydia/gonorrhea	All sexually active women aged 25 years and younger, and other women at increased risk for infection
Screen for hepatitis B virus	Pregnant women at first prenatal visit
Screen for human immunodeficiency virus	All pregnant women, and adults at increased risk of infection
Screen for syphilis	All pregnant women, and adults at increased risk of infection
Screen for latent tuberculosis infection	Adults with increased risk of infection
Screen/counsel for alcohol use	All adults
Screen/counsel for tobacco use	All adults
Screen for depression	All adults
Screen for iron deficiency anemia	All pregnant women
Screen/counsel for obesity	All adults
Screen for osteoporosis	All women aged 65 or older, women aged 60 or older who are at increased risk for osteoporosis fractures
Screen for Rh(D) incompatibility	All pregnant women at first prenatal visit; repeat screening at 24 to 28 weeks gestation unless biological father is known to be Rh(D) negative

radical methods, screening attempts to diagnose occult illnesses at the earliest possible stage. However, early diagnosis also depends on targeting more intensive evaluation to higher-risk individuals and the prompt evaluation of patients with suggestive symptoms or signs. A list of cancer prevention strategies recommended by the USPSTF is shown in Table 129.4 and a list of USPSTF recommendations for noncancer prevention interventions is listed in Table 129.5.

CHAPTER 130

Smoking Cessation

Robert Maglio

Cigarette smoking is the preferred method of tobacco consumption, rapidly delivering high nicotine concentrations to the central nervous system. The tobacco curing process enhances absorption of nicotine through the lungs, thus maximizing the addictive potential of cigarettes. Indeed, 90% of those exposed to nicotine become addicted, in contrast to 50% of heroin users and 10% of alcohol users.

Smoking is the major preventable cause of disease in the United States, where it results in over 440,000 deaths annually (20% of total deaths), and at least 5 million deaths annually worldwide. Since the 1964 Surgeon General's report, the dangers of tobacco have been widely disseminated. The prevalence of smoking in the United States has subsequently declined from 42% in the mid-1960s to its current levels of 23% of men and 21% of women.

ETIOLOGY

Nicotine causes addiction to tobacco. Nicotine acts on dopaminergic neurons to cause sensations of pleasure, hunger suppression, arousal with memory and other cognitive enhancement, plus reduced tension and anxiety.

CLINICAL MANIFESTATIONS

While nicotine causes the physical dependence on cigarette smoking, other constituents of burning tobacco cause the smoking illnesses. Smoking is responsible for nearly 90% of lung cancer; seven other malignancies are secondary to or linked to smoking including those arising from the oral cavity, larynx, esophagus, stomach, pancreas, bladder, and cervix. Smoking increases the incidence of coronary heart disease between two and four times, and doubles the risk of stroke. Cigarette smoking is the most important risk factor for Chronic Obstructive Pulmonary Disease (COPD), and is also linked to pulmonary hemorrhage, Histiocytosis-X, spontaneous pneumothorax, idiopathic pulmonary fibrosis, invasive pneumococcal infection, and tuberculosis. Smoking is associated with accelerated osteoporosis and peptic ulcer disease. In addition, smoking is the most important modifiable cause of poor pregnancy outcome. Several major birth defects occur more frequently in children of smoking mothers, as do complications of pregnancy. Smoking-related intrauterine growth retardation increases perinatal mortality. Secondhand smoke causes a similar spectrum of negative health consequences.

With chronic nicotine use, neuronal function is changed. Nicotine absence then causes a withdrawal syndrome with strong cigarette cravings, increased appetite, anxiety, anger, restlessness, difficulty concentrating, and depression. The physical syndrome usually resolves by three to four weeks of complete abstinence, but prolonged intermittent cravings will persist.

Smoking cessation brings benefits to those with all degrees of smoking history, at all ages, with decreased mortality from all causes. Quitters' risk of cardiovascular events decreases rapidly, while risks of other complications from atherosclerotic disease decrease more slowly. Smokers' accelerated decline of Forced Expiratory Volume in 1 second (FEV) returns to the rate of nonsmokers; only supplemental oxygen and smoking cessation have been found to extend survival in COPD. Chronic cough and sputum production improve in the first year following cessation. Risk of developing and dying from tuberculosis and invasive pneumococcal disease declines. Although never quite returning to the risk of lung cancer in lifelong nonsmokers such that by 10 to 20 years of abstinence, smoking induced risk is decreased by 92% to 96%. Negative reproductive effects and accelerated osteoporosis remit, whereas peptic ulcer disease improves.

DIAGNOSIS

The U.S. Preventive Services Task Force strongly recommends that all adults be screened for tobacco use. This screen should record a cigarette smoking history typically measured as pack years (number of packs per day × number of years smoking), a patient's willingness to quit smoking, and their experience with prior quit attempts. History should also screen for the risk and presence of smoking-related health problems.

Assessing the degree of nicotine addiction is vital in matching the smoker to a cessation program. Two factors—time to first morning cigarette <30 minutes and total daily cigarettes smoked >25 (1 pack)—quickly identify the heavily dependent smoker. Presence in serum of the nicotine metabolite cotinine at levels >250 mg/mL can also be used to identify the heavily dependent smoker. The widely used Fagerstrom Test for Nicotine Dependence (Table 130.1) has six questions that stratify

TABLE 130.1 Fagerstrom Test for Level of Nicotine Dependence

Question	Answer/points	
How soon after waking do you smoke the first cigarette?	<5 minutes	3 points
	5 to 30 minutes	2 points
	31 to 60 minutes	1 point
Do you find it difficult to refrain from smoking in places where it is forbidden?	Yes	1 point
	No	0 points
Which cigarette would you most hate to give up?	First one in morning	1 point
	Any other	0 points
How many cigarettes do you smoke per day?	>30 per day	3 points
	21 to 30 per day	2 points
	11 to 20 per day	1 point
Do you smoke more frequently during the first hours after waking than during the rest of the day?	Yes	1 point
	No	0 points
Do you smoke if you are so ill that you are in bed most of the day?	Yes	1 point
	No	0 points

Score

5 to 6 points = heavy dependence
3 to 4 points = moderate dependence
0 to 2 points = light dependence

nicotine addiction into three levels of severity. Greater dependency indicates greater difficulty in cessation. However, older age, higher income, lower alcohol intake, initiation of smoking at age >20 years, past attempts at cessation, and being the only smoker in the household suggest greater success.

TREATMENT

The directive that smoking be assessed and documented at every health care visit (outpatient or inpatient) increases the likelihood of smoking-related discussions. A physician recommendation to quit doubles cessation rates compared with no counseling. The opportunity to achieve success is high as most smokers are interested in quitting and 40% of current smokers have made a serious quit attempt in the previous year. A personalized health message (e.g., decline in pulmonary function tests) further increases chances of successful cessation. Societal pressure and removal of enablers (e.g., nonsmoking bars) also serve the purpose of cessation. If quitting is not desired, be sure to raise the matter at the next visit. If contemplated, set a quit date preferably within the next 2 weeks. If motivated to stop soon, begin a cessation program. The National Cancer Institute recommends these five "A"s to facilitate smoking cessation: Ask about smoking and readiness to quit, Advise quitting, Assess motivation, Assist quitting, and Arrange follow-up visits. No "magic bullet" treatment or technique exists.

When patients are ready to stop smoking, have them enlist social assistance by asking family, friends, and associates to support their quit efforts. Patients should minimize or eliminate exposure to smokers, smoking behaviors, and other cues to smoke. Ashtrays, cigarette products, and lighters should be removed from the patient's surroundings. Continuation of the counseling already initiated by the physician is necessary to enhance coping skills. More intensive counseling increases rates of success. Most systems or institutions will offer programs that range from telephone help lines to individual or group psychotherapy sessions. Initial and follow-up visits should explore lessons learned from past unsuccessful attempts and factors that allowed relapse. Quit rates at 1 year in those completing smoking cessation programs are close to 20%.

Quit rates can be enhanced with use of pharmacologic treatments to reduce nicotine withdrawal symptoms or cigarette cravings. Nicotine withdrawal symptoms usually last 3 to 4 weeks. Nicotine replacement therapy (NRT) will alleviate most if not all of these symptoms. Its use is safe and effective, with quit rates three times that of placebo. The response is dose-dependent and is greater than that achieved with intensive counseling alone. NRT has not been associated with increased risks of acute myocardial infarction, stroke, peripheral artery disease, or malignancy; however, it should not be used in pregnancy, within 1 month of myocardial infarction, in unstable angina, and with "serious" arrhythmia. The British Medical Association and the Agency for Healthcare Research and Quality both recommend NRT be given to all those attempting cessation. Nicotine replacement comes in several modalities; chewing gum, lozenges, and transdermal patch are available without a prescription, whereas the inhaler and nasal spray are prescription items. Near equal efficacy in quit rates at 1 year are demonstrated in comparison studies, ranging from 15% to 25%.

Oral nicotine is available as a gum or lozenge and consists of a resin (Polacrilex) to which nicotine is bound. Twelve to 24 pieces of gum or 10 lozenges are recommended daily. The gum is intermittently chewed, then "parked" in the cheek; the lozenges are allowed to dissolve in the mouth. Nicotine levels achieved are 40% of those produced by smoking, quelling a major portion of the withdrawal symptoms. Those who smoke <25 cigarettes daily are given 2-mg products, with the 4-mg size reserved for heavier smokers and those whose first cigarette is <30 min after arising. Gum and lozenge are recommended for 12 weeks.

Transdermal patches provide 40% to 50% of nicotine levels attained with smoking 1 to 1.5 packs per day. They are designed to be worn for either 16 or 24 hours. Dose is based upon the Fagerstrom Test for Nicotine Dependence, with 21 mg given to the heavily dependent, 14 mg to those moderately dependent, and 7 mg to those lightly addicted. Treatment is for at least 8 weeks, with long-term success best in the high-dose group.

The nicotine inhaler with absorption through the buccal mucosa produces levels roughly one third those of cigarette smoking. The nasal spray produces the rapid rise seen with smoking and the highest levels of any NRT.

Bupropion slows central nervous system reuptake and breakdown of dopamine, thereby suppressing and possibly relieving withdrawal. It replaces the antidepressant effects of nicotine in baseline depressed individuals and prevents the depression sometimes seen with nicotine withdrawal. With nicotine receptor antagonist properties, it reduces the reinforcing properties of nicotine. It must be started 1 week prior to quitting. When used alone, the quit rate at 1 year was 23%.

Combination therapy, using both bupropion and high-dose patches as controllers combined with "rescue" nicotine replacement therapy (gum, lozenge, spray, or inhaler), results in a 50% cessation rate at 1 year.

Varenicline, a partial necotinic acetylcholine receptor agonist, is recently FDA approved. Randomized, comparison trials with buproprion and placebo demonstrated higher rates of both 9–12 week (44%) and 12–52 week (23%) abstinence. Varenicline, however, was more commonly associated with disturbing dreams, and almost 30% experienced nausea. Treatment should be started one week prior to a quit date, and if successful at 12 weeks, continued to 24 weeks.

CHAPTER 131

Substance Abuse

Kimberly Stoner and William Anderson

According to the Substance Abuse and Mental Health Services Administration 2004 survey of Americans aged 12 years and older, 18.2 million Americans met criteria for alcohol abuse or dependence. In addition, 19.1 million respondents had used illicit drugs during the month prior to being surveyed. More than one fourth of hospital admissions are related to the medical sequelae of substance abuse. Detection and effective treatment can significantly reduce the morbidity, mortality, and societal costs related to substance abuse.

Alcohol is the most commonly abused substance in the United States. Estimates of the lifetime risk of alcohol dependence range from 10% to 20% for males and 3% to 9% for females. Alcohol is associated with more than 200,000 deaths annually in the United States. Due to its high prevalence and associated serious morbidity and mortality, all physicians should familiarize themselves with the detection and treatment of alcohol dependence.

Other commonly abused drugs include sedatives, opiates, and stimulants. Although heroin was the most commonly abused opiate, prescription narcotics such as oxycodone are becoming more prominent. Likewise, methamphetamine abuse is becoming more popular among stimulant abusers, increasing as the growth of cocaine abuse wanes.

ETIOLOGY

Addiction is most accurately conceptualized as a chronic medical disease. Substance dependence is a condition that is managed rather than "cured," with relapse being a common occurrence. Genetic research and studies of the brain indicate that addiction has a biological basis. Environmental factors, as well as the properties of the substances themselves, also contribute to the development of addiction.

CLINICAL MANIFESTATIONS

When alcohol abuse or dependence is suspected (Table 131.1), the history should include the type and quantity of alcoholic beverages consumed as well as the frequency of drinking behavior. Clinicians should inquire about interpersonal, occupational, or legal problems stemming from alcohol consumption. Inquiring about alcohol use is particularly important in patients presenting with medical diagnoses that can be caused or exacerbated by alcohol use, including insomnia, depression, peripheral neuropathy, seizures, Wernicke-Korsakoff syndrome, upper gastrointestinal bleeding, pancreatitis, cirrhosis, hepatitis, aspiration pneumonia, osteopenia, gout, hypertension, atrial fibrillation, and cardiomyopathy. Physical examination findings may include Dupuytren's contractures, hepatomegaly, abnormal cerebellar testing, nystagmus, altered consciousness or slurred speech in acute intoxication, or signs of chronic liver disease including gynecomastia, splenomegaly, spider angiomas, palmar erythema, jaundice, ascites, and caput medusae. It is important to remember that only 15% to 30% of alcoholics develop cirrhosis and many alcoholic patients may have a normal physical examination.

TABLE 131.1 *Diagnostic and Statistical Manual of Mental Disorders, Fourth Revision* criteria for substance abuse and dependence

Substance abuse	Substance dependence
A pattern of use that causes impairment or distress and one or more of the following: 1. Substance use results in failure to fulfill obligations at work, school, or home 2. Substance use in physically hazardous situation 3. Substance-related legal problems 4. Continued use despite social or interpersonal problems 5. Criteria for dependence are not met	Three or more of the following: 1. Tolerance 2. Withdrawal 3. Use of more for longer than intended 4. Unable to cut down 5. Substantial time devoted to substance-related activities 6. Important activities are given up 7. Use despite adverse physical or psychological consequences

Opiate abuse should be suspected in patients with a history of multiple physicians for pain complaints, demands for early refills, and requests for specific narcotics for conditions in which nonnarcotic analgesics are generally adequate. Intravenous drug abusers commonly present with infectious complications including skin infections, endocarditis, hepatitis C virus, and human immunodeficiency virus. Physical examination during opiate effects may demonstrate pinpoint pupils. Narcotic overdose can present with somnolence and life-threatening respiratory depression and coma. In contrast, opiate withdrawal presents with symptoms and signs of rhinorrhea, lacrimation, piloerection, diarrhea, myalgias, nausea, vomiting, and yawning, but is generally not a life-threatening condition.

Cocaine abusers commonly present to the healthcare system with medical complications. Cocaine use may precipitate angina, myocardial infarction, ventricular dysrhythmias, rhabdomyolysis with secondary renal failure, pulmonary edema, seizures, cerebral vascular accidents, aortic dissection, malignant hypertension and respiratory distress. Chronic cocaine users may have perforated nasal septums from snorting cocaine or "track" marks from injections. "Crack" (smokable cocaine) users may have burns on fingers or lips.

The symptoms of other drugs of abuse are listed in Table 131.2.

DIAGNOSIS

The U.S. Preventive Services Task Force recommends screening adults for alcohol abuse in the primary care setting. The most commonly used screening instrument is the four-item CAGE questionnaire:

1. Have you ever felt the need to **C**ut down on your drinking?
2. Have you ever been **A**nnoyed by others criticizing your drinking?
3. Have you ever felt **G**uilty about your drinking?
4. Have you ever had an **E**ye-opener (drink first thing in the morning)?

Two positive responses predict alcoholism with a sensitivity of 75% and a specificity of 95%.

Alcohol levels may be measured in the blood or through the use of a breathalyzer and may also be detected on a urine drug screen. While elevated transaminases with an increased aspartate transaminase to alanine transaminase ratio may be seen, increases in gamma-glutamyl transferase or carbohydrate-deficient transferrin are more sensitive markers. Complete blood count abnormalities

TABLE 131.2 Signs and symptoms of selected drugs of abuse

Drug class/drugs	Intoxication	Withdrawal
MDMA/Ecstasy	Hallucinations, tachycardia, nystagmus, ataxia, tremor, hyperthermia	Not reported
Barbiturates	Somnolence, slurred speech, disinhibition, nystagmus, diplopia, vertigo	Restlessness, tremor, tachycardia, insomnia, hyperpyrexia, hyperreflexia
Gamma-hydroxybutyrate/ date rape drug	Sedation, respiratory depression	Not reported
Benzodiazepines/ Rohypnol	Sedation, blackouts (antegrade amnesia), slurred speech, incoordination	Anxiety, insomnia, hallucinations, irritability, tremors, seizures, tachycardia
Stimulants: cocaine, methamphetamine	Anorexia, insomnia, psychosis, increased energy, mydriasis, tachycardia, hypertension	Fatigue, dysphoria, increased appetite, hypersomnia
Marijuana/cannabis hashish	Conjunctival injection, increased appetite, dry mouth, tachycardia, inattention, altered perception	Controversial whether there is a withdrawal syndrome
Hallucinogens: LSD, mescaline/peyote, mushrooms	Distortion of senses, psychosis	No withdrawal syndrome, patients may experience flashbacks after discontinuation
Phencyclidine	Euphoria, hypertension, tachycardia, nystagmus, hyperthermia, agitation	Not reported in humans
Inhalants: nitrous oxide	Altered perception, impaired coordination, nystagmus, dizziness, slurred speech, lethargy, depressed reflexes	Not reported, long-term use may lead to dementia

such as macrocytosis with or without anemia, leukopenia, thrombocytopenia, hypomagnesaemia, and hypophosphatemia are possible.

Urine drug screens are also helpful in confirming abuse of other drugs. Opiates can be detected in the urine for 1 to 3 days after use. Not all opiates are included in all urine drug screens; clarification with the toxicology laboratory is needed to verify what is being tested. Cocaine metabolite can be detected in the urine drug screen for 48 to 72 hours after use.

TREATMENT

Substance dependence should not be viewed as a character defect nor attributed to a lack of will power or self-control. An empathetic and nonjudgmental approach is not only appropriate for a physician confronting any illness, but is essential for the development of an effective treatment alliance.

Once a physician has identified a patient with alcohol abuse or dependence, a brief intervention is appropriate. The patient should be educated about the risks associated with excess alcohol use and counseled to quit or reduce their intake. However, the cardinal feature of dependency is loss of control and complete cessation of use is preferred.

There are several community 12-step programs, in addition to professionally directed rehabilitation treatment, to which patients may be referred: Alcoholics Anonymous, Narcotics Anonymous, Cocaine Anonymous, and others. Self-help groups such as Alcoholics Anonymous have been shown to reduce the risk of relapse for those who can make use of them. They are an adjunct to therapy and support sobriety maintenance, not actual directed therapy.

Naltrexone, disulfiram, and acamprosate are U.S. Food and Drug Adminstration–approved medications that some alcohol-dependent patients find helpful in reducing relapse. The importance of abstinence should be reinforced at follow-up visits. Patients should also be evaluated for depression and anxiety, which are common comorbid disorders.

Alcohol withdrawal is a potentially life-threatening diagnosis. Withdrawal syndromes most commonly occur in alcoholics who consume a large quantity of alcohol daily, over a number of years. However, the diagnosis of alcohol withdrawal should be considered for all patients presenting with tachycardia, hypertension, and elevated temperature. Alcohol withdrawal occurs along a spectrum ranging from mild anxiety to seizures (which generally occur 6 to 48 hours after cessation) to delirium tremens (which usually occurs 2 to 3 days after the patient's last drink and carry a 20% to 40% mortality if untreated). First-line treatment of alcohol withdrawal is symptom-based benzodiazepine dosing according to the severity of alcohol withdrawal measured by the Clinical Institute Withdrawal Assessment Scale for Alcohol, Revised (CIWA-Ar). The CIWA-Ar is a 10-item scale that scores: nausea/vomiting, paroxysmal sweats, anxiety, agitation, tremor, headache, auditory disturbances, visual disturbances, tactile disturbances, and orientation/clouding of sensorium over a range of severity. A similar rating scale called Modified Selected Severity Assessment for Alcohol Withdrawal is used in some locales. Sedation is given to control withdrawal symptoms, except in cases where a true delerium has developed, in which case the titration end point is that the patient can achieve a light sleep.

Sedative withdrawal and treatment, such as benzodiazepine or barbiturate withdrawal, is similar to alcohol withdrawal, but the time frames are extended depending on the particular drug's pharmacology.

Withdrawal symptoms of opiate withdrawal may be ameliorated with use of a replacement opiate, such as methadone, buprenorphine, or by use of clonidine, but special regulations governing treatment with replacement opiates may apply. For the chronically opiate-addicted patient, opioid maintenance therapy is preferred. Buprenorphine or methadone clinics are effective treatment options for maintaining return to normal functioning. Because dose and tolerance match, patients essentially feel normal. Harm reduction counseling (e.g., cleaning needles) is helpful for patients who are chronically opiate addicted.

CHAPTER 132

Obesity

Jennifer Zebrack

Obesity is the most common nutritional disorder in the developed world and the second most preventable cause of death after smoking. With the incidence of obesity increasing in epidemic proportions, it is estimated that more than 65% of U.S. adults are overweight or obese. Obesity has also become an increasing problem for children and adolescents. The U.S. Preventive Services Task Force recommends that all adults be screened for obesity using the body mass index (BMI) with or without a waist circumference (WCf) at least every 2 years.

Obesity is defined by the body mass index (BMI), or body weight in kilograms divided by the height in meters squared (kg/m^2). The BMI correlates well with total body fat. Obesity is a BMI $\geq$30 kg/m^2. Morbid obesity is a BMI $\geq$40 kg/m^2 (Table 132.1).

ETIOLOGY

Obesity has multiple causes and pathophysiologic mechanisms. Genetic, behavioral, environmental, and metabolic factors contribute to an energy imbalance. Most commonly, overeating (the ingestion of an amount of energy exceeding the body's needs) and a sedentary lifestyle contribute to the development of obesity. Hormones such as ghrelin, leptin, and peptide YY3-36 are felt to play an important role in maintaining body adiposity and body weight. Their clinical implications are still unclear.

Secondary causes of weight gain may include endocrinopathies (e.g., hypothyroidism, Cushing's disease), psychiatric disorders (e.g., depression, anxiety, binge eating disorders), medications (e.g., steroids, antipsychotics, antidepressants, insulin, sulfonylureas), and smoking cessation.

CLINICAL MANIFESTATIONS

Obesity is associated with many medical complications (Table 132.2). BMI correlates directly with the risk for hypertension, diabetes, stroke, coronary artery disease, and death. Hypertension occurs three to five times more often in obese persons. Obesity often coexists with lipid abnormalities, including elevated total cholesterol, reduced high-density lipoprotein (HDL) cholesterol, and increased triglyceride levels. The combination of central obesity with hypertension, hyperglycemia, and lipid abnormalities suggests the metabolic syndrome and is associated with a particularly high risk for coronary artery disease (Table 132.3).

Respiratory abnormalities, including hypoventilation and sleep apnea, are more frequent in obese patients. Liver abnormalities often include abnormal liver tests, liver steatosis (fatty liver), and nonalcoholic steatohepatitis (NASH). Cholelithiasis is strongly associated with obesity, with a prevalence of 30% among obese women. Overweight women are also more likely to experience menstrual disorders, infertility, and pregnancy complications, and the risk of breast and endometrial

TABLE 132.1 Classification of weight based on body mass index

Classifications	Body mass index (kg/m^2)
Underweight	<18.5
Normal weight	18.5 to 24.9
Overweight	25 to 29.9
Obese	
Class 1	30 to 34.9
Class 2	35 to 39.9
Class 3	>40

cancers is enhanced; excess estrogens may be partly responsible. Obese men may have decreased libido and impotence; total testosterone levels are often low. Obese patients commonly report musculoskeletal and joint pain, especially in the lumbosacral spine, hips, knees, and ankles. Excess weight contributes to the evolution of degenerative joint disease. Depression and other psychiatric disorders are prevalent in obese patients.

Data gathered from the history should include onset of weight problem, eating habits, physical activity, previous attempts at weight loss, and the patient's desire and motivation to lose weight. Clinicians should also review all medications, discuss if there is family history of weight problems, and screen for eating disorders. Comorbid conditions should be noted (e.g., diabetes, hypertension, dyslipidemia, sleep apnea).

On physical exam, the BMI should be calculated, and the patient's general appearance should be carefully noted for signs of secondary causes. Clinicians should also evaluate patients for nonfat

TABLE 132.2 Medical complications associated with obesity

Organ system	Associated medical conditions
Cardiovascular	Coronary artery disease Cerebrovascular accident Diabetes mellitus Hypertension
Respiratory	Obstructive sleep apnea Hypoventilation syndrome
Endocrine	Diabetes mellitus Hyperlipidemia Decreased libido
Hepatic	Fatty liver Nonalcoholic steatohepatitis Cholelithiasis
Musculoskeletal	Osteoarthritis
Psychiatric	Depression

TABLE 132.3 Criteria for metabolic syndrome

Risk factor	Defining level
Waist circumference	
Men	>40 inches
Women	>35 inches
Triglycerides	≥150 mg/dL
High-density lipoprotein cholesterol	
Men	<40 mg/dL
Women	<50 mg/dL
Blood pressure	≥130/85 mmHg
Fasting glucose	≥110 mg/dL

Three or more of these risk factors are needed to meet the criteria for metabolic syndrome.

weight gain, such as edema. The BMI does not account for body fat distribution. Therefore, measurement of the WCf can determine if the patient has abdominal obesity (i.e., central, visceral, or "male-type" fat distribution). This is done in the horizontal plane at the level of the iliac crest. A high waist circumference is >40 inches (102 cm) in men and >35 inches (88 cm) in women. A central fat distribution results in greater health risks than a peripheral (gluteofemoral) fat distribution. Abdominal obesity is often associated with the metabolic syndrome.

TREATMENT

Although short-term weight loss often is achieved, long-term weight reduction commonly fails. Only 20% of obese persons maintain their weight loss 5 to 15 years after initial treatment. Thus, obesity should be considered a chronic medical condition requiring lifelong therapy. Obesity due to a medical cause should receive specific therapy. However, most of the time obesity is not the result of an underlying medical disorder or secondary cause.

Initial patient counseling should include recommending weight loss, discussing the risks of obesity, and determining the patient's desire and readiness to attempt weight loss. Patients with multiple comorbid conditions and/or severe obesity should be more aggressively counseled.

A weight loss of only 5% to 10% of body weight significantly improves the metabolic profile and reduces cardiovascular risk. A reasonable initial weight loss goal is 5% to 10% weight loss from baseline in 6 months (or, at most, 1 to 2 pounds per week).

Dietary Therapy, Physical Activity, and Behavioral Therapy

The cornerstone of obesity therapy is a combined, three-part approach: dietary therapy, physical activity, and behavioral modifications. Although a variety of dietary approaches exist, a low-calorie diet is known to be successful and is the diet most well studied. To attain a loss of 1 pound per week, dietary restriction should be individualized to produce a calorie deficit of 500 to 1,000 kcal/day (3,500 kcal = 1 pound) below his/her daily caloric needs to maintain current weight. A simple way to estimate the daily caloric intake needed to lose 1 pound per week is to take the patient's weight (lb) × 10. Diets with extreme restriction in macronutrients (e.g., low-carbohydrate diets) are difficult to maintain and the long-term risks are unclear. Consultation with a dietician to review dietary changes in more detail may be beneficial.

Physical activity is an important part of any weight loss program and is most helpful in the prevention of regain. Physical activity should be initiated gradually with the goal to attain 30 to 45 minutes of exercise at least 5 days per week. An activity should be recommended that the patient enjoys, can fit into his/her daily life, and maintain long term. Whether a pre-exercise cardiopulmonary evaluation is needed depends on the patient's age, symptoms, and risk factors for cardiovascular disease. An emphasis should also be placed on decreasing sedentary time, such as TV watching and computer use. In severely obese persons, some weight loss may be necessary before exercise can be initiated.

Long-term success in therapy also requires behavioral modifications. These behavioral changes often include self-monitoring of weight, calories, and activity; control of eating stimuli; stress management; social support; and healthier attitudes toward socializing and entertaining. Dietary behavioral changes include increasing water and fiber intake, eating slower, keeping healthy snacks available, and limiting alcohol, regular sodas, dining out, and fast food.

Pharmacotherapy

Drug therapy is sometimes used as an adjunct to dietary therapy, physical activity, and behavioral modifications. Guidelines recommend drug therapy only for individuals with a BMI $\geq$30 kg/m^2, or a BMI $\geq$27 kg/m^2 if the patient has at least one of the following: diabetes, dyslipidemia, hypertension, cardiovascular disease, or sleep apnea.

Currently, only two prescription medications are approved for use for longer than 12 weeks, sibutramine and orlistat. Sibutramine inhibits the reuptake of serotonin and norepinephrine to suppress appetite. Side effects include palpitations and increased blood pressure, so regular monitoring of pulse and blood pressure is required. Sibutramine is contraindicated in patients with a history of heart disease, stroke, arrhythmias, and uncontrolled blood pressure. Orlistat is an inhibitor of gastric and pancreatic lipase that results in reduced absorption of fat. Orlistat is typically administered at each meal. Side effects are primarily gastrointestinal. A multivitamin is recommended at bedtime to replace fat-soluble vitamins. In research studies, the efficacy of sibutramine and orlistat is fairly similar. The mean weight loss attributable to these medications is approximately 6 to 10 lbs when compared to placebo at 1 year of use.

The use of fenfluramine and dexfenfluramine for weight loss were found to be associated with valvular heart disease and are no longer available. Thyroid hormone and diuretics should be used only when medically indicated. Amphetamines should never be prescribed to treat obesity.

Surgery

Occasionally, morbid obesity requires surgical treatment. It is considered in patients with a BMI >40 kg/m^2 or a BMI >35 kg/m^2 if significant comorbid conditions are present. The most common procedures are gastric bypass (Roux-en-Y) and gastric restriction (gastroplasty). Both procedures cause patients to limit food intake by delaying gastric emptying and causing the sensation of fullness after a small meal. The gastric bypass also reduces the absorption of food by bypassing a portion of the small bowel. Patients who undergo bariatric surgery have the potential to lose large amounts of weight (e.g., 100 to 200 lbs in 6 to 12 months). Surgery should be combined with behavior modifications to prevent regain. Patients should be monitored for late complications, such as dumping syndrome, vitamin deficiencies (i.e., iron, B12, folate), and weight loss failure.

CHAPTER 133

Hypertension

Jeff Whittle

The designation of blood pressure (BP) above a certain level as a disease called hypertension (HTN) is based on epidemiologic data that shows that a certain level of blood pressure elevation is associated with increased risk for adverse events. In practice, the term HTN designates a BP elevation at which there is consensus that reduction of BP with pharmacologic agents reduces the risk of events. Currently, the Joint National Committee on Prevention, Detection, Evaluation, and Treatment of High Blood Pressure (JNC) considers all persons with systolic blood pressure (SBP) of 140 mm Hg or more or diastolic blood pressure (DBP) of 90 mm Hg and above to have HTN.

The term "prehypertension" is used for people whose pressure is 120–139/80–89 because they are at high risk of eventually developing HTN, and because they are at higher risk of cardiovascular events than persons with lower BP. When either only the systolic or the diastolic BP is elevated, the severity classification is based on the higher of the two. The JNC VII report notes that persons with systolic BP >160 or diastolic BP >100 will almost certainly require two or more antihypertensive drugs to achieve goal BP, but otherwise makes no distinction in treatment recommendations between different degrees of blood pressure elevation within the hypertensive range. Hypertensive emergencies (Table 133.1) occur when markedly elevated blood pressure causes acute complications or when HTN exacerbates another clinical condition. Patients with BP greater than 180/130 mm Hg are typically referred to as having hypertensive urgency if they do not have a hypertensive emergency.

"White-coat hypertension" is a term for the situation when BP is elevated in the doctor's office but not in other settings. White-coat HTN is a special case of "labile" HTN, in which BP is elevated to the hypertensive range some of the time but is in the normal range at other times. Persons with labile HTN are likely to develop persistent HTN if followed over time. Moreover, they have a risk for cardiovascular events (e.g., stroke, myocardial infarction) that is intermediate between persons with persistently elevated BP and those with normal BP. It is unclear whether treatment of persons with labile HTN decreases the rate of cardiovascular events.

Hypertension is the most common cardiovascular disease and one of the greatest public health problems in developed countries. In the United States, the prevalence of HTN is increasing, at least in part because of the aging of the population and the increasing prevalence of obesity. Estimates from the ongoing National Health and Nutrition Examination Survey suggests that in the year 2000 there were 63 million Americans with a systolic BP of 140 mm Hg or higher and/or a diastolic BP of 90 mm Hg or higher or who were taking medications for HTN.

ETIOLOGY

Nonmodifiable risk factors for hypertension include increasing age, sex, African American race, and family history. The prevalence of HTN increases with age, from 9% in persons 20 to 39 years of age, to 30% in persons 40 to 59 years old, to 60% in those more than 60 years old. Among individuals less than 60 years of age, HTN is more common among men than among women. Among persons 70 years of age and older, women are more likely than men to have HTN. African Americans are

TABLE 133.1 Hypertensive emergencies

Clinical condition	Reason BP needs to be lowered
Aortic dissection	Increased shear stress increases the likelihood of propagation of the dissection and/or rupture
Ongoing myocardial ischemia with markedly elevated BP (myocardial infarction or unstable angina)	Increased cardiac work exacerbates ischemia
Acute congestive heart failure/pulmonary edema	Increased afterload leads to decreased cardiac output
Acute intracranial hemorrhage including acute subarachnoid hemorrhage[a]	Increased BP leads to resumption of or accelerated bleeding[a]

[a]The possibility of exacerbating ischemia must be considered in both of these situations, which may be associated with impaired cerebral autoregulation. However, unlike ischemic stroke, in which BP typically is not treated, these situations may call for judicious lowering of the BP, even in the acute phase.
BP, blood pressure.

more likely than whites to be hypertensive at all ages, although the incidence (i.e., the chance of developing HTN for someone who does not have it) is similar for African Americans and whites after the age of 65 years. The presence of one or two parents with HTN is said to double the risk of HTN, compared to someone with no family history. However, only a small fraction of HTN is due to monogenetic conditions (e.g., congenital adrenal hyperplasia).

Modifiable risk factors for hypertension include high sodium intake, obesity, physical inactivity, other dietary elements (low potassium, calcium, fiber, and fish intake; or higher protein intake), and consumption of more than two alcoholic drinks daily.

Studies of societies where sodium consumption is typically less than 1,200 mg daily find that HTN is rare at all ages. As sodium consumption rises, HTN becomes progressively more common, particularly as the population ages.

The relative risk of HTN approximately doubles with each 5-point increase in body mass index (BMI) in the range from 20 to 35 kg/m^2. Postulated mechanisms for the association are: (a) the increased cardiac output of obesity, which for a given level of systemic vascular resistance results in an increased BP; and (b) associated sleep apnea, which causes reactive increases in sympathetic tone that eventually lead to persistently increased vascular resistance. However, obesity is associated with HTN independent of the presence or absence of sleep apnea.

Regular physical activity is associated with a lower risk of HTN, beyond that explained by the lower BMI that is associated with regular activity.

Patients with a low potassium intake appear to have an increased risk of HTN in epidemiologic studies. Similarly, there is an inverse relationship between calcium, fiber, and fish intake and risk of HTN in epidemiologic studies. Conversely, increased intake of protein is associated with higher risk of HTN. Because of the complexity of diet, it is hard to separate the effects of these different dietary elements. Even with short-term intervention studies, it is difficult to identify the specific dietary components responsible for these observed associations.

Essential HTN

More than 95% of patients with elevated BP have essential (idiopathic, primary) HTN. A comprehensive discussion of the pathophysiology of essential HTN is beyond the scope of this book. It is important to note that BP is directly related to cardiac output and peripheral resistance. Cardiac output is the volume of blood ejected by the left ventricle into the aorta per minute. It, along with the elasticity of the aorta, is the major determinant of SBP. Vascular resistance in the arterioles primarily determines DBP. Cardiac output and peripheral resistance are directly and indirectly affected by such factors as blood volume, blood viscosity, sympathetic nervous system activity, the renin-angiotensin-aldosterone system, arginine vasopressin (AVP), insulin, and vasodilator substances such as nitric oxide, prostaglandins, bradykinin, and atrial natriuretic peptide (ANP). It is likely that one or more of these processes is dominant for some people who have essential HTN. However, it has not been possible to separate these groups in a way that is useful in usual clinical practice. Therefore, regardless of underlying predominant pathophysiology, patients without identified secondary causes of hypertension are classified as having essential hypertension.

Although the pathophysiologic sequence varies, cardiac output usually is elevated in earlier stages of essential HTN. As the blood pressure rises further, cardiac output falls and the elevated BP becomes a reflection of increased peripheral resistance. Over time, atherosclerosis leads to decreased elasticity of the aorta (and other large arteries), resulting in a relatively greater rise in BP in response to the bolus of blood ejected during cardiac systole, and a more rapid drop in pressure as the blood distributes peripherally. This phenomenon plays a comparatively greater role in HTN among elderly individuals, leading to a greater prevalence of isolated systolic HTN among elderly persons.

Secondary HTN

A specific cause of high BP can be identified in fewer than 5% of people with HTN. HTN with an identifiable cause is called secondary HTN. One classification divides these causes into renal parenchymal disease, renovascular disease, endocrine diseases, and miscellaneous causes. These causes and their estimated frequency in primary care populations are listed in Table 133.2. The prevalence and relative proportions of these underlying causes vary with population demographics. A physician whose practice includes primarily young people will find a larger number with uncommon secondary causes, and fewer with sleep apnea, renal parenchymal disease, or essential HTN, conditions that increase in prevalence with age.

Secondary HTN usually results from underlying conditions causing increased cardiac output, increased peripheral resistance, and/or volume expansion. Renal parenchymal disease can cause HTN through fluid retention, activation of the renin-angiotensin system, and possibly accumulation of vasopressors that normally are metabolized or excreted by the kidney, or deficiency of certain vasodilators such as prostaglandins and kinins that are normally produced by the kidney. In patients with renovascular HTN, reduced renal blood flow due to stenosis of one or both renal arteries secondary to atherosclerosis or fibromuscular dysplasia leads to activation of the renin-angiotensin-aldosterone system. Coarctation of the aorta causes HTN by a similar mechanism. The increased glucocorticoids of Cushing's syndrome increase cardiac output, activate the renin-angiotensin system through increased hepatic production of angiotensinogen, and reduce synthesis of vasodilatory prostaglandins. Mineralocorticoid excess and acromegaly increase sodium and fluid retention. Estrogen, androgens, and fludrocortisone also increase sodium retention. Hypothyroidism increases blood pressure through extracellular volume expansion and increased peripheral resistance, while hyperthyroidism increases cardiac output. Cyclosporine causes renal vasospasm with secondary activation of the renin-angiotensin-aldosterone system. Adrenergic agonists cause HTN via increased cardiac output and peripheral vasoconstriction. Alcohol increases cardiac output, but the association with blood pressure is complex and poorly understood. Sleep apnea is also postulated to cause HTN through sustained increases in sympathetic nervous system activation. The mechanism linking hypercalcemia to HTN is unclear because there is no direct correlation between blood pressure and either elevated parathyroid hormone or calcium levels.

CLINICAL MANIFESTATIONS

HTN diagnosis and treatment decisions should be based on measurements taken in a standardized fashion. The BP should be measured with the patient in a seated position with the feet on the floor

TABLE 133.2 Secondary causes of hypertension

Secondary cause of hypertension	Frequency among patients with hypertension in a primary care practice
Renal parenchymal disease	2%–3%
Renovascular disease	
Atherosclerotic renal artery stenosis	1%–2%
Fibromuscular dysplasia	0.1%
Endocrine causes	
Pheochromocytoma	<0.1%
Cushing's syndrome (excess production or consumption of glucocorticoids)	<0.1%
Mineralocorticoid excess	0.3%
Primary hyperaldosteronism	Most common cause of this syndrome
17-alpha hydroxylase defects	Rare
11-beta hydroxylase defects	Rare
Excess consumption of licorice	Rare
Acromegaly (excessive growth hormone)	<0.1%
Hypothyroidism	10%–12% (most not related to the hypertension)
Hyperthyroidism	1%–2% (most not related to the hypertension)
Hypercalcemia (hyperparathyroidism)	1% (most not related to the hypertension)
Miscellaneous	
Coarctation of the aorta	<0.1%
Exogenous vasoconstrictor drugs	<0.1%
Chronic alcohol use in high doses	3%–5%
Sleep apnea syndrome	10% (treatment usually does not resolve hypertension)
Exogenous estrogens	0.5%–1%

and arm supported, after a period of 5 minutes of rest. The cuff bladder should encircle 80% of the arm. First, the examiner palpates the pulse either near the antecubital fossa where it will be auscultated, or at the radial artery, which is simpler. The examiner inflates the cuff beyond the point where the pulse can no longer be felt. Then the cuff is deflated until the pulse returns, establishing the approximate SBP. Then the cuff is fully deflated and the brachial pulse located. The cuff is reinflated to a pressure 20 mm Hg higher than the estimated SBP. Cuff pressure is slowly reduced (2 mm Hg per second is recommended) while the examiner auscultates the brachial artery (using the bell, since the Korotkoff sounds are low frequency). Systolic BP is the point at which the first of two or more sounds is heard (phase 1) and diastolic BP is the point where the sounds are last heard (phase 5). The cuff is then fully deflated and a second measure is obtained. The average of the two is used for clinical decision-making. Since an individual's BP varies widely from day to day and during the day, repeated BP measurements are required to establish the patient's "usual" BP.

At the initial evaluation, BP should be measured in both arms to determine whether they yield readings that reliably differ by more than 5 mm Hg. If this is the case, the arm with the higher BP is the more correct one and should be used in the future. BP should also be measured in both the seated and standing position, to confirm that BP remains elevated when the patient is erect. The standing BP should be measured after the person has been erect for 3 minutes, to give the homeostatic mechanisms time to compensate for any change in BP. If there is a marked fall in BP it may affect the decision to treat, and it may suggest some forms of secondary HTN. In general, the higher, seated measure is recommended for decision-making, although side effects due to low erect BPs may limit treatment decisions. Finally, if the person is relatively young (most suggest 30 years of age as a cutoff), a thigh cuff should be used to measure the BP in one leg as a screen for coarctation of the aorta.

Essential Hypertension

The manifestations of essential HTN can be nonspecific symptoms, asymptomatic physical examination findings, or clinical events that may cause enduring disability or death.

Certain symptoms including headache, epistaxis, dizziness, fatigue and weakness may each be seen with very severe HTN, particularly if it is of relatively new onset. However, in population-based studies, these symptoms are no more common in persons with than those without elevated BP. Thus, these symptoms in the presence of mild to moderate HTN are likely due to something other than HTN. Similarly, cardiac symptoms such as palpitations, chest pain, and shortness of breath may be more likely among persons with HTN, but this reflects a greater risk for arrhythmia, ischemic heart disease, or congestive heart failure rather than a direct effect of HTN.

The initial history and physical examination must determine the risk for, and presence of, target organ damage. Does the past medical history include heart disease, stroke or transient ischemic attack, renal disease, diabetes mellitus, or peripheral arterial disease? Does the medication list include drugs that may increase BP, or suggest the presence of another risk factor? Besides the standard Framingham cardiovascular risk factors, obesity (BMI >30 kg/m^2), physical inactivity, and renal disease (microalbuminuria or glomerular filtration rate <60 mL/min) are associated with increased risks of HTN complications. The social history must identify the presence of smoking and alcohol, the former because it increases the risk of complications, the latter because it may cause HTN. The family history may give clues to secondary causes of HTN (polycystic kidney disease, multiple endocrine neoplasia, or congenital heart disease) or suggest that a patient is at increased risk for HTN complications, such as a family history of stroke or heart disease. A family history of diabetes or hyperlipidemia makes these comorbidities more likely but appropriate laboratory tests must be obtained regardless of the family history.

The review of systems should focus on manifestations of cardiovascular disease: dyspnea on exertion, orthopnea, claudication, angina, or palpitations. Also important are signs of renal disease: nocturia, change in urine color or quality, or signs of prostatism. Finally, a review for symptoms of cerebrovascular disease might be useful, as a previously healthy patient may not have attributed a minor sensory or motor loss to a transient ischemic attack or subtle stroke.

In patients with markedly elevated BP, the clinician should also search for clues of HTN emergency including blurred vision, altered level of consciousness, headache, nausea, vomiting, seizures, or focal neurologic signs.

The clinician should also identify factors that may influence the choice of treatment. This goal requires the clinician to identify conditions for which there is evidence that certain antihypertensive agents have activity independent of their BP-lowering effect. In addition, it is important to know of baseline problems that might be exacerbated by side effects of a specific drug. Moreover a thorough history may identify factors that will help the patient and clinician identify the nonpharmacologic approaches that are most likely to be feasible, successful, and effective.

Because of the many complications of HTN and the many causes of secondary HTN, a thorough examination should be done for a patient with newly diagnosed HTN. Moreover, a thorough examination gives the patient the sense that this diagnosis is important, even though they typically have no symptoms that would suggest a serious disease. Particular attention should be paid to the cardiovascular system, and the examiner should search for target organ damage. In patients with markedly elevated BP, the physical examination should search for signs of acute complications such as pulmonary edema, altered mental status, and capillary leak (i.e., retinal hemorrhages, exudates, and papilledema). Important clues to secondary causes of HTN are presented in the next section.

In all patients with HTN, the retina should be examined for papilledema, hemorrhages, and exudates. Hemorrhages can be shaped like blots, flames, or lines (splinters). Exudates can be soft (also called cotton wool spots) or hard, based on their edges. All of these findings suggest more severe HTN and in themselves demand immediate attention, although a number of other conditions can cause them. The retinal vessels should be examined for focal spasm, arteriole-to-venule (AV) ratio, AV nicking, and abnormal arteriolar light reflex. The normal AV ratio (ratio of widths of retinal arterioles and veins) is somewhere between 2:3 and 4:5; but with HTN the ratio progressively decreases. Ordinarily, veins appear to gradually taper throughout their course, even where they cross the path of arteries, but with chronic HTN the vein becomes depressed on either side of the artery (AV nicking). With advanced hypertensive retinopathy, there can be dilation of the vein distal to the crossing point. The normal artery is a thick red line with a fine yellow line centrally (the light reflex). With arteriosclerosis, this light reflex gets progressively wider, eventually merging with the red column to be an entirely orange (or copper) structure, hence, this finding is called copper wiring. As the vessel wall gets thicker, the red blood makes a smaller contribution and the artery is nearly white, a finding that is called silver wiring. These retinal vessel changes can be difficult to reliably ascertain on examination. However, they can provide a measure of the severity of target organ damage.

The cardiovascular exam may be normal in patients with HTN. The thickening of the muscular arterial walls, loss of elasticity of the larger arteries, and endothelial dysfunction that cause most of the sequelae of chronic HTN typically do not cause detectable changes in the physical examination. Late sequelae of arterial wall hypertrophy can include reduced peripheral pulses or bruits of the abdominal aorta, femoral, or carotid arteries, but these are manifestations of atherosclerosis rather than HTN per se, and can be seen in its absence. Similarly, chronic HTN can lead to a prominent abdominal aortic impulse associated with an aortic aneurysm. Longstanding HTN can lead to wall thickening and enlargement of the left ventricle, which may be evidenced by a fourth heart sound, lateral displacement of the point of maximal impulse, and a more prominent apical impulse.

Secondary Hypertension

Most persons do not require extensive testing for secondary causes of HTN. However, patient characteristics that suggest secondary HTN and therefore warrant a battery of screening tests for secondary causes include prepubertal onset, onset before the age of 30 years in a nonobese person without a family history of HTN, evidence of severe HTN (based on BP >180/110 mm Hg or fundoscopic abnormalities), or new onset after age 50 years in someone whose BP had been regularly measured and known to be in the normal range.

Renovascular disease can be suggested by new-onset HTN in a young woman (suggesting fibromuscular dysplasia) or by the new appearance or sudden worsening of HTN in a person with evident atherosclerosis (suggesting atherosclerotic renovascular stenosis). These individuals are prone to sudden exacerbations of BP, which may precipitate flash pulmonary edema, and may develop hypotension in response to initial treatment with angiotensin converting enzyme (ACE) inhibitors. Physical examination may reveal renal bruits.

Coarctation of the aorta is typically asymptomatic except for the HTN, but can be suspected with onset of HTN in childhood or young adulthood. Physical examination findings can include delayed or reduced femoral pulses compared to brachial pulses, and an audible (primarily) systolic murmur best heard in the posterior chest. A detailed examination will detect a discrepancy in BP between arms and legs. There may be classic finding on chest x-ray (rib notching from increased flow in the intercostal arteries, or a 3 sign in the silhouette of the aorta). Most aortic coarctations are distal to the take off of the left subclavian artery, so that BP is similar in the right and left arm, but as many as a third of patients have coarctation that affects flow to the left subclavian artery, resulting in a lower BP when measured using the left arm.

Pheochromocytoma is suggested by episodic rises and falls of BP. Other manifestations include signs of adrenergic excess (e.g., arrhythmias) and episodic "crises" with flushing, headache, sweating, palpitations, and/or a sense of apprehension. Because of a chronically vasoconstricted state, these patients are more likely to have significant orthostatic BP drops. Neurofibromatosis and café-au-lait spots may be seen in patients with pheochromocytoma, particularly in the context of one of the multiple endocrine neoplasia syndromes.

Typical history and examination findings in patients with Cushing's syndrome, acromegaly, hypothyroidism, and hyperthyroidism are discussed in Chapters 66 and 67.

Sleep apnea is sometimes not considered in the list of secondary causes of HTN because it is associated so closely with obesity, another known contributor to HTN. However, HTN can be seen even in nonobese persons with sleep apnea, so a careful sleep history should be obtained in all hypertensive persons. If the history is suggestive, a sleep study serves as both the screening and definitive diagnostic test.

Exogenous substances are among the most common secondary causes of HTN. Adrenergic agents including appetite suppressants (dextroamphetamine, sibutramine) and decongestants (pseudoephedrine, phenylephrine) can be associated with HTN. Although effect on BP of these drugs is undetectable for most patients, they can raise BP substantially in individual patients. Some herbal supplements also have adrenergic properties, including ma huang and ephedra. Drugs of abuse including cocaine and amphetamines are also potent vasoconstrictors that can raise BP. Exogenous estrogens in the form of oral contraceptives or postmenopausal hormone replacement therapy can also raise BP through fluid retention.

Hypertension Complications

The complications of HTN are primarily cardiovascular. The presence of other cardiovascular risk factors as well as the level of BP elevation determines the risk of complications (called target organ damage).

Chronic HTN increases the work of the left ventricle, which initially causes ventricular hypertrophy, then dilation, and eventually left ventricular failure. Although still considered one of the major causes of systolic heart failure, elevated BP can also cause heart failure by leading to a noncompliant ventricle that impairs diastolic filling, even though systolic function as measured by ejection fraction is preserved. Moreover, in the setting of heart failure caused by other conditions, the increased afterload generated by HTN can further inhibit emptying of the ventricle and increase symptoms.

Chronic HTN causes progressive arteriolar thickening that contributes to congestive heart failure and peripheral arterial disease. In the elastic arteries, chronic BP elevation leads to aneurysmal dilation, typically in the context of atherosclerosis.

Chronic HTN accelerates loss of renal function in diseased kidneys. It causes progressive thickening of the walls of the renal arterioles with subsequent progressive loss of glomerular and tubular function. Indeed, the most important step in slowing the progression of diabetic nephropathy is not glucose control, but rather BP control.

HTN predisposes to arterial thrombosis, presumably via direct adverse effects on endothelial function and by altered blood flow related to increased wall thickness, decreased elasticity, and increased tortuosity of arteries. The association of HTN with thrombotic events varies with the vascular bed. HTN is strongly associated, in a graded relationship, with cerebrovascular infarcts, but is only weakly associated with infarcts of the limbs, gastrointestinal system, and myocardium. This may reflect differences in the sensitivity of the beds to the effect of HTN, or differences in the tendency of small infarcts to cause clinically noticeable events.

Abrupt or severe elevations of BP can rapidly cause acute complications. In the presence of sustained high BP, there is arteriolar vasoconstriction, which maintains relatively constant end organ perfusion and protects the less muscular distal vasculature from very high BPs; this phenomenon is called autoregulation. Failure of autoregulation contributes to the development of hypertensive emergencies. When autoregulation fails, the distal vessels are faced with markedly elevated BP that can lead to so-called "breakthrough" vasodilation. In the brain, this can lead to cerebral edema and the syndrome of hypertensive encephalopathy. In multiple organ beds, the markedly elevated pressures can precipitate endothelial cell damage, leading to vasoconstriction, extravasation of plasma constituents, and thrombosis. In the kidneys, this phenomenon can precipitate glomerular damage, causing acute renal failure associated with hematuria and proteinuria. In the brain, these phenomena may precipitate microinfarcts that further contribute to the encephalopathy. Not surprisingly, the effects may not be completely reversible, even with rapid BP control.

This sequence occurs most commonly in the setting of chronic poorly controlled HTN. The factors that precipitate acute decompensation are not well characterized. It rarely occurs at a DBP below 130 mmHg. Occasionally, this decompensation occurs at modestly elevated BPs that represent an abrupt change for the individual (abrupt rises in BP may follow discontinuation of therapy or may occur for unknown reasons). Thus, a pregnant woman who develops pre-eclampsia may develop signs of hypertensive crisis with a BP of 150/95 mm Hg.

DIAGNOSIS

The initial diagnosis of HTN requires that elevated BP be documented on two separate visits. However, because of the potential for damage with extreme elevations of BP, one would likely consider treatment based on measures taken at a single visit if there was evidence of ongoing target organ damage or if the BP was very high (greater than 180/110 mm Hg).

Certain laboratory investigations are routinely performed as part of the initial evaluation of a hypertensive patient (Table 133.3). They are ordered for the purpose of ruling out some of the more common causes of secondary HTN and for identifying important comorbidities or target organ damage, either of which would warrant more aggressive treatment. Although echocardiography is a more sensitive screen for left ventricular hypertrophy (LVH), it is not routinely used because the bulk of literature supporting a screen for LVH is based on electrocardiogram-diagnosed LVH. Chest x-ray should be performed in most patients with markedly elevated BP. In patients with HTN emergency or urgency, detection of crenated red blood cells, red blood cell casts, or significant proteinuria suggests acute glomerular injury.

Evaluation for secondary causes of HTN should be based on clues detected in the history, physical examination, or basic screening laboratory tests mentioned above. Renal parenchymal disease is suggested by an elevation of serum creatinine or abnormal urine sediment. Renal ultrasound is indicated whenever urinary tract obstruction is suspected, when there is a family history of polycystic kidney disease, and to further evaluate hematuria.

Renal artery magnetic resonance angiography and Doppler ultrasonography are sensitive tests for anatomic stenoses, but not all detected stenoses are physiologically significant. Further testing can give clues regarding whether the stenosis is physiologically significant, but can be associated with complications or give misleading information. Ultimately, the most reliable approach is to dilate the stenosis using angioplasty with or without stenting and assess whether the BP improves subsequent

TABLE 133.3 Laboratory evaluation of newly diagnosed hypertension

Test	Goals
Hematocrit	Anemia can increase cardiac work and blood pressure. Polycythemia can suggest secondary causes of hypertension including renal artery stenosis or pheochromocytoma.
Creatinine and/or blood urea nitrogen	Both are signs of parenchymal renal disease, both a cause and consequence of hypertension. An elevated creatinine is associated with increased cardiac risk.
Urinalysis	Active sediment or significant proteinuria suggest renal parenchymal causes of hypertension. Proteinuria is also a marker for increased cardiac risk.
Fasting lipid profile	Dyslipidemia increases the risk of renal and cardiac complications of hypertension.
Fasting blood glucose	Diabetes mellitus increases the risk of complications of hypertension.
Thyroid stimulating hormone	Screen for hyper- or hypothyroidism, both of which can contribute to hypertension.
Calcium	Screen for hyperparathyroidism, which is associated with hypertension. Calcium levels may rise with thiazide diuretics.
Potassium	Screen for mineralocorticoid excess, a cause of hypertension.
Electrocardiogram	Screen for left ventricular hypertrophy, an early sign of target organ damage.

to the procedure. Specialty consultation is often helpful in assessing persons with HTN and renal artery stenosis detected on noninvasive testing.

There are a number of effective screening tests for pheochromocytoma (Chapter 69). Measuring metanephrine in a 24-hour urine collection is one highly sensitive yet parsimonious approach.

Mineralocorticoid excess is suggested by hypokalemia. Because hypokalemia is neither sensitive nor specific, one should have a low threshold to perform biochemical screening if BP is difficult to control, or if there is a marked fall in potassium with use of thiazide diuretics. The ratio of plasma aldosterone concentration to plasma renin activity is an appropriate screening test that can effectively rule out the diagnosis, unless the pretest probability is unusually high. It is best performed in the morning in an ambulatory patient who has not received an aldosterone receptor antagonist during the last 6 weeks. The most common causes of mineralocorticoid excess are primary aldosteronism due to either adrenal hyperplasia or an adrenocortical adenoma. Defects in synthetic enzymes are rare and may be suspected by suppression of both renin and aldosterone. Primarily because it is a question that commonly arises during attending rounds, it is important to know that glycyrrhizinic acid, a "natural" licorice flavoring that has been used in both chewing tobacco and candies, affects cortisol metabolism in a way that increases mineralocorticoid activity.

Hypercalcemia (most often due to hyperparathyroidism) can be associated with HTN prior to any clinical manifestations of the hypercalcemia. For these reason, a serum calcium level is typically obtained during the initial evaluation of a person with HTN. If elevated, testing directed at determining the etiology of the hypercalcemia should be performed.

TREATMENT

Lifestyle changes are recommended for all patients with HTN. These often reduce cardiac risk to an extent greater than would be predicted from their impact on BP alone. Table 133.4 presents the JNC VII summary of the effects on BP seen in randomized trials of recommended lifestyle changes. Almost all of these trials reflect short-term studies and the effect of sustained changes are less well established. However, the magnitude of changes seen in these randomized controlled trials is consistent with estimates of the impact on BP of these lifestyle factors from observational data, suggesting the benefit will be sustained as long as the lifestyle change is maintained.

In studies of dietary sodium restriction among normotensive persons, the short-term drop in BP with a reduction from 4 to 5 g of sodium daily (as seen with a typical American diet) to 2 grams (88 mEq) of sodium is only 1 to 2 mm Hg. However, that reduction attenuates the usual age-related increase in BP prevalence. There are further drops in BP with further sodium restriction; SBP drops up to 8 mm Hg in persons with HTN (less in normotensive persons) with a decrease in sodium

TABLE 133.4 Lifestyle modifications to manage hypertension

Modification	Recommendation	Approximate systolic blood pressure reduction, range
Weight reduction	Maintain normal body weight (body mass index, 18.5–24.9)	5–20 mm Hg/10-kg weight loss
Adopt dietary approaches to stop hypertension (DASH) eating plan	Consume a diet rich in vegetables, fruits, and low-fat dairy products with a reduced content of saturated and total fat	8–14 mm Hg
Dietary sodium reduction	Reduce dietary sodium intake to no more than 100 mEq/L (2.4 g sodium or 6 g sodium chloride)	2–8 mm Hg (if starting at a 4–5 gram sodium diet); greater reductions are possible with lower sodium intake
Physical activity	Engage in regular aerobic physical activity such as brisk walking (at least 30 minutes per day, most days of the week)	4–9 mm Hg
Moderation of alcohol consumption	Limit consumption to no more than 2 drinks per day (1 oz or 30 mL ethanol [e.g., 24-oz beer, 10-oz wine, or 3-oz 80-proof whiskey]) in most men and no more than 1 drink per day in women and lighter-weight persons	2–4 mm Hg

For overall cardiovascular risk reduction, stop smoking. The effects of implementing these modifications are dose and time dependent and could be higher for some individuals.

intake to 50 mEq per day. In patients who are overweight, SBP and DBP both drop an estimated 1 mm Hg for each 1 kg of acute weight loss. This drop may be attenuated over time, so that a sustained drop in weight of 1 kg may have half the effect of the short-term drop. Among hypertensive individuals who do not exercise regularly, regular exercise reduces SBP by up to 4 mm Hg. It appears that both aerobic and resistance exercise are effective. Exercise that is more intensive is more effective, and intensity may be more important than duration. Randomized trials comparing the Dietary Approaches to Stop Hypertension (DASH) diet, which is rich in low-fat dairy products, fruits, and vegetables, and reduced in total and saturated fats compared to a usual American diet, have shown a substantial drop in BP (as much as 12 mm Hg for persons with HTN). The effect of the DASH diet on BP is additive to sodium restriction.

Current recommendations suggest early initiation of one or even two drugs, unless there are compelling indications to *not* initiate drug therapy. To minimize the total time with inadequate control of HTN, experts recommend simultaneously initiating drug treatment and lifestyle changes, maintaining the option of later stopping drugs if lifestyle changes are successful. This approach also avoids the potentially demoralizing scenario in which significant lifestyle changes are made, but the follow-up BP is no better than the baseline.

Experts almost uniformly endorse a treatment goal of reducing the BP below 140 mm Hg systolic and below 90 mm Hg diastolic for average-risk adults. Although there is less agreement on the precise goals for all higher-risk persons most experts, including, JNC VII suggests a target of 130/80 mm Hg for patients with diabetes or chronic kidney disease (i.e., glomerular filtration rate less than 60 ml/min or microalbuminuria). Some experts recommend a lower goal for other high risk groups, but there is limited urepiric support for this.

In general, pharmacotherapy should always be initiated with a thiazide diuretic, since only a very few trials have suggested an advantage of other agents over thiazides, even in specific populations. For each of these special cases (e.g., the use of ACE inhibitors in diabetics), there are studies that suggest that diuretics are as effective as the putatively superior agent at reducing cardiovascular events. Although experts disagree over how firmly the "thiazide diuretic first" rule should be followed, there is consensus that in situations where an alternative agent is thought to be the best first choice, a diuretic should be the drug that is added if a second drug is used. Similarly, experts agree that the benefit of choosing one agent over another is not as great as the benefit from achieving adequate BP control. Current recommendations do not suggest choosing a drug based on patient demographics, in part because diuretics are effective in all population groups, and also because differences in response between patients within a group are much greater than differences in response between demographic groups. The JNC VII guidelines suggest beginning two drugs simultaneously when starting from an untreated BP of 160/90 mm Hg or greater.

Antihypertensive drugs are typically classified by their mechanism of action. Table 133.5 presents the most commonly used agents grouped in clinically coherent classes, with a summary of their most important side effects. Not surprisingly, patients have been shown to be more likely to take medicine they can afford, so choosing a medicine that is inexpensive is preferable to choosing an expensive medicine that may be marginally less likely to have a particular side effect. Because of evidence that once-daily dosing is associated with better patient adherence, such agents are preferred.

Many antihypertensive drugs have proven benefits in other conditions and in many cases should be used in the treatment of persons with those conditions, irrespective of the presence or absence of HTN. ACE inhibitors and angiotensin-receptor blockers (ARBs) are both indicated to slow the progression of renal disease in persons with diabetic nephropathy demonstrated by microalbuminuria or proteinuria. Beta-adrenergic blocking agents (beta-blockers) reduce the risk of death following myocardial infarction. ACE inhibitors, ARBs, and beta-blockers each have been shown to reduce the risk of adverse outcomes in persons with left ventricular systolic dysfunction. Peripherally acting alpha-adrenergic blocking agents (alpha-blockers) ameliorate the symptoms of benign prostatic hypertrophy; however, they are less effective than diuretics in preventing stroke and congestive heart failure.

TABLE 133.5 Drugs commonly used in the treatment of hypertension

Class of drug	Commonly used agents	Contraindications	Selected side effects and comments
Diuretics	*Thiazide-type diuretics* Hydrochlorothiazide Chlorthalidone Indapamide *Potassium-sparing diuretics* Triamterene Amiloride Spironolactone *Loop diuretics* Furosemide	Gout	*Thiazide and thiazide-like diuretics*: More likely to cause impotence at starting doses Hypokalemia, except indapamide *Potassium-sparing Agents*: Hyperkalemia Triamterene raises creatinine without decreasing glomerular filtration rate Spironolactone can cause gynecomastia *Furosemide*: Less effective than thiazides, but it is effective even in presence of markedly reduced creatinine clearance
Beta-blockers	Atenolol Metoprolol Propranolol Bisoprolol Combined alpha- and beta-blockers Labetolol Carvedilol	Reactive airways Heart block Peripheral vascular disease Athletes and physically active patients	Bronchospasm Bradycardia May be more likely to cause fatigue than alternatives Withdrawal hypertension if at high doses Combined alpha- and beta-blockers may be more likely to cause postural hypotension, less likely to cause fatigue
Calcium antagonists	Verapamil Diltiazem *Dihydropyridine-type* Nifedipine Amlodipine Felodipine	Heart block, congestive heart failure (*nondihydropyridine*)	*Nondihydropyridines*: Conduction defects Constipation *Dihydropyridines*: Ankle edema Headache Avoid short-acting formulations

Angiotensin-converting enzyme (ACE) inhibitors	Captopril Enalapril Lisinopril Ramipril Fosinopril	Pregnancy Hyperkalemia Bilateral renal artery stenosis	Significant cough in up to 10% Angioedema Hyperkalemia ↑ fetal loss if given in second or third trimester
Angiotensin-receptor blockers	Valsartan Losartan Telmisartan Irbesartan	Pregnancy Bilateral renal artery stenosis Hyperkalemia	Similar to ACE inhibitors but do not cause cough and rarely cause angioedema
Alpha-blockers	Doxazosin Terazosin	Pregnancy Orthostatic hypotension	Orthostatic hypotension common with first dose Effective therapy for benign prostatic hypertrophy Inferior to diuretics as first-line therapy to prevent cardiovascular events
Direct vasodilators	Hydralazine Minoxidil		Common: headaches, fluid retention, tachycardia, hypertrichosis (with minoxidil) Rare: lupus-like syndrome with hydralazine
Centrally acting sympathetic inhibitors	Clonidine Alpha-methyl-dopa Reserpine		Sedation Dry mouth Withdrawal hypertension, primarily seen at high doses

With the availability of many effective drugs, it is surprising that more than one third of hypertensive patients are still not controlled. Common causes include poor patient adherence to treatment, drug-induced resistance to typical antihypertensive medicines (e.g., nonsteroidal anti-inflammatory drugs attenuate the effects of ACE inhibitors and can cause fluid retention), failure to recognize concomitant secondary HTN (especially related to prescription, over-the-counter, and illicit drugs or alcohol), or inadequate doses or inappropriate choices or combination of medications.

HYPERTENSIVE URGENCIES AND EMERGENCIES

Because persons with markedly elevated BP are at risk for developing a hypertensive crisis as long as the BP remains markedly elevated, they need urgent lowering of BP. But complications may be more likely to occur from overrapid correction of BP than from persistence of a well-tolerated, although frightening, BP. Thus, patients with hypertensive urgencies should receive prompt treatment

TABLE 133.6 Intravenous drugs used in the treatment of hypertensive emergencies

Agent	Description/advantages	Side effects/comments
Nicardipine	Vasodilating dihydropyridine calcium channel blocker. Administered as infusion. Relatively short half-life (15–30 minutes).	May have prolonged effect. Headaches frequent; can exacerbate ischemia by increasing cardiac work.
Labetalol	Mixed alpha-/beta-adrenergic blocker. Readily administered as bolus. Has oral equivalent.	Long half-life means it cannot be readily reversed.
Nitroprusside	Direct acting vasodilator. Very short half-life (1–2 minutes) allowing for rapid titration of blood pressure.	Compensatory tachycardia requires beta blockade if cardiac ischemia is a concern.
Enalaprilat	Angiotensin-converting enzyme inhibitor, so may have special role in high renin states or congestive heart failure.	Long half-life; unpredictable effect based on etiology of hypertension.
Nitroglycerin	Primarily venodilator so unlikely to increase cardiac work.	Less effective as monotherapy. Headache; tolerance/methemoglobinemia with prolonged use.
Fenoldopam	Dopamine receptor agonist; i.e., vasodilator, especially renal, leading to enhanced renal perfusion, diuresis.	Can increase cardiac work; can increase intraocular pressure, hypokalemia.
Esmolol	Nonselective, short-acting beta-blocker. Can use with direct acting vasodilator to control reflex tachycardia—especially used with nitroprusside.	Can exacerbate heart failure; bronchospasm; heart block. Not effective as monotherapy.
Hydralazine	Direct-acting vasodilator; many years of use, including use in pregnancy.	Can increase cardiac work via reflex tachycardia; headache.

aimed at gradually reducing mean arterial pressure by 20% to 25% over 24 hours. A low initial dose of an oral medication may be given immediately, with monitoring of the response. Favorite choices include centrally acting agents (clonidine or alpha-methyldopa) and captopril (an ACE inhibitor with a short duration of action). Short-acting vasodilators (in particular nifedipine) should be avoided because of the risk of abruptly lowering BP and precipitating ischemia. Otherwise, drug therapy appropriate for long-term use should be initiated. Reassessment should occur in 1 to 3 days. In this setting, thiazide diuretic monotherapy, which typically takes several days to have its effect, is probably not a good choice, although thiazides should be started if a multidrug regimen is elected.

If a hypertensive emergency is diagnosed, then the time course for BP lowering must be short, despite the risk of precipitating ischemia. Short-acting agents are preferred, and they are administered with constant monitoring of the BP. In almost all cases, this would involve admission to an intensive care setting and use of an intra-arterial line. An intravenous (IV) line may be placed to allow for a rapid response to a change in condition, and to allow for IV therapy if needed. Typical IV agents are presented in Table 133-6.

CHAPTER 134

Dyslipidemias

Karen Fickel

Coronary heart disease (CHD) remains the leading cause of death for both males and females in the United States. While many factors play a role in CHD, dyslipidemia represents a major modifiable risk. Dyslipidemia describes a wide range of lipid disorders. The most clinically important lipid disorders are elevated total cholesterol, low-density lipoprotein cholesterol (LDL-C), triglyceride, apolipoprotein (apo)-B or lipoprotein a (Lp[a]) levels above the 90th percentile, and low high-density lipoprotein (HDL) level or apo A-1 below the 10th percentile compared to the general population.

These disorders have diverse manifestations, but perhaps most important is the close linkage to CHD. In particular, increasing levels of LDL-C are strongly related to increased risk of atherosclerosis and CHD, while HDL has an inverse relationship with CHD because it pulls cholesterol out of the circulation. Many treatments have been identified that reduce CHD morbidity and mortality. A 10% decrease in cholesterol is associated with a 15% decrease in CHD mortality and an 11% decrease in total mortality.

ETIOLOGY

The two major circulating lipids are triglycerides and cholesterol. Triglycerides, composed of three fatty acids esterified to glycerol, are stored in adipose tissue in the fed state and are mobilized during fasting; they provide the body's primary fuel reserves. Cholesterol serves several functions. It is a major structural component of the cell membrane and the synthetic precursor of steroid hormones and bile salts.

Lipids, such as cholesterol and triglycerides, are transported in the plasma by lipoproteins. Lipoprotein particles are comprised of a nonpolar lipid core, surrounded by a polar coat of phospholipids, nonesterified cholesterol, and apolipoproteins. The two main lipid transport pathways are the exogenous and endogenous pathway.

The exogenous pathway (Fig. 134.1) begins with the intestinal absorption of dietary fats. These fats are assembled into large particles called chylomicrons. The chylomicrons are secreted into the intestinal lymph and then pass into the systemic circulation. While in the circulation, they are exposed to the enzyme lipoprotein lipase, which hydrolyzes the triglyceride component of the chylomicrons into fatty acids and glycerol. The triglyceride-depleted chylomicrons are removed from circulation by the liver and catabolized. Through this process, the triglycerides go to the adipose tissue and skeletal muscle and the cholesterol goes to the liver.

The endogenous pathway begins when triglycerides are made in the liver after ingestion of excess carbohydrate. They are secreted as very low-density lipoprotein (VLDL) and are transported to the systemic circulation (Fig. 134.2). VLDL contains mostly triglycerides, but some cholesterol esters as well. The VLDL particles are hydrolyzed by the same enzyme, lipoprotein lipase. Fatty acids are once again deposited in the adipose tissue and skeletal muscle. The VLDL remnants are termed intermediate density lipoprotein (IDL), which in turn are transformed into LDL.

LDL receptors are present on the liver as well as the gonads and adrenal cortex, allowing for

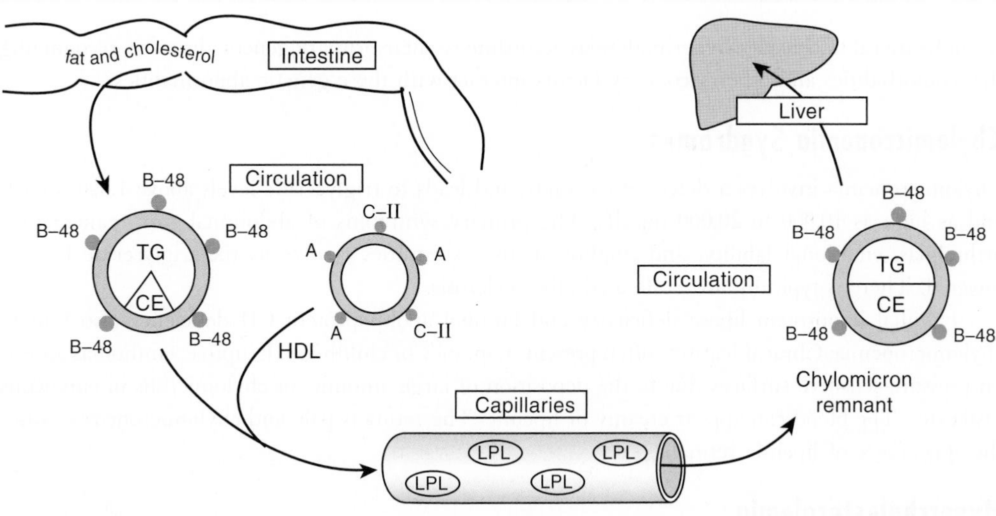

Figure 134.1 • Absorption of dietary fat and its assembly into chylomicrons.

steroid production. LDL uptake also occurs by a scavenger cell system involving macrophages. However, the uptake of LDL by these mechanisms is fairly inefficient and allows high levels of LDL to be left circulating in the plasma. HDL, in a reverse transport process, can take free cholesterol from the peripheral tissues and esterify it with the enzyme lecithin: cholesterol acyltransferase. This action decreases the free cholesterol in the tissue and the plasma.

Dyslipidemias result from abnormalities of lipid metabolism: either increased synthesis or decreased degradation of lipoproteins. These diseases can be primary genetic disorders or secondary to environmental or other factors.

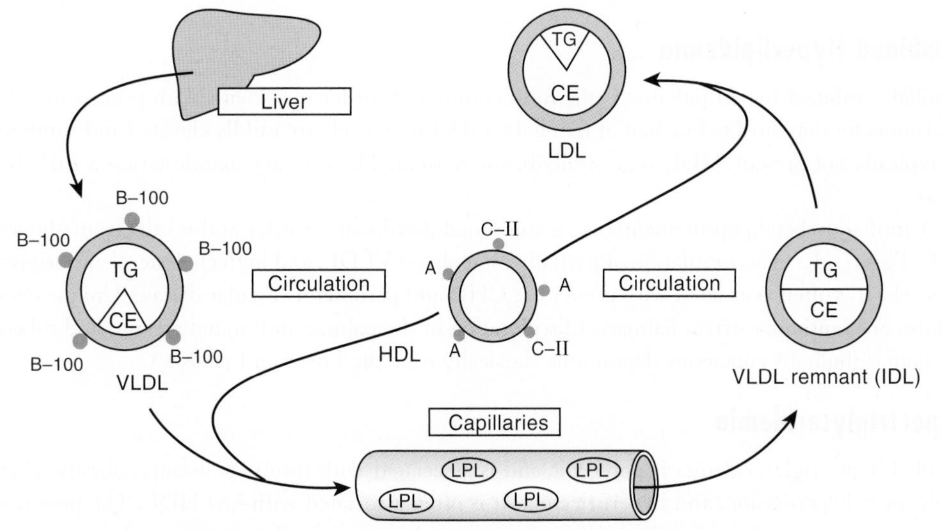

Figure 134.2 • Formation of very-low-density lipoproteins.

CLINICAL MANIFESTATIONS

It can be useful to consider hyperlipidemias according to their primary genetic disorder, recognizing that comorbidities and other secondary factors interact with these genetic abnormalities.

Chylomicronemia Syndromes

Chylomicronemia involves a defect in clearance and leads to triglyceride levels above 1,000 mg/dL and as high as 10,000 to 20,000 mg/dL. The primary symptoms of abdominal pain, pancreatitis, arthralgias, emotional lability, and tingling in the extremities resolve as the triglyceride level is lowered. There is typically no accelerated atherosclerosis.

Familial lipoprotein lipase deficiency and familial apolipoprotein CII deficiency also lead to chylomicronemia. Clinical features often present in infancy or childhood. Eruptive xanthomas appear on pressure-sensitive surfaces due to the deposition of large amounts of chylomicrons in cutaneous histocytes. The blood can appear creamy or lipemic. The retina is pale and chylomicronemia causes the appearance of lipemia retinalis.

Hypercholesterolemia

The cholesterol and LDL disorders have both single gene and multifactorial causes. These disorders include: familial hypercholesterolemia, familial combined hyperlipidemia, polygenic hypercholesterolemia, and familial hyperalphalipoproteinemia. Xanthomas (lipid accumulations in the skin and tendons) as well as xanthelasmas (raised, yellow plaques along the eyelids) are common. However, the depositions do not correlate directly with the severity of disease.

Familial hypercholesterolemia is very common, occurring in as many as 1 in 500 people. In familial hypercholesterolemia, heterozygotes have cholesterol levels in the 300 to 500 mg/dL range. Homozygotes (rare, 1 in 1 million) often have cholesterol levels higher than 800 mg/dL. These patients often develop symptoms in childhood. They have tendon and plantar xanthomas and severe CHD as well as aggressive aortic atherosclerosis, which can lead to supravalvular aortic stenosis. Most die before the age of 20 years. The heterozygotes, however, do not typically develop symptoms until the third or fourth decade when they have myocardial infarctions and accelerated coronary atherosclerosis.

Combined Hyperlipidemia

Familial combined hyperlipidemia is the most common disorder in patients with premature CHD. It accounts for one third to one half of familial CHD. Lipid levels are mildly elevated and xanthomas are typically not present. HDL is generally below normal. The primary manifestation is early heart disease.

Familial dysbetalipoproteinemia is an autosomal dominant disorder and results from abnormal apoE. This results in accumulation of partially catabolized VLDL, and high cholesterol and triglyceride levels. It is often associated with premature CHD and peripheral vascular disease. Unique clinical features are xanthoma striata palmaris (discoloration of the palmar and digital creases) and tuberous xanthomas (bulbous cutaneous depositions classically over the knees and elbows.)

Hypertriglyceridemia

Familial hypertriglyceridemia is polygenic and is associated with insulin resistance, obesity, glucose intolerance, hypertension, and hyperuricemia. It is often associated with low HDL. The presence of secondary factors such as diabetes, obesity, and alcohol can markedly increase triglycerides in this disorder.

TABLE 134.1 Secondary causes of dyslipidemia

Diabetes mellitus
Obesity
Nephrotic syndrome, chronic renal insufficiency
Obstructive liver disease
Alcohol
Estrogens
Glucocorticoid excess

Secondary Hyperlipidemias

Secondary hyperlipidemias are common. They are typically due to medications or coexisting diseases (Table 134.1). They can present as any of the phenotypic syndrome categories. In hypothyroidism or significant insulin deficiency, lipoprotein lipase activity is reduced. Estrogens and alcohol elevate triglycerides. HDL is lowered by beta-blockers and anabolic steroids. Patients with obstructive liver disease produce an abnormal lipoprotein (lipoprotein X).

History and Physical Examination

Key elements of the medical history include questions about dietary history, family history of heart disease, and medications (especially alcohol, steroids, and estrogens). The review of systems should ask about symptoms of atherosclerosis including claudication, angina, and other cardiac symptoms. The physical examination must include evaluation of the eyes (lipemia retinalis or corneal arcus), skin (xanthomas), and the cardiovascular system (carotid or femoral bruits, decreased peripheral pulses, elevated blood pressure, S3/S4, and abdominal aneurysm).

DIAGNOSIS

Clinically important lipid disorders are typically diagnosed with a fasting lipoprotein profile, which includes total cholesterol, HDL cholesterol, and triglycerides; LDL levels may be obtained using either the Friedewald equation: LDL = Total Cholesterol − (HDL + Triglycerides/5) when triglyceride levels are less than 400 mg/dL, or by direct measurement of LDL when triglyceride levels are greater than 400 mg/dL.

The most commonly cited guidelines specifying which patient groups to screen and how often are those of the National Cholesterol Education Panel (NCEP). The most recent NCEP guidelines recommend screening all adults 20 years or older with a fasting (12 to 14 hours) lipid profile every 5 years. First-degree relatives of people with premature CHD (men with events prior to age 55 years and women with events prior to age 65 years) should be screened as well. Guidelines do not address whether to further screen family members of people with premature CHD with more specific lipoprotein analyses to uncover other lipid abnormalities that may confer additional atherogenic risk.

In addition to a fasting lipid profile, other lab tests such as glucose, thyroid-secreting hormone, creatinine, urinalysis, liver function, and blood count are helpful to look for secondary causes of dyslipidemia.

TREATMENT

Dyslipidemias represent an important opportunity for primary prevention of CHD. There is clear evidence that total cholesterol, high LDL, and low HDL are independent risk factors for CHD.

TABLE 134.2 Major risk factors for coronary heart disease that modify low-density lipoprotein goals

Risk factor	Description
Cigarette smoking	Any cigarette use in the past month
Hypertension	Blood pressure >140/90 mmHg or on antihypertensive medications
Low high-density lipoprotein[a]	<40 mg/dL
First-degree relative with premature coronary heart disease	Age: male <55 years, female <65 years
Patient age	Male >45 years, female >55 years
Diabetes	National Cholesterol Education Panel Adult Treatment Panel III considers diabetes as a CHD equivalent

[a]High HDL (>60 mg/dL) is considered a "negative" risk factor due to its cardioprotective nature.

Triglycerides and other lipoproteins are also likely risks. It is vital to identify and treat patients with dyslipidemia in order to decrease CHD morbidity and mortality.

LDL remains the primary target of intervention. Triglycerides and low HDL are also receiving more attention as targets of therapy. The NCEP Adult Treatment Panel III (ATP III) focused on intensive treatment for patients with CHD while broadening its scope to include an emphasis on primary prevention for people with multiple risk factors.

TABLE 134.3 National Cholesterol Education Panel Adult Treatment Panel III target levels for low-density lipoprotein cholesterol (LDL-C)

Risk	LDL-C goal (mg/dL)	LDL-C level for lifestyle changes (mg/dL)	LDL-C level to consider medications (mg/dL)
Coronary heart disease or its risk equivalents of diabetes mellitus, peripheral vascular disease, cerebrovascular disease (10-year risk >20%)[a]	<100[b]	>100	>130
2+ risk factors (10-year risk <20%)	<130	>130	10-year risk 10%–20%: >130 10-year risk <10%: >160
0–1 risk factor[c]	<160	>160	>190

[a]10-year risk is based on Framingham risk factor score.
[b]In patients with active coronary artery disease, it may be prudent to lower LDL to <70.
[c]People with 0–1 risk factor almost always have <10% risk of coronary heart disease event in 10 years, so formal analysis with Framingham data is not necessary.

TABLE 134.4 Major groups of lipid-lowering drugs

Drug class	Lipid effects	Side effects	Contraindications
HMG CoA reductase inhibitors (statins)	LDL down 18%–55% HDL up 5%–15% TG down 7%–30%	Myopathy, elevated liver enzymes	Active/chronic hepatic disease, drug interactions with cytochrome p450[a]
Fibric acids	LDL down 5%–20% HDL up 10%–20% TG down 20%–50%	Dyspepsia, gallstones, myopathy	Renal and hepatic disease
Nicotinic acid	LDL down 5%–25% HDL up 15%–35% TG down 20%–50%	Flushing, hyperglycemia, hyperuricemia, GI distress, hepatotoxicity	Hepatic disease, severe gout; relatively contraindicated with diabetes, peripheral vascular disease
Bile acid sequestrants	LDL down 15%–30% HDL up 3%–5% TG no change, occasional increase	GI distress, constipation, decreased absorption of other medications	Elevated TG
Ezetimibe	LDL down 10%–20% HDL up 3%–5% TG down 5%–10%	GI side effects	

[a]Medications such as macrolide antibiotics, cyclosporine, antifungals. Niacin and fibrates, use with caution.
GI, gastrointestinal; HDL, high-density lipoprotein; LDL, low-density lipoprotein; TG, triglycerides.

Risk Assessment and Identification of Cholesterol Goals

CHD risk assessment is the first step in dyslipidemia management. It is important to identify not only the measured LDL-C, but correlate it with the other CHD risk factors (Table 134.2).

After the LDL and other risk factors are identified, a risk calculator based on the Framingham data is used to estimate the 10-year risk of a CHD event. This is used to determine the goal for LDL-C (Table 134.3).

Lifestyle Interventions

Initial treatment of hypercholesterolemia includes limiting saturated fats to <7% of daily calories, and increasing polyunsaturated fats up to 10% and monounsaturated fats up to 20% of daily calories. Plant stanols and sterols are encouraged (2 g/day) as is soluble fiber (10 to 25 g/day). Weight reduction and increased activity are also key components. Diet rarely reduces LDL levels more than 25%, so often patients require additional treatments.

Drug Therapy

Typically, if the goal LDL is not met in 6 to 12 weeks, a medication is initiated. However, even with the initiation of medications, lifestyle modifications must be continued. Diet is particularly important for chylomicronemia; restriction of dietary fat to less than 20% of daily calories is the only effective therapy because the triglycerides within chylomicrons originate from dietary fat.

The LDL-lowering drugs have been widely studied and have been shown to decrease overall mortality, CHD events, CHD procedures, and cerebrovascular accident (Table 134.4). They are effective in both short- and long-term therapy. About 4 to 6 weeks after drug therapy is started, lipid levels must be checked to insure achievement of goal LDL; monitoring is recommended every 4 to 6 months thereafter once at a stable dose. Liver function testing (alanine aminotransferase) is recommended for patients on a 3-hydroxy-3-methyl-glutaryl-CoA (HMG CoA) reductase inhibitor.

Typically, for elevated LDL, an HMG CoA-reductase inhibitor is started. If adequate control is not achieved, further treatment with ezetimibe or fibrate is added. However, the combination of an HMG CoA reductase inhibitor and fibrate should be used with caution because of the potential risk of severe muscle toxicity.

Reduction of elevated triglycerides are a secondary goal, unless they are >500 mg/dL. In this case, the patient is at risk for pancreatitis and a fibrate is generally started first, prior to addressing the LDL goal. Treatment of the non-HDL cholesterol and low HDL levels are secondary as well. Low HDL can be raised with smoking cessation, weight loss, and exercise. Alcohol and estrogen also raise HDL, but are not recommended therapeutic approaches for cholesterol treatment. Niacin causes the largest increases in low HDL levels.

CHAPTER 135

Osteoporosis

Joan Neuner

Osteoporosis is the most prevalent metabolic bone disease. It is a common disorder defined as reduced bone mass and microarchitectural deterioration of bone tissue, leading to enhanced bone fragility and a consequent increase in fracture risk.

Osteoporosis can occur at any age, but becomes very common by the eighth decade. Thirty-eight percent of white women age 75 years and older have osteoporosis. Hispanic women appear to have a similar risk of osteoporosis, whereas black women have approximately half the risk of white women. Men are less likely to have osteoporosis, but their risk also becomes substantial with age.

Uncomplicated osteoporosis is asymptomatic. Symptoms, when they occur, are related to fractures and their complications. At least 40% of postmenopausal women in the United States will have a fracture during their remaining lifetime. Approximately 300,000 women are hospitalized with hip fracture in the United States each year, and less than half of them ever regain their prefracture level of function. Morbidity and mortality are high following hip fractures, particularly from venous thromboembolism.

ETIOLOGY

Bone is composed of matrix, mineral, and cells. The matrix is the intercellular substance of bone tissue, consisting of collagen fibers, ground substance, and inorganic bone salts. Minerals, primarily calcium salts such as hydroxyapatite, determine the rigidity of bone. Three specialized cells form, regulate, and continuously turn over the bone matrix and its minerals: the osteoblast, osteoclast, and osteocyte. The osteoblast synthesizes the enzymes involved in bone formation as well as most of the proteins of the bone matrix. Osteocytes, a mature form of osteoblasts, become embedded within the bone structure. Osteoclasts, giant multinucleated cells, are primarily responsible for bone resorption.

In osteoporosis, bone matrix and bone mineral are proportionally decreased as bone resorption occurs at a higher rate than formation. Most osteoporosis is primary and believed to be age related, although the key mechanisms involved are not clear. The higher rate of osteoporosis in women is believed to occur because of both lower peak bone mass and the rapid drop in estrogen at the menopause. After peak bone mass in women is reached in the 20s to early 30s, there is a very slow decline in bone mass until menopause. Bone density then declines 1% to 3% per year over 3 to 5 years after the last menstrual period. After a period of slower decline, bone density then again rapidly declines, reaching 1% to 2% per year in women over 80 years old.

Many risk factors have been identified for both primary osteoporosis and fractures. A few of these risk factors are particularly common and also easy to identify in the office (Table 135.1). Most fracture risk factors appear to work by lowering bone density. A few fracture risk factors, however, such as poor balance or tall height, make patients more prone to fracture through hip anatomy or an increased risk of falls.

Secondary osteoporosis can be triggered by a number of factors including factors that increase bone turnover, decrease calcium absorption, or infiltrate the bone matrix (Table 135.2). Endocrine

TABLE 135.1 Major risk factors for primary osteoporosis and related fractures in white postmenopausal women

Personal history of fracture as an adult
History of fragility fracture in a first-degree relative
Low body weight (less than ~127 lbs)
Current smoking
Use of oral corticosteroid therapy for more than 3 months
Additional risk factors
Impaired vision
Estrogen deficiency at an early age (<45 years)
Dementia
Poor health/frailty
Recent falls
Low calcium intake (lifelong)
Low physical activity
Alcohol in amounts >2 drinks per day

Adapted from the Nelson HD, Helfand M. Screening for Postmenopausal Osteoporosis. Rockville, MD: Agency for Healthcare Research and Quality; 2002 Sep. (Systematic evidence review; no. 17). Available online at www.ahrq.gov/clinic/3druspstf/osteoporosis

problems including hyperthyroidism, Cushing's disease, and hypogonadism are examples. Several medications, most notably corticosteroids, can lead to or accelerate osteoporosis.

CLINICAL MANIFESTATIONS

Fractures most commonly involve the thoracic or lumbar vertebral bodies, the ribs, the proximal femur, and the distal radius. They generally result from minimal trauma, particularly falls. Chronic pain from vertebral body collapse is especially common; it may be unremitting and disabling. Physical

TABLE 135.2 Common causes of secondary osteopenia and osteoporosis

Endocrine
Hyperthyroidism
Cushing's syndrome
Primary hyperparathyroidism
Hypogonadism
Gastrointestinal disease, malabsorption
Drugs
Anticonvulsants
Glucocorticoids
Levothyroxine (overreplacement)
Neoplastic disease
Multiple myeloma
Diffuse metastatic disease

examination may demonstrate an exaggeration of the normal thoracic kyphosis related to loss of anterior height of the vertebral bodies. Hip and vertebral fractures in particular can lead to functional disabilities, but even wrist fractures may heal poorly.

DIAGNOSIS

Approximately one third of skeletal mass must be lost before it is appreciable on standard radiographs, so radiographs are not sensitive indicators of bone loss. Bone mass can be more accurately quantified by specific bone densitometry techniques. Central dual-energy x-ray absorptiometry (DEXA) measures bone density in the spine and hip with minimal radiation exposure. There is no clear threshold for where low bone mineral density goes from "normal" to a "disease." Using DEXA, the World Health Organization currently defines osteoporosis as a bone density T-score (measured in standard deviations below mean young adult peak bone mass) of −2.5 or lower. Currently osteopenia is defined as a T-score of −1 to −2.5.

Peripheral DEXA and ultrasound are also commonly used to measure bone mass. All bone density tests can predict fracture, but there is significant variability in bone density between peripheral and central sites. Experts recommend a follow-up central DEXA for any patient with a peripheral densitometer T score less than −1.0. Similarly, central DEXA is recommended on any patient with a T-score <0 on a peripheral ultrasound test.

Bone densitometry is indicated in all women aged 65 years and older, in patients with evidence of osteopenia on routine radiographs, and in most patients with diseases listed as secondary causes of osteoporosis. Other risk factors should prompt testing before age 65, either around the time of menopause or perhaps at age 60 years.

Secondary forms of bone loss, especially vitamin D deficiency, should be excluded before primary osteoporosis is diagnosed. A careful review of systems can suggest the need for workup for most other conditions, but some experts advocate a few screening tests for anyone diagnosed with osteoporosis (Table 135.3).

TREATMENT

Prevention and treatment of osteoporosis must include calcium and vitamin D supplementation to reach an intake of 1,200 mg elemental calcium and 600 to 800 IU vitamin D/day, and at least 30

TABLE 135.3 Workup for causes of secondary osteoporosis

Basic tests
Calcium levels
Renal function
Liver function (including albumin and total protein)
Thyroid stimulating hormone
Complete blood count
25-OH vitamin D level
Optional additional tests (generally used only if history suggestive of disorder)
24-hour urinary calcium
Celiac sprue antibody testing
Erythrocyte sedimentation rate
Serum protein electrophoresis

minutes 3 times per week of a combination of weight-bearing high-impact or low-impact aerobic activity and muscle strengthening exercise. In frail, elderly patients, it is critical to assess for risk of falls (Chapter 143) and to undertake any appropriate interventions. However, multiple studies indicate that these nonprescription treatments are not enough for most women with osteoporosis already established.

Bisphosphonates are generally considered first-line pharmacologic therapy. Bisphosphonates are stable analogues of pyrophosphate, and act as inhibitors of bone resorption, reducing osteoclast recruitment and activity and increasing osteoclast apoptosis (programmed cell death). Oral bisphosphonates including alendronate, risedronate, and ibandronate reduce the risk of vertebral fractures by one half and the risk of nonvertebral fractures by one third to one half in patients with osteoporosis. Alendronate and risedronate can be given weekly, and ibandronate can be given monthly.

Raloxifene is a selective estrogen receptor modulator (SERM) that competitively inhibits the action of estrogen in the breast and endothelium, but acts as an agonist on bone and on lipid metabolism. One large trial of this medication has shown it to be effective in preventing vertebral fractures in women with low bone density. No effect has been shown upon nonvertebral fractures.

Synthetic salmon calcitonin increases calcium absorption into bone. It is administered intranasally, usually 1 nasal puff once daily. It has been shown to reduce bone loss and decrease vertebral fracture risk. However, it is less effective than alendronate and there are no studies on clinical or nonvertebral fractures. Parathyroid hormone (PTH or teriparatide) has been approved for treatment of severe osteoporosis as a recombinant 1,34 fragment given once-daily subcutaneously. While either the excess secretion of hyperparathyroidism or a continuous infusion of PTH results in increased bone resorption and overall bone loss, this intermittent daily use in women with prevalent vertebral fractures reduced recurrent vertebral fractures by 65%. Intermittent parathyroid hormone works through osteoblast stimulation and appears to increase bone formation. PTH is generally reserved for patients who fracture or continue to lose large amounts of bone mass on other therapies.

CHAPTER 136

Back Pain

Kendall Novoa-Takara

About 25% of adults have low back pain each year. Low back pain affects nearly 80% of the population at some time in their lives. Low back pain is the fifth most common reason for physician visits. Fortunately, most patients (75% to 90%) with acute low back pain seen in primary care improve within 1 month; although 25% to 50% of patients will have further episodes of back pain in the following year. Chronic low back pain occurs in 6% to 10% of patients with low back pain.

ETIOLOGY

The majority of low back pain is mechanical pain (87%). Most mechanical back pain is due to strains and sprains (70%). Other mechanical causes are degenerative processes of the spine, herniated discs, spinal stenosis, fractures, and congenital disease. Nonmechanical spinal conditions comprise about 1% of back pain, such as neoplasia, infection, and inflammatory arthritis. Visceral disease accounts for 2% of back pain.

CLINICAL MANIFESTATIONS

Local pain is caused by stretching the pain sensitive structures or compressing sensory nerve endings. This pain is near the affected part of the back. Pain may also be referred to the back from the abdomen and pelvis. This type of referred pain is not usually affected by posture. Lumbar spine diseases tend to refer pain to the lumbar region, groin, or anterior thighs. Lower lumbar disease may result in pain of the buttocks, posterior thighs, calves, or feet. Radicular pain is sharp and is felt in the structures supplied by the nerve root. Coughing, sneezing, and contraction of the abdominal muscles may reproduce the pain. Pain may also come from muscle spasm. The spasms are accompanied by abnormal posture, tight paraspinal muscles, and dull pain.

Red Flags

Most back pain is lower or lumbar pain that is acute and self-limited. However, there are signs and symptoms of serious etiologies of back pain requiring urgent or emergent evaluation, which are referred to as "red flags" (Table 136.1). For example, isolated thoracic spine pain is more concerning for serious conditions such as aortic dissection, spinal epidural abscess, vertebral osteomyelitis, or malignancy. Constitutional symptoms such as fever, night sweats, fatigue/malaise, or weight loss; and pain worsened by lying down or awakening patients at night are concerning for malignancy or infection.

Most patients with back pain have paraspinal discomfort. Midline back pain is more likely to be due to serious pathology such as fracture, spinal epidural abscess, vertebral osteomyelitis, or malignancy. Back pain following trauma should raise concerns for possible fracture. Minimal trauma

TABLE 136.1 Signs and symptoms that should raise clinical concern in patients with back pain

Age >50 years
Constitutional symptoms: fever, night sweats, malaise
History of malignancy
Hypotension or hypertension
Immunocompromised patient
Intravenous drug abuse
Midline back pain
Neurologic deficits
Pain awakens patient at night
Pain worsened by lying down
Recent procedure that could cause bacteremia
Taking large doses of pain medication
Trauma
Urinary or fecal incontinence

in osteoporotic patients can cause a vertebral fracture. Intravenous drug abusers are at risk of spinal epidural abscesses. Back pain following a recent procedure should raise concerns for infection due to bacteremia and hematogenous seeding of the spine. Immunocompromised patients (those with human immunodeficiency virus, on steroids, with diabetes, and organ transplant recipients) are also at increased risk for infection.

Back pain in older patients (>50 years of age) is more likely to be caused by malignancy, compression fracture, and other serious conditions. Patients with prior history of malignancy must be evaluated for spinal epidural metastases. Patients with back pain and urinary or fecal incontinence must be evaluated for spinal cord compression. Smokers and patients with uncontrolled hypertension are at risk for aortic dissection or rupturing abdominal aortic aneurysm.

Young patients with serious back pain are more likely to have a congenital abnormality. Pain improved by flexion or sitting implies spinal stenosis. Patients taking large doses of pain medications should be evaluated for more serious causes of back pain.

Examination

Patients should have an examination that includes abdomen and rectum as well as the back and a neurologic examination. Vital signs and general appearance of the patient should not be overlooked. A pale, diaphoretic, hypotensive patient must be considered to have a rupturing abdominal aortic aneurysm. Severe thoracic back pain and hypertension is concerning for aortic dissection. Fever is a red flag for infection but not all patients with spinal infections have fever. Patients with complaints of urinary incontinence should have a postvoid residual. Lumbar muscle spasm results in flattening of the lumbar lordosis. Scoliosis may also be seen on back examination.

Pain of bony spine origin is often reproduced by palpation or percussion over the affected vertebra. Forward bending is often limited in patients with paraspinal muscle spasm. Lateral bending to the side opposite the injury worsens pain and limits motion. Hyperextension of the spine is limited with nerve root compression or bony spine disease. Pain from the hips can be differentiated from back pain by internal and external rotation of the hips in flexion and by tapping the heel with the examiner's palm while the leg is extended. With the patient lying flat, passive flexion of the extended leg at the hip stretches the L5 S1 nerve roots and the sciatic nerve. Normally, flexion to 80 degrees

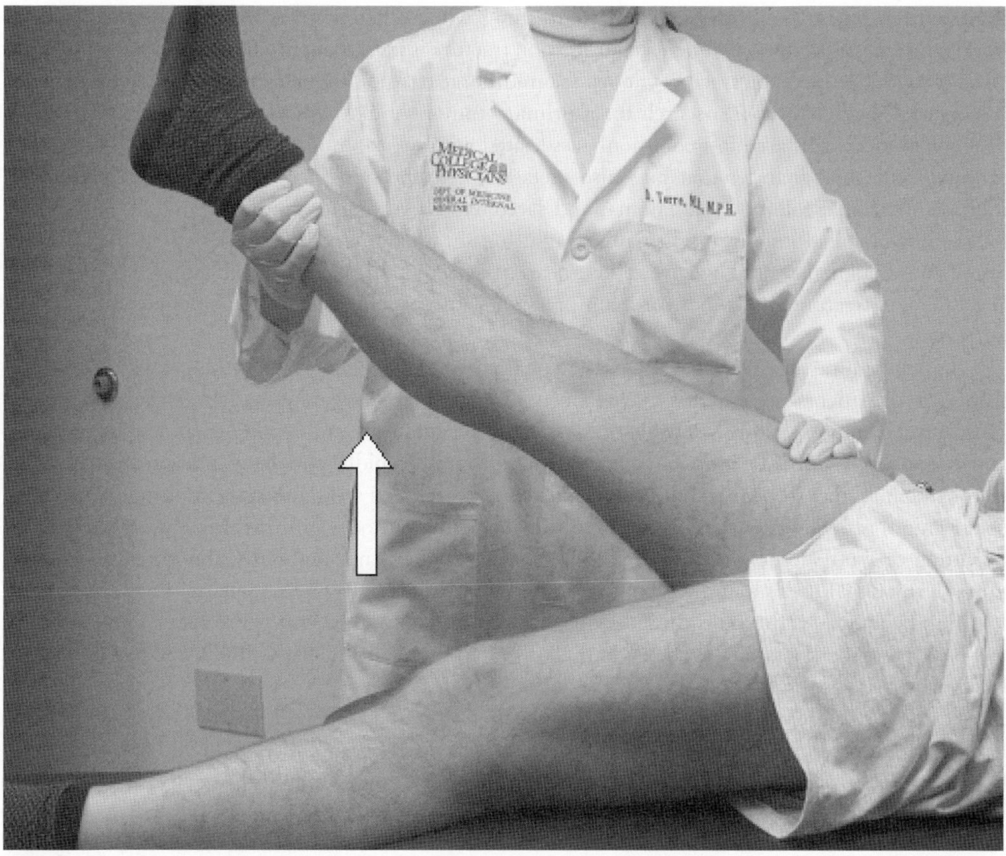

Figure 136.1 • Straight leg raising test. The leg is raised with the knee fully extended. Pain radiating below the knee when the leg is raised between 15 and 60 degrees suggests lumbar nerve root compression.

is possible without pain. The straight leg raising (SLR) test is positive if the maneuver causes the patient's usual back or limb pain (Fig. 136.1). Crossed SLR is positive when flexion of the leg causes pain in the opposite leg or buttock. The crossed SLR sign is less sensitive but more specific for disc herniation than the SLR sign. The nerve or nerve root lesion is always on the side of the pain. The neurologic examination should be focused on weakness, muscle atrophy, focal reflex changes, decreased sensation in the legs, and signs of spinal cord injury.

Common Conditions Causing Back Pain

Back strains and sprains refer to self-limited soft-tissue injury resulting from minor trauma such as lifting a heavy object, fall, or accident. The pain is localized to the lower back and there is no radiation of the pain to the buttocks or legs. There are no neurologic deficits.

Lumbar disc herniation usually occurs in the lower lumbar region. Minimal trauma such as coughing or sneezing may cause the nucleus pulposus to prolapse through a rent in the annulus fibrosis. Symptoms include back pain, abnormal posture, limitation of spine motion (especially flexion), or radicular pain. A dermatomal pattern of sensory loss or absent deep tendon reflex suggests location of the root lesion. Motor changes such as weakness, atrophy, or fasciculation occur less frequently. Vertebral compression fracture is usually due to osteoporosis. Minimal trauma may cause the fractures. These can present as localized aching while other patients may have radicular pain. Focal tenderness is common. When a compression fracture is identified, modifiable risk factors should be addressed. Compression fractures above the midthoracic region suggest malignancy. If malignancy is suspected, bone biopsy or a search for a primary tumor should be done.

Spinal metastases are most commonly associated with breast, lung, prostate, thyroid, and kidney cancers. Other malignancies that may also metastasize to the spine are non-Hodgkin's lymphoma, multiple myeloma, colorectal carcinoma, and sarcoma. The thoracic spine is the most common site for malignant spinal lesions. Night pain, weight loss, gradual onset of pain, persistent pain, history of previous malignancy, and age over 50 years are risk factors for malignancy. Diagnosis is important as pathologic fracture and spinal cord compression with permanent neurologic deficits can result if untreated.

Spinal epidural abscess classically presents with fever, back pain, and neurologic defects, but less than 20% of patients present this way. Pain is usually severe and midline. Tenderness of spinous process is a common finding. Neurologic symptoms are common and include weakness, paresthesia, and bowel or bladder dysfunction; patients can progress rapidly and have irreversible paralysis. Lumbar spinal stenosis pain is more diffuse; it typically worsens on standing or walking (neurogenic claudication) or hyperextension of the back, radiates to the buttocks or down the legs, and decreases on sitting or with supine position. Straight-leg raise usually is not markedly abnormal, and one or more dermatomal levels may be involved.

Cauda equina syndrome is caused by injury to multiple lumbosacral nerve roots. Symptoms are low back pain, weakness, and areflexia in the lower extremities, saddle anesthesia, and loss of bladder function.

Chronic low back pain is defined as pain lasting more than 12 weeks. Risk factors are obesity, female, older age, prior history of back pain, restricted spinal mobility, pain radiating into leg, high levels of psychological stress, poor self-rated health, minimal physical activity, smoking, and widespread pain.

DIAGNOSIS

Routine blood tests and x-rays are not usually needed for acute back pain. Imaging and blood tests should be reserved for those patients presenting with red flag signs or symptoms, and patients with prolonged back pain. The complete blood count may show elevated white blood cell count in patients with spinal infection; erythrocyte sedimentation rate is elevated in patients with spinal infection, inflammatory etiologies of spine pain, and malignancy; however, it is nonspecific.

Plain spine x-ray films are inexpensive and readily available. They are best for viewing bony structures. Oblique and flexion/extension views are not routinely recommended. Plain radiographs are useful in identifying fractures and metastases; however, other imaging modalities are more sensitive in detecting these.

Computed tomography (CT) is useful in identifying herniated discs, central canal stenosis, nerve root impingement/compression, and defects in cortical bone. Magnetic resonance imaging (MRI) offers several advantages over CT: soft-tissue contrast, visualization of the vertebral marrow, and contents of the spinal canal are better. MRI is best for characterizing spinal infections. MRI does not visualize cortical bone. Traditional myelography required injection of contrast medium into the subarachnoid space and was used to assess the nerve roots and spinal cord. CT and MRI may also be used for myelography and are usually superior to conventional myelography.

Bone scans use intravenous injection of technetium-99m-labelled phosphate to detect occult fractures, infections, or bony metastases and can differentiate these from degenerative changes. It can also identify old versus new fractures.

Electromyelogram (EMG) can be used to assess nerve function. EMG provides objective information about motor nerve injury. EMG and nerve conduction studies are normal when sensory nerve root injury or irritation are present.

TREATMENT

The majority of acute low back pain resolves spontaneously within 6 weeks. Treatment is conservative. Nonsteroidal anti-inflammatory drugs and acetaminophen are effective. Therapeutic exercises such as Williams' flexion exercises (knees brought up to chest) may help reduce muscle tightness and spasm. Muscle relaxants on a short-term basis are helpful but drowsiness often limits their use. Prolonged bed rest (>2 days) is not indicated for back pain. A short course of spinal manipulation or physical therapy is often helpful. Education about symptoms is an important part of treatment. Routine imaging studies are not indicated unless there are risk factors for serious etiology.

Disc herniation can be treated nonsurgically. Indications for surgery are:

1. Progressive motor weakness
2. Bowel or bladder disturbance or other signs of spinal cord compression
3. Incapacitating nerve root pain with conservative treatment of at least 4 weeks
4. Recurrent incapacitating pain despite conservative treatment

The usual treatment is partial hemilaminectomy. Epidural corticosteroid injection may be tried in refractory cases before surgical intervention.

Treatment of spinal epidural abscess is surgical drainage and decompression followed by appropriate antibiotics.

Treatment options of cauda equina syndrome include surgical decompression to restore or preserve motor or sphincter function. Treatment of spinal metastases requires a multidisciplinary approach with medical oncology, radiation oncology, and spine surgeons.

CHAPTER 137

Knee, Shoulder, and Other Regional Musculoskeletal Syndromes

Jerome Van Ruiswyk

Acute or chronic musculoskeletal pain is a frequent cause of ambulatory care visits. Pain frequently originates from intraarticular or periarticular structures of a single or a few joints, but patients with fibromyalgia may present with widespread pain with associated trigger points. Fibromyalgia (fibrositis) is second only to osteoarthritis in frequency. Primary care or emergency department physicians typically do the initial evaluation and treatment of these complaints. Recognition and accurate diagnosis of these conditions is important to prevent misdiagnosis of regional musculoskeletal syndromes as systemic illnesses (e.g., shoulder bursitis as angina, ruptured Baker's cyst as calf deep venous thrombosis, or tibial stress fracture as claudication).

ETIOLOGY

Pain is commonly caused by injury from trauma or overuse syndromes, inflammation, and altered structure or mechanics, but no specific etiology is found in many cases. Bursitis, which is inflammation of a saclike structure that facilitates sliding of one tissue over another, usually presents with pain, tenderness, or local swelling after overuse or trauma. Tendon inflammation (tendonitis, which typically occurs at sites of tendon insertion to bone or another point of tendon friction) and tenosynovitis (which is inflammation of a tendon sheath and typically occurs at sites where a tendon passes through a fibrous ring) are usually due to strain or injury. However, bursitis and tenosynovitis may sometimes be due to local (e.g., staphylococcal or streptococcal) or systemic (e.g., gonococcal) infections, or inflammatory arthritis such as rheumatoid arthritis or gout. In addition, symptoms are sometimes due to neurologic problems such as radiculopathy and spinal stenosis, or vascular problems such as peripheral vascular disease.

CLINICAL MANIFESTATIONS

Diagnosis of specific conditions is based mostly on the history and physical findings. Because patients typically present with pain, a careful pain history should be obtained including onset, duration, frequency, quality, intensity, radiation, and aggravating and alleviating factors. The response to prior interventions should be determined. Usual activity level and activity just prior to or at the onset of pain should be ascertained. History should determine function of the involved area and the impact of the pain on the patient's activities.

Physical examination should encompass the area of pain plus adjacent joints or the spine since these structures may cause pain referred to the same area. Examination should search for areas of tenderness or muscle spasm, articular and periarticular deformity or swelling, range of motion or signs of instability, and impaired function. For pain localized to the limbs, it is useful to compare the affected and unaffected sides.

Knee Pain

Patients with knee problems often report pain, stiffness, swelling, locking, instability, or weakness. Symptoms of ligament or tendon injury include trauma followed by swelling and instability. Symptoms that begin after a twisting injury suggest possible meniscal tear.

Examination of the knee should include inspection of standing alignment looking for varus (bowing) or valgus (knock-kneed) deformity; atrophy or asymmetry of the thigh muscles, and inspection of the popliteal fossa for swelling. Gait should be observed; patellar tracking should be observed while palpating for crepitus. The suprapatellar pouch should be "milked" toward the joint, followed by ballottement or lateral palpation in the space posterior to the patella to allow detection of small effusions. The joint line should be palpated and range of motion measured. Medial and lateral collateral ligament integrity should be determined by applying lateral and medial stress, respectively, while the knee is flexed to 25 degrees (Figs. 137.1 and 137.2). The integrity of the anterior cruciate ligament is determined by pulling the tibia anterior relative to the femur, while the knee is in 25 degrees of flexion (known as the Lachman's test).

Alternatively, the knee can be flexed to 90 degrees with the foot slightly medially deviated. The examiner grasps the posterior leg just below the knee and pulls forward firmly feeling for laxity (known as the anterior drawer test; Fig. 137.3). The posterior cruciate ligament is assessed by placing the thumbs on the anterior tibial plateau with the knee flexed to 90 degrees (known as the posterior

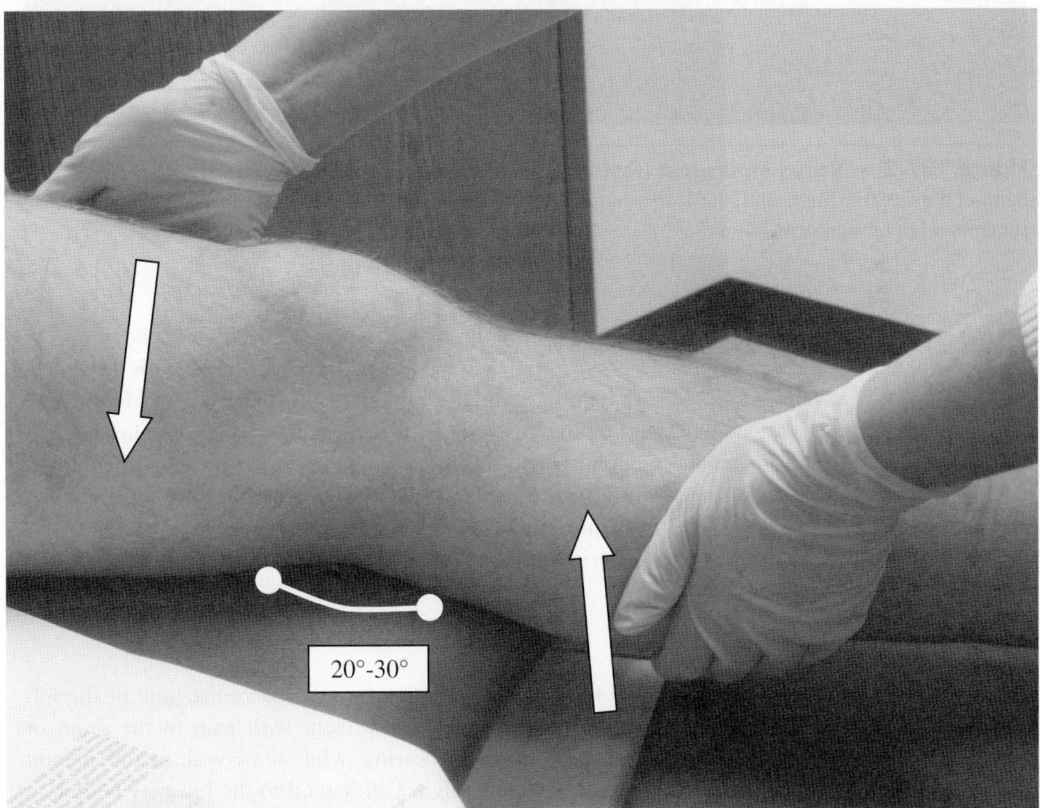

Figure 137.1 • Valgus stress test (test integrity of collateral medial ligament). After placing the patient's knee at a 25-degree angle, the upper hand stabilizes the thigh and the lower hand applies pressure outward. Pain or looseness of the knee indicates a medial ligament lesion.

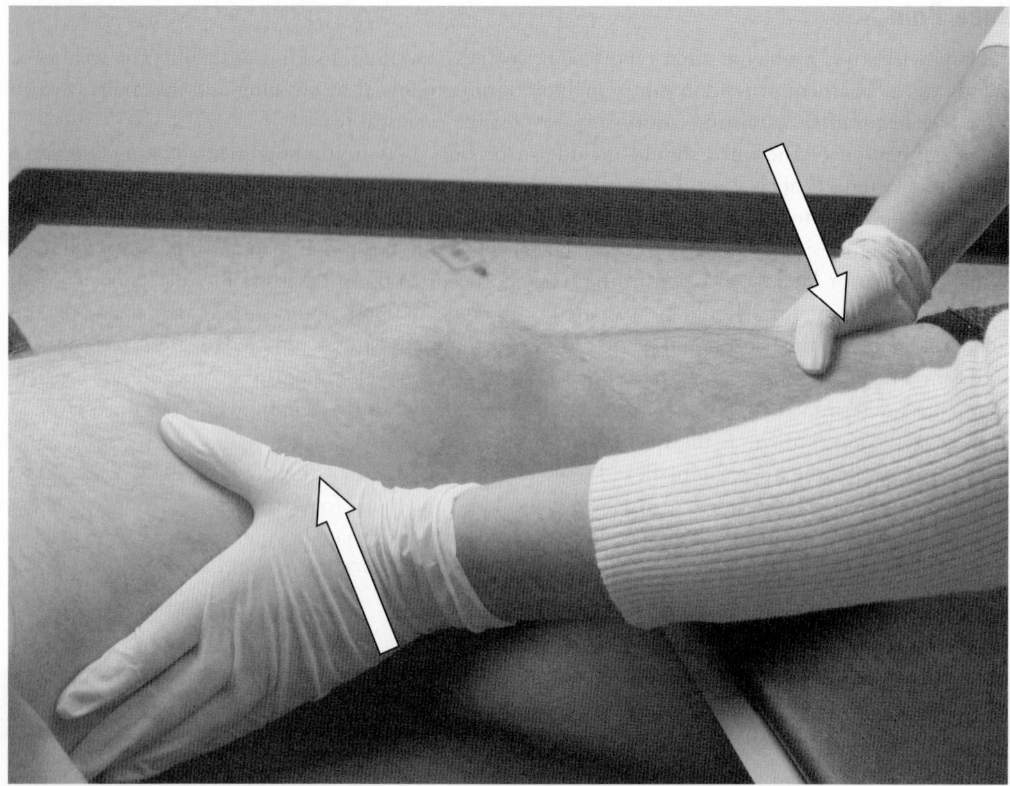

Figure 137.2 • Varus stress test (test integrity of lateral collateral ligament). The upper hand stabilizes the thigh and the lower hand applies inward pressure. Pain or loosening of the knee suggests a lateral ligament lesion.

drawer test). Normally the tibial plateau sits 1 cm anterior to the femoral condyles (known as the thumb sign), but the proximal tibia falls posteriorly when the posterior cruciate ligament is disrupted. Meniscal tears are usually associated with joint line tenderness plus clicking or pain with McMurray's test (Fig. 137.4), which is done by extending the knee from a fully flexed position while holding the foot in external rotation for medial meniscus tears and internal rotation for lateral meniscal tears. Patellar instability can be evaluated by pushing the patella laterally and flexing the knee to 30 degrees; apprehension is a sign of possible patellar instability. Tenderness at the medial flare of the tibia just below the tibial plateau suggests pes anserine bursitis, whereas swelling and tenderness over the patella suggests prepatellar bursitis.

Hip Pain

Hip joint problems must be differentiated from pain originating from the sacroiliac joint or the soft tissues around the hip. Patients with hip joint problems often present with pain in the groin or anterior thigh that is increased with ambulation or weightbearing, while those with sacroiliac joint problems often report pain in the buttock or posterior thigh. Pain lateral to the hip may be due to trochanteric bursitis or iliotibial band irritation from "snapping" over the greater trochanter, while hamstring injuries typically cause pain in the posterior thigh or buttock. Pain in the hip region sometimes represents referred pain from the lumbar spine, while hip pain is sometimes referred to the knee.

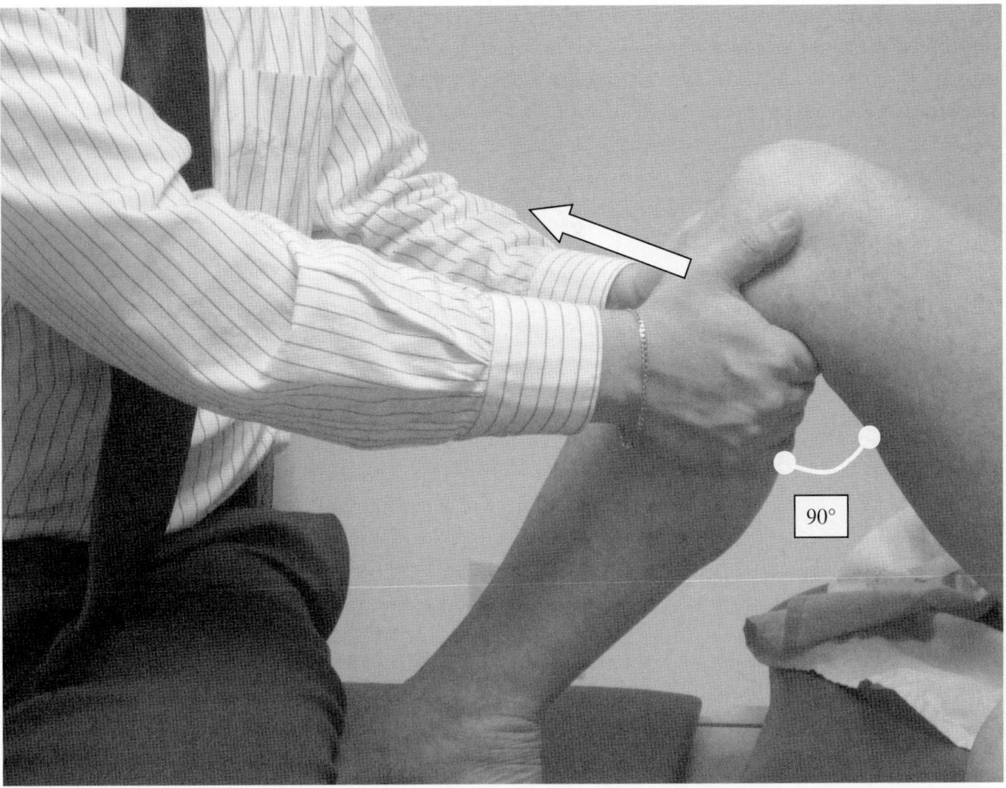

Figure 137.3 • The knee is flexed to 90 degrees with the examiner sitting on the foot, which is slightly medially deviated. The lower leg is firmly pulled toward the examiner at the knee. Laxity indicates an anterior cruciate tear.

Physical examination of the hip should include observation for alignment of the hip, leg, and foot in the lying posture, and observation for tilting of the iliac crests and asymmetry of the anterior or posterior thigh musculature in the standing posture. Slight shortening of the leg with external rotation of the foot in a patient who cannot bear weight on the affected leg is seen with intertrochanteric hip fracture. For patients with chronic hip pain, the strength of the hip abductors should be tested by having the patient stand on one leg; with normal abductor strength, the pelvis remains level, but with decreased strength the iliac crest drops on the opposite side (Trendelenburg's test). Lateral tenderness over the greater trochanter suggests underlying bursitis; tenderness over the ischial tuberosity with a history of pain with sitting on a hard surface suggests ischial bursitis. Range of motion including flexion, extension, abduction, adduction, internal and external rotation should be recorded. Decrease in internal rotation is often the first sign of hip osteoarthritis.

Shoulder Pain

Common traumatic injuries of the shoulder include humeral or clavicular fracture, acromioclavicular joint separation, and anterior shoulder dislocation. Nontraumatic shoulder pain is most commonly from periarticular structures since osteoarthritis of the glenohumeral, acromioclavicular, or sternoclavicular joints is relatively uncommon. Pain with overhead activity suggests impingement syndrome related to rotator cuff pathology or subacromial bursitis, while pain with adduction suggests acromioclavicular joint pathology. Pain in a radicular pattern or in the distribution of a peripheral nerve,

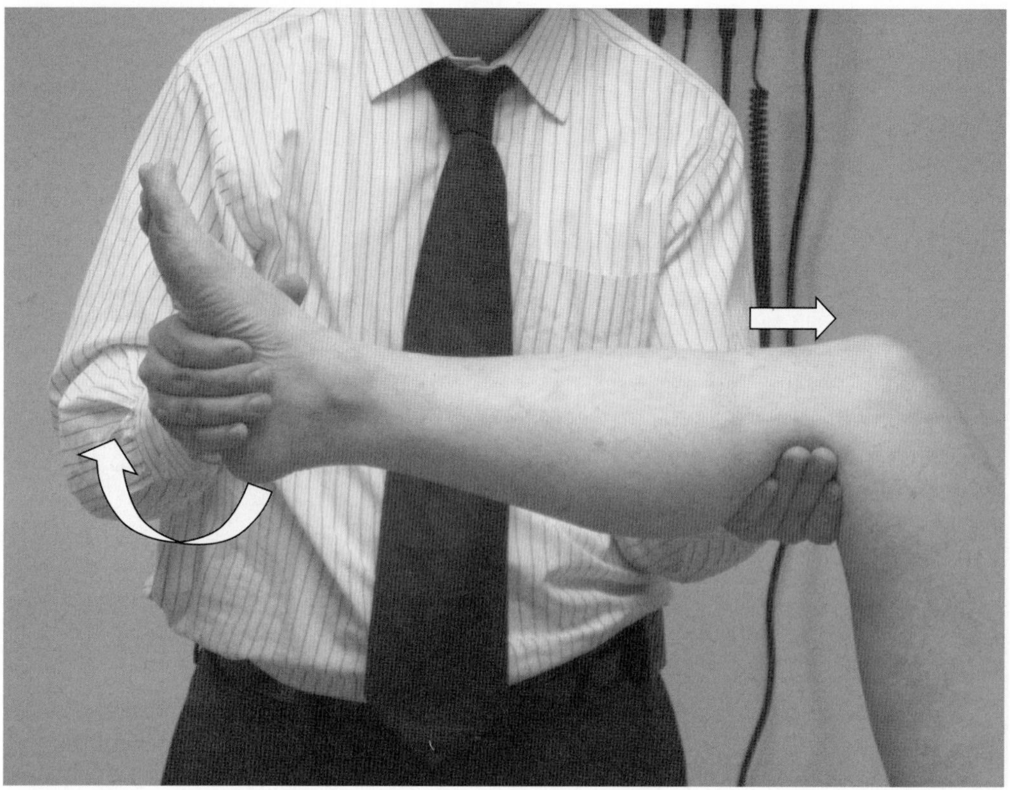

Figure 137.4 • McMurray's test. The knee is flexed and the tibia is rotated internally and externally. While the tibia is rotated, a valgus stress is placed on the knee and the knee is slowly extended. The presence of pain and a "click" suggests a meniscal tear.

with associated numbness or weakness in the arm or hand, suggests cervical radiculopathy or brachial plexus/peripheral nerve injury, respectively.

Physical examination of the shoulder should include inspection for joint swelling and bony or muscular asymmetry. Anterior, inferior, and medial displacement of the humeral head suggests anterior dislocation; a bulge in the lower arm suggests rupture of the long head of the biceps with retraction of the muscle belly. The clavicle, humerus, scapula, periarticular muscles, acromioclavicular joint, anterolateral subacromial space, and humeral bicipital groove should be palpated for deformity or tenderness. Inferior displacement of the acromion suggests acromioclavicular joint separation; tenderness over the bicipital groove and pain with resisted supination of the hand (Yergason's maneuver) suggests bicipital tendonitis (Fig. 137.5). Shoulder flexion, abduction, internal and external rotation should be recorded; internal rotation is typically recorded by recording the highest spinous process that can be reached by the upturned thumb. Inability to reach the top of the head with associated lack of glenohumeral abduction is indicative of frozen shoulder. Reduced function of the rotator cuff muscles suggests either tendonitis or tear. Supraspinatus strength is tested by having the patient place the arm in 90 degrees of abduction and 30 degrees of flexion with the thumb pointed downward (Fig. 137.6). Strength of the infraspinatus and teres minor is tested by applying resistance to adduction with the arm at the side and held in 30 degrees of internal rotation. Subscapularis strength is tested by having the patient "lift off" against resistance while their hand is behind their back.

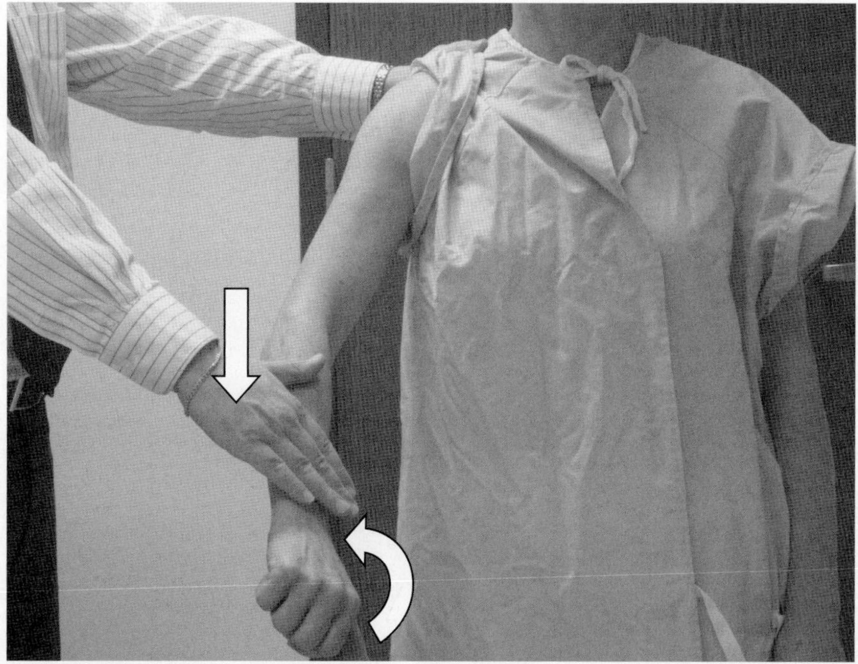

Figure 137.5 • Yergason's maneuver for biceps tendinitis. With the shoulder at rest, the hand is supinated against resistance. Pain indicates biceps tendinitis.

Neck Pain

Acute neck pain, often with muscle spasm, can be triggered by ligamentous sprain (e.g., whiplash secondary to motor vehicle accidents, falls, or athletic injuries), tension, activities involving repetitive neck movement, or nerve root irritation. Chronic neck pain may result from disc degeneration, apophyseal joint arthritis, or radiculopathy. It is important to remember that neck pain may also be referred from other areas and therefore may represent thoracic outlet syndrome, brachial plexus injury or compression, intrathoracic lesions (Pancoast's tumor), diaphragmatic irritation (subphrenic abscess, splenic or gallbladder disease), or coronary disease.

The physical examination often reveals limitation of neck motion, tenderness to palpation, and paracervical muscle spasm. Careful neurologic examination should be done searching for upper extremity weakness, and sensory or reflex loss in a dermatomal distribution.

Other Sites

Tendonitis, bursitis, and enthesopathies (diseases of tendon or ligament attachment points) can occur at several other sites around the body (Table 137.1).

Fibromyalgia

Patients with fibromyalgia report stiffness, weakness, and diffuse, poorly localized pain involving the neck, back, and extremities. Symptoms are worse in the morning and with weather changes, stress, fatigue, or cold, and improve with heat, massage, or a vacation. Patients are chronically exhausted because of waking frequently, often due to pain. Fibromyalgia is a generalized-pain and symptom-amplification syndrome so that its coexistence with irritable bowel syndrome and spastic bladder, and its overlap with chronic fatigue syndrome, are not uncommon.

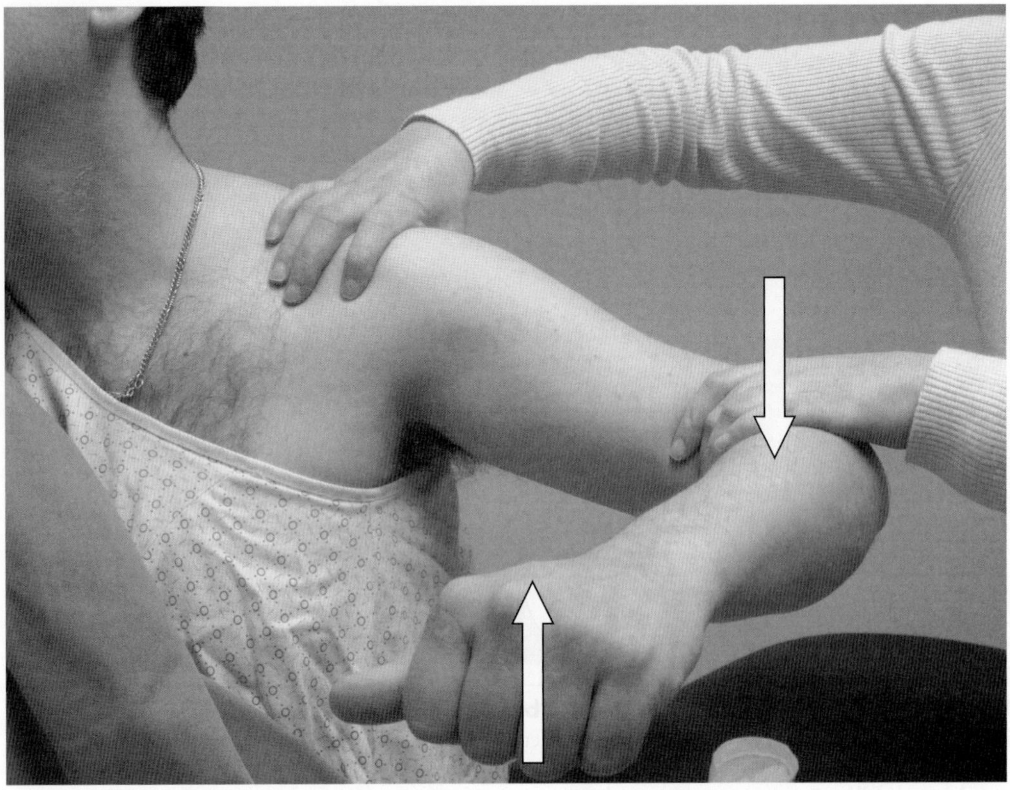

Figure 137.6 • Testing the supraspinatus. After placing the patient arm at 90 degrees, the patient is asked to abduct the arm against resistance. Discomfort indicates inflammation of the muscle tendon and a rotator cuff injury.

On physical examination, patients have a remarkably similar distribution of tender points, which are sites exquisitely sensitive on palpation; some of these tender points may not correlate with described areas of pain and thus may surprise the patient. The diagnosis of fibromyalgia (per the American College of Rheumatology) rests on finding 11 of 18 tender points, both above and below the waist and on both sides of the body, which have been present for at least 3 months (Fig. 137.7). Pain in only one or a few localized areas is termed myofascial pain; this is more likely to resolve over time.

DIAGNOSIS

Plain radiographs in patients with regional musculoskeletal syndromes may be helpful to confirm clinically suspected bony pathology, and in those cases which cannot be diagnosed on history and physical examination. Plain films may also reveal conditions such as calcific tendonitis, chondrocalcinosis, degenerative disc disease, foraminal impingement, or diffuse idiopathic skeletal hypertrophy. Magnetic resonance imaging may be necessary to confirm intraarticular or periarticular soft-tissue abnormalities such as meniscal tear, ligament, or tendon injuries such as anterior cruciate ligament or rotator cuff tear, nerve root impingement, and certain other conditions such as avascular necrosis or osteomyelitis. When inflammatory arthritis or infection are possible explanations, diagnostic aspiration of bursa or joint fluids for crystal analysis, gram stain, and culture should be performed. In

TABLE 137.1 Other common regional musculoskeletal disorders

Disorder	Findings
Elbow	
Lateral epicondylitis	Lateral elbow and forearm pain, increased with arm use ("tennis elbow"), tenderness over the lateral epicondyle
Medial epicondylitis	Medial elbow and forearm pain, increased with use, tenderness over the medial epicondyle ("golfer's elbow")
Olecranon bursitis	Usually caused by pressure or trauma, may have fluid accumulation over olecranon
Wrist	
De Quervain's tenosynovitis	Radial wrist pain; tenderness over the distal radius; pain near base of thumb (over abductor pollicis longus, extensor pollicis brevis tendons)
Hand	
Flexor tendonitis	May affect any of the flexor tendons, finger may lock in flexion and snap with extension ("trigger finger"), flexor tendon may be tender in distal palm, may click with finger movement
Ankle	
Achilles' tendonitis	Tenderness at the insertion of the Achilles' tendon on the calcaneus
Achilles' bursitis	Swelling anterior to the Achilles' tendon
Peroneal tenosynovitis	Pain posterior and inferior to the lateral malleolus
Foot	
Plantar fasciitis	Pain at medial aspect and anterior to calcaneus that is worse on initially standing or with maneuvers that stretch the plantar fascia

patients with unclear etiologies of symptoms, if infection has been ruled out, a diagnostic injection of local anesthetic and/or steroid may help localize the source of pain. Electrodiagnostic studies may be indicated in some cases to rule out referred pain from an underlying radiculopathy or plexopathy.

In patients with fibromyalgia, a complete blood count, erythrocyte sedimentation rate, and thyroid function should be done. In selected cases, further laboratory, imaging, or electrodiagnostic studies may need to be done to exclude rheumatic, endocrine, hematologic, musculoskeletal, and neurologic disorders.

TREATMENT

Treatment of most regional musculoskeletal disorders is initially conservative with a combination of rest and/or immobilization followed by graded increase in activity, and use of nonsteroidal anti-inflammatory drugs. Patients with impaired function will often benefit from appropriate physical therapy; some patients may benefit from additional physical modalities such as local application of heat or cold, or ultrasound. Local corticosteroid injections are often helpful in patients who do not

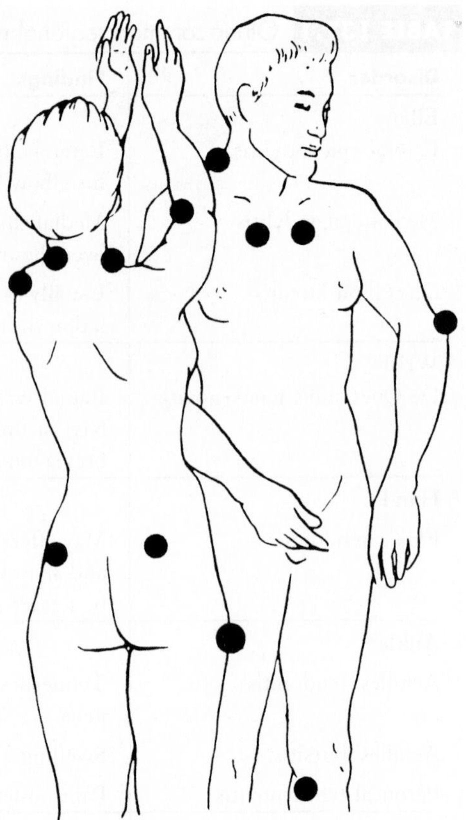

Figure 137.7 • Location of 18 typical tender points in fibromyalgia. Tender points appear symmetrically in the body. The suboccipital muscle insertions onto the base of the skull; the lower lateral neck muscles; the midpoint of the trapezii; the medial supraspinata; the second costochondral junctions; 2-cm distal to the lateral epicondyles; the upper outer glutei; the posterior aspect of the greater trochanters of the femur; and the medial proximal tibiae.

improve with initial conservative treatment. Patients with syndromes due to infection or systemic illnesses should be treated with antibiotics and other appropriate measures and may require referral to appropriate specialists.

Treatment of fibromyalgia is often frustrating. Patients may be defensive because they feel threatened by their symptoms and by physicians who dismiss their nonspecific symptoms as psychogenic or emotional. Explanation of a "vicious cycle" of sleep deprivation and pain magnification is the first step. Drug therapy is controversial. Many patients respond to tricyclic antidepressants (e.g., amitriptyline) taken at bedtime to improve sleep, although side effects may limit their use. Exercise, particularly aerobics (e.g., swimming or bicycling 4 to 6 days a week), should be started gradually and increased as tolerated. Stress management and other relaxation techniques may be important for some patients. Presented in a positive, concerned manner, these measures may alleviate the patient's fears and make symptoms more tolerable.

CHAPTER 138

Upper Respiratory Tract Infection

Robert Maglio

The "common cold" is the most frequently acquired acute illness. Not severe, with a limited course and sequelae, the two to three yearly adult episodes are estimated to cost the U.S. economy $40 billion annually. Familiarity with its conundrums of prevention, diagnosis, and effective treatment is essential for anyone who cares for patients in the ambulatory setting.

ETIOLOGY

This condition is viral inflammation of the nose, pharynx, tracheobronchial tree, sinuses, and middle ear. Three viruses cause 70% of colds. These are the rhinoviruses (40%), corona viruses (20%), and respiratory syncytial virus (RSV; 10%). They characteristically cause inflammation, but do not damage infected epithelium. Other viral species cause typical upper respiratory infection (URI)-type colds, but are more commonly known for systemic effects and lower respiratory tract infection. With them, damage to epithelium results. These include influenza, parainfluenza, and adenovirus. The enteroviruses Echo and Coxsackie occasionally produce cold symptoms. When studied, up to one third of adults with colds have no discernible etiologic agent.

The high incidence of URI is secondary to the many viral etiologies and their ability to cause reinfection upon reexposure. Seasonal variation is present worldwide. The annual epidemic of colds occurs in tropical and temperate areas, during the rainy season in the former and the colder months in the latter. U.S. winter incidence is roughly twice that seen in summer. This rise comes in late summer and early fall, with decline in spring. Viral agents demonstrate individual seasonal patterns of activity: coronaviruses, RSV, and adenovirus in winter; rhinoviruses in fall; Echo in the spring; and Coxsackie in late summer.

The upper airway of younger children is the main reservoir of respiratory viruses. Domestic pigs may also serve as a reservoir for coronavirus. Where children are present, spread occurs (e.g., home, school, daycare). Secondary infection in adults then results from contact with young children. Viral shedding itself is of short duration: 3 weeks with rhinoviral infections and 2 weeks with coronaviruses, with a slightly longer duration in children. In experimental rhinovirus infection, peak viral shedding occurs with peak symptoms, predominantly from the nose. Asymptomatic shedding in adults is uncommon.

Two mechanisms of viral spread have been described; direct contact and aerosol (large and small droplet). Close contact is the most effective way rhinovirus is spread, with hand-to-hand transmission effecting viral transfer and secondary infection arising from autoinoculation of the nose and conjunctiva. Rhinovirus is viable in dried nasal mucous on human skin for at least 2 hours. Virus capable of producing illness has been recovered from the hands of 40% to 90% of those suffering from colds and from 6% to 15% of objects in their proximity, including environmental surfaces. It is currently felt that coronavirus and RSV transmission are similar. Aerosol spread of rhinoviral infection has been demonstrated experimentally, but has not been confirmed as a clinical mechanism of spread, as is the case with RSV.

Salivary viral content is nil in 90% of symptomatic patients with colds, which suggests that kissing can be considered unlikely to spread illness. However, caution is advised because the act implies other close contact likely to spread illness. Although experimental evidence shows that rhinovirus can be spread by aerosol, a recent study found no difference in cold symptoms occurring subsequent to commercial airline flights in airframes with fresh and recirculated cabin air. Porous cotton handkerchiefs are not hospitable for viral persistence. Virucidal hand wash and home cleansers effectively limit transmission.

Neither tonsillectomy nor cigarette smoking influence the frequency of colds. Persons in cold climates do not suffer colds with any greater frequency than those in warm climates. As noted above, adults have on average two to three episodes of colds per year. Children, however, have up to nine colds per year; this likely explains the increased incidence of colds in their adult caregivers.

CLINICAL MANIFESTATIONS

Cardinal symptoms arise characterizing the common cold following a brief incubation period, usually 12 to 72 hours. Their presence and magnitude varies among patients and causative viral agents. Rhinitis, nasal stuffiness, cough, and sore throat are most common. Fever is usually slight in adults affecting less than 30% and, when present, is usually low grade. Conjunctival irritation and burning is common, but overt conjunctivitis is seen only with the pharyngoconjunctival syndrome produced by enteroviruses and adenovirus infections. In general, sore throat is present early on with nasal symptoms, but then resolves with the latter predominating on the second and third day of illness. Nasal symptoms diminish by day 4 with cough becoming most vexing over the next few days. This cough is the "bronchitis" that brings so many patients to seek care. Physical findings are meager, although patient discomfort is not. Resolution usually occurs by 1 week, but in one quarter of patients, it persists up to 14 days or more. Infections due to rhinovirus and coronavirus infections are felt to exhibit similar content and progression. No URI characteristics allow for differentiation of the viral etiologies.

TREATMENT

Treatment at present is symptomatic. No curative therapy exists and no effective vaccine is available. "Nontraditional" therapies have been studied without evidence of clear benefit, including echinacea, vitamins E and C, as well as zinc. Inhalation of heated, humidified air decreased nasal resistance, but little else. A single dose of topical or oral decongestant was found to be effective, but not repeated doses, although they were tolerated in well-controlled hypertensives. Codeine and dextromethorphan commonly are used to control cough, but their efficacy is not demonstrated. Bronchodilators are helpful only in those with airway obstruction.

Sneezing, rhinorrhea, and cough are decreased with first-generation antihistamines, but second-generation agents do not effect sneezing. Nonsteroidal anti-inflammatory drugs decrease fever, headache, other systemic complaints, and possibly cough. Used together, nasal obstruction is diminished and may obviate the need for decongestants. Cromolyn sodium, by inhalation or intranasally, brought decreased symptoms and quicker resolution. Ipratropium is also helpful.

Acute Bronchitis

The cough component of the common cold may last up to 3 weeks. Initially due to nasal obstruction and postnasal drip, it later persists from mucosal inflammation. In late stages, it is assumed to be bacterial because the previously dry cough comes to produce purulent sputum. However, no study has demonstrated benefit from antibiotics in purulent cough lasting <3 weeks. Although *Mycoplasma, Chlamydia pneumoniae*, and *Chlamydophila psittaci* infections cause bronchitis, the disease is mild, self limited, and resolves spontaneously. The Centers for Disease Control and Prevention recommends that only bronchitis due to *Bordetella pertussis* be treated with antibiotics.

Influenza

Influenza should be suspected in anyone presenting with rapid onset of fever, chills, rigors, prominent myalgias, and malaise during "flu" season, especially in the epidemiologic setting of a known outbreak. Initial dry cough and tender anterior cervical nodes accompany rhinorrhea. Neither marked pharyngeal erythema nor exudates are described with influenzal infection. The rapid antigen test now available requires 30 minutes and has excellent specificity. If positive early within the course of illness antivirals, oseltamivir or zanamivir are indicated.

Streptococcal Pharyngitis

Streptococcal pharyngitis may be a consideration early in URI, as sore and scratchy throat complaints are frequently described with initial cold symptoms. In a viral cold, sore throat is neither the only complaint nor is the pharynx remarkable for the marked erythema or exudates usually seen with streptococcal infection. In addition, other findings are present such as posterior and anterior nasal discharge. In streptococcal pharyngitis, severity varies with some cases presenting only mild symptoms and findings. This overlap makes it difficult to clinically distinguish the two entities (Table 138.1).

Group A streptococcal pharyngitis needs antibiotic treatment. Although the most common bacterial etiology of pharyngitis, it causes only 10% of adult cases. Invasive and cytopathic inflammation

TABLE 138.1 Clinical features of major causes of pharyngitis

Organism	Major associated clinical symptoms	Clinical syndrome or associated diseases
Group A streptococci (*S. pyogenes*)	Fever, tonsillar exudate, tender cervical nodes	May lead to rheumatic fever or glomerulonephritis
Rhinoviruses	Mild pharyngeal discomfort, rhinorrhea	Common cold
Influenza viruses	Fever, myalgia, headache, cough	Influenza
Epstein-Barr virus	Fever, tonsillar exudate, tender cervical nodes, palatal petechiae, atypical lymphocytosis	Infectious mononucleosis
Coxsackie virus	Fever, soft palate vesicles	Herpangina
Adenoviruses	Fever, malaise, tonsillar exudate, conjunctivitis	Pharyngoconjunctival fever
Herpes simplex virus	Soft palate vesicles	Immunosuppression
Candida albicans	White plaquelike lesions	Predisposing factors include acquired immunodeficiency virus, corticosteroids, antibiotics
Mixed anaerobes and spirochetes	Membrane, tonsillar exudate, foul odor	Vincent's angina

of the pharynx, tonsils, and surrounding lymphatics results from infection. The typical consequence is rapid onset of fever, sore throat, tender cervical adenopathy, tonsillar exudate, pharyngeal erythema, and edema. Serious complications are less common in adults but include local suppurative peritonsillar abscess and nonsuppurative rheumatic fever, both prevented by antibiotic administration (the latter if treatment is started by 9 days following onset). Decreased duration and symptoms severity also occurs. Identifying those individuals appropriate for antibiotics is therefore very important. The Centor criteria (fever, exudates, adenopathy, no cough) are felt to result in 50% antibiotic overtreatment, although they have an 80% negative predictive value when absent. Although throat cultures are highly accurate, they take 24 to 48 hours for results. Consequently, the rapid antigen test (RAT) is performed. Accuracy approaches cultures, although many authorities recommend simultaneous culture if RAT is negative.

The treatment of choice is penicillin. Oral dosing (500 mg four times daily for 10 days) is effective but presents compliance issues. Benzathine penicillin (1.2 million units intramuscularly) "guarantees" compliance and maintains bactericidal levels for 3 to 4 weeks. Amoxicillin is a suitable alternative. For those patients who are penicillin allergic, a macrolide is recommended.

Acute Sinusitis

Acute sinusitis is a frequent development, noted in 39% to 90% of colds by plain films and computed tomography imaging, respectively (many refer to the URI as "rhinosinusitis"). Blowing the nose pushes nasal secretions into the sinuses and middle ear, likely seeding them, whereas sneezing and coughing do not. Viral disease has been detected in 82% of patients, with episodes resolving by day 21 without antibiotics. Purulent nasal discharge is characteristic of sinusitis, but does not differentiate between viral and bacterial disease. Neither does computed tomography imaging. Rather, failure to improve by days 7 to 10, unilateral pain, and tenderness accompanied by maxillary "toothache" pain are suggestive of bacterial disease. This develops in 0.5% to 2.5% of colds.

Acute Otitis Media

Acute otitis media occurs with similar frequency, complicating about 2% of adult viral colds. Fluid in the middle ear is a hallmark of the illness and is best detected by pneumatic otoscopy. If fluid accompanies the presence of acute illness, otalgia, tympanic membrane erythema, and thickening, treatment is indicated, covering *Streptococcus pneumoniae, Branhamella catarrhalis,* and *Haemophilus influenzae*. The drug of initial choice is amoxicillin as the resistance of the latter two bacteria is not high enough to warrant other antibiotics.

CHAPTER 139

Sexually Transmitted Diseases

Christopher Sobczak

Sexually transmitted diseases (STDs) are a substantial health problem. This diverse collection of infections is grouped together because sexual contact is one of their major methods of transmission. Major chronic sequelae of STDs include genital and other cancers, reproductive health problems, pregnancy-related problems including transmission to offspring, and a variety of other complications related to chronic infection such as chronic liver disease, acquired immune deficiency syndrome (AIDS), and tertiary syphilis.

STDs tend to occur in younger patients, and the adolescent population from 15 to 19 years of age has higher rates of STDs than any other age group in the United States. STDs are a reportable infection to public health services. It is essential to be familiar with state regulations regarding ages of confidential treatment of STDs in adolescents, and mandatory reporting of any suspected abuse of those under the age of 18 years.

All patients diagnosed with a sexually transmitted disease warrant close follow-up. Although a test of cure is often not recommended, those with persistent symptoms should be tested again. Sexual partners should be treated and patients should abstain from sex until both the patient and their partner have completed treatment and they are both asymptomatic.

ETIOLOGY

STDs may be caused by various infectious agents, such as bacteria, viruses, and protozoa (Table 139.1). Patients who present with STDs can be classified by syndromes of presenting symptoms or signs, or by sexual practices. STDs may have different manifestations in men and women, and a significant proportion of STDs in women may not cause recognizable symptoms.

Clinicians must be aware that many STDs occur as coinfections. Up to one half of all cases of gonorrhea are associated with concurrent chlamydia infection. Any STD can increase the transmission of human immunodeficiency virus (HIV) by 2 to 9 times. Likewise, HIV can increase susceptibility to STDs. STDs should be viewed as a reflection of "high-risk" behavior, rather than a sporadic disease.

CLINICAL MANIFESTATIONS

A thorough sexual history should be obtained in all patients with STDs. The clinician should inquire about history of intercourse and sexual practices, gender preference, number of sex partners, route of penetration, and contraceptive or condom use. The review of systems in both sexes should elicit information about genital pain, discharge, dysuria, pruritus, and skin rashes, and in women a menstrual history should be obtained. Patients should be asked about prior history of STDs, in addition to history of STDs, symptoms, or high-risk behavior in sexual contacts.

TABLE 139.1 Sexually transmitted diseases

Syndrome	Common etiologies
Urethritis	*Neisseria gonorrhea, Chlamydia trachomatis, Mycoplasma genitalium, Ureaplasma urealyticum*
Vaginitis	*Neisseria gonorrhea, Chlamydia trachomatis, Trichomonas vaginalis,* anaerobic bacteria (*Gardnerella vaginalis*)
Pelvic inflammatory disease	*Neisseria gonorrhea, Chlamydia trachomatis*, polymicrobial aerobic-anaerobic bacteria
Genital ulcers	Herpes simplex virus, *Treponema pallidum, Haemophilus ducreyi, Chlamydia trachomatis* strains L1-3, *Calymmatobacterium granulomatis*
Nonulcerative genital lesions	Human papillomavirus, *Molluscum contagiosum*
Other	Human immunodeficiency virus, hepatitis B virus, *Phthirus pubis*

The genital examination should include inspection of the inguinal region and pubic hair. In men, the penis and scrotum should be examined for lesions and discharge, and the testes and epididymis should be palpated. In women, the vulva and vagina should be inspected, the presence and character of vaginal discharge should be noted, and bimanual examination should be done to search for cervical motion tenderness and adnexal mass or tenderness. In both sexes, pharyngeal or anal examination may be indicated depending on the patient's symptoms and sexual practices.

The common STD syndromes include urethritis, vaginitis, pelvic inflammatory disease (PID), genital ulcers, and nonulcerative genital lesions.

Patients with urethritis typically present with discharge and dysuria, although epidemiologic studies suggest a significant prevalence of asymptomatic infections. Examination may yield discharge, which should be sent for Gram stain to allow classification into gonococcal versus nongonococcal urethritis.

Gonorrhea is the most common cause of urethritis in men. *Neisseria gonorrhoeae* is a gram-negative diplococcus. It is a facultative intracellular bacterium that produces an endotoxin. Symptoms will manifest 2 to 5 days after exposure; women are more likely to have asymptomatic infection. Complications can occur including epididymitis, prostatitis, conjunctivitis, and disseminated disease. Disseminated gonorrhea occurs in 0.5% to 3% of those infected and includes fever, chills, arthralgias, septic joints, or skin lesions. Rarely, it may spread to the central nervous system (CNS) or cardiac system causing meningitis or endocarditis.

Common causes of nongonococcal urethritis are *Chlamydia*, *Trichomonas*, *Mycoplasma genitalium*, and *Ureaplasma urealyticum*. *Chlamydia trachomatis* is a gram-negative, obligate intracellular bacterium. Chlamydia is asymptomatic in 90% of males and up to 75% of females. As a result, the Centers for Disease Control and Prevention (CDC) recommends annual screening of sexually active adolescents and women 20 to 25 years of age. Trichomoniasis is caused by the protozoan *Trichomonas vaginalis*. Most often this is an asymptomatic infection, but men may complain of dysuria and women may have symptoms of vaginitis with a yellow malodorous discharge and vulvar irritation. *Mycoplasma genitalium* and *Ureaplasma urealyticum* infection are believed to cause urethritis because they are found more frequently or in higher numbers in patients with urethritis than in asymptomatic controls.

Vaginitis is a general vulvar or vaginal irritation that typically presents with an increase in the amount, odor, or color of vaginal discharge, irritation of the vulva, vaginal soreness, or dyspareunia.

It may be caused by gonorrhea, chlamydia, or trichomonas infection (discussed under urethritis), bacterial vaginosis, or fungal infection.

Bacterial vaginosis follows replacement of the normal vaginal *Lactobacillus* flora with anaerobes (*Peptostreptococcus*, *Peptococcus*, and *Bacteroides*). Despite a correlation with heightened sexual activity and the number of sexual partners, not all forms of bacterial vaginosis are sexually transmitted. Patients report a fetid discharge and occasionally pruritus. Dyspareunia is quite uncommon. The major diagnostic aids are the examination of the vaginal discharge for pH (>4.7) and potassium hydroxide or whiff test noting a fishy odor.

Candidal vaginitis, although frequently encountered, is not an STD. It is caused by an overgrowth of *Candida albicans* and may occur following treatment of an STD with antibiotics. Here a white thick vaginal discharge is noted. Itching is a common symptom. Commonly an underlying process such as diabetes mellitus, corticosteroid therapy, broad-spectrum antibiotic therapy, or pregnancy is readily identifiable.

Pelvic inflammatory disease is an inflammatory disorder of the upper genital tract in women and includes endometritis, salpingitis, and tubo-ovarian abscess. Approximately 1 million women or 1% of sexually active young women acquire PID annually. Causative agents are *N. gonorrhea*, *C. trachomatis*, and the anaerobic-aerobic vaginal flora. The clinical presentation may vary from subtle with mild abdominal pain to frank peritonitis. Regrettably, the clinical diagnosis is unreliable, with laparoscopy confirming the diagnosis in only two thirds of suspected cases. Minimal diagnostic criteria include lower abdominal tenderness, adnexal tenderness, or cervical motion tenderness. Additional supportive criteria include a temperature over 38.3°C, abnormal cervical or vaginal discharge, elevated sedimentation rate, and laboratory documentation of *N. gonorrhea* or *C. trachomatis*. In a small percentage of PID cases, right upper quadrant abdominal pain results from perihepatitis (known as Fitz-Hugh-Curtis syndrome).

The most classic presentation of an STD is a genital lesion. Genital lesions can be classified into ulcerative and nonulcerative lesions.

Herpes simplex virus (HSV) is the most common cause of genital ulcers in the United States. Many of these infections are asymptomatic or have nonspecific symptoms; only 20% patients with HSV have classic clinical findings. Genital herpes is caused by herpes simplex virus type I or type II. Historically type I has been associated with oral infections and type II with genital infections, but either can be sexually transmitted. Genital HSV causes over 400,000 episodes of primary infection each year in the United States. Up to 90% of these infections are with HSV type II. The risk of transmission is more likely to occur when lesions are present, but most spread of the virus is occurring in the general population with no lesions by a process of asymptomatic viral shedding or subclinical infection.

The incubation period from the time of infection to the first clinical manifestation is usually 2 to 7 days. The virus manifests as painful genital papules that progress to vesicles and ulcers. Tender inguinal lymphadenopathy is often noted on examination. Approximately 60% of women and 40% of men have constitutional symptoms including fever, headache, malaise, urinary retention, and myalgias with the first clinical episode. CNS complications include aseptic meningitis, sacral radiculopathy, and transverse myelitis. After the initial acquisition of herpes simplex virus, the virus resides indefinitely in a latent state in neuronal bodies. Recurrences of HSV may be symptomatic or asymptomatic. Symptomatic recurrences may have a prodrome of tingling or shooting pain in the genital region.

Syphilis is caused by the spirochete *Treponema pallidum*. The lesions of syphilis are clinically painless but tender with palpation. The disease is classified into primary, secondary, latent, and tertiary phases; primary and secondary syphilis affect 40,000 persons annually in the United States. The primary stage is an ulcer or chancre at the site of inoculation. The incubation period is 10 to 90 days. Without treatment the chancre can heal in 1 to 12 weeks in 60% of patients. The secondary stage begins approximately 6 weeks after the primary syphilis in untreated patients. This is the bacteremic phase when dissemination to other organs occurs. The signs and symptoms are flu-like fever, malaise, myalgias, headache, and anorexia. Secondary syphilis classically presents as a "coppery" rash on the palms and the soles. Condyloma lata can occur as a wart-like lesion associated with secondary syphilis. After the secondary phase, a latent or subclinical phase can occur; here the only evidence of infection is serologic testing. Finally, a tertiary phase can occur with progressive involvement of the CNS or cardiovascular system. It is this stage where granulomatous lesions or gumma can develop in any organ.

In contrast to syphilis, the ulcers of chancroid are painful. Chancroid is caused by *Haemophilus ducreyi*, which is a fastidious coccobacillary gram-negative bacterium. The incubation period is 4 to 7 days. An initial papule progresses to a pustule and then an ulcer within a few days. Multiple ulcers may coalesce to form a large ulcer. Inguinal lymphadenopathy, which may become fluctuant and rupture, develops in about one half of affected patients.

Lymphogranuloma venereum (LGV) may also cause suppurative lymphadenitis after an initial transient ulcer that heals without scarring. LGV is caused by *C. trachomatis* strains L1, L2, and L3. Acute infection is often associated with fever. From the primary site of infection, the organism spreads via regional lymphatics, and represents 2 to 6 weeks later with constitutional symptoms and painful adenopathy that eventually develops multiple fistulas. Late complications include persistent fistulas, lymphatic obstruction, and rectal strictures.

Donovanosis is a chronic, progressive bacterial infection caused by *Calymmatobacterium granulomatis*, which is an intracellular gram-negative encapsulated bacterium. It can occur in epidemics, but currently is rarely seen in the United States. After a usual incubation period of 1 to 4 weeks, it begins as a subcutaneous nodule that erodes through the skin to produce a painless ulcer.

The most clinically important nonulcerative genital lesions are genital warts and cervical cancer related to human papillomavirus (HPV) infection. This virus is likely the most common sexually transmitted infection, although numbers are inaccurate because most people will clear the infection spontaneously. Besides genital warts and cervical cancer, the infection may also cause oral malignancies and recurrent respiratory papillomatosis. HPV is a member of the *Papillomaviridae* family. At least 100 types of papillomaviruses infect humans and approximately 40 types infect human genitalia. High-risk types that are associated with cancer include 16, 18, 31, 33, 35, 39, 45, 51, 52, 56, 58, 59, 68, 73, and 82. It is important to note that 99% of cervical cancers contain at least one high-risk type of papillomavirus, and approximately 70% contain HPV types 16 or 18. Low-risk types not associated with cancer include types 6 and 11. After exposure to the virus, those who manifest symptoms have lesions within 6 to 12 weeks. The lesions start as small bumps or pedunculated skin-colored lesions. The lesions often progress to become large, fleshy cauliflower-like excrescences that are referred to as condylomata acuminata. The lesions are rarely painful. The diagnosis of HPV is made with clinical examination. Excision of a wart-like lesion for pathologic evaluation can be confirmatory. Identification of the virus can also be noted on Pap smears. Genotyping is done to aid in treatment and determine the aggressiveness of cervical intraepithelial malignancy.

A final common STD is pubic lice. Affected patients present with intense pruritus due to infestation with *Phthirus pubis*. This ectoparasite is a bloodsucking louse that tends to be limited to the pubic area, and is usually transmitted via sexual contact. Physical examination, sometimes aided by a magnifying loupe, reveals lice attached to the skin and lice eggs (nits) attached to the hair shafts.

Variants and different etiologies of these syndromes can be seen in patients with different host factors such as immunosuppression, different STD coinfections, and different sexual practices. In particular, anorectal infections are more prevalent in men who have sex with men.

DIAGNOSIS

Diagnostic testing should be done in all patients who present with STD symptoms or a sexual contact with a confirmed STD. Because STDs are a sign of high-risk sexual behavior and given the high rate of coinfections, many experts recommend that all patients with STD symptoms or exposure, regardless of specific suspected etiologies based on clinical syndrome, should be screened for gonorrhea, chlamydia by polymerase chain reaction (PCR) or ligase chain reaction, rapid plasma reagin (RPR), and HIV serology. In women of child-bearing potential, a pregnancy test should routinely be obtained.

Patients with urethritis, vaginitis, or PID should be tested for gonorrhea by direct culture or by nucleic acid amplification testing. DNA probes have sensitivities of 90% to 97%. In those with symptoms of disseminated infection, the culturing of blood, synovial fluid, and cerebrospinal fluid is advised. Testing for chlamydia can occur by direct culture of the cervix or urethral discharge or by nucleic acid amplification testing. The later tends to be more sensitive and specific and allows for added testing of the urine as well as cervical or urethral specimens. It is important to note that nucleic acid amplification testing measures nucleic acid, and not viable organisms; thus tests can remain positive for up to 3 weeks after effective treatment of the infection. Diagnosis of trichomoniasis is by direct visualization of the organism under the microscope or culture. Many times, *Trichomonas* will be noted on Pap smear or even found on microscopic urinalysis. In patients with PID, ultrasonography is recommended in patients who are suspected of having a tubo-ovarian abscess.

In patients with genital ulcers, HSV can be diagnosed by direct culture of a vesicle. Polymerase chain reaction assays for HSV DNA are highly sensitive, but their role in the diagnosis of genital ulcer disease is not well defined; it is the preferred test for cerebrospinal fluid analysis. Serologic testing for antibody is available, but is of little clinical value, as it cannot distinguish current, recent, or remote infection. The CDC recommends glycoprotein G tests, which have a high sensitivity to 98% and specificity to 96%. Examples of this test are the POCkit HSV2 test, HerpeSelect-1 and 2 ELISA, and HerpeSelect 1 and 2 Immunoblot.

Dark field examination allows direct visualization of the syphilis spirochetes and should be performed in patients with a chancre of primary syphilis or condylomata lata of secondary syphilis. Serologic tests include nontreponemal tests and a specific antitreponemal antibody test. The former tests are nonspecific and include the Venereal Disease Research Laboratory (VDRL) or the RPR. These tests measure immunoglobulin (Ig) M and IgG antibodies directed against a lipid antigen formed by interaction of *T. pallidum* and the host, and are used for screening or following up disease activity. A fourfold change (two dilutions) is considered significant. Because of the frequent false-positive results, a confirmatory test is usually done using treponemal tests, such as the fluorescent treponemal antibody absorption (FTAABS) or the microhemagglutination assay for antibody to *T. pallidum* (MHATP).

Diagnostic testing for other causes of genital ulcers varies with the suspected etiology. Chancroid can be diagnosed by culture, or the use of a new multiplex PCR that tests for *H. ducreyi*, *T. pallidum*, and HSV. The confirmatory tests of choice for LGV are isolation of the *C. trachomatis* LGV strain from an involved lymph node, or elevated complement fixation or immunofixation titers. Donovanosis is best diagnosed by smears or biopsies of lesions showing typical intracellular Donovan bodies within large mononuclear cells.

TREATMENT

Treatment of uncomplicated *N. gonorrhea* urethritis/cervicitis includes cefixime 400 mg orally as a single dose or ceftriaxone 125 mg intramuscularly in a single dose. Disseminated disease warrants more aggressive treatment with ceftriaxone 1 g intravenous (IV) daily for 7 days. Meningitis often requires ceftriaxone 1 gram IV twice daily for 10 to 14 days; endocarditis will require 4 weeks of the same IV regimen.

Recommended treatment for uncomplicated chlamydia urethritis/cervicitis is azithromycin 1 gram orally once or doxycycline 100 mg orally twice a day for 7 days. Alternatively, levofloxacin

500 mg once a day for 7 days or erythromycin base 500 mg orally four times a day for 7 days may be used.

Antimicrobial therapy is essential for treatment of PID. Coverage should include treatment for *N. gonorrhea* and *C. trachomatis*. Outpatient treatment includes ceftriaxone 250 mg intramuscularly and doxycycline 100 mg twice a day for 10 to 14 days. Inpatient therapy is recommended when outpatient treatment has failed, the patient is pregnant, the patient is nulligravid or an adolescent, the patient cannot tolerate oral therapy or is toxic, the patient has HIV or is immunosuppressed, or the patient has a pelvic abscess. Inpatient treatment is with cefoxitin 2 g every 6 hours IV or cefotetan 2 g every 12 hours IV, plus doxycycline 100 mg IV or orally every 12 hours. Another regimen is clindamycin 900 mg every 8 hours IV plus gentamicin IV. When an abscess is identified, consultation with a gynecologist should be sought. In patients with tubo-ovarian abscess, approximately 43% respond to IV broad-spectrum antibiotics alone. Others may require surgical drainage or removal of an infected tube or abscess.

Treatment of trichomoniasis is with 2 g of metronidazole orally once or 500 mg orally twice a day for 7 days. Success with oral treatment is 95%, but a vaginal gel can be used with a cure rate less than 50% for those who cannot tolerate the oral regimen. Studies have now shown metronidazole to be safe in pregnant women.

Bacterial vaginosis is treated with metronidazole 500 mg orally twice daily for 5 to 7 days or clindamycin vaginal cream. Candidal vaginitis is treated with nystatin or one of the topical azoles; fluconazole 150 mg orally once is also an effective treatment.

Treatment of recurrent HSV lesions can begin with the prodrome symptoms. Suppressive therapy can reduce the frequency of recurrences by 70% to 80%, and transmission to unaffected partners is cut in half. Medications used are oral acyclic nucleoside analogs (Acyclovir, Valacyclovir, Famciclovir). Because HSV infection may initially be asymptomatic, a symptomatic episode does not necessarily mean that the patient's current partner is not monogamous. The diagnosis of genital herpes is emotionally devastating and the fear of transmission can affect sexual functioning. Management includes counseling that genital ulcer disease increases the risk of transmission of HSV. Acyclovir-resistant HSV has been seen among immunosuppressed persons and should be suspected when a response is lacking, especially to intravenous therapy; intravenous Foscarnet is then indicated.

Penicillin remains the drug of choice for all stages of syphilis. The treatment for each stage is best outlined in Table 139.2. Penicillin-allergic patients should be desensitized.

The CDC recommends treating chancroid with a single 1 g oral dose of azithromycin; antimicrobial susceptibility should be checked in patients who do not rapidly respond to treatment. LGV is

TABLE 139.2 Treatment of primary, secondary, and latent syphilis

Stage	Treatment regimen	Comments
Primary, secondary, and early latent	Benzathine penicillin 2.4 MU intramuscularly	If penicillin allergic, doxycycline 100 mg orally twice daily for 14 days for all stages; desensitize for syphilis complicating pregnancy
Late latent or unknown duration; tertiary syphilis (excluding neurosyphilis)	As above, except benzathine penicillin weekly for 3 weeks or doxycycline 100 mg orally twice daily for 28 days	

treated with a 3-week course of doxycycline 100 mg orally twice daily. Donovanosis is treated with doxycycline, azithromycin, or Bactrim, continued until lesions have healed (typically 3 to 5 weeks).

Curative therapy is not available for HPV. Warts respond to topical podofilox 0.5% solution or gel applied to the visible warts twice daily for 3 days followed by 4 days of no therapy. The provider can also treat warts with cryotherapy every 2 weeks until gone, surgical resection, or trichloroacetic acid 85% applied to the wart and allowed to dry with washing off after 6 hours. The latest research has involved prevention. HPV vaccines have been developed to elicit a cell-mediated cytotoxic T-cell response, leading to elimination of cells expressing nonstructural viral proteins. Studies of HPV vaccines have shown that they are well tolerated, highly immunogenic, and prevent both acquisition of HPV infection and HPV-related disease.

Women's Health Issues

CHAPTER 140

Menstrual Concerns and Menopause

Julie Mitchell and Jennifer Zebrack

The menstrual cycle starts and ends with the first day of menstrual bleeding, and a normal cycle length is between 21 to 35 days (average 28 days). The normal duration of bleeding is 2 to 6 days (average 4 days), and is typically accompanied by some menstrual cramping. Figure 140.1 graphs the levels of pituitary and ovarian hormones along with ovarian and endometrial activity by the day of the menstrual cycle, where the ovary is illustrated as first recruiting follicles and developing a dominant follicle (follicular phase), then ovulating, and finally housing the corpus luteum, which is the remnant of the follicle after ovulation (luteal phase).

The relevant pituitary hormones are follicle-stimulating hormone (FSH) and luteinizing hormone (LH); they are stimulated by the hypothalamic hormone GnRH. FSH develops the ovarian follicles, whereas LH induces ovulation. The ovarian follicle makes 17-β estradiol, which primes the uterus for progesterone action and thins the cervical mucus. The corpus luteum induces endometrial secretory activity, proliferates the endometrium, thickens the cervical mucus, and increases basal body temperature.

From menarche (first menstrual period) to menopause (cessation of menses), most women have regular, monthly menstrual cycles. The average age of menarche is 11 years (range 10 to 15 years). Menopause is a natural process, where the ovaries cease to produce estrogen and progesterone despite increased pituitary stimulation. The age of menopause is defined as 12 months without menses, and the average age is 51 years (range 43 to 56 years). The time preceding and including frank menopause is termed the perimenopause. Postmenopause is the time after the menopause.

Common menstrual concerns are defined in Table 140.1. Primary amenorrhea is the absence of menarche in women age 16 years or older. Secondary amenorrhea is the absence of 3 months of menses in women with previously regular cycles. Abnormal uterine bleeding includes heavy, frequent, or irregular bleeding; postcoital bleeding (bleeding after sexual intercourse); and intermenstrual bleeding (bleeding between menses).

Uterine cramping is part of the normal process of menses, but it can often be severe (primary dysmenorrhea). Typically, the pain is colicky or crampy, felt in the pelvis or low abdomen, begins with menses, and lasts 1 to 3 days. Premenstrual syndrome (PMS) is a symptom complex including dysmenorrhea, malaise, and fatigue.

ETIOLOGY

Amenorrhea and Oligomenorrhea

Pregnancy (in the younger woman) and menopause (in the older woman) are the most common causes of amenorrhea. The differential diagnosis of amenorrhea or oligomenorrhea not related to pregnancy is classified by ovarian and pituitary hormone levels.

LOW GONADOTROPINS AND LOW ESTROGEN (HYPOTHALAMIC HYPOGONADISM)

The most common cause is psychosocial stress, followed closely by low body weight, particularly in competitive athletes or in women with eating disorders. High prolactin, which inhibits GnRH release,

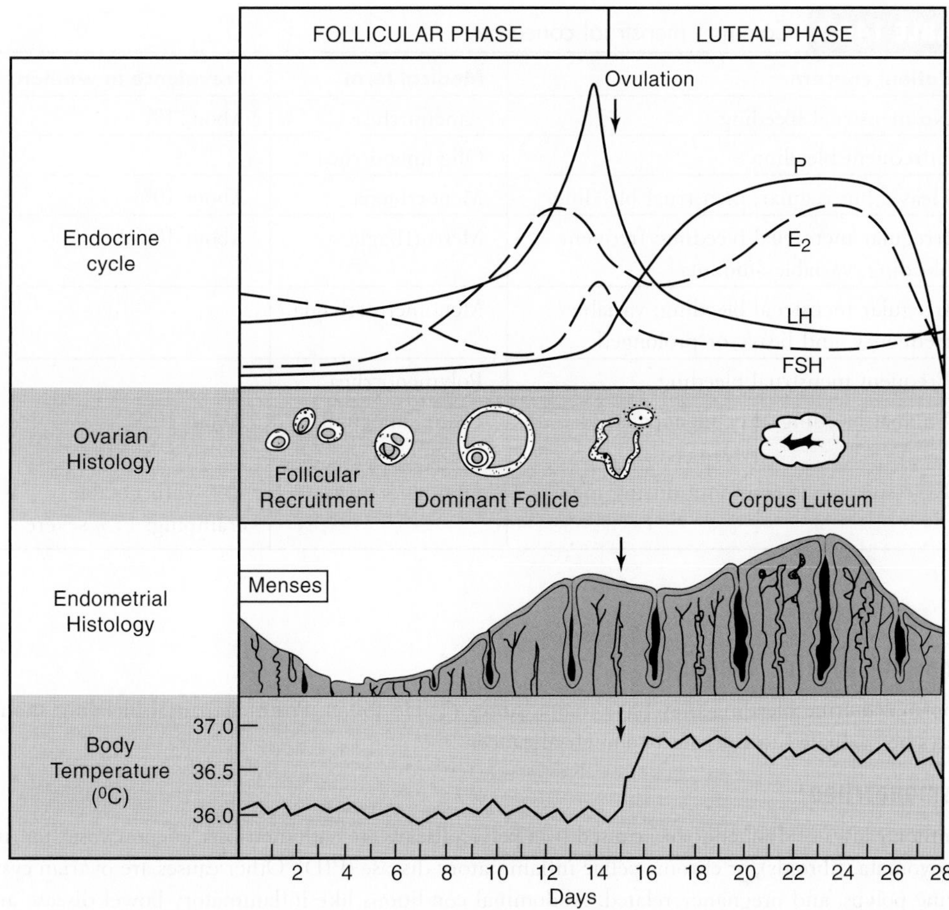

Figure 140.1 • Normal menstrual cycle: hormonal, ovarian, and endometrial activities according to the day of cycle. E2, estrogen; FSH, follicle stimulating hormone, LH, luteinizing hormone; P, progesterone.

is the cause of 15% of amenorrhea cases (Chapter 67). Tumors, infections, or sarcoidosis in or around the hypothalamus or pituitary also can disrupt gonadotropin production. The most common tumor is a pituitary adenoma.

HIGH GONADOTROPINS AND LOW ESTROGEN (HYPERGONADOTROPIC HYPOGONADISM)

The most common cause is gonadal dysgenesis or Turner's syndrome. Turner's syndrome is a condition caused by a defect or absence of one of the two X chromosomes and occurs in about 1 in 2,000 female births. Typical characteristics are short stature, webbing of the neck, low-set ears with low posterior hairline, and underdeveloped secondary sexual characteristics. Less frequent causes are ovarian enzymatic deficiencies and premature ovarian failure (early menopause).

NORMAL OR NEAR-NORMAL ESTROGEN

Causes include polycystic ovary syndrome (Chapter 141), adult-onset congenital adrenal hyperplasia, Cushing's syndrome, and hypothyroidism or hyperthyroidism. Primary amenorrhea may occur with congenital anatomic abnormalities of the reproductive tract.

TABLE 140.1 Common menstrual concerns

Patient concern	Medical term	Prevalence in women
No menstrual bleeding	Amenorrhea	About 1%
Infrequent bleeding	Oligomenorrhea	
Heavy, but regular, menstrual bleeding	Menorrhagia	About 10%
Irregular menstrual bleeding: frequent bleeding, variable amounts	Metrorrhagia	About 10%
Irregular menstrual bleeding: variable frequency, and heavy or prolonged	Menometrorrhagia	
Frequent menstrual bleeding	Polymenorrhea	
Vaginal bleeding after menopause	Postmenopausal bleeding	About 10%
Excessive pelvic cramping during menses	Dysmenorrhea	75% with notable cramping; 15% severe

Abnormal Uterine Bleeding

Abnormal uterine bleeding may have many causes (Table 140.2). Postmenopausal bleeding should always be evaluated to rule out endometrial cancer.

Dysmenorrhea

Common causes of dysmenorrhea caused by a pelvic disease are endometriosis, adenomyosis, uterine leiomyomata (fibroids), or chronic pelvic inflammatory disease (PID). Other causes are ovarian cysts, uterine polyps, and pregnancy related. Abdominal conditions like inflammatory bowel disease and irritable bowel syndrome can also mimic dysmenorrhea.

CLINICAL MANIFESTATIONS

Menstrual Concerns

Careful questioning about the patient's bleeding pattern is essential. First, be sure any abnormal bleeding is vaginal in origin (i.e., not rectal or urethral). Ask the patient to diary the bleeding. Ask about how frequently a pad or tampon is changed (normal is more than every 3 hours, although this varies to some degree with patient's preferences), how many pads or tampons are used in the cycle (normal is less than 21), and whether pads or tampons are changed at night (rare is normal).

The history should include sexual activity and contraceptive use, risk factors for sexually transmitted infections, psychosocial stress, domestic violence, weight loss and exercise, vasomotor symptoms (hot flashes), headaches, fever, visual field changes, galactorrhea, bowel patterns, symptoms of thyroid disorders, medical conditions, and medications. Anovulation may be suspected if the patient does not have typical ovulatory cycle symptoms of breast tenderness, changing cervical mucus, and uterine cramping. If uterine cramping is prominent, characterize the pattern and severity. Ask about features of endometriosis: severe chronic pelvic pain with regular menstrual cycles, dyspareunia, and infertility.

Important elements of the physical examination are the body habitus, skin (looking for striae of Cushing's, hirsutism, and acne), visual fields, thyroid, and breasts (Tanner staging and milky discharge). The pelvic examination should include particular attention to the vulva and vagina for

TABLE 140.2 Causes of abnormal uterine bleeding

Category	Examples	Epidemiology comment
Pregnancy or its complications	Normal pregnancy, threatened abortion, ectopic pregnancy	
Vulvar, vaginal, or cervical abnormality	Infection, polyp, cancer, skin lesions	Cervical cancer rate: 5/100,000 women-years
Uterine abnormality	Fibroids, infection, polyp, hyperplasia, cancer	Uterine cancer incidence: 20/100,000 women-years (when aged 40–50 years); 75/100,000 women-years (when aged 50–60 years)
Anovulation (often called dysfunctional uterine bleeding)	Perimenarchal and perimenopausal bleeding, polycystic ovarian syndrome, congenital adrenal hyperplasia, estrogen-secreting tumor	Outside of pregnancy, anovulation is the most common cause of abnormal bleeding
Bleeding diathesis	Von Willebrand's disease, platelet dysfunction, anticoagulants	Bleeding diathesis is cause of abnormal bleeding in about 20% of cases in adolescents
Metabolic or systemic problem	Thyroid, adrenal, hepatic, or renal disease	Thyroid disorders are cause of abnormal bleeding in 1%–2% of cases
Medication	Phenytoin, digoxin, exogenous estrogen or progesterone, steroids, antipsychotics	
Injury	Domestic violence	Prevalence of current or past domestic violence is about 25% of women in internal medicine clinics

signs of trauma, vaginal atrophy or loss of rugae, vaginal discharge, and congenital anomalies, the size and shape of the uterus, and the presence of any adnexal masses or tenderness.

Menopause

Perimenopausal women typically have variable cycles and vasomotor symptoms, such as episodic, transient, and intense hot flushing ("hot flashes") and night sweats. Vasomotor symptoms occur in 75% to 90% of perimenopausal women and about 10% to 25% will continue to have vasomotor symptoms well past the menopause. In postmenopausal women, clinicians should carefully and sensitively ask about symptoms of vaginal and vulvar atrophy such as vaginal irritation or discharge, vaginal dryness, and dyspareunia because they may not be voluntarily reported; there are effective therapies. Physical examination may reveal thin mucosa of the vulva, the vagina may lack rugae, and the vaginal discharge may be scant and possibly serosanguineous (atrophic vaginitis).

DIAGNOSIS

Menstrual Concerns

In general, it is good practice to order a pregnancy test in all cases of amenorrhea or abnormal uterine bleeding. In women with amenorrhea or oligomenorrhea, thyroid and prolactin abnormalities are also common enough to warrant universal thyroid-stimulating hormone and prolactin testing, and 17-β estradiol, FSH, and LH will help define whether the problem is due to low ovarian hormones, low stimulating hormones, or both. A progesterone challenge test determines whether there is adequate circulating estrogen, functional endometrial lining, and integrity to the cervix-vaginal outflow tract.

In women with abnormal uterine bleeding, check for anemia, test for gonorrhea and chlamydia, and do a Pap test. Additional tests include evaluation for bleeding diathesis with prothrombin time, partial thromboplastin time, or possibly factor VIII or von Willebrand factor antigen (especially if adolescent or with family history), endometrial biopsy (especially in women older than 35 years, who are obese, or with a history of prescription estrogens without progesterone), or pelvic ultrasound (if uterine abnormalities are suspected). Endometrial biopsy is necessary in postmenopausal women. Anovulation is the likely diagnosis once other causes are excluded.

In patients with dysmenorrhea, pelvic ultrasound can diagnose fibroids, uterine polyps, and ovarian cysts. Cervical swabs for gonorrhea and chlamydia can rule out PID. If endometriosis is suspected, laparoscopy is often required for the diagnosis. As primary dysmenorrhea is common, it is often reasonable to empirically treat, and then to suspect a benign cause if treatment is effective.

Menopause

Diagnosis of menopause is clinical; it is based on the absence of menses or altered menstrual cycles and the presence of vasomotor symptoms. A high FSH level (e.g., more than 30 to 40 mIU/mL) can confirm the diagnosis or suggest it in women on oral contraceptives (who will generally continue menstrual cycles despite the end of ovarian hormone production).

TREATMENT

Menstrual Concerns

The treatment of amenorrhea depends on the diagnosis and on patient goals. Influential patient factors include desire for fertility or contraception, potential risks of long-term estrogen deprivation (such as osteoporosis) or estrogen without progesterone (such as endometrial cancer with unopposed estrogen), and satisfaction with feminine appearance.

The treatment of abnormal uterine bleeding is also based on the cause. Oral contraceptives are the treatment of choice in chronic anovulation.

The treatment for primary dysmenorrhea is nonsteroidal anti-inflammatory drugs and oral contraceptives. Women who do not respond should be referred for endometriosis evaluation.

Menopause

The best treatment for the vasomotor symptoms of menopause is hormone therapy. Women without a uterus (i.e., after hysterectomy) can be given estrogen-alone, but women with a uterus require estrogen and progesterone because unopposed estrogen confers a high risk of endometrial cancer.

TABLE 140.3 Risks and adverse effects of menopausal hormone therapy

Absolute contraindications	Relative contraindications	Risks of estrogen	Risks of estrogen-progestin	Adverse effects
Pregnancy or undiagnosed bleeding	Strong family history of breast cancer, VTE, or CHD	Stroke	Estrogen risks plus CHD	Vaginal bleeding (common in first 6 months of therapy)
Personal history of breast or endometrial cancer	Provoked VTE	Dementia	Breast cancer	Breast tenderness
Unprovoked VTE, CHD	Hypertriglyceridemia Gallstones	DVT		

CHD, coronary heart disease; DVT, deep vein thrombosis; VTE, venous thromboembolism.

Initiation of hormone therapy should be done only after reviewing risks with the patient (Table 140.3). Hormone therapy can be prescribed as pills or patches, and cyclically, continuously, or with a combination product.

Alternatives to hormone therapy should be considered in women with a contraindication, intolerance, or reluctance to accept the risks. Alternatives include antidepressants such as venlafaxine, paroxetine, fluoxetine, and gabapentin. Herbal supplements do not have established efficacy, but are generally safe and may be tried.

CHAPTER 141

Polycystic Ovary Syndrome and Hirsutism

Jennifer Zebrack and Julie Mitchell

POLYCYSTIC OVARY SYNDROME

Polycystic ovary syndrome (PCOS), also known as Stein-Leventhal syndrome, is a disorder characterized by chronic anovulation and hyperandrogenism. It is one of the most common hormonal disorders in women and affects approximately 5% to 10% of reproductive age women. More than 90% of adult women presenting with clinical androgen excess have PCOS.

Etiology

The exact cause of PCOS is unclear. Studies have found more frequent surges of gonadotropin-releasing hormone (GnRH) and luteinizing hormone (LH), resulting in increased androgen production by the ovary and anovulatory cycles. Emerging evidence suggests that insulin resistance plays a central role in the pathophysiology of PCOS. Genetic factors may also be relevant since PCOS is more common in women with a family history.

Clinical Manifestations

Women with PCOS may exhibit some or all of the following symptoms: amenorrhea or oligomenorrhea (<9 menses per year), hirsutism, infertility, and obesity. However, approximately 50% of women with PCOS are not obese. PCOS is associated with the metabolic syndrome. Insulin resistance is common and an important marker of cardiovascular risk in patients with PCOS. Among women with PCOS, 40% have impaired glucose tolerance and 10% have type 2 diabetes. PCOS is also associated with lipid abnormalities, hypertension, and sleep apnea. Women with PCOS have a higher risk for endometrial hyperplasia and endometrial cancer, likely due to chronic estrogen stimulation of the uterus.

History should include attention to menstrual history, obstetric history, and family history of PCOS, diabetes, and cardiovascular disease. The blood pressure and body mass index (BMI) should be noted. Physicians should consider evaluating women with PCOS for lipid disorders, impaired glucose tolerance, and diabetes. Physical examination may reveal signs of androgen excess (i.e., acne, seborrhea, hirsutism, male pattern alopecia, and central or abdominal obesity) and insulin resistance (e.g., acanthosis nigricans: a diffuse, velvety, dark brown or black skin pigmentation chiefly on the back of the neck, axillae, and other body folds). Pelvic examination may reveal enlarged cystic ovaries. Patients with signs of excess androgens should also be examined for virilization, defined as a decrease in feminine secondary sexual characteristics (i.e., breast and vaginal mucosal atrophy), and an increase in masculine secondary sexual characteristics (i.e., hirsutism, deepening voice, temporal balding, increased muscle mass, clitoromegaly), which would alert one to a possible androgen-secreting tumor rather than PCOS.

Diagnosis

Because PCOS is a heterogeneous disorder with variable presentations, it is often difficult to diagnose. Women with PCOS may not exhibit all of the classic signs and symptoms, but the majority present to their physician because of menstrual concerns or infertility. Most experts agree that the diagnosis can be made after excluding other medical causes of androgen excess and/or irregular menses and at least two of three criteria are present: amenorrhea or oligomenorrhea (<9 menses per year), hyperandrogenism (clinical signs of elevated androgens) or hyperandrogenemia (elevated androgen levels), and polycystic ovaries by ultrasound. Despite the name, cystic ovaries are not essential for diagnosis, and, in fact, 25% of women with PCOS have normal-appearing ovaries. Conversely, women with cystic ovaries may not have PCOS. Transvaginal ultrasound is not always necessary but may be performed if there is diagnostic uncertainly or a concern for endometrial hyperplasia.

Other endocrine disorders need to be excluded when PCOS is suspected. An evaluation for the following disorders should be considered based on the patient's clinical presentation: Cushing's syndrome, hypothyroidism, hyperprolactinemia, premature ovarian failure, congenital adrenal hyperplasia (partial 21-hydroxylase deficiency), acromegaly, and virilizing adrenal or ovarian neoplasm. Therefore, exclusionary labs may include 24-hr urinary free cortisol, thyroid-stimulating hormone, prolactin, FSH, 17-hydroxyprogesterone, insulin-like growth factor 1, DHEA-S, and free and total testosterone, respectively. Androgen levels typically are extremely elevated in virilizing neoplasms. Although PCOS patients may have an abnormally high LH-to-FSH ratio of 2 or greater, this test lacks sensitivity and specificity for the diagnosis. If amenorrhea is present, a pregnancy test should be performed. Women who have not had a menses for 12 months should be referred for endometrial biopsy.

Treatment

The core treatment of PCOS should involve interventions to improve insulin sensitivity, which will likely result in lowered circulating androgens, improved metabolic profile, and a return to ovulatory cycles. These interventions include lifestyle modifications such as weight reduction, diet, and exercise. Insulin-sensitizing agents such as metformin and thiazolidinediones or spironolactone for its antiandrogen properties are sometimes used. If the patient is interested in becoming pregnant and initial interventions, such as weight loss and/or metformin, are unsuccessful, stimulation of the ovaries with fertility agents such as clomiphene may be necessary. If pregnancy is not currently desired, additional treatment with an estrogen-progestin combination oral contraceptive protects the endometrium from unopposed estrogen and decreases androgen production. Selection of a nonandrogenic progestin is preferred (e.g., drospirenone, norgestimate, desogestrel).

HIRSUTISM

Hirsutism is excessive terminal body hair in women growing in a masculine pattern. There are two types of hair: vellus and terminal. Vellus hair is fine, soft, generally unpigmented hair that is not androgen-stimulated and is found diffusely over the body. Terminal hair is coarse, pigmented, androgen-dependent, and normally localized to the back, face, chest, abdomen, axilla, and pubic area. Hirsutism should be distinguished from hypertrichosis, which is an androgen-independent, generalized increase in growth of vellus-type hair. Hypertrichosis may be hereditary or a result of starvation (e.g., anorexia nervosa) or drugs (e.g., phenytoin, minoxidil, glucocorticoids, cyclosporine). Approximately 5% of reproductive-age women have hirsutism.

Etiology

Hirsutism typically is due to excessive adrenal or ovarian androgen production or to increased hair follicle sensitivity to androgen. Most cases of hirsutism are due to PCOS or are idiopathic. Other infrequent causes include congenital adrenal hyperplasia, Cushing's syndrome, hyperprolactinemia, acromegaly, thyroid disorders, androgen-secreting ovarian or adrenal tumors, and androgenic-medications.

Clinical Manifestations

History and physical examination should focus on onset, rate of progression, and distribution of hirsutism. Abrupt onset or rapidly progressive hirsutism suggests a serious disease. Medications should be reviewed for use of androgenic drugs; it is important to inquire about anabolic steroid use, especially in athletes. History should also include the elements listed above under clinical manifestations of PCOS. Abdominal and pelvic examination should be performed to evaluate for masses and clitoromegaly.

Diagnosis

The primary goal in the diagnostic evaluation is to exclude a serious underlying cause. Laboratory evaluation is typically not necessary in a woman with mild hirsutism, regular menses, and no other characteristics to suggest a secondary cause, all of which would suggest idiopathic hirsutism. If moderate or severe hirsutism is present or there are signs of virilization or a secondary cause, androgen levels are indicated. Adrenal tumors primarily produce DHEA and DHEA-S; ovarian tumors primarily produce testosterone. A serum testosterone level above 200 ng/mL usually suggests a virilizing ovarian tumor. If the DHEA-S level is more than twice normal, a virilizing adrenal tumor is suspected. Features of other endocrinologic disorders (i.e., congenital adrenal hyperplasia, Cushing's syndrome, hyperprolactinemia, acromegaly, thyroid disorders) should be worked up accordingly.

TREATMENT

Therapy for idiopathic hirsutism is primarily cosmetic, with medical therapy sometimes used as an adjunct. Cosmetic therapies include shaving, bleaching, electrolysis, and laser hair removal. Topical eflornithine hydrochloride cream (Vaniqa), a cell-cycle inhibitor, can be tried but is contraindicated in pregnancy. Spironolactone is the antiandrogen drug of choice for treating moderate to severe hirsutism. Spironolactone is contraindicated in pregnancy and usually used in conjunction with an oral contraceptive. Oral contraceptives with nonadrogenic progestins (e.g., drospirenone, norgestimate, desogestrel) will not reverse hirsutism but may prevent progression. It usually takes at least 6 months to evaluate the efficacy of any given oral agent. Lifelong therapy usually is required to prevent recurrence.

CHAPTER 142

Contraception

Jennifer Zebrack and Julie Mitchell

The most widely used contraceptive method is combination estrogen-progestin oral contraceptives (OCs), although several other alternatives are available and may be preferred based on a woman's preferences and medical history.

ETIOLOGY

Most unplanned pregnancies are caused by contraceptive failure due to improper use. Physicians can help women choose the method they are most likely to use consistently and correctly.

CLINICAL MANIFESTATIONS

Taking a contraceptive history is essential for all premenopausal women, especially those at risk for an unwanted pregnancy. History should assess a woman's current contraceptive method, reproductive plans, previous contraceptive experiences, preferences, cost limitations, and religious and cultural beliefs.

DIAGNOSIS

Ask about menstrual history, sexual activity, and contraceptive use to determine risk of current pregnancy; pregnancy testing may be necessary. A pelvic examination can be done to screen for cervical cancer and test for sexually transmitted infections (STIs). However, to optimize access to contraception, a pelvic examination and STI screening should not be required prior to providing contraception.

TREATMENT

A variety of contraceptive options are available. Table 142.1 compares contraceptive products and methods. All hormonal contraceptive formulations contain a progestin, which typically works by inhibiting peak luteinizing hormone (LH) release and thus ovulation. Progestin also thickens cervical mucus, thins the endometrium, and decreases fallopian tube motility. Many hormonal contraceptives also contain estrogen, which inhibits ovulation by inhibiting FSH, thus decreasing follicle development. Cyclic estrogen allows for predictable menstrual bleeding.

The most commonly prescribed contraceptive is the combination OC, which contains both estrogen (30 to 35 μg ethinyl estradiol: low dose) and progestin, and is typically given for 3 weeks

TABLE 142.1 Contraceptive options

Product	Advantages compared to low-dose OC	Disadvantages compared to low-dose OC	Comments
Estrogen-progestin products			
OC with 30–35 μg ethinyl estradiol (low dose)	—	—	Most common OC
OC with 20–25 μg ethinyl estradiol (ultra-low dose; e.g., Loestrin, Alesse)	May reduce side effects (i.e., nausea, breast tenderness)	Slightly less effective than low-dose pills Breakthrough bleeding more common	Often used during the menopausal transition or in women with side effects on low-dose pills Less preferred option in obese women
OC extended 91-day regimen (Seasonale, Seasonique)	4 menses per year 84 days of active pills then 1 week of placebo for menses (Seasonale) or 1 week 10 μg ethinyl estradiol (Seasonique)	Breakthrough bleeding more common	Consider in PMS, dysmenorrhea, menorrhagia, anemia, menstrual migraines
OC with the progestin drospirenone (a spironolactone-analogue; e.g., Yasmin, Yaz)	May further improve acne and limit progression of hirsutism Decreases fluid retention	Possible hyperkalemia	Contraindications: renal and adrenal insufficiency; caution with angiotensin-converting enzyme inhibitors and other potassium-sparing diuretics
Transdermal patch (Ortho Evra)	May improve compliance (1 patch per week for 3 weeks, then remove for menses)	60% higher total estrogen exposure than low-dose OC	Uncertainty about possible risks related to higher estrogen levels Less preferred option in obese women
Vaginal ring (Nuvaring)	Lowest dose of estrogen available; fewer side effects May improve compliance (self-insert, wear continuously for 3 weeks, remove for menses)	Rare expulsion <5% May be noticed during intercourse	One size fits all, no need to be fitted Contraindicated with cystocele and uterine prolapse

Injectable (Lunelle)	Monthly injection Highly effective (0.3% failure rate)	More irregular bleeding Weight gain (4 lb at 1 year, 6 lb at 2 years of use) Delayed return to fertility	Need medical personnel for injection Monthly withdrawal bleed occurs
Progestin-only products			
Injectable Medroxyprogesterone acetate (DMPA; Depo-Provera)	Injection every 3 months Highly effective (0.3% failure rate) One of the least expensive methods	Irregular bleeding Weight gain (5 lb at 1 year, 8 lb at 2 years, 14 lb at 4 years) Decreases bone mineral density Delayed return to fertility, up to 2 years May cause or worsen depression	Need medical personnel for injection Ensure adequate calcium/vitamin D intake; consider bone mineral density testing, especially if prolonged use (>2 years) 50% of users are amenorrheic at 1 year
Progestin-only OC or "mini-pill" (i.e., norethindrone or norgestrel)	Rapidly reversible	Less effective (5%–13% failure rate) More breakthrough bleeding Must be taken at same time daily for best effectiveness	Best suited for women who already have reduced fertility (i.e., older women and lactating women) No placebo week; must take all pills in the pack
Intrauterine system (secretes the progestin levonorgestrel; Mirena)	FDA approved for up to 5 years of use Highly effective (0.1% failure rate) Rapidly reversible Reduction in dysmenorrhea and menorrhagia	Requires trained physician for insertion Initial cramping and irregular bleeding, but less than copper intrauterine device	Contraindications: at risk for STI, HIV infection, pregnancy Caution: nulliparity 20%–50% amenorrheic at 1 year

(*continued*)

TABLE 142.1 Contraceptive options (*continued*)

Product	Advantages compared to low-dose OC	Disadvantages compared to low-dose OC	Comments
Subdermal implant (Implanon)	FDA approved for up to 3 years of use <1% failure rate	Requires trained physician for insertion Irregular bleeding Weight gain (3 lb at 1 year)	Faster return to fertility than DMPA
Nonhormonal products			
Intrauterine device (Copper T 380A)	FDA approved for up to 10 years of use Highly effective (0.8% failure rate) Rapidly reversible	Requires trained physician for insertion Cramping and irregular bleeding, especially first 6 months	Contraindications: at risk for STI, HIV infection, pregnancy Caution: nulliparity
Diaphragm	Spontaneous use	Failure rate 12% to 20%	Must be fitted Used with spermicide
Cervical cap	Spontaneous use	Failure rate 20%; less effective in parous women	Must be fitted Used with spermicide
Sponge	Spontaneous use	Failure rate 15% to 30% Less effective in parous women	Available OTC Contains spermicide
Male and female condoms	Spontaneous use Best protection from STIs and cervical cancer (i.e., HPV)	Male condom: 10% to 20% failure rate Female condom: 20% failure rate	Available OTC More effective if used with spermicide
Spermicide	Variety of forms (foam, cream, jelly, film, suppository)	Failure rate 20% to 50% when used alone	Available OTC
Surgical sterilization			
Tubal ligation	Highly effective (0.5% failure rate)	Permanent method	May not be reversible
Vasectomy	Highly effective (0.1% failure rate)	Permanent method	May not be reversible

HPV, human papillomavirus; OC, oral contraceptive; OTC, over-the-counter; PMS, premenstrual syndrome; STI, sexually transmitted infection.

TABLE 142.2 Contraindications to combination estrogen-progestin oral contraceptives and other estrogen-containing contraceptives

History of thrombophlebitis or thromboembolic disease, or known thrombophilia
History of stroke or coronary artery disease
Smoker >35 years of age
Uncontrolled blood pressure
Diabetes, if associated with vascular disease or end-organ damage
Complex migraines with focal symptoms
History of, current, or suspected breast cancer
History of or current endometrial cancer
Undiagnosed abnormal vaginal bleeding
Liver tumors or liver failure
Known or suspected pregnancy
Breastfeeding

followed by placebo (or no pills) for 1 week to stimulate withdrawal bleeding. A progestin is combined with the estrogen in a monophasic (same daily dose) or biphasic or triphasic pattern (varying doses to mimic more closely the normal menstrual cycle). There is clinically little difference between monophasic and multiphasic formulations. The failure rate is 3% to 8% at 1 year for typical use but less than 1% for perfect use.

The benefits of combination OCs include improvement in dysmenorrhea (painful menses) and menorrhagia (heavy menses); OCs are often prescribed for these reasons. The risk for pelvic inflammatory disease is also decreased, probably due to the inhibition of organism ascension through thickened cervical mucus. Combination OC use is associated with a reduction in benign breast disease and helps prevent osteoporosis. Most combination OCs improve acne. Combination OCs can also limit the progression of hirsutism if less androgenic progestins—such as norgestimate, desogestrel, and drospirenone—are used. Combination OCs reduce the risk for ovarian cancer (50% risk reduction with 5 years of use) and endometrial cancer.

Postcoital emergency contraception (EC or Plan B; the progestin levonorgestrel) should be offered to women who experienced a contraceptive failure, used no method during intercourse, or were victims of a sexual assault. EC inhibits pregnancy by preimplantation effects (delays ovulation and interferes with sperm function and fertilization). EC can be taken up to 5 days after unprotected intercourse but is most effective (up to 80%) if taken within 72 hours.

The most frequent reason for stopping combination OCs is side effects, and the 1-year continuation rate is only 50%. Therefore, new users should be counseled to call before stopping their OC and seen or contacted in follow-up to assess tolerability. Common side effects of combination OCs include nausea, breast tenderness, fluid retention, spotting, and increased blood pressure. Blood pressure should be checked before prescribing and followed periodically thereafter. Several medications, including antibiotics, antiseizure medications, and herbal products, can decrease the effectiveness of OCs, and women should be counseled to use back-up contraception (e.g., condoms) when using these medications.

The most serious adverse effect associated with combination OCs is the prothrombotic effect associated with the estrogen component; estrogen-containing contraceptive agents are contraindicated in some women (Table 142.2). Whether combination OCs increase the risk for breast cancer is an area of uncertainty, but they are generally contraindicated in women with a history of breast cancer.

Geriatrics

CHAPTER 143

Falls

Marcos Montagnini

Falls are events in which an individual inadvertently comes to rest on the ground or a lower level in the absence of an overwhelming force, syncope, or stroke. Falls cause significant morbidity and mortality in older adults. The incidence of falls increases with age and varies according to living situation, affecting 30% to 40% of community-dwelling older adults and approximately 50% of nursing-home residents. Falls are indicators of poor functional status and are a contributing factor to long-term care placement.

ETIOLOGY

Falls in older adults are often multifactorial and caused by changes in balance and gait, cognitive impairment, medications, acute and chronic medical conditions, and environmental factors (Table 143.1). Several age-related changes in vision (reductions in visual acuity, depth perception, contrast sensitivity), vestibular function (loss of labyrinthine hair cells, vestibular ganglion cells, and nerve fibers), and proprioception (loss of proprioceptive sensitivity) increase fall risk in older adults.

Orthostatic hypotension is a common cause of falls in older adults. It is caused by the combined effects of venous pooling, relative hypovolemia, and probably some degree of lowered sensitivity of the baroreceptor system. Several drugs (sedatives, antihypertensives, vasodilators, and antidepressants) and disorders (e.g., autonomic dysfunction, hypovolemia, low cardiac output) contribute to orthostatic hypotension.

CLINICAL MANIFESTATIONS

Elderly patients should be screened for falls at least once a year. Patients who experience two or more falls within 12 months (recurrent fallers), those who present for medical attention due to fall, and patients who demonstrate gait and/or balance disorder should undergo a complete fall assessment. The elements of the fall assessment include a thorough history, physical examination, diagnostic testing, and identification of possible environmental factors that may have contributed to the fall.

Important components of the history include the circumstances of a fall: where and when the fall occurred and the activity of the faller at the time of the incident. Information on footwear and environmental factors such as lighting, floor covering, door thresholds, railings, and furniture may add important clues. Information on previous falls should also be collected. The presence of premonitory symptoms such as dizziness, unsteadiness, palpitations, and lightheadedness should be determined; loss of consciousness prior to the fall leads to a syncope workup rather than a fall workup.

It is important to review patient's past medical and surgical history to identify chronic diseases that are associated with an increased fall risk. A complete medication history—with particular attention to vasodilators, diuretics, and sedative hypnotic drugs—is critical. Questions about dizziness,

TABLE 143.1 Common risk factors of falls in older adults

Common risk factors of falls in older adults
Age-related physiologic changes in gait and balance
Acute medical conditions
Delirium
Arrhythmia
Sepsis/infection
Seizures
Hypoglycemia
Dehydration
Bleeding
Transient ischemic attack
Chronic medical conditions
Arthritis
Orthostatic hypotension
Anemia
Diabetes mellitus
Drugs
Benzodiazepines
Phenothiazine
Tricyclic antidepressants
Opioids
Diuretics
Antihypertensives
Neurologic disorders
Peripheral neuropathy
Vestibular dysfunction
Parkinson's disease
Hemiparesis
Dementia
Myelopathy
Myopathy
Normal pressure hydrocephalus
Cerebellar disorders
Visual loss
Footwear
Environmental factors
Clutter
Electrical cords in pathways
Poor lighting
Throw rugs
Low or soft chairs
Uneven or slippery surfaces
Stairs

paresthesia, weakness, joint pain, and memory loss help to identify the extent of vestibular, neurological, orthopedic, and cognitive disease. Urinary urgency may increase the risk of a fall. Leg pain from several etiologies increases the likelihood of falls. Information on patient's capacity to do activities of daily living and alcohol intake of more than 2 drinks per day are highly relevant because functional dependence and alcohol use increase the risk of falls.

The physical examination begins with an assessment of the postural vital signs to rule out postural hypotension. Blood pressure and heart rate are checked with the patient supine, then immediately after standing and at least two minutes of standing. Visual acuity should be checked with and without glasses. Hearing may be assessed using the whisper test or a handheld audiometer. The precordium and neck are auscultated for rhythm, murmurs, and bruits. Examination of the lower extremities for joint deformities, limitations of range of motion, calluses, and bunions is also important.

A complete neurological examination is mandatory and should include an evaluation of gait, muscle tone and strength, cerebellar function, deep tendon reflexes, and peripheral nerves. Parkinson's disease increases the risk of falls by causing bradykinesia, tremor, rigidity, postural instability, festinating gait, and stooped posture. Peripheral neuropathy causes decreased proprioception, sensory loss, and muscle weakness. Myelopathy impairs strength and sensation of lower extremities leading to an ataxic gait. Myopathic diseases will present with progressive muscle weakness and gait instability. Vestibular and cerebellar disorders cause a broad-based gait with irregular steps. The gait in normal pressure hydrocephalus is broad-based with short, slow, and shuffling steps; the person assumes a forward-flexed posture, and at times, the feet appear glued to the floor.

Screening for cognition using the Short Portable Mental Status Questionnaire and depression using the Geriatric Depression Scale are advocated (Chapter E34). Dementia increases the risk of falls by impairing judgment, visual-spatial perception, apraxia, and ability to orient oneself geographically. Falls also happen when dementia patients wander, attempt to get out of wheelchair, or climb over bed rails.

The Timed Up and Go test is a performance-based test for gait that can be easily administered in the office setting. The patient is asked to rise from a sitting position, walk 10 feet, turn, and return to the chair to sit. A Timed Up and Go test over 14 seconds suggests an increased fall risk.

History and examination should also search for potential acute causes of falls (Table 143.1). Delirium manifests with acute mental status changes, poor attention, psychomotor agitation, cognitive loss, perceptual disturbances, and changes in the sleep-wake cycle. It is always related to an underlying acute medical condition. The course of delirium tends to fluctuate during the day. Confusion, agitation, distraction, impaired judgment, and lack of awareness of the environment contribute to falls in a delirious patient.

Arrhythmia symptoms include dizziness, palpitations, heart racing, sweats, and chest discomfort. Patients can lose their balance and fall due to postural hypotension or brain hypoperfusion caused by the underlying arrhythmia. Both tachycardias and bradycardias can contribute to falls. Examination may be normal if the arrhythmia is episodic, or may reveal an irregular pulse and hypotension.

Sepsis presents with fever, chills, confusion, dizziness, and weakness. Other symptoms will depend on the source of infection. Physical examination reveals hypotension, fever, diaphoresis, confusion, and generalized weakness. Other examination findings will depend on the source of infection.

Seizures when generalized (tonic-clonic seizures) present with an arrest of activity and sudden loss of consciousness, followed by shaking, tonic extension of the arms and legs, and then clonic rhythmic limb jerking, followed by flaccidity, stupor, and labored, deep breathing. Incontinence commonly accompanies a generalized seizure. Seizures of the motor cortex (focal seizures) present with involuntary and repetitive movements of a limb or trunk. During a focal seizure patients retain some degree of consciousness.

Hypoglycemia presents with hunger, palpitations, sweats, anxiety, and generalized weakness. If prolonged, patients will lose consciousness and develop coma. Seizures and incontinence commonly happen in severe hypoglycemic episodes. Examination reveals lethargy or coma, pallor, cold and clammy extremities, and tachycardia.

Decreased intravascular volume caused by salt or water loss, or bleeding present with weakness, lethargy, and postural symptoms. Examination reveals orthostatic hypotension, dry mucosa, tachycardia, diminished skin turgor, and pallor when bleeding is present.

Symptoms of a transient ischemic attack (TIA) depend on the vascular territory involved. When the carotid artery territory is involved, symptoms may include paresis, sensory loss, speech or language disturbances, loss of vision in one eye, homonymous hemianopsia, and cognitive impairment. Vertebrobasilar ischemia often includes vertigo, diplopia, dysarthria, paresis, sensory loss or ataxia, and homonymous hemianopsia.

DIAGNOSIS

Diagnostic testing may be indicated based on the history and the physical examination. Laboratory tests such as hemoglobin level, serum urea and creatinine, and serum glucose can help identify causes of falls such as anemia, dehydration, and hypoglycemia. An infection workup including a complete blood cell count, urinalysis, and chest x-ray should be performed in a patient with acute change in mental status, fever, and falls. An electrocardiogram should be obtained in patients with irregular heart rate. An echocardiogram and a carotid Doppler can be considered when there is evidence of heart murmur or carotid bruit. Brain computed tomography scan or magnetic resonance imaging may be considered in patients with mental status changes or focal neurological findings. Electrodiagnostic studies should be considered when there is evidence of peripheral neuropathy. Spine x-rays or magnetic resonance imaging may be useful in patients with gait disorders, abnormalities on neurological examination, lower extremity spasticity, or hyperreflexia to rule out cervical spondylosis or spinal cord lesions.

TREATMENT

Treatment and strategies to prevent future falls should be targeted to identified underlying causes. An individual plan should be developed for each patient taking into consideration the risk factors and the patient's functional level. Studies have shown that exercise (such as balance training), correct use of assistive devices, medication review, environmental hazard elimination, treatment of postural hypotension, and cardiovascular disorders are effective in prevention of falls in community-dwelling older adults. In long-term care facilities, the key component is staff and resident education in addition to gait training, correct use of assistive devices, and medication review.

CHAPTER 144

Delirium and Dementia

Jerome Van Ruiswyk and Edmund Duthie

Delirium and dementia are significant geriatric concerns. The physician should approach dementia and delirium as brain failure. Just as with any other major organ failure (cardiac, renal, or hepatic), the physician must determine whether the problem is acute or chronic and whether it is fully or partially reversible.

Acute reversible brain failure, referred to as delirium, is present in about 30% of elderly patients admitted to general medical and surgical wards. The prognosis of delirium depends on the underlying cause. Given a mortality risk as high as 25%, delirium is a true medical emergency, requiring skillful evaluation to define the underlying cause.

Dementia is the chronic form of brain failure, afflicting roughly 10% of the population older than 65 years and almost half of those older than 85 years. Alzheimer's disease, the most common form of dementia, progresses through mild, moderate, and severe stages. Patients with mild disease exhibit mild changes in memory and language. In the moderate stage, many behavioral domains are involved and the classic syndrome is identifiable. Severe Alzheimer's disease is characterized by marked impairment of all intellectual abilities. Motor dysfunction may emerge. Death may be caused by aspiration pneumonia, sepsis from pressure ulcers or urinary tract infection, or concomitant medical illnesses.

ETIOLOGY

The search for a cause of delirium can be painstaking in view of the many possibilities (Table 144.1). Although delirium may be due to metabolic, toxic, infectious, or structural causes, drug side effects are the most common cause in elderly patients. Drugs notorious for precipitating delirium are the sedative-hypnotics, minor tranquilizers, major tranquilizers, and tricyclic antidepressants; some of the other common agents are listed in Table 144.2.

The major causes of dementia are primary degenerative dementia (Alzheimer's disease or senile dementia of the Alzheimer's type), vascular dementia, and a combination of these two. Together, these causes account for three fourths or more of all cases of dementia. Other causes are listed in Table 144.3.

As noted, Alzheimer's disease (primary degenerative dementia) is the most common form of dementia, but its cause remains obscure. Data from twin studies indicate the importance of both genetic and nongenetic factors in the development of this illness. Chromosome 21 controls production of the precursor to beta-amyloid protein which accumulates in the brain of patients with Alzheimer's disease. Chromosome 19 generates apolipoprotein E alleles ϵ1-4, which modulate risk for Alzheimer's disease. Putative nongenetic factors include slow-acting viral agents, environmental toxins and trace metals, and deficiencies of neurotrophic hormones. Acetylcholine deficits in the central nervous system have been noted. Microscopic hallmarks of the illness include selective neuronal death, neurofibrillary tangles, and neuritic plaques.

TABLE 144.1 Common causes of delirium

Drugs (see text and Table 144.2)
Intoxication or withdrawal (alcohol, other)
Infections
Hypoxemia/hypercarbia
Hypoglycemia or hyperglycemia
Fluid and electrolyte abnormalities (e.g., sodium, calcium, phosphorous)
Acid/base disturbances
Renal failure
Hepatic failure
Anemia
Thyroid disease
Hypotension
Hypothermia or hyperthermia
Central nervous system structural lesion
Seizure
Sensory deprivation (intensive care unit psychosis)

CLINICAL MANIFESTATIONS

It is important to differentiate delirium and dementia because delirium must be rapidly evaluated to prevent immediate morbidity or mortality (Table 144.4).

However, patients with brain failure are difficult to evaluate. History must be obtained from family, friends, or the nursing staff. History should focus on premorbid level of functioning and new symptoms of systemic illness. The patient's history of chronic illnesses will help stratify their risks for acute complications that might present as delirium. A complete medication history is essential because the foremost consideration in differential diagnosis should be a drug-induced delirium.

The physical examination of the delirious patient is hindered by their uncooperativeness. Vital

TABLE 144.2 Additional drugs reported to cause delirium in the aged

Antiadrenergic agents (e.g., β-blockers and central α-blockers)
Anticholinergic agents
Antihistamines
Antiparkinsonian drugs
Cimetidine
Digoxin
Lithium
Muscle relaxants
Opioids
Nonsteroidal antiinflammatory agents
Corticosteroids
Theophylline

TABLE 144.3 Causes of dementia

Alzheimer's disease Vascular (cerebrovascular accident, anoxia) Drugs (alcohol, others) Posttraumatic
Degenerative central nervous system diseases (Lewy-body, Parkinson, progressive multifocal leukoencephalopathy, Huntington, Pick)
Space-occupying lesion (tumor, infection) Normal pressure hydrocephalus Vitamin deficiencies (vitamin B_{12}, thiamine) Infectious (human immunodeficiency virus, neurosyphilis, Creutzfeldt-Jakob,) Vasculitis

TABLE 144.4 Clinical features differentiating delirium from dementia

Characteristic	Delirium	Dementia
Onset	Sudden	Insidious
Course over 24 hours	Fluctuating, with nocturnal exacerbation	Stable
Consciousness	Reduced	Clear
Attention	Globally disordered	Normal, except in severe cases
Cognition	Globally disordered	Globally impaired
Hallucinations	Usually visual	Often absent
Delusions	Fleeting, poorly systematized	Often absent
Orientation	Usually impaired, at least for a time	Often impaired
Psychomotor activity	Increased, reduced, or shifting unpredictably	Often normal
Speech	Often incoherent, slow or rapid	Difficulty finding words, perseveration
Involuntary movements	Often asterixis or coarse tremor	Often absent
Physical illness, or drug toxicity	One or both are present	Often absent, especially in senile dementia of the Alzheimer's type

Adapted from Lipowski ZJ. Delirium in the elderly patient. *N Engl J Med* 1989;320:578–582.

signs should be reviewed for irregularities including arrhythmias, abnormal blood pressure, temperature, or respiratory rate, and pulse oximetry should be obtained. The cardinal features of delirium are a decreased awareness of the environment and impaired attention span (clouding of consciousness), perceptual disturbance (e.g., visual hallucinations and illusions), incoherent speech, sleep-wake disturbance, increased or decreased psychomotor activity (e.g., tachycardia, diaphoresis, mydriatic pupils, and fever), disorientation and memory impairment, rapid onset with fluctuating course, and the presence of some underlying organic factors.

The history of the patient with suspected dementia should first confirm the presence of dementia. Dementia has several main features: loss of intellectual abilities of sufficient severity to interfere with social or occupational functioning; memory impairment, impairment of abstract thinking (e.g., concrete proverb interpretation or the inability to find similarities and differences between related words); impaired judgment; disturbances of higher cortical function (e.g., aphasia, apraxia, agnosia, and an inability to copy three-dimensional figures); personality change; normal level of consciousness; and an organic factor judged to be causative. Isolated memory loss, especially short-term memory, differs from dementia and in some cases can be termed mild cognitive impairment.

The history should also search for clues to differentiate among the possible causes of dementia. A history of hypertension, transient ischemic attack, stroke, abrupt onset, and stepwise deterioration indicates vascular dementia. Patients should be screened for depression and substance abuse. Family history should inquire about dementia. Hallucinations and Parkinson's features suggest Lewy body dementia. Incontinence and ataxia might prompt evaluation for normal pressure hydrocephalus.

Physical examination in dementia patients should begin with a mental status examination to confirm and help grade the severity of the cognitive impairment. The examiner should also search for focal neurologic deficits that would suggest localized central nervous system pathology or extrapyramidal features seen in Lewy body or Parkinson's dementias.

DIAGNOSIS

Basic laboratories should be obtained in the evaluation of delirium and dementia, but more specialized testing or imaging should be tailored to the individual clinical clues obtained from the history and physical examination (Table 144.5). While delirium is by definition typically reversible, a completely reversible cause of dementia is found in only a small proportion of dementia cases. However, the human suffering that could be alleviated and cost savings achieved by reducing needless institutionalization through such an evaluation cannot be discounted.

The association of dementia and depression is important because depression is usually treatable. Depression is suggested when the patient is actively seeking medical attention; the onset is more rapid and is known with precision; the patient is aware of cognitive loss; depressed affect is present with vegetative signs; "don't know" answers are given to questions on the mental status examination; and behavior is observed that is not congruent with the severity of the cognitive loss. Neuropsychological testing, referral to a psychiatrist, or an empiric trial of antidepressant therapy may help differentiate depression from dementia in cases in which the diagnosis is in doubt.

TREATMENT

Therapy of delirium requires a gentle approach that optimizes sensory function, diminishes extraneous environmental stimuli, and incorporates familiar people, such as family members. Restraints should be used sparingly and caution exercised to avoid pressure ulcers, peripheral nerve damage, and aspiration. Restraints are potentially injurious to agitated patients. Sedation should be used

TABLE 144.5 Evaluation of delirium and dementia

Laboratory
- Complete blood count
- Glucose, electrolytes
- Renal function
- Hepatic function
- Thyroid function
- Vitamin B_{12}, folate
- Calcium, phosphate

Other studies may be appropriate in certain clinical situations
- Chest x-ray
- Electrocardiogram
- Neuroimaging (CT scan, MRI, PET, SPECT)
- Human immunodeficiency virus, syphilis serology
- Lumbar puncture
- Electroencephalogram
- Neuropsychological evaluation
- Speech/language evaluation

CT, computed tomography; MRI, magnetic resonance imaging; PET, positron emission tomography; SPECT, single photon emission computed tomography.
Adapted from Knopman DS, DeKosky ST, Cummings JL, et al. Practice parameter: diagnosis of dementia (an evidence-based review): report of the Quality Standards Subcommittee of the American Academy of Neurology. *Neurology* 2001; 56:1143–1153.

TABLE 144.6 Managing patients with dementia

Optimize function by treating medical conditions and providing ongoing medical care, treating with appropriate medical therapies (e.g., cholinesterase inhibitors), avoiding medications with central nervous system side effects, optimizing sensory function (e.g., glasses, hearing aids), encouraging physical and social activity, and assessing the home environment and recommending adaptations (i.e., occupational therapy home safety evaluation)

Identify and manage complications such as psychosis, agitation and aggressiveness, depression, wandering, incontinence

Educate patients and families about the nature of the disease, prognosis, new treatments, and research protocols

Provide social service and legal information about community resources, respite or institutional care, advance directives, legal and financial issues

Adapted from Confusion. Kane RL, Ouslander JG, Abrass IB. *Essentials of Clinical Geriatrics.* 5th ed. New York: McGraw-Hill; 2004:125–153.

sparingly, especially in cases in which a drug is the suspected cause. Adding a second agent may only complicate matters further, because many of the same agents used to treat delirium may also produce it. However, in instances in which the patient is a danger to self or others and cannot be managed with nonmedical measures alone, drug therapy may be necessary. One approach in using drug therapy is to use a major tranquilizer to sedate the patient and then gradually wean him or her off the drug. Management of such patients is further complicated by the possibility that delirium may be superimposed on dementia, with the premorbid mental status abnormal as well.

A comprehensive approach is needed in the management of patients with dementia, who often require the coordination of many resources. Management of patients with dementia focuses on optimizing function, managing complications, educating patients and families, and providing social service and legal information (Table 144.6). Treatment can also include therapies targeted at the underlying etiology of the patient's dementia. Therapies for Alzheimer's disease include the cholinesterase inhibitors donepezil, rivastigmine, and galantamine, and the N-methyl-D-aspartate receptor antagonist memantine. Combination therapy with memantine plus a cholinesterase inhibitor has been found to be superior to single-agent therapy. These agents have demonstrated efficacy in slowing/delaying the progression of mental status decline. Specific therapy for patients with vascular dementia should include management of cardiovascular risk factors and prophylactic therapies to prevent further strokes. Since no cure currently exists for dementia, physicians caring for these patients should help patients and their family cope with the illness.

CHAPTER 145

Urinary Incontinence

Mary Cohan and Kathryn Denson

Involuntary voiding of urine is common in elderly persons and is underreported to physicians. An estimated 15% to 30% of elderly community dwellers and up to 50% of institutionalized elderly patients suffer from this condition. Transient incontinence should be excluded before evaluating this problem in depth. The mnemonic DIAPPERS is helpful in recalling causes of transient incontinence (Table 145.1). Correction of these conditions may cure the incontinence. Incontinence that is chronic and persistent should then be evaluated.

ETIOLOGY

The basic types and causes of persistent urinary incontinence are listed in Table 145.2. Urge incontinence and mixed (stress and urge) incontinence are most common in older women, whereas urge and overflow incontinence are most common in men.

TABLE 145.1 Common causes of transient incontinence

Delirium or confusional state
Infection, urinary (symptomatic)
Atrophic urethritis or vaginitis
Pharmaceuticals Sedatives or hypnotics, especially long-acting agents Loop diuretics Anticholinergic agents (antipsychotic agents, antidepressants, antihistamines, antiparkinsonian agents, antispasmodics, antidiarrheal agents) Alpha-adrenoceptor agonists and antagonists Opiates Calcium-channel blockers Vincristine
Psychological disorder (especially depression)
Endocrine disorder (hypercalcemia or hyperglycemia)
Restricted mobility
Stool impaction

Adapted from Resnick NM. Urinary incontinence in the elderly. *Medical Grand Rounds* 1984;3:281–290, with permission.

TABLE 145.2 Basic types and causes of persistent urinary incontinence

Type	Definition	Common causes
Stress	Involuntary loss of urine (usually small amounts) with increases in intraabdominal pressure (e.g., cough, laugh, or exercise)	Weakness and laxity of pelvic floor musculature, bladder outlet, or urethral sphincter weakness
Urge	Leakage of urine (usually larger volumes) because of inability to delay voiding after perceiving sensation of bladder fullness	Detrusor motor or sensory instability, isolated or associated with one or more of the following: • Local genitourinary condition (cystitis, urethritis, tumors, stones, diverticula, and outflow obstruction) • Central nervous system disorders (stroke, dementia, Parkinsonism, suprasacral spinal cord injury or disease[a])
Overflow	Leakage of urine (usually small amounts) resulting from mechanical forces on an overdistended bladder or from other effects of urinary retention on bladder and sphincter function	• Anatomic obstruction by prostate, stricture, cystocele • Noncontractile bladder associated with diabetes mellitus or spinal cord injury • Neurogenic (detrusor-sphincter dyssynergy), associated with multiple sclerosis and other suprasacral spinal cord lesions
Functional	Urinary leakage associated with inability to toilet because of impairment of cognitive or physical functioning, psychological unwillingness, or environmental barriers	• Severe dementia and other neurological disorders • Psychological factors such as depression, regression, anger, and hostility

[a]When detrusor motor instability is associated with a neurological disorder, it is termed "detrusor hyperreflexia" by the International Continence Society.

From Kane RL, Ouslander JG, Abrass IB, eds. *Essentials of Clinical Geriatrics*. 4th ed. New York: McGraw-Hill; 1999: 181–230.

CLINICAL MANIFESTATIONS

History taking is the initial step in urinary incontinence evaluation and will help determine the type of incontinence present. Frequency, severity, duration, volume, and timing of urine loss, as well as fluid intake, can be recorded in a "bladder diary." This allows for better definition of incontinence type and identification of any associated factors (e.g., medications, caffeine use). It is essential to understand the impact of the incontinence on the patient's functional status and quality of life.

Physical examination begins with a general medical examination that includes pelvic and rectal examinations to evaluate for contributing causes of incontinence including atrophic vaginitis/urethritis, pelvic muscle laxity (cystocele/rectocele), enlarged prostate, and fecal impaction. Neurologic examination is needed to evaluate mental status, sacral reflexes, and perineal sensation. Measurement of the postvoid residual volume helps categorize the type of incontinence. The patient is instructed to urinate and empty the bladder as completely as possible. Next, any urine volume remaining in the bladder is measured by bladder ultrasound or catheterization. Patients with large residual volumes (>150 mL) need evaluation for anatomic obstruction or detrusor dysfunction. Incontinence with a small residual volume can mean a normally functioning bladder (functional incontinence) or detrusor instability (involuntary detrusor muscle contractions). It may also occur in patients (primarily women) with stress incontinence.

DIAGNOSIS

Laboratory studies include urine analysis and culture to exclude infection, measurement of electrolytes, calcium, glucose, and urea nitrogen to uncover any other contributing or causative factors.

The type of incontinence and any contributing factors can often be identified after the initial office evaluation, but urologic consultation for cystoscopy and urodynamic testing may be required in some instances.

TREATMENT

Treatments for incontinence fall into three main categories: behavioral interventions, drug therapy, and surgery. Therapy depends on the cause of the incontinence. Stress incontinence is managed by weight loss for obese patients, pelvic floor exercises (Kegel exercises), and topically administered estrogens in women. Failures of conservative measures or improper urethral anatomy may warrant surgical correction of the anatomic problem. Pads and adult diapers are helpful for refractory nonoperative patients or patients with a poor surgical result. Treatment of detrusor instability may include behavioral measures such as adequate fluid intake, scheduled voiding every 2 hours, and pelvic floor muscle exercises. Drug therapy using oxybutynin, tolterodine, and anticholinergic agents have been used with varying results. Overflow incontinence is initially treated medically using an alpha-blocker and/or 5α-reductase inhibitors. However, if this is ineffective and a high postvoid residual volume of urine remains in the bladder, transurethral resection of the prostate or intermittent urinary catheterization may be necessary.

Indwelling Foley catheter use should be avoided because of the high risk of infectious complications and the possibility of meatal damage, bladder stones, and urosepsis. Catheterization may be necessary in patients with anatomic obstruction who cannot be managed surgically or for patients with an underactive detrusor who cannot be intermittently catheterized. Patients with indwelling catheters should receive antibiotics only for symptomatic urinary tract infections, because these patients rapidly develop resistant organisms. The frequency of catheter change is empirical. Although monthly changes have been advocated, there are few data to support this practice.

CHAPTER 146

Benign Prostatic Hypertrophy

Jerome Van Ruiswyk

Benign prostatic hypertrophy (BPH) is a common cause of morbidity in older men. The histologic findings of BPH are epithelial and stromal proliferation, which result in the formation of large, fairly discrete nodules in the periurethral region of the prostate. The prevalence of histologic BPH increases with age from 25% of men in their 40s to 85% of men in their 80s. However, the degree of histologic BPH is only poorly correlated with the presence or severity of lower urinary tract symptoms.

Complications of BPH include urinary tract infection, acute urinary retention, and occasionally obstructive uropathy. It is the most common cause of bladder outlet obstruction, defined as increased bladder detrusor pressure relative to the rate of urine flow, in men over age 50 years. However, bladder outlet obstruction is due to a combination of static obstruction related to urethral anatomic deformity from nodules, and dynamic obstruction related to smooth muscle tone within the prostate. Fortunately, the incidence of acute urinary retention in men with BPH is only about 1% per year.

ETIOLOGY

BPH is largely related to the action of androgens. Dihydrotestosterone (DHT) is formed from testosterone by 5α-reductase type 2, which is located primarily in the prostatic stromal cells; DHT stimulates growth and division of prostatic stromal and epithelial cells. This cell growth eventually coalesces into discrete nodules that are visible on cross section of the prostate.

Other trophic factors, including estrogen and local peptide growth factors, also play a role in the development of BPH. The role of genetics in the development of BPH is incompletely understood, but BPH incidence is higher in men with certain mutations in the androgen receptor gene.

CLINICAL MANIFESTATIONS

Symptomatic patients typically present with nocturia, frequency, straining to urinate, hesitancy, sense of incomplete bladder emptying, double voiding, and reduced force of urinary stream. Those who develop complications may complain of dysuria, overflow dribbling, or inability to void. However, only about half of men with prostatic enlargement will develop lower urinary tract symptoms. Likewise, lower urinary tract symptoms are often caused by other lower urinary tract problems, comorbid conditions, or medications.

History should search for other causes of these urinary symptoms. Urinary frequency may be due to poorly controlled diabetes mellitus, diuretics, or increased fluid intake. Nocturia may be indicative of heart failure or redistribution of peripheral edema. Urinary retention may be caused by autonomic neuropathy, stroke, or spinal cord injury. Urethral stricture could develop after prior sexually transmitted diseases, trauma, or urethral instrumentation. Symptoms may also be caused or exacerbated by medications such as alpha-adrenergics or anticholinergics.

The severity of symptoms should be quantified using a standardized instrument such as the American Urologic Association (AUA) symptom score (Table 146.1), which measures the frequency of seven voiding symptoms on a scale from 0 to 5. A total score of less than 8 reflects mild symptoms, 8 to 18 moderate symptoms, and 19 to 35 severe symptoms. In individual patients, a change in symptom score of 5 points has an 80% probability of representing a true clinical change. Serial measurement of AUA score allows monitoring of symptom stability and response to therapy within an individual patient. In addition, patients should be asked how bothered they are by their symptoms because some patients tolerate severe symptoms quite well, whereas other patients are aggravated by moderate symptoms.

On examination, the abdomen should be palpated for a suprapubic mass suggesting enlarged bladder with urinary retention. Digital rectal exam (DRE) is insensitive and nonspecific for BPH because hypertrophy largely involves the medial and lateral lobes, rather than the posterior lobes, which are accessible on DRE. However, it can reveal asymmetry or hard nodules suggestive of prostatic carcinoma, or tenderness that may implicate prostatitis as the etiology of the patient's symptoms.

Sitting and standing blood pressures should be obtained in patients with possible autonomic neuropathy, or who may be treated with alpha-blocker therapy. Examination should also search for clues of congestive heart failure and underlying neurologic disease.

DIAGNOSIS

Routine testing in men with BPH symptoms should include a urinalysis to look for hematuria, glucosuria, or signs of infection. Hematuria should prompt further investigation to rule out genitourinary cancer (e.g., urine cytologies and cystoscopy to rule out bladder cancer).

A prostate-antigen test (PSA) test is typically obtained in men with lower urinary tract symptoms since prostate cancer can coexist with BPH. However, prostate cancer screening studies do not confirm that patients with BPH symptoms are more likely to harbor prostate cancer. In addition, the positive predictive value of PSA testing is lower in men with BPH due to lower test specificity. Nevertheless, patients with elevated PSA require further evaluation, especially when PSA values are greater than 10 ng/mL and the man is a candidate for definitive treatment of prostate cancer. PSA testing can also help predict which patients will progress to urinary retention, as well as which patients are more likely to respond to therapy with a 5α-reductase inhibitor.

Postvoid residual should be checked by bladder ultrasound or urinary catheterization for patients with moderate to severe symptoms or coexistent neurologic disease. However, elevated residual volume may be due to a weak detrusor (e.g., due to anticholinergics), rather than bladder outlet obstruction. Likewise, inability to pass a urethral catheter is more often due to sphincter spasm than prostatic obstruction.

Office testing of urinary flow rates may be helpful in confirming the diagnosis. About 90% of men with urinary flow rates of $<$10 mL per second have bladder outlet obstruction. However, there is significant intrapatient variability in urinary flow rates; low flow rates may be seen with inadequate voided volumes (i.e., $>$150 mL is needed for reliable results) or weak detrusor activity. Consequently, low flow rates are sensitive but not specific for bladder outlet obstruction.

TREATMENT

Patients with acute urinary retention or obstructive uropathy require prompt bladder drainage, typically via urethral catheter. Other causes for the patient's symptoms, such as medication side

TABLE 146.1 American Urologic Association symptom score

	Not at all	Less than 1 time in 5	Less than half the time	About half the time	More than half the time	Almost always
Over the past month or so, how often have you had a sensation of not emptying your bladder completely after you finished urinating?	0	1	2	3	4	5
Over the past month or so, how often have you had to urinate again less than 2 hours after you finished urinating?	0	1	2	3	4	5
Over the past month or so, how often have you found you stopped and started again several times when you urinated?	0	1	2	3	4	5
Over the past month or so, how often have you found it difficult to postpone urination?	0	1	2	3	4	5
Over the past month or so, how often have you had a weak urinary stream?	0	1	2	3	4	5
Over the past month or so, how often have you had to push or strain to begin urination?	0	1	2	3	4	5
Over the last month, how many times did you most typically get up to urinate from the time you went to bed at night until the time you got up in the morning?	0	1	2	3	4	5

effects, urinary tract infection, poorly controlled diabetes, or congestive heart failure, should also be promptly treated to allow a determination of the remaining symptoms that may be related to BPH. Treatment of any remaining BPH symptoms is undertaken mostly to improve quality of life or to prevent complications. Therefore, it requires a discussion with the patient about how much they are bothered by their symptoms, the natural history of the disease, and the risks and benefits of treatment.

Treatment of BPH symptoms can begin with lifestyle changes such as limiting fluid intake in the evening or a bladder retraining program. Patients should be counseled to avoid common medications, such as cold remedies with sympathomimetics or anticholinergic agents, which may cause urinary retention or worsening of symptoms.

Alpha-adrenergic blockers are the current first line therapy for patients with BPH symptoms. Prostatic smooth muscle contraction is largely mediated via alpha 1 adrenergic receptors. Alpha-blockers work within 2 to 4 weeks to reduce this dynamic component of bladder outlet obstruction. There is no difference in efficacy among available alpha-blockers, but the selective alpha-1 blockers tamsulosin and alfuzosin may cause less dizziness and orthostatic hypotension than nonselective alpha blockers prazosin, terazosin, and doxazosin. The decrease in blood pressure with these agents tends to be greater in patients with elevated blood pressures. Despite improving BPH symptoms, these agents do not appear to reduce the risk of BPH complications such as urinary retention or the need for surgery.

The 5α-reductase inhibitors finasteride and dutasteride block the conversion of testosterone to DHT. This blockade leads to a 25% reduction in prostate size in the first year of treatment. Finasteride has been shown to significantly reduce the risks of urinary retention and the need for BPH surgery. Higher baseline PSA values predict a higher likelihood of response to the 5α-reductase inhibitors. In addition, treatment with these medications will reduce PSA levels by about 50%, so it is recommended that PSA cancer screening thresholds for referral or biopsy be halved in patients who are treated with 5α-reductase inhibitors. Finasteride was associated with a slightly lower risk of prostate cancer, but a slightly higher risk of aggressive prostate cancer, in a large prostate cancer prevention trial.

Various surgical options are available to relieve BPH symptoms. Transurethral resection of prostate (TURP) remains the standard operation for BPH. Indications for surgery are acute urinary retention, obstructive uropathy, and recurrent urinary tract infections. The main complications of TURP are bleeding, infection, and initial difficulty voiding. A rare unique complication is hyponatremia due to systemic absorption of hypotonic bladder irrigation used during the procedure. Newer surgical techniques including transurethral incision of the prostate, laser prostatectomy, transurethral microwave therapy, and transurethral needle ablation may lead to fewer complications but sometimes at the expense of reduced efficacy; in addition, there are few long-term studies on the durability of their treatment responses.

INDEX

Page numbers in *italics* indicate figures; page numbers followed by a "t" indicate tables; page numbers followed by a "b" indicate boxes; numbers preceded by CP indicate color plate figures.

A
Abatacept, 284t
Abdominal distress, panic attack, 703t
Abdominal pain, 2–6, *3,* 3t, 4t, 118t. *See also* Peptic ulcer
- adrenal neoplasm, 437t
- appendicitis, 2, 5
- biliary colic, 2, 5
- cholecystitis, 2–3, 5–6, 459–460
- colitis, 15–16, 490–496, 491t, *492,* 493t
- diabetic ketoacidosis, 3, 8t, 9, 378, 386–387
- diarrhea with, 45, 45t
- diverticulitis, 3, 6, 15
- endocarditis, 344t, 349–357, *350,* 351f, *353,* 354t, 355t, 364t
- gastroenteritis, 2, 5, 117t
- glomerulonephritis, 520–527, *521,* 521t, 522t, 523t, 525t, 526t, 527t
- mesenteric ischemia, 4–5, 6, 711–715, 713t, 714t
- pancreatitis, 3, 6
- peptic ulcer disease, 442–449, *445, 446,* 447t
- rheumatic disease causing, 113–115, 113t, 115t
- ruptured abdominal aortic aneurysm, 5, 6
- small bowel obstruction, 4, 6

Abilify, 710t
Abscess
- lung, 98, 99–100, 99t, 327
- pelvic, 78t
- splenic, endocarditis complication, 356
- visceral, glomerulonephritis from, 520–527, *521,* 521t, 522t, 523t, 525t, 526t, 527t

ACC. *See* American College of Cardiology
ACE inhibitors. *See* Angiotensin-converting enzyme inhibitors
Acetaminophen, 303
- headache from overuse of, 81
- hyperbilirubinemia from, 102t
- liver disease from, 469t, *470*
- osteoarthritis treatment, 276–277

Acetazolamide, 538
Acetylcholinesterase inhibitors, 693
Acetylcysteine, 242, 508–509
Achilles' tendonitis/bursitis, 799t
Acid-base disorders, 7–12, 8t–9t, *11,* 12t, 311t
- chronic kidney disease causing, 515–516, 515t
- common causes of, 8t–9t
- metabolic acidosis, 7, 9–10, *11,* 12t, 57, 511t, 711–715, 713t, 714t
- metabolic alkalosis, 10, *11,* 12t
- pH range, 11, *11,* 12t
- renal failure causing, 519
- respiratory acidosis, 10, *11,* 12
- respiratory alkalosis, 10–11, *11,* 12

Acidosis
- diabetic ketoacidosis, 3, 8t, 9, 378, 386–387
- metabolic, 7, 9–10, *11,* 12t
- renal tubular, 10
- respiratory, 10, *11,* 12

Acne, 728–731, 729t. *See also* Lesion
- rosacea, 730–731
- vulgaris, 728–730

Acoustic neuroma, 51
Acquired immunodeficiency syndrome (AIDS), 366–375, *367, 368, 369,* 369t, *370,* 370t, 371t, 372t, 373t. *See also* Human immunodeficiency virus
- clinical manifestations, 367–370, *368, 369,* 369t, 370t
- complications, 373–375, 373t
- conjugated hyperbilirubinemia with, 102t, 103
- diagnosis, *370,* 370–372, 371t
- etiology, 366–367
- prevalence, *367*
- treatment, 372–373, 372t

ACR. *See* American College of Rheumatology
Acromegaly, 419–420, 419t, *420*
Actinic keratosis, 733
Acute inflammatory demyelinating polyradiculoneuropathy (AIDP), 686
Acute interstitial nephritis (AIN), 531–532, 532t
Adalimumab, 284t
Adefovir, 465
Adenosine, *210*
ADH. *See* Antidiuretic hormone
ADPKD. *See* Autosomal dominant polycystic kidney disease
Adrenal gland diseases, 427–440
- adrenal insufficiency, 389t, 427–429, 428t
- androgens and estrogens, 427–429
- congenital adrenal hyperplasia, 435–436
- Cushing's syndrome, 429–434, *430,* 431t, *432, 433,* 433t
- incidental mass, 439–440, 439t, 440t
- pheochromocytoma, 436–439, 437t, 438t
- primary hyperaldosteronism, 434–435, 435t

Adrenal insufficiency, 389t, 427–429, 428t. *See also* Adrenal gland diseases
  hypoglycemia from, 389t
Adrenal neoplasm, 437t
Adrenocorticotropic hormone, gout treatment, 313
Adult respiratory distress syndrome (ARDS), 348, 486
Aerosol propellants, myocarditis from, 184t
AHA. *See* American Heart Association
AIDP. *See* Acute inflammatory demyelinating polyradiculoneuropathy
AIDS. *See* Acquired immunodeficiency syndrome
AIN. *See* Acute interstitial nephritis
Albuterol, 236t
  asthma treatment, 230t, 235t, 236, 236t
  hyperkalemia treatment, 548
Alcohol abuse. *See also* Substance abuse
  dyslipidemia associated with, 779t
  heart failure risk, *175*
  hepatitis from, 468–469
  leading cause of cirrhosis, 468
  as obstructive sleep apnea risk, 251t
  recommendations for prevention, 747t
  syncope from, 132t, 133
  tuberculosis activation factor, 262t
Aldosterone antagonist, heart failure therapy, *175,* 176
Alfuzosin, 846
Alkalosis
  metabolic, 10, *11,* 12t
  respiratory, 10–11, *11,* 12
Allergies, cough associated with, 37, *38*
Allopurinol, 538
  acute interstitial nephritis from, 531–532, 532t
  gout prophylaxis, 313
Alopecia, rheumatic diseases, 113–115, 113t, 115t
Alpha thalassemia, 26t, 27t, *29,* 30t, *581,* 582–584
Alpha-adrenergic blockers, 846
Alpha-glucosidase inhibitors, diabetes mellitus treatment, 383t, 384
Alprazolam, 706t
ALS. *See* Amyotrophic lateral sclerosis
Altered mental status, 19–24, 20t, 22t–23t, 24t, 118t. *See also* Confusion; Delirium; Psychiatric abnormality
  dialysis for, 511t
  drugs or medications causing, 20t, 21, 24t
  eating disorder causing, 711–715, 713t, 714t
  hepatic encephalopathy, 477t
  kidney disease, 513t
  laboratory and imaging evaluation of, 23–24, 24t
  metabolic abnormality, 20t, 21, 22t
  neurological abnormality, 19, 20t, 22t
  psychiatric abnormality causing, 20t, 21
  systemic abnormality, 20t, 21
Alzheimer's disease, 742t
Amantadine, multiple sclerosis treatment, 683
Amenorrhea, 814–816, 816t. *See also* Menstrual irregularities
  uremia causing, 515t
American College of Cardiology (ACC), 174, *175*
American College of Rheumatology (ACR)
  criteria for rheumatoid arthritis, 283t
  criteria for systemic lupus erythematosus, 289t
American Heart Association (AHA), 174, *175*
American Urologic Association (AUA), benign prostatic hypertrophy symptom scoring, 845t
Aminoglycosides, cellulitis treatment, 334t
Aminophylline, 236t
  asthma treatment, 235t, 236, 236t
Amiodarone, 218, 219
  connective tissue disease treatment complication, 240t
  liver disease from, 469t
Amoxicillin-clavulanic acid, bite wound infection therapy, 335t
Amphetamines, 760
  seizures from, 124t
Amphotericin B, autoimmune hemolytic anemia from, 590t
Ampicillin
  endocarditis treatment, 355t
  meningitis therapy, 341t
Amylase, diseases associated with elevated, 484t
Amyloidosis, renal involvement, 525t
Amyotrophic lateral sclerosis (ALS), 684–685
  Guillain-Barré syndrome v., 690t
Anakinra, 284t
Analgesics, choledocholithiasis treatment, 460
ANCA. *See* Antineutrophilic cytoplasmic antibody
Androgens, 427–429, 568. *See also* Adrenal gland diseases
Anemia, 25–30, 26t, 27t, 28t, *29,* 30t. *See also* Cryoglobulinemia; Jaundice; Myelodysplastic syndrome
  autoimmune hemolytic, 588–592, 589t, 590t, 592t
  chronic disease, 26t, 575–576, 575t, 576t
  diagnosis of, 28t, *29*
  dizziness from, 48, 49t, 51
  dyspnea from, 57, *58,* 59
  eating disorder causing, 711–715, 713t, 714t
  edema from hypoalbuminemia, 69, 70, 71
  exogenous erythropoietin for, 568
  hemolytic, 22, 27, 27t, 28t
    Wilson's disease manifestation, 473t
  macrocytic, 27–28, 28t, *29*
  megaloblastic, 569–572, 570t, 571t
  microcorpuscular volume classification, 26t
  microcytic, 26, 26t, *29*
    chronic disease causing, 515t, 516
    iron deficiency, 26t, *29,* 569–572, 570t, 571t, 576t, 747t
    sideroblastic (medications, toxins, lead poisoning), 26t
    thalassemia, 26t, 27t, *29,* 30t, 580–584, *581*
  myelofibrosis with myeloid metaplasia, 567–568, 567t
  normocytic, 26–27, 26t, *29*
  primary bone marrow disorders, 27

Aneurysm. *See also* Stroke
  cerebral, 661, 663
  mycotic, endocarditis complication, 356
  ruptured abdominal aortic, 5, 6
Angina
  chronic stable, 150–156, 151t, 153t, 155–156
  medication side effect, 553t
  shock leading to, 127t
  unstable, 157–162, 158t–159t
  variant, 162
Angiotensin receptor blockers (ARB), 174, *175*
  heart failure risk management, 174, *175*
Angiotensin-converting enzyme (ACE) inhibitors, 39, 40, 518, 527
  anginal symptoms treatment, 156
  cardiac chest pain management, 161
  heart failure risk v., *175*
  kidney disease treatment, 519t
  pancreatitis associated with, 483t
  polyarteritis nodosa treatment, 309
  scleroderma with renal crisis treatment, 297
Anion gap
  calculation formula, 12
  definition, 7
  dialysis for, 511t
  elevated, 12
  increased, uremia causing, 515t
Anisocytosis, 30t
Ankylosing spondylitis, 300–302, 301t
Anorexia
  cyclic vomiting, 117t
  endocarditis, 344t, 349–357, *350,* 351f, *353,* 354t, 355t, 364t
  glomerulonephritis, 520–527, *521,* 521t, 522t, 523t, 525t, 526t, 527t
  hypercalcemia, 393, 394t
  kidney disease, 513t, 514t
  metabolic acidosis, 7, 9–10, *11,* 12t, 57, 511t, 711–715, 713t, 714t
  uremic, 513t, 514t, 519
Anovulation, 818
Antacids, 449
Anterior pituitary diseases. *See* Pituitary diseases
Anthracycline, 559
  endocarditis from, 182t
Antiarrhythmia drug therapy, 218–219. *See also* Arrhythmia
Antibiotics, 526, 579, 810
  acute interstitial nephritis from, 531–532, 532t
  bacterial meningitis, 338–340, *339,* 339t
  choledocholithiasis treatment, 460
  endocarditis treatment, 344t, 349–357, *350,* 351f, *353,* 354t, 355t, 364t
  fever from, 78
  glomerulonephritis treatment, 520–527, *521,* 521t, 522t, 523t, 525t, 526t, 527t
  infectious arthritis, 317, 317t
  macrolide, 781t
  osteomyelitis treatment, 361
  pneumonia treatment, 326
  sepsis syndrome treatment, 347
  urinary tract infection, 332t
  vomiting/nausea from, 117t
Anticholinergic agents, 231, 842
  altered mental status from, 21
  inhaled, asthma treatment, 230t
  urinary incontinence associated with, 840t
Anticoagulation therapy
  atrial fibrillation treatment, 219
  pulmonary embolism treatment, 257
  stroke management, 658
Antidepressant medications, 679, 699t
  migraine headache management, 669
  myocarditis from, 184t
  syncope from, 132t, 133
  weight loss from, 142t
Antidiuretic hormone (ADH), 421, 425–426, 425t
Antiepileptic drugs, 679
  multiple sclerosis treatment, 683
  seizure treatment, 666
  weight loss from, 142t
Antifungal medications, 720, 781t
Antihypertensive medications
  migraine headache management, 669–670
  orthostatic hypotension from, 132t, 133
Antineutrophilic cytoplasmic antibody (ANCA), glomerulonephritis from, 520–527, *521,* 521t, 522t, 523t, 525t, 526t, 527t
Antinuclear antibody (ANA), 114, 115t
Antipsychotic medications, 710t
Antithrombotic agents, stroke management, 658
Anxiety
  acute chest pain associated with, 35
  adrenal neoplasm, 437t
  disorders, 702–706, 703t, 705t, 706t
    selective serotonin reuptake inhibitors for, 704–705, 706t
  Wilson's disease manifestation, 473t
Aorta
  aneurysm, ruptured, 5, 6
  dissection, 220–223
    diagnosis, 221–222, 222t
    etiology, 220–221, 221t
    treatment, 22–223
  regurgitation, 188–191, 189t, 190t
    causes of, 189t
    physical signs of, 190t
  stenosis, 186–188
Aortoenteric fistula, 14t, 15
Appendicitis, 2, 5
ARB. *See* Angiotensin receptor blockers
ARDS. *See* Adult respiratory distress syndrome
Arrhythmia, *58,* 59, *204,* 204–215, *205,* 206t–207t, *208, 209, 210, 211, 212, 213, 214,* 214t, 215t. *See also* Coronary artery disease; Tachycardia
  antiarrhythmia drug therapy, 218–219
  classifications of, 206t–207t
  clinical manifestations/treatments, 206t–207t

Arrhythmia (*contd.*)
  diagnosis, 160, 208
    atrial flutter, *209*
    bigeminy, *211*
    Torsades de pointes, *213*
    ventricular pre-excitation ECG, *211*
  dizziness and vertigo with, 48, 49t, 51
  eating disorder causing, 711–715, 713t, 714t
  etiology, *204,* 204–205, *205*
  Guillain-Barré syndrome, *58,* 59
  heart failure complication, 176–177
  medication side effect, 553t
  myocardial infarction complication, 167t
  syncope from, 133
  treatment, 208–214
    Estes criteria for left ventricular hypertrophy, 214t
    pacemaker code, 215t
Arthralgia, 109, *110*. *See also* Joint pain
  differential diagnosis, 112
Arthritis, 109–115, *110, 111,* 111t, 112t, 113t, 115t. *See also* Joint pain; Rheumatoid arthritis
  infectious, 113, 314–318, 317t
  inflammatory bowel disease with, 301t, 303–304
  inflammatory v. noninflammatory, 109, *110, 111,* 111t
  mono-, 110–111, *111*
    myelofibrosis with myeloid metaplasia, 567–568, 567t
  osteo-, *110,* 111, 111t, 274–278, *275,* 275t, 276t, *277*
    diagnosis, 276, 276t
    etiology, 274, 275t
    Heberden's nodes, *275,* 275–276, 276t
    treatment, 276–278
  peripheral, seronegative spondyloarthropathies, 300–304, 301t
  poly-, 110–111, *111*
    causes of, 112t
  psoriatic, 301t, 303
  reactive, 301t, 302–303
  refractory, 303
  rheumatoid, *110*
Arthrocentesis, 114
Arthropathy, seronegative spondylo-, 300–304, 301t
Arthrosclerosis, 221
5-ASA, 496
Asbestosis, 259–260
Ascorbic acid, 509t
Aspirin
  anginal symptoms treatment, 156
  atrial fibrillation treatment, 219
  chronic stable angina treatment, 155
  headache from overuse of, 81
  intolerance to, 155
  pericardia disease treatment, 200
  systemic lupus erythematosus treatment, 293
Asthma, 37, *38,* 39t, 40. *See also* Bronchial asthma
  COPD v., 233t
  dyspnea with, 54–56, 55t
Ataxia, 50t
  cerebellar hemorrhage, 660
  Fredreich's, dilated cardiomyopathy from, 179t
  multiple sclerosis, 680–683, 681t, *682*
  Wilson's disease manifestation, 473t
Atherosclerosis, 148–168, *149,* 149t, 151t, 153t, 158t–159t, 166t, 167t. *See also* Coronary artery disease
  heart failure risk, *175*
  risk factors for, 149t
Atonic seizures, 122t
Atorvastatin, myocardial infarction risk treatment, 156
Atrial fibrillation, 216–219. *See also* Stroke
  diagnosis, 217
  etiology, 216
  treatment, 217–219
AUA. *See* American Urologic Association
Aura/flashing lights. *See also* Visual disturbance
  seizure premonition, 123t
Auranofin (oral gold), rheumatoid arthritis treatment, 284
Autoimmune hemolytic anemia, 588–592, 589t, 590t, 592t
Autoimmune hepatitis, 467–468
Autosomal dominant polycystic kidney disease (ADPKD), 533–534
Azathioprine, 242, 268, 468
  pancreatitis associated with, 483t
  polyarteritis nodosa treatment, 309
  refractory arthritis treatment, 303
  rheumatoid arthritis treatment, 284
  systemic lupus erythematosus treatment, 293
Azithromycin, acquired immunodeficiency syndrome treatment, 372–373, 372t
Azotemia, 711–715, 713t, 714t

B
Babesia, 27t
Babinski's sign, Parkinson's disease, 674, 675t
Back pain, 787–791, 788t, *789*
  common conditions causing, 789–790
Bacterial vaginitis, 65t. *See also* Vaginitis
Balloon valvotomy, 187–188
  mitral stenosis treatment, 192
Bárány's maneuver, *52,* 52–53
Barbiturates. *See also* Substance abuse
  migraine headache management, 669
  seizure treatment, 666
Bartonella, 27t
Basal cell carcinoma, 732
Behavioral therapy, obesity treatment, 759–760
Behçet's syndrome, 61, 63t, *66*
Benign dizziness and vertigo, 48, 49t, 50
Benign paroxysmal positional vertigo (BPPV), 50–53, *52*
Benign prostatic hypertrophy, 61, 63t, 64, *66,* 95t, 843–846, 845t. *See also* Dysuria; Prostate cancer; Prostatitis
  American Urologic Association symptom score, 845t

Benzathine penicillin, syphilis treatment, 365, 810
Benzodiazepines, 666, 706t
  commonly prescribed, 706t
Beta blockers, 552
  anginal symptoms treatment, 156
  aortic dissection treatment, 223
  asthma symptoms worsened by, 227t
  atrial fibrillation treatment, 219
  cardiac chest pain management, 161
  cardiomyopathy treatment, 181
  heart failure risk management, 174, *175*
  heart failure risk v., *175*
  migraine headache management, 669–670
  mitral stenosis treatment, 192
  nausea and vomiting from, 117t
  syncope from, 132t, 133
Beta thalassemia, 26t, 27t, *29,* 30t, 580–582, *581*
Beta-lactam agents, 326
Biguanides, diabetes mellitus treatment, 383, 383t
Bile acid sequestrants, 781t
Biliary colic, 2, 5
Biliary disease, 454–462, 455t, *456,* 456t, 457t
  acute cholecystitis, 2–3, 5–6, 459–460
  choledocholithiasis and cholangitis, 460
  cholestasis, 454–457, 455t, *456,* 456t
  gallstone disease, 457–459, 457t
    risk factors for, 457t
  primary cirrhosis, 461
  primary sclerosing cholangitis, 461–462
Bilirubinemia. *See* Jaundice
Binge eating. *See* Eating disorders
Bisoprolol, heart failure risk management, 174, *175*
Bisphosphonates
  joint pain from, 113
  osteoporosis treatment, 786
Bite wound infection therapy, 335t
Bitolterol, asthma treatment, 230t
Bladder cancer, 61, 63t, *66,* 95t
Bleeding disorder, uremia causing, 515t, 516
Bleomycin, dilated cardiomyopathy from, 179t
Blood pressure. *See also* Hypertensive emergencies; Obesity
  altered mental status with low/high, 22t
  hypertensive emergency, 775
Blood urea nitrogen (BUN)
  causes of low/elevated, 509t
  dialysis for elevated, 511t
Bloody stools, rheumatic disease causing, 113–115, 113t, 115t
Bone disease. *See also* Calcium; Metabolic bone disease; Osteomyelitis; Parathyroid disorders
  uremia causing, 515t
Bowel obstruction, 4, 6, 500–502, 501t, *502*
BPPV. *See* Benign paroxysmal positional vertigo
Bradycardia, as medication side effect, 553t
Bradykinesia, Parkinson's disease, 674, 675t
Breast cancer, 624–630, 625t, *626,* 627t, 628t, 629t
  menopausal hormone therapy causing, 819t
  recommendations for prevention, 747t
Breathing, abnormal, reduced alertness with, 22t
Breathing discomfort, 54–60, 55t, *58*. *See also* Dyspnea
Bronchial asthma, 226–231, 227t, 228t, 229t, 230t. *See also* Asthma
  clinical manifestations, 226, 227t
  diagnosis, 227–228, 228t
  management, 228–231, 229t, 230t
Bronchitis, 39, 802–803, 803t
Bronchodilators, 236
  asthma treatment, 235t, 236, 236t
Brudzinski sign, 119t
  bacterial meningitis, 338–340, *339,* 339t
Budd-Chiari syndrome, 473–474
Bulimia. *See* Eating disorders
BUN. *See* Blood urea nitrogen
Busulfan, endocarditis from, 182t
Butalbital-caffeine, headache from overuse of, 81
B_{12} deficiency, 26t, *29,* 573–574

C
Calcification, atherosclerosis risk from, *149*
Calcium. *See also* Dietary therapy; Hypercalcemia; Hypocalcemia; Metabolic bone disease
  kinetics, *392*
  physiologic functions of, 391
Calcium channel blockers, 663
  anginal symptoms treatment, 156
  atrial fibrillation treatment, 217
  cardiac chest pain management, 161
  cardiomyopathy treatment, 181
  migraine headache management, 669–670
  mitral stenosis treatment, 192
  syncope from, 132t, 133
Calcium gluconate, hyperkalemia treatment, 548
Calcium pyrophosphate disease (CPPD), 112
Calcium stones. *See* Nephrolithiasis
Calcium supplements, 538, 548
Calcium-channel blockers
  edema from, 69–70, 69t
  urinary incontinence associated with, 840t
Cancer. *See also* Asbestosis; Malignancy; Smoking cessation; Tumor
  adrenocortical, 329–430, *430*
  bladder, 61, 63t, *66,* 95t
  breast, 624–630, 625t, *626,* 627t, 628t, 629t
    menopausal hormone therapy causing, 819t
    recommendations for prevention, 747t
  cervical, 639–646, 640t, 641t, 747t
  colon, 631–634, 632t, 633t, 634t
  colorectal, 747t
  lung, *58,* 59, 635–638, *636,* 636t, *637*
  metastatic, to liver, 78t
  ovarian, 642–646, 643t, 644t, 645t
  prevention recommendations, 747t
  prostate, 95t, 647–650, 649t (*See also* Benign prostatic hypertrophy)
  treatment options for, 732
Candidal vaginitis, 806t, 807
Capsaicin, osteoarthritis treatment, 276–277
Captopril, nephrotic syndrome from, 529t

Carbamazepine, 679
  liver disease from, 469t
  multiple sclerosis treatment, 683
  seizure treatment, 666
Carbon monoxide, dilated cardiomyopathy from, 179t
Carbromal, autoimmune hemolytic anemia from, 590t
Cardiac arrhythmia. *See* Arrhythmia
Cardiac disorder. *See also* Valvular heart diseases
  chest pain from, 31, 32t, 34, 35
  dyspnea from, 56–57
  syncope from, 131, 131t, 132t
Cardiac tamponade, 200–202, 201t, *202*
Cardiogenic shock, 126t, 127–129, *128*
Cardiomyopathies, 178–185, 179t, 182t, 184t
  dilated cardiomyopathy, 178–180, 179t
    known causes of, 179t
  eating disorder causing, 711–715, 713t, 714t
  hypertrophic, 180–182
  myocarditis, 183–185, 184t
  restrictive, 182–183, 182t
Cardiopulmonary disease, vomiting from, 117t
Carvedilol, heart failure risk management, 174, *175*
Cataracts, Wilson's disease manifestation, 473t
Cation exchange resin sodium polystyrene sulfonate, hyperkalemia treatment, 548–549
CCP. *See* Cyclic protein antibodies
Cefotaxime, cellulitis treatment, 334t
Cefoxitin, 509t
Ceftriaxone, 326
  meningitis therapy, 341t
Celiac sprue, *46*
Cellulitis, 333–336, 334t, 335t
  diagnosis, 335–336
  etiology, 333, 334t, 335t
  treatment, 336
Central nervous system (CNS). *See also specific disease*
  infection, vomiting from, 117t
Cephalosporins, autoimmune hemolytic anemia from, 590t
Cerebellar infarction, 48, 49t. *See also* Ischemia; Stroke
Cerebral aneurysm, 661, 663
Cerebrovascular accident, 742t
  uremia causing, 515t, 517
Cervical cancer, 639–646, 640t, 641t
  recommendations for prevention, 747t
Chagas disease, 183, 184t
Chancroid ulcers, 806t, 808, 810
Charcot's triad, 103
Chemotherapy agents, 559, 646
  connective tissue disease treatment complication, 240t
  dilated cardiomyopathy from, 179t
  nausea and vomiting from, 117t
  restrictive cardiomyopathy treatment, 183
  weight loss from, 142t
Chest pain, 31–36, 32t, 33t. *See also* Coronary artery disease; Hypertension
  adrenal neoplasm, 437t
  cardiac disorder, 31, 32t, 34, 35
  endocarditis, 344t, 349–357, *350,* 351f, *353,* 354t, 355t, 364t
  evaluation
    biochemical markers, 160
    ECG, 152, 158t–159t, 160
  gastrointestinal disorder, 32t, 34, 36
  musculoskeletal disorder, 32t, 34, 36
  panic attack, 703t
  psychosomatic, 35, 36
  pulmonary disorder, 32t, 33t, 34, 36
    pneumothorax, 32t, 33t, 34, 56
  pulmonary embolism symptom, 254t
Cheyne-Stokes breathing, reduced alertness with, 22t
CHF. *See* Congestive heart failure
Child-Turcotte Pugh classification of liver disease, 476t
Chills/rigors
  bacteremia, 346t
  endocarditis, 344t, 349–357, *350,* 351f, *353,* 354t, 355t, 364t
  panic attack, 703t
Chlamydia, 64t, 747t, 806, 806t. *See also* Dysuria; Sexually transmitted disease
  doxycycline for, 302
Chloramphenicol, cellulitis treatment, 334t
Chlordiazepoxide, 706t
Chloroquine, 268
Chlorpromazine, 455t
Chlorpropamide, autoimmune hemolytic anemia from, 590t
Choking sensation, panic attack, 703t
Cholangitis, 460. *See also* Biliary disease
Cholecalciferol (vitamin D_3). *See also* Parathyroid disorders
  calcium kinetics involving, *392*
  physiologic functions of, 391
Cholecystitis. *See also* Biliary disease
  acute, 2–3, 5–6, 459–460
Choledocholithiasis, 460. *See also* Biliary disease
  pancreatitis associated with, 483t
Cholestasis, 454–457, 455t, *456,* 456t. *See also* Biliary disease
Cholesterol
  hypercholesterolemia, atherosclerosis risk from, 149t
  lowering of LDL, anginal symptoms treatment, 156
  target levels for, 780t, 782
Cholestyramine, 462, 538
Cholinesterase inhibitors, 838t, 839
Chondroitin sulfate, osteoarthritis treatment, 276–277
Chronic disease anemia, 26t, 575–576, 575t, 576t
Chronic kidney disease (CKD), 512–519, 513t–514t, 515t, 518t, 519t
  clinical manifestations, 515–517
  etiology, 512–515, 513t–514t, 515t
  treatment and prevention, 518–519, 519t
Chronic myelogenous leukemia (CML), 561–563, 562t, 563t
Chronic obstructive pulmonary disease (COPD), 37, *38,* 54–56, 55t, *58,* 59, 232–238, 233t, *235,* 236t